Unit 6
Assisting With Diagnostic Tests and Therapeutic Procedures for Common Disorders *503*

29
Introduction to Anatomy and Physiology *504*

30
Caring for Patients With Integumentary Disorders *516*

31
Caring for Patients With Musculoskeletal Disorders *542*

32
Caring for Patients With Neurologic Disorders *580*

33
Caring for Patients With Sensory Disorders *606*

34
Caring for Patients With Endocrine Disorders *640*

35
Caring for Patients With Cardiovascular Disorders *656*

36
Caring for Patients With Immune Disorders *690*

37
Caring for Patients With Respiratory Disorders *706*

38
Caring for Patients With Gastrointestinal Disorders *726*

39
Caring for Patients With Urinary Disorders *750*

40
Caring for Patients With Disorders of the Male Reproductive System *764*

41
Caring for Patients With Gynecologic and Obstetric Disorders *778*

Unit 7
Performing Laboratory Procedures *817*

42
Introduction to the Clinical Laboratory *818*

43
Microbiology *840*

44
Urinalysis *866*

45
Phlebotomy *894*

46
Hematology *922*

47
Serology and Immunohematology *950*

48
Clinical Chemistry *966*

Unit 8
Working With Special Patient Populations *985*

49
Pediatric Patients *986*

50
Geriatric Patients *1016*

Section IV
Career Strategies **1033**

Unit 9
Competing in the Job Market *1035*

51
Externship *1038*

52
Employment *1048*

Appendices *A-1*
Appendix I
1990 DACUM Analysis of the Medical Assisting Profession *A-2*

Appendix II
Key English-to Spanish Health Care Phrases *A-4*

Appendix III
Two Letter State and profession Abbreviations *A-10*

Appendix IV
Abbreviations Commonly Used in Documentation *A-11*

Appendix V
Metric measurements *A-14*

Appendix VI
Celciuos—Farenheit Temperature Conversion Scale *A-15*

Appendix VII
Laboratory Tests *A-16*

Glossary *G-1*

Index *I-1*

LIPPINCOTT'S
Textbook for
Medical
Assistants

LIPPINCOTT'S
Textbook for
Medical Assistants

Julie B. Hosley, RN, CMA
Medical Assisting Curriculum Coordinator
Carteret Community College
Morehead City, North Carolina

Shirley A. Jones, MSEd, MHA
Program Director
Allied Health Education
Methodist Hospital
Indianapolis, Indiana

Elizabeth A. Molle-Matthews, RN, CEN
Clinical Research Nurse
Middlesex Hospital
Middletown, Connecticut
Formerly Director, Medical Assisting Program
Morse School of Business
Hartford, Connecticut

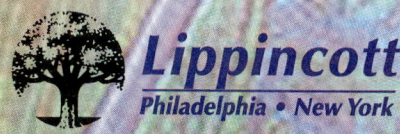

Lippincott
Philadelphia • New York

Acquisitions Editor: Andrew Allen
Editorial Assistant: Patricia Moore
Project Editor: Sandra Cherrey Scheinin
Production Manager: Helen Ewan

Production Coordinator: Nanette Winski
Design Coordinator: Doug Smock
Indexer: Ellen Murray

Library of Congress Cataloging in Publication Data

Hosley, Julie B.
    Lippincott's textbook for medical assistants / Julie B. Hosley,
  Shirley A. Jones, Elizabeth Molle-Matthews.
        p.   cm.
    Includes bibliographical references and index.
    ISBN 0-397-55096-0
    1. Medical assistants.   I. Jones, Shirley A.   II. Molle-Matthews,
  Elizabeth.   III. Title.
    [DNLM: 1. Physician Assistants.   2. Clinical Medicine—methods.
  3. Practice Management, Medical.   W 21.5 H826L   1997]
  R728.8.H66   1997
  610.69'53—dc20
  DNLM/DLC
  for Library of Congress   96-34495
                                                         CIP

The material contained in this volume was submitted as previously unpublished material, except in the instances in which credit has been given to the source from which some of the illustrative material was derived.

Any procedure or practice described in this book should be applied by the health-care practitioner under appropriate supervision in accordance with professional standards of care used with regard to the unique circumstances that apply in each practice situation. Care has been taken to confirm the accuracy of information presented and to describe generally accepted practices. However, the authors, editors, and publisher cannot accept any responsibility for errors or omissions or for any consequences from application of the information in this book and make no warranty, express or implied, with respect to the contents of the book.

The authors and publisher have exerted every effort to ensure that drug selection and dosage set forth in this text are in accordance with current recommendations and practice at the time of publication. However, in view of ongoing research, changes in government regulations, and the constant flow of information relating to drug therapy and drug reactions, the reader is urged to check the package insert for each drug for any change in indications and dosage and for added warnings and precautions. This is particularly important when the recommended agent is a new or infrequently employed drug.

Materials appearing in this book prepared by individuals as part of their official duties as U.S. Government employees are not covered by the above-mentioned copyright.

9 8 7 6 5 4 3 2 1

Selected figures (illustrations) in this text were reproduced with permission from the following Lippincott-Raven sources: Taylor C, Lillis C, LeMone P: Fundamentals of Nursing, Second Edition; Craven RF, Hirnle CJ: Fundamentals of Nursing, Second Edition; Smeltzer SC, Bare B: Brunner and Suddarth's Textbook of Medical-Surgical Nursing, Eighth Edition; Memmler RL, Cohen BJ, Wood DL: The Human Body in Health and Disease, Eighth Edition; Burton GRW, Engelkirk PG: Microbiology for the Health Sciences, Fifth Edition; Lotspeich-Steininger CA, Steine-Martin EA, Koepke JA: Clinical Hematology; Timby BK: Fundamental Skills and Concepts in Patient Care, Sixth Edition; Kurzen CR: Contemporary Practical/Vocational Nursing, Second Edition; Jones SA, Weigel A, White RD, McSwain NE, Breiter M: Advanced Emergency Care for Paramedic Practice; Bates B, Bickley LS, Hoekelman RA: A Guide to Physical Examination and History Taking, Sixth Edition; Ellis JR, Nowlis EA, Bentz PM: Modules for Basic Nursing Skills, Volume I, Sixth Edition; Bullock BL: Pathophysiology, Fourth Edition; Porth CM: Pathophysiology, Fourth Edition; David D: How to Quickly and Accurately Master ECG Interpretation, Second Edition; Reeder SJ, Martin LL, Griffin DK: Maternity Nursing, Eighteenth Edition; Bishop ML: Clinical Chemistry, Third Edition; Koneman EW, Allen SD, Janda WM, Schreckenberger PC, Winn WC: Color Atlas and Textbook of Diagnostic Microbiology, Fourth Edition; Harvey RA, Champe PC: Lippincott's Illustrated Reviews: Microbiology; McCall RE, Tankersley CM: Phlebotomy Exam Review; Broadwell JD, Saunders RB: Child Health Nursing.

This book is dedicated to my long-suffering husband who assured me that I could do this, but who thought it would never end; to my parents who always helped me believe I could do anything I set out to do; to my sons who cheered me on; to my friends and co-workers who put up with me when I was distracted and frantic; and to my boss who always believed in me.

JULIE HOSLEY

To my sister, Dr. Virginia Kelleher, for her invaluable contribution to the field of medicine; to my trusted companion, Zachary; and to my editor, Andrew Allen, for his encouragement and support.

SHIRLEY JONES

I would like to dedicate this book to my husband, Kevin; my son, Benjamin; my mother; and my two sisters for their love and support. In addition, I would like to dedicate this book to three health care professional role models—Karen, Carol, and Sharon.

BETTY MOLLE-MATTHEWS

Contributors

Beverly A. Baker, DA, CST
Program Director and Instructor, Surgical Technology
Western Iowa Technical and Community College
Sioux City, Iowa
Chapter 43: Microbiology

Rita-Ann Boegel, ADN, RN, CGRN
Charge Nurse
Gastroenterology Diagnostic Center
Veterans Administration Medical Hospital
San Francisco, California
*Chapter 38: Caring for Patients With
Gastrointestinal Disorders*

Barbara Marie Boor, RN
Office Manager
Office of John William Boor, MD
Riddle Memorial Hospital Health Care Center
Media, Pennsylvania
Chapter 16: Accounts Payable and Payroll

Sharon Brill, RN, BSN, PHN
Associate Instructor, Health Care Technologies
West Valley College
Saratoga, California
Chapter 49: Pediatric Patients

Lisa A. Bruno, BSN, CCRC
Clinical Research Coordinator
Department of Family Practice
Middlesex Hospital
Middletown, Connecticut
Chapter 11: Computers in the Medical Office

Harriette Cooper, LPN
Carteret Surgical Associates
Morehead City, North Carolina
Chapter 23: Instruments and Equipment

Toni M. Crowell, CMA
Program Coordinator, Medical Assisting and Medical
    Office Administration
Sussex County Community College
Newton, New Jersey
Instructor, Medical Assisting and Medical Office
    Administration
Berdan Institute
Totowa, New Jersey
*Chapter 10: Medical Records and Record
    Management*

Laura G. Cullen, RN, CMA, AA, PARALEGAL
Nurse–Paralegal
Law Office of Kathleen C. Cresson
New Orleans, Louisiana
Chapter 24: Assisting With Minor Office Surgery
*Chapter 34: Caring for Patients With Endocrine
    Disorders*

Phyllis Davis, CMA-AC, AA
Administrative Medical Assistant
Office of Harold A. Rosenfield, MD
Torrance, California
Chapter 8: Appointments

Theresa P. Ford, MT(ASCP), MEd
Hematology Supervisor
Craven Regional Medical Center
New Bern, North Carolina
Chapter 47: Serology and Immunohematology

Barbara Gierach-Lato, RN, BSN, CMA
Medical Assistant Program Director
Mid-State Technical College
Marshfield, Wisconsin
Chapter 5: Patient Education
*Chapter 6: Teaching Patients About Maintaining
    Health*

Loretta M. Hamilton, AOS, CMA, RMLA, RPT
Paramedical Examiner
Portamedic
Metairie, Louisiana
Chapter 25: Pharmacology
*Chapter 26: Preparing and Administering
    Medications*
*Chapter 34: Caring for Patients With Endocrine
    Disorders*
*Chapter 36: Caring for Patients With Immune
    Disorders*

Judy White Harris, RN, CMA-C
J.W. Harris Publications
Sarasota, Florida
*Chapter 33: Caring for Patients With Sensory
    Disorders*

Diane Herschfelt, RN, CMA, BS, MAHB
Department Chair, Health Care Technologies
West Valley College
Saratoga, California
> *Chapter 4: Fundamental Communication Skills*

Julie B. Hosley, RN, CMA
Medical Assisting Curriculum Coordinator
Carteret Community College
Morehead City, North Carolina
> *Chapter 39: Caring for Patients with Urinary*
> *Disorders*
> *Chapter 40: Caring for Patients with Disorders of*
> *the Male Reproductive System*
> *Chapter 50: Geriatric Patients*

Shirley A. Jones, MSEd, MHA
Program Director
Allied Health Education
Methodist Hospital
Indianapolis, Indiana
> *Chapter 28: Medical Office Emergencies*

David E. Kelleher
President
HealthCare Options, Inc.
Indianapolis, Indiana
> *Chapter 18: Health Insurance*

Anne Kirby, MA
Instructor, Medical Assisting Program
Carteret Community College
Morehead City, North Carolina
> *Chapter 7: The First Contact: Telephone*
> *and Reception*

Lauri A. Kollross, CMA
Operations Manager, Marshfield Clinic
Advisor and Coordinator, Medical Assistant Program
Mid-State Technical College
Marshfield, Wisconsin
> *Chapter 35: Caring for Patients With*
> *Cardiovascular Disorders*

Pauline Leventry, ADN, CMA
Medical Assistant Department Chairman
Mount Aloysius College
Cresson, Pennsylvania
> *Chapter 19: Asepsis and Infection Control*

Tibby Loveman, BSN
Former Medical Assistant Instructor
Gadsden Business College
Gadsden, Alabama
> *Chapter 22: Physical Examination*
> *Chapter 30: Caring for Patients With*
> *Integumentary Disorders*

Larry H. Miller, RT(R)
Radiography Curriculum Coordinator
Carteret Community College
Morehead City, North Carolina
> *Chapter 27: Diagnostic Imaging*

Elizabeth A. Molle-Matthews, RN, CEN
Clinical Research Nurse
Middlesex Hospital
Middletown, Connecticut
Formerly Director, Medical Assisting Program
Morse School of Business
Hartford, Connecticut
> *Chapter 1: Medicine and Medical Assisting*
> *Chapter 2: Medical Ethics and Bioethical Issues*
> *Chapter 3: Medicine and the Law*
> *Chapter 9: Written Communications*
> *Chapter 32: Caring for Patients with Neurologic*
> *Disorders*

Sue Overstreet
Operations Improvement, Provider Relations
Pro Health
Community Hospitals of Indianapolis
Indianapolis, Indiana
> *Chapter 18: Health Insurance*

Peter J. Quinn, Sr., BA
Advisor, Business and Accounting
Commonwealth College
Richmond, Virginia
> *Chapter 52: Employment*

Susan Ravagni, MT(ASCP)
Medical Technologist
Hematology Laboratory
Brigham and Women's Hospital
Boston, Massachusetts
> *Chapter 44: Urinalysis*
> *Chapter 46: Hematology*
> *Chapter 48: Clinical Chemistry*

Midge Noel Ray, MSN, RN
Associate Professor, Health Information Management
 Program
Health Services Administration
School of Health Related Professions
University of Alabama at Birmingham
Birmingham, Alabama
> *Chapter 41: Caring for Patients With Disorders of*
> *the Female Reproductive System*

Cynthia M. Reed, MT (ASCP)
School Director
Georgia Medical Institute
Atlanta, Georgia
> *Chapter 42: Introduction into the Clinical*
> *Laboratory*

Dory Rincon, BA, CMA
Instructor, Medical Assisting Program
City College of San Francisco
San Francisco, California
Chapter 15: Bookkeeping and Banking

Nora Mae Sanborn, BSMT(ASCP)
Curriculum Coordinator, Phlebotomy Program
Instructor, Medical Assisting Program
Carteret Community College
Morehead City, North Carolina
Chapter 45: Phlebotomy

Janet R. Sesser, RMA(AMT), CMA
Corporate Training Director, Allied Health Programs
High-Tech Institute, Inc.
Phoenix, Arizona
Chapter 51: Externship

Kasey Coal Summer, BA, TED, RMA
Director, Career Services
Ultrasound Diagnostic Schools
Atlanta, Georgia
Chapter 12: Quality Improvement and Risk Management
Chapter 13: Management of the Medical Office Team
Chapter 20: Medical History and Patient Assessment
Chapter 21: Anthropometric Measurements and Vital Signs

Kimberly D. Summer
Senior Account Coordinator
Vanstar Corporation
Kennesaw, Georgia
Chapter 14: Credit and Collections

Patricia E. Taglianetti, RRA, BS, MBA
Coordinator, Health Information Technology Program
Northern Essex Community College
Haverhill, Massachusetts
Chapter 17: Diagnostic and Procedural Coding

Barbara S. Thomas, RRT, BA, BS, MPH
Curriculum Coordinator, Respiratory Care Technology
Carteret Community College
Morehead City, North Carolina
Chapter 37: Caring for Patients with Respiratory Disorders

Natalie Uebele, RN, BSPA
Instructor, Nursing Department
Carteret Community College
Morehead City, North Carolina
Chapter 29: Introduction to Anatomy and Physiology

Louise D. Yurko, MAPT
President, Carteret Physical Therapy Associates, Inc.
Morehead City, North Carolina
Adjunct Professor, School of Physical Therapy
East Carolina University
Greenville, North Carolina
Chapter 31: Caring for Patients With Musculoskeletal Disorders

Reviewers

Stefanie O. Ardoin, RRA
Business Manager
Office of Bradley J. Chastant, MD, FACS
Lafayette, Louisiana

Ursula Backner, AAS, CMA
Program Coordinator, Medical Assisting
Methodist Hospital
Indianapolis, Indiana

Cathy A. Below, CMA
Medical Assisting Program Director; Instructor
Professional Careers Institute
Indianapolis, Indiana

Kathy Boyle, BA, MEd
Adjunct Instructor, Aquinas College
The Boyle Company
Manchester, Massachusetts

Judy D. Breuker, CPC
Allied Health - Medical Insurance Instructor
Baker College of Muskegon
Muskegon, Michigan
President - Medical Reimbursement Service, Inc.
Jenison, Michigan

Sharon Brill, RN, BSN, PHN
Associate Instructor
Department of Healthcare Technologies
West Valley College
Saratoga, California

Elizabeth Christoff, RN, BSEd
Medical Coordinator
Medical Assistant Program
Business Institute of Pennsylvania
Sharon, Pennsylvania

Bob Degaetano, RMT
Instructor
Pima Medical Institute
Tucson, Arizona

Bonnie Lou Deister, MS, BSN, CMA-C
Chairperson - Medical Assisting/Paramedic
Broome Community College
Binghamton, New York

Irene Figliolona, CMA
Program Director
Berdan Institute
Totowa, New Jersey

Linda Fulton, CMA
Instructor and Executive Assistant
North Hills School of Health Occupations
Pittsburgh, Pennsylvania

Christine Goehner
Instructor and Clinical Supervisor
Pima Medical Institute
Mesa, Arizona

Michelle A. Green, MPS, RRA, CMA
Associate Professor
Alfred State College
Alfred, New York

Rebecca Hageman, ART
Instructor
Health Information Technology Program
Hutchinson Community College
Wichita, Kansas

Debra E. Hampton, LPN, BSPH
Medical Office Procedures Instructor
Medical Assisting Program
Methodist Hospital
Indianapolis, Indiana

Sue Hunt, MA, RN, CMA
Coordinator, Medical Assisting
Middlesex Community College
Lowell, Massachusetts

Marie A. James, ART
Instructor and Technical Assistant
Health Information Technology Program
Firelands College/Bowling Green State University
Huron, Ohio

Lori Jasper, CMT
Instructor
Mid-State Technical College
Plover, Wisconsin

Gertrude Kenny, BSN, RN, CMA
Associate Dean of Allied Health
Baker College of Muskegon
Muskegon, Michigan

Anne Kirby, MA
Part-time Instructor
Carteret Community College
Morehead City, North Carolina

Barbara Geirach-Lato, RN, BSN, CMA
Program Director
Medical Assisting Program
Mid-State Technical College
Marshfield, Wisconsin

Pauline Leventry, ADN, CMA
Medical Assistant Department Chairman
Mount Aloysius College
Cresson, Pennsylvania

Mary B. Lewis, MA
Instructor and Nursing Resource Laboratory Coordinator
Department of Nursing
Essex County College
Newark, New Jersey

Tibby Loveman, BSN
Former Medical Assistant Instructor
Gadsden Business College
Gadsden, Alabama

Paula Podein, CMA
Instructor
Baker College
Muskegon, Michigan

Vicki Prater, CMA, RMA, RAHA
Medical Assistant and Director of Medical Office
  Management Program
Concorde Career Institute
San Bernardino, California

Gracia Riedell, RN, BA, MA
Instructor, Director
Medical Assisting Program
Northeast Metro Technical College
Woodbury, Minnesota

Barbara R. Rockwell
Career Development Director
Pima Medical Institute
Tucson, Arizona

Vicki Scott, BA, MLT(ASCP), CMA
Program Director
Medical Assisting
Medical Institute of Minnesota
Bloomington, Minnesota

Patricia Suminski, RN, BSN, CMA
Instructor Coordinator of Medical Assistant Program
Milwaukee Area Technical College
Racine, Wisconsin

Janette B. Thomas, MPS, RRA
Director, Health Information Technology Program
Alfred State College
Alfred, New York

Mary Wahl, RN, BSN, MEPD, CMA
Health Occupations Instructor
Mid-State Technical College
Marshfield, Wisconsin

Jean Wheeler, RT, ASPT, RMA
Instructor
Andon College
Modesto, California

Wilma Yarnal, MT(ASCP)
Instructor, Medical Assistant Program
Business Institute of Pennsylvania
Masury, Ohio

Preface

This is an exciting and challenging time to enter the field of medical assisting. As emphasis shifts from hospital-based patient care to ambulatory care in the medical office, health care workers in office settings will be required to possess greater skills to care for patients with more complex needs. These changes have expanded the role of the office professional, requiring a higher degree of training and professionalism. The medical assistant is uniquely poised to function as the most versatile professional in the medical office and to continue to fill the need for a multiskilled health professional to address rapidly changing medical needs as technology races into the twenty-first century.

Lippincott's Textbook for Medical Assistants is designed to introduce the student to both administrative and clinical medical assisting practice. Foremost in the minds of the authors and contributors was the need to foster caring, compassion, and professionalism in the student. The text is based on the American Association of Medical Assisting (AAMA) DACUM, but is also designed to be applicable to American Medical Technologist programs. It may stand alone as a comprehensive text or may be used in conjunction with more specialized texts.

► ORGANIZATION OF THE TEXT

The text is organized to lay the groundwork for building an understanding of the practice of medical assisting and its origins. Administrative duties required to efficiently manage the medical office are examined with considerations for future technological needs. Clinical skills are arranged to flow from those more easily mastered to those that are relatively complex.

The text is divided into four main sections.

Section I, **Introduction to Medical Assisting,** provides a background for understanding medical practice and medical assisting and covers the legal and ethical issues that will impact the profession. The second unit of this section focuses on communicating with the patient and patient education to ensure a rapid return to optimum health.

Section II, **The Administrative Medical Assistant,** explores the administrative and financial operation of the medical office. Emphasis is placed on the expanding technological advances in office management. The student is introduced to appointment scheduling, medical records, computers, management and quality improvement, office finances, insurance, and coding.

Section III, **The Clinical Medical Assistant,** acquaints the student with the clinical aspects of medical assisting. Protection of the patient and assistant is emphasized throughout, with a focus on the practice of Standard Precautions to prevent the spread of disease. General procedures common to all practices, such as patient history and physical assessment, vital signs, physical examination, and instruments and equipment are covered in this section. In addition, chapters on pharmacology and medication administration, minor office surgery, diagnostic imaging, and medical office emergencies introduce the student to procedures found in many medical offices.

A unique systems approach to diagnostic testing and therapeutic procedures was written by contributors who are medical assisting instructors or practitioners in the medical specialties. These chapters begin by explaining normal function and progress to altered function with diagnostic tests, treatment, and the medical assistant's role and responsibilities in each medical specialty. Laboratory procedures performed in the medical office are covered comprehensively to provide the student with the skills required to perform diagnostic testing in a physician's office laboratory.

Pediatric and geriatric populations are presented separately to address the needs of special populations in this age of specialization.

Finally, Section IV, **Career Strategies,** prepares the student for externship to ease the transition to the lifelong challenge and rewards of a medical career.

► KEY FEATURES

In an effort to make this text as student-friendly as possible, many features have been incorporated that should also assist the instructor in presenting the information in a clear and understandable manner.

Learning and performance objectives are listed at the beginning of each chapter to alert the student and instructor to the purpose of the chapter and the skills that will be acquired upon mastering the information.

Key Terms are listed at the beginning of each chapter and are introduced within the chapter in boldface type. A glossary at the back of the book defines all key terms.

Standard Precautions are explained and are indicated in procedures that present a risk for exposure to blood and body fluids. An icon representing a glove is included as a visual reminder in procedures requiring Standard Precautions.

Step-by-step procedures explain the progression required to accomplish medical tasks. Many steps include the purpose for performance to help the student understand the importance of established protocol. Full color photographs are included where appropriate.

Charting Examples are included throughout to instruct the student in proper procedures for recording patient information.

Patient Education boxes alert the student to opportunities to assist the patient in acquiring health care knowledge that will help ensure compliance with prescribed treatment or lead to health oriented life-style changes.

What if . . . situations remind the student that medical challenges are rarely textbook perfect, and that many will require research and collaboration with other health care professionals for the best possible response.

Legal and Ethical Tips are included to alert the student to potential areas of concern and to help avoid litigation or ethical stumbling blocks.

Focus on the Patient boxes remind the student that every action in the medical office is directed at assisting the patient in the return to health.

Critical Thinking Challenges urge the student to think through situations that require a logical progression of thought processes, using information and skills acquired through the course of study. These exercises also encourage the student to analyze and evaluate problems that may be encountered in the medical office setting and to determine what actions to take. In addition, a number of these exercises promote the performance of advanced-level skills, such as developing educational materials, as defined by

the DACUM analysis of the medical assisting profession.

Full color illustrations clarify concepts and add visual appeal.

Charts, boxes, and tables are included for clarity and easy access to information.

DACUM relevance for each chapter is included for those programs associated with the AAMA to ensure that all entry-level skills required of the graduate are addressed within the text.

➤ TEACHING-LEARNING PACKAGE

Lippincott's Textbook for Medical Assistants has an extensive ancillary package, designed with both the student and instructor in mind.

— A student *Study Guide* augments the text and provides a means of student self-evaluation. The Study Guide contains numerous exercises including chapter reviews, critical thinking practice, charting documentation, and patient teaching. Performance checklists are included for every procedure in the textbook. A unique feature is the *Interactive Self-Study Computer Disk* in the back of the Study Guide, which contains multiple choice questions.

— An *Instructor's Manual* offers tips for expanding learning opportunities in the classroom.

— *Four-color Transparencies Acetates* help clarify and enhance lecture materials.

— *A Printed and Computerized Testing Program* facilitates instructor-designed queries and examinations and prepares the student for the certification examination.

We hope this textbook will serve to introduce the student to the knowledge needed to excel in this most exciting health care profession. As educators, it is our hope that this text will make it easier for other instructors to share with their students the joy and rewards we have found in medical assisting.

Julie B. Hosley, RN, CMA
Shirley A. Jones, MSEd, MHA
Elizabeth A. Molle-Matthews, RN, CEN

Acknowledgments

No book of this length and complexity is possible without the help of many people—from its inception to its completion. Thanks go out to the photography models from Carteret Community College, who bring visual clarity to the text, and to Trey Shepard for his time and patience in setting up scenes for the photography. We would also like to thank the great people at Dr. Donald L. Myers' office, the instructors and students at the Crafts Institute, and the entire staff at Philadelphia Health Associates—thank you all for helping us with and modeling for the photographs in this book. Thanks to Mia Carter, who helped transfer manuscripts onto compatible software. The reviewers are to be commended for making sure that what was written was factual and current. They made valuable suggestions for improving the quality of this book. We would like to thank Marilyn Costanza for the incident report illustration and Stefanie O. Ardoin, RRA, and Dr. Bradley J. Chastant for the discipline record illustration.

Rose Foltz, our developmental editor, molded continuity and logical flow into the contributor manuscripts that had been crafted by experts in all fields of clinical medicine and administrative office management. Laura Dover and Patty Moore, Andrew Allen's editorial assistants, kept us all encouraged, on track, and in touch. And finally, we wish to extend our gratitude to Andrew Allen, Executive Editor. Andrew's vision of the text was the goal toward which all of us worked to bring to the profession of medical assisting a text that will set the standard for quality education.

Contents

Expanded Contents *xvii*

Procedures *xxiv*

Summary of Recurring Displays *xxvii*

Section I
Introduction to Medical Assisting 1

Unit 1 *Understanding the Profession* 3

1 Medicine and Medical Assisting 4

2 Medical Ethics and Bioethical Issues 18

3 Medicine and the Law 32

Unit 2 *Communicating With Patients* 53

4 Fundamental Communication Skills 54

5 Patient Education 70

6 Teaching Patients About Factors Influencing Health 80

Section II
The Administrative Medical Assistant 97

Unit 3 *Performing Administrative Duties* 99

7 The First Contact—Telephone and Reception 100

8 Appointments 112

9 Written Communications 126

10 Medical Records and Records Management 142

11 Computers in the Medical Office 156

12 Quality Improvement and Risk Management 168

13 Management of the Medical Office Team 180

Unit 4 *Managing Finances in the Practice* 195

14 Credit and Collections 196

15 Bookkeeping and Banking 204

16 Accounts Payable and Payroll 216

17 Diagnostic and Procedural Coding 228

18 Health Insurance 242

Section III
The Clinical Medical Assistant 263

Unit 5 *Performing Clinical Duties* 265

19 Asepsis and Infection Control 266

20 Medical History and Patient Assessment 288

21 Anthropometric Measurements and Vital Signs 300

22 Physical Examination 334

23 Instruments and Equipment 352

24 Assisting with Minor Office Surgery 374

25 Pharmacology 414

26 Preparing and Administering Medications 426

27 Diagnostic Imaging 468

28 Medical Office Emergencies 482

Unit 6 *Assisting With Diagnostic Tests and Therapeutic Procedures for Common Disorders* 503

29 Introduction to Anatomy and Physiology 504

30 Caring for Patients With Integumentary Disorders 516

31 Caring for Patients With Musculoskeletal Disorders 542

32 Caring for Patients With Neurologic Disorders 580

33 Caring for Patients With Sensory
     Disorders   *606*

34 Caring for Patients With Endocrine
     Disorders   *640*

35 Caring for Patients With Cardiovascular
     Disorders   *656*

36 Caring for Patients With Immune
     Disorders   *690*

37 Caring for Patients With Respiratory
     Disorders   *706*

38 Caring for Patients With Gastrointestinal
     Disorders   *726*

39 Caring for Patients With Urinary
     Disorders   *750*

40 Caring for Patients With Disorders of the Male
     Reproductive System   *764*

41 Caring for Patients With Gynecologic and
     Obstetric Disorders   *778*

Unit 7 *Performing Laboratory
Procedures*   *817*

42 Introduction to the Clinical Laboratory   *818*

43 Microbiology   *840*

44 Urinalysis   *866*

45 Phlebotomy   *894*

46 Hematology   *922*

47 Serology and Immunohematology   *950*

48 Clinical Chemistry   *966*

Unit 8 *Working With Special Patient
Populations*   *985*

49 Pediatric Patients   *986*

50 Geriatric Patients   *1016*

Section IV
Career Strategies   **1033**

Unit 9 *Competing in the Job Market*   *1035*

51 Externship   *1038*

52 Employment   *1048*

Appendices   *A-1*

Appendix I: 1990 DACUM Analysis of the
        Medical Assisting Profession   *A-2*

Appendix II: Key English-to-Spanish Health
        Care Phrases   *A-4*

Appendix III: Two-Letter State and Possession
        Abbreviations   *A-10*

Appendix IV: Abbreviations Commonly Used
        in Documentation   *A-11*

Appendix V: Metric Measurements   *A-14*

Appendix VI: Celsius–Fahrenheit Temperature
        Conversion Scale   *A-15*

Appendix VII: Laboratory Tests   *A-16*

Glossary   *G-1*

Index   *I-1*

Expanded Contents

Section I
Introduction to Medical Assisting 1

Unit 1 *Understanding the Profession* 3

  1 Medicine and Medical Assisting 4
- History of Medicine 6
- The Medical Assisting Profession 9
- Duties of a Medical Assistant 11
- Characteristics of a Professional Medical Assistant 12
- Members of the Health Care Team 13
- Employment Opportunities 14

  2 Medical Ethics and Bioethical Issues 18
- History of Medical Ethics 20
- American Medical Association (AMA) Code of Ethics 20
- American Association of Medical Assistants (AAMA) Code of Ethics 21
- Medical Assistant's Role in Ethics 21
- Bioethics 23
- American Medical Association Council on Ethical and Judicial Affairs 23

  3 Medicine and the Law 32
- The American Legal System 34
- Physician–Patient Relationship 35
- Specific Laws and Statutes That Apply to Health Professionals 43
- Specific Medical Law 47
- The Litigation Process 49
- Defenses to Professional Liability Suits 49
- A Defense for the Medical Assistant 50

Unit 2 *Communicating With Patients* 53

  4 Fundamental Communication Skills 54
- Basic Communication Flow 56
- Forms of Communication 56
- Active Listening 59
- Interviewing Techniques 59
- Factors Affecting Communication 61
- Establishing Positive Patient Relationships 66
- Patient Teaching 68

  5 Patient Education 70
- The Patient Education Process 72
- The Patient's Ability to Learn 75
- Patient Teaching Plans 76

  6 Teaching Patients About Factors Influencing Health 80
- Teaching Patients About Nutrition 82
- Teaching Patients About Exercise 89
- Teaching Patients to Cope with Illness and Stress 90
- Teaching Patients About Substance Abuse 92
- Teaching Patients About Medication Therapy 94

Section II
The Administrative Medical Assistant 97

Unit 3 *Performing Administrative Duties* 99

  7 The First Contact—Telephone and Reception 100
- Professional Image 102
- Reception 103
- Telephone 105

  8 Appointments 112
- Patient Office Visits 114
- Scheduling Appointments 114
- Factors That Affect Scheduling 117
- Scheduling Guidelines 118
- Preparing a Daily or Weekly Schedule 120
- Patient Reminders 120

➤ **Adapting the Schedule** *121*

➤ **Cancellations** *123*

➤ **Making Appointments for Patients in Other Facilities** *123*

➤ **When the Appointment Schedule Does Not Work** *124*

9 Written Communications *126*

➤ **Letter Development** *128*

➤ **Memorandum Development** *135*

➤ **Sending Written Communication** *135*

➤ **Receiving and Handling Incoming Mail** *138*

➤ **Composing Agendas and Minutes** *139*

➤ **Transcription** *140*

10 Medical Records and Records Management *142*

➤ **Standard Medical Records** *144*

➤ **Medical Record Organization** *144*

➤ **Documentation Forms** *145*

➤ **The Medical History** *147*

➤ **Medical Record Entries** *147*

➤ **Worker's Compensation Records** *149*

➤ **Filing Procedures** *150*

Procedure 10-1: Preparing a Medical Record File *150*

➤ **Filing Systems** *151*

➤ **Classifying Medical Records** *153*

➤ **Storing Medical Records** *153*

➤ **Releasing Medical Records** *154*

➤ **Reporting Obligations** *155*

11 Computers in the Medical Office *156*

➤ **Computer Components** *158*

➤ **Care and Maintenance of the System and Equipment** *161*

➤ **Operating a Computer** *162*

➤ **Training Options** *163*

➤ **Computer Applications** *163*

➤ **Automated Front Desk** *165*

➤ **Purchasing a Computer** *165*

12 Quality Improvement and Risk Management *168*

➤ **Quality Improvement Programs in the Medical Office Setting** *170*

➤ **Developing a Quality Improvement Program** *172*

➤ **Risk Management** *174*

➤ **Putting It All Together: A Case Review** *178*

13 Management of the Medical Office Team *180*

➤ **Overview of Medical Office Management** *182*

➤ **Responsibilities of the Medical Office Manager** *183*

➤ **Legal Issues Regarding Office Management** *193*

Unit 4 *Managing Finances in the Practice* **195**

14 Credit and Collections *196*

➤ **Fees** *198*

➤ **Credit** *199*

➤ **Collections** *199*

15 Bookkeeping and Banking *204*

➤ **Bookkeeping Systems** *206*

➤ **Banking** *212*

➤ **Petty Cash** *214*

16 Accounts Payable and Payroll *216*

➤ **Accounting Cycle** *218*

➤ **Record-Keeping Components** *218*

➤ **Accounts Payable** *219*

➤ **Payroll** *221*

➤ **Preparation of Reports** *227*

➤ **Assisting With Audits** *227*

17 Diagnostic and Procedural Coding *228*

➤ **Diagnostic Coding** *230*

➤ **Procedural Coding** *232*

➤ **Reimbursement** *238*

➤ **Fraud and Coding** *239*

18 Health Insurance *242*

➤ **Health Benefit Plans** *246*

➤ **Filing Claims** *250*

➤ **Managed Care** *255*

➤ **Policies in the Practice** *261*

Section III
The Clinical Medical Assistant 263

Unit 5 *Performing Clinical Duties* **265**

19 Asepsis and Infection Control *266*

➤ **Microorganisms and Normal Flora** *268*

➤ **Conditions That Favor the Growth of Pathogens** *269*

➤ **The Infection Cycle** *269*

➤ **Modes of Transmission** *270*

➤ **Medical Asepsis** *270*

➤ **Maintaining Medical Asepsis** *271*

➤ **Isolation Precautions** *271*

Procedure 19-1: Handwashing for Medical Asepsis 272

➤ **Surgical Asepsis** 276

➤ **Surgical Scrub** 276

➤ **Infection Control** 276

Procedure 19-2: Performing a Surgical Scrub 277

Procedure 19-3: Sterile Gloving 280

Procedure 19-4: Removing Gloves After a Procedure 283

20 Medical History and Patient Assessment 288

➤ **The Medical History** 290

➤ **Conducting a Patient Interview** 293

Procedure 20-1: Interviewing the Patient to Obtain a Medical History 294

➤ **Assessing the Patient** 295

21 Anthropometric Measurements and Vital Signs 300

➤ **Weight** 302

➤ **Height** 302

➤ **Temperature (T)** 302

➤ **Pulse (P)** 308

➤ **Respiration (R)** 310

➤ **Blood Pressure (BP)** 312

➤ **Charting Vital Signs in the Hospital Setting** 314

Procedure 21-1: Measuring Weight 317

Procedure 21-2: Measuring Height 318

Procedure 21-3: Measuring Oral Temperature Using a Glass Mercury Thermometer 319

Procedure 21-4: Measuring Rectal Temperature Using a Glass Mercury Thermometer 321

Procedure 21-5: Measuring Axillary Temperature Using a Glass Mercury Thermometer 323

Procedure 21-6: Measuring Temperature Using an Electronic Thermometer 324

Procedure 21-7: Measuring Temperature Using a Tympanic Thermometer 325

Procedure 21-8: Disinfecting a Glass Thermometer 325

Procedure 21-9: Measuring the Radial Pulse 326

Procedure 21-10: Measuring the Apical Pulse 327

Procedure 21-11: Counting Respirations 329

Procedure 21-12: Measuring Blood Pressure 329

22 Physical Examination 334

➤ **Components of the Physical Examination** 336

➤ **Basic Instruments and Supplies** 336

➤ **Special Instruments and Supplies** 338

➤ **Examination Techniques** 341

➤ **Responsibilities of the Medical Assistant** 341

➤ **Physical Examination Format** 342

Procedure 22-1: Assisting With the Physical Examination 345

➤ **General Health Guidelines and Checkups** 350

23 Instruments and Equipment 352

➤ **Instruments** 354

➤ **Instruments and Equipment Used by Specialists** 359

➤ **Care and Handling of Instruments** 359

➤ **Principles and Practices of Asepsis** 363

➤ **Sanitation** 363

➤ **Disinfection** 363

Procedure 23-1: Sanitizing Equipment for Sterilization or Disinfection 364

➤ **Sterilization** 365

➤ **Boiling** 370

Procedure 23-2: Operating an Autoclave 371

➤ **Storage and Recordkeeping** 372

➤ **Maintaining Surgical Supplies** 372

24 Assisting with Minor Office Surgery 374

➤ **Preparing and Maintaining a Sterile Field** 376

➤ **Preparing the Patient for Minor Office Surgery** 379

➤ **Local Anesthetics** 381

➤ **Scalpels and Blades** 381

➤ **Wound Closure** 382

➤ **Assisting with Suture Removal** 384

➤ **Assisting with Staple Removal** 385

➤ **Sterile Dressings** 386

➤ **Bandaging** 386

➤ **Commonly Performed Office Surgical Procedures** 389

➤ **Electrosurgery** 391

➤ **Laser Surgery** 392

➤ **Specimen Collection During Office Surgery** 393

➤ **Postsurgical Procedures** 393

Procedure 24-1: Opening Sterile Surgical Packs 395

Procedure 24-2: Using Sterile Transfer Forceps 397

Procedure 24-3: Adding Sterile Solution to the Field 397

Procedure 24-4: Performing Skin Preparation and Hair Removal 399

Procedure 24-5: Removing Sutures 400

Procedure 24-6: Removing Staples 402

Procedure 24-7: Applying a Sterile Dressing 403

Procedure 24-8: Changing an Existing Sterile Dressing 405

Procedure 24-9: Applying a Tubular Gauze Bandage 407

Procedure 24-10: Assisting with Excisional Surgery 411

Procedure 24-11: Assisting with Incision and Drainage (I&D) 412

25 Pharmacology 414

➤ **Medication Names** 416

➤ **Legal Regulations** 416

➤ **Prescriptions** 420

➤ **Sources of Drugs** 420

➤ **Pharmacodynamics** 420

➤ **Pharmacokinetics** 421

➤ **Drug Interactions** 423

➤ **Medication Allergies** *424*
➤ **Sources of Information in Pharmacology** *424*

26 Preparing and Administering Medications *426*
➤ **Common Abbreviations** *428*
➤ **Safety Guidelines** *428*
➤ **Seven Rights for Correct Medication Administration** *429*
➤ **Systems of Measurement for Medication Administration** *429*
➤ **Converting Measurements** *431*
➤ **Calculating Adult Dosages** *432*
➤ **Calculating Pediatric Dosages** *433*
➤ **Medication Routes** *434*
➤ **Oral Administration** *435*
➤ **Mucosal Administration** *435*
➤ **Dermal Administration** *437*
➤ **Parenteral Administration** *438*
➤ **Equipment Needed for Giving Injections** *438*
➤ **Types of Injections and Injection Sites** *441*
➤ **Other Medication Routes** *445*
Procedure 26-1: Administering Oral Medications *446*
Procedure 26-2: Administering Sublingual or Buccal Medications *449*
Procedure 26-3: Applying Transdermal Medications *450*
Procedure 26-4: Applying Topical Medications *451*
Procedure 26-5: Preparing an Injection *452*
Procedure 26-6: Administering an Intradermal Injection *458*
Procedure 26-7: Administering a Tine or Mantoux Test *460*
Procedure 26-8: Administering a Subcutaneous Injection *462*
Procedure 26-9: Administering an Intramuscular Injection *464*
Procedure 26-10: Administering an Intramuscular Injection Using the Z-Track Method *466*

27 Diagnostic Imaging *468*
➤ **X-rays and X-ray Machines** *470*
➤ **Principles of Radiography** *471*
➤ **Patient Positioning** *471*
➤ **Examination Sequencing** *471*
➤ **Radiation Safety** *472*
➤ **Diagnostic Procedures** *474*
➤ **Teleradiology** *478*
➤ **Interventional Radiologic Techniques** *478*
➤ **Radiation Therapy** *479*
➤ **The Medical Assistant's Role in Radiologic Procedures** *479*
➤ **Transfer of Radiographic Information** *480*

28 Medical Office Emergencies *482*
➤ **Emergency Medical Services System** *484*

➤ **Medical Office Emergency Procedures** *484*
➤ **Patient Assessment** *486*
Procedure 28-1: Managing an Adult Patient With a Foreign Body Airway Obstruction *489*
Procedure 28-2: Performing Cardiopulmonary Resuscitation (One Rescuer) *490*
➤ **Types of Emergencies** *493*

Unit 6 *Assisting With Diagnostic Tests and Therapeutic Procedures for Common Disorders* *503*

29 Introduction to Anatomy and Physiology *504*
➤ **Organization of the Body** *506*
➤ **General Plan of the Body** *511*
➤ **Homeostasis** *514*

30 Caring for Patients With Integumentary Disorders *516*
➤ **Function of the Integumentary System** *518*
➤ **Structure of the Integumentary System** *518*
➤ **Common Integumentary Disorders** *520*
➤ **Common Diagnostic Procedures and the Medical Assistant's Role** *529*
➤ **Warm and Cold Applications** *531*
Procedure 30-1: Applying Cold *534*
Procedure 30-2: Applying a Warm or Cold Compress *536*
Procedure 30-3: Using a Hot Water Bottle or Commercial Hot Pack *536*
Procedure 30-4: Assisting With Therapeutic Soaks *538*

31 Caring for Patients With Musculoskeletal Disorders *542*
➤ **Structure and Function of the Musculoskeletal System** *544*
➤ **Common Musculoskeletal Disorders** *556*
➤ **Common Diagnostic Procedures** *570*
➤ **Ambulatory Aids and the Medical Assistant's Role** *570*
Procedure 31-1: Measuring a Patient for Axillary Crutches *572*
Procedure 31-2: Teaching a Patient Crutch Gaits *574*

32 Caring for Patients With Neurologic Disorders *580*
➤ **Structure and Function of the Nervous System** *582*
➤ **Central Nervous System** *583*
➤ **Peripheral Nervous System** *587*
➤ **Autonomic Nervous system** *587*
➤ **Common Nervous System Disorders** *590*
➤ **Common Diagnostic Tests for Nervous System Disorders** *598*
Procedure 32-1: Assisting With a Lumbar Puncture *602*

33 Caring for Patients With Sensory
Disorders   *606*

➤ **The Eye**   *608*

➤ **The Ear**   *615*

➤ **The Nose**   *622*

➤ **Other Senses**   *625*

Procedure 33-1: Measuring Distance Visual
Acuity   *628*

Procedure 33-2: Measuring Color Perception   *629*

Procedure 33-3: Instilling Eye Medications   *630*

Procedure 33-4: Irrigating the Eye   *631*

Procedure 33-5: Removing a Foreign Object
From the Eye   *633*

Procedure 33-6: Irrigating the Ear   *634*

Procedure 33-7: Instilling Ear Medication   *636*

Procedure 33-8: Instilling Nasal Medication   *637*

34 Caring for Patients With Endocrine
Disorders   *640*

➤ **Structure and Function of the
Endocrine System**   *642*

➤ **Common Endocrine Disorders**   *647*

➤ **Common Laboratory Tests and Diagnostic
Procedures and the Medical Assistant's Role**   *654*

35 Caring for Patients With Cardiovascular
Disorders   *656*

➤ **Structure and Function of
the Cardiovascular System**   *658*

➤ **Common Cardiovascular Disorders**   *664*

➤ **Common Diagnostic Procedures and the Medical
Assistant's Role**   *673*

Procedure 35-1: Performing a 12-Lead
Electrocardiogram   *679*

Procedure 35-2: Mounting the ECG Strip for
Reading   *683*

Procedure 35-3: Applying a Holter Monitor   *686*

36 Caring for Patients With Immune
Disorders   *690*

➤ **Structure and Function of
the Lymphatic System**   *692*

➤ **Common Lymphatic Disorders**   *695*

➤ **Functions of the Immune System**   *696*

➤ **Common Immune Disorders**   *700*

➤ **Common Diagnostic Procedures and the Medical
Assistant's Role**   *704*

37 Caring for Patients With Respiratory
Disorders   *706*

➤ **Structure and Function of
the Respiratory System**   *708*

➤ **Organs of the Respiratory System**   *709*

➤ **Ventilation**   *712*

➤ **Respiration**   *713*

➤ **Defense Mechanisms of
the Respiratory System**   *714*

➤ **Common Respiratory Disorders**   *715*

➤ **Common Diagnostic Procedures and the Medical
Assistant's Role**   *719*

Procedure 37-1: Collecting a Specimen for
a Throat Culture   *722*

Procedure 37-2: Collecting a Sputum Specimen   *723*

38 Caring for Patients With Gastrointestinal
Disorders   *726*

➤ **Structure and Function of the Gastrointestinal
System**   *728*

➤ **Organs of the Gastrointestinal System**   *730*

➤ **Accessory Organs**   *732*

➤ **Common Gastrointestinal Disorders**   *733*

➤ **Common Diagnostic Procedures and the Medical
Assistant's Role**   *742*

Procedure 38-1: Preparing the Patient for
Colon Procedures   *744*

Procedure 38-2: Collecting a Stool Specimen   *747*

Procedure 38-3: Testing Stool for Occult Blood   *748*

39 Caring for Patients With Urinary
Disorders   *750*

➤ **Structure and Function of
the Urinary System**   *752*

➤ **Organs of the Urinary System**   *754*

➤ **The Voiding Reflex**   *756*

➤ **Common Urinary Disorders**   *756*

➤ **Common Diagnostic Studies and the Medical
Assistant's Role**   *760*

40 Caring for Patients With Disorders of the Male
Reproductive System   *764*

➤ **Evolution and Differentiation of the Male
Reproductive System**   *766*

➤ **Organs of the Male Reproductive System**   *766*

➤ **Common Disorders of the Male Reproductive
System**   *769*

➤ **Common Diagnostic Procedures and the Medical
Assistant's Role**   *776*

➤ **Preparing the Patient for Procedures**   *776*

41 Caring for Patients With Gynecologic and
Obstetric Disorders   *778*

➤ **Organs of the Female Reproductive System**   *780*

➤ **The Menstrual Cycle**   *781*

➤ **Gynecologic Disorders**   *784*

➤ **Common Gynecologic Tests and Therapeutic
Procedures and the Medical Assistant's Role**   *789*

Procedure 41-1: Assisting With a Pelvic Examination
With a Pap Smear   *792*

Procedure 41-2: Assisting With Colposcopy With
Cervical Biopsy   *796*

➤ **Obstetric Care**   *797*

➤ **Obstetric Disorders**   *803*

➤ **Onset of Labor**   *806*

➤ **Postpartum Care**   *806*

➤ **Common Obstetric Tests and Therapeutic
Procedures and the Medical Assistant's Role**   *808*

➤ **Contraception** *809*

Procedure 41-3: Assisting With the Insertion of an Intrauterine Device (IUD) *811*

➤ **Menopause** *812*

Procedure 41-4: Assisting With the Removal of an Intrauterine Device (IUD) *813*

Procedure 41-5: Assisting With the Insertion of Hormonal Subdermal Implants *814*

Unit 7 *Performing Laboratory Procedures* 817

42 Introduction to the Clinical Laboratory *818*

➤ **Laboratory Types** *820*

➤ **Laboratory Departments** *823*

➤ **Laboratory Personnel** *824*

➤ **Physician's Office Laboratory Testing** *824*

➤ **Laboratory Equipment** *824*

➤ **Laboratory Safety** *828*

➤ **Clinical Laboratory Improvement Amendments** *834*

43 Microbiology *840*

➤ **Microbiologic Life Forms** *842*

➤ **Microbiologic Testing: The Medical Assistant's Role** *845*

➤ **Specimen Collection and Handling** *845*

➤ **Microscopic Examination of Microorganisms** *848*

Procedure 43-1: Preparing the Specimen for Transport *853*

Procedure 43-2: Preparing a Dry Smear *854*

Procedure 43-3: Gram Staining a Smear Slide *856*

Procedure 43-4: Inoculating a Culture *861*

44 Urinalysis *866*

➤ **Specimen Collection Methods** *868*

➤ **Physical Properties of Urine** *869*

➤ **Chemical Properties of Urine** *870*

➤ **Urine Sediment** *874*

➤ **Urine Pregnancy Testing** *877*

Procedure 44-1: Obtaining a Clean-catch Midstream (CCMS) Urine Specimen *877*

Procedure 44-2: Obtaining a 24-Hour Urine Specimen *879*

Procedure 44-3: Determining Color and Clarity of Urine *880*

Procedure 44-4: Determining Specific Gravity of Urine Using the Urinometer *881*

Procedure 44-5: Determining Specific Gravity of Urine Using the Rafractometer *882*

Procedure 44-6: Performing Chemical Reagent Strip Analysis *883*

Procedure 44-7: Performing a Copper Reduction Test for Glucose *885*

Procedure 44-8: Performing Nitroprusside Reaction (Acetest) for Ketones *887*

Procedure 44-9: Performing an Acid Precipitation Test for Protein *888*

Procedure 44-10: Performing Diazo Tablet Test (Ictotest) for Bilirubin *889*

Procedure 44-11: Preparing a Urine Sediment *890*

Procedure 44-12: Preparing Urine Sediment for a Microscopic Examination *890*

45 Phlebotomy *894*

➤ **Blood Collection Sites** *896*

➤ **General Blood Drawing Equipment** *897*

➤ **Venipuncture Equipment** *898*

➤ **Blood Collection Systems** *899*

➤ **Order of Draw** *901*

➤ **Skin Puncture (Microcollection) Equipment** *901*

➤ **Patient Preparation** *903*

➤ **Performing a Venipuncture** *905*

Procedure 45-1: Obtaining a Blood Specimen by Venipuncture *906*

➤ **Performing a Skin Puncture** *913*

Procedure 45-2: Obtaining a Blood Specimen by Skin Puncture *914*

46 Hematology *922*

➤ **Formation of Blood Cells** *924*

➤ **Hematologic Testing** *925*

➤ **Complete Blood Count** *925*

➤ **Erythrocyte Sedimentation Rate (ESR or SED Rate)** *930*

➤ **Coagulation Tests** *930*

Procedure 46-1: Performing a Manual WBC Count *932*

Procedure 46-2: Making a Peripheral Blood Smear *936*

Procedure 46-3: Staining a Peripheral Blood Smear *939*

Procedure 46-4: Performing a WBC Differential *940*

Procedure 46-5: Performing a RBC Count *941*

Procedure 46-6: Performing a Hemoglobin Determination *942*

Procedure 46-7: Performing a Microhematocrit Determination *944*

Procedure 46-8: Performing a Wintrobe ESR *946*

Procedure 46-9: Determining Bleeding Time *947*

47 Serology and Immunohematology *950*

➤ **Antigens and Antibodies** *952*

➤ **Serology Test Methods and Principles** *952*

➤ **Specimen Collection and Handling** *954*

➤ **Reagent and Kit Storage and Handling** *955*

➤ **Following Test Procedures** *956*

➤ **Quality Assurance and Quality Control** *956*

➤ **Serology Tests** *957*

➤ **Immunohematology** *961*

➤ **Blood Supply** *963*

48 Clinical Chemistry *966*

➤ **Special Instruments and Methods** *968*

➤ **Renal Function** *968*

➤ **Liver Function** *971*

➤ **Thyroid Function** *972*

➤ **Cardiac Function** *973*

➤ **Lung Function** *973*

➤ **Pancreatic Function** *974*

Procedure 48-1: Determining Blood Glucose Using the Glucometer *976*

Procedure 48-2: Glucose Tolerance Testing (GTT) *978*

➤ **Lipids and Lipoproteins** *981*

Unit 8 *Working With Special Patient Populations* **985**

49 Pediatric Patients *986*

➤ **The Pediatric Practice** *988*

➤ **The Office Environment** *988*

➤ **Psychological Aspects of Care** *989*

➤ **Physiologic Aspects of Care** *990*

➤ **The Physical Examination** *998*

Procedure 49-1: Restraining a Child *1002*

Procedure 49-2: Measuring Height *1003*

Procedure 49-3: Measuring Length *1003*

Procedure 49-4: Measuring Head Circumference *1004*

Procedure 49-5: Measuring Chest Circumference *1005*

Procedure 49-6: Weighing an Infant *1006*

Procedure 49-7: Measuring Pediatric Blood Pressure *1010*

➤ **Administering Medications** *1010*

➤ **Collecting a Urine Specimen** *1011*

➤ **Understanding Child Abuse** *1011*

Procedure 49-8: Applying a Pediatric Urine Collection Device *1012*

50 Geriatric Patients *1016*

➤ **Concepts of Aging** *1018*

➤ **Memory Enhancement to Reinforce Medical Compliance** *1018*

➤ **Reinforcing Mental Health** *1019*

➤ **Coping With Aging** *1020*

➤ **Long-Term Care** *1021*

➤ **Elder Abuse** *1021*

➤ **Medications and the Elderly** *1022*

➤ **Systemic Changes in the Elderly** *1023*

➤ **Diseases of the Elderly** *1023*

➤ **Maintaining Optimum Health** *1029*

Section IV

Career Strategies *1033*

Unit 9 *Competing in the Job Market* **1035**

51 Externship *1036*

➤ **Externship Scheduling** *1038*

➤ **Types of Facilities** *1038*

➤ **Site Selection** *1038*

➤ **Benefits of Externship** *1039*

➤ **Responsibilities of Externship** *1039*

➤ **Student Evaluation Criteria for the Preceptor** *1040*

➤ **Guidelines for a Successful Externship** *1042*

➤ **Time Records and Site Evaluations for the Student** *1043*

52 Employment *1048*

➤ **Establish the Job for You** *1050*

➤ **Finding the Right Job** *1051*

➤ **Applying for the Job** *1051*

➤ **Interviewing** *1055*

➤ **Follow-up** *1058*

➤ **Keep the Job or Move On?** *1059*

Appendices A-1

Appendix I: 1990 DACUM Analysis of the Medical Assisting Profession *A-2*

Appendix II: Key English-to-Spanish Health Care Phrases *A-4*

Appendix III: Two-Letter State and Possession Abbreviations *A-10*

Appendix IV: Abbreviations Commonly Used in Documentation *A-11*

Appendix V: Metric Measurements *A-14*

Appendix VI: Celsius–Fahrenheit Temperature Conversion Scale *A-15*

Appendix VII: Laboratory Tests *A-16*

Glossary *G-1*

Index *I-1*

Procedures

10

Medical Records and Records Management **142**

Procedure 10-1: *Preparing a Medical Record File* 150

19

Asepsis and Infection Control **266**

Procedure 19-1: *Handwashing for Medical Asepsis* 272

Procedure 19-2: *Performing a Surgical Scrub* 277

Procedure 19-3: *Sterile Gloving* 280

Procedure 19-4: *Removing Gloves After a Procedure* 283

20

Medical History and Patient Assessment **288**

Procedure 20-1: *Interviewing the Patient to Obtain a Medical History* 294

21

Anthropometric Measurements and Vital Signs **300**

Procedure 21-1: *Measuring Weight* 317

Procedure 21-2: *Measuring Height* 318

Procedure 21-3: *Measuring Oral Temperature Using a Glass Mercury Thermometer* 319

Procedure 21-4: *Measuring Rectal Temperature Using a Glass Mercury Thermometer* 321

Procedure 21-5: *Measuring Axillary Temperature Using a Glass Mercury Thermometer* 323

Procedure 21-6: *Measuring Temperature Using an Electronic Thermometer* 324

Procedure 21-7: *Measuring Temperature Using a Tympanic Thermometer* 325

Procedure 21-8: *Disinfecting a Glass Thermometer* 325

Procedure 21-9: *Measuring the Radial Pulse* 326

Procedure 21-10: *Measuring the Apical Pulse* 327

Procedure 21-11: *Counting Respirations* 329

Procedure 21-12: *Measuring Blood Pressure* 329

22

Physical Examination **334**

Procedure 22-1: *Assisting With the Physical Examination* 345

23

Instruments and Equipment **352**

Procedure 23-1: *Sanitizing Equipment for Sterilization or Disinfection* 364

Procedure 23-2: *Operating an Autoclave* 371

24

Assisting with Minor Office Surgery **374**

Procedure 24-1: *Opening Sterile Surgical Packs* 395

Procedure 24-2: *Using Sterile Transfer Forceps* 397

Procedure 24-3: *Adding Sterile Solution to the Field* 397

Procedure 24-4: *Performing Skin Preparation and Hair Removal* 399

Procedure 24-5: *Removing Sutures* 400

Procedure 24-6: *Removing Staples* 402

Procedure 24-7: *Applying a Sterile Dressing* 403

Procedure 24-8: *Changing an Existing Sterile Dressing* 405

Procedure 24-9: *Applying a Tubular Gauze Bandage* 407

Procedure 24-10: *Assisting with Excisional Surgery* 411

Procedure 24-11: *Assisting with Incision and Drainage (I&D)* 412

26

Preparing and Administering Medications **426**

Procedure 26-1: *Administering Oral Medications* 446

Procedure 26-2: *Administering Sublingual or Buccal Medications* 449

Procedure 26-3: *Applying Transdermal Medications* 450

Procedure 26-4: *Applying Topical Medications* 451

Procedure 26-5: *Preparing an Injection* 452

Procedure 26-6: *Administering an Intradermal Injection* 458

Procedure 26-7: *Administering a Tine or Mantoux Test* 460

Procedure 26-8: *Administering a Subcutaneous Injection* 462

Procedure 26-9: *Administering an Intramuscular Injection* 464

Procedure 26-10: *Administering an Intramuscular Injection Using the Z-Track Method* 466

28

Medical Office Emergencies **482**

Procedure 28-1: *Managing an Adult Patient With a Foreign Body Airway Obstruction* 489

Procedure 28-2: *Performing Cardiopulmonary Resuscitation (One Rescuer)* 490

30

Caring for Patients With Integumentary Disorders **516**

Procedure 30-1: *Applying Cold* 534

Procedure 30-2: *Applying a Warm or Cold Compress* 536

Procedure 30-3: *Using a Hot Water Bottle or Commercial Hot Pack* 536

Procedure 30-4: *Assisting With Therapeutic Soaks* 538

31

Caring for Patients With Musculoskeletal Disorders **542**

Procedure 31-1: *Measuring a Patient for Axillary Crutches* 572

Procedure 31-2: *Teaching a Patient Crutch Gaits* 574

32

Caring for Patients With Neurologic Disorders **000**

Procedure 32-1: *Assisting With a Lumbar Puncture* 602

33

Caring for Patients With Sensory Disorders **606**

Procedure 33-1: *Measuring Distance Visual Acuity* 628

Procedure 33-2: *Measuring Color Perception* 629

Procedure 33-3: *Instilling Eye Medications* 630

Procedure 33-4: *Irrigating the Eye* 631

Procedure 33-5: *Removing a Foreign Object From the Eye* 633

Procedure 33-6: *Irrigating the Ear* 634

Procedure 33-7: *Instilling Ear Medication* 636

Procedure 33-8: *Instilling Nasal Medication* 637

35

Caring for Patients With Cardiovascular Disorders **656**

Procedure 35-1: *Performing a 12-Lead Electrocardiogram* 679

Procedure 35-2: *Mounting the ECG Strip for Reading* 683

Procedure 35-3: *Applying a Holter Monitor* 686

37

Caring for Patients With Respiratory Disorders **706**

Procedure 37-1: *Collecting a Specimen for a Throat Culture* 722

Procedure 37-2: *Collecting a Sputum Specimen* 723

38

Caring for Patients With Gastrointestinal Disorders **726**

Procedure 38-1: *Preparing the Patient for Colon Procedures* 744

Procedure 38-2: *Collecting a Stool Specimen* 747

Procedure 38-3: *Testing Stool for Occult Blood* 748

41

Caring for Patients With Gynecologic and Obstetric Disorders **778**

Procedure 41-1: *Assisting With a Pelvic Examination With a Pap Smear* 792

Procedure 41-2: *Assisting With Colposcopy With Cervical Biopsy* 796

Procedure 41-3: *Assisting With the Insertion of an Intrauterine Device (IUD)* 811

Procedure 41-4: *Assisting With the Removal of an Intrauterine Device (IUD)* 813

Procedure 41-5: *Assisting With the Insertion of Subdermal Hormonal Implants* 814

43

Microbiology **840**

Procedure 43-1: *Preparing the Specimen for Transport* 853

Procedure 43-2: *Preparing a Dry Smear* 854

Procedure 43-3: *Gram Staining a Smear Slide* 856

Procedure 43-4: *Inoculating a Culture* 861

44

Urinalysis **866**

Procedure 44-1: *Obtaining a Clean-catch Midstream (CCMS) Urine Specimen* 877

Procedure 44-2: *Obtaining a 24-Hour Urine Specimen* 879

Procedure 44-3: *Determining Color and Clarity of Urine* 880

Procedure 44-4: *Determining Specific Gravity of Urine Using the Urinometer* 881

Procedure 44-5: *Determining Specific Gravity of Urine Using the Refractometer* 882

Procedure 44-6: *Performing Chemical Reagent Strip Analysis* 883

Procedure 44-7: *Performing a Copper Reduction Test (Clinitest) for Glucose* 885

Procedure 44-8: *Performing Nitroprusside Reaction (Acetest) for Ketones* 887

Procedure 44-9: *Performing an Acid Precipitation Test for Protein* 888

Procedure 44-10: *Performing Diazo Tablet Test (Ictotest) for Bilirubin* 889

Procedure 44-11: *Preparing a Urine Sediment* 890

Procedure 44-12: *Preparing Urine Sediment for a Microscopic Examination* 890

45

Phlebotomy **894**

Procedure 45-1: *Obtaining a Blood Specimen by Venipuncture* 906

Procedure 45-2: *Obtaining a Blood Specimen by Skin Puncture* 914

46

Hematology **922**

Procedure 46-1: *Performing a Manual WBC Count* 932

Procedure 46-2: *Making a Peripheral Blood Smear* 936

Procedure 46-3: *Staining a Peripheral Blood Smear* 939

Procedure 46-4: *Performing a WBC Differential* 940

Procedure 46-5: *Performing a RBC Count* 941

Procedure 46-6: *Performing a Hemoglobin Determination* 942

Procedure 46-7: *Performing a Microhematocrit Determination* 944

Procedure 46-8: *Performing a Wintrobe ESR* 946

Procedure 46-9: *Determining Bleeding Time* 947

48

Clinical Chemistry **966**

Procedure 48-1: *Determining Blood Glucose Using the Glucometer* 976

Procedure 48-2: *Glucose Tolerance Testing (GTT)* 978

49

Pediatric Patients **998**

Procedure 49-1: *Restraining a Child* 1002

Procedure 49-2: *Measuring Height* 1003

Procedure 49-3: *Measuring Length* 1003

Procedure 49-4: *Measuring Head Circumference* 1004

Procedure 49-5: *Measuring Chest Circumference* 1005

Procedure 49-6: *Weighing an Infant* 1006

Procedure 49-7: *Measuring Pediatric Blood Pressure* 1010

Procedure 49-8: *Applying a Pediatric Urine Collection Device* 1012

Summary of Recurring Displays

1

Medicine and Medical Assisting **4**

Patient Education: **The Health Care System** 12

2

Medical Ethics and Bioethical Issues **18**

Focus on the Patient: **Respecting Other Viewpoints** 21

3

Medicine and the Law **32**

Patient Education: **Legally Required Disclosures** 43

4

Fundamental Communication Skills **54**

Focus on the Patient: **Using the Right Tone of Voice** 57

Ethical Tips 68

5

Patient Education **70**

Patient Education: **General Teaching Topics** 72

Focus on the Patient: **Helping Patients Feel at Ease** 74

6

Teaching Patients About Factors Influencing Health **80**

Patient Education: **Diet and the Diabetic Patient** 85

7

The First Contact—Telephone and Reception **100**

Patient Education: **Television as a Teaching Tool** 105

8

Appointments **112**

Legal Tips 117

Charting Example 122

10

Medical Records and Records Management **142**

Legal Tips 154

11

Computers in the Medical Office **156**

Ethical Tips 165

13

Management of the Medical Office Team **180**

Legal Tips 192

14

Credit and Collections **196**

Legal Tips 202

15

Bookkeeping and Banking **204**

Ethical Tips 211

17

Diagnostic and Procedural Coding **228**

Legal Tips 239

18

Health Insurance **242**

Focus on the Patient: **Ensuring Fair Treatment** 249

Ethical Tips 250

Legal Tips 255

19

Asepsis and Infection Control **266**

Patient Education: **Basic Aseptic Technique** 274

20

Medical History and Patient Assessment **288**

Legal Tips 290

Focus on the Patient: **Helping Patients Feel At Ease** 293

Charting Example 294

Patient Education: **General Teaching Topics** 295

21

Anthropometric Measurements and Vital Signs **300**

Patient Education: **Fever** 304

Charting Example 313
Charting Example 315

22

Physical Examination **334**
Patient Education: **The Body's Warning Signals** 342
Charting Example 350

24

Assisting with Minor Office Surgery **374**
Charting Example 381
Charting Example 385
Charting Example 386
Charting Example 388
Charting Example 391
Patient Education: **Instructions Following Minor Surgery** 392

25

Pharmacology **414**
Ethical Tips 420
Focus on the Patient: **Understanding Drug Dependence** 424

26

Preparing and Administering Medications **426**
Charting Example 435
Charting Example 435
Patient Education: **Insertion of Suppositories** 438
Charting Example 438
Charting Example 442
Charting Example 443
Charting Example 443
Charting Example 444

27

Diagnostic Imaging **468**
Focus on the Patient: **Invading Personal Privacy?** 474
Legal Tips 480

28

Medical Office Emergencies **482**
Focus on the Patient: **Recognizing Groups at High Risk for Hypothermia** 500

30

Caring for Patients With Integumentary Disorders **516**
Focus on the Patient: **Dealing with Adolescents** 520
Charting Example 531
Charting Example 533
Charting Example 533
Patient Education: **Heating Pads** 533
Charting Example 540

31

Caring for Patients With Musculoskeletal Disorders **542**
Legal Tips 562
Patient Education: **Cast Care** 562
Focus on the Patient: **Living With Carpal Tunnel Syndrome** 568
Patient Education: **Tips for Crutch Walking** 571
Charting Example 571

32

Caring for Patients With Neurologic Disorders **580**
Focus on the Patient: **Coping With Febrile Seizures** 595
Patient Education: **Spinal Cord and Traumatic Brain Injuries** 598
Charting Example 601

33

Caring for Patients With Sensory Disorders **606**
Focus on the Patient: **Assisting the Sight-Impaired Patient** 611
Charting Example 613
Charting Example 615
Charting Example 615
Patient Education: **Preventive Eye Care** 616
Charting Example 616
Charting Example 617
Patient Education: **Otologic Disorders** 621
Charting Example 622
Charting Example 622
Charting Example 625
Patient Education: **Nasal Disorders** 625

34

Caring for Patients With Endocrine Disorders **640**
Patient Education: **Diabetes Mellitus** 652
Focus on the Patient: **Monitoring Elderly Diabetic Patients** 653

35

Caring for Patients With Cardiovascular Disorders **656**
Focus on the Patient: **Handling Cardiovascular Complaints** 665
Patient Education: **Nitroglycerin** 666
Charting Example 678
Charting Example 685

36

Caring for Patients With Immune Disorders **690**
Patient Education: **AIDS Prevention** 703
Legal Tips 704

37

Caring for Patients With Respiratory Disorders **706**
Legal Tips 715

Focus on the Patient: **Living with COPD**   718

Charting Example   721

Charting Example   724

38

Caring for Patients With Gastrointestinal Disorders   726

Patient Education: **Maintaining Good Bowel Habits**   739

Charting Example   745

Charting Example   748

39

Caring for Patients With Urinary Disorders   750

Patient Education: **Urinary Tract Health**   759

40

Caring for Patients With Disorders of the Male Reproductive System   764

Focus on the Patient: **Reducing Anxiety**   769

Patient Education: **Testicular Self-examination**   775

41

Caring for Patients With Gynecologic and Obstetric Disorders   778

Patient Education: **Kegel Exercises**   786

Charting Example   791

Charting Example   795

Charting Example   810

Charting Example   812

Charting Example   812

42

Introduction to the Clinical Laboratory   818

Patient Education: **Specimen Collection**   820

Ethical Tips   823

43

Microbiology   840

Patient Education: **Lyme Disease**   845

Charting Example   848

Charting Example   849

Charting Example   851

44

Urinalysis   866

Patient Education: **Urine Specimen Collection**   868

Charting Example   869

Charting Example   871

Charting Example   871

Charting Example   872

Charting Example   872

Charting Example   873

Charting Example   874

45

Phlebotomy   894

Charting Example   905

Charting Example   913

46

Hematology   922

Patient Education: **Iron Deficiency Anemia**   928

Charting Example   929

Charting Example   930

Charting Example   932

47

Serology and Immunohematology   950

Patient Education: **Expectant Mothers and RhoGAM**   961

48

Clinical Chemistry   966

Charting Example   975

Charting Example   980

Patient Education: **Using a Glucometer**   980

49

Pediatric Patients   986

Legal Tips   988

Focus on the Patient: **Communicating With Children**   989

Patient Education: **Middle Ear Infections**   998

Charting Example   1009

50

Geriatric Patients   1016

Focus on the Patient: **Communicating With the Hearing Impaired**   1019

Introduction to Medical Assisting

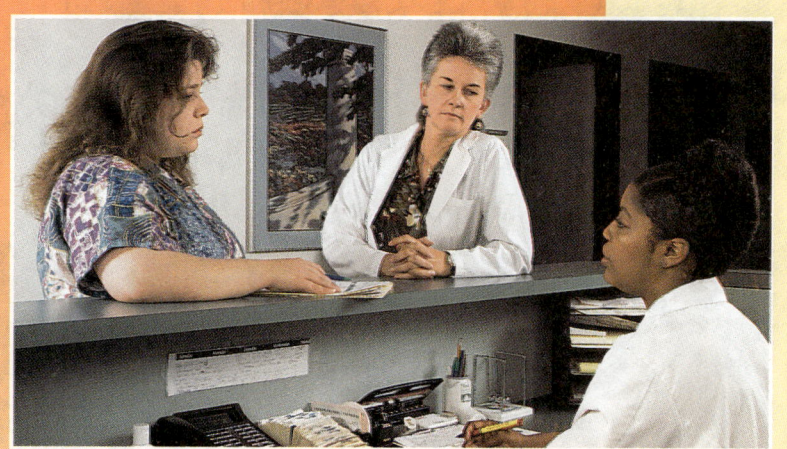

Unit 1

Understanding the Profession

The history of medicine, from prehistory to today's advanced technology, is a fascinating progression from superstition and magical illnesses and cures to an understanding of diseases and their effects on the body. With this knowledge and our mastery of many of the illnesses that continue to plague humankind, we have encountered concerns that pit legally accepted medical treatment against what is considered to be ethical by current standards. Our expanding technology will continue to outpace our written laws and our religious concepts about life and death. In this section, we attempt to provide a broad perspective on these issues affecting the practice of medicine.

Medicine and Medical Assisting

1

Chapter Outline

History of Medicine
    Ancient Medical History
    Modern Medical History
The Medical Assisting Profession
    What Is a Medical Assistant?
    The History of Medical Assisting
    Medical Assisting Associations
    Medical Assisting Education
    Medical Assisting Certification
    Association Membership
Duties of a Medical Assistant

    Administrative Duties
    Clinical Duties
Characteristics of a Professional Medical Assistant
Members of the Health Care Team
Employment Opportunities
Summary
Critical Thinking Challenges
Answers to Checkpoint Questions
Suggestions for Further Reading

DACUM Components

1.1   Project a positive attitude
1.2   Perform within ethical boundaries
1.5   Work as a team member
1.9   Promote the profession

Chapter Competencies

Learning Objectives

Upon successfully completing this chapter, you will be able to:

1. Spell and define the Key Terms
2. Outline a brief history of medicine.
3. Identify the key founders of medical science.
4. Explain the four pathways of education for medical assistants.
5. List the duties of a medical assistant.
6. Describe the desired characteristics of a medical assistant.
7. List the benefits of certification.
8. List the benefits of membership in a professional organization.
9. Identify members of the health care team.
10. List settings in which medical assistants may be employed.

Key Terms

(See Glossary for definitions.)

administrative
American Association of Medical
   Assistants (AAMA)
American Medical Technologists
   Institute for Education (AMTIE)
caduceus
clinical
DACUM

externship
inpatient
medical assistant
multidisciplinary
multiskilled health professional
outpatient
proprietary

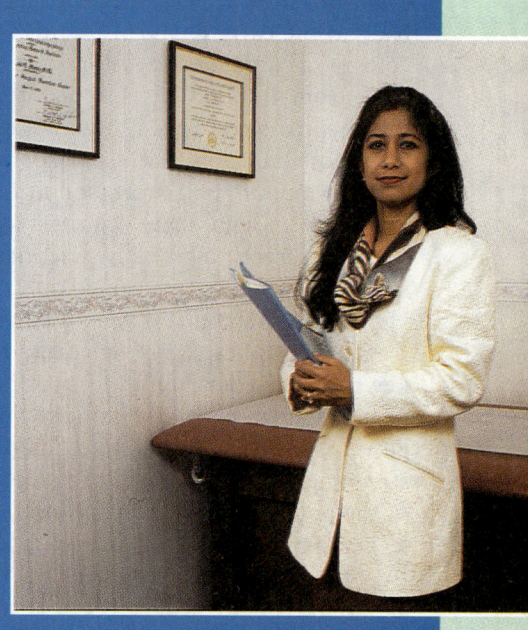

Welcome to the field of medicine and to the medical assisting profession! You have selected a fascinating and challenging career, one of the fastest growing specialties in the medical field. The need for the **multiskilled health professional**—an individual with versatile training in the health care field—will continue to grow within the foreseeable future and you are about to become a part of this exciting career direction.

To understand the significance of the medical knowledge and skills you will receive during your course of study, we begin by taking a chronological look at the history of medicine and then exploring the profession of medical assisting.

➤ HISTORY OF MEDICINE

Tremendous achievements in the general health, comfort, and well-being of patients have been made just within the past 100 to 150 years, with the greatest advances occurring in this century. It is difficult to imagine health care without antibiotics, x-ray machines, or anesthesia, but these developments are fairly new to the world of medicine. For example, penicillin was not produced in large quantities until World War II, and surgery was performed without anesthesia until the mid 1800s!

Ancient Medical History

The earliest recorded evidence of medical history dates back to the early Egyptians. Papyrus records of tuberculosis, pneumonia and arteriosclerosis are still in existence from 4000 B.C. It is evident that during this time the Egyptians performed surgeries, including brain surgery! Fossil remains have shown patients with fractures (broken bones) that were splinted and subsequently healed. Although many cultures practiced primitive forms of surgery, most early practitioners used a combination of religion and superstition to heal ailments. Herbs, roots, and plants were used as medications.

Some of these early "medications" have played a key role in the development of our modern pharmacology. Digitalis, from the common garden plant foxglove, is still in use today for its original purpose of strengthening the heart's action. Opium, from the pods of the poppy plant, is still used to induce stupor and a level of painlessness. Supplemental iron as a method of treating anemia was recognized by the Chinese as early as 2500 B.C. Medical research is constantly uncovering evidence that previously used treatment methods were based on sound theory and are being incorporated into our modern arsenal against illness.

More than a thousand years before Christ, Moses was appointed the first public health officer. He wrote rules for sanitation. He stated that all people preparing and serving public food must be neat and clean. In the days long before refrigeration, it became a religious law that only freshly slaughtered animals could be eaten. Moses also required that serving dishes and cooking utensils be washed between customers at public restaurants.

Aesculapius, a mythical Greek god of healing and the son of Apollo, had many followers who used massage and exercise to treat patients. This god is also believed to have used the magical powers of a yellow, nonpoisonous serpent to lick the wounds of surgical patients. Aesculapius was often pictured holding the serpent wrapped around his staff or wand; this staff is a symbol of medicine. Another medical symbol is the **caduceus**, the staff of the Roman god Mercury, shown as a winged staff with two serpents wrapped around it (Fig. 1-1).

Around 400 B.C., Hippocrates practiced medicine and set high behavioral standards for practicing physicians. Hippocrates, called the "Father of Medicine," turned medicine into a science and erased the element of mysticism that it once held. He wrote the "Oath of Hippocrates," which is still part of medical school graduation ceremonies.

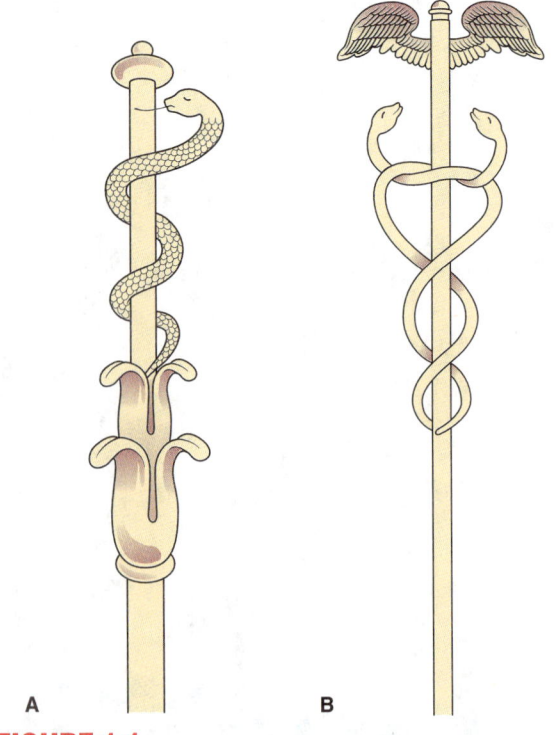

FIGURE 1-1
(**A**) Staff of Aesculapius. (**B**) Caduceus.

The Greek physician, Galen (131–201 A.D.), became known as the "Father of Experimental Physiology." He was the first physician to document a patient's pulse, although he did not know that the pulse was related to the heart. Galen identified many parts of the body. However, his anatomic findings were mostly incorrect because they were based on the dissection of apes and swine. Postmortem human dissections were illegal and were considered sacrilegious until the Renaissance period (1350–1650).

The rule of the Roman Empire, from about 200 B.C. until its dissolution several centuries later, brought great strides in public health. Water was brought from clean mountain streams by way of raised aqueducts that were regularly cleaned and maintained, sewers carried wastes away from the cities, and personal cleanliness was encouraged. One Roman physician, Marcus Varro (116–21 B.C.), even suggested that there might be creatures too small to be seen that caused illness. This was 1800 years before the invention of the microscope.

During the Dark Ages (400–800 A.D.) and through the Middle Ages (800–1400 A.D.), few advances were made in the medical field. Medicine was practiced primarily in convents and monasteries and consisted of simply caring for patients rather than trying to find a cure for the illness. The population became more mobile, ranging away from traditional homelands for war, crusades, and exploration. Each venture exposed whole cultures to diseases against which they had no immunity. Cities grew larger with none of the Roman technology for maintaining sanitation. It was during this period that ignorance, crowded conditions, and poor health practices led to the eruption of the bubonic plague that twice swept through Europe and Asia killing approximately 20 million people. This deadly disease, the greatest killer in our history, was spread from rat fleas to humans, killing approximately one-half the known population within a few years.

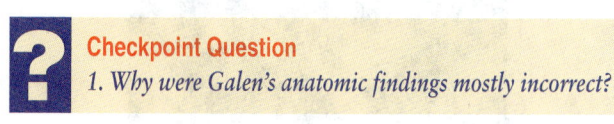

Checkpoint Question

1. Why were Galen's anatomic findings mostly incorrect?

Modern Medical History

The Renaissance was a period of enlightenment in all areas of art, science, and education and fostered great strides in medicine. The advent of the printing press and the establishment of great universities made the practice of medicine more accessible to larger numbers of practitioners. Clusters of learning worked to advance medical and scientific theories and allowed great minds to collaborate on experiments that led to discoveries of enormous benefit in the fight against disease.

During this period, Andreas Vesalius, 1514–1564, became known as the "Father of Modern Anatomy." He corrected many of Galen's errors and wrote the first relatively correct anatomy textbook. Shortly after Vesalius' writings, William Harvey identified the pumping action of the heart. He described circulation as a continuous circuit pumped by the heart to carry blood through the body. However, Harvey studied the action of the heart using dogs, not humans.

The next significant contribution to medicine was the invention of the microscope in the mid 1660s by a dutch lens maker, Anton von Leeuwenhoek. He was the first person to observe bacteria under a lens although he had no idea of the significance of the microorganisms to human health. His instrument also allowed him to accurately describe a red blood cell.

John Hunter (1728–1793) became known as the "Father of Scientific Surgery." He developed many surgical techniques that are still used today. Hunter developed and inserted the first artificial feeding tube into a patient in 1778. He also was the first person to classify teeth in a scientific manner.

In 1796, Edward Jenner, a physician in England, overheard a young milkmaid explain that she would not catch smallpox because she had already had the very mild cowpox caught while milking her cows. Jenner experimented with a small boy by inoculating him with crusts from the cowpox. Several weeks later, Jenner inoculated the boy with smallpox crusts. When the boy did not contract the disease, the prevention for smallpox was discovered. Today, smallpox has been eradicated and the vaccine is no longer administered. Jenner's discovery of the smallpox vaccine opened the door to an emphasis on prevention of disease rather than simply trying to cure preventable illnesses.

At this time, the importance of the mind as a part of the health care process was becoming a recognized field of medicine. The first extensive work and writing in the field of mental health was published in 1812 by Benjamin Rush, entitled *Medical Inquiries and Observations upon Diseases of the Mind*. He advocated humane treatment of the mentally ill at a time when most were imprisoned, chained, starved, exhibited like animals, or simply killed. Rush's influence began a separate field of study into the working of the mind that became modern psychiatry.

The mid 1880s experienced the greatest surge in the recognition of disease transmission. At this time, Louis Pasteur (1822–1895) became famous for his work with bacteria. Pasteur discovered that wine turned sour because of the presence of bacteria. He found that when the bacteria were eliminated, the wine lasted longer. Pasteur's discovery that bacteria in liquids could be eliminated by heat led to the process that is known as pasteurization. This finding led to using heat to sterilize surgical instruments. Pasteur was labeled the "Father of Bacteriology" for this accomplishment. Pasteur also focused on preventing the transmission of anthrax and discovered the rabies vaccine. Pasteur was also honored with the title "Father of Preventive Medicine" for this work.

In the mid 1880s, Ignaz Semmelweiss, a Hungarian physician, noticed that women whose babies were born at home with a midwife in attendance had fewer incidences of childbed fever than those who delivered in well-respected hospitals with prestigious physicians at the bedside. He was ridiculed by the medical establishment and was fired from his position when he required handwashing in a solution of chlorinated lime before the manual vaginal examinations of maternity patients. He was right, of course, and handwashing is still the most important factor in the fight against disease transmission.

At about the same time, Joseph Lister began to apply antiseptics to wounds to reduce the incidence of infection. The concept was not clearly understood, but before Lister's practices, as many patients died of infection as died from the primitive surgical techniques of the early part of the century.

Anesthesia was discovered in 1842 by Dr. Crawford Williamson Long. The effects of nitrous oxide were known by the mid 1700s but the therapeutic use was discovered by accident when he observed a group of chemistry students inhaling it for amusement purposes. Before this time, anesthesia consisted of large doses of alcohol or opium, leather straps for patient restraint, or unconsciousness from the pain. Ether and chloroform were also coming into use at about this time.

X-rays were discovered in 1895 by Wilhelm Konrad Roentgen when he observed that a previously unknown ray generated by a cathode tube was able to pass through soft tissue and outline underlying structures. Medical diagnosis was revolutionized, earning Roentgen a Nobel Prize in 1901 for his discovery. The therapeutic uses of x-rays were recognized much later.

In 1928, Sir Alexander Fleming, a bacteriologist, accidentally discovered penicillin when his assistant forgot to wash the Petri dishes Fleming had used for experiments. When he noticed the circles of non-growth around areas of a certain mold, he was able to extract the prototype for one of our most potent weapons against disease. He won the Nobel Prize in 1945 for this accomplishment.

Jonas Edward Salk and Albert Sabin discovered the vaccine for polio in the 1950s and eradicated one of the 20th century's greatest killers.

Although "wise women" throughout history practiced the medical arts as midwives and gatherers of healing herbs, the first notable records of the contribution of women to the medical field began in the 1800s.

Florence Nightingale (1820–1910) was the founder of modern nursing. She set standards for nurses to follow and developed educational requirements for nurses (Fig. 1-2).

Clara Barton (1821–1912) founded the American Red Cross in 1881 and was its first president. She identified the need for psychological support as well as physical support for soldiers during the Civil War. Barton also noted that no records were kept on soldiers who were injured or killed. She formed the Bureau of Records in Washington, DC, which still keeps records of killed or injured soldiers.

Elizabeth Blackwell (1821–1910) became the first woman to complete medical school in the United States when she graduated from Geneva Medical College in New York. In 1869, Blackwell established her own medical school in Europe for women only, opening the door for a rapidly expanding role for women in the medical field.

Marie Curie (1867–1934), a brilliant scientific student, married Pierre Curie and together they discovered polonium and radium. Their discovery revolutionized the principles of energy and radioactivity. Madame Curie shared the Nobel Prize for chemistry with her husband in 1903. She continued the research after his death and won the Nobel Prize for physics in 1911.

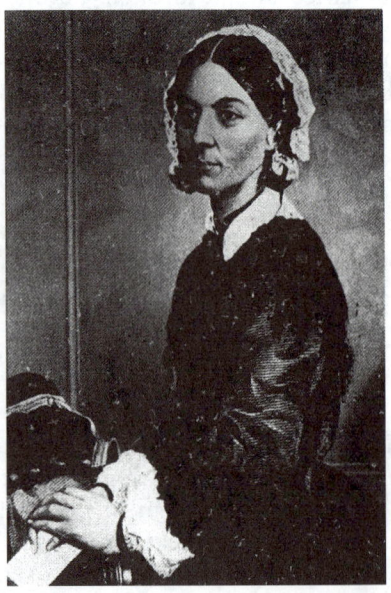

FIGURE 1-2
Florence Nightingale.

Lillian Wald (1867–1940), a nurse and social worker, founded and operated the first visiting nurse service in New York City. In 1902, she opened the first public school nursing system.

Unimaginable discoveries will continue to expand the parameters of medicine as research in recombinant DNA, transplantation, immunizations, diagnostic procedures, and so forth push back the boundaries of health care and make our current therapies seem as primitive as those we have just covered. You will be a part of this fascinating evolution of health care. Within the next decade *expect* to see immunization against or cures for many of the illnesses that continue to plague us.

Your role as a medical assistant, the ultimate multiskilled health care professional, will expand as the need for highly trained, versatile medical personnel keeps pace with the ever-changing practice of medicine. Today heart bypass surgeries and organ transplants are routine occurrences. Research continues to search for the cures for cancer, acquired immunodeficiency syndrome, and many other ailments. As a medical assistant, you play a key role in advancing the medical profession into the 21st century.

Checkpoint Question

2. What did Louis Pasteur discover about bacteria found in liquids?

➤ THE MEDICAL ASSISTING PROFESSION

What Is a Medical Assistant?

A medical assistant is a multiskilled health professional who performs a variety of clinical and administrative duties in a medical setting. Clinical tasks generally involve direct patient care; administrative tasks usually focus on office-related procedures. Medical assistants are employed in physician's offices, hospitals, health insurance companies, public health agencies, and ambulatory care settings. Salaries, hours, and working conditions for medical assistants vary greatly based on experience, location, employer, and job responsibilities.

The History of Medical Assisting

Medical assisting as a separate profession dates from the 1930s. In 1934, Dr. M. Mandl recognized the need for a medical professional possessing skills required in an office environment and opened the first school for medical assistants in New York City. Although medical assistants were employed before 1934, no formal schooling was available. Office assistants were trained on the job to perform medical procedures or nurses were trained to perform administrative procedures. The need for a highly trained professional with a background in secretarial sciences and clinical skills led to the formation of an alternate field of health care. The medical assistant has since grown into a independent and highly respected member of the health care team.

Medical Assisting Associations

American Association of Medical Assistants

In 1955, the **American Association of Medical Assistants (AAMA)**, the professional organization for medical assistants, was founded during a meeting of medical assistants in Kansas City, Kansas. The resolutions adopted by the group were accepted and commended by the American Medical Association (the professional association of licensed physicians). In 1959, Illinois recognized the AAMA as a not-for-profit educational organization. The first national office was established in Chicago with state and local chapters throughout the United States. A professional journal is published and distributed to members of the organization and accredited continuing education opportunities are available through the national organization. Professional benefits, such as insurance, are also made available to AAMA members. Figure 1-3 displays the insignia of the AAMA.

The accrediting body of the AAMA is the educational branch of the American Medical Association. Quality of education is maintained by program reviews conducted at intervals to ensure the educational level of the courses offered. Program accreditation is based on adherence to the **DACUM** (Developing a Curriculum), a list of the areas of competence expected of the graduate (see Appendix I).

In 1963, a certification examination for Certified Medical Assistant (CMA) was developed that would set the standards required for medical assistant educa-

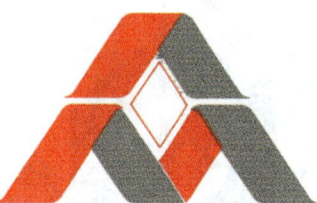

FIGURE 1-3
Affiliate of the American Association of Medical Assistants (AAMA) insignia.

tion. The first AAMA examinations were given in Kansas, California, and Florida. Certification examinations are discussed in detail later in the chapter.

 **Checkpoint Question**
3. What prompted the establishment of a school for medical assistants?

American Medical Technologists

The Accrediting Bureau of Health Education Schools (ABHES) accredits schools that offer the Registered Medical Assistant (RMA) certification through a program review process conducted by the **American Medical Technologists Institute for Education (AMTIE)**. This body has also accredited medical technicians, medical laboratory technicians, and dental technicians since the late 1930s but offered its first medical assisting examination in 1972. The organization and its governing body are set up similarly to the AAMA with local, state, and national affiliations, opportunities for continuing education, professional benefits, and a professional journal. Figure 1-4 displays the insignia of the American Medical Technologists.

Medical Assisting Education

Medical assistants have traditionally been educated and trained by four different methods: on-the-job training, vocational schools, **proprietary** schools (private schools with preset curricula) and community colleges.

On-the-job training, the most common method used until approximately 20 years ago, still occurs in small offices; however, the potential for personal growth and expansion is limited.

Medical assisting training programs offered by *vocational schools* are frequently part of a high school curriculum, allowing the student to gain hands-on experience in the senior grade level.

Proprietary schools may be accredited by the AAMA or the AMTIE, indicating that they have met

basic curriculum development standards. Programs offered by proprietary schools vary in length and may offer job placement services along with **externships**. An externship is an educational course offered in the last module or semester during which the student works in the field gaining hands-on experience. It varies in length and is a noncompensated position. (See Chap. 51, Externship, for more detailed information.)

Medical assisting programs offered by *community colleges* tend to be 1 to 2 years in length. One-year programs offer a certificate of graduation or a diploma, and 2-year programs award the graduate an associate degree. Externships are also included in these programs, and the college can be accredited by the AAMA or AMTIE.

Schools are accredited to offer medical assisting programs by the AAMA or AMTIE based on the curriculum offerings, faculty qualifications, laboratory facilities, job placement statistics, and many other factors. The school's curriculum must meet the governing body's written requirements. After January 1998, only graduates of an accredited school will be allowed to sit for certification examinations for the AAMA.

This book is designed to follow the AAMA's DACUM. At the beginning of each chapter, you will see the DACUM components that the chapter will cover.

After completing school, your education should not stop. You should continue to take courses on various related topics. These may include new computer programs, new clinical procedures, new laws and regulations, or pharmaceutical updates. Some employers will pay for conferences. In some situations, conference costs may be listed for tax credit when filing your income tax.

 **Checkpoint Question**
4. What are the four educational paths that a medical assistant may take?

Medical Assisting Certification

The AAMA and the AMTIE have developed certification examinations that signify that a graduate has meet entry level competency. After passing the examination, the initials CMA (Certified Medical Assistant) or RMA (Registered Medical Assistant) may be used after your name (Fig. 1-5). Recertification may be obtained by either retesting or completing a number of continuing education units (CEUs). CEUs are awarded for attendance at approved seminars and through the completion of guided study courses. Both organizations publish journals with articles of interest to the medical assistant to keep knowledge and skills current and to provide notice of upcoming events with opportunities for continuing education.

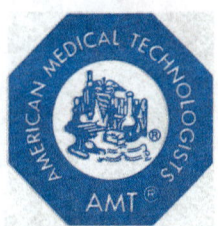

FIGURE 1-4
American Medical Technologists (AMT) insignia.

Medical assistants who pass the AAMA certification examination become Certified Medical Assistants and may use the designation CMA after their names. Those who pass the AMTIE certification examination become Registered Medical Assistants and may use the designation RMA after their names. (See examples below.)

4/25/97   9:30 a.m.   Patient complaining of sore throat. Throat culture taken and sent to the laboratory. Dr. Rogers in to see patient. -------- Paula Jones, CMA

4/25/97   1130   Amoxicillin 250 mg po given to patient. ------------------------------- Andrea Charlton, RMA

FIGURE 1-5
Using the CMA or RMA designation.

There are many advantages to obtaining certification. First and foremost, it is the mark of a professional. Certification indicates to potential employers, patients, and colleagues that you have succeeded in meeting the educational requirements for medical assisting. The certification gives you a hiring edge over other applicants and shows your employer that you take your career seriously and that you are a competent professional. Your hourly wage should reflect your certification and increase your earning potential.

Association Membership

You are not required to join a national organization to work as a medical assistant or to be eligible to take the certification examination. However, the associations have many benefits for members. These benefits include:

- Access to educational seminars
- Access to continuing education units
- Subscription to the professional journals that alert you to new procedures and trends in medicine
- Access to the annual conventions
- Group insurance plans
- Networking opportunities

For further information on the organization associated with your certification, contact your local chapter or speak with your instructor for the procedure for applying for membership.

➤ DUTIES OF A MEDICAL ASSISTANT

The duties of a medical assistant are divided into two categories: administrative and clinical. The ratio of administrative to clinical duties will vary based on your job description. For example, if you work in a family practice office, you may do mostly clinical work; a psychiatric practice will probably require primarily administrative duties.

Administrative Duties

Administrative tasks that are performed correctly and in a timely manner will make the office more efficient and productive. Conversely, an office that is not managed correctly can result in loss of business, poor patient service, and loss of revenue. Following is a partial list of standard administrative duties:

- Managing and maintaining the waiting room, office and examining rooms
- Handling telephone calls
- Using written and oral communication
- Maintaining medical records
- Bookkeeping
- Scheduling appointments
- Ensuring good public relations
- Maintaining office supplies
- Screening sales representatives
- Filing insurance forms
- Processing employees payroll
- Arranging patient hospitalizations
- Sorting and filing mail
- Instructing new patients regarding office hours and procedures
- Applying computer concepts to office practices
- Implementing ICD-9 and CPT coding for insurance claims (See Chap. 17, Diagnostic and Procedural Coding.)
- Completing medical transcriptions

Clinical Duties

Clinical responsibilities will vary among employers. Following is a partial list of clinical duties:

- Preparing patients for examinations/treatments
- Assisting other health care providers with procedures
- Preparing and sterilizing instruments
- Obtaining urine and blood specimens
- Performing laboratory tests (pregnancy tests, urinalyses)
- Completing electrocardiograms
- Applying Holter monitors
- Obtaining medical histories
- Assisting with radiographs (laws vary by state)
- Administering medications/immunizations
- Obtaining vital signs (blood pressure, pulse, temperature, respirations)
- Obtaining height and weight measurements
- Documenting in the medical record

Patient Education: The Health Care System

As a medical assistant, you play a key role in educating patients not only about their health, but also about the health care system. A number of patients become confused and are overwhelmed by the number and variety of health care workers. You can help by providing the answers to these common questions:

- What is a multidisciplinary team?
- Who will conduct the examination (physician, nurse practitioner, or physician's assistant)?
- What is a medical assistant?
- What do medical assistants do?
- What kind of training is required for medical assistants?
- What does certification or registration mean for a medical assistant?

Patients who understand the health care field and are well educated regarding the care they will receive seem to recover more quickly and are more comfortable asking questions that will have an impact on their return to health.

- Performing eye or ear irrigations
- Recognizing and treating medical emergencies
- Initiating and implementing patient education

Checkpoint Question

5. What are five administrative duties and five clinical duties that a medical assistant may perform?

➤ CHARACTERISTICS OF A PROFESSIONAL MEDICAL ASSISTANT

Medical assistants play a key role in creating and maintaining a professional image for their employers. Medical assistants must always appear neat and well groomed. Clothing should be clean, pressed and in good condition. Footwear should be neat, comfortable, and professional. (Sneakers should not be worn unless approved by your supervisor.) Only minimal makeup

and jewelry should be worn. Fingernails should be clean and at a functional length. If polish is worn, it should be pale or clear.

Medical assistants must be dependable and punctual (Fig. 1-6). Tardiness and frequent sick calls are not acceptable. If you are not at work, someone must fill in for you. Medical assistants must be flexible and adaptable to meet the constantly changing needs of the office. Weekend and holiday hours may be required in some specialties.

Additional characteristics vital to the profession include:

- Excellent written and oral *communications skills*. You will be required to interact with patients and other health care members on a professional basis. Only the best grammar skills are acceptable. (Communication skills are covered in appropriate sections of this text.)
- *Maturity*. Remaining calm in an emergency or during stressful situations and being able to calm others is a key skill. You must also be able to accept criticism without resentment.
- *Accuracy*. The physician must be able to trust you to pay close attention to detail because the health and well-being of the patients are at stake. Careless errors could cause harm to the patient and result in legal action against the physician.
- *Honesty*. If errors are made, they must be admitted and corrective procedures must be initiated immediately. Covering up errors or blaming others is dishonest. So is using office property for personal business, making telephone calls on the employer's time, or falsifying time records. Such practices can ruin your career and are to be strictly avoided.

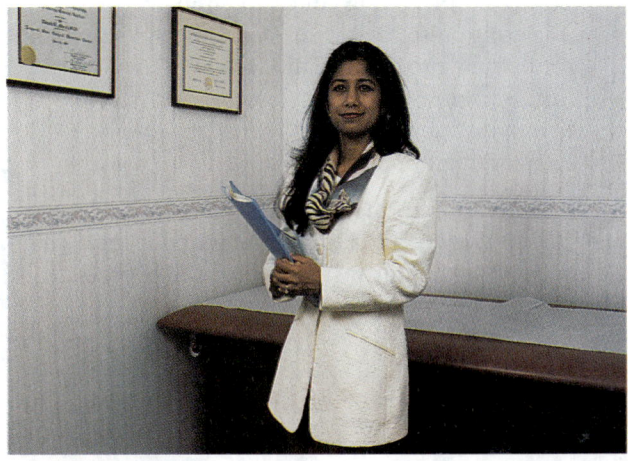

FIGURE 1-6
Medical assistants play a key role in creating and maintaining a professional image for their employers.

- The ability to *respect patient confidentiality*. Few issues in health care can damage your career as profoundly as divulging confidential patient information.
- *Empathy*. The ability to care deeply for the health and welfare of your patients is the heart of medical assisting.
- *Courtesy*. Every patient who enters the office must be treated with respect and gracious manners.
- Good *interpersonal skills*. Tempers may flare in stressful situations; learn to keep yours in check and work well with all levels of interaction.
- The ability to project a *positive self-image*. If you are confident in your abilities as a professional, this attitude will reflect in all of your relationships.
- The ability to *work as a team player*. The patient's return to health is the most important objective of the office. Each staff member must work toward this goal.
- *Initiative* and *responsibility*. The entire team expects each of its members to perform assigned responsibilities.
- *Tact and diplomacy*. The right word at the right moment can calm and soothe anger, depression, and fear and relieve a potentially unsettling situation.
- *High moral and ethical standards*. Project for your profession the highest level of professionalism.

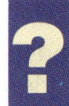

Checkpoint Question

6. *What are eight characteristics that a professional medical assistant should have?*

What If?

What if you do not currently have all of the skills and characteristics of a professional medical assistant? Will you make a good medical assistant?

Yes! One of the most important characteristics a medical assistant can have is a caring and empathic attitude. Many of the other skills can be learned with practice or training, but being empathic is a special trait. It allows you to share the feelings of others, such as the joy of a baby's birth or the sadness and grief of losing a loved one or friend. It is extremely important for medical assistants to understand and be supportive of patients as well as colleagues in the medical office.

➤ MEMBERS OF THE HEALTH CARE TEAM

As a medical assistant you will work with a variety of health care workers. Today's health care team must be **multidisciplinary**. A multidisciplinary team is a group of specialized professionals who are brought together to meet the needs of the patient. Some patients will need the assistance of many individuals, whereas other patients may only need one or two members of the team. The team may be broken into three groups: physicians, nurses, and allied health care providers.

Physicians will generally be the team leaders. They are responsible for diagnosing and treating the patient. Minimum education for a physician consists of a 4-year undergraduate degree, often consisting of pre-medical studies, 4 years of medical school, followed by a residency program usually concentrating on a certain specialty. The residency program can vary from 2 to 6 years based on the field of study. Physicians must pass a licensure examination for the state in which they wish to practice. Table 1-1 lists and describes physician specialties. Table 1-2 lists and describes the most common surgical specialties.

Physician's Assistants (PAs) are specially trained and are usually licensed. They work closely with a physician and may perform many of the tasks traditionally done by physicians. Preliminary physical examinations and basic diagnostic and treatment procedures that do not require an intense medical background may be assigned to a physician's assistant. Their educational levels vary from several months to 2 years depending on the program and the individual's background in medicine. National certification is available through the American Association of Physician Assistants.

Nurses work with physicians and implement various patient care needs. There are several levels of nursing education.

Registered Nurses (RNs) have 2 years (ADN—Associate Degree in Nursing) or 4 years (BSN—Bachelor of Science in Nursing) of education. Their job descriptions vary based on their experiences, specialties, and certifications. Three-year, hospital-based nursing programs are also available for a diploma in nursing but are increasingly rare.

Licensed Practical Nurses (LPNs) or *Licensed Vocational Nurses* (LVNs) generally have 1 year of education. LPNs report to RNs.

Nurse Practitioners (NPs) may practice medicine independently. In some states, NPs can write prescriptions, operate their own offices, and admit patients to hospitals. In other states, an NP may work more closely with a physician. All NPs are experienced RNs

Table 1-1
Physician Specialties

Allergist—Performs tests to determine the basis of allergic reactions to eliminate or counteract the offending allergen.

Anesthesiologist—Determines the most appropriate anesthesia for the patient's situation

Cardiologist—Diagnoses and treats disorders of the cardiovascular system

Dermatologist—Diagnoses and treats skin disorders

Emergency Care Physicians—Usually works in emergency or trauma centers with immediate care

Endocrinologist—Diagnoses and treats disorders of the endocrine system

Family Practitioner—Serves a variety of patient age levels, also known as Primary Care physicians

Gastroenterologist—Diagnoses and treats disorders of the gastrointestinal system.

Gerontologist—Limits practice to disorders of the aging population

Gynecologist—Diagnoses and treats disorders of the female reproductive system; may also be an obstetrician or limit the practice to gynecology

Hematologist—Diagnoses and treats disorders of the blood-forming organs

Immunologist—Concentrates on disease incidence, transmission, and prevention

Internist—Limits practice to treatment of disorders of internal organs by medical means

Neonatologist—Limits practice to the care and treatment of infants to about 6 weeks of age

Nephrologist—Diagnoses and treats disorders of the kidneys

Obstetrician—Limits practice to care and treatment of pregnancy and the postpartum period

Occupational Physician—Treats and works to prevent disorders caused by the working environment

Oncologist—Diagnoses and treats tumors, both benign and malignant

Ophthalmologist—Diagnoses and treats disorders of the eyes

Orthopedist—Diagnoses and treats disorders of the musculoskeletal system

Otorhinolaryngologist—Diagnoses and treats disorders of the ear, nose, and throat

Pathologist—Diagnoses abnormalities in tissue samples or specimens from surgery or autopsies

Pediatrician—Limits practice to childhood disorders; may be further divided as early childhood or adolescent pediatricians

Podiatrist—Diagnoses and treats disorders of the feet

Proctologist—Limits practice to disorders of the colon, rectum, and anus

Psychiatrist—Diagnoses and treats mental disorders

Pulmonologist—Diagnoses and treats disorders of the respiratory system

Radiologist—Diagnoses and treats by using forms of radiation

Rheumatologist—Diagnoses and treats disorders of mobility

Urologist—Diagnoses and treats disorders of the urinary system

Table 1-2
Types of Surgeons

Surgical Specialty	Description
Cardiovascular	Repairs dysfunctions of the cardiovascular system
Cosmetic, reconstructive, plastic	Restores, repairs, or reconstructs body parts
General	Performs repairs on a variety of body parts
Maxillofacial	Repairs disorders of the face and mouth (a branch of dentistry)
Neurologic	Repairs disorders of the nervous system
Orthopedic	Corrects deformities and treats disorders of the musculoskeletal system
Thoracic	Repairs organs within the rib cage
Trauma	Limited to correcting traumatic wounds
Vascular	Repairs disorders of vessels, usually excluding the heart

and in most cases have a Master's Degree in Nursing with the addition of specialized training as an NP.

Allied health care professionals make up a large section of the health care team. Table 1-3 lists and describes some of these team members. The educational requirements and responsibilities vary greatly among these professionals. Medical assistants fall into this category.

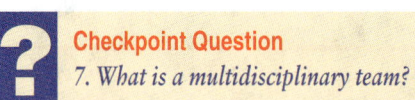

Checkpoint Question
7. What is a multidisciplinary team?

➤ EMPLOYMENT OPPORTUNITIES

The outlook for medical assisting employment is highly promising. Health care is being restructured to be more productive and cost effective. Medical assistants are the most cost-effective employees in health care today because of the flexible, multiskilled nature of their education. Medical assistants can work in a variety of health care settings performing many different functions.

Medical assistants can work in either **inpatient** or **outpatient** settings. An inpatient setting is a facility that admits patients for diagnostic, rehabilitative, or treatment purposes. Outpatient settings are sites that

Table 1-3
Allied Health Care Professionals

Chiropractor—Manipulates the musculoskeletal system and spine to relieve symptoms

Dental Hygienist—Trained and licensed to work with a dentist by providing preventive care

Dietitian—Trained nutritionist who addresses dietary needs associated with illness

Electrocardiograph Technician—Assists with the performance of diagnostic procedures for cardiac electrical activity

Electroencephalograph Technician—Assists with the diagnostic procedures for brain wave activity

Emergency Medical Technician—Trained in techniques of administering emergency care enroute to trauma centers

Histologist—Studies cells and tissues for diagnosis

Infection Control Officer—Identifies situations at risk for transmission of infection and implements preventive measures

Laboratory Technician—Trained in performance of laboratory diagnostic procedures

Medical Secretary—Trained in secretarial sciences with an emphasis on medical applications

Medical Transcriptionist—Trained in secretarial sciences to make typed records of dictated medical information

Nuclear Medical Technician—Specializes in diagnostic procedures using nuclear devices

Occupational Therapist—Evaluates and plans programs to relieve disorders that interfere with activities

Paramedic—Trained in advanced rescue and emergency procedures

Pharmacist—Prepares and dispenses medications by the physician's order

Phlebotomist—Trained to perform venipunctures

Physical Therapist—Plans and conducts rehabilitation procedures to relieve musculoskeletal disorders

Psychologist—Trained in methods of psychological assessment and treatment

Radiographer—Works with a radiologist or physician to operate radiologic equipment for diagnosis and treatment

Respiratory Therapist—Trained to preserve or improve respiratory function

Risk Manager—Identifies and corrects potential high-risk situations within the health care field

Social Worker—Trained to evaluate and correct social, emotional, and environmental problems associated with the medical profession

Speech Therapist—Treats and prevents speech and language disorders

Unit Clerk—Performs the administrative duties in a hospital patient care unit

---

- Hospital admissions department
- Patient care units
- Hospital radiology department
- Hospital laboratory department
- Skilled nursing facilities
- Hospital medical records department
- Psychiatric institutions
- Drug or alcohol rehabilitation centers

Examples of outpatient settings may include:

- Ambulatory care centers
- Walk-in care centers
- Physician offices
- Adult day-care centers
- Insurance companies
- Research centers
- Clinics
- Offices of Planned Parenthood

Checkpoint Question

8. What are five inpatient settings and five outpatient settings in which medical assistants may be employed?

 SUMMARY

Medicine is a constantly changing science that grows more complex with each new medical discovery. The well trained medical assistant will be a part of the most exciting and challenging era of medical advances in the history of patient care. By ensuring that educational levels are constantly enhanced and by continuing to grow professionally, the medical assistant graduate will be poised for the challenge of a lifelong career that is both fascinating and rewarding.

 CRITICAL THINKING CHALLENGES

1. Review the list of characteristics for medical assistants. Which characteristics do you already have? How will you acquire the others? Are there additional characteristics that you have that will make you a good medical assistant?

2. Look at the list of physician specialties. Which type of physician would you want to work for and why? Which physician specialties would you least want to work with? Explain your response.

3. How do you feel that you can make a contribution to the medical field? What kind of contribution can you make to the medical assisting profession?

---

provide care to patients for procedures or tests that will not require admission. Generally, outpatient policies limit the patient stay to less than 24 hours.

Following are examples of inpatient settings where a medical assistant may work with a variety of responsibilities:

ANSWERS TO CHECKPOINT QUESTIONS

1. Galen's anatomic findings were mostly incorrect because they were based on the dissection of apes and swine, not humans.
2. Pasteur discovered that bacteria in liquids could be destroyed by heating the liquid.
3. The first school for medical assistants was established because of the need for a highly trained professional with secretarial and clinical skills.
4. A medical assistant may be educated through on-the-job training or through programs offered by vocational schools, proprietary schools, or community colleges.
5. Examples of administrative duties include managing the medical office, handling telephone calls, preparing written communications, bookkeeping, scheduling, filing, and sorting mail. Examples of clinical duties include preparing patients for examinations, collecting and processing urine and blood specimens, completing electrocardiograms, and applying Holter monitors.
6. Examples of professional characteristics include punctuality, dependability, honesty, showing respect for patient confidentiality, courtesy, diplomacy, and having high ethical and moral standards.
7. A multidisciplinary team is a group of specialized professionals working together to meet the needs of the patient.
8. Inpatient settings include hospitals, skilled nursing facilities, psychiatric institutions, and drug and alcohol rehabilitation centers. Outpatient centers include physician offices, ambulatory care centers, walk-in care centers, Planned Parenthood offices, insurance companies, and research centers.

SUGGESTIONS FOR FURTHER READING

Encyclopedia Americana, International Edition. (1993). Danbury, CT. Grolier, Inc.

Hamann, B. (1994). *Disease: Identification, Prevention, and Control.* St. Louis: Mosby-Yearbook.

Lyons A. S., & Petrucelli, R. J. (1978). *Medicine: An Illustrated History.* St. Louis: C. V. Mosby.

Taylor, C., Lillis, C., LeMone, P. (1993). *Fundamentals of Nursing: The Art and Science of Nursing Care,* 2nd ed. Philadelphia: J.B. Lippincott.

World Book Encyclopedia. (1995). Chicago: World Book International.

Medical Ethics and Bioethical Issues

Chapter Outline

History of Medical Ethics
American Medical Association (AMA)
Code of Ethics
American Association of Medical Assis-
tants (AAMA) Code of Ethics
Principles
Medical Assistants' Creed
Medical Assistant's Role in Ethics
Patient Advocacy
Maintaining Ethical Standards in
the Medical Office
Examining Ethical Dilemmas
Issues of Unprofessional Conduct

Bioethics
American Medical Association Council
on Ethical and Judicial Affairs
Social Policy Issues
Professional Conduct and Behavior
Office Management Issues
Summary
Critical Thinking Challenges
Answers to Checkpoint Questions
Suggestions for Further Reading

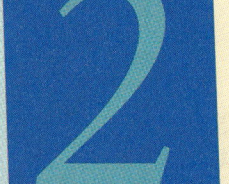

DACUM Components

1.2 Perform within ethical boundaries
1.3 Practice within the scope of education, training, and personal capabilities
1.6 Conduct oneself in a courteous and diplomatic manner

Chapter Competencies

Learning Objectives

Upon successfully completing this chapter, you will be able to:

1. Spell and define the Key Terms.
2. Differentiate between legal issues and ethical issues.
3. Describe the difference between medical ethics and bioethics.
4. List the seven American Medical Association principles of ethics.
5. List the ethical principles stated by the American Association of Medical Assistants.
6. Describe the steps that you can use to resolve an ethical dilemma.
7. Describe the opinions of the American Medical Association (AMA) Council on Ethical and Judicial Affairs on social policy issues.
8. List 10 opinions of the American Medical Association's Council pertaining to administrative office procedures.

Key Terms

(See Glossary for definitions.)

advance directives	expulsion
artificial insemination	Hippocratic Oath
bioethics	institutional review boards
censure	staff privileges
confidentiality	surrogate mother
due process	suspension
ethics	withdrawing treatment
euthanasia	withholding treatment

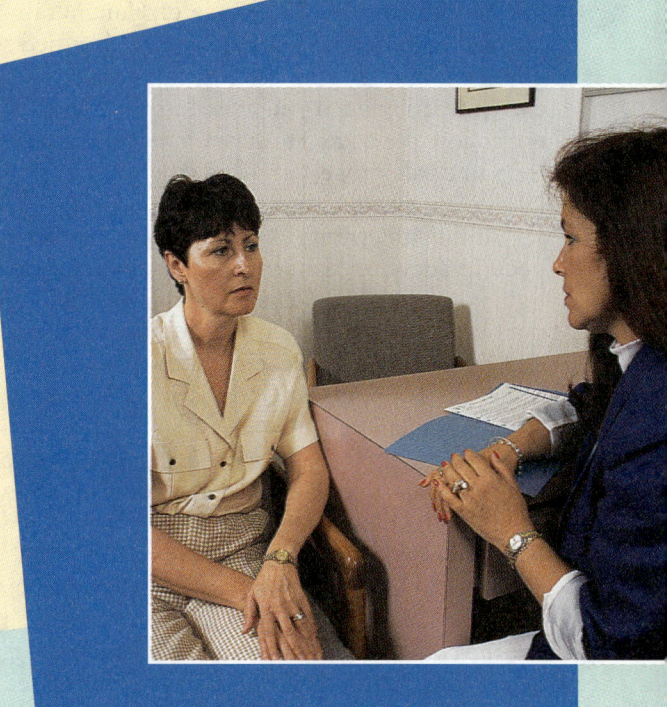

Medical **ethics** are principles of ethical and moral conduct that govern the behavior and conduct of health professionals. These principles define proper medical etiquette, customs, and professional courtesy. Ethics are guidelines specifying what should be done from a moral standpoint and are enforced by peer review and professional organizations. Laws, on the other hand, are regulations or sets of rules that must be adhered to and are enforced by the government. **Bioethics** are moral issues and problems that affect a patient's life; many bioethical issues have arisen due to the advances of modern medicine (see the section "Bioethics," below).

As a medical assistant, you will be confronted with situations in the practice of medicine that will require moral decisions. An important part of your responsibility as a health care professional is that you apply ethical standards as you perform your duties as a medical assistant.

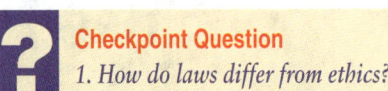

Checkpoint Question
1. How do laws differ from ethics?

➤ HISTORY OF MEDICAL ETHICS

The first ethical guidelines were written in 2500 B.C. by the Babylonians. The Code of Hammurabi was a detailed manuscript that specifically identified what a physician may or may not do and what fees could be charged. It included penalties for physicians who did not follow the code. However, it was not adaptable to the standards of western civilization and it slowly fell into disuse through the ages.

In the 4th century B.C., the Greek physician, Hippocrates, developed an ethical code that focused on the rights of patients and encouraged physicians to follow their moral instincts. There were, however, no penalties imposed for noncompliance. This ethical code, called the **Hippocratic Oath**, is still a part of medical school graduation ceremonies.

In 1803, a physician named Thomas Percival published a code that identified the conduct a physician must maintain in hospital settings and stated physician requirements for charitable work.

In 1847, the American Medical Association's (AMA) code of ethics was drafted in Philadelphia, using the codes of Percival and Hippocrates as its foundation for ethical standards. It has been revised many times since then to reflect contemporary issues and language. It was last revised in 1980. It was at this time that references to gender were removed from the code.

➤ AMERICAN MEDICAL ASSOCIATION (AMA) CODE OF ETHICS

A code of ethics is a collective statement from a professional organization that depicts the behavioral expectations of its members. Additionally, a code of ethics allows the organization to set standards by which it may discipline its members. The AMA's code of ethics has two sections: the preamble and the principles.

The preamble clearly states that physicians must recognize and accept their responsibilities for both patients and society. It also states that these are not laws, but *standards of conduct* by which a physician's professional behavior will be assessed.

Seven principles in the AMA's code of ethics state that the physician shall:

1. Practice competent medical care with compassion while respecting human dignity.
2. Remain honest in dealings with patients and colleagues, expose colleagues with character deficiencies or who are incompetent or who engage in fraud or deception.
3. Adhere to all laws and, when needed, be a voice to lawmakers in the best interest of patient care.
4. Respect the rights of patients and other health care professionals, safeguard patient **confidentiality** (privacy), except within the provisions of the law.
5. Continue appropriate education to remain current; request consultation and obtain the knowledge and skills of other health professionals when needed.
6. Be free to select whom to treat, where to establish a practice, and whom to associate with, except in emergency situations.
7. Participate in activities to enhance the community.

Violations of these AMA principles may result in **censure, suspension,** or **expulsion.** Censure is the least punitive action and is a verbal or written reprimand from the association indicating their negative feelings regarding a specific incident. Suspension is the temporary removal of privileges and association with the organization. Expulsion is a formal discharge from the professional organization and is the maximum punishment. It is important to note, however, that many of these issues deal with laws and the patient's rights as established by law. When violations of laws are involved, physicians may lose their license to practice, may be fined, or may be imprisoned. Serious consequences can arise for a breach of this code of ethics.

Checkpoint Question
2. What are the three penalties that physicians may face for violation of ethical principles? Briefly describe each.

► AMERICAN ASSOCIATION OF MEDICAL ASSISTANTS (AAMA) CODE OF ETHICS

Principles

The AAMA has published a set of five principles of ethical and moral conduct that all medical assistants must follow in the practice of the profession. They state that the medical assistant must always strive to:

1. Render services with respect for human dignity.
2. Respect patient confidentiality, except when information is required by the law.
3. Uphold the honor and high principles set forth by the AAMA.
4. Continually improve knowledge and skills for the benefit of patients and the health care team.
5. Participate in community services that promote good health and welfare to the general public.

Medical Assistants' Creed

The AAMA also has a written creed for medical assistants to follow. It is generally recited as a group during graduation or pinning services. The creed of the AAMA is:

I believe in the principles and purposes of the profession.
I endeavor to be more effective.
I aspire to render greater service.
I protect the confidence entrusted to me.
I am dedicated to the care and well-being of all patients.
I am loyal to my physician-employer.
I am true to the ethics of my profession.
I am strengthened by compassion, courage, and faith.*

► MEDICAL ASSISTANT'S ROLE IN ETHICS

Patient Advocacy

Your primary responsibility as a medical assistant is to be a patient advocate at all times. Advocacy requires that you consider the best interests of the patient above all other concerns. You may be asked to speak out in defense of the patient's rights and wishes in bioethical issues or situations. This often means setting aside your own personal beliefs, values, and biases and looking at a given situation in an objective manner. How-

*Reprinted with the permission of the American Association of Medical Assistants, Inc.

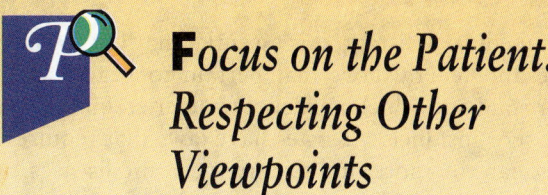

Focus on the Patient: Respecting Other Viewpoints

A patient's views on ethical issues will vary based on age, gender, culture, religion, and personal background. As a medical assistant, your role is to respect each patient's personal viewpoints. You can show support by listening to the patient's concerns, providing a reassuring or caring touch, and being nonjudgmental.

ever, you should never be asked or forced to compromise your own value system.

Maintaining Ethical Standards in the Medical Office

As an agent of the physician in the medical office, you are governed by ethical standards and are responsible for:

- Protecting patient confidentiality
- Following all state and federal laws
- Being honest in all your actions

Patient Confidentiality

Confidentiality of patient information is one of the most important ethical principles to be observed by the medical assistant. Information obtained in the care of the patient may not be revealed without the permission of the patient unless required by law. Whatever you say to, hear from, or do to a patient is confidential. Patients will reveal some of their innermost thoughts, feelings, and fears. This information is not for public knowledge. Family members, friends, pastors, or others may call the physician's office to inquire about a patient's condition. Many of these calls are made with good intentions; however, NO INFORMATION should be released to anyone—friends, family, media, or insurance companies—without prior written approval from the patient. Most offices have a standard disclosure form that must be signed by the patient before any information may be released. The only exception to releasing patient information without consent is when it is required by law. (See Chap. 3, Medicine and the Law, for information on reporting obligations.)

State and Federal Laws

As a medical assistant, it is essential that you know the state and federal laws that pertain to health care in your state and which incidences you are required to report. For instance, all states have laws that require the physician to report vital statistics, certain diseases, and acts of violence. These are discussed in detail in Chapter 3, Medicine and the Law, but are also considered to be ethical standards.

Honesty

One of the most important character traits for a medical assistant to possess is honesty. We all make mistakes at times; how we handle our mistakes is the indication of our ethical standards. If you make a mistake (eg, giving the wrong medication) you **must** immediately report the error to your supervisor and the attending physician. The mark of a true professional is the ability to admit mistakes and take full responsibility for all actions. When speaking to patients concerning medical issues, be honest; give the facts in a straightforward manner. Never offer false expectations or hope. Never minimize or exaggerate the risks or benefits of a procedure. If you do not know the answer to a question, say "I don't know, but I will find out for you" or refer the question to the physician. Treating the patient with dignity, respect, and honesty in all interactions will build trust in you and your professional abilities.

Checkpoint Question
3. What are three primary ethical standards that must be maintained in the medical office?

Examining Ethical Dilemmas

Medical-ethical issues may involve patients, their families, or your professional colleagues. The formation of office policy, including ethical concerns, is usually set by the physician in charge. You may be asked to give your opinion regarding the issues to be addressed, or you may be required to abide by ethical standards set by others. If office policy is a joint decision, the steps listed below will help to reach a consensus; if policy is in place when you are hired or if you are not allowed input into standards, you must examine the issues from your own set of values and arrive at a solution for handling issues that may oppose your ethical standards. No matter what the issue or course of action, the steps to resolving the problem remain the same.

1. *Identify the problem.* Determine exactly what the problem is: Who are the principal persons involved (eg, patients, health care workers)? What are the individuals' views of the problem (eg, who is for and who is against the issue)? Determine *your* feelings regarding the issue and the feelings of any other health care professionals involved.
2. *Gather additional data.* Determine if any laws or regulations govern the problem at hand. Determine *your* state's laws. Are there administrative agencies (eg, local health department, child and elder protective services) that have rules or regulations that apply to the particular issue. For instance, the allowed reporting time for child and elder abuse varies from state to state; research your state laws for the period of time within which abuse must reported. Check also for the method of reporting and to whom it should be reported. If you are employed in a hospital setting, is there a special policy written by your institution relating to this issue?
3. *Formulate options.* Make a list of alternative solutions because problems always have more than one solution. With each option, determine potential risks related to that option.
4. *Implement the decision and then evaluate it.* Often the implementation of an action is the easiest step. Review and evaluate the decision after it has been implemented. If the issue involved the office policy, evaluate the decision from the perceptions of the other members of the health care team. Did the policy work for all involved? Were ethical standards appropriate for all parties? If the issue was personal for you, will you be uncomfortable with the policy? What are your options if the specific situation arises again?

What If?
What if you are unable to think of any options to solve a particular problem? Where should you turn?

Many professionals can help you and the team explore options. These include members of the clergy, social workers, peers, and psychologists. Often, support groups have trained personnel on staff who can help as well.

Issues of Unprofessional Conduct

Dealing with ethical issues that involve unprofessional conduct of a peer or a physician can be extremely difficult. It is your obligation as a professional and a patient advocate to report unethical

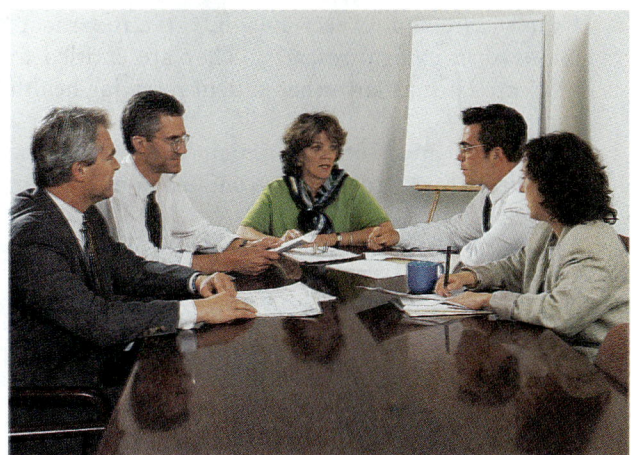

FIGURE 2-1
Meeting of an Institutional Review Board (IRB).

behaviors. Reports can be made to state, federal, or professional organizations, depending on the situation and the health care worker involved. Some institutions have an ethics committee or an **institutional review board** (IRB) (Fig. 2-1). The role of these committees is to "police" themselves internally. They can consist of employees of the institution or facility or independent persons, who are required to investigate and oversee claims or risks of violations of patients' rights. It is important to remember that everyone is entitled to **due process**. Due process is a formal proceeding in which the accused is considered not guilty until substantial evidence supports a verdict of guilty. A formal proceeding is usually conducted by a subcommittee of the organization or by the IRB.

Checkpoint Question
4. What steps should you follow when examining ethical dilemmas?

➤ BIOETHICS

Bioethics are patient centered and deal specifically with the moral issues and problems that affect human life. As a result of advances in medicine and research, many situations have developed in our society that require moral decisions for which there are no clear answers. Abortion and genetic engineering are two examples. The goal is to make the right decision in each specific instance as it applies to an individual's specific circumstances. What may be right for one patient may be wrong for another; that is the foundation of bioethics.

➤ AMERICAN MEDICAL ASSOCIATION COUNCIL ON ETHICAL AND JUDICIAL AFFAIRS

Because of the broad scope of medical ethics and bioethical issues, a subcommittee was formed within the American Medical Association (AMA) to review the principles set forth by the AMA and to interpret them as they apply to everyday clinical situations. This subcommittee is called the Council on Ethical and Judicial Affairs. The council has formulated a series of opinions on various medical and bioethical issues that are intended to provide the physician with *guidelines* for professional conduct and responsibilities. These opinions were most recently revised in 1992 and are divided into four general categories:

- Social policy issues
- Relations with colleagues and hospitals
- Administrative office procedures
- Professional rights and responsibilities

The following discussion provides a summary of these opinions, most of which include a case scenario and discussion questions. These issues are not within the scope of decisions for medical assistants, but you will be faced with their consequences at some time in your career. The purpose of these questions is to promote your ability to use reasoning to examine difficult issues.

Social Policy Issues

The social policy section deals with various issues of societal importance and provides guidelines to aid the physician in making ethical choices. Five common societal topics and the opinion statements from the AMA Council on Ethical and Judicial Affairs follow.

Allocation of Resources

The term allocate means to set aside or to designate for a purpose. Allocation of resources in the medical profession may refer to many different health needs:

- Organs for transplantation. Who gets this heart, the college professor or the young recovering addict whose heart was damaged by his life-style? Should life-style or perceived worth be considered in the decision?
- Funds for research. Which disease deserves the greatest funding, cancer or acquired immunodeficiency syndrome (AIDS)?
- Funds for health care. Where should the money be spent, for keeping alive extremely premature infants or making preventive health care available for a greater number of poor children?

- Hospital beds and professional care. With hospital care at a premium, who will pay for the indigent? How is it decided which patient is entitled to the last bed in the intensive care unit?

The council's viewpoint states that:

- When resources are limited, decisions for allocating health care materials should be based on fair and socially acceptable criteria. Economic or social position should not be a factor in the decision.
- Priority care is given to the person or persons who are more likely to receive the greatest long-term benefit from the treatment. Patients with other disease processes or who are not good candidates for treatment for whatever reason will be less likely to receive treatment than otherwise healthy patients. For instance, a patient with cancer in other sites would not be considered for a liver transplant, whereas a patient whose liver was damaged by trauma but who has no other involvement would probably be a good candidate.
- An individual's societal worth must not be a deciding factor during the decision process. The socially or politically prominent patient should not be considered a better recipient of treatment options than the young mother on welfare.
- Age must not be considered in the decision process. If the age of the patient is not a contraindication for the treatment, all ages should be considered on an even basis for most medical resources.

Clinical Investigations and Research

Physicians are frequently involved in studying the effectiveness of new procedures and medications, often called clinical investigations or research. When a drug or treatment has been through the preliminary trials, usually involving animal testing, and is considered safe for human testing, guidelines have been established by the council.

The council's viewpoint on research investigation of new drugs and procedures states that:

- A physician may participate in clinical research as long as the project is part of a systematic program with controls for patient evaluation during all phases of the research. At all stages of the testing and at the completion of the study, a protocol must be in place to evaluate the immediate and the long-term effects of the study.
- The goal of the research must be to obtain scientifically valid data. The objectives of the study must be available to the physician and the patient, results must be provided to all participants on request, and the testing must serve a medically sound purpose to provide better patient care.

- Utmost care and respect must be given to patients involved in clinical research. They are entitled to be treated just as any other patient receiving health care.
- Physicians must obtain patient permission or consent before enrolling the patient in a research project.
- The patient's decision to participate in the program must be completely voluntary.
- The patient must be advised of any potential risks, side effects, and benefits of participating in the project.
- The patient must be advised that this procedure or drug is experimental. Patients must be made aware that research is not complete, that this is the purpose of the trials, and that risks and benefits are not fully known at this time.
- The physician and the institution must have a check and balance system in place to ensure that quality care is always given and ethical standards are followed. Documentation of patient education and instruction for following testing guidelines and patient response to the treatment must be ongoing and thorough.

Scenario: A pharmaceutical company has developed a new drug to treat depression. It is now ready to be tested on humans. The company contacts a psychiatrist at a psychiatric facility who agrees to conduct a clinical trial on depressed patients at the facility. The patients are fully informed of the drug's potential benefits and possible side effects. Only five patients agree to take the medication; the others refuse to participate. The company and the psychiatrist feel strongly that all patients suffering from depression would benefit from this medication and might recover sufficiently to be discharged and to live independently. The psychiatrist feels that the patients refusing to participate in the research should be counseled and strongly encouraged to take the new drug.

Discussion questions: Should these patients be encouraged against their wishes to take this medication? What if a patient's spouse wants the patient to receive the medication—should the spouse be allowed try to persuade the patient to make this decision? If patients are under age 18, should parents have the right to enroll their children in research programs?

Obstetric Dilemmas

Advances in technology have created legal and ethical situations that have polarized opinions and are difficult to bring to consensus. Issues such as the beginning of life, genetic testing and engineering, sex determination, the rights of the fetus, ownership of the fertilized egg, and so forth will not be easily answered. The council formulated an opinion regarding obstetric issues as fairly as possible and states the following:

Abortion: As the law now stands, a physician may perform an abortion as long as state and federal laws are followed regarding the trimester in which an abortion may be performed. A physician who does not want to perform abortions cannot be forced to perform the procedure; however, that physician should refer the patient to other health care professionals who can assist the patient (Fig. 2-2).

Scenario: While you are working for an obstetrician, Mrs. Bryant comes into the office for a regular pregnancy checkup. It is determined that the Bryant's baby has many congenital abnormalities. The baby will probably be blind and mentally retarded. Mr. Bryant wants his wife to have the pregnancy terminated, but Mrs. Bryant refuses.

Discussion questions: Should Mrs. Bryant be counseled and strongly encouraged against her wishes to have an abortion? Because the baby's care is only partially covered by Mr. Bryant's insurance plan, should his decision be more important? Should a pregnancy be terminated because of genetic problems? Does a fetus have rights? Who should decide these questions—the physician, the mother, the father, or the courts?

Genetic Testing: If an amniocentesis is performed on a mother and a genetic defect is found, both parents must be told. The parents may request or refuse to have the pregnancy terminated. (An amniocentesis is a procedure in which a needle is inserted in a pregnant woman's abdomen to remove and test amniotic fluid. Many abnormalities and disorders can be diagnosed early in pregnancy by this procedure.)

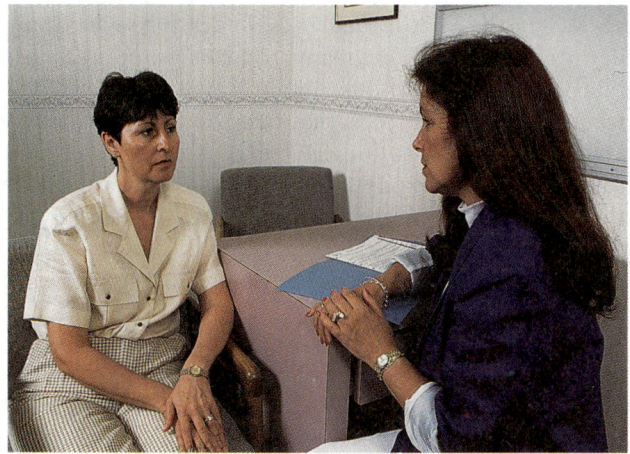

FIGURE 2-2
Counseling a patient regarding pregnancy alternatives.

Scenario: Carol Smith is a 15-year-old unwed mother on public assistance. A sonogram (a type of x-ray) suggests extensive fetal abnormalities that are confirmed by amniocentesis. She is uncertain about terminating her pregnancy.

Discussion questions: Should Carol be counseled to keep or to terminate the pregnancy? Consider her age and her ability to care for a baby with multiple handicaps. What about the long-term costs to our already overburdened public assistance? What about the rights of the fetus?

Artificial Insemination: This procedure involves the insertion of sperm into a woman's vagina for the purpose of conception. The donor may be the husband (artificial insemination-husband, or AIH) or an anonymous donor (artificial insemination-donor, or AID). The council states that both the husband and wife must consent to this procedure. If a donor is used, the sperm must be tested for infectious and genetic disorders. Complete confidentiality for the donor and recipient must be maintained.

Scenario: There is currently a repository for sperm from donors who test in the highest intellectual percentiles or who are outstanding in other areas, such as sports or music. In an effort to have a baby who might grow up to excel in an area of the parents' interest, some couples are choosing to search for donors among this group. Infertility of the male partner is not always an issue; the choice may simply be to ensure the best possible offspring.

Discussion questions: What are the ethics of choosing a donor solely on intellectual or athletic abilities? Suppose the choice was based on issues such as heroism, bravery, or kindness—would these choices make the selection more acceptable?

Surrogate Mothers: According to the council, the use of surrogate (or substitute) mothers to carry a pregnancy to term is ethically permissible; however, both parties must have legal and medical counseling before the insemination. The surrogate mother can be paid for medical and housing expenses along with an inconvenience fee.

Recent court cases have brought this issue to the attention of the public. Surrogate mothers may contract to carry a pregnancy to term for a couple who may be the donors of both the egg and the sperm or just the father's sperm using the surrogate's egg. In several instances, surrogate mothers have decided that they are unwilling to release the baby after delivery.

Scenario: Mrs. Brown has a scarred uterus and cannot carry a fetus to term; her eggs are not affected. Mr. Brown has no fertility problems. Mr. and Mrs. Brown have contracted through an attorney to pay Jane Jones to carry their fertilized egg to maturity. They will pay all of her medical and housing bills and will donate a substantial fee for her inconvenience. At time of delivery, Ms. Jones decides that she cannot part with the baby she has carried for 9 months and refuses to relinquish the baby to the Browns.

Discussion questions: Should Ms. Jones be bound by her contract to give the baby to the Browns? Would it matter if the egg had been Ms. Jones's rather than Mrs. Brown's? How do you feel about "renting" a uterus?

Organ Transplantation

Organ transplantation became a medical option in the mid 1950s although at that time there were many problems with rejection of the organs by the recipient's immune system. As this postoperative complication was corrected by antirejection drugs, the practice became more common. Organs are viable (able to support life) for varying lengths of time but most can be used successfully if transplanted within 24 to 48 hours. An organization called the United Network of Organ Sharing in Richmond, Virginia, coordinates local organ procurement teams that will fly to areas having organs to be harvested to assist with the surgery if needed and to ensure the integrity of the organ. There are far fewer organs available than are needed and every year thousands of patients die who could have lived if an organ had been available. Most states now have listed on driver's license forms whether or not the driver wishes to be an organ donor (Fig. 2-3). The scarcity of organs has caused many third world countries to become sources of organs as poor people sell parts of their bodies for basic needs.

The use of organs from a baby born without a brain (anencephaly) raises many serious ethical issues. The council states that everything must be done for the infant until the determination of death can be made. For infant organs to be transplanted, both parents must consent.

The council's views on transplantation state that:

- **The rights of the donor and organ recipient must be treated equally.** The imminent death of the donor does not release the medical personnel from observing all rights that every patient is due.
- **Organ donors must be given every medical opportunity for life.** Life support cannot removed until all criteria have been met that life has ended. These criteria usually involve the loss of brain wave activity and the inability to support life without artificial aids.
- **Death of the donor must be determined by a physician who is not on the transplant team** to avoid a charge of conflict of interest.
- **Consent (permission) must be received from both the donor, if possible, and recipient before the transplant. Family members may give consent if the donor is unable to do so.**

Signed by the donor and the following two witnesses in the presence of each other:

Sophie Cyzewski — Signature of Donor; 5/10/66 — Date of Birth of Donor

12/6/91 — Date Signed; Pittsburgh, PA — City and State

Dave Jarrett — Witness; Debbie Smith — Witness

This is a legal document under the Uniform Anatomical Gift Act or similar laws in all 50 states

For further information call

Delaware Valley TRANSPLANT PROGRAM

800 KIDNEY-1
2401 Walnut St., Suite 404
Philadelphia, PA 19103

UNIFORM DONOR CARD

Sophie Cyzewski
Print or type name of donor

In the hope that I may help others, I hereby make this anatomical gift, if medically acceptable, to take effect upon my death. The words and marks below indicate my desires.
I give: a) ✓ any needed organs or parts
b) ______ only the following organs or parts

Specify the organ(s) or part(s)

for the purpose of transplantation, therapy, medical research or education;
c) No my body for anatomical study if needed

Limitations or special wishes, if any

FIGURE 2-3
A sample organ donor card.

- **Transplants can only be performed by surgeons who are qualified to perform this complex surgery and who are affiliated with institutions that have adequate facilities for the surgery and postoperative care.**

Scenario: Charlie Rogers is on death row for murdering five women. He wants to be executed in a hospital setting so that his organs can be donated for transplantation. He feels that this will help repay society for what he has done. An execution in a hospital setting will cost taxpayers more money. The families of the murdered women do not want him to be allowed to do this. They feel it is a privilege to donate organs and that he should be executed in jail without special treatment or press attention.

Discussion questions: Should Mr. Rogers be allowed to donate his organs? Who should pay for the extra expenses if Mr. Rogers is allowed to donate his organs? Due to the shortage of available organs, should prisoners on death row be required to donate their organs?

Withholding or Withdrawing Treatment

Physicians have a professional and ethical obligation to promote quality of life, which means sustaining life and relieving suffering. Sometimes these obligations conflict with a patient's wishes. For instance, it may not be possible for the physician to alleviate the pain and suffering of a terminally ill cancer patient. Patients have the right to refuse medical treatments and to request that life support or life-sustaining treatments be withheld or withdrawn. **Withholding treatment** means that certain medical treatments may not be initiated. For example, a patient may request to withhold a feeding tube or cardiopulmonary resuscitation in the event of cardiac arrest. **Withdrawing treatment** is terminating a treatment that has already begun. For example, a patient or his family may request that a ventilator be withdrawn or removed even if it means that respirations will cease. The wishes of a patient concerning specific medical treatment are noted in a written request form called an **advance directive**. Advance directives are discussed in more detail in Chapter 3, Medicine and the Law.

Scenario: Mrs. Rodriguez has bone cancer (osteosarcoma). Her doctor has estimated she has 6 months to live. Mrs. Rodriguez wants the physician to withhold all medical treatments. She does not want chemotherapy or any life-sustaining measures. Her family wants her to be provided with all medical treatments.

Discussion questions: Should her family have any input into her health care decisions? As her condition deteriorates, she asks her physician for a prescription for pain medication that she could take to end her life. She states the pain is unbearable. Should the physician give her a prescription for pain, knowing that she may use it as a means of suicide? Is the physician justified in denying her pain relief for fear she will use it to kill herself? Should her family be involved in the decision? Do patients have the right to end their lives?

Box 2-1 presents a further discussion of end-of-life ethical issues such as euthanasia and assisted suicide.

Checkpoint Question

5. *What is the difference between withholding and withdrawing treatment?*

Professional Conduct and Behavior

The council feels that all health care team members *must* work together in the best interest of patient care. The council states that all health care profes-

---

BOX 2-1   End-of-Life Ethical Issues

Although authorities vary the terminology, **euthanasia** generally refers to allowing a patient to die a quiet death, as pain free as possible and with minimal medical intervention. This may also be called *passive euthanasia*. Examples include medication adequate to relieve pain, intravenous fluids to maintain hydration, and various other comfort measures.

Performing an act that causes or hastens death is usually considered to be *mercy killing* or *active euthanasia*. Examples may involve administering an overdose of medication or removing life support when brain wave activity is present and death is not imminent.

Recent media coverage has alerted us to another option: *assisted suicide* or *voluntary euthanasia*. A patient may choose to end his life with another person or a professional in attendance who will help ease the transition from life to death.

Special circumstances are involved if the helper is a physician. Proponents of physician-assisted suicide feel that the goal of medical care is the relief of suffering, not necessarily the extension of life. They stress that

careful regulation must be in place that includes review procedures, consultations, and so on. They feel it should be considered as a last resort for competent patients who have decided that extended medical care is not their choice. Those opposed to the practice feel that involving a physician conflicts with the right to life of all persons and the most basic principles of medicine.

Although the general consensus in our country supports the rights of competent adults to make health care decisions, hastening death is understandably a concern to many. Voters in several states have demonstrated the public's ambivalence about the issue by allowing it in some states and forbidding it in others.

This issue is not new. Hippocrates indicated that this was a concern by including in his oath: "I will neither give a deadly drug to anyone if asked for it, nor will I make a suggestion to that effect." If the conflict has not been resolved in 2400 years, it is unlikely that current medical ethics will finally settle the issue to the satisfaction of all.

sionals are responsible for reporting unethical practices to the appropriate agencies. No health care professional should engage in any act that he or she feels is ethically or morally wrong. Additionally, the council states that:

- A physician must never assist or allow an unlicensed person to practice medicine.
- Hospitals and physicians must jointly work together for the best care for patients. Hospitals should allow physicians **staff privileges** based on the ability of the physician, educational background, and the needs of the community. (Staff privileges allow physicians to admit their patients into a given hospital). Issues of a personal nature must never be considered when accepting or declining a physician's application for privileges.

- It is unethical for physicians to admit patients into the hospital or to order excessive treatments for the sole purpose of financial rewards.

Office Management Issues

The council's guidelines regarding administrative issues include:

- Physicians must seek consultations for patients when their care exceeds the physician's ability or training. For instance, an ophthalmologist should not treat gynecologic disorders.
- The physician must not accept gifts from private industries in return for promoting products. For example, a physician cannot accept a trip to Europe from a pharmaceutical company and in re-

---

BOX 2-2 Ethical Dilemma

Here is a sample medical-ethical issue that could occur in a medical office. How would you solve it?

Scenario

You are working in a clinic administering influenza vaccines. You have two vaccines left, but there are six patients waiting. No more vaccines are available from the pharmaceutical company. A $20 donation is requested from each patient. The Centers for Disease Control and Prevention expect this year's influenza outbreak to reach record levels.

Patients

Patient #1 is a 54-year-old healthy man. He exercises on a regular basis and is considered to be at low risk for acquiring flu. Because of his healthy condition, if he did acquire the flu, his chances for a quick recovery would be good. He knows that there is a shortage of vaccines and offers you a $100 donation. (He is a member of the Board of Directors for this clinic.)

Patient #2 is a 20-year-old man with AIDS. He has a history of drug abuse. He is considered high risk for the flu, and his prognosis for surviving the flu would be unlikely because of his history of AIDS-related pneumonia. He does not have the $20 donation.

Patient #3 is a 60-year-old woman with cancer. Because of the large doses of chemotherapy she has received, her immunity is low and she is at high risk for the flu. She has less than a 20% chance of surviving her cancer due to extensive metastasis.

Patient #4 is an 80-year-old nursing home patient. He has severe lung disease due to smoking. Last winter he developed pneumonia and almost died. He weeps as he tells you the story and adds that he is afraid of dying. He begs you for the vaccine. Payment will be made through Medicare.

Patient #5 is a 72-year-old retired general from the armed services. He lost one lung from a gunshot wound during combat. He is otherwise healthy. Money is not a concern for him.

Patient #6 is a 38-year-old man. He has a long history of psychiatric problems. He is presently institutionalized for suicidal tendencies. He does not have the money for the donation.

Questions

- Which two people would you choose to receive the vaccines and why?
- What if one of the patients were a relative? Would that change your decision?
- What if one of the patients were a convicted murderer? Would that affect your decision?
- Should the ability to pay make a difference?

Discussion

Each person who reads the above scenario will select a different combination of patients, for different reasons. The solution will vary based on each reader's family background, past experiences, and value system. This problem is like many medical-ethical problems; the solution is neither black nor white, it is often shades of gray.

turn only prescribe that company's medications to patients. Promotional gifts must be of small value (eg, note pads or pens) or educational in nature, such as videos or booklets that are not explicitly for the purpose of promoting the product.

- Physicians must never practice medicine under the influence of drugs or alcohol.
- Physicians must treat patients equally without religious, ethnic, or racial biases.
- Financial interests must never come above patient care. Ordering the most expensive tests or not ordering needed tests based on the patient's ability to pay is not acceptable.
- If a physician's office routinely charges patients for canceling appointments within 24 hours of the actual scheduled appointment, a warning must be posted to advise patients of this charge.
- The medical record must never be held against nonpayment of a bill.
- In relation to fees, the council states that:

> Fees cannot be excessive. They must be based on fair and standard charges for all patients. Guidelines for charges should consider the difficulty and unique nature of the services involved and the use of medical equipment.
>
> Interest on past due accounts can be charged in accordance with state laws and with *prior* notification to the patient.
>
> No fees can be charged for physician referrals or for admitting a patient into the hospital.
>
> A fee should not be charged to the patient for completing or filing a simple insurance form. If the form is extensive, a minimal fee may be charged.
>
> Caution must be used with computers to maintain patient confidentiality. If patient data are sent via fax machine, utmost care must be used to ensure that the material is received by only the correct recipient.

- If the physician advertises his or her practice, it must be done with the utmost honesty. Misrepresentation of information is never appropriate.
- If a physician closes the practice (or dies), all patients must be notified that the office is closing and must be given instructions for retrieving their medical records. Generally, copies of medical records are transferred to another local physician. The originals are stored as directed by state law.

Scenario: You have graduated from school and passed your certification examination. Jobs are hard to find. After almost 6 months of job hunting, you finally find a job working for a prestigious and well known surgeon. When you first begin, everything seems perfect. Within 2 weeks you find many unethical procedures being performed in the office by the surgeon and the staff. You approach another medical assistant working there and voice your concerns. She admits that "they do things wrong here" but adds "I need this job so I keep quiet." She suggests that you keep quiet and do your job or be fired.

Discussion questions: What should you do? Who would you go to with this problem? You decide to confront the issue with the surgeon. He tells you that if you report these procedures, he will make it impossible for you to work at any nearby offices. What should you do now?

Box 2-2 describes a medical-ethical dilemma that might occur in a medical office. Read it carefully, then analyze how you would handle the problem.

SUMMARY

Medical ethics and bioethics involve complex issues and controversial topics. There will be no easy or clear cut answers to questions raised by these issues. As a medical assistant, your first priority must be to act as your patients' advocate with their best interests and concerns foremost in your actions and interactions. You must always maintain ethical standards in your actions and report the unethical behaviors of others.

CRITICAL THINKING CHALLENGES

1. The United States Congress has attempted to reorganize the health care system to provide health care insurance to all Americans. Do you think the government should be involved in regulating who receives medical care and what medical care is given? Do you think all U.S. citizens should be provided with health care insurance? Who should pay for it? Would you be willing to pay higher taxes so that everyone would have coverage? Explain your response.
2. Medications are tested on laboratory animals before being tested on humans. Should animals be used for research? If your answer is no, should the first subject to test a medication be a human? Explain your response. Now consider the question if the drug is a prospective cure for AIDS: Should AIDS patients be allowed to try the drug before all preliminary testing is complete?
3. Should physicians assist in terminating a pregnancy? What if the woman's life is in danger if she carries a baby to term—is that grounds for terminating a pregnancy? Explain your response.
4. Many young children die each year waiting for transplant organs. Considering the shortage of organs for

transplantation, should anencephalic babies be used as organ donors? Should research continue exploring the possibility of replacing human organs with animal organs? Explain your response.

ANSWERS TO CHECKPOINT QUESTIONS

1. Laws are regulations that must be adhered to and that are enforced by governmental agencies. Ethics are standards of moral conduct and behavior and are enforced by professional organizations.

2. Physicians who violate ethical principles may face these penalties: censure (reprimand), suspension (removal or privileges and association with the professional organization), and expulsion (formal discharge from the professional organization).

3. In the medical office, the medical assistant must maintain patient confidentiality, follow state and federal laws, and be honest.

4. When examining an ethical dilemma, you should identify the problem, gather information, formulate options, and implement and evaluate the decision. Institutional review boards (IRBs) should be used as necessary.

5. Withholding treatment is not initiating certain medical treatments. Withdrawing treatment is terminating medical treatment that has already been initiated.

SUGGESTIONS FOR FURTHER READING

American Medical Association. (1992). *Code of Medical Ethics, Current Opinions*. Chicago: AMA.

Flight, M. (1993). *Law, Liability and Ethics*, 2nd ed., Albany, NY: Delmar Publishers.

Levin, C. (1995). *Taking Sides: Clashing Views on Controversial Bioethical Issues*, 6th ed. Guilford, CT: The Dushkin Publishing Group.

Lewis, M. A., & Tamparo, C. D. (1993). *Medical Law, Ethics and Bioethics in the Medical Office*, 3rd ed. Philadelphia: F. A. Davis.

Perlin, T. M. (1992). *Clinical Medical Ethics: Cases in Practice*. Boston: Little, Brown.

Purtilo, R. (1993). *Ethical Dimensions in the Health Professions*, 2nd ed. Philadelphia: W. B. Saunders.

Rodwin, M. A. (1995). *Medicine, Money and Morals*. New York: Oxford University Press.

Snell, M. (1991). *Bioethical Dilemmas in Health Occupations*. Peoria, IL: Glencoe Division of McGraw-Hill.

Medicine and the Law

Chapter Outline

The American Legal System
    Sources of Laws
    Branches of the Law
    The Rise in Medical-Legal Cases
Physician–Patient Relationship
    Contracts
    Consent
    Legally Required Disclosures
Specific Laws and Statutes That Apply to Health Professionals
    Medical Practice Acts
    Controlled Substances Act
    Good Samaritan Act
    Uniform Anatomical Gift Act
    Self-Determination Act (Advance Directives)
    Consolidated Omnibus Budget Reconciliation Act (COBRA)

Specific Medical Law
    Tort Law
The Litigation Process
Defenses to Professional Liability Suits
    Medical Records
    Statutes of Limitation
    Assumption of Risk
    Res Judicata
    Contributory Negligence
    Comparative Negligence
    Immunity
A Defense for the Medical Assistant
    Respondeat Superior or Law of Agency
Summary
Critical Thinking Challenges
Answers to Checkpoint Questions
Suggestions for Further Reading

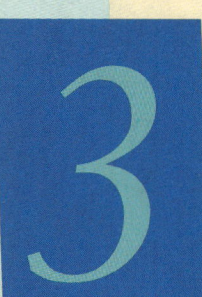

DACUM Components

5.1   Document accurately
5.2   Determine needs for documentation and accurate reporting
5.4   Follow established policy in initiating or terminating medical treatment
5.5   Dispose of controlled substances in compliance with government regulations
5.6   Monitor legislation related to current health care issues and practices

Chapter Competencies

Learning Objectives

Upon successfully completing this chapter, you will be able to:

1. Identify the two branches of the American legal system.
2. Identify reasons for the escalation of medical malpractice cases.
3. Describe the difference between implied and expressed contracts.
4. List four items that must be included in a contract termination or withdrawal letter.
5. List six items that must be included in an informed consent form.
6. Explain who may sign consent forms.
7. List five incidents that must be reported to specified authorities.
8. Describe the purpose of the Self-Determination Act.
9. Give four examples of intentional torts.
10. Describe the four elements that must be proven in a medical-legal suit.
11. Describe four possible defenses against litigation for the medical professional.
12. Explain the theory of *respondeat superior* or law of agency and how it applies the medical assistant.
13. List ways that a medical assistant can assist in the prevention of a medical malpractice suit.

Key Terms

(See Glossary for definitions.)

age of majority
appeal
assault
battery
bench trial
certification
civil law
coerce
common law
comparative negligence
consent
consideration
contract
contributory negligence
cross examination
damages
defamation of character
defendant

deposition
direct examination
durable power of
   attorney
duress
emancipated minor
expert witness
expressed consent
fee-splitting
fraud
implied consent
informed consent
libel
licensure
litigation
malpractice
negligence
non compos mentis

plaintiff
precedent
registered
res ipsa loquitur
res judicata
*respondeat
   superior*
slander
stare decisis
statutes
statutes of
   limitation
subpoena
subpoena *duces
   tecum*
tort
verdict

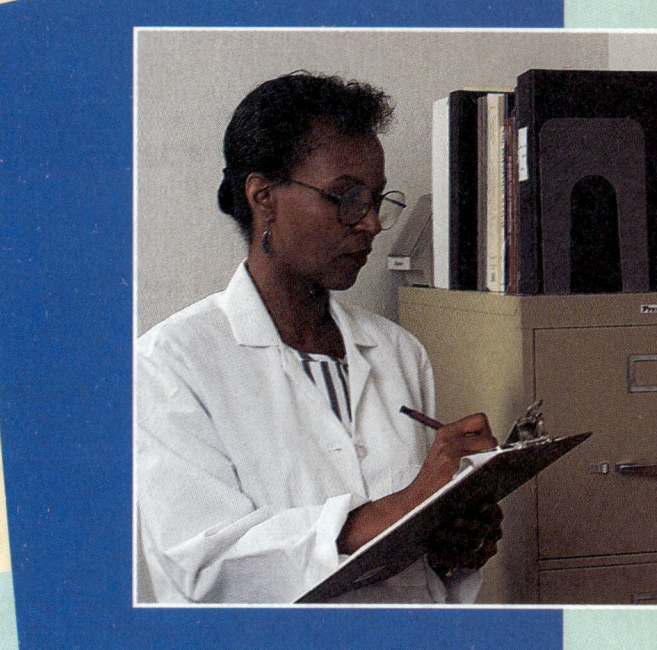

During your career as a medical assistant, you will be involved in many medical situations with potential legal implications. Physicians may be sued for a variety of reasons, including significant clinical errors (eg, removing the wrong limb, ordering a toxic dose of medication), claims of improperly touching a patient without consent, or failure to properly diagnosis or treat a disease. Medicare **fraud** (concealing the truth) and falsifying medical records can also result in a lawsuit. Medical assistants and other health care workers are frequently included in many of the suits brought to court. You may help to prevent many of these claims against your physician, and also protect yourself, by complying with medical laws, keeping abreast of medical trends, and maintaining a high level of professionalism at all times.

➤ THE AMERICAN LEGAL SYSTEM

Even in the best physician–patient relationships, **litigation** (lawsuits) between patients and physicians may occur. Litigation may result from a single medication error or a mistake that costs a person's life. It is essential that you have a basic understanding of the American legal system to protect yourself and to protect patients and physicians from errors. You must know your legal duties and understand the legal nature of the physician–patient relationship and your role and responsibilities as the physician's agent.

Sources of Law

Laws are rules of conduct and principles established by custom, by agreement, or by authority set to govern the affairs of a community with provisions made for enforcement by appointed authorities. The foundation of our legal system was based on our rights outlined in the Constitution and on the laws established by our founding fathers, which were based primarily on the English legal system. These traditional laws are known as **common law**.

Common law principles are based on the theory of **stare decisis**. This term means "the previous decision stands." Judges follow these **precedents** (previous court decisions) until the decision is outdated or overruled.

Another source of law is the establishment of **statutes**. Statutes are laws that are formulated by federal, state, or local legislators. Statutes pertaining to Medicare, Medicaid, and the Food and Drug Administration are common examples in the medical profession.

The third source of law is administrative. These laws are passed by governmental agencies, such as the Internal Revenue Service.

Branches of the Law

The two main branches of the legal system are public law and private (or civil) law.

Public Law

Public law is the branch of law that focuses on issues between the government and its citizens. It can be divided into four subgroups:

1. *Criminal law* is concerned with issues of citizen welfare and safety. Examples include arson, burglaries, murder, and rape. Practicing medicine without a license is also an example.
2. *Constitutional law* is commonly called the "law of the land." The United States government has a constitution and each state has a constitution of its own with laws and regulations voted on by its citizens. State laws may be more restrictive than federal laws but may not be more lenient. Two examples of constitutional law include laws involving abortion and civil rights issues.
3. *Administrative law* pertains to the regulations set forth by governmental agencies. This category includes laws pertaining to the Food and Drug Administration, the Internal Revenue Service, and Board of Medical Examiners.
4. *International law* pertains to treaties between countries. Related issues include trade agreements, extradition, boundaries, and international waters.

Private or Civil Law

Private law, or **civil law**, is the branch of the law that focuses on issues between private citizens. The medical profession is primarily concerned with private law. The subcategories that pertain to the medical profession are contract, commercial, and **tort** law. Contract and commercial laws concern the rights and obligations of those who enter into contracts, as in a physician–patient relationship. Tort law governs the righting of wrongs or injuries suffered by someone because of another person's wrongdoing or misdeeds resulting from a breach of legal duty. Tort law is the basis of most lawsuits against physicians and health care workers. These branches will be discussed in detail later in the chapter. Other civil law branches include property, inheritance, and corporation law.

> **Checkpoint Question**
> 1. *What are the two branches of the law? Briefly describe each. Which branch is the medical professional primarily concerned with?*

The Rise in Medical-Legal Cases

Since World War II, the number of medical **malpractice** cases brought to court has increased significantly. Malpractice refers to an action by a professional health care worker that causes harm to a patient. A government task force found four primary reasons for the rise in malpractice claims. These reasons were:

1. Scientific advances—As new and improved medical technology becomes available, the potential risks and complications of these procedures escalate, making physicians more vulnerable to litigation.
2. Unrealistic expectations—Some patients expect miracle cures and will often file lawsuits because recovery was not as they hoped or expected, even if the physician is not at fault.
3. Economic factors—Some patients may view lawsuits as a means to obtain "quick cash." (In fact, an increase in the number of lawsuits filed has been noted during economic recessions.)
4. Poor communication—Statistics show that when patients do not feel a bond with their physicians, they are more likely to sue.

➤ PHYSICIAN–PATIENT RELATIONSHIP

Contracts

A **contract** is an agreement between two or more parties to do or not do an act with certain factors agreed on among all parties. The physician–patient relationship is reinforced by the formation of a contract. All contractual agreements have three components:

1. **Offer** (contract initiation)
2. **Acceptance** (both parties agree to the terms)
3. **Consideration** (the exchange of fees for service)

The offer is initiated by the patient's presence. The patient asks either literally or by his presence: "Will you treat me?" The physician responds "yes" by accepting the patient, again either literally or by beginning treatment. Both have expressed acceptance of the relationship. Consideration in the medical profession implies the mutual agreement that the physician will perform a given task and that the patient will pay the physician for that care. A contract is not valid unless all three elements are present.

A contract offer is made when a patient calls the office to request an appointment. The implication is made that if the offer is accepted, payment for services will be made. The offer is accepted when you make an appointment for the patient. You have formed a con-

tract that implies that for a fee, the physician will do all in his or her power to address the health concerns of the patient.

The two types of contracts between physicians and patients are implied and expressed, as discussed below.

Implied Contracts

Implied contracts, the most common kinds of contracts between physicians and patients, are not written but are assumed by the actions of the parties. *Example*: A patient calls the office and requests to see Dr. Smith for an earache. The patient arrives for the appointment, is seen by the physician, and a prescription is given. It is "implied" that because the patient came on his own and requested care that he wants this physician to care for him. The physician's action of accepting the patient for care "implies" that he acknowledges responsibility for his part of the contract. The patient "implies" by accepting the services that he will render payment even though the price was not discussed.

Expressed Contracts

Expressed contracts are either written or oral and consist of specified details. A mutual sharing of responsibilities is always stated in an expressed contract. These kinds of contracts are not used as often in the medical setting as implied contracts.

Checkpoint Question
2. What is a contract and what three components must it include?

Rights and Responsibilities of the Patient and Physician

In any contractual relationship, both parties have certain rights and responsibilities. The patient's rights and responsibilities are considered first.

The patient has the right to:

1. Consult the physician of his or her choice
2. Receive respectful and considerate care
3. Expect confidentiality and privacy
4. Receive information regarding the condition, including diagnosis, treatment, and prognosis
5. Receive information regarding treatments including the risks, benefits, cost, and other alternatives to the recommended treatment
6. Make decisions regarding medical care
7. Refuse treatment
8. Refuse to participate in research projects

9. Expect continuity of care
10. Obtain copies of medical records, according to the physician's policy and applicable state laws

The American Hospital Association, among other organizations, has prepared a Patient's Bill of Rights (Fig. 3-1).

Responsibilities of the patient are to:

1. Provide the physician with accurate data about the duration and nature of symptoms
2. Provide a complete and accurate past medical history to the physician
3. Follow the physician's instructions for diet, exercise, medications, and follow-up appointments
4. Compensate the physician for services rendered

A physician in private practice has the right to:

1. Accept or decline new patients into the practice
2. Accept or decline former patients with new problems, even though no other physician is available
3. Designate the type of services that he or she will provide
4. Specialize in a given field
5. Select office hours, vacation schedules, and time availability
6. Relocate the office
7. Select substitute physician coverage in his or her absence

Physicians may also refuse to treat an emergency patient, unless the physician is assigned to emergency room duty. Although this is not considered ethical, it is legal.

Responsibilities of the physician are to:

1. Respect the patient's confidential information
2. Provide reasonable skill, experience, and knowledge in treating the patient
3. Continue treating the patient until the contract has been withdrawn or as long as the condition requires treatment
4. Inform patients of their condition, treatments, and prognosis
5. Give complete and accurate instructions
6. Provide competent coverage for the practice during time away from the practice
7. Obtain **informed consent** before performing procedures (Informed consent is a statement of approval from the patient for the physician to perform a given procedure after the patient has been educated about the risks and benefits of the procedure.)
8. Caution against unneeded or undesirable treatment or surgery

Termination or Withdrawal of the Contract

The ideal resolution of a contract occurs when the patient is satisfactorily cured of the illness and the physician has been paid for the services. The patient may end the contract at any time, but the physician must follow legal protocol to dissolve the contract if the patient still seeks treatment and the physician wishes to end the relationship.

PATIENT-INITIATED TERMINATION

If the patient chooses to terminate the relationship, a letter should be written to the physician stating reasons for the termination. This letter must be kept in the medical record for legal purposes. Following the receipt of this letter, a letter should be sent from the physician to the patient stating that:

- The physician accepts the termination
- Medical records are available on written request
- Medical referrals are available if needed

If the patient verbally asks to end this relationship, the physician should send a letter to the patient documenting the conversation and again offering references and access to the medical records. Clear documentation is essential. When a patient is unhappy, the potential for litigation escalates. Efforts must be made to comply with patient requests to ease any patient dissatisfaction.

PHYSICIAN-INITIATED TERMINATION

The physician may also want to end the relationship. Physicians may wish to stop caring for a patient if payment is not rendered, if patient compliance is poor, if appointments are not kept, or for personal reasons. The physician must send a letter of withdrawal or termination intent. The letter must include:

- A statement of intent to terminate the relationship
- A brief explanation stating the reasons for this action
- The termination date (the date should include a reasonable time frame)
- A statement indicating the availability of medical records that can be transferred to another physician on patient request
- A recommendation that the patient seek additional medical care as warranted

As the medical assistant, you may be responsible for creating these letters at the request of the physician and for posting them properly. They are sent by certified mail with a return receipt requested. A copy of the termination letter and the return receipt are placed in the patient's record (Fig. 3-2).

text continues on page 39

Introduction

Effective health care requires collaboration between patients and physicians and other health care professionals. Open and honest communication, respect for personal and professional values, and sensitivity to differences are integral to optimal patient care. As the setting for the provision of health services, hospitals must provide a foundation for understanding and respecting the rights and responsibilities of patients, their families, physicians, and other caregivers. Hospitals must ensure a health care ethic that respects the role of patients in decision making about treatment choices and other aspects of their care. Hospitals must be sensitive to cultural, racial, linguistic, religious, age, gender, and other differences as well as the needs of persons with disabilities.

The American Hospital Association presents *A Patient's Bill of Rights* with the expectation that it will contribute to more effective patient care and be supported by the hospital on behalf of the institution, its medical staff, employees, and patients. The American Hospital Association encourages health care institutions to tailor this bill of rights to their patient community by translating and/or simplifying the language of this bill of rights as may be necessary to ensure that patients and their families understand their rights and responsibilities.

Bill of Rights*

1. The patient has the right to considerate and respectful care.
2. The patient has the right to and is encouraged to obtain from physicians and other direct caregivers relevant, current, and understandable information concerning diagnosis, treatment, and prognosis.

   Except in emergencies when the patient lacks decision-making capacity and the need for treatment is urgent, the patient is entitled to the opportunity to discuss and request information related to the specific procedures and/or treatments, the risks involved, the possible length of recuperation, and the medically reasonable alternatives and their accompanying risks and benefits.

   Patients have the right to know the identity of physicians, nurses, and others involved in their care, as well as when those involved are students, residents, or other trainees. The patient also has the right to know the immediate and long-term financial implications of treatment choices, insofar as they are known.
3. The patient has the right to make decisions about the plan of care prior to and during the course of treatment and to refuse a recommended treatment or plan of care to the extent permitted by law and hospital policy and to be informed of the medical consequences of this action. In case of such refusal, the patient is entitled to other appropriate care and services that the hospital provides or transfer to another hospital. The hospital should notify patients of any policy that might affect patient choice within the institution.
4. The patient has the right to have an advance directive (such as a living will, health care proxy, or durable power of attorney for health care) concerning treatment or designating a surrogate decision maker with the expectation that the hospital will honor the intent of that directive to the extent permitted by law and hospital policy.

   Health care institutions must advise patients of their rights under state law and hospital policy to make informed medical choices, ask if the patient has an advance directive, and include that information in patient records. The patient has the right to timely information about hospital policy that may limit its ability to implement fully a legally valid advance directive.
5. The patient has the right to every consideration of privacy. Case discussion, consultation, examination, and treatment should be conducted so as to protect each patient's privacy.
6. The patient has the right to expect that all communications and records pertaining to his/her care will be treated as confidential by the hospital, except in cases such as suspected abuse and public health hazards when reporting is permitted or required by law. The patient has the right to expect that the hospital will emphasize the confidentiality of this information when it releases it to any other parties entitled to review information in these records.

These rights can be exercised on the patient's behalf by a designated surrogate or proxy decision maker if the patient lacks decision-making capacity, is legally incompetent, or is a minor.

(*continues*)

FIGURE 3-1
The American Hospital Association's Patient's Bill of Rights.

7. The patient has the right to review the records pertaining to his/her medical care and to have the information explained or interpreted as necessary, except when restricted by law.

8. The patient has the right to expect that, within its capacity and policies, a hospital will make reasonable response to the request of a patient for appropriate and medically indicated care and services. The hospital must provide evaluation, service, and/or referral as indicated by the urgency of the case. When medically appropriate and legally permissible, or when a patient has so requested, a patient may be transferred to another facility. The institution to which the patient is to be transferred must first have accepted the patient for transfer. The patient must also have the benefit of complete information and explanation concerning the need for, risks, benefits, and alternatives to such a transfer.

9. The patient has the right to ask and be informed of the existence of business relationships among the hospital, educational institutions, other health care providers, or payers that may influence the patient's treatment and care.

10. The patient has the right to consent to or decline to participate in proposed research studies or human experimentation affecting care and treatment or requiring direct patient involvement, and to have those studies fully explained prior to consent. A patient who declines to participate in research or experimentation is entitled to the most effective care that the hospital can otherwise provide.

11. The patient has the right to expect reasonable continuity of care when appropriate and to be informed by physicians and other caregivers of available and realistic patient care options when hospital care is no longer appropriate.

12. The patient has the right to be informed of hospital policies and practices that relate to patient care, treatment, and responsibilities. The patient has the right to be informed of available resources for resolving disputes, grievances, and conflicts, such as ethics committees, patient representatives, or other mechanisms available in the institution. The patient has the right to be informed of the hospital's charges for services and available payment methods.

The collaborative nature of health care requires that patients, or their families/surrogates, participate in their care. The effectiveness of care and patient satisfaction with the course of treatment depend, in part, on the patient fulfilling certain responsibilities. Patients are responsible for providing information about past illnesses, hospitalizations, medication, and other matters related to health status. To participate effectively in decision making, patients must be encouraged to take responsibility for requesting additional information and instructions. Patients are also responsible for ensuring that the health care institution has a copy of their written advance directive if they have one. Patients are responsible for informing their physicians and other caregivers if they anticipate problems in following prescribed treatment.

Patients should also be aware of the hospital's obligation to be reasonably efficient and equitable in providing care to other patients and the community. The hospital's rules and regulations are designed to help the hospital meet this obligation. Patients and their families are responsible for making reasonable accommodations to the needs of the hospital, other patients, medical staff, and hospital employees. Patients are responsible for providing necessary information for insurance claims and for working with the hospital to make payment arrangements, when necessary.

A person's health depends on much more than health care services. Patients are responsible for recognizing the impact of their life-style on their personal health.

Conclusion

Hospitals have many functions to perform, including the enhancement of health status, health promotion, and the prevention and treatment of injury and disease; the immediate and ongoing care and rehabilitation of patients; the education of health professionals, patients, and the community; and research. All these activities must be conducted with an overriding concern for the values and dignity of patients.

A patient's Bill of Rights was first adopted by the American Hospital Association in 1973. This revision was approved by the AHA Board of Trustees on October 21, 1992.

FIGURE 3-1
The American Hospital Association's Patient's Bill of Rights. *(continued)*

Carolyn Gleason, M.D.
Miami Family Practice
220 NW 3rd Avenue
Miami, FL 33015

August 22, 1999

Maria Seffern
Jones Hill Road
Nutley, NJ 07110

Dear Ms. Seffern:

I will be retiring from practicing medicine on October 31, 1999. Dr. Trent will be accepting my patients. His office is located at 622 Terrace Avenue in Miami.

I will forward your medical records to his office.

If you would prefer a different physician, please advise my office of the physician's name and address and I will be happy to forward your records there.

Thank you for being my patient for ten years.

Sincerely,

Carolyn Gleason, M.D.

CG/srd

FIGURE 3-2
Physician's letter of termination intent.

ABANDONMENT

If a contract is not properly terminated, the physician can be sued for abandonment. Abandonment may be charged if the physician withdraws from the contractual relationship without proper notification while the patient still needs treatment.

If the physician is not available when needed by the patient, an abandonment suit is possible. Physicians must always arrange coverage during absences from the office, such as vacations, conferences, and so on. Patients may sue for abandonment in any instance that a suitable substitute is not available for care.

Other examples of abandonment include:

- The physician abruptly and without reasonable notice stops treating a patient whose condition requires additional or continued care.

- The physician fails to see a patient as often as the condition requires or incorrectly advises the patient that further treatment is not needed.

Checkpoint Question
3. What five elements must be in the physician's termination intent letter?

Consent

Consent is an agreement by the patient that he may be touched, examined, or treated by the physician or by agents of the physician with whom he has entered into a contractual agreement. No treatment may be made without a consent given either orally, nonverbally by behavior, or clearly in writing.

Implied Consent

In the typical visit to the physician's office, the presence of the patient and the body language act as **implied consent** (informal agreement) for care to be given. A patient who raises her sleeve to receive an injection is implying that she agrees to the treatment. Implied consent also occurs in an emergency situation. If a patient is in a life-threatening situation and is unable to give verbal permission for treatment, it is implied that the patient would consent to treatment if possible. As soon as possible, informed consent should be signed by either the patient or family members in this type of situation. In nonemergency situations, implied consent should be used only if the procedure poses no risk to the patient.

Informed or Expressed Consent

An *informed consent* is the responsibility of the physician and is required whenever the treatment involves an invasive procedure such as surgery, use of experimental drugs, potentially dangerous procedures such as stress tests, or any treatment that poses a high risk to the patient. Informed consent may also be referred to as **expressed consent**.

Informed consent is based on the patient's right to know every possible benefit, risk, or alternative to the suggested treatment and the possible outcome if *no* treatment is initiated. The patient must voluntarily give permission and must understand the implications of consenting to the treatment. This requires that the physician and patient communicate in a manner understandable to the patient. Educating patients during the informed consent process encourages rational decision making and helps the patient to become an active participant in personal health care decisions.

A consent (Fig. 3-3) must include the following information:

1. Name of the procedure to be performed
2. Name of the physician who will perform the procedure
3. Name of the person administering the anesthesia (if applicable)
4. Any potential risks from the procedure
5. Anticipated result or benefit from the procedure
6. Alternatives to the procedure and their risks
7. Any exclusions that the patient requests
8. Statement indicating that all patient questions or concerns regarding the procedure have been answered
9. Patient and witness signatures and the date

As the medical assistant, you will frequently be required to witness consent signatures.

It is important to note that the informed consent form supplied for the patient's signature must be in the language that the patient speaks. Most physicians who treat multicultural patients will have consent forms available in a variety of languages. A patient should never be asked to sign a consent form if he or she:

- Does not understand the procedure
- Has questions regarding the procedure
- Is unable to read the consent form

Never **coerce** a patient (force or compel against his wishes) into signing a consent form.

WHO MAY SIGN A CONSENT FORM?

An *adult* (usually someone over the age of 18) who is mentally competent and not under the influence of medication or other substances may sign a consent form. It is permissible for a *minor* to sign a consent form if he or she is:

- In the armed services
- Requesting treatment for communicable diseases (including sexually transmitted diseases)
- Pregnant
- Requesting information regarding birth control, abortion, or drug or alcohol abuse counseling
- Emancipated

An **emancipated minor** is under the **age of majority** but is either married or self-supporting and responsible for his or her debts. The age of majority varies from state to state and ranges from 18 to 21. Minors may give consent if just one of the above-listed criteria is present.

Legal guardians may also sign consent forms. A legal guardian can be appointed by a judge when the court has ruled the individual to be **non compos mentis** (*Non compos mentis* is a general legal term referring to any mental incompetence). *Health care surrogates* may also sign consent forms. Health care surrogates are discussed later in the chapter.

Checkpoint Question
4. Under what circumstances should a patient never be asked to sign a consent form?

Refusal of Consent

Patients may refuse consent for treatments based on religious or personal beliefs and preferences. For instance, a Jehovah's Witness may refuse a blood transfusion on religious grounds, or an elderly person may not want to undergo serious surgery because the potential complica-

I hereby authorize Dr. _Doe_____, and such assistants as may be designated, to perform:

_____endoscopy_____

(Name of treatment/procedure)

and any other related procedures or forms of treatment, including appropriate anesthesia, transfusions that they deem necessary for the welfare of:

William Brown

(Name of patient)

I consent to the administration of anesthesia and/or such drugs as may be necessary. I understand that all anesthetics invovle risks of complication, serious injury, or rarely death from both known and unknown causes.

I consent to the examination and retention for educational, scientific and research purposes by the University of Washington Medical Staff of all body fluids, tissues and organs removed during the course of the above treatment/procedure with privilege of ultimate use and disposal resting with said medical staff.

I understand that the expected results of said treatment cannot be guaranteed. The physicians, surgeons, or dentists of the University of Washington have discussed to my satisfaction the following:

A. The nature and character of the proposed treatment/procedure.

B. The anticipated results of the proposed treatment/procedure.

C. The recognized alternative forms of treatment/procedure.

D. The recognized serious possible risks and complications of the treatment/procedure and of the recognized alternative forms of treatment/procedure, including non-treatment.

E. The anticipated date and time of the proposed treatment/procedure.

Additional M.D. comments: _____

My physician has offered to answer all inquiries concerning the proposed treatment/procedure. I understand that I am free to withhold or withdraw consent to the proposed treatment/procedure at any time.

Witness	Signature of Person Giving Consent
Jane White	William Brown

Date Signed	Time	☒ A.M.	Relationship to Patient (if applicable)
11/15/97	700	☐ P.M.	

❏ Please check if this is a telephone monitored consent.
   No treatment will be performed until this consent has been executed. This consent will be permanently filed in the patient's medical record.

Pt. No.	**Gastroenterology Associates** Anytown, CA
Name	**Special Consent to Treatment** (Diagnostic & Surgical Procedures, Anesthesia, Medical Treatment & Other Procedures)
D.O.B.	

FIGURE 3-3
Example of a consent form.

tions may limit future life-style options. In this situation a refusal of consent should be signed indicating that the patient was instructed regarding the potential risks and benefits of the procedure as well as the risks if the transfusion is not allowed. The physician has a legal right to refuse to perform elective surgery on a patient who refuses to receive blood if needed. If the patient is a minor, the courts may become involved at the request of the physician or hospital and may award consent for the child. In this situation, the physician should follow legal counsel and document the incident carefully. In any instance that the patient refuses treatment, full documentation must be made to protect the physician.

Legally Required Disclosures

Physicians and medical assistants have a joint responsibility to report certain events to governmental agencies. The following situations must be reported to the state health department.

Vital Statistics

All states maintain records of births, deaths, marriages, and divorces. The medically applicable reports include:

- *Birth* certificates must be filed within 5 days of the birth and information regarding both parents must be completed. Should the identity of the father be unknown, the record is marked as such.
- *Death* certificates must be signed by a physician. The cause and time of death must be included. *Stillbirths* must also be reported. A stillbirth is the birth of a baby who never takes a breath. If a baby breathes at the time of birth and then dies, both a birth and a death certificate must be completed. Some states have separate stillbirth forms; other states use a regular death certificate.

These reports are almost always made through the hospital involved. In an office setting, you will probably only be responsible for filing the finished report on the patient's chart.

Medical Examiner's Reports

Each state has laws pertaining to which deaths must be reported to the medical examiner's office. Generally these include:

- Death from an unknown cause
- Violence-related deaths or vehicular deaths
- Deaths from suspected criminal or violent acts
- Any death outside the hospital setting when the deceased was not attended by a physician at the

time of death or for a reasonable period of time preceding the death
- When death occurs within 24 hours of hospital admission

Infectious or Communicable Diseases

These reports are made to the local health department. The information is used for statistical purposes and for preventing or tracking the spread of these diseases. Although state guidelines vary, there are usually three categories of reports:

- *Telephone reports* are required for these diseases: diphtheria, cholera, meningococcal meningitis and plague. Telephone reports are always followed by written reports.
- *Written reports* are made for these diseases: anthrax, hepatitis, leprosy, malaria, rubeola, polio, rheumatic fever, tetanus, and tuberculosis. Sexually transmitted diseases must also be reported.
- *Trend reports* are used when your office notes an unusually high occurrence of influenza, streptococcal infections, or any other infectious diseases.

Abuse, Neglect, or Maltreatment

All states require that suspected child abuse or neglect be reported. Each state has a 24-hour hotline for these reports. All verbal reports must be followed by written documentation. Abuse, neglect, or maltreatment of any person who is incapable of self-protection usually falls under this category and may include the elderly or the mentally incompetent. Reports are usually filed by the physician, but the medical assistant should relay suspicions to the physician. Local police departments should be notified in these cases.

Violent Injuries

Life-threatening injuries caused by violence must also be reported. Domestic violence injuries, such as spousal abuse, do not have to be reported in some states unless the injuries are life- threatening. Reports of severe injuries, or at the request of the victim, are made to your local police department.

Other Reports

A diagnosis of *cancer* must be reported in some states to assist in tracking environmental carcinogens. Some states also require that *epilepsy* (a seizure condition) be reported to local motor vehicle departments. The testing of all newborns for *phenylketonuria (PKU)* is required in all states. Some states require positive PKU results to be reported to the health department so that

Patient Education: Legally Required Disclosures

Patients who have conditions that require legal disclosure should be informed about the applicable law. Patients should be assured that all steps to ensure their confidentiality will be followed. Patients should be educated about why the disclosure is necessary, who receives the information, what particular forms will be completed, and any anticipated follow-up from the organization. For example, patients with sexually transmitted diseases will usually be followed by the state health department in an attempt to alert and advise the patients' sexual partners. Patients who are educated about these legally required disclosures will be more understanding and accepting of the need to file official reports.

close observation and follow-up care can be ensured to prevent serious complications for the infant. Infantile hypothyroidism is also a reportable condition in some states.

Each state has its own regulations regarding what must be reported. You and your employer should check with local regulatory agencies. Patient confidentiality rights are waived when the law requires you to report certain conditions.

Checkpoint Question

5. What situations or conditions are you legally required to report?

➤ SPECIFIC LAWS AND STATUTES THAT APPLY TO HEALTH PROFESSIONALS

Medical Practice Acts

Although each state has its own medical practice act, the following elements are usually included:

- Definition of the practice of medicine
- Prohibition forbidding citizens from practicing medicine
- Requirements stating that the physician must have graduated from an accredited medical school and

residency program and have passed the state medical examination
- Description of the procedure for licensing
- Description of the conditions for which a license can be suspended or revoked
- Description of the renewal process for licensure— Most states require the physician to have attended a certain number of continuing education hours.
- Enumeration of the personal requirements to become a licensed physician—Generally, a licensed physician must be a state resident, of good moral character, a United States citizen, and 21 years of age or older.

A physician may have his or her license revoked or suspended for a variety of reasons, including criminal offenses, unprofessional conduct, fraud, or professional or personal incompetence. Criminal offenses include, but are not limited to, murder, manslaughter, robbery, or rape. Examples of unprofessional conduct may include invasion of patient privacy, excessive use of alcohol or illegal drugs, and **fee-splitting** (sharing fees for the referral of patients to certain colleagues). Fraud is a common reason for revoking licenses. Fraud may include filing of false Medicare or Medicaid claims, falsifying of medical records, or professional misrepresentation. Examples of misrepresentation or fraud include advertising a medical cure that does not exist, guaranteeing 100% success of a treatment, or falsifying medical credentials. Incompetence is often a hard charge to prove. The three most common examples include insanity, senility, or other documented mental incompetence.

Negligence and malpractice are also examples of incompetence, but for conviction, repeated charges must be brought against the physician.

Other medical professions have similar acts. For example, states have nurse practice acts, which state the requirements to become a registered nurse and the conditions under which a nurse's license may be revoked.

Medical professionals can be *licensed*, *registered*, or *certified*. **Licensure** is the strictest form of professional accreditation and is regulated by governmental agencies. The term **registered** indicates that a professional has met basic requirements, usually for education and standard testing, and has been approved by a governing body to perform given tasks within a state. **Certification** is a voluntary process regulated through professional organizations. Standards for certification are set by the organization issuing the certificate.

As a medical assistant, you are not licensed, and presently do not have to be certified for employment. However, certification indicates that you have achieved baseline, or entry level, competency. Some states have strict regulations regarding tasks that you can perform only if you are certified. Should you be sued in a professional capacity or called to testify in a medical court case, certification will give you credibility.

Controlled Substances Act

The Controlled Substances Act of 1970 is a federal law regulated by the Drug Enforcement Agency (DEA). The act regulates the manufacture, distribution, and dispensing of narcotics or nonnarcotic drugs considered to have a high potential for abuse. (A narcotic is a chemical agent that can cause physical or psychological dependence.) This act was designed to decrease the use of controlled substances by unauthorized persons and to prevent substance abuse by medical professionals. The law states that any physician who dispenses, administers, or prescribes narcotics or other controlled substances must be registered with the DEA.

Physicians who maintain a stock of controlled substances in the office for dispensing or administering must obtain the substances through the DEA with a special triplicate order form. A narcotic inventory record must be kept for 2 to 3 years. The record must be available for inspection by the DEA at any time.

The act requires that all controlled substances be kept in a locked cabinet and that close security of the keys be maintained. Prescription pads used for prescribing controlled substances must remain in a safe place at all times. Box 3-1 lists steps you can take to keep these prescription pads safe.

This act also requires a physician to return all registration certificate(s) and any unused order forms to the DEA if the practice is closed or sold. Violation of this act is a criminal offense. Penalties range from fines to imprisonment. (See Chap. 25, Pharmacology, for additional information.)

Good Samaritan Act

As the number of lawsuits against physicians began to rise, physicians feared that giving emergency care to strangers outside the office setting could lead to malpractice suits. To combat that fear, California passed the first Good Samaritan Act in 1959. All states now have similar acts. Good Samaritan acts ensure that caregivers are immune from liability suits as long as the care was given in good faith and in a manner that a reasonable and prudent person would have done in a similar situation. Each state has specific guidelines written into the Good Samaritan Act; some even set standards for various professional levels, such as standards for a physician versus others for emergency medical technicians. Your state's Good Samaritan Act will **not** protect you if you are grossly negligent or willfully perform negligent acts.

You are not covered by the Good Samaritan Act while you are working at your profession, nor does it cover physicians in the performance of their duties. If you render emergency care and accept compensation for that care, the act does not apply.

The provisions only cover acts outside of the formal practice of the profession.

Uniform Anatomical Gift Act

Many citizens die each year while waiting for an organ transplant. Many organs can be transplanted, including livers, kidneys, corneas, hearts, lungs, and the skin. To meet the growing need for organs and to allay the concern over donor standards, the National Conference of Commissioners for Uniform State Laws passed legislation known as the Uniform Anatomical Gift Act.

Generically, all acts include the following clauses:

- Any mentally competent person over the age of 18 may donate all or part of his or her body for transplantation or research.
- The donor's wishes supersede any other wishes except when state laws require an autopsy.
- Physicians accepting donor organs in good faith are immune from lawsuits against harvesting organs.
- Death of the donor must be determined by a physician **not** involved in the transplant team.
- Financial compensation may not be given to the donor or survivors.

BOX 3-1	**Prescription Pad Safety Tips**

- Keep only one prescription pad in a cabinet in the examining room. All other pads should be locked away. Do not leave prescription pads for controlled substances unattended.
- Keep a limited supply of pads. It is better to re-order on a regular basis than to overstock.
- Keep track of the number of pads in the office. If a burglary occurs, you will be able to advise the police regarding the number of missing pads.
- Report any prescription pad theft to the police and alert local pharmacies of the theft. If the theft involves the loss of narcotic pads, the Drug Enforcement Agency must be notified.

- Persons wishing to donate organs can revoke permission or change their minds at any time.

Most states have provisions for the Department of Motor Vehicles to query applicants for drivers' licenses about organ donation and to indicate their wishes on their licenses. In addition, an individual may designate the wish to donate all or parts of the body in a will or any legal document, including a Uniform Donor Card.

Self-Determination Act (Advance Directives)

A federal law passed in December 1991 gives all hospitalized patients the right to make health care decisions on admission to the hospital. These decisions may be referred to as advance directives. An advance directive is a statement of wishes prior to a critical event (Fig. 3-4). Advance directives may include specific patient wishes, such as whether or not a ventilator can be used, whether or not cardiopulmonary resuscitation (CPR) should be initiated, or whether or not a feeding tube should be inserted. Advance directives may also identify a health care surrogate who may make health care decisions when the patient is unable to make them. A health care surrogate may be a spouse, a friend, a pastor, or an attorney.

A **durable power of attorney** for health care form (Fig. 3-5) may be signed that gives the patient's representative the ability to make health care decisions as the health care surrogate. The law states that each patient must be questioned regarding advance directives

DECLARATION

I, *Mildred Jones*, being of sound mind, willfully and voluntarily make this declaration to be followed if I become incompetent. This declaration reflects my firm and settled commitment to refuse life-sustaining treatment under the circumstances indicated below.

I direct my attending physician to withhold or withdraw life-sustaining treatment that serves only to prolong the process of my dying, if I should be in a terminal condition or in a state of permanent unconsciousness.

I direct that treatment be limited to measures to keep me comfortable and to relieve pain, including any pain that might occur by withholding or withdrawing life-sustaining treatment.

In addition, if I am in the condition described above, I feel especially strongly about the following forms of treatment. **I realize that if I do not specifically indicate my preference regarding any of the forms of treatment listed below, I may receive that form of treatment.**

- Cardiac resuscitation: I do want (✗)   I do not want( )
- Mechanical respiration: I do want ( )   I do not want (✗)
- Tube feeding or any other artificial or invasive form of nutrition (food): I do want ( )   I do not want (✗)
- Any artificial or invasive form of hydration (water): I do want ( )   I do not want (✗)
- Blood or blood products: I do want ( )   I do not want (✗)
- Any invasive diagnostic tests: I do want ( )   I do not want (✗)
- Any form of surgery: I do want ( )   I do not want (✗)
- Kidney dialysis: I do want ( )   I do not want (✗)
- Antibiotics: I do want (✗)   I do not want ( )

Other instructions:

I(✗) do ( ) not want to designate another person as my surrogate to make medical treatment decisions for me if I should be incompetent and in a terminal condition or in a state of permanent unconsciousness.

Name and address of surrogate (if applicable):

Jonathan Jones
423 Main Street
Crossroads SC

Name and address of substitute surrogate (if surrogate designated above is unable to serve):

Trudy Conover
619 Wyoming Drive
Crossroads SC

I made this declaration on the *21* day of *10/95* (month, year).

Declarant's signature: *Mildred Jones*
Declarant's address: *423 Main Street*
Crossroads SC

The declarant or the person on behalf of and at the direction of the declarant knowingly and voluntarily signed this writing by signature or mark in my presence.

1. Witness's signature: *Mary Martin*
   Witness's address: *818 Hill Drive*
   Bayside GA

2. Witness's signature: *Rosa Díaz*
   Witness's address: *1043 River Road*
   Summit SC

FIGURE 3-4
Sample of an advance directive.

DURABLE POWER OF ATTORNEY FOR HEALTH CARE*

I, _____

hereby appoint:

name _____

home address _____

_____

home telephone number _____

work telephone number _____

as my agent to make health care decisions for me if and when I am unable to make my own health care decisions. This gives my agent the power to consent to giving, withholding or stopping any health care, treatment, service, or diagnostic procedure. My agent also has the authority to talk with health care personnel, get information, and sign forms necessary to carry out those decisions.

If the person named as my agent is not available or is unable to act as my agent, then I appoint the following person(s) to serve in the order listed below.

1. _____

name _____

home address _____

_____

home telephone number _____

work telephone number _____

2. _____

name _____

home address _____

_____

home telephone number _____

work telephone number _____

By this document I intend to create a power of attorney for health care that shall take effect upon my incapacity to make my own health care decisions and shall continue during that incapacity.

*Check requirements of individual state statute.

My agent shall make health care decisions as I direct below or as I make known to him or her in some other way.

(a) STATEMENT OF DESIRES CONCERNING LIFE-PROLONGING CARE, TREATMENT, SERVICES, AND PROCEDURES:

_____

_____

_____

_____

_____

_____

_____

_____

(b) SPECIAL PROVISIONS AND LIMITATIONS:

_____

_____

_____

_____

_____

_____

_____

_____

BY SIGNING HERE I INDICATE THAT I UNDERSTAND THE PURPOSE AND EFFECT OF THIS DOCUMENT.

I sign my name to this form on _____ (date)

My current home address: _____

_____

(You sign here)

WITNESS

I declare that the person who signed or acknowledged this document is personally known to me, that he/she signed or acknowledged this durable power of attorney in my presence, and that he/she appears to be of sound mind and under no duress, fraud, or undue influence. I am not the person appointed as agent by this document, nor am I the patient's health care provider or an employee of the patient's health care provider.

First Witness

Signature: _____

Home Address: _____

Print Name: _____

Date: _____

Second Witness

Signature: _____

Home Address: _____

Print Name: _____

Date: _____

(AT LEAST ONE OF THE ABOVE WITNESSES MUST ALSO SIGN THE FOLLOWING DECLARATION.)

I further declare that I am not related to the patient by blood, marriage, or adoption, and, to the best of my knowledge, I am not entitled to any part of his/her estate under a will now existing or by operation of law.

Signature: _____

Signature: _____

I further declare that I am not related to the patient by blood, marriage, or adoption, and, to the best of my knowledge, I am not entitled to any part of his/her estate under a will now existing or by operation of law.

Signature: _____

Signature: _____

FIGURE 3-5
Durable power of attorney form.

---

by the admitting representative in the hospital. The law does not require that patients have advance directives; it only alerts them to their rights. It is good practice to keep a copy of a patient's advance directive in the medical record.

What If?

What if a patient asks you how to prepare an advance directive? How should you respond?

In most states, advance directives can be written by the patient in long hand and signed along with a witness's signature. However, the best and most accurate response is to direct the patient to his or her personal attorney for help and guidance.

Consolidated Omnibus Budget Reconciliation Act (COBRA)

This Medicare law was designed to prevent "patient dumping" in emergency rooms. Before this regulation, hospital emergency rooms could refuse to treat patients who did not have insurance, causing larger, publicly owned, inner city hospitals to be "dumped" on. This act requires any hospital that receives Medicare funds to provide a screening examination for all who request care, *before* determining insurance or ability to pay. If the screening indicates an emergency situation, the hospital must stabilize the patient. Patients can then be transferred to other facilities. The act also stipulates that a specialized hospital (burn center, trauma center) must accept any transfer from a nonspecialized hospital, providing that beds are available. Hospitals that do not comply can face severe fines and may lose Medicare provider status.

➤ SPECIFIC MEDICAL LAW

Tort Law

A *tort* is a wrongful act or injury that results in harm for which restitution must be made. Two forms of torts are *intentional* and *unintentional*. An allegation of an unintentional tort means that the accuser (the **plaintiff**) believes that a mistake has been made; however, the plaintiff believes that the caregiver or the party that is accused (the **defendant**) was operating in good faith and did not intend for the mistake to occur. Most suits against physicians fall into this category.

Negligence and Malpractice (Unintentional Torts)

Unintentional torts are commonly referred to as **negligence**. These are the most common forms of medical malpractice suits. Negligence is performing an act that a reasonable health care worker or physician would not have done or the omission of an act that a reasonable professional or physician would have done. Any instance in which there is a failure to take reasonable precautions to prevent harm to a patient is termed negligence. If the medical professional involved is a physician, the term usually used is malpractice. Malpractice is said to have occurred when the patient is harmed by the professional's actions. The three types of malpractice are:

- Malfeasance—incorrect treatment
- Misfeasance—treatment performed incorrectly
- Nonfeasance—treatment delayed or not attempted

What a reasonable professional would do is based on the standard of care. Standards of care are written by various professional agencies to clarify what the reasonable and prudent physician or health care worker would do in a given situation.

Example: A patient comes into the emergency department after falling from a horse and complains of arm pain. The standard of care for emergency physicians would require a radiograph of the injured extremity after trauma.

Standard of care will vary with the level of the professional. A registered nurse will not be held to the same standards as a physician, nor will the medical assistant be expected to perform by the same standards as the registered nurse. Each must practice within the scope of their training.

Standards of care are explained through expert testimony. Experts are retained by the representing attorney and state under oath the standards of care for a specific situation. **Expert witnesses** may be physicians, nurses, physical therapists, or other specialized practitioners who have excellent reputations in their field.

Expert witnesses are always used in malpractice cases, except when the doctrine of *res ipsa loquitur* is tried. This doctrine means "the thing speaks for itself." In other words, it is obvious that the physician's actions, or negligence, caused the injury. A judge must preapprove the use of this theory in pretrial hearings. Examples of these cases could include a sponge left in an abdomen after surgery or a fracture that occurred when the patient fell from an examining table.

For negligence to be proved, the plaintiff's attorney must prove four elements: duty, dereliction of duty, direct cause, and **damages**. These elements were written by the American Medical Association to help clarify the points of the suit. (Note that the courts place the burden of proof on the plaintiff; the physician is assumed to have given proper care.)

DUTY

Duty is present when the patient and the physician have formed a contract. This is usually straightforward and the easiest of the elements to prove.

DERELICTION OF DUTY

The patient must prove that the physician did not meet the standard of care guidelines, either by performing an act inappropriately or by omitting an act.

DIRECT CAUSE

The plaintiff must prove that the derelict act directly caused the injury. This can be difficult to prove if the patient has a extensive medical history that may have contributed to the injury.

DAMAGES

The plaintiff must prove that an injury or damage occurred. There are three types of awards for damages:

1. Nominal—Minimal injuries or damages occurred and compensation is small.
2. Actual (compensatory)—Money may be awarded for the injury, disability, mental suffering, loss of income, or the anticipated future earning loss. This payment is moderate to significant.
3. Punitive—These awards are seldom given. They are only given to "punish" the practitioner for reckless or malicious wrongdoing. Punitive damages are the most costly. (Note: A physician may have committed a major medical error, but if the

patient suffered no injuries or damages, he or she cannot win the suit. Also, if the outcome was not as expected but the physician cannot be shown to be at fault, the patient will not be compensated.)

? **Checkpoint Question**
7. What are the four elements that must be proved in a negligence suit?

Intentional Torts

An intentional tort means that the accuser believes that the alleged incident occurred with malice and with the intent of causing harm. Intentional torts are the deliberate violation of another person's legal rights. Examples of intentional torts are: assault and battery, invasion of privacy, **defamation of character**, false imprisonment, fraud, tort of outrage, undue influence. These are described below.

ASSAULT AND BATTERY

Assault is the unauthorized attempt or threat to touch another person without consent. **Battery** is the actual physical touching of a patient without consent; this includes beating or physical abuse. By law, a conscious adult has the right to refuse medical care. An example of battery might be suturing a laceration that the patient refuses to have sutured or grabbing and forcefully restraining a child who is uncooperative during a routine examination.

If a patient is coerced into an act, then the patient can possibly sue for the tort of **duress**. Following is a situation in which a patient may be able to sue for assault, battery, and duress. *Example*: A 22-year-old woman arrives at a pregnancy center. She is on public assistance and has five children. Her pregnancy test is positive. The staff persuades her to have an abortion. She signs the consent and the abortion is performed. Later she sues, stating that she was verbally coerced into signing the consent form (duress) and that the abortion was performed against her wishes (assault and battery).

INVASION OF PRIVACY

Patients have the right to privacy. Written permission must be obtained from the patient to:

- release medical records or personal data
- publish case histories in medical journals
- make photographs of the patient (exception: suspected cases of abuse or maltreatment)
- allow observers in examination rooms

Example: A 57-year-old woman is seen in your office for a skin biopsy. Her insurance company calls asking for information regarding the bill and also asks for the biopsy report. You give the requested information and then find that the patient never signed a release form. She has a valid case for invasion of privacy.

DEFAMATION OF CHARACTER

Making malicious or false statements about a person's character or reputation is *defamation of character*. **Libel** refers to written statements and **slander** refers to oral statements. *Example*: A patient asks for a referral to another physician. She states that she has heard "Dr. Rogers is a good surgeon." You know his history of alcoholism and know that he is not respected among his peers. You tell the patient that he is probably not a good choice because of his reputation. That is defamation of his character.

FALSE IMPRISONMENT

Unlawfully detaining or restraining a person is false imprisonment. Committing a person to a mental hospital or psychiatric ward may also be false imprisonment. Patients cannot be held against their will unless they are declared mentally incompetent or a danger to themselves. *Example*: An intoxicated patient comes into your walk-in center and requests that a wound on his left arm be sutured. After suturing the arm, the physician begins to suture a facial laceration. The patient refuses and security is called. The patient is restrained and the facial laceration is sutured. The physician has falsely restrained the patient and can be sued. (There is potential for a charge of battery and for treatment without consent.)

FRAUD

Fraud is any deceitful act with the intention to conceal the truth, such as:

- Intentionally raising false expectations regarding recovery
- Not properly instructing the patient regarding possible side effects of a procedure
- "Readjusting" patient bills for reimbursement purposes

TORT OF OUTRAGE

This is the intentional infliction of emotional distress. For this tort to be proven, the plaintiff's attorney must prove that the physician:

- **Intended** to inflict emotional distress
- **Acted** in a manner that is not morally or ethically acceptable
- **Caused** the emotional distress by his actions
- Caused distress that was **severe** in nature

UNDUE INFLUENCE

Improperly convincing another to act in a way contrary to that person's free will is termed undue influence. For instance, preying on the elderly or the mentally incompetent is a common type of undue influence. Unethical practitioners who gain the trust of these persons and convince them to submit to expensive and unnecessary medical procedures are practicing undue influence.

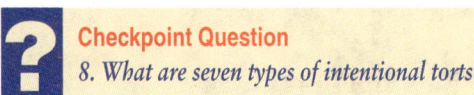

Checkpoint Question

8. What are seven types of intentional torts?

➤ THE LITIGATION PROCESS

The litigation process begins when an alleged patient incident occurs or the patient becomes aware of a prior possible injury. Next, the patient (plaintiff) or the patient's family members consult an attorney. The plaintiff's attorney obtains the medical records, which are reviewed by medical-legal consultants. (Such consultants may be nurses or physicians who are considered experts in their field.) Then the plaintiff's attorney files a *complaint*—a written statement that lists the claim against the defendant and the remedy desired, usually monetary compensation.

The defendant and his or her attorney answer the complaint. The discovery phase begins with interrogatories and depositions. During this phase, attorneys for both parties gather relevant information. Box 3-2 describes the discovery process.

Next, the trial phase begins. A jury is selected unless the parties agree to a **bench trial**. In a bench trial, the judge hears the case without a jury and renders a **verdict** (decision or judgment). Opening statements are given, first by the plaintiff's attorney, then by the defendant's attorney. The plaintiff's attorney presents the case. Expert witnesses are called and the evidence is shown. Examination of the witnesses begins. **Direct examination** involves questioning by one's own attorney; **cross examination** is questioning by the opposing attorney. When the plaintiff's attorney is finished, the defense presents the opposing arguments. The plaintiff's attorney may cross examine the defendant's witnesses. Closing arguments are heard. Finally, a verdict is made.

If the defendant is found guilty, damages are awarded. If the defendant is not guilty, the charges are dismissed. The decision may be appealed to a higher court. (An **appeal** is a process by which the higher court reviews the decision of the lower court.)

BOX 3-2 Understanding the Discovery Phase of a Lawsuit

During the discovery phase of a lawsuit, attorneys for the defendant and the plaintiff gather information and medical data. The information can be obtained by the following methods:

- **Deposition**—Process in which one party questions the other party under oath. A court reporter is present and records every word of both the questions and answers. Lying in a deposition can bring a charge of perjury and will carry significant consequences. Before attending a deposition, you should review the medical record and rehearse possible lines of questioning with your own attorney.
- **Interrogatory**—A written set of questions sent to one party of a lawsuit that requires a written response. You are considered to be under oath when completing this form.
- **Subpoena**—A court order requiring that you appear in court at a given date and time. If you do not appear as ordered, you may be charged with contempt of court. A subpoena is delivered in person by an officer of the court.
- **Subpoena** *Duces Tecum*—A court order to submit to the court a set of medical records by a given date and time. The physician must be made aware of this request as soon as it is received. Whenever possible, a photocopied set of the records should be submitted. Before submission, the records should be reviewed for content to ensure that all components are present. A representative of the medical office should accompany the records when the originals must be submitted to court.

➤ DEFENSES TO PROFESSIONAL LIABILITY SUITS

There are many defenses that the health care worker can use to win a lawsuit. These include the medical record, **statutes of limitation**, assumption of risk, *res judicata*, **contributory negligence**, or **comparative negligence** (see below).

Medical Records

The best and most solid defense the caregiver has is the medical record. Every item in the record is considered to be a part of a legal document. Juries may believe a medical record regardless of testimony. Juries tend to believe these records because they are tangible items from the actual time the injury occurred. They refresh the memory of the defendant and provide documentation of care given. As a medical assistant, you must make sure that all of your documentation is timely, accurate, and legible. (See Chap. 10, Medical Records and Records Management, for specific information regarding charting practices.)

Statutes of Limitation

Each state has a statute that defines the length of time during which a patient may file a suit against a caregiver. Once the statute of limitation has expired, the patient loses the right to file a claim. Generally, the limits vary from 1 to 3 years following the alleged occurrence. Some states allow 1 to 3 years following the patient's *discovery* of the occurrence. States vary greatly when an alleged injury involves a minor. The statute may not take effect until the minor reaches the age of majority and then may extend 2 to 3 years past this time. Some states have longer claim periods in wrongful death action suits.

Assumption of Risk

In this defense, the physician will claim that the patient was aware of the risks involved before the procedure and fully accepted the potential for damages. *Example*: A patient is instructed regarding the adverse effects of chemotherapy. The patient fully understands these risks, receives the chemotherapy, and wants to sue for alopecia (hair loss). Alopecia is a given risk with certain forms of chemotherapy.

Res Judicata

The doctrine of *res judicata* means "the thing has been decided." Once the suit has been brought against the physician or patient and a settlement has been reached, the losing party may not countersue. If, for instance, the physician sues a patient for not paying his bills and the court orders the patient to pay, the patient cannot then sue the physician for malpractice. The opposite may occur as well. If the physician is sued for malpractice and loses, he cannot countersue for defamation of character.

Contributory Negligence

With the defense of contributory negligence, the physician usually admits that negligence has occurred; however, he will claim that the patient aggravated the in-

jury or assisted in making the injury worse. *Example*: The patient's laceration is sutured with only three sutures when ten were needed. The patient is discharged from the emergency room with instructions to limit movement of the arm. The patient plays baseball and the laceration reopens causing infection to occur and, subsequently, the formation of extensive scar tissue. Both the patient and the physician contributed to the postoperative damages. Most states do not grant damage awards for contributory negligence. If an award is granted, the courts assess comparative negligence.

Comparative Negligence

The damages awarded are based on a percentage of the contribution to the negligence. If the patient contributed to 30% of the damage, then the damage award would be 30% less than what was granted. In the above example, the courts may decide that the negligence by both parties is shared at 50%. Therefore, if the court granted an award of $20,000, the physician would be responsible for $10,0000.

In the past, contributory negligence, such as not returning for appointments, was seen as absolute defense for the physician. However, since the 1970s, the trend has been toward comparative negligence with the responsibility shared between the physician and the patient.

Immunity

The Federal Tort Claim Act of 1946 prohibits suits against any United States governmental facility such as veterans' hospitals or military bases. This provides immunity to all of their employees for ordinary negligence but not for intentional torts.

➤ A DEFENSE FOR THE MEDICAL ASSISTANT

Respondeat Superior or Law of Agency

The doctrine of **respondeat superior** literally means "let the master answer." This may also be called "Law of Agency." This doctrine implies that physicians are liable for the actions of their employees. The physician is responsible for your actions, as a medical assistant, as long as your actions are within your scope of practice and you practice the standard of care required for your assigned duties and responsibilities. If your actions exceed your abilities or training, the physician is not generally responsible for any error that you make. You must understand that you **can** be sued in this instance and that *respondeat superior* does not guarantee immunity for your actions.

Example: Mrs. Smith is a chronic complainer, calling your office frequently with minor concerns. Today she calls complaining of "tingling in her arms." The physician has left for the day, so you tell Mrs. Smith, "Don't worry about this; take your medication and call us tomorrow." During the night a blood vessel in Mrs. Smith's brain bursts. She suffers a cerebral hemorrhage (bleeding inside the brain) and dies. The family sues. The physician claims that you were instructed not to give advice over the telephone. You are not covered by *respondeat superior* because you acted outside of your scope of practice.

To protect yourself from situations such as this, have your job description in written format and always practice within its guidelines. Do not perform tasks that you have not been trained to do. Never hesitate to seek clarification from a physician. If you are not sure about something, such as a medication order, **ask!** Box 3-3 provides some additional tips for preventing lawsuits.

To further protect yourself from professional liability claims, you can purchase malpractice insurance. When purchasing a policy, keep these points in mind:

- Purchase insurance from a reputable firm.
- Keep records of your policy numbers and registration forms.

- Read the entire policy before purchasing, making sure you understand the "fine print."
- Be aware of the two types of policies: **occurrence** or **claims made**. An occurrence policy will cover a claim whenever the claim is made, even if the policy has expired when the claim is reported. A claims made policy only covers the claim if it is made while the policy is current. Claims made policies tend to be less expensive.
- If you are to be included under your employer's policy, request to see the policy. Make sure the policy is current and note the expiration date. (Recheck with your employer on the expiration date to see if the policy has been renewed).

SUMMARY

The fields of medicine and law are linked in common concern for the patient's rights and the patient's health. Increasingly, health care professionals are the object of medically oriented lawsuits. You must keep abreast of medical-legal issues to protect yourself and other health care professionals from legal action. You can help prevent medical malpractice by acting professionally, maintaining clinical competency, and properly documenting in the medical record. By promoting good public relations between the patient and the health care team, suits can be avoided and attention and energy can be directed toward optimum health care.

CRITICAL THINKING CHALLENGES

1. Because of the rising number of malpractice cases, the United States Congress has debated legislation that would limit the amount of monetary damages that can be awarded. Do you approve of threshold caps on damage awards, and if so, what dollar amount would you choose?

2. A patient asks your opinion of a particular surgeon. From your experiences, you know that his skills are below the standard of care and that his privileges at a nearby hospital have been revoked for incompetency. How would you answer her question to avoid defamation of character?

3. The physician you are working for gives you false billing information for a Medicare patient. What should you do? Who would you tell?

4. A patient in your office trips over an electrical wire on the floor and sustains a fractured (broken) arm. You document the incident and the physician asks you to "rewrite" what happened to state that the patient tripped over her shoelaces. What should you do?

5. You suspect that a new employee in the office is misusing narcotics. Would you approach the employee? If so, what would you say?

BOX 3-3 **Tips for Preventing Lawsuits**

- Keep medical records neat and organized. Always document and sign legibly.
- Stay abreast of new laws and medical technology.
- Become a Certified or Registered Medical Assistant.
- Keep your CPR and First Aid certification current.
- Never give any information over the telephone unless you are sure of the caller's identity and you have patient consent.
- Keep the office neat and clean. Make sure that children's toys are clean and in good condition to avoid office-related injuries. Perform safety checks frequently.
- Limit waiting time for patients. If an emergency arises, causing a long wait, explain this to the patients in a timely and professional manner.
- Practice good public relations. Always be polite, smile, and show genuine concern for your patients and their families.

ANSWERS TO CHECKPOINT QUESTIONS

1. The two branches of law are public and private or civil law. Public law involves issues between government and citizens; private (or civil) law involves issues between private citizens. Medical professionals are concerned with private or civil law.

2. A contract is an agreement between two or more parties to do or not to do a given act. The three components of a contract are the offer, the acceptance, and the consideration.

3. The following elements must be in a physician's termination intent letter: statement of intent, explanation of reasons, termination date, availability of medical records, and a recommendation that the patient seek medical help as needed.

4. Never ask a patient to sign a consent form if the patient does not understand the procedure, has questions about the procedure, or is unable to read the consent form.

5. The six situations or conditions legally requiring disclosure are vital statistics, medical examiner reports, infectious diseases, abuse or maltreatment, violent injuries, and others according to state laws.

6. The six acts that the medical assistant must be aware of include the Medical Practice Act, the Controlled Substance Act, the Uniform Anatomical Gift Act, the Self-Determination Act, and the Consolidated Omnibus Budget Reconciliation Act (COBRA).

7. The four elements that must be proved in a negligence suit are duty, dereliction of duty, direct cause, and damages.

8. The seven types of intentional torts are assault and battery, invasion of privacy, defamation of character, false imprisonment, fraud, tort of outrage, and undue influence.

SUGGESTIONS FOR FURTHER READING

Flight, M. (1993). *Law, Liability and Ethics for the Medical Professional*, 2nd ed. Albany, NY: Delmar.

Lewis, M. A., & Tamparo, C. D. (1993). *Medical Law, Ethics, and Bioethics in the Medical Office*, 3rd ed. Philadelphia: F. A. Davis.

Rosdahl, C. B. (1993). *Textbook of Basic Nursing*, 6th ed. Philadelphia: J.B. Lippincott.

Taylor, C., Lillis, C., LeMone, P. (1993). *Fundamentals of Nursing: The Art and Science of Nursing Care*, 2nd ed. Philadelphia: J.B. Lippincott.

Unit 2

Communicating With Patients

Communication is basic to human interaction. Nowhere is it more vital than in providing treatment for patients and interpreting their health care needs. Understanding how information is exchanged in normal situations will enhance our ability to adjust to the many factors that can impede the exchange necessary for successful medical practice.

Fundamental Communication Skills

Chapter Outline

Basic Communication Flow
Forms of Communication
    Verbal Communication
    Nonverbal Communication
Active Listening
Interviewing Techniques
    Reflecting
    Paraphrasing or Restatement
    Asking for Examples
      or Clarification
    Asking Open-ended Questions
    Summarizing
    Allowing Silences
Factors Affecting Communication
    Cultural Differences

Language Barriers
Special Communication Challenges
Stereotyping and Biased Opinions
Establishing Positive Patient Relationships
    Proper Form of Address
    Professional Distance
    Empathy Versus Sympathy
    Providing Grief Support
Patient Teaching
Summary
Critical Thinking Challenges
Answers to Checkpoint Questions
Suggestions for Further Reading

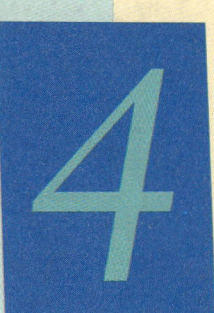

DACUM Components

1.1   Project a positive attitude
1.2   Perform within ethical boundaries
1.6   Conduct oneself in a courteous and diplomatic manner
2.1   Listen and observe
2.2   Treat all patients with empathy and impartiality
2.3   Adapt communication to individuals' abilities to understand
2.4   Recognize and respond to verbal and non-verbal communication
2.5   Serve as liaison between physician and others
2.6   Evaluate understanding of communication
2.9   Interview effectively
2.10 Use medical terminology appropriately

Chapter Competencies

Learning Objectives

Upon successfully completing this chapter, you will be able to:

1. Spell and define the Key Terms.
2. List two major forms of communication.
3. Explain how various components of communication can affect the meaning of verbal messages.
4. Define active listening.
5. List and describe the six interviewing techniques.
6. Give an example of how cultural differences may affect communication.
7. Discuss how to handle communication problems caused by language barriers.
8. List several special communication challenges and how to handle them.
9. Explain how stereotyping and biased opinions can affect patient care.
10. Give two ways to establish positive patient relationships.
11. Explain what is meant by professional distance.
12. Explain what causes grief and how you can support a grieving patient.

Key Terms

(See Glossary for definitions.)

belief	message
bias	mourning
clarification	nonlanguage
culture	paralanguage
demeanor	paraphrasing
denial	proxemics
discrimination	reflecting
empathy	stereotyping
feedback	summarizing
grief	sympathy
kinesics	therapeutic
	values

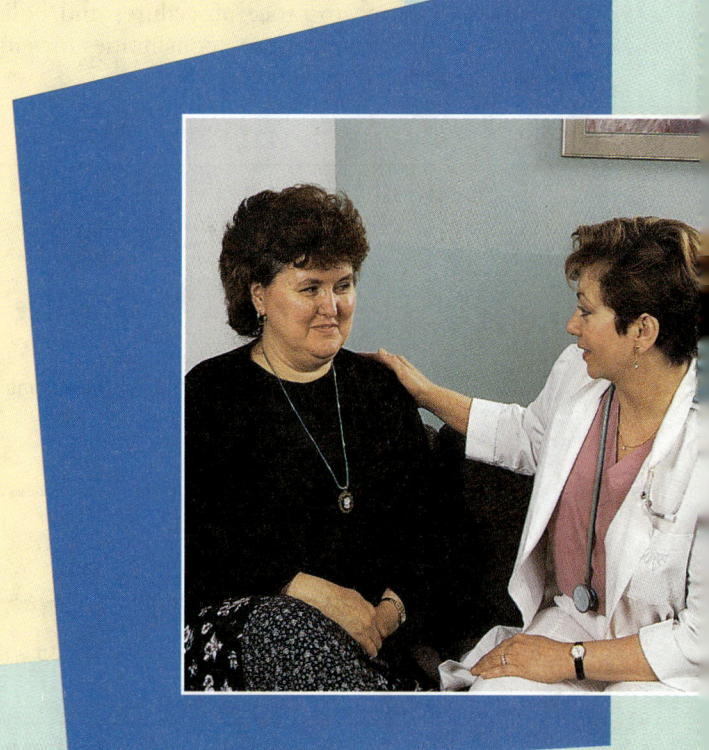

Communication involves sending and receiving **messages** (information), either verbally or nonverbally. The ability to communicate effectively is a crucial skill for medical assistants. In your role, you must accurately and appropriately share information with physicians, other professional staff members, and patients. The medical assistant is usually the first person the patient meets in the medical office. Thus, your positive attitude, pleasant presentation, and use of good communication skills will set the tone for future interactions.

➤ BASIC COMMUNICATION FLOW

Communication requires the following elements:

a message to be sent
a person to send the message
a person to receive the message

During the act of communicating, both persons will alternate roles as sender and receiver as they seek **feedback** (responses) and **clarification** (understanding) regarding the message. The process of message exchange is akin to a swing moving back and forth between two people. Figure 4-1 illustrates the flow of communication and its common components.

As a medical assistant, you are responsible for keeping conversations with patients focused on pertinent topics relating to office procedures and policies and patient care. Your other responsibilities for ensuring good communication include:

- Clarifying confusing messages
- Validating (confirming) the patient's perceptions
- Adapting messages to the patient's level of understanding
- Asking for feedback to make sure that the messages sent were received as intended

Checkpoint Question
1. What three elements must be present for communication to occur?

➤ FORMS OF COMMUNICATION

Verbal Communication

Verbal communication requires the exchange of messages using words, or language; it encompasses both oral and written communication. You will need good verbal communication skills when performing such tasks as making appointments, instructing patients, sharing information with the physician, or documenting in medical records.

Oral communication involves sending or receiving messages using spoken language. As a professional, your manner of speaking should be pleasant and polite. Use proper English and grammar at all times; lapsing into local slang and colloquialisms projects an unprofessional image. Gear your conversation to the patient's educational level. A well educated patient

---

Person A   **Person B**
Message/Question -->>
<<--- Response/Feedback
Clarification/Verification --->>
<<---Response/Feedback

In a conversation with a patient, the communication flow might go something like this:

Patient   **Medical Assistant**
Why do I need blood drawn? --->>
(Message/Question)
<<------------------------------------- The doctor wants to check your cholesterol level.
                (Response/Feedback)
Is this just a routine check?--->>
(Clarification/Verification)
<<--------------------------Yes, this is done as part of the complete physical examination.
                (Response/Feedback)

FIGURE 4-1
Flow of communication.

Focus on the Patient: Using the Right Tone of Voice

To understand the influence of paralanguage, consider how differently a patient might interpret a simple statement such as *"I'll be with you in a minute"* when spoken in different voice tones. For example, when spoken in short, clipped tones, this statement implies impatience and a lack of interest in listening to the patient's concerns. In contrast, when this statement is spoken in a soft, low-pitched voice, it can project a more calm and soothing attitude to a patient who may be upset.

treatment and recovery. Even the most clearly outlined instructions can sometimes be misunderstood, particularly by those with deficient hearing or reading abilities. As a medical assistant, you are responsible for asking questions to verify that the patient has correctly understood the information received.

Checkpoint Question
2. List the five examples of paralanguage.

may resent your using other than the correct terms, yet a less educated patient may be confused and intimidated by the same phrases. Avoid using elaborate medical terminology if you think it might confuse or frighten a patient. Will this patient understand myocardial infarction or should you use heart attack? Do not "talk down" to the patient, but do phrase your communication appropriately.

Be aware, too, that the meaning of spoken messages may be affected by other components of oral communication, including **paralanguage** and **nonlanguage sounds**. Paralanguage includes voice tone, quality, volume, pitch, and range. Nonlanguage sounds include laughing, sobbing, sighing, grunting, and so on. Other nonlanguage clues to understanding can be found in a speaker's grammatic structure, pronunciation, and general articulation, which can indicate regional or cultural background and level of education. Knowing this information can help you adapt responses and explanations to the patient's level of understanding.

Written communication is limited to the use of written language to exchange messages. The ability to write clearly, concisely, and accurately is important in the health care profession (see Chap. 9, Written Communications, for a detailed discussion). Typically, patients receive verbal instructions first, as you or the physician explain points of concern. These verbal instructions are then reinforced with written instructions (Fig. 4-2).

If the instructions, verbal or written, are not clear, the patient may misinterpret the meaning and hinder

Nonverbal Communication

Nonverbal communication—exchanging messages without using words—is sometimes called "body language." Body language includes several types of behaviors such as **kinesics**, **proxemics**, and the use of touch (Table 4-1).

Kinesics refers to body movements, including facial expressions, gestures, and eye movements. A patient's face can sometimes reveal inner feelings—such as sadness, happiness, fear, or anger—that may not be mentioned explicitly during a conversation (Fig. 4-3). Gestures also carry various meanings. For instance, shrugging the shoulders can mean simple disinterest or hopeless resignation. Eyes can often hint at what a person may be thinking or feeling. For example, a patient whose eyes wander away from you while you are talking may be impatient, lack interest, or may not understand what you are saying.

Nonverbal communication may more accurately reflect a person's true feelings and attitude than verbal communication. Many patients will mask their feelings, so you must learn to read their actions and nonverbal clues in addition to what they tell you. Be aware also that patients are acutely attuned to your facial and nonverbal reactions to what they say. Responding with expressions of disgust or shaking your head in a negative way can jeopardize communication and rapport between you and the patient.

How and where individuals physically place themselves in relation to others can affect communication as well. Proxemics refers to spatial relationships or physical proximity tolerated by humans. Generally, the area within a 3-foot radius around a person is considered personal space and is not to be invaded by strangers, although this area varies among individuals and people of various **cultures** (societies). To deliver care to a patient, physicians and medical assistants must enter a patient's personal space. Because some individuals may become uncomfortable when their space is invaded, it is essential to approach the patient in a professional man-

```
Paul Brown, MD
55 Main Street
New London, Connecticut


Patient Discharge Instructions


Patient's Name: Christina Sefferin
Address: 140 Scott Drive, New London, CT
Date: October 24, 1997



You have been diagnosed with: Otitis Media—Right ear


Definition: Otitis Media is an infection of the inner ear with the presence
of fluid.
Instructions:
1. Finish all your antibiotics. Follow the accompanying medication in-
   struction sheet.
2. Call the physician if the ear pain persists, if blood appears in the
   ear canal, or if fever or other symptoms do not resolve in 72 hours.
3. Avoiding swimming or any other contact in which water will enter the
   ear canal.



Patient's Signature                      Physician's Signature


_____                  _____
```

FIGURE 4-2
Example of written patient instructions.

Table 4-1	
Forms of Communication	

Form	Description
• Verbal communication	Communication using words
Oral communication	Spoken messages
	Paralanguage: voice quality, pitch, volume, tone, range
	Nonlanguage sounds: laughing, sobbing, sighing, grunting
Written communication	Written messages
• Nonverbal communication	Behaviors or physical expressions ("body language")
	Kinesics: facial expressions, gestures, eye movements
	Proxemics: physical proximity comfortably tolerated by humans ("personal space")
	Touch: gentle physical contact with another person

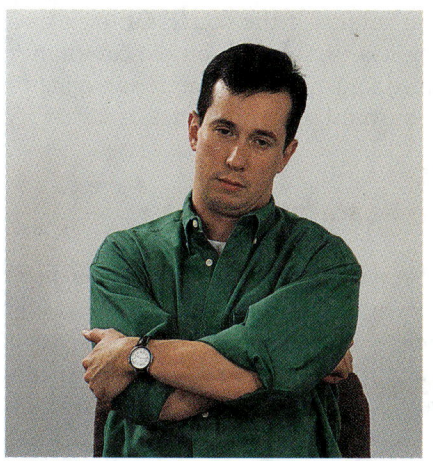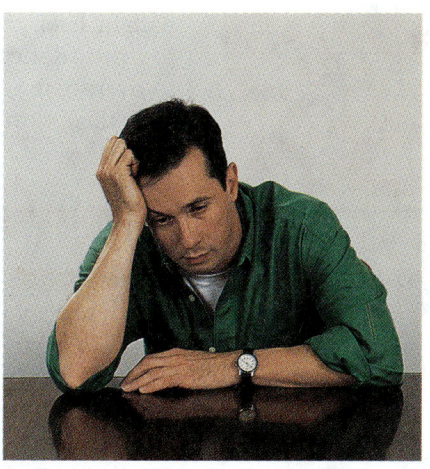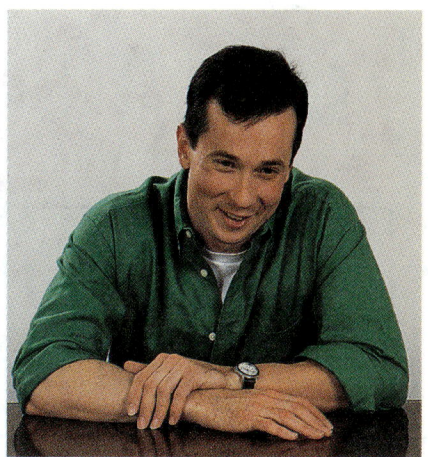

FIGURE 4-3
Different facial expressions convey different meanings.

ner and explain what you plan to do. Explanations help ease patient anxiety about what will happen.

Related to proxemics is the use of touch, which can be **therapeutic** (beneficial) for some patients. It can indicate emotional support and convey concern and feeling. For some patients, however, being touched by a stranger is an uncomfortable or even a negative experience. Many patients perceive touch in a medical setting as a prelude to something unpleasant such as injections. To change this negative perception, try offering a comforting touch when nothing invasive or painful is imminent (Fig. 4-4). Before comforting a patient by touching, assess the patient's **demeanor** (expressions and behavior) for clues indicating that touch would be acceptable.

 **Checkpoint Question**
3. How would you describe kinesics and proxemics?

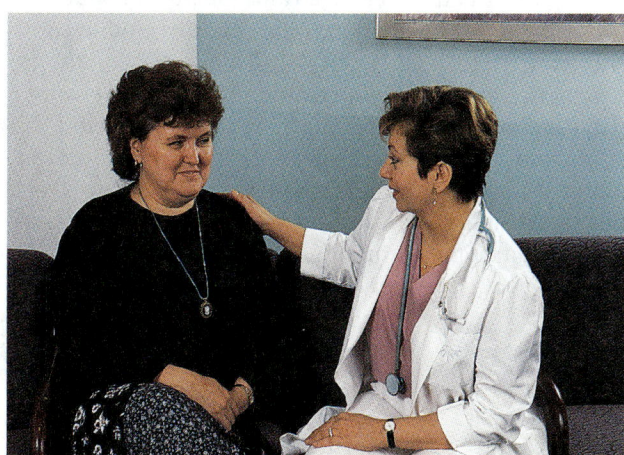

FIGURE 4-4
Using therapeutic touch.

ACTIVE LISTENING

To actively listen, you must give your full attention to the patient with whom you are speaking. Interruptions should be kept to a minimum. You need to focus not only on what is being said, but also on what is being conveyed through paralanguage, body language, and other aspects of communication. Occasionally, a patient's verbal messages may seem to conflict with the nonverbal messages. For example, a patient who is wringing his hands while telling you "everything is fine" is sending conflicting signals that require further exploration. If a patient's verbal response does not correspond to your observations, convey your concern to the physician.

Active listening is a skill that develops with practice. To test your current listening ability, try this exercise:

Ask another student to speak continuously for 1 to 2 minutes while you listen. (The student should discuss a topic with which you are unfamiliar.) When he or she finishes, wait silently for the same amount of time. Then try to repeat back verbatim what you just heard.

If you have trouble doing this exercise, you need to consciously practice listening.

INTERVIEWING TECHNIQUES

As a medical assistant, you typically will be responsible for gathering initial patient information. This task is accomplished by interviewing, that is, asking questions and talking directly to the patient. A patient interview includes a review of past and current medical history. The main goal is to obtain accurate and pertinent information (see Chap. 20, Medical History and Patient Assessment, for a more detailed discussion). To do this, you must use effective interview techniques, listen actively, and record the answers. Box 4-1 provides sug-

---

BOX 4-1 Setting the Stage for Successful Communication

Before you begin the interview, set the stage for successful communication by observing the following suggestions.

1. Review the patient's chart before beginning. Being knowledgeable about the patient's background and medical history will show interest and concern and will suggest directions for your questions.
2. Sit at the patient's level, eye-to-eye, and maintain eye contact if it is culturally acceptable to this patient.
3. Assume a comfortably relaxed and open posture; crossed arms signal closure, rigid posture is intimidating, and slouching is unprofessional.
4. Indicate interest by appropriate facial and nonverbal expressions such as smiling, nodding, and so on.
5. Listen attentively and stay centered on the conversation. Patients are aware when your interest is elsewhere.
6. Phrase your questions to elicit an extended response unless specific information is required.
7. Remember that many responses may be subjective. For instance, what is described as "pain" by one patient may be "discomfort" to another, or what one patient may describe as "a small amount of blood" another might describe as a "hemorrhage." Open-ended questions may help clarify responses.
8. Indicate when the interview is over by stressing points of concern to the patient for clarification. Ask for additional questions before terminating the interview.

---

gestions for successful communication. In addition, the following discussion explains several effective interview techniques, which are summarized in Table 4-2.

Reflecting

Repeating back what you have heard, using open-ended statements, is called **reflecting**. With this technique, you do not complete a sentence, but leave it up to the patient to do so. For example, you might say, "*Mrs. Rivera, you were saying that when your back hurts you....*" Reflection encourages the patient to make further comments. It also can help bring the

patient back to the subject if the conversation begins to drift. (Reflecting is a useful tool, but be careful not to overuse it because some patients find it annoying to have their words constantly parroted back.)

Paraphrasing or Restatement

To **paraphrase** or restate is to repeat what you have heard, using your own words or phrases. Paraphrasing can help verify that you have accurately understood the meaning of what was said. It also allows patients the opportunity to clarify their thoughts or statements. Typically, a paraphrased statement begins with "*You are saying that...,*" or "*It sounds as if...,*" followed by the rephrased content.

Asking for Examples or Clarification

If you are confused about some of the information you have received, ask the patient to give an example of the situation being described. For instance, "*Can you describe one of these dizzy episodes?*" The example should help you better understand what the patient is saying. It also may give you an insight into how the patient perceives the situation.

Asking Open-ended Questions

The best way to obtain specific information is to ask open-ended questions that require the patient to formulate an answer and elaborate on the response. Open-ended questions usually begin with "what," "when," or "how." Be careful about asking "why" questions because they can often sound judgmental or accusing. For example, asking "*Why did you do that?*" or "*Why didn't you follow directions?*" may imply to patients that you have already made a negative value judgment about their behavior, and they could become defensive and uncooperative. Instead, you might ask "*What part of the instructions did you not understand?*" "*When did you take the medication?*" or "*How did you clean the wound?*"

Avoid closed-ended questions that allow the patient to answer with one word (eg, "yes" or "no") or a few words unless you want a yes or no answer or very specific bits of information. For example—"*Are you allergic to any medications? What are they?*"

Summarizing

Briefly restating the information you have obtained, or **summarizing**, gives the patient another chance to clarify statements or correct misinformation. This tech-

Table 4-2	
Interviewing Techniques	
Techique	**Purposes**
Reflecting	• Encourages the patient to make additional comments
	• Helps redirect the conversation
Paraphrasing	• Verifies understanding
	• Allows for correction and clarification
Asking for examples	• Aids understanding
	• Offers insight into the patient's perceptions
Asking questions	• Aids information gathering
	• Encourages the patient to elaborate
Summarizing	• Allows for clarification or correction
	• Helps organize complex information or events
Allowing silences	• Aids thought formation, reconstruction of events, and evaluation of feelings

nique can also help you organize complex information or events in sequential order. For example, if the patient has been feeling dizzy and stumbling a lot, you might summarize by saying, *"You told me that you have been feeling dizzy for the last 3 days and that you frequently stumble as you are walking...."*

Allowing Silences

Periods of silence will sometimes occur during the patient interview and these can be beneficial. Some people are uncomfortable with prolonged silences and feel a need to quickly break the silence with words in an effort to "jump start" a stalled conversation. Keep in mind that silences are natural parts of conversations and can give patients time to formulate their thoughts, reconstruct events, evaluate their feelings, or assess what has already been said. Silences can often help you gather information during the interview, so do not discourage them.

 **Checkpoint Question**

4. What are six techniques that can be used when interviewing patients?

➤ FACTORS AFFECTING COMMUNICATION

Sometimes, despite your best efforts, messages may not be received accurately. There are many reasons for miscommunications. For example:

1. The message may have been unclear or inappropriate to the situation.
2. The person receiving the message may have been distracted, anxious, or confused.
3. Environmental elements, such as noise or interruptions, may have distorted the message.

In addition to these factors, the specific factors described below may affect communication.

Cultural Differences

The way a person perceives situations and other people is greatly influenced by cultural, social, and religious **beliefs,** or firmly held convictions. Personal **values** (principles or ideals) are commonly developed from these same beliefs. As a medical assistant, you will interact with people from varied ethnic backgrounds and cultural origins who bring with them beliefs and values that may differ from your own. Understanding those differences can aid communication and thereby improve patient care (Table 4-3).

The value of being on time or timeliness, for example, varies widely among cultures. Americans typically tend to value promptness; for instance, showing up on time for an appointment is considered to be good manners. But in some countries where life-styles are somewhat more relaxed, being several minutes late for an appointment is not considered unmannerly or disrespectful.

Some cultures may be offended by the types of intensely personal questions necessary for a medical history and may perceive them as an inexcusable invasion

text continues on page 64

Table 4-3
Cultural Factors That Affect Patient Care

White Middle Class

Family
- Nuclear family is highly valued.
- Elderly family members may live in a nursing home when they can no longer care for themselves.

Folk and Traditional Health Care
- Self-diagnosis of illnesses
- Use of over-the-counter drugs (especially vitamins and analgesics)
- Dieting (especially fad diets)
- Extensive use of exercise and exercise facilities

Values and Beliefs
- Youth is valued over age.
- Cleanliness
- Orderliness
- Attractiveness
- Individualism
- Achievement
- Punctuality

Common Health Problems
As a resullt of the high value placed on achievement:
- Cardiovascular diseases
- Gastrointestinal diseases
- Some forms of cancer
- Motor vehicle accidents
- Suicides
- Mental illness
- Chemical abuses

African American

Family
- Close and supportive extended-family relationships
- Develop strong kinship ties with nonblood relatives from church or organizational and social groups
- Family unity, loyalty, and cooperation are important.
- Frequently matriarchal

Folk and Traditional Health Care
- Varies extensively and may include spiritualists, herb doctors, root doctors, conjurers, skilled elder family members, voodoo, faith healing

Values and Beliefs
- Present oriented
- Members of the African American clergy are highly respected in the black community.
- Frequently highly religious

Common Health Problems
- Hypertension (precise cause unknown, may be related to diet)
- Sickle cell anemia
- Skin disorders; inflammation of hair follicles, various types of dermatitis and excessive growth of scar tissue (keloids)
- Lactose enzyme deficiency resulting in poor toleration of milk products
- Higher rate of tuberculosis
- Diabetes mellitus
- Higher infant mortality rate than in the white population

Asian

(Beliefs and practices vary, but most Asian cultures share some characteristics.)

Family
- Welfare of the family is valued above the person.
- Extended families are common.
- A person's lineage (ancestors) is respected.
- Sharing among family members is expected.

Folk and Traditional Health Care
- Theoretical basis is in Taosim, which seeks a balance in all things.
- Good health is achieved through the proper balance of yin (feminine, negative, dark, cold) and yang (masculine, positive, light, warm).

Values and Beliefs
- Strong sense of self-respect and self-control
- High respect for age
- Respect for authority
- Respect for hard work
- Praise of self to others is considered poor manners.
- Strong emphasis on harmony and the avoidance of conflict

(continued)

Table 4-3
Cultural Factors That Affect Patient Care (Continued)

Asian

Folk and Traditional Health Care

- An imbalance in energy is caused by an improper diet or strong emotions.
- Diseases and foods are classified as hot or cold and a proper balance between them will promote wellness (eg, treat a cold disease with hot foods).
- Many Asian health care systems use herbs, diet, and the application of hot or cold therapy. Also, many Asians believe that there are points on the body that are located on the meridians or energy pathways. If the energy flow is out of balance, treatment of the pathways may be necessary to restore the energy equilibrium.
  Acumassage—Technique of manipulating points along the energy pathways
  Acupressure—Technique for compressing the energy pathway points
  Acupuncture—Technique by which fine needles are inserted into the body at energy pathway points

Common Health Problems

- Tuberculosis
- Communicable diseases
- Malnutrition
- Suicide
- Various forms of mental illness
- Lactose enzyme deficiency

Hispanic, Mexican American

Family

- Familial role is important.
- *Compadrazgo:* special bond between a child's parents and his or her grandparents
- Family is the primary unit of society.

Folk and Traditional Health Care

- *Curanderas(os):* frequently folk healers who base treatments on humoral pathology—basic functions of the body are controlled by four body fluids or "humors":
  - Blood—hot and wet
  - Yellow bile—hot and dry
  - Black bile—cold and dry
  - Phlegm—cold and wet
- The secret of good health is to balance hot and cold within the body; therefore, most foods, beverages, herbs, and medications are classified as hot (*caliente*) or cold (*fresco, frio*) (a cold disease will be cured with a hot treatment).

Values and Beliefs

- Respect is given according to age (older) and sex (male).
- Roman Catholic Church may be very influential.
- God gives health and allows illness for a reason; therefore, may perceive illness as a punishment from God. An illness of this type can be cured through atonement and forgiveness.

Common Health Problems

- Diabetes mellitus and its complications
- Poverty and resultant problems, such as poor nutrition, inadequate medical care, poor prenatal care
- Lactose enzyme deficiency

Hispanic, Puerto Rican

(Since the Jones Act of 1917, all Puerto Ricans are American citizens.)

Family

- *Compadrazgo*—same as in Mexican-American culture

Folk and Traditional Health Care

- Similar to that of other Spanish-speaking cultures

Common Health Problems

- Parasitic diseases, such as dysentery, malaria, filariasis, and hookworms
- Lactose enzyme deficiency

Values and Beliefs

- Place a high value on safeguarding against group pressure to violate a person's integrity (may be difficult for Puerto Ricans to accept teamwork)
- Reticent about personal and family affairs (psychotherapy may be difficult to achieve at times because of this belief)
- Proper consideration should be given to cultural rituals such as shaking hands and standing up to greet and say goodbye to people.

(continued)

Table 4-3
Cultural Factors That Affect Patient Care (Continued)

Hispanic, Puerto Rican

Values and Beliefs

- Time is a relative phenomenon; little attention is given to the exact time of day.
- *Ataques*—culturally acceptable reaction to situations of extreme stress, characterized by hyperkinetic seizure activity

Native Americans

(Each tribe's beliefs and practices vary to some degree.)

Family

- Families are large and extended.
- Grandparents are official and symbolic leaders and decision makers.
- A child's namesake may assume equal parenting authority with biological parents.

Folk and Traditional Health Care

- Medicine men (shaman) are frequently consulted.
- Heavy use of herbs and psychological treatments, ceremonies, fasting, meditation, heat, and massages

Common health problems

- Alcoholism
- Suicide
- Tuberculosis
- Malnutrition
- Communicable diseases
- Higher maternal and infant mortality rates than in most of the population
- Diabetes mellitus
- Hypertension
- Gallbladder disease

Values and Beliefs

- Present oriented. Taught to live in the present and not to be concerned about the future. This time consciousness emphasizes finishing current business before doing something else.
- High respect for age
- Great value is placed on working together and sharing resources.
- High respect is given to a person who gives to others. The accumulation of money and goods often is frowned on.
- Some Native Americans practice the Peyotist religion in which the consumption of peyote, an intoxicating drug derived from mescal cacti, is part of the service. Peyote is legal if used for this purpose. It is classified as a hallucinogenic drug.

(From Taylor, C., Lillis, C., & LeMone, P., [1996]. Fundamentals of Nursing, 2nd ed., pp. 122–125. Philadelphia: Lippincott-Raven.)

---

of privacy. If this occurs, your physician may be required to intervene to allay the patient's concerns.

Looking someone else directly in the eyes or eye contact is also perceived differently by people of various backgrounds. Eye contact occurs more often among friends and family members than among acquaintances or strangers. In the United States, someone who maintains good eye contact is usually perceived as being honest, believable, and concerned. In contrast, in some Asian and Mideastern cultures, direct eye contact is perceived as sexually suggestive or disrespectful. In other cultures, such as Native Americans, *lack* of eye contact or casting the eyes downward is a sign of respect.

In addition to cultural differences in values, many differences occur among individuals. Some people are just more reserved or shy than others and may feel less comfortable in medical settings. To help avoid miscommunication and offending patients, you must be sensitive to these differences in all of your patient interactions.

Language Barriers

Effective communication is based on the use of language. But sometimes a patient may be unable to speak or understand English well enough for good communication to occur. Because it is crucial for you to give and receive accurate information, you will need to use an interpreter to help bridge any language barriers. A staff person might serve as the interpreter. Or an English-speaking member of the patient's family could help. In either case, be sure the interpreter fully understands what is being discussed. In the absence of a reliable interpreter, a phrase book of common medical questions with lists of possible answers may be helpful. If your area has a large population of non–English-speaking patients, your office should be equipped with an appropriate phrase book (See Appendix II for a list of key health care phrases in English and Spanish).

When seeking an interpreter, it might be best to seek someone of the same sex as the patient because certain cultures prohibit members of the opposite sex (even family members) from discussing personal issues about the body. Also, some cultures have religious guidelines dictating how members of the opposite sex should interact with one another (Fig. 4-5).

The following suggestions can be used for communicating with non–English-speaking patients:

1. Do not shout. Raising your voice will *not* increase understanding.
2. Demonstrate or pantomime as needed. Gestures are usually relatively universal.
3. If using an interpreter, speak directly to the patient, with the interpreter in your line of vision, so that the patient can read your facial expressions.
4. Speak slowly with simple sentences and phrases that require simple answers. The patient may comprehend small amounts of English.
5. Avoid slang; it may not translate well.
6. Avoid distractions and provide a relaxed, quiet interview space.

7. Learn some basic phrases of the most common language required in your area. Patients appreciate your effort.

Special Communication Challenges

Many patient situations present special communication challenges. For instance, hearing- or sight-impaired patients, young children, patients with limited understanding, those who are too ill or sedated to comprehend, and those who are frightened or anxious require particular attention. In each instance, you will need to assess the situation and the patient's ability to comprehend on any level. In some cases, a responsible family member will be with the patient and can be included in the communication process. Never exclude the patient from the exchange, but do ensure that all needed information is communicated, whether you obtain the information through questions about the patient's condition or you give instructions for further care. Patients must feel a part of the process but conditions may require involvement by caregivers.

Hearing-Impaired Patients

Forms of hearing impairment are discussed in Chapter 33, Caring for the Patient With Sensory Disorders. To communicate with patients who are unable to hear what you are saying will require tact, diplomacy, and patience. These suggestions may help.

1. Touch the patient gently to gain his attention.
2. Talk directly face-to-face to him, not at an angle and certainly not with your back to him.

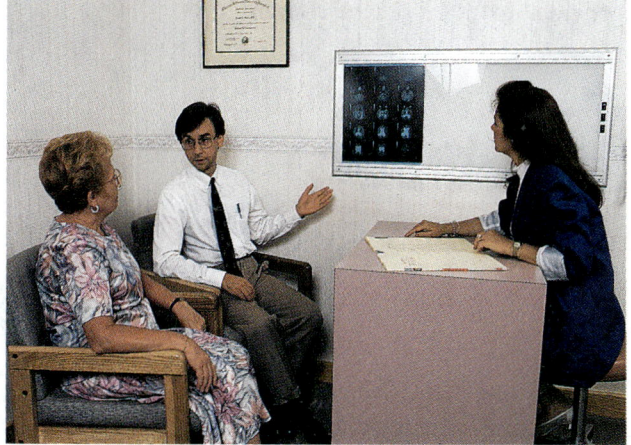

FIGURE 4-5
An interpreter can help you and the patient overcome language barriers.

What If?

What if you need to call a hearing-impaired patient? How can this be accomplished?

Hearing-impaired patients can make and receive calls using a special telephone with a service called Converse Communication Center, which uses a system called Telecommunication Device for the Deaf (TDD). If your office has a TDD telephone, you would call the patient and type in your verbal message. The patient would read your message, then type a response. If your office does not have a TDD telephone, your local telephone company can communicate with TDD users and non-TDD users. Check your telephone directory for more information.

3. Turn to the most prominent light so that your face is illuminated.
4. Lower the pitch of your voice; higher pitches are frequently lost with nerve impairment, but speak distinctly and with force. In most instances, shouting does not help and will only distort what might be heard.
5. Use note pads, demonstration, and pantomime as needed.
6. Use short sentences with short words. Enunciate clearly but do not exaggerate your facial movements.
7. Eliminate all distractions. Extraneous noises may confuse the patient.

Sight-Impaired Patients

Patients who cannot see can usually hear, however, they miss the vitally important nonverbal language. To increase access to communication with these patients, try these suggestions.

1. Identify yourself by name each time the patient comes into the office.
2. Do not raise your voice; the patient is not hearing impaired.
3. Let the patient know exactly what you will be doing at all times and alert him before touching.
4. Orient the patient spatially by having him touch the table, the chair, the counter, and so forth.
5. Assist him by having him take your arm and escorting him to the interview room.
6. Tell him when you are leaving the room and knock before entering.
7. Explain the sounds of machines to be used in the examination (eg, buzzing, whirring) and what each will do.

Children

Levels of comprehension vary greatly during childhood and will need to be addressed to the specific child. In most instances these suggestions will help facilitate communication.

1. Children are responsive to eye-level contact. Either lift them to your height or lower yourself to theirs.
2. Keep your voice low pitched and gentle.
3. Make your movements slow and keep them visible. Tell children when you need to touch them.
4. Rephrase your questions until you gain comprehension.
5. Expect children to regress to a lower level of development during an illness.
6. Use play to phrase your questions and to gain the child's cooperation.

7. Allow the child to express fear, to cry, and so on.
8. If the patient is an adolescent, expect a resentment for authority. During the interview process, some teenagers may not want a parent in the room. Assess the situation before including the parent.
9. Never show shock or judgment when dealing with adolescents; to do so will immediately close communication.

Stereotyping and Biased Opinions

Medical assisting is a profession that deals with people of differing ages, races, cultures, and sexual orientation. Sometimes your values may be in stark contrast to those held by a patient, but you should not let your personal values or **bias** (opinions) affect your treatment of a patient. All patients must be treated fairly, respectfully, and with dignity, regardless of their cultural, social, or personal values. To treat them in any other fashion would be considered **discrimination**.

Stereotyping is holding an opinion of all members of a particular culture, race, religion, or age group based on oversimplified or negative characterizations. It is a form of prejudice. Examples of negative stereotypes include: "All old people are frail and senile" or "Those people are always dirty and never bathe." Stereotyping and prejudice are deterrents to establishing therapeutic relationships because they do not allow for patient individuality and can prevent quality care from being given to everyone on an equal basis.

As a health care professional, you are expected to treat all patients impartially. To guard against discriminatory practices, remain nonjudgmental, avoid stereotypes, and display a professional demeanor. By doing so, you communicate to patients that you accept human differences and that quality health care will be provided to all those who seek it.

Checkpoint Question
5. What are four main factors that can affect communication with patients?

➤ ESTABLISHING POSITIVE PATIENT RELATIONSHIPS

Your approach to patients conveys a message about who you are and how you feel about yourself and your profession. Medical assistants can be role models, earning the trust and admiration of patients. To establish—and maintain—positive patient relationships, speak respectfully and exhibit an appropriate demeanor during all interactions.

Proper Form of Address

The way you address patients provides clues about your attitude and the way you will likely provide care. When greeting patients, use a proper form of address— for example, "*Good morning, Mr. Jones.*" or "*How are you feeling, Mrs. Smith?*" This type of address shows respect and sets a professional tone. In contrast, calling patients "sweetie," "granny," "gramps," or "honey" can be offensive. These terms denigrate the individual's dignity and put the interaction on a personal, not professional, level.

Other inappropriate forms of address include referring to the patient as a medical condition—for example, "the gallbladder in room 2" or "the broken arm in the waiting room." Patients often come to the medical office feeling anxious, so they may be particularly sensitive to everything they see and hear (or overhear). Addressing the patient as a medical condition sends the message that the staff values the patient as nothing more than an illness, which can lead to heightened anxiety.

Professional Distance

How people interact with each other is influenced by the level of emotional involvement between them. For instance, communication between a husband and wife is more intimate than the personal level of communication between friends or the social level of communication between acquaintances. In the health care setting, you must establish an appropriate level of communication to deliver direct patient care, make objective assessments, and provide quality patient teaching. You should not become too personally involved with patients because doing so may jeopardize your ability to make objective assessments. Keeping a "professional distance" allows you to deal objectively with patients while creating a therapeutic environment. To keep this distance, avoid revealing intimate information about yourself (eg, marital woes, financial troubles, family conflicts) that might shift the dynamics of the relationship to a more personal level.

Empathy Versus Sympathy

Closely linked to professional distance are the concepts of **sympathy** and **empathy**. Many psychologists describe sympathy as feeling *for* someone and empathy as feeling *with* someone. In the health care setting, empathy means trying to understand what patients are feeling so you can help them. Empathizing can help you recognize a patient's fear and discomfort so you can do everything possible to provide support and reassurance. Sympathy or pitying your patient may compromise your professional distance and cause you to become personally involved.

Checkpoint Question

6. What is the difference between showing sympathy and showing empathy to your patients?

Providing Grief Support

Occasionally, you will need to support patients who are experiencing **grief**, or great sadness caused by a loss. This entails an understanding of what the patient is going through and feeling and is different from offering sympathy.

The grieving process starts when a person experiences a significant loss such as the loss of a loved one through death, or the loss of a relationship, a body part, or personal health. The loss may be either perceived or real. Grief includes such emotional responses as anger, sadness, and depression, and each emotion may trigger certain behaviors. For example, anger may result in outbursts, sadness could cause crying, and depression may lead to unusual quietness or isolation.

The grieving process occurs in stages: shock, disbelief or **denial** (refusal to acknowledge something), anger, awareness of reality, and, finally, acceptance of the loss. A person experiences these stages over a period of months or years. Sometimes, the collective signs of grief are referred to as **mourning** (Box 4-2).

In the medical practice, expect to see grief displayed in many different ways. Know, too, that several factors can influence how a patient demonstrates grief and that different cultures and individuals demonstrate grief in a variety of ways ranging from stoic, impassive responses to loud, prolonged wailing and fainting. Other responses may reflect religious beliefs about the meaning of death. Grieving is a unique and personal process. There is no set time period for grieving to be completed, and there is no one "right" way to grieve.

Grieving patients may want to talk about their feelings and review events. Terminally ill patients may want to discuss their fears of dying and concerns for surviving loved ones. To support grieving patients, allow time for them to express themselves and actively listen to what they say. When appropriate, consider using touch to convey your understanding. If patients'

BOX 4-2 Dealing With Grief

Patients and families faced with great loss must be helped to feel that they need not handle this alone. Most communities have resources to help make the loss less devastating. The workers in hospice situations and volunteer grief counselors are trained to answer the questions, acknowledge the fears and anger, ease the transition, and offer respite for caregivers. The knowledgeable medical assistant will, with the physician's permission, direct the patient and the family to the proper organization.

Patients and families must be allowed to grieve in their own way and at their own pace. Much has been written about the process of dealing with loss. Theories vary regarding the number of stages, and the titles and sequences of stages, but all authorities agree that for healing to begin, the process must be allowed to run its course.

With variations, the stages include those outlined by Elizabeth Kübler-Ross:

1. *Denial*—Refusal to accept that loss has occurred or will soon occur
2. *Anger*—Lashing out at caregivers, physicians, a Supreme Being
3. *Bargaining*—An effort to gain time, bargaining with self or Supreme Being
4. *Depression*—Withdrawal, weeping, isolation
5. *Acceptance*—Coming to realize and accept what has happened and feeling tranquility and readiness

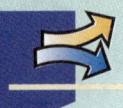

Ethical Tips

All patient communication is confidential. However, patient information is sometimes discussed unintentionally. To avoid breaching confidentiality, follow these guidelines:

- Do not discuss patient problems in office lunch rooms or break rooms.
- Do not discuss patient problems in public places, such as elevators or parking lots. A patient's friends or family members might overhear your conversation and misinterpret what is said.
- When calling coworkers over the office intercom, do not use a patient's name or reveal other information. Avoid saying something like, "Bob Smith is on the phone and wants to know if his strep throat culture came back." Instead, say "There's a patient phone call on line one."
- Before going home, destroy any slips of paper in your uniform pockets that contain patient information (eg, reminder notes from verbal reports).

concerns stem from a lack of understanding about their condition, provide pertinent education for them and for their caregivers (if appropriate). You should also become familiar with available community resources, such as grief or other counseling services and hospice care, so you can suggest these services when necessary.

➤ PATIENT TEACHING

One of the most fundamental communication skills you will need is the ability to teach patients about their medical conditions. Patient teaching might involve something as relatively simple as explaining how often a medication should be taken to instructing a newly diagnosed diabetic patient about self-injection. The guidelines listed below incorporate such key communication skills as interviewing and active listening. Follow these to provide effective patient education. (See Chap. 5, Patient Education, for a more detailed discussion.)

1. Be knowledgeable about current medical issues, discoveries, or trends.
2. Be aware of special services available in your local area.
3. Have pertinent handouts or information sheets available.
4. Allow an appropriate amount of teaching time so that you are not interrupted or rushed.
5. Find a quiet room away from the main office flow if at all possible.
6. Give information in a clear, concise, sequential manner; provide written instructions as a follow-up.
7. Allow the patient time to assimilate this new information.
8. Encourage the patient to ask questions.
9. Ask questions in a way that will allow you to know if the patient has correctly understood what is to be learned.
10. Invite the patient to call the office with additional questions that may arise.

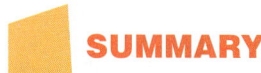

SUMMARY

Communication is a complex and dynamic process involving the sending and receiving of messages. It includes verbal and nonverbal forms of expression and is influenced by personal and societal values, individual beliefs, and cultural orientation. In the medical practice, important aspects of patient communication involve interviewing and active listening. To communicate effectively, you must understand the various factors that can affect the exchange of messages and use the communication techniques that are most appropriate for each individual patient situation.

CRITICAL THINKING CHALLENGES

1. Dr. Roberts has just told a patient that she has breast cancer. Describe the kinesics that you would expect to see. Write three sample questions that you could ask the patient to promote open communication about her feelings.
2. Dr. Rodriguez has just discharged a patient with specific instructions for wound care. How would you determine the patient's understanding of these instructions? Are there any nonverbal clues that can help you determine if the patient is confused?
3. Review the difference between sympathy and empathy. How would you demonstrate empathy?

ANSWERS TO CHECKPOINT QUESTIONS

1. For communication to occur, these three elements must be present: a message to be sent, a person to send the message, and a person to receive the message.
2. Voice tone, quality, volume, pitch, and range are five examples of paralanguage.

3. Kinesics refers to body movements (facial expressions, gestures, eye movements). Proxemics refers to spatial relationships.
4. When interviewing patients, you can use six different techniques. These include reflecting, paraphrasing or restatement, asking for examples or clarification, asking open-ended questions, summarizing, and allowing for silences.
5. The four main factors that affect communication are cultural differences, language barriers, special communication challenges, and stereotyping and biased opinions.
6. Sympathy means to feel sorry for someone. Empathy means to show an understanding for what someone is experiencing.

SUGGESTIONS FOR FURTHER READING

Craven, R. F., & Hirnle, C. J. (1996). *Fundamentals of Nursing: Human Health and Function*, 2nd ed. Philadelphia: Lippincott-Raven.

Galanti, G. A. (1991). *Caring for Patients from Different Cultures*. Philadelphia: University of Pennsylvania Press.

Lipkin, G., & Cohen, R. (1992). *Effective Approaches to Patient Behavior*, 4th ed. New York: Springer.

Long, L. (1992). *Understanding/Responding*, 2nd ed. Boston: Jones and Bartlett.

Purtilo, R. (1990). *Health Professional and Patient Interaction*, 4th ed. Philadelphia: W. B. Saunders.

Samarel, N. (1991). *Caring for Life and Death*. Bristol, PA: Hemisphere Publishing.

Taylor, C., Lillis, C., & LeMone, P. (1996). *Fundamentals of Nursing: The Art and Science of Nursing Care*, 2nd ed. Philadelphia: Lippincott-Raven.

Timby, B. K., & Lewis, L. W. (1992). *Fundamental Skills and Concepts in Patient Care*, 5th ed. Philadelphia: J. B. Lippincott.

Patient Education

Chapter Outline

The Patient Education Process
    Assessment
    Planning
    Implementation
    Evaluation
    Documentation
The Patient's Ability to Learn
    Maslow's Hierarchy of Needs
    Factors That Promote Learning
    Factors That Hinder Learning

Patient Teaching Plans
    Developing a Plan
    Selecting and Adapting Teaching
      Material
    Developing Your Own Material
Summary
Critical Thinking Challenges
Answers to Checkpoint Questions
Suggestions for Further Reading

5

DACUM Components

1.1   Project a positive attitude
1.3   Practice within the scope of education, training, and personal capabilities
1.6   Conduct oneself in a courteous and diplomatic manner
2.2   Treat all patients with empathy and impartiality
2.3   Adapt communication to individuals' abilities to understand
2.5   Serve as liaison between physician and others
2.6   Evaluate understanding of communication
3.6   Locate resources and information for patients and employers
7.2   Instruct patients with special needs
7.3   Teach patients methods of health promotion and disease prevention
      Advanced-level skill:
      Develop educational materials

Chapter Competencies

Learning Objectives

Upon successfully completing this chapter, you will be able to:

1. Spell and define the Key Terms.
2. Explain the medical assistant's role in patient education.
3. Define the five steps in the patient education process.
4. Describe what is necessary before learning can be accomplished.
5. Explain Maslow's hierarchy of human needs.
6. List five factors that may facilitate patient learning.
7. List five factors that may hinder patient learning.
8. Describe how to prepare a teaching plan.
9. List potential sources of patient education materials.

Key Terms

(See Glossary for definitions.)

assessment
documentation
evaluation
implementation
learning goal
learning objectives
noncompliance
patient education
planning

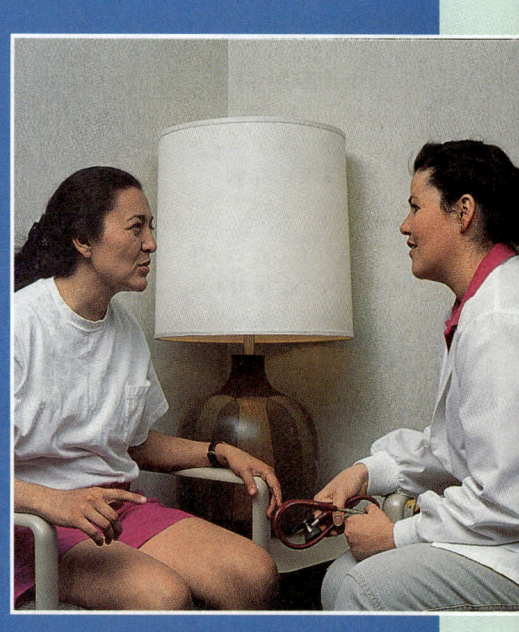

In the current health care climate of shorter hospital stays, patients seen in the medical office typically have more acute conditions requiring more intensive and extensive education through their health care provider. This may be one of your most challenging and rewarding roles. Of course, you will not be responsible for teaching patients everything they need to know about health care. However, you will be expected to treat **patient education**—a process in which the patient actively participates and that results in a behavior change—as seriously as you do your other clinical duties. Patient education is performed under the direction of the physician. To protect yourself and your physician, make sure you know exactly what information your physician wants conveyed to each patient. In addition, have the physician review and approve all patient teaching materials before you provide them to patients.

> ### ➤ THE PATIENT EDUCATION PROCESS

Patient education involves more than telling patients which medications need to be taken or which life-style behaviors need to be changed, and expecting them to blindly follow these instructions. To educate patients effectively, you need to involve them in the process of gaining knowledge about their condition and care. Ultimately, that knowledge should lead to a change in behavior or attitude.

The process of patient education is divided into five major steps:

- Assessment
- Planning
- Implementation
- Evaluation
- Documentation

You must carry out each of these steps to achieve effective patient teaching.

Checkpoint Question
1. What must you do to educate patients effectively?

Assessment

Before you begin to teach, you must assess your feelings and attitudes about the patient and the topic to be taught. Sometime in your career as a medical assistant, you may encounter situations or patients that make you feel uncomfortable. You must remember, however,

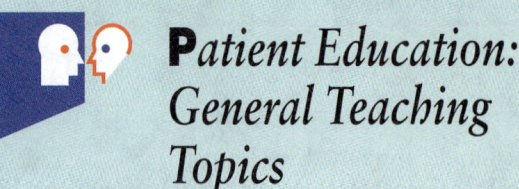

Patient Education: General Teaching Topics

What clinical topics might patients need to learn about? Here are some suggestions:

- Etiology, treatment, and complications of diagnosed disease(s)
- Prescribed medications (eg, when to take them, what they are for, side effects, dosages, food interactions)
- Wound care procedure
- Nutrition/diet management
- Exercise programs
- Preventive health measures (eg, mammogram, self-examination of the testicles or breasts)
- Child and home safety
- Laboratory and radiograph procedures (eg, preparations, results, purpose of test)
- Community resources
- Substance abuse help programs

In addition to the topics listed above, you may also need to educate the patient about the administrative aspects of the medical practice (eg, office hours and policies, filing insurance claims, obtaining copies of medical records).

that your role as educator requires you to set aside your own personal feelings and life experiences and to instruct the patient objectively and to the best of your ability. Always consider how your responses and actions will affect the patient, and be sure to treat each patient impartially.

Assessment requires gathering information about the patient's present health care needs and abilities. This includes:

- Past and present health experiences
- Current understanding of health problems
- Additional information required
- Feelings about the effects of any health problems
- Factors such as sedation or hearing impairment that might hinder learning

You can obtain this information from a number of sources, including the patient (see Chap. 20, Medical History and Patient Assessment), the patient's record, the physician, the patient's family members or significant others, and other members of the health care team. When you have collected all the assessment data, you are ready to start the next step of the education process—planning (Fig. 5-1).

Planning

Planning involves using the information gathered during the assessment phase to determine the patient's particular learning needs. If possible, allow the patient to be involved in this part of the process. Learning goals and objectives that are established with input from the patient are often more meaningful. A patient's **learning goal** is what the patient and educator feel will be the outcome of the educational program. The patient's **learning objectives** include procedures or tasks that will be discussed or performed at various points in the educational program to help achieve the goal. Make certain the objectives you establish are specific for each individual patient and measurable in some manner.

For example, consider a patient who needs to limit fluid intake. Which of these objectives would be more specific and allow for evaluation of progress? *Patient will understand why he should limit his fluid intake* or *Patient will be able to prepare a schedule for daily fluid intake and explain why it is important that he limit his fluid intake.* The second objective is more specific and not only evaluates the patient's understanding, but it also requires the patient to demonstrate understanding. Having the patient prepare his own schedule gets him involved in his own health care. It also allows him to customize the schedule to fit his life-style, which is likely to increase compliance.

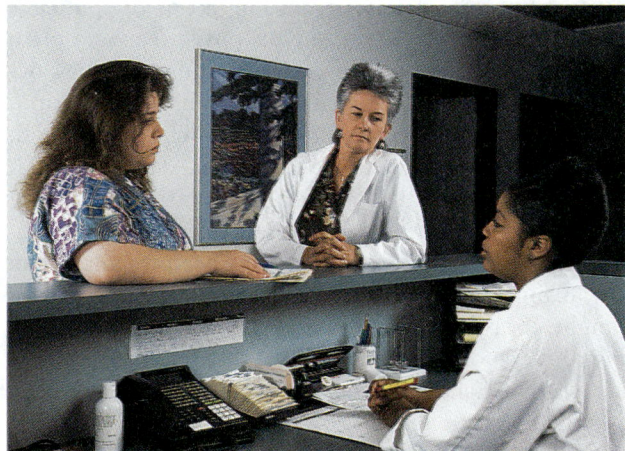

FIGURE 5-1
The medical assistant may obtain information regarding the patient's condition from the physician and other members of the health care team.

Checkpoint Question
2. What two things should you keep in mind when writing learning objectives for patient education?

Implementation

After you establish the need for patient teaching and agree on the goals and objectives, you begin implementation. **Implementation is the process used to carry out the agreed on teaching plan.** This plan can usually be carried out in several ways. For example, you may be able to instruct the patient through discussion, either one-on-one or in a group setting. Box 5-1 presents other implementation methods. Patients also benefit from the use of teaching aids (eg, drawings, charts, graphs, pamphlets) that can be taken home and used as references. You can also use filmstrips, videos, and audio cassettes to supplement the implementation pro-

BOX 5-1   Implementation Methods

Implementing the learning process should be individualized to the patient's best method of comprehension and retention. These may include:

1. Lecture and demonstration—This method presents the information in the most basic form but requires no patient participation for reinforcement and retention.
2. Role playing and demonstration—The patient watches you perform a medical procedure, then performs it to ensure understanding. Information is more likely to be recalled if the patient actively participates in the process.
3. Discussion—This is a two-way exchange of information and ideas and works well for life-style changes (eg, making dietary changes to lower cholesterol) rather than for medical procedures.
4. Audiovisual material—This works well for patients who are not motivated to read or who have reading problems; however, a method for assessing the level of individual understanding must be established. The patient may take the material home to review as needed.
5. Printed material and programmed instructions—All information should be discussed with the patient to clarify points and to elicit questions before assuming that the instructions are understood.

cess. Keep in mind, too, that other members of the health care team or community support group members are usually willing to assist as needed during this process.

Occasionally, you may need to demonstrate a procedure to a patient. Try to make demonstrations as realistic as possible to ensure that patients are aware of all that will be expected of them when they are caring for themselves at home. Miscommunication or misinterpretation can lead to serious complications or injury (Fig. 5-2).

No matter how the plan is implemented, it will not be effective if the patient does not understand what is important and why. That is the reason evaluation, the next step in the teaching process, is so important.

Evaluation

Is the patient progressing? Is the teaching plan working? Does the plan need any changes? These are a few of the questions that you must ask yourself when you begin to evaluate. Evaluation is the process that indicates how well the patient is adapting to the information learned. This can be the most difficult part of the education process.

In the medical office setting, where patient contact is limited, part of the evaluation may need to be done by the patients at home. For example, in cases in which office visits for direct observation are not scheduled, patients will be responsible for telephoning and reporting their status. You can help by planning a time schedule for the patient to call to give progress reports. If you do not hear from the patient, make sure to call and document the progress.

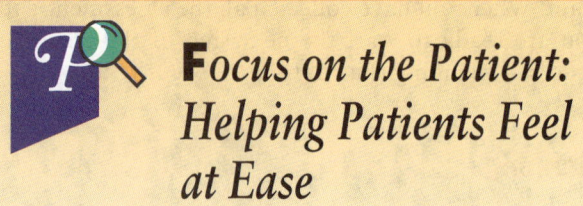

Focus on the Patient: Helping Patients Feel at Ease

Everyone responds well to positive reinforcement. As you evaluate the patients' understanding and compliance, tell them how well they are doing on those points performed or followed correctly. Most patients genuinely want to take charge of their health care. Try statements such as, "You understood (or performed) that quickly and well. Now let's go over the next point."

Patients must be adequately informed about what health care points need to be documented and when to seek medical help. If problems do arise, reevaluate the educational plan. If you discover **noncompliance** (a patient's inability or refusal to follow prescribed orders), first check for understanding. If the concepts and consequences are understood but the patient refuses to comply, the physician must be notified. A patient has the right to refuse any treatment, even self-treatment, but this *must* be documented.

Remember: Evaluation is an ongoing process, so you should expect to update and modify your plan periodically.

Documentation

Documentation includes recording all of the patient's agreed on learning needs, the proposed teaching plan, and the implementation and evaluation that has occurred. Document any written or verbal information, such as telephone conversations or teaching aids used, in the patient record. In a society that demands high-quality care from all of its health professionals, documenting services provided is essential because it establishes a written record of what has been taught, when it was taught, how it was taught, and by whom it was taught. If problems arise or the patient does not follow instructions or is noncompliant, the documentation is a record of what information and teaching has been supplied so far.

To stress the importance of documentation, it has been listed as a single step. However, continual documentation must be done throughout the teaching process. Documentation is essential because proce-

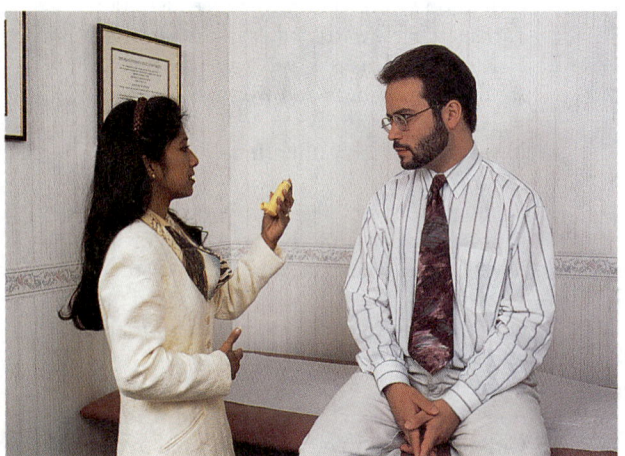

FIGURE 5-2
Be as realistic as possible when demonstrating a procedure to a patient.

dures are considered not to have been done if they are not recorded.

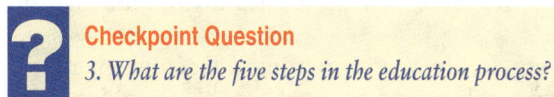

Checkpoint Question

3. What are the five steps in the education process?

➤ THE PATIENT'S ABILITY TO LEARN

Learning is the knowledge, wisdom, or skill acquired through studying or instruction. The same type of factors that influence how well *you* learn also affect how well your patients will learn what you are trying to teach them. Learning cannot occur without motivation or a perceived need to learn.

Maslow's Hierarchy of Needs

Abraham Maslow, an American psychiatrist, recognized that people are motivated by needs, and certain basic needs must be met before people can progress to the level of taking personal responsibility for their health (self-actualization). Maslow arranged his theory of needs in the form of a pyramid, with the most basic needs at the bottom and the higher needs progressing up to the top (Fig. 5-3). The patient follows this progression upward, fulfilling the levels of needs toward the highest level, which results in a state of health and well-being. In your responsibility as educator, you must be aware that patients must have all the more basic needs satisfied before they are willing and able to learn to take care of their own health.

Physiologic needs are the basic needs for air, food, water, rest, and comfort. If these basic needs are unmet, the patient cannot begin to progress.

Safety needs include the need to live in a safe environment and to be free from fear and anxiety. Patients are particularly susceptible to the fear and anxiety that accompany many medical conditions. For example, a patient diagnosed with cancer may be so frightened as to be unable to think of anything else but dying. Also, patients who have experienced some sort of trauma or disaster (eg, hurricane, fires, motor vehicle accident) may place the need to feel safe above all other needs.

Affection needs or the need for love and belonging are essential for feeling connected and important to others. A sense of love or belonging can often be a powerful motivation for patients to try to regain good health.

Esteem needs are our needs to feel self-worth. Esteem can be self-generated or it can come from those who admire us. If others value us or if we value ourselves, we are more likely to strive to maintain good health.

Self-actualization is the pinnacle of the pyramid at which a person has satisfied all the other basic needs and feels personal responsibility and control over his or her own life and an obligation to others in society. Self-actualized patients will strive to control their state of wellness by following all health directives and may even help others to achieve wellness.

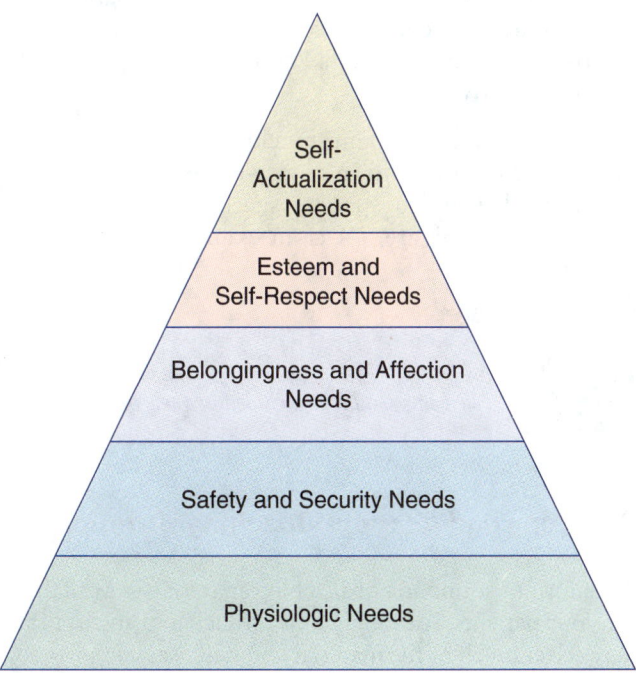

FIGURE 5-3
This scheme of Maslow's hierarchy of human needs shows how a person moves from basic need fulfillment to higher levels of needs.

Factors That Promote Learning

To ensure that the patient is, indeed, capable of learning what is being taught, consider the following questions:

- Is the patient emotionally or physically able to learn?
- Does the patient perceive the information to be important?
- Is the atmosphere friendly, uninterrupted, free of distractions, and conducive to learning?
- Is the material organized in a simple-to-complex, familiar-to-unfamiliar fashion?
- Are different types of media used to repeat and reinforce the important information?

- Is information available that the patient can take home to use as a reference?
- Can the information be used by the patient or demonstrated immediately?
- Are other community services available that could supplement or assist with the information the patient needs?
- Is the patient wearing needed sensory aids such as glasses or hearing aids?
- Have you allowed time for questions and answers?
- Can the information be divided into manageable portions?

Factors That Hinder Learning

If the patient is having trouble learning, use these questions to determine what might be affecting the education process:

- Is the patient in intense pain or physically unable to learn because of fatigue or weakness?
- Is the patient emotionally upset or overwhelmed and unable to handle another concept at the present time?
- Does the patient have any physical impairments that might hinder communication abilities?
- Does the patient speak the same language you speak?
- Does the patient have the same cultural or ethical background that you do? If not, will it affect how the concept is perceived?
- Does the patient perceive you as condescending?
- Are you well prepared?
- Are you using too many technical words?

You should consider the potential factors that can promote and hinder learning before teaching even begins, during the assessment phase. However, you can use these questions at any time during the patient education process to help determine the reasons for any learning difficulties.

Checkpoint Question
4. What are three factors that promote learning and three that hinder learning?

➤ PATIENT TEACHING PLANS

Developing a Plan

Because medical assistants are usually allotted only minimal time for patient teaching, you may often find yourself teaching with no written plan. To ensure teaching is done logically, always use the education process to help you formulate a plan in your mind. Also remember to document in the patient record whatever teaching you perform and the patient's response.

Many facilities use preprinted teaching plans for common problem areas, such as "Controlling Diabetes," "Living With Multiple Sclerosis," "Coping With Hearing Loss," and so on. Although these save time, they are not individualized for each patient. If you use preprinted teaching plans, be sure to adapt them to your particular patient's learning needs and abilities.

If preprinted plans are not an option, consult teaching plan resource books, which contain the necessary information in outline form. You can take the plans from these sources and transfer them as needed to your facility-approved teaching plan format, adding your own comments to fit the patient's needs.

All teaching plans, no matter what the design, should contain the following elements:

- Learning goal—description of what the patient should learn from implementation of the teaching plan
- Material to be covered—all major topics to be discussed
- Learning objectives—steps or procedures the patient must understand or demonstrate to accomplish the learning goal
- Evaluation—appraisal of the patient's progress
- Comments—remarks concerning circumstances that may have prohibited successful completion of the objectives

Teaching plans also must include an area for documenting when the information was presented to the patient and when the patient successfully completed each objective. Figure 5-4 is an example of a patient teaching plan.

Checkpoint Question
5. What elements should be included in a teaching plan?

Selecting and Adapting Teaching Material

An enormous amount of teaching material is available for your patients. Although your physician or institution may select much of the material you will use, you may be responsible for selecting some teaching aids. Assess your patients' general level of understanding so you can choose appropriately. When selecting preprinted material, consider the format, headings, illustrations, vocabulary, and writing style for overall clarity and readability.

Teaching Plan: 32-year-old female with Iron Deficiency Anemia
Patient Learning Goal: Increase patient's knowledge of Iron Deficiency Anemia, its complications, and treatments
Material to be Covered: Description of disorder, complications, diet, medications, procedures

Learning Objectives Comments	Teaching Methods/ Tools	Procedure Explained/ Demonstrated Date/Initial	PT Demonstrated/ Objectives Met Date/Initial

1. Patient describes what happens when body's demand for oxygen is not met.
  a. oxygen and hgb concentration decrease
  b. patient develops signs/symptoms of anemia
  c. anemia occurs only after body stores of iron are depleted
	Instruction		

2. Patient describes complications caused by decrease of oxygen concentration
  a. chronic fatigue
  b. dyspnea
  c. inability to concentrate, think
  d. decrease in tissue repair
  e. increase of infection
  f. increase in heart rate
	Instruction		

3. Patient discusses importance of diet in prevention of iron deficiency anemia
  a. including iron-rich foods in diet (beef, poultry, green vegetables)
  b. including foods that contain ascorbic acid to assist in absorbing iron in body (fruits)
  c. importance of limiting large meals if fatigued; stress importance of several small meals
	Instruction/Video: "Your Diet: Why It Is Important"		

4. Patient describes prescribed medication, its purpose, dosage, route, and side effects	Instruction/Pamphlet: *Taking Your Oral Iron Supplements*		
5. Patient aware of importance of follow up appointments for evaluation of prescribed plan of treatment	Instruction/Appointment slip with next scheduled appointment		

FIGURE 5-4
Example of a teaching plan that may be used when preparing your own material.

Also, ensure that the information provided on commercial materials is truthful and in agreement with the policies and procedures of your facility (Fig. 5-5).

Many patient education textbooks are available from your clinic library. If you do not have access to a library, you usually can order most texts from local bookstores. Many of these sources list addresses for other patient education materials that can be acquired from companies or associations. These materials commonly include printed items as well as videos, audio cassettes, filmstrips, and slides. Use commercially prepared materials to start a patient teaching library in the physician's office so you will have information at your fingertips when needed.

Developing Your Own Material

Sometimes, you may need to create your own teaching materials. Review available resources and teaching aids and adapt the information to benefit your patients. When developing patient teaching material, remember to do the following:

- Indicate the objective of the information.
- Personalize the information so the patient wants to learn.
- Make sure information is clear and well organized.
- Use lists and outlines, which are easier to read and remember than paragraphs.

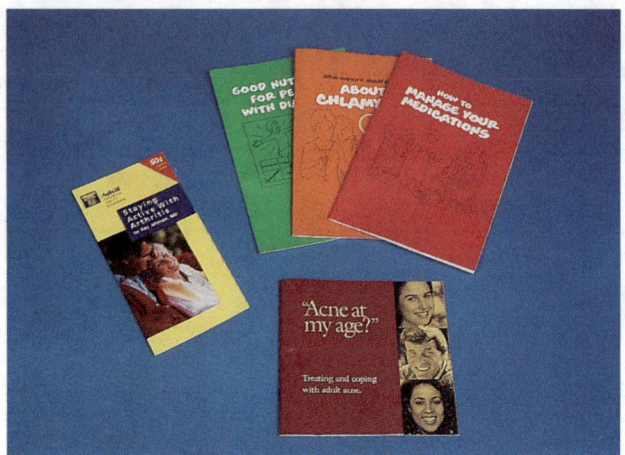

FIGURE 5-5
A wide variety of preprinted teaching materials are available.

- Avoid as much medical jargon as possible.
- Focus on the key points.
- Select appropriate printing type.
- Use diagrams that are simple, clear, and well labeled.
- Include the names and telephone numbers of people or organizations that patients can call with further questions or concerns.

After patients have been using the material for awhile, periodically evaluate its effectiveness and modify as needed.

Keep in mind that not all of the patient teaching materials you create need to be in print form. Patients must be motivated to read, but many will be more receptive to audiovisual instruction. Take advantage of

any opportunity to develop teaching materials in other media.

SUMMARY

Your role in patient teaching depends on the clinical setting in which you work. Some facilities hire professional staff to perform patient teaching duties. If that is the case in your facility, your patient teaching experience may be limited. Even so, never pass up an opportunity to teach. Encourage questions and always provide a number that patients can call with additional questions. Periodically check to ensure that your teaching has been effective.

Remember: Do not overstep your role as the medical assistant. The patient teaching you provide should clarify and complement information provided by the physician. A well planned patient education program helps ensure that patients receive the high-quality health care they deserve.

CRITICAL THINKING CHALLENGES

1. Review the factors that hinder learning. How can you, as a medical assistant, eliminate these factors?
2. Make a list of preprinted educational materials that every office should have available. How would you get these materials? What professional agencies (eg, American Heart Association, American Cancer Society) could help you?
3. Select a disease that you would like to learn more about. Develop a list of educational topics concerning this disease, then create learning objectives for each topic.

ANSWERS TO CHECKPOINT QUESTIONS

1. To educate patients effectively, you must get them involved in the education process.
2. Learning objectives must be specific to the patient's needs and must be measurable.
3. The five steps in the education process are assessment, planning, implementation, evaluation, and documentation.
4. Factors that promote learning include emotional and physical readiness, information that is important to the patient, a friendly atmosphere, and media available for review. Factors that hinder learning include severe pain, physical impairments, language barriers, ethnic barriers, and an unprepared educator. (Answers will vary.)
5. All teaching plans should include a learning goal, material to be covered, learning objectives, evaluation, and comments.

What If?
What if a patient is not ready or willing to learn?

Often, a patient may need more time to comprehend the diagnosis; until that occurs, teaching may be ineffective and should be postponed. For example, a patient who has not accepted the diagnosis of diabetes will not be ready to learn how to give himself insulin injections. You should never push a patient to learn a procedure. Instead, notify the physician, who may write an order for a social worker to become involved. Support groups can also help a patient begin to accept a diagnosis so learning can begin.

SUGGESTIONS FOR FURTHER READING

Craven, R. F., & Hirnle, C. J. (1996). *Fundamentals of Nursing: Human Health and Function*, 2nd ed. Philadelphia: Lippincott-Raven.

Redman, B. Klug. (1993). *The Process of Patient Education.* St. Louis: Mosby-Yearbook.

Roe, C. (1992). The muddy waters of clinical teaching, patient education segment. *American Journal of Nursing, (7),* 20.

Smeltzer, S., & Bare, B. (1995). *Brunner and Suddarth's Textbook of Medical-Surgical Nursing*, 8th ed. Philadelphia: Lippincott-Raven.

Taylor, C., Lillis, C., & LeMone, P. (1993). *Fundamentals of Nursing: The Art and Science of Nursing Care*, 2nd ed. Philadelphia: J. B. Lippincott.

Timby, B. K., & Lewis, L. W. (1992). *Fundamental Skills and Concepts in Patient Care*, 5th ed. Philadelphia: J. B. Lippincott.

Teaching Patients About Factors Influencing Health

Chapter Outline

Teaching Patients About Nutrition
    The Food Guide Pyramid
    Dietary Guidelines
    Physician-Ordered Diets
Teaching Patients About Exercise
Teaching Patients to Cope with Illness and Stress
    Positive and Negative Stress
    Relaxation Techniques

Teaching Patients About Substance Abuse
Teaching Patients About Medication Therapy
Summary
Critical Thinking Challenges
Answers to Checkpoint Questions
Suggestions for Further Reading

DACUM Components

1.3   Practice within the scope of education, training, and personal capabilities
1.6   Conduct oneself in a courteous and diplomatic manner
2.2   Treat all patients with empathy and impartiality
2.3   Adapt communication to individuals' abilities to understand
2.5   Serve as liaison between physician and others
2.6   Evaluate understanding of communication
7.2   Instruct patients with special needs
7.3   Teach patients methods of health promotion and disease prevention

Chapter Competencies

Learning Objectives

Upon successfully completing this chapter, you will be able to:

1. Spell and define the Key Terms.
2. List five main factors that play important roles in patient health.
3. Identify the components of a healthy diet.
4. Describe how to perform range-of-motion exercises.
5. Discuss the difference between positive and negative stress.
6. List and explain relaxation techniques.
7. Identify commonly abused substances.
8. Explain the kinds of information that should be included in patient teaching about medication therapy.

Key Terms

(See Glossary for definitions.)

coping mechanisms
exercise
negative stress
nutrition
positive stress
range of motion
visualization

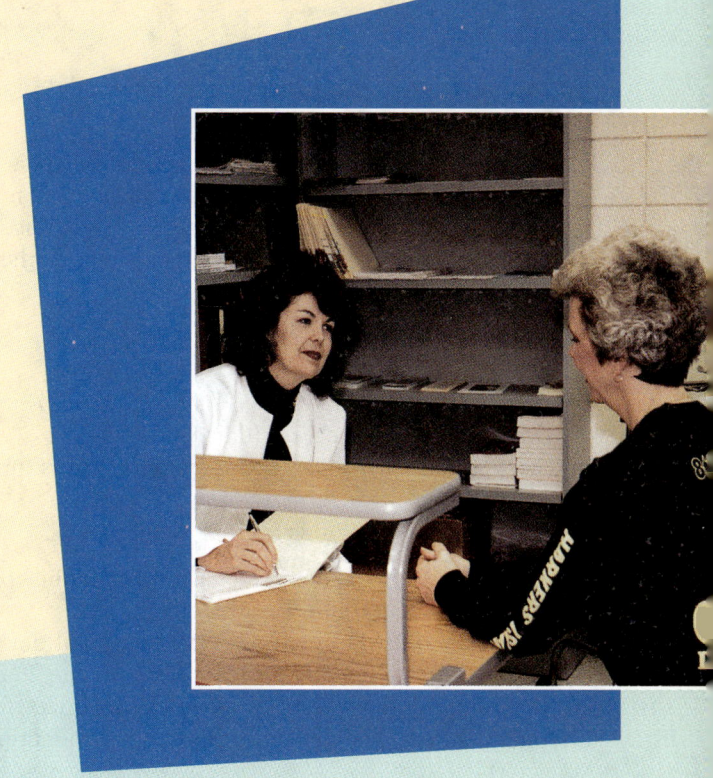

A number of factors can influence the health of your patients. By understanding what these factors are and how to handle them, patients can work toward achieving optimum health. The range of potential teaching topics is varied; the selected topics discussed here are those that medical assistants may frequently need to address including nutrition, exercise, illness and stress, substance abuse, and medication therapy.

➤ TEACHING PATIENTS ABOUT NUTRITION

Patients seen in the medical office have numerous reasons for being concerned about their **nutrition**. Nutrition is not only what people eat, but how the body uses the food it ingests to maintain and repair itself. The need for education about nutrition is a concern for everyone, not just people who are ill. People who care about healthy eating often turn to the medical profession to sort out the large amount of media "hype" pertaining to diet that bombards them each day. Whether the information pertains to "fast food" to keep up with the fast pace of life, or fad diets to keep thin, the media should not be the only source of guidelines for your patients. Materials are available to help you instruct patients on healthy eating.

The Food Guide Pyramid

In 1992, the U.S. Department of Agriculture updated its basic food group system and changed to the new Food Guide Pyramid (Fig. 6-1). The pyramid consists of five main food group categories and one "other" category. These categories are:

1. Bread, cereal, grains, and pasta
2. Vegetables
3. Fruits
4. Milk, yogurt, and cheese (dairy)
5. Meat, poultry, fish, dry beans, eggs, and nuts (protein)
6. Fats, oils, sweets (other)

This pyramid is a good reference for anyone concerned about maintaining a healthy diet.

Also in 1992, the National Dairy Council developed a nutritional guide to complement the Food Guide Pyramid (Fig. 6-2). It stresses the fact that anyone can eat healthy by following two simple steps:

1. Eat food from all five food groups every day.
2. Eat different foods from each food group every day.

This guide also takes the pyramid one step further by showing pictures of the types of foods that are acceptable in each category and listing the number of servings of each group the patient should eat. It assists in clarifying the "other" category because it shows pictures of foods almost everyone loves to eat, but should only eat in moderation. Using this guide, patients should have no doubts about which foods fall into each category.

Checkpoint Question
1. What are the five main food groups?

Dietary Guidelines

The U.S. Department of Agriculture and U.S. Department of Health and Human Services also have guidelines that are intended to improve our diets. Their recommendations are:

1. Eat a variety of foods from each of the five food groups.
2. Maintain a healthy weight by balancing the food you eat with physical activity.
3. Choose a diet low in fat, saturated fat, and cholesterol.
4. Choose a diet with plenty of vegetables, fruits, and grain products.
5. Use sugar and salt (sodium) in moderation.
6. Drink alcoholic beverages in moderation.

If your patient has no health concerns and is interested in preparing healthy meals at home, a pamphlet entitled *Dietary Guidelines for Americans* as well as other useful information on diets can be acquired at local public health offices. Encourage patients to read the labels on food containers; these labels provide important information on the nutritional value of the food, specific ingredients used, or any additives. After discussing healthy foods, give patients information about healthy food preparation. Instead of frying, encourage patients to broil, boil, bake, roast, or grill. Doing this will help reduce the amount of grease and oil that patients consume.

If an appropriately balanced diet is maintained, adequate vitamins and minerals will be included in the foods consumed. Tables 6-1 and 6-2 list minerals and vitamins needed to sustain body functions.

text continues on page 86

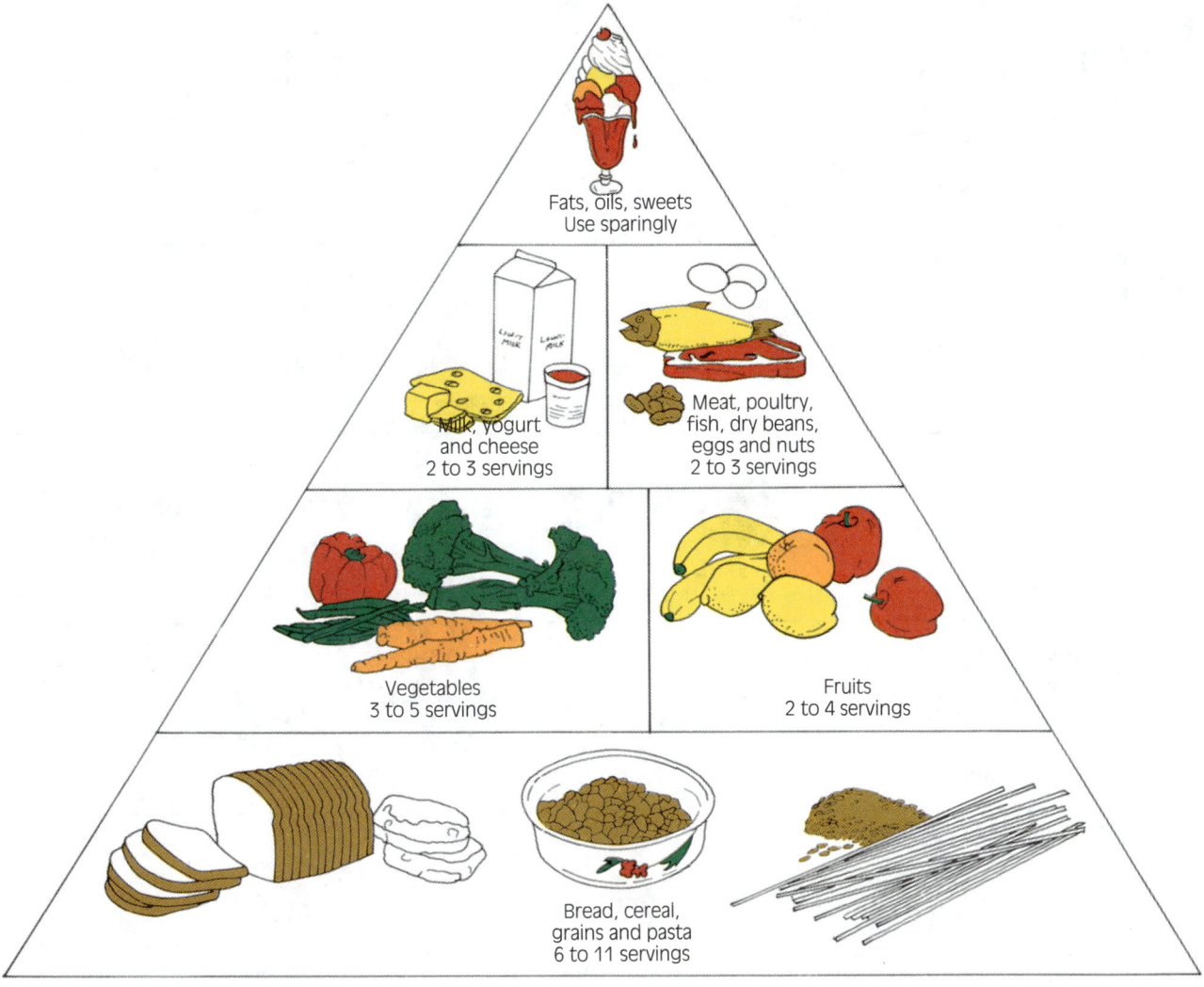

What Counts as 1 Serving?

The amount of food that counts as 1 serving is listed below. If you eat a larger portion, count it as more than 1 serving. For example, a dinner portion of spaghetti would count as 2 or 3 servings of pasta.

Be sure to eat at least the lowest number of servings from the five major food groups listed below. You need them for the vitamins, minerals, carbohydrates, and protein they provide. Just try to pick the lowest fat choices from the food groups. No specific serving size is given for the fats, oils, and sweets group because the message is USE SPARINGLY.

Food Groups

Milk, Yogurt, and Cheese

1 cup of milk or yogurt	1½ ounces of natural cheese	2 ounces of process cheese

Meat, Poultry, Fish, Dry Beans, Eggs, and Nuts

2–3 ounces of cooked lean meat, poultry, or fish	½ cup of cooked dry beans, 1 egg, or 2 tablespoons of peanut butter count as 1 ounce of lean meat

Vegetable

1 cup of raw leafy vegetables	½ cup of other vegetables, cooked or chopped raw	¾ cup of vegetable juice

Fruit

1 medium apple, banana, orange	½ cup of chopped or cooked, or canned fruit	¾ cup of fruit juice

Bread, Cereal, Rice, and Pasta

1 slice of bread	1 ounce of ready-to-eat cereal	½ cup of cooked cereal, rice, or pasta

FIGURE 6-1

The Food Guide Pyramid emphasizes food from the five major food groups shown in the three lower sections of the pyramid. Each of these food groups provides some, but not all, of the nutrients you need. Foods in one group cannot replace those in another. None of these major food groups is more important than another. (Source: U.S. Department of Agriculture/U.S. Department of Health and Human Services.)

GUIDE TO GOOD EATING

Anyone can eat for good health. Just follow these 2 simple steps:

1. *Eat foods from all Five Food Groups every day.* Each food group provides you with different nutrients.

2. *Eat different foods from each food group every day.* Some foods in a food group are better sources of a nutrient than others. By eating several foods from each food group, you increase your chance of getting all the nutrients you need.

Every day eat: | *Suggested Serving Sizes*

MILK
Group for calcium

2-4 servings*

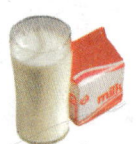 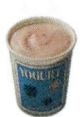  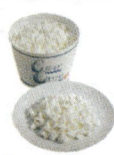 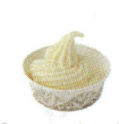

| Milk 1 cup | Yogurt 1 cup | Cheese 1½ – 2 oz | Cottage cheese ½ cup | Ice cream, ice milk, frozen yogurt ½ cup |

MEAT
Group for iron

2-3 servings

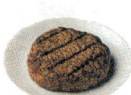 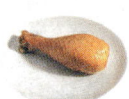 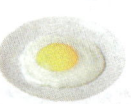 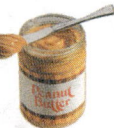 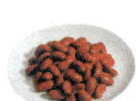

| Cooked, lean meat 2-3 oz | Cooked, lean poultry, fish 2-3 oz | Egg 1 | Peanut butter 2 tbsp | Cooked, dried peas, dried beans ½ cup |

VEGETABLE
Group for vitamin A

3-5 servings

 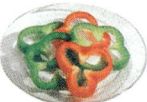 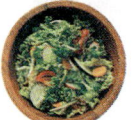 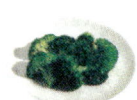 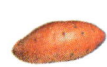

| Juice ¾ cup | Raw vegetable ½ cup | Raw leafy vegetable 1 cup | Cooked vegetable ½ cup | Potato 1 medium |

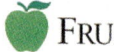

FRUIT
Group for vitamin C

2-4 servings

 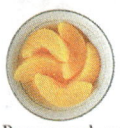 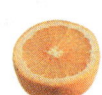 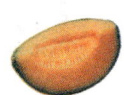

| Juice ¾ cup | Raw, canned, or cooked fruit ½ cup | Apple, banana, orange, pear 1 medium | Grapefruit ½ | Cantaloupe ¼ |

GRAIN
Group for fiber

6-11 servings

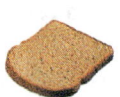 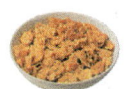 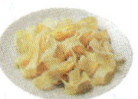 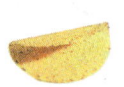

| Bread 1 slice | English muffin, hamburger bun ½ | Ready-to-eat cereal 1 oz | Pasta, rice, grits, cooked cereal ½ cup | Tortilla, roll, muffin 1 |

Some foods don't have enough nutrients to fit in any of the Five Food Groups. These foods are called "Others." These foods are okay to eat in moderation. They should not replace foods from the Five Food Groups.

USDA recommends 2–3 servings of Milk Group foods. Four servings are recommended on the Guide to Good Eating for teens, adults under 25 years of age, and pregnant and lactating women due to their higher needs for calcium.

"OTHERS"
Category

Fats and oils, sweets, salty snacks, alcohol, other beverages, and condiments

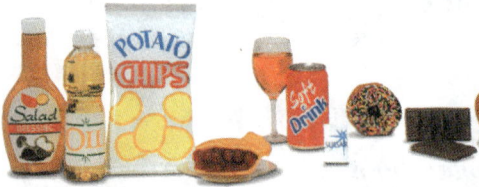

 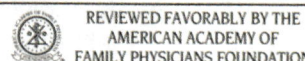

REVIEWED FAVORABLY BY THE AMERICAN ACADEMY OF FAMILY PHYSICIANS FOUNDATION

FIGURE 6-2
Guide to Good Eating from the National Dairy Council

Table 6-1

Common Minerals Needed by the Body, Their Chief Functions, and Dietary Sources

Mineral	Chief Functions	Common Dietary Sources
Sodium	Maintenance of water and electrolyte balance	Table salt Processed meat
Potassium	Maintenance of electrolyte balance Neuromuscular activity Enzyme reactions	Bananas Oranges Potatoes
Chloride	Maintenance of fluid and electrolyte balance	Table salt Processed meat
Calcium	Formation of teeth and bones Neuromuscular activity Blood coagulation Cell wall permeability	Milk Milk products
Phosphorus	Buffering action Formation of bones and teeth	Eggs Meat Milk
Iodine	Regulation of body metabolism Promotion of normal growth	Seafoods Iodized salt
Iron	Component of hemoglobin Assistance in cellular oxidation	Liver Egg yolk Meat
Magnesium	Neuromuscular activity Activation of enzymes Formation of teeth and bones	Whole grains Milk Meat
Zinc	Constituent of enzymes and insulin	Seafoods Liver

From Timby, B. K. (1996). Fundamental Skills and Concepts in Patient Care, 6th ed., p. 230. Philadelphia: Lippincott-Raven Publishers.

Patient Education: Diet and the Diabetic Patient

For diet education to be effective, the patient must understand that diet, medications, and the body are all interdependent. Any changes in diet or medication could have a serious effect on the disease process. Because food intake needs to match the body's ability to metabolize carbohydrates and other nutrients, the patient may need to weigh food to comply with the prescribed diet. You may be responsible for instructing the patient about the correct methods for weighing and measuring prescribed amounts of food.

The American Diabetes Association has developed a standard diet model for diabetic patients to follow. It divides the food into groups that are similar to those of the pyramid system: vegetables, fruit, bread, meat, fat, and milk. These groups are called ex-

changes because they allow the patient to choose from a variety of foods in each category. The exchange list allows patients to easily determine accurate intake requirements for the calories, proteins, and fats ordered by the physician. The patient must be told how to use the food exchange groups to prepare a daily menu. Using the exchange list, an example of a planned meal for a diabetic patient may include: 2-vegetable, 2-fruit, 3-bread, 2-fat, and 2-meat exchanges.

You must stress that only foods appearing on the exchange lists should be eaten. Because the diet is prescribed to coincide with the medications that are taken, meals should not be missed and the entire serving must be eaten to avoid an insulin–glucose imbalance.

Table 6-2

Common Vitamins Needed by the Body, Their Chief Functions, and Common Dietary Sources

Vitamin	Chief Functions	Common Dietary Sources

A (Retinol)
  Not destroyed by
  ordinary cooking
  temperatures
	Growth of body cells
	Promotion of vision, healthy hair and skin, and integrity of
	  epithelial membranes
	Prevention of xerophthalmia, a condition characterized by
	  chronic conjunctivities
		Animal fats: butter, cheese, cream,
		  egg yolk, whole milk
		Fish liver oil and liver
		Green leafy and yellow fruits and
		  vegetables

B₁ (Thiamine)
  Not readily destroyed
  by ordinary cooking
  temperatures
	Carbohydrate metabolism
	Functioning of nervous system
	Normal digestion
	Prevention of beriberi, a condition characterized by
	  neurologic involvement
		Fish
		Lean meat and poultry
		Glandular organs
		Milk
		Whole grain cereals
		Peas, beans, and peanuts

B₂ (Riboflavin)
  Not destroyed by heat
  except in presence of
  alkali
	Formation of certain enzymes
	Normal growth
	Light adaptation in the eyes
		Eggs
		Green leafy vegetables
		Lean meat
		Milk
		Whole grains
		Dried yeast

B₃ (Niacin)	Carbohydrate, fat, and protein metabolism Enzyme component Prevention of appetite loss Prevention of pellagra, a condition characterized by cutaneous, gastrointestinal, neurologic, and mental symptoms	Lean meat and liver Fish Peas, beans Whole grain cereals Peanuts Yeast Eggs Liver

B₆ (Pyridoxine)
  Destroyed by heat,
  sunlight, and air
	Healthy gums and teeth
	Red blood cell formation
	Carbohydrate, fat, and protein metabolism
		Whole grain cereals and wheat
		  germ
		Vegetables
		Yeast
		Meat
		Bananas
		Black strap molasses

B₉ (Folic acid)	Protein metabolism Red blood cell formation Normal intestinal-tract functioning	Green leafy vegetables Glandular organs Yeast
B₁₂ (Cyanocobalamin)	Protein metabolism Red blood cell formation Healthy nervous system tissues Prevention of pernicious anemia, a condition characterized by decreased red blood cells	Liver and kidney Dairy products Lean meat Milk Saltwater fish and oysters

(continued)

Physician-Ordered Diets

The majority of time spent on nutritional education will probably be for patients who need to be instructed regarding new or modified diets. Table 6-3 shows examples of modified diets commonly prescribed by the physician. Your role is to clarify the information provided about each diet and to help the patient construct a workable meal schedule.

As with any patient teaching, many factors must be considered before sending the patient home with a preprinted diet form. Be aware that the patient's age, culture, religion, geographic background, and social and financial circumstances may all play a part in whether or not the patient has difficulties complying with the diet modification. (Table 6-4 presents a discussion of cultural variations on nutrition.) If necessary, the physician may refer the patient to a dietitian or someone more skilled in assisting with the nutritional needs of individuals on modified diets. Remember to check your patient's progress during each return visit.

Table 6-2

Common Vitamins Needed by the Body, Their Chief Functions, and Common Dietary Sources (continued)

Vitamin	Chief Functions	Common Dietary Sources

C (Ascorbic acid)
  Readily destroyed
  by cooking tempera-
  tures
	Healthy bones, teeth, and gums
	Formation of blood vessels and capillary walls
	Proper tissue and bone healing
	Facilitation of iron and folic acid absorption
	Prevention of scurvy, a condition characterized by hemor-
	  rhagic condition and abnormal bone and teeth formation
		Citrus fruits and juices
		Tomato
		Berries
		Cabbage
		Green vegetables
		Potatoes

D (Calciferol)
  Relatively stable
  with refrigeration
	Absorption of calcium and phosphorus
	Prevention of rickets, a condition characterized by weak
	  bones
		Fish liver oils, salmon, tuna
		Milk
		Egg yolk
		Butter
		Liver
		Oysters
		Formed in the skin by exposure to sunlight

E (α-Tocopherol)
  Heat stable in ab-
  sence of oxygen
	Red blood cell formation
	Protection of essential fatty acids
	Important for normal reproduction in experimental animals
	  (*i.e.*, rats)
		Green leafy vegetables
		Wheat germ oil
		Margarine
		Brown rice

Pantothenic acid	Metabolism	Liver Egg yolk Milk
H (Biotin) Heat sensitive	Enzyme activity Metabolism of carbohydrates, fats, and proteins	Egg yolk Green vegetables Milk Liver and kidney Yeast
K (Menadione)	Production of prothrombin	Liver Eggs Green leafy vegetables Synthesized in the gastrointestinal tract by bacteria

From Timby, B. K. (1996). Fundamental Skills and Concepts in Patient Care, *6th ed., p. 231–232.* Philadelphia: Lippincott-Raven Publishers.

Table 6-3

Examples of Physician-Ordered Modified Diets

Name of Diet Ordered	Reason Ordered
Soft diet	Difficulties chewing
Clear diet	Preparation for tests, acute diarrhea
Full liquid	Recovery from procedures, recovery from diarrhea
Low calorie	Weight reduction
Restricted carbohydrate	Weight reduction
High carbohydrate	Liver and gallbladder disease
High fiber	Constipation
BRAT (bananas, rice, applesauce, and toast)	Pediatric patients with gastrointestinal disturbances
Low fat	Weight reduction, gallbladder disease, gastrointestinal disturbances
Restricted sodium	Cardiac, liver, pancreas, and gallbladder disease

Table 6-4
Cultural Variations on Nutrition

Culture	Milk	Meat	Bread and Cereals	Fruits and Vegetables	Additional Variations
Italian	Seldom use milk; cheese is calcium source	Chicken, beef, veal, fish—baked, simmered, or browned in olive oil	Bread and pasta basic foods	Squash, tomatoes, salad; fruit used as dessert	Drink red or white wine with dinner; use garlic for seasoning
Chinese	Use little milk or cheese	Pork, lamb, chicken, fish—cooked in combination with vegetables	Rice with most meals	Cabbage, snow peas, squashes, mushrooms; fruit usually eaten fresh	Fresh foods prepared by stir-frying; unsweetened green tea
Japanese	Little milk or cheese	Seafood main protein source, especially raw fish	Rice is basic grain; white and wheat bread being increasingly used	Steamed and served with soy sauce; tray of fruit served at main meal	Soy sauce main seasoning; soybean oil main cooking fat; traditionally, dinners follow specific sequence of courses; tea is main beverage
Greek	Little milk; yogurt popular; cheese a favorite food	Lamb favorite meat; little beef eaten	Bread center of every meal; rice commonly served	Large amounts of vegetables, cooked and seasoned, preferably fresh; large quantities of fresh fruit	Meal is family ritual; holidays are special occasions with great variety of foods
Puerto Rican	Little milk	Most cannot afford meat; may use dried codfish; legumes good protein source	Rice	Almost all eat viandas, which are starchy vegetables and fruits, such as plantain and green bananas; other fruits and vegetables used in limited quantity	Simple daily diet that contrasts with holiday meal; economy major factor in food selection
Mexican	Little milk	Little meat used	Corn basic grain used in bread and cereal; oatmeal popular cereal	Corn, fresh or canned, and chili peppers; fruit use depends on availability	Drink large amounts of coffee; common seasonings chili pepper, onions, and garlic; lard basic cooking fat
African American	Low intake of milk and dairy foods	Diet usually high in protein; favorite meats pork and chicken; most meats fried or barbecued	Sweet potatoes and hominy grits	High intake of dark, leafy green vegetables; fruits used in limited quantity	Diet high in fat and sodium because of methods of preparation

From Taylor, C., Lillis, C., & LeMone, P., (1989) Fundamentals of Nursing, *2nd ed., p. 812. Philadelphia: J. B. Lippincott.*

Your patients may want to try many of the fad diets, but patients need to be educated in the potential dangers of these diets. Some of these diet plans can produce cardiac, renal, and digestive complications. Patients who want to lose weight should be instructed about eating regular, small, balanced meals; counting calories; monitoring fat intake; and reading food package labels. Patients must also be taught that diet modification alone will not result in a significant long-term weight loss; regular exercise must also be included in any weight reduction plan.

➤ TEACHING PATIENTS ABOUT EXERCISE

Exercise is defined as performed activity of the muscles, voluntary or otherwise, to maintain fitness. It is beneficial to the body for several reasons. If done in moderation until endurance levels are reached, exercise can help relieve stress, maintain healthy body weight, and increase circulation and muscle tone. All patients should actively participate in some form of exercise daily. Box 6-1 describes the benefits of exercise, and Box 6-2 discusses various types of exercise.

Patients who are under age 35 and in good health usually do not need a medical clearance before starting a routine exercise program. However, a physician con-

---

BOX 6-1 Benefits of Regular Exercise

Benefits of a regular program of exercise include:

- Weight reduction
- Improved cardiac and pulmonary function
- Restored motion, function, and strength after a musculoskeletal surgery or injury or after neurologic damage
- A feeling of well-being and increased self-esteem
- Improved rest and sleep patterns
- Stress reduction
- Increased energy
- More manageable diabetes

BOX 6-2 Types of Exercise

An effective exercise program incorporates elements of body alignment, posture, balance, coordination, and endurance. For maximum benefits, programs should be performed at least three times a week for a sustained 30-minute period to increase the heart rate. A warm up and a cool down period should be included. At no time should you exercise through pain or fatigue; these are the body's warning signs. Cross-training, with various methods that are enjoyable and challenging, is more likely to result in the achievement of long-term exercise goals than trying to perform difficult routines that are not fun. Many beneficial programs are available through health clubs and personal trainers approved by the physician.

- Aerobics: Vigorous, continuous motion such as dancing, running, cycling, rapid walking
- Anaerobic: Short-term use of stored oxygen; used for strength and endurance training such as weight lifting
- Isotonic: Constant muscle tension and contraction; many aerobic movements are isotonic.
- Isometric: Muscle tension changes but no movement or change in the length occurs, as in pressing the palms of the hands together
- Stretching: Gentle stretching of the muscle fibers through range of motion; yoga is an example

---

sultation is recommended for patients age 35 or older who have not been active in several years. Patients with known medical disorders (eg, hypertension, cardiovascular problems, or a family history of stroke) should first check with the physician before exercising.

The American Heart Association (AHA) offers patient education information on exercise. The AHA has numerous, frequently updated pamphlets available on various exercise activities and programs such as swimming, running, jogging, walking, and biking. Each pamphlet covers the following information:

- Benefits of the specific exercise
- How to get started
- How to choose a time to exercise
- How to choose a partner
- What clothing is best suited for the exercise
- How to warm up
- What a target heart rate zone is and how to achieve it

Table 6-5
Calorie Use Chart for Exercise

Activity	75-lb Person	100-lb Person	150-lb Person
Walking, 2 mph	125	160	240
Walking, 3 mph	175	210	320
Walking, 4½ mph	245	295	440
Jogging, 5½ mph	365	440	740
Jogging, 7 mph	510	610	920
Swimming 25 yd/min/h	155	185	275
Swimming 50 yd/min/h	270	325	500

Adapted from calorie use charts in patient teaching materials provided by the American Heart Association.

- Training program
- Calories used (Table 6-5)
- Checklist (a review of highlights from all of the above topics)

After being cleared by the physician (if needed), patients should be able to take the information learned in the AHA pamphlets and continue exercising on their own.

If patients are unable to perform exercises without assistance, it may be necessary to instruct them or their family members on range-of-motion (ROM) exercises. To perform ROM exercises, the patient moves the affected limb and joint through all of the movements that the joint is capable of making, until resistance is met. (See Chap. 31, Caring for the Patient With Musculoskeletal Disorders, for more information.) In most cases, ROM exercises are ordered by the physician to prevent further loss of motion or disfigurement after a musculoskeletal injury, surgery, or neurologic damage.

When a stroke or other type of paralyzing injury is involved, ROM exercises are performed several times a day on each involved joint. If the patient is unable to perform the exercise on the affected area, passive ROM is performed. This requires someone else to perform the exercises on the patient. You can instruct family members to do these exercises. Remember, ROM exercises are needed to promote circulation and maintain muscle tone. If not performed as ordered, the patient may not be able to regain use of the affected area.

? Checkpoint Question

2. What are the four benefits of exercise? What is the specific purpose of passive ROM exercises?

➤ TEACHING PATIENTS TO COPE WITH ILLNESS AND STRESS

During a lifetime, almost everyone is affected by some type of illness or injury. Along with this often comes stress. Stress is defined as forces such as fear, anxiety, crises, and joy. When faced with illness or injury, a patient usually must confront:

- Physical and psychological pain
- Inability to perform self-care
- Stress of treatments, procedures, and possible hospitalization
- Changes in role identity and self-image
- Loss of control and independence
- Changes in relationships with friends and family

Patients with chronic conditions may need more time to adjust than patients with acute illnesses. If patients are able to deal with the factors listed above, they are more likely to adapt and adjust to life-style changes.

Many other causes besides illness or injury can place patients under stress. The best way to cope is living a healthy life-style. When the body is healthy, it can handle stress more easily. Unfortunately, most of the same reasons that hinder learning (see Chap. 5, Patient Education) are the same factors that hinder patients' ability to comply with patient education. Patients who are not capable of coping with stress on their own or with the help of instruction provided by the medical office may need professional counseling.

Positive and Negative Stress

Two types of stress affect all of us daily: **positive stress** and **negative stress**. Positive stress allows individuals to work efficiently and perform to the best of their abilities. Examples of positive stress include working on a challenging new job or assignment, getting married, or giving a speech or performance. In fact, many people work best when under positive stress. Once the job (or wedding) is over, though, time must be taken to relax and prepare for the next project. If relaxation techniques are not incorporated into the daily routine, positive stress can become negative stress.

Negative stress is the inability to relax after a stressful encounter. Left unchecked, it can lead to physiologic responses such as:

- Headache
- Upset stomach
- Sweating palms
- Rapid heart rate

Long-term physical effects of unrelieved stress include increases in blood pressure, glucose levels, metabolism, intraocular pressure, and finally exhaustion. If the stress is not relieved, patients will progress to higher anxiety levels requiring all of their energy and attention to focus solely on the problem at hand. Most mental and physical activity will be directed at relief of the stress to avoid the ultimate anxiety level known as panic—a sudden, overwhelming state of anxiety or terror.

Most people have developed methods of alleviating intense stressors called **coping mechanisms**, which are usually beyond our conscious ability to direct. Coping mechanisms are our psychological defense against unpleasant situations. Common coping mechanisms are listed and explained in Table 6-6.

It may be difficult to escape completely from stress-causing factors, but management of them is possible. For a patient suffering from the physiologic affects of negative stress, you can offer the following coping strategies:

- Attempt to reduce irritants, but do not try to make the thing perfect (perfectionism adds its own stress).
- Organize and limit as many activities as possible.
- Try to lessen your fear of failure and just do the best you can.
- When feeling anxious, talk to someone about the problem and "let off steam."

Any one of these tips may help patients to regain control over stressors.

 Checkpoint Question
3. What are eight physiologic effects of negative stress?

Table 6-6
Common Coping Mechanisms

Coping Mechanism	Definition	Example
Repression	Forgetting about situations that produced stress	Being unable to remember the circumstances of a tragic traffic accident
Denial	Refusing to believe information	Not accepting a diagnosis despite medical evidence
Rationalization	Minimizing a disappointment by finding something positive in the outcome	Believing that it was better to have been passed over for a job promotion because the raise would have placed one in a higher tax bracket
Compensation	Redirecting a desire for something unobtainable into efforts toward achieving or acquiring something similar	Being unsuited to be a great athlete and becoming a sports journalist instead
Displacement	Redirecting anger toward one person onto an object or different person	Kicking a wastebasket after being criticized by a supervisor at work

From Timby, B. K., Lewis, L. W. (1992). Fundamental Skills and Concepts in Patient Care, 5th ed., p. 25. Philadelphia: J. B. Lippincott.

Relaxation Techniques

Several types of relaxation techniques are available to patients. To determine what works best for them, they must first consider the time available and the type of relaxation needed. Five examples of relaxation techniques follow.

Relieving Muscle Tension

Stretching is the most common way to relieve muscle tension. Think about it: If you have been sitting and reading for a long period of time, the first thing you may need to do when taking a break is stretch. Stretching exercises can be performed for the neck, shoulders, back, arms, upper body, and legs. Stretching exercises take only a few minutes and can be performed during break or lunch periods. These can be as simple as reaching high overhead and stretching through the body or as involved and choreographed as yoga. Many sources of stretching exercises are available through bookstores and libraries.

Breathing Techniques

Breathing exercises can be done anywhere. Most people are shallow breathers and need to be instructed on deep-breathing techniques. To perform these breathing exercises, the patient should sit up straight with hands placed on the stomach. The patient then takes a deep breath in through the nose, feeling the hands being pushed away by the stomach. (This may feel awkward because most people do just the opposite.) The patient holds his breath for a few seconds, then exhales through pursed lips as the hands are felt being pulled in. Doing this allows for better control of the exhalation rate. Sometimes getting the oxygen flowing through the body at a faster rate is all that is needed to relieve boredom, tension, and stress.

Visualization

Visualization is a relaxation technique that involves allowing the mind to wander and the imagination to run free and focus on positive and relaxing situations. It is similar to daydreaming. It can "remove" the patient from a stressful situation and put him in a place where, if nothing else, the mind can relax. Remind the patient that it is important to choose appropriate times for this daydreaming technique. For example, it would be dangerous to use this technique when driving a car or operating heavy equipment.

Clearing the Mind (Meditation)

This technique involves setting aside 5 to 10 minutes each day with no interruptions. To do this, the patient should find a comfortable location to sit, close their eyes, then take a few deep breaths. The mind should focus on one peaceful word, thought, or image. Encourage the patient to avoid having other thoughts during this time. When the allotted time is finished, the patient should stretch, exhale, and feel more refreshed.

Physical Exercise

There is no better tranquilizer than physical exercise. Most people who exercise regularly say that it helps them reduce tension and relax and rest better at night. See the section "Teaching Patients About Exercise," above.

Checkpoint Question

4. *What are five relaxation techniques? Briefly describe each.*

➤ TEACHING PATIENTS ABOUT SUBSTANCE ABUSE

Substance abuse is excessive use of and dependency on drugs. Some abused substances are legal (eg, alcohol, nicotine), whereas others are illegal (eg, marijuana, cocaine). Initial teaching contact with patients affected by commonly abused substances is usually made by trained specialists or counselors. Following is a partial discussion of abused drugs and some of the consequences of using them. Substance abuse can be highly detrimental to your patients' health, so it is important that you give them information about substance abuse if they should ask.

Alcohol is the most frequently abused drug in our society. Alcohol is chemically classified as a mind-altering substance because it contains ethanol and the chemical power to depress the action of the central nervous system. This depression affects motor coordination, speech, and vision. In large amounts, alcohol can affect respiration and heart rate control. Death can result when the level of blood alcohol exceeds 0.40% Prolonged abuse of alcohol can lead to alcoholism, malnutrition, and cirrhosis of the liver.

Nicotine is highly addictive, whether ingested by smoking or chewing. This drug reaches the brain in 6 seconds, damages the lungs, decreases heart strength, and is associated with many cancers. The withdrawal

Table 6-7
Commonly Abused Drugs: Uses and Effects

Drug	Street Name (Trade Name)	Route of Ingestion	Duration of Effect (h)	Effects
Stimulants				
Cocaine	Coke, crack, snow, flake	Nasal, oral, IV, smoked	1–2	Anesthesia, euphoria, confusion, depression, convulsions, cardiotoxicity
Amphetamine	Bennies, dexies, uppers	Oral, IV	2–4	Insomnia, anorexia, euphoria, tolerance and dependence, paranoid psychosis
Methamphetamine	Meth, speed, crystal	Oral, IV	2–4	Euphoria, agitation, psychosis, depression, exhaustion
Narcotics				
Heroin	Horse, smack, white lady, scag	IV, nasal, smoked	3–6	Euphoria, drowsiness, respiratory depression, convulsions, coma
Codeine		Oral, IV, IM	3–6	Sedation, convulsions, respiratory failure
Morphine	Junk, white stuff, morpho, M	IV, IM, oral, smoked	3–6	Analgesia, euphoria, nausea, respiratory coma
Methadone	Methadose	Oral, IV, IM	12–24	Analgesia, sedation, respiratory depression, coma
Meperidine	(Demerol)	IV, oral	3–6	Analgesia, stupor, respiratory depression, hypotension, coma
Propoxyphene	Yellow footballs (Darvon)	Oral	1–6	Analgesia, stupor, respiratory depression, coma
Hallucinogens				
Phencyclidine (PCP)	PCP, angel dust, hog, killer weed	IV, oral, nasal, smoked	2–4; psychoses may last weeks	Dissociative anesthesia, depression, psychosis, stupor, coma, seizures
LSD	Acid, LSD-25, white lightning, microdots	Oral	8–12	Hallucinations, flashbacks, psychosis, vomiting, paralysis, respiratory depression
Marijuana, hashish	Pot, THC, mary jane, grass, hash	Oral, smoked, IV	2–4	Altered perception, memory loss, disorientation, psychosis
Benzodiazepines				
Chlordiazepoxide	(Librium)	Oral, IM	4–8	Drowsiness, muscle relaxation, coma
Diazepam	(Valium)	Oral, IV, IM	4–8	Drowsiness, dizziness, muscle relaxation
Sedatives/ Depressants				
Pentobarbital	Yellow, nembies, yellow jackets	Oral, IV, IM	3–6	Sedation, respiratory collapse
Amobarbital	Rainbows, blues, bluebirds	Oral, IV, IM	3–24	Exhilaration, sedation, disorientation, respiratory depression, coma
Secobarbital	Reds, seccies, red devils, M & M's	Oral, IV, IM	3–6	Sedation, lethargy, coma, respiratory collapse
Ethanol		Oral	2–6	Slurred speech, loss of equilibrium, drowsiness, coma, respiratory collapse
Methaqualone	Ludes, soapers	Oral	4–8	Sedation, dizziness, paresthesias, convulsions, respiratory and circulatory depression
Chloral hydrate	Joy juice	Oral, rectal	5–8	Sedation, GI distress, hypotension, respiratory depression

Adapted from Bishop, M. L., Duben-Engel Kirk, J. L., & Fody, E. D. (1996). *Clinical Chemistry,* 3rd ed., pp. 709–710. Philadelphia: Lippincott-Raven.

symptoms include anxiety, progressive restlessness, irritability, and sleep disturbance.

Marijuana and *hashish* impair the short-term memory and comprehension of the user. They alter the sense of time and reduce the ability of the user to perform tasks requiring concentration and coordination. They also increase the heart rate and appetite. Long-term users may develop psychological dependence that can produce paranoia and psychosis. Because these drugs are inhaled as unfiltered smoke, users intake more cancer-causing agents and experience more damage to the respiratory system than from regular, filtered tobacco smoke.

Cocaine and *crack cocaine* stimulate the central nervous system and are extremely addictive. "Crack" cocaine is particularly dangerous because this pure form of cocaine is usually smoked and absorbed rapidly in the bloodstream and can cause sudden death. Use of cocaine can cause psychological and physical dependency. Side effects include dilated pupils, increased pulse rate, elevated blood pressure, insomnia, loss of appetite, paranoia, and seizures. It can also cause death by disrupting the brain's control of the heart and respiration.

Stimulants and *amphetamines* can have the same effect as cocaine, causing increased heart rate and blood pressure that can result in stroke or heart failure. Symptoms include dizziness, sleeplessness, and anxiety; these substances and can cause psychosis, hallucinations, paranoia, and even a physical collapse.

Depressants and *barbiturates* can cause physical and psychological dependence. Abuse of these drugs can lead to respiratory depression, coma, and death, especially when used simultaneously with alcohol. Withdrawal can lead to restlessness, insomnia, convulsions, and death.

Hallucinogens such as lysergic acid diethylamide (LSD), phencyclidine (Angel dust or PCP), mescaline, and peyote all interrupt brain messages that control the intellect and keep instincts in check. Large doses can produce seizures, coma, and heart and lung failure. Chronic users complain of persistent memory problems and speech difficulties for up to a year after discontinued use. Because hallucinogens stop the brain's pain sensors, drug experiences may result in severe self-inflicted injuries.

Narcotics such as heroin, codeine, morphine, and opium are addictive drugs. An overdose, which is likely with increased dependence, can lead to seizures, coma, and death.

Table 6-7 lists the medical uses and effects of controlled substances. You and your patients who are substance abusers need to be aware of this information.

? Checkpoint Question
5. What are nine commonly abused substances?

➤ TEACHING PATIENTS ABOUT MEDICATION THERAPY

With the number of medication therapies available to patients increasing daily, patient teaching possibilities in this area are virtually endless. Pharmaceutical companies offer in-depth medication information for health care providers concerning the chemical makeup of the drug, physiologic reactions in the body, prescribed dosage and route, and possible side effects. However, information provided by these companies specifically for patient education is limited. If this information is not available, the patient may not understand the importance of the medication therapy and this could lead to noncompliance. You may be responsible for gathering the information needed and preparing teaching materials for your patients to help prevent noncompliance.

When preparing a medication therapy teaching tool, you must consider such factors as the patient's financial abilities, social or cultural demands, physical disabilities, and age. Be sure to include the following information in any teaching:

- Medication name (generic/brand)
- Dosage
- Route
- What the medication is used for
- Why the medication needs to be taken as prescribed
- Normal changes in bodily functions (eg, colored urine)
- Possible side effects
- Other medications (including over-the-counter ones) that might interfere with the action of this medication
- Foods or liquids to be avoided
- Activities to be avoided
- Telephone number to call for any questions or concerns

Figure 6-3 shows an example of a medication therapy teaching tool that incorporates all of these elements.

After assessing the patient's knowledge base, you may find that scheduling is a prime concern. For example, the patient may be taking several types of medications and may need to schedule them at different times of the day or week. Before developing a medication schedule, evaluate the daily routine to see how adhering to the schedule may affect the patient's life-style. For instance, you might ask the patient:

- How long do you sleep each morning?
- What time do you go to bed?
- When do you usually eat?

Once you have collected this information, consider using a scheduling tool such as the one displayed in Figure 6-4.

Medication Therapy Teaching Tool

Trade name/Brand name: _____

Circle the one that applies:

Take by mouth	Apply to affected area	Drop into ear
Insert rectally	Place under tongue	Insert vaginally
Drop in eye	Other _____	

The dosage of this medication is:

This medication was ordered for you because:

It may cause:

You should not take this medication if:

If you notice any of the following, you should call Dr. Smith's office at 123-4567.

The above information has been explained to me and I understand the importance of following the prescribed treatment.

_____   _____
          (patient's signature)   (date)

_____
    (signature of person teaching patient)

FIGURE 6-3

Medication therapy teaching tool used for teaching patients about their medications.

Medication Schedule for the Week of _____

	Sunday	Monday	Tuesday	Wednesday	Thursday	Friday	Saturday
6:00							
7:00							
8:00							
9:00							
10:00							
11:00							
12:00							
1:00							
2:00							
3:00							
4:00							
5:00							
6:00							
7:00							
8:00							
9:00							
10:00							

FIGURE 6-4

Use this medication schedule form for patients who are taking multiple medications or having trouble remembering when to take their medications.

Another patient education area that falls under the category of medication therapy includes how to administer medications, whether orally, vaginally, rectally, etc. (see Chap. 26, Preparing and Administering Medications).

For more patient teaching information regarding safe and effective use of medications, you can contact the National Council on Patient Information and Education (NCPIE), a nonprofit organization, at 666 Eleventh Street, NW, Suite 810, Washington, DC 20001. NCPIE can provide you with literature and referrals to other sources.

SUMMARY

Patients can exert greater control over their well-being when they have the proper knowledge about healthy living. As a medical assistant, you may be responsible for teaching patients about ensuring proper nutrition, staying fit with exercise, dealing with illness and stress, understanding the effects of substance abuse, and adhering to a medication regimen. Your responsibility as a medical assistant is to be prepared with the pertinent teaching tools and to ensure that they are appropriate for each individual patient. This often means considering the patient's age, culture, religion, educational level, and social and financial circumstances.

CRITICAL THINKING CHALLENGES

1. Using the Medication Therapy Teaching Tool in Figure 6-3 and the *Physician's Desk Reference*, prepare a patient teaching tool for Peter Dorrance, a 75-year-old man suffering from congestive heart failure. Mr. Dorrance's physician has prescribed digoxin, one 0.25-mg tablet per day. Mr. Dorrance has no difficulty hearing, reading, or understanding English.

2. Create a patient education brochure about constipation. Consider the information in Figures 6-1 and 6-2 (Food Guide Pyramid and National Dairy Council recommendations). Refer back to Chapter 5, Patient Education, for tips on developing teaching tools.

3. Review the types of relaxation techniques. How can you implement these in the office setting to help relax your patients?

ANSWERS TO CHECKPOINT QUESTIONS

1. The five main food groups are: (1) bread, cereal, grains, and pasta; (2) vegetables; (3) fruits; (4) meat, poultry, fish, dry beans, and eggs; (5) milk, yogurt, and cheese.

2. Exercising will relieve stress, help maintain a healthy body weight, increase circulation, and promote muscle tone. Passive ROM exercises will prevent further loss of motion and dysfunction of an extremity.

3. Eight physiologic effects of negative stress include headache, upset stomach, sweaty palms, and elevations in heart rate, blood pressure, glucose levels, metabolism, and intraocular pressure.

4. Five relaxation techniques include relieving muscle tension (stretching), breathing deeply, visualizing (focusing on a positive and relaxing situation), meditating (focusing on one peaceful word, thought, or image for 5–10 minutes daily), and exercising.

5. Nine commonly abused substances include alcohol, nicotine, marijuana, hashish, cocaine, stimulants, depressants, hallucinogens, and narcotics.

SUGGESTIONS FOR FURTHER READING

Lecy, K. (1993). *Students' Right to Know: Alcohol and Other Drug Abuse, Sexual Assault and Harassment, and Campus Security and Crime*. Marshfield, WI: Mid-State Technical College.

Merkatz, R., & Coruig, M. P. (1992). Helping America take its medicine. *American Journal of Nursing*, (6), 58-62.

Redman, B. K. (1993). *The Process of Patient Education*. St. Louis: Mosby-Year Book.

U.S. Department of Agriculture and Health and Human Services. (1990). *Dietary Guidelines for Americans*. Washington, DC: Author.

U.S. Department of Health and Human Services, Public Health Service. (1995). *Healthy People 2000: Midcourse Review and 1995 Revisions*. Washington, DC: Author.

U.S. Department of Health and Human Services, Office of the Inspector General. (1990, June). *Medication Regimens: Causes of Non-Compliance*. Washington, DC: Author

The Administrative Medical Assistant

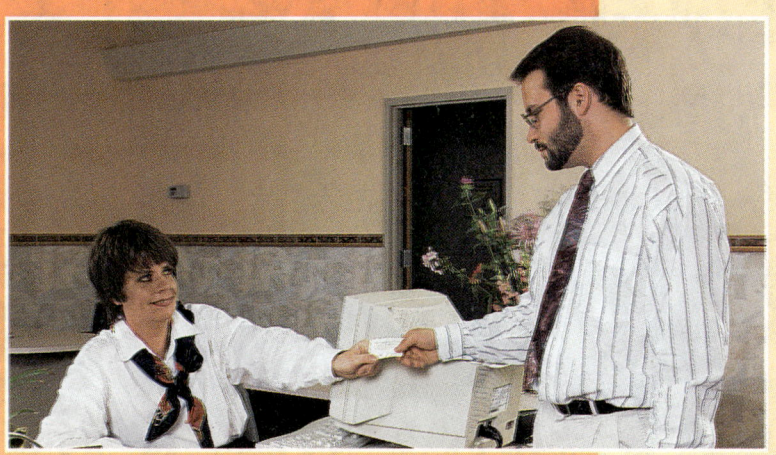

Unit 3

Performing Administrative Duties

A well-run medical office requires that all departments work to support the physician in the effort to deliver premium health care. Cooperation between the administrative and clinical areas is vital. From the first phone call, to the stocking of supplies and the coordination of office staff, teamwork and professionalism will ensure that progression through the office departments is smooth and reassuring to the patient.

The First Contact— Telephone and Reception

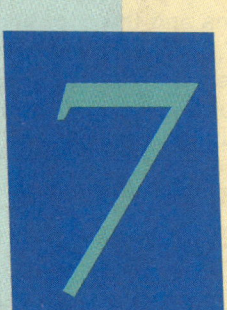

Chapter Outline

Professional Image
The Medical Assistant as an Attitude Transmitter
The Medical Assistant as a Role Model
Courtesy and Diplomacy in the Medical Office
First Impressions

Reception
Duties and Responsibilities of the Receptionist
The Reception Environment

The End of the Patient Visit
Telephone
Importance of the Telephone in the Medical Office
Basic Guidelines for Telephone Use
Incoming Calls
Outgoing Calls
Services and Special Features
Summary
Critical Thinking Challenges
Answers to Checkpoint Questions
Suggestions for Further Reading

DACUM Components

1.1 Project a positive attitude
1.4 Maintain confidentiality
1.5 Work as a team member
1.6 Conduct oneself in a courteous and diplomatic manner
1.7 Adapt to change
1.8 Show initiative and responsibility
2.1 Listen and observe
2.2 Treat all patients with empathy
2.3 Adapt communication to individuals' abilities to understand
2.4 Recognize and respond to verbal and nonverbal communication
2.5 Serve as liaison between physician and others
2.6 Evaluate understanding of communication
2.8 Use proper telephone technique
7.1 Orient patients to office polices and procedures

Chapter Competencies

Learning Objectives

Upon successfully completing this chapter, you will be able to:

1. Spell and define the key terms.
2. Discuss how the medical assistant influences the patient.
3. List seven duties of the medical office receptionist.
4. Discuss the basic guidelines for telephone use.
5. Describe the types of incoming telephone calls received by the medical office.
6. Discuss how to identify medical emergencies.
7. Place an outgoing call.
8. Describe the types of telephone services and special features.

Key Terms

(See Glossary for definitions.)

cellular telephone
conference call
diction
diplomacy

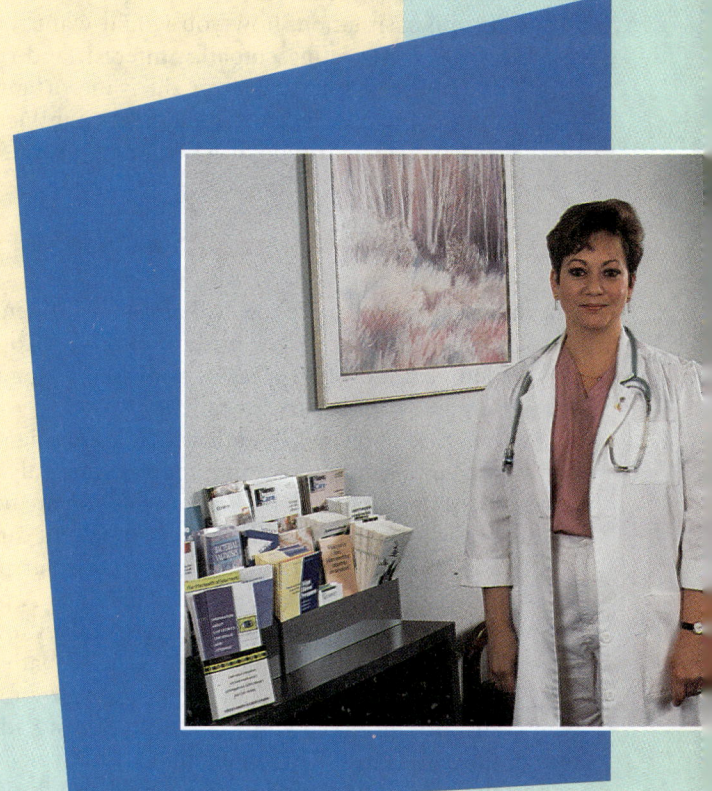

As a medical assistant, you are the patient's primary contact with the physician. In certain situations, the patient may spend more time with you than with the physician. Your interaction with the patient sets the tone for the visit and directly influences the patient's perception of the office and the quality of care the patient will receive. Therefore, it is vital that you project a caring and competent professional image at all times.

➤ PROFESSIONAL IMAGE

The Medical Assistant as an Attitude Transmitter

An attitude is a state of mind or feeling regarding some matter and can be either positive or negative. Attitudes can be formed by past experiences or they can be transmitted from one person to another. How you *feel* influences how you act; thus, your *attitude* shapes your *behavior*. You transmit your attitude to others through your behavior, thereby influencing their attitudes and behaviors.

The medical assistant must be able to transmit a positive attitude to the patient. This requires acceptance of the patient as a unique individual who has the right to be treated with dignity and compassion in a nonjudgmental manner. Ask yourself how you would feel in a similar situation, how you would want to be treated. By demonstrating empathy, interest, and concern, you tell the patient that he or she is important to you and that you care. This exerts a positive influence on the patient's own attitude, behavior, and response.

The Medical Assistant as a Role Model

Another way in which the medical assistant influences the patient's perception of the medical office is through personal appearance. Good health and good grooming present a positive image to the patient.

Taking care of oneself by eating well, exercising regularly, and getting enough rest is important not only for appearance but also for job performance. If you are tired or sluggish, you cannot provide the proper patient care.

You need to pay particular attention to your personal hygiene to avoid offending your patients. A person who is ill may be acutely sensitive to odors, even ones normally considered pleasant. A daily bath or shower is essential, followed by application of an unscented deodorant. Keep your hair clean and styled so that it does not touch your collar. Good oral hygiene is important, and during the day you should avoid foods that may create an offensive odor. Keep your fingernails clean and trimmed, with clear or neutral polish.

Long nails polished with vivid colors are not appropriate for the medical office! If you wear makeup, keep it natural and apply it lightly. Do not wear perfume, cologne, scented lotions, hair sprays, and the like.

Most offices will have a dress code defining what is appropriate apparel. Whether you wear uniforms or street clothes, they should be clean, neat, pressed, and in good repair. Wrinkles, missing buttons, split seams, torn hems, and stains project a negative image. Always wear clean, polished shoes. Your stockings should be full length, of a neutral shade, and free from runs and holes. Jewelry such as dangling earrings, large rings, long chains, and ornate or multiple bracelets are not appropriate in the health care environment (Fig. 7-1).

Courtesy and Diplomacy in the Medical Office

Being a medical assistant requires excellent human relations skills. In the course of a day you will interact with a variety of personalities in a variety of situations, and you must be able to maintain a positive professional attitude regardless of how difficult the encounter may be. Courtesy and diplomacy are fundamental to successful human relations.

Courtesy is based on sensitivity to the needs and feelings of others and demands that everyone be treated with respect and dignity. It is disrespectful to refer to the physician by first name or title only—always use the title and last name. Be courteous to your coworkers as well as your employer and your patients. Do not borrow supplies or use desks without asking permission. Always knock before entering an office, even if the door is open.

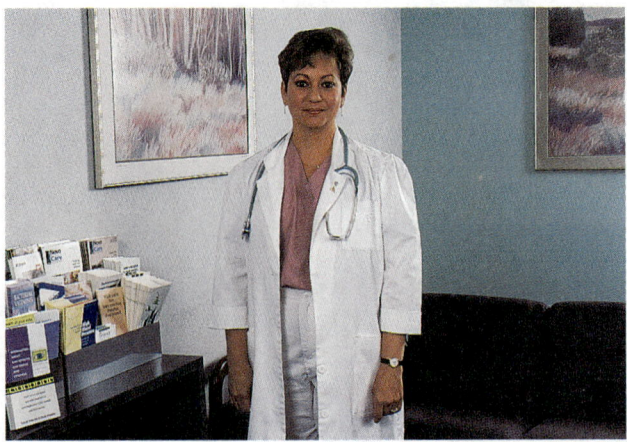

FIGURE 7-1
The properly dressed medical assistant presents a positive image to patients.

Diplomacy is the art of handling people with tact and genuine concern. Use diplomacy in difficult situations. Patients may be curious about other patients, family members may want to know what the doctor said to the patient—such questions must be met with a polite refusal to disclose confidential information. Pain, worry, and waiting can make a patient unreasonable or irritable. You must exercise self-control and understanding and maintain your professional attitude. Never argue with a patient. Try to calm the patient and communicate your desire to help.

First Impressions

First impressions are lasting ones. Remember, you have only one chance to make a first impression. The patient's perception of the medical office is based on the impression you create. A negative perception can adversely affect the patient's health and can also result in lost business. A positive perception can establish a successful doctor–patient relationship, facilitate the patient's compliance with the treatment regimen, and boost the practice.

Checkpoint Question

1. What are four ways that a medical assistant can display a professional image?

➤ RECEPTION

Duties and Responsibilities of the Receptionist

The duties of the receptionist begin long before the first appointment of the day. Each morning you should review the appointment schedule and place one copy of it on the physician's desk and one copy at the clinical assistant's station (see Chap. 8, Appointments). You then need to prepare the charts and the office before patients begin to arrive.

PREPARE THE CHARTS

Gather the charts and put them in chronological order by appointment. You need to review each chart to ensure that it is complete and up to date and that adequate clinical data sheets are available for the doctor to record any notes. Test results received since the patient's last appointment and any other new information are placed in the front of the chart for the doctor's review. Make up a chart for each new patient (see Chap. 10, Medical Records and Records Management) and

have the appropriate registration forms ready for the patient to complete. Once the charts are prepared, they are usually kept at the reception desk and given to the doctor or the clinical assistant as the patients arrive, although some doctors prefer to have all the charts placed on their desks at the start of the day.

PREPARE THE OFFICE

The receptionist is at least partly responsible for preparing the office for the patients' arrival. Check the reception/waiting area and make sure it is clean and tidy. Because the reception desk is in full view of the patients, you need to keep it free from clutter and ensure that confidential material is safely out of sight. Restock your desk with necessary forms and office supplies before the patients arrive. In smaller offices you may be responsible for stocking and setting up the examination rooms.

WELCOME PATIENTS AND VISITORS

You should make every attempt to greet patients personally and by name. A smile and cheerful greeting promote a positive image and make the patient feel welcome. Try to remember something personal about each patient, such as hobbies, pets, or special interests that you can ask about. There will be instances when you are not at your desk when a patient arrives. Therefore, some offices have a log for patients to sign, but this is not a preferred system because it breaches confidentiality. Many offices install a bell or chime on the door and post a sign requesting patients to check in with the receptionist.

REGISTER AND ORIENT PATIENTS

Patients who are new to the office will need to complete a registration form, also called a patient information sheet. The information gathered includes the patient's name, address, and telephone number; the name, address, and telephone number of the party responsible for payment; employer names and addresses; the patient's marital status; spouse's name; the Social Security numbers of the patient and responsible party; insurance information; and by whom the patient was referred. Some patient information sheets include questions about the patient's medical history. You may complete the form while interviewing the patient; most offices allow the patients to fill in the forms and consult the receptionist if they have any questions.

Once the new patient has been registered, you should orient the patient to the office. Informational brochures that give the names of the doctor(s) and staff, office hours, telephone numbers, and so on, are most helpful to the new patient. Explain the office policies and procedures and ask if the patient has any questions. Show the patient where the water fountain and restrooms are located, but caution the patient against using the restroom without checking to determine if a specimen is needed for the examination. Escort the patient to the examination room.

MANAGE WAITING TIME

Patients expect to be seen at an appointed time. They have allotted time in their schedules to see the doctor and do not want to be kept waiting. One of the major complaints of patients is the length of time they must wait to see the physician. Be sure to tell the patients if the doctor is behind schedule. If you expect the wait to be prolonged, offer the waiting patients some choices. Perhaps several would like to come back in an hour, or some may choose to reschedule the appointment for a more convenient time. If patients elect to wait, offer a magazine and a cup of coffee (if fluids are not contraindicated for the examination) to help alleviate the situation. If a patient wants to talk, let the patient pick the subject matter but avoid discussing controversial subjects such as politics and religion.

PICK UP MESSAGES

Another responsibility of the receptionist is acquiring messages that were left while the office was closed. Messages may be left with the answering service or in a voice mail box. A voice mail box is a type of answering machine in which the caller can leave a detailed message. You will need to know the security access code to obtain messages. After obtaining the messages, they should be deleted on the recorder, unless otherwise directed by office policy. Messages should be checked as soon as the office opens, at midday, after breaks, after other times when the telephone is unattended, and before the office closes.

Other duties of the receptionist include answering the telephone and scheduling appointments, which are discussed later.

Checkpoint Question
2. What are six responsibilities of a receptionist?

The Reception Environment

The reception area should be designed for the comfort, safety, and enjoyment of the patients. It should be kept clean and uncluttered, and the furniture arranged to allow ample room for walking. A coat rack and umbrella stand should be provided. Restrooms and a water fountain should be easily accessible. There should be a sign in the restrooms stating that patients should not urinate until they have checked with the medical staff to determine if a urine specimen is needed.

A low-key color scheme is advisable—muted pastels are preferable to bright primary colors although the latter work well in pediatric offices. Lighting should be bright but not harsh. The room should be well ventilated and kept at a comfortable temperature. Many offices provide soothing background music.

Furniture should be aesthetically pleasing, comfortable, and durable. Chairs are preferable to sofas because most people find sharing a sofa with strangers uncomfortable. Chairs allow patients to maintain a degree of privacy and personal space. There should be a variety of soft chairs and firm chairs and chairs with or without arms. Some patients will find it hard to stand from a soft chair; others will need the comfort. Some will need the chair arms to rise; others will be more comfortable without chair arms (Fig. 7-2).

Landscapes, waterscapes, floral, and animal pictures work better as wall decor than abstract art. Lamps and plants can add interest to corners. Keep plants in good condition and remove any that are dead. An office with dead or dying plants does not project a comforting image.

A good selection of reading material should be available. It is best to have a variety of current magazines appropriate to the specialty, such as children's books and parenting magazines for a pediatrician's office. The doctor's professional journals should not be included. The reception area is a good place to set out patient education materials. Some offices provide television for patients who prefer not to read. A writing desk will give the patients an opportunity to catch up on work or correspondence while waiting (Fig. 7-3).

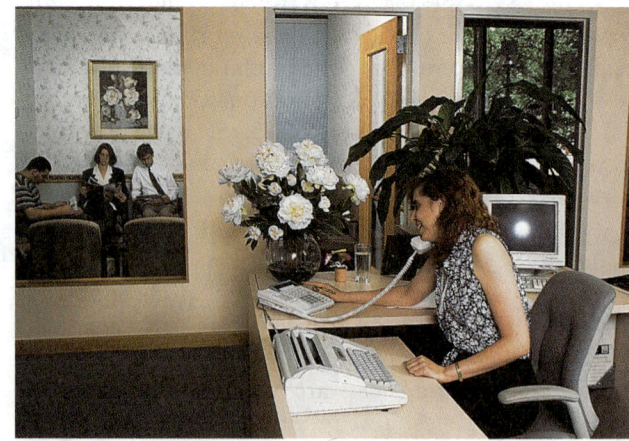

FIGURE 7-2
The reception area should be designed for the comfort, safety, and enjoyment of the patients.

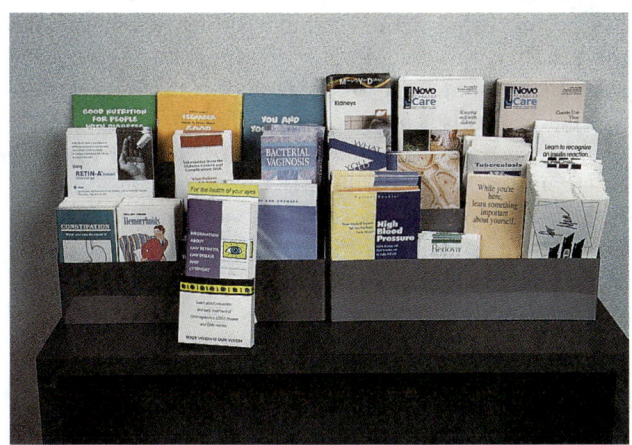

FIGURE 7-3
The reception area is a good place to set out patient education materials.

Many offices include a children's play area in the reception room. This should be kept away from the seating area. Toys should be unbreakable and easy to clean and have no sharp edges. A small table and chairs will give children a place to read or color. Most pediatric offices will have the reception area divided into two areas: well child and sick child areas. (In some offices, the receptionist may be responsible for checking sick children for communicable diseases such as chickenpox or measles. In this situation, you would be educated by the physician in identifying various childhood rashes.)

The medical assistant is at least partly responsible for keeping the reception area neat. You should check it several times during the day to make sure it is clean and tidy.

The End of the Patient Visit

When the doctor has completed the examination, the patient is directed back to the reception desk. The assistant will calculate the patient's bill and collect any fees that are due. At this time the assistant checks the patient's understanding of the treatment recommended by the physician. Make sure the patient understands the dosage and frequency of prescribed medications. If the doctor has requested a follow-up visit, schedule the appointment before the patient leaves. Be sure to give the patient an appointment reminder card. Before the patient leaves, ask if there are any questions. You should bid the patient goodbye in a warm and friendly manner. As patients leave the office, they should feel they have been well cared for by a competent and courteous staff.

➤ TELEPHONE

Importance of the Telephone in the Medical Office

The medical office is filled with expensive scientific equipment used in the diagnosis and treatment of disease, but one of the most important instruments is the ordinary telephone. It allows the patient round-the-clock access to medical care. A patient can schedule an appointment, seek medical advice, request prescription refills, obtain test results, question a bill, or report an emergency simply by picking up the telephone. The telephone also links the physician's office to the rest of the medical community (eg, hospitals, pharmacies, and other doctors).

You must be able to communicate a positive image of the physician and staff while speaking on the tele-

---

*P*atient Education: Television as a Teaching Tool

A television in the reception area can entertain patients while they wait for an appointment, but it can also be a patient education tool. By using a television in conjunction with a VCR, you can play a variety of educational videos. Here are some points to keep in mind:

- Be sure all videos have been previewed by the physician.
- Select videos that are geared toward the specialty of the practice (eg, a video about heart attacks would be appropriate for a cardiologist's office but not for a rheumatologist's).
- Carefully assess the graphic nature of certain videos. (A picture of the birth of a child may be of interest to you, but it may be too much for certain patients.)
- Keep in mind the age of the patients and family members that will be in the waiting room. Caution must be used if small children are often in the area. For example, a video about preventing sexually transmitted diseases may provide information appropriate for a family practice, but it would not be appropriate to show it in the reception area.
- Keep the volume on the television at a reasonable level. It should serve only as background, not as a main attraction.

phone, without the aid of nonverbal cues such as appearance, facial expressions, body language, and gestures. You must rely solely on the tone and quality of your voice and speech to project a competent and caring attitude over the telephone.

Basic Guidelines for Telephone Use

Telephone communication is not effective if either party does not fully understand what is being said. Misunderstandings can be embarrassing, frustrating, or even life-threatening. The medical assistant must be able to overcome obstacles to effective telephone communication, such as a noisy environment, poor telephone connection, emotional distress, and hearing and speech impairments.

DICTION

Diction is the style of speaking and enunciating words. You should speak clearly and distinctly. Talk clearly into the speaker—do not prop the handset between your chin and shoulder. Never chew gum or eat while you speak on the telephone. Speak at a moderate pace to avoid slurring your words.

PRONUNCIATION

Make sure you pronounce words correctly to avoid misunderstandings. Avoid using unfamiliar words, slang, and idiomatic expressions. Most patients do not understand medical terminology, so it is best to use lay terms whenever possible.

EXPRESSION

Put a smile in your voice by sitting up straight and putting a smile on your lips. Speak in a well modulated pitch and volume. Use proper inflection to avoid a droning, monotonous speaking style.

LISTENING

Be an attentive listener. Focus on the conversation and ignore outside distractions. Do not interrupt the speaker. You may need to have a message clarified by asking the caller to repeat what was said. Verify your understanding by repeating the message.

COURTESY

Always speak politely and courteously. Address the caller by title and last name. Although many telephone calls interrupt your work, do not allow your voice to betray impatience or irritation. Remember that you are there to help the patient.

Never answer the telephone and put the caller on hold immediately. If you need to answer another line or finish a task before you can engage in conversation,

ask if the caller would mind holding. Courtesy demands that you wait for an answer before you place the call on hold. Also of great importance—you must determine if this is an emergency. If you are still unable to take the call after 90 seconds, check back with the caller and ask if he would like to continue holding. Again, wait for an answer before you place the call on hold. If the hold exceeds 3 minutes, you should apologize to the caller for the delay and offer to return the call as soon as you are available.

If you are already engaged in a telephone conversation and need to answer another line, ask the party with whom you are speaking if he would mind holding. Again, wait for a reply before answering the second call. Explain to the second caller that you are on the other line and need to complete that call. Do not handle the second call while the first party waits unless the second call is an emergency, a long distance call that cannot be referred to another worker, or a physician calling to speak with your physician.

Checkpoint Question
3. *What are six important guidelines to remember when using the telephone?*

Incoming Calls

An incoming call should be given the same courtesy and attention as an arriving visitor. Just as you would not keep a patient waiting without acknowledging his or her presence, so you must acknowledge an incoming call promptly. Answer the telephone by the second ring if at all possible. Identify both the office and yourself to assure the caller that the correct number has been reached, and offer the caller your assistance.

Types of Calls

The medical assistant screens incoming calls to make sure they are handled appropriately. Many calls do not require the physician's personal attention and can be handled competently by the medical assistant.

SCHEDULING APPOINTMENTS

New patients will call to make appointments and established patients will call to schedule return visits. (See Chap. 8, Appointments, for the processes for handling these types of calls.)

BILLING INQUIRIES

In some offices the medical assistant is responsible for handling routine inquiries concerning billing, fees, services, and insurance. You may be asked to give specific information concerning the cost of services; do not quote exact prices but tell the patient that costs depend on the type of examination and diagnostic tests performed. Sometimes third-party callers will request information about the patient; remember that confidential information cannot be divulged without a specific release from the patient.

DIAGNOSTIC TEST REPORTS

Many laboratory and x-ray reports are called to the physician's office before the written copy is sent. The medical assistant records the information and posts it on the front of the chart for the physician to review. If the results were needed stat, the information must be brought to the physician's attention immediately on receiving the report. Having at hand blank laboratory slips or specially designed forms listing the most frequently ordered reports for your office will save time and will make it easier to accurately record the results as they are relayed from the laboratory. These will be replaced with the official report when it is received.

ROUTINE AND SATISFACTORY PROGRESS REPORTS

At the end of an office visit a patient may be told to call in a progress report within a few days. If the report is satisfactory you may take down the information, record it in the patient's chart, and place it on the physician's desk for review. You may also handle routine progress reports from hospitals, home health agencies, and other allied health professionals.

TEST RESULTS

Patients often call for test results, and many doctors allow the medical assistant to report favorable test results. The office should have a specific policy regarding the handling of this issue. Unless you are certain that the caller is the patient, it may be a good idea to explain that you will call back with the results after checking with the physician and using the patient's telephone number listed in the chart. It is illegal to give information to anyone other than the patient without the patient's specific consent.

UNSATISFACTORY PROGRESS REPORTS AND TEST RESULTS

The doctor will need to speak with a patient whose progress is unsatisfactory during treatment. The urgency of the patient's condition will determine whether the call requires the physician's immediate attention. The physician will discuss unsatisfactory test results of a serious nature with the patient. In less serious cases,

the physician may ask you to speak with the patient. Never discuss unsatisfactory test results with a patient unless the doctor directs you to do so.

PRESCRIPTION REFILLS

The medical assistant can handle requests for prescription refills if they are indicated on the chart. If there is any doubt, tell the pharmacy or the patient that you will check with the doctor and call back.

Other calls ordinarily handled by the medical assistant are requests for referrals to other physicians, clarifying instructions for patients, and calls concerning routine administrative matters.

Certain calls are handled personally by the physician. You will need to screen these calls to determine whether they should be put through to the physician immediately or returned at a more convenient time. If your physician receives a number of calls during the day that you are unsure how to handle, ask which calls he or she prefers to have referred immediately and which can be returned later. Calls from other physicians should be directed to the physician immediately or according to office policy.

Problem Callers

UNIDENTIFIED CALLERS

Sometimes callers who ask to speak with the physician will refuse to state their names or the nature of their business. In such instances you should politely but firmly tell the caller that you cannot interrupt the physician and politely explain that you would be happy to leave a message. If the caller persists, ask the caller to call back at a specific time when the physician will be available. Alert the physician that there will be a call for him at the specified time. Unidentified callers tend to be sales representatives.

What If?

What if the caller is a sales representative?

Question sales representatives about the nature of their products (eg, surgical supplies, medications, office equipment). If the products are used in your office, ask the sales representative to mail printed materials. Explain that after the physician has reviewed the printed material, an appointment may be scheduled if the products appear appropriate for the office. Do not put sales representatives through to the physician unless the physician tells you otherwise.

IRATE PATIENTS

The physician should always be made aware of complaints about fees or care. When the caller is angry, you must be careful to keep your own temper in check. Try to calm the patient and offer assurance that you want to help. Listen carefully and take notes. If you cannot resolve the situation, let the patient know you must consult with the physician and offer to call back. The physician will probably want to speak with the patient personally.

MEDICAL EMERGENCIES

As a medical assistant, you must be able to differentiate between routine, nonemergency, and emergency situations. To do this you must try to calm the caller and ask specific questions concerning the patient's condition. Severe pain, profuse bleeding, respiratory distress, chest pain, loss of consciousness, severe vomiting or diarrhea, or a temperature greater than 102°F are all considered emergency situations and you should put the call through to the physician immediately. Determine the patient's name, location, and telephone number as quickly as possible in case you are disconnected or the patient is unable to continue the conversation. This will allow you to direct emergency personnel to the patient's aid. The office should have a policy on how to handle emergency calls when the doctor is not in the office.

Ask your physician to list instances that might constitute an emergency in this specialty and describe how they should be handled. Listing these in a prominent place near the telephone will help you, and your replacement in your absence, to most appropriately assist the patient in receiving care as quickly as possible.

Personal Calls

The physician will receive personal calls from friends, family, and business associates. Your employer will advise you which calls should be put through immediately. Otherwise, take a message and tell the caller that the doctor will return the call.

Taking Messages

Recording messages for the physician or clinical assistant will be a large part of your daily responsibilities. This will be easier if you have at hand note pads that are designed for this task. Office supply companies have an assortment of pads that can be used, or your physician may choose to design his own (Fig. 7-4). Having carbonless copies will give you a record of the messages taken during the day and the action taken. The minimum information needed for a telephone message includes: the name of the caller, date and time of the call, the telephone number where the caller can be reached, a short description of the caller's concern, and the person to whom the message is routed. When the call has been handled, the action taken must be recorded. Some message pads are designed to be added to the progress notes on the patient's chart when the call is complete; in other instances the information will be transferred by writing or transcribing in the patient's progress notes.

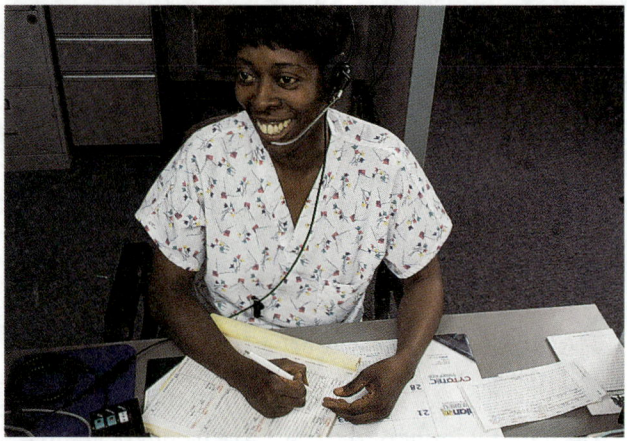

FIGURE 7-4
Your daily responsibilities may include recording messages for the physician or clinical assistant.

Checkpoint Question
4. *What elements must be included in a telephone message?*

Outgoing Calls

The medical assistant is responsible for placing outgoing calls as well as receiving incoming calls. Most offices will set a specific time each day for returning calls, but other calls will be placed throughout the day. You should prepare your calls carefully—have all the information gathered and know what you want to say before you dial the number. When placing a call for the physician, make sure that all the needed information is at hand and that he or she is prepared to receive the call. If you are calling to reschedule an appointment, be able to explain why the change is necessary and be prepared to offer a new appointment time.

At times you may need to place long distance calls. Keep in mind the difference in time zones; if you do not know the time zone of the city you are calling, check the front of your telephone directory. Long distance calls may be either dialed directly or operator assisted. If you do not need to speak with a particular person, it is less expensive to dial the number directly. You will need operator assistance to place a person-to-person call, bill the call to a third number, reverse the charges, or obtain time and charges on the call. If you are connected to a wrong number or disconnected during the call, notify the long distance operator immediately to avoid charges or to be reconnected.

Your employer may ask you to place a **conference call**, a call about a designated topic involving two or more people. These calls can connect up to 14 points. Notify all parties of the date and time the call will be made to ensure everyone will be available to participate. At the appointed time, give the operator the names and numbers of the participants and say you want to place a conference call. The operator will call you when the call is ready.

Services and Special Features

The recommended telephone service to a medical office is two incoming lines per medical assistant and one private line per physician. A wide variety of communication equipment is available today, and communications consultants can help determine the appropriate services and equipment for your office.

The standard six-button telephone with several lines, an intercom, and a hold button is in common use. A multiline speaker telephone with last number redial, volume control, intercom, call forwarding, call back, and caller identification is also popular (Fig. 7-5). Whatever style equipment is used, telephones should be placed in easily accessible areas that afford privacy for the user.

With a **cellular telephone** and a pager, a physician can remain accessible while away from the office. (A cellular telephone works by electronic signals and does not require attachment to a telephone plug.) Answering services and answering machines handle incoming calls after hours. An answering machine will have a pre-recorded message giving the office hours and instructions for emergency situations and will allow the caller to leave a message if desired. Answering services employ operators to pick up calls coming in to the office or physician's home. The operator will relay messages to the physician, but usually will not connect the caller or give out the physician's number.

The features available in each telephone system will vary considerably. In almost all instances, the sales representative will assist you in the initial operations and will be available for questions as they arise. All units are supplied with owner's manuals for quick reference until you are familiar with all or most of the office system functions.

 SUMMARY

As the receptionist, you are the most immediately visible or accessible representative of the medical practice. Your telephone manner and your interpersonal skills will be the first and last encounters for all patients passing through the office or making contact by telephone. You must practice all the tact and diplomacy required of your profession to ease the patient's anxiety and to ensure that the best and most confident image of the practice is projected.

 CRITICAL THINKING CHALLENGES

1. How would you assist in calming an irate patient on the telephone? Identify some phrases that you might use.
2. Assume that you are working in an obstetrician's office. What kinds of educational videos might be appropriate for the waiting room? What if you were working in an orthopedic office or for a surgeon?

 ANSWERS TO CHECKPOINT QUESTIONS

1. Medical assistants can display a professional image by transmitting a positive attitude, acting as a role model, using courtesy and diplomacy, and making a positive first impression.

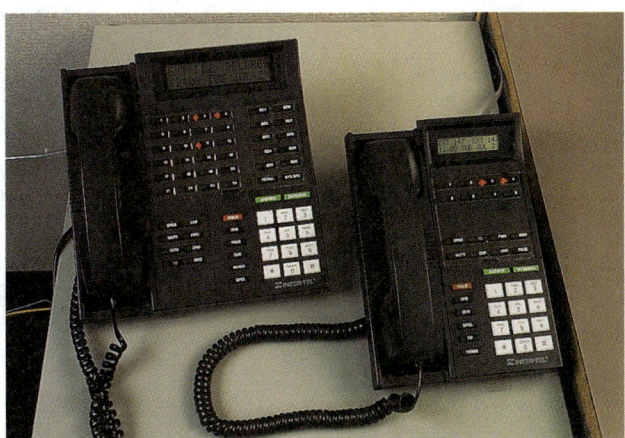

FIGURE 7-5
Various telephone systems.

2. The receptionist is responsible for preparing charts, preparing the office, welcoming patients and visitors, registering and orienting patients, managing waiting time, and obtaining messages.

3. When using the telephone, be sure to speak clearly, pronounce words correctly, have a positive expression, listen attentively, be courteous, and never place callers on hold immediately.

4. When taking a telephone message, be sure to include the name of the caller, date and time of the call, the telephone number where the caller can be reached, a short description of the caller's concern, and the person to whom the message is routed.

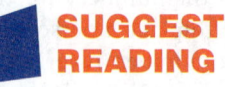

SUGGESTIONS FOR FURTHER READING

Becklin, K. J., & Sunnarborg, E. M. (1992). *Medical Office Procedures*, 3rd ed. New York: Glencoe/McGraw-Hill.

Humphrey, D. D. (1990). *Contemporary Medical Office Procedures*. Cincinnati: South-western Publishing.

Appointments

Chapter Outline

Patient Office Visits
    Scheduled Appointments
    Flexible Hours
    Open Hours
Scheduling Appointments
    The Appointment Book
    Computerized Scheduling
Factors That Affect Scheduling
    Patients' Needs
    The Physician's Preferences and
        Needs
    Physical Facilities
Scheduling Guidelines
    New Patients
    Double Bookings
    Return Appointments
Preparing a Daily or Weekly Schedule
Patient Reminders
    Appointment Cards
    Telephone Reminders
    Mailed Reminder Cards

Adapting the Schedule
    Emergencies
    Patients Who Are Acutely Ill
    Walk-in Patients
    Late Patients
    Physician Delays
    Missed Appointments
Cancellations
    Cancellations by the Office
    Cancellations by the Patient
**Making Appointments for Patients in
    Other Facilities**
    Referrals and Consultations
    Laboratory Tests or X-rays
    Surgery
**When the Appointment Schedule Does
    Not Work**
Summary
Critical Thinking Challenges
Answers to Checkpoint Questions
Suggestions for Further Reading

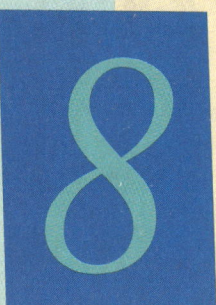

DACUM Components

1.1   Project a positive attitude
1.3   Practice within the scope of education, training, and personal capabilities
1.5   Work as a team member
1.6   Conduct oneself in a courteous and diplomatic manner
2.2   Treat all patients with empathy and impartiality
2.5   Serve as liaison between physician and others
2.7   Receive, organize, prioritize, and transmit information
3.2   Schedule and monitor appointments
3.4   Apply computer concepts for office procedures
5.1   Document accurately
5.3   Use appropriate guidelines when releasing records or information
6.6   Exercise efficient time management

Chapter Competencies

Learning Objectives

Upon successfully completing this chapter, you will be able to:

1. Spell and define the Key Terms.
2. Describe the various systems for patient office visits.
3. Identify the factors that affect appointment scheduling.
4. Explain guidelines for scheduling appointments for new patients and return visits.
5. List three ways to remind patients about appointments.
6. Describe how to handle patient emergencies, acutely ill patients, walk-in patients, late patients, and patients who miss their appointments.
7. Explain what to do if the physician is delayed.
8. Discuss how to handle appointment cancellations made by the office or by the patient.

Performance Objectives

Upon successfully completing this chapter, you will be able to:

1. Schedule an appointment for a new patient.
2. Schedule an appointment for a patient's return visit.

Key Terms

(See Glossary for definitions.)

matrix
tickler file
wave scheduling

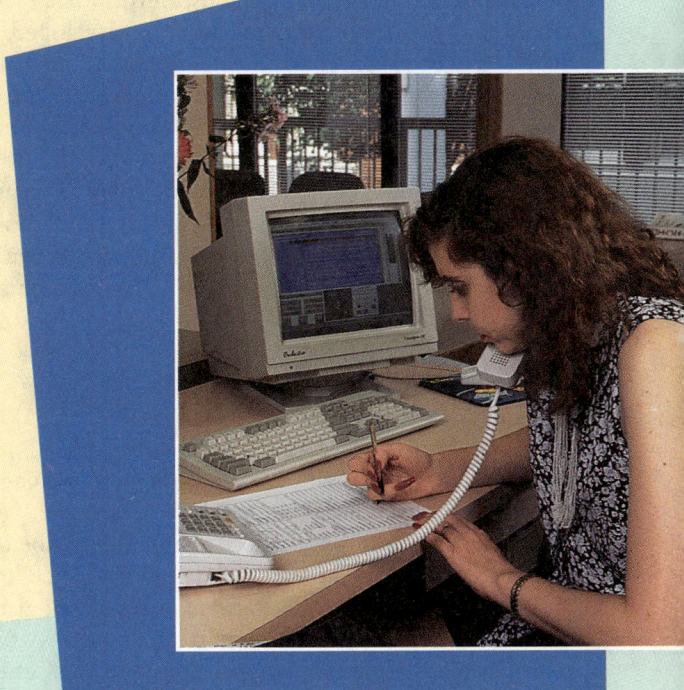

Responsibility for the appointment desk in a medical office or clinic can be the most important duty assigned to a medical assistant. You might provide the first, last, and most durable impression that the patient has of your office and, by extension, of the physician. Depending on your demeanor, that impression can be favorable or unfavorable. If properly used, the appointment system helps maintain a well run office. If improperly used, it can mean confusion and chaos; more importantly, it can waste precious time for the physician and the patient.

To use the office facilities and the physician's availability most efficiently, you must determine which patients will be seen, when they will be seen, and how much time to allot to each of them depending on their problems. Of course, every practice will have occasional delays and emergencies. Your responsibility is to manage all of this while maintaining a calm, efficient, and polite attitude.

➤ PATIENT OFFICE VISITS

Scheduled Appointments

Many medical offices use a system of scheduled appointments for patient office visits. Each patient is assigned a time on the schedule and allotted a specific period for examination and treatment.

The advantages of this system include better daily time management and optimum use of the office facility. Additionally, a daily schedule may be developed and charts may be prepared in advance of patient arrival.

A disadvantage of this system is that a patient may need more of the physician's time than you have scheduled. Therefore, it is important that you ask the proper questions at the time the appointment is made to reasonably evaluate the time needed. Keep in mind, though, that the patient may have different complaints when seeing the physician, requiring even more (or less) time for the actual visit.

Flexible Hours

Offices that operate with flexible hours are open at different times throughout the week. For example, Monday, Wednesday, and Friday office hours might be from 8 AM to 5 PM, and Tuesday and Thursday office hours might be from 8 AM to 8 PM. Some offices may also be open on Saturdays for all or part of the day. Patients still have scheduled appointments, but this greater range of available appointment times available accommodates work and family schedules. Your main challenge with flexible hours is to determine which patients really need to be scheduled for these special times. For

example, Saturday appointments may be reserved only for patients whose work schedules do not permit weekday appointments. Flexible hours are most often used by clinics, group practices, or family physicians.

Open Hours

A medical office that operates with open hours for patient visits is open for specified hours during the day or evening. Patients may arrive at any time during those hours to be seen by the physician in the order of their arrival; there are no scheduled appointments. This system does eliminate such patient complaints as "I had an appointment at 2 PM but had to wait until 3 PM to be seen." However, it has some clear disadvantages:

- Effective time management is almost impossible.
- The facilities may be overloaded at some times and empty at other times.
- Charts must be pulled and prepared as each patient arrives.

So that patients are seen in the order in which they arrive, some offices use "sign-in sheets." When using sign-in sheets, keep in mind that they are considered to be legal documents and are subject to subpoena. Also, patients signing in will see the names of other patients on the sheets; this may present a breach of confidentiality.

Checkpoint Question
1. What are the three systems that can be used for patient office visits?

➤ SCHEDULING APPOINTMENTS

The Appointment Book

If your medical office uses a system of scheduled appointments for patient office visits, you will need an appointment book. An appointment book provides space for noting appointments for an entire year. Some offices prefer an appointment book with pages showing only one day at a time; others may want to see a whole week at a glance. A different color page for each day may also be desired.

When deciding which kind of book will work best for your office, make sure that it has enough space in which to write all pertinent information (eg, patient name, telephone number, reason for visit), is divided into time units appropriate for your practice (eg, 10- or 15-minute intervals), can open flat on the desk where it will be used, and fits easily into its storage place when not in use (Fig. 8-1).

THURSDAY, APRIL 11

HOUR	Dr. North	Dr. South	Dr. East	Dr. West
8 00				
8 15				
8 30				
8 45				
9 00				
9 15				
9 30				
9 45				
10 00				
10 15				
10 30				
10 45				
11 00				
11 15				
11 30				
11 45				
12 00				
12 15				
12 30				
12 45				
1 00				
1 15				
1 30				
1 45				
2 00				
2 15				
2 30				
2 45				
3 00				
3 15				
3 30				
3 45				
4 00				
4 15				
4 30				
4 45				
5 00				
5 15				
5 30				
5 45				
6 00				
6 15				
6 30				
6 45				
7 00				
NOTES				

FIGURE 8-1

An appointment book provides space for noting appointments.

Before you begin using the appointment book, you will need to set up a **matrix**. This involves crossing off all times that will not be used for patient visits. Note the reasons for crossing off the space (eg, vacations, meetings, hospital rounds). Some practices cross off specific times or even days for certain activities, such as physical examinations and surgery. Also, it is advisable to block off 15 to 30 minutes of time each morning and afternoon to accommodate emergencies, late arrivals, or other patient delays. Some physicians may wish to have notations of professional or personal obligations made on the appointment schedule so that patients are not booked up to the last minute (Fig. 8-2).

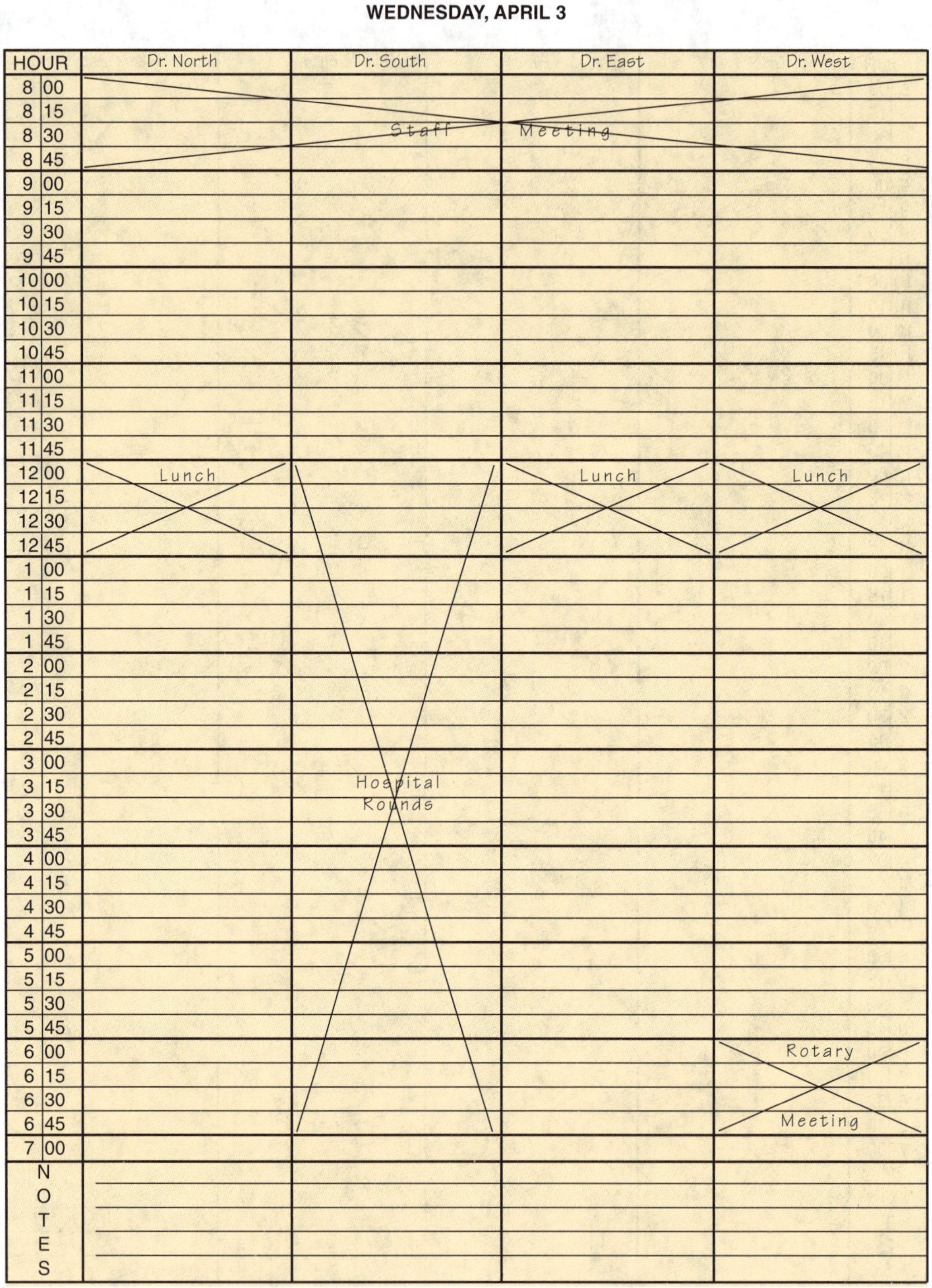

WEDNESDAY, APRIL 3

HOUR	Dr. North	Dr. South	Dr. East	Dr. West
8 00				
8 15				
8 30	Staff		Meeting	
8 45				
9 00				
9 15				
9 30				
9 45				
10 00				
10 15				
10 30				
10 45				
11 00				
11 15				
11 30				
11 45				
12 00	Lunch		Lunch	Lunch
12 15				
12 30				
12 45				
1 00				
1 15				
1 30				
1 45				
2 00				
2 15				
2 30				
2 45				
3 00				
3 15		Hospital		
3 30		Rounds		
3 45				
4 00				
4 15				
4 30				
4 45				
5 00				
5 15				
5 30				
5 45				
6 00				Rotary
6 15				
6 30				
6 45				Meeting
7 00				
NOTES				

FIGURE 8-2

An appointment book matrix involves crossing off all times that will not be used for patient visits.

Once you have acquired and prepared an appointment book, it is not enough to just schedule a time and date for a patient visit and hope everything will run smoothly. Before actually making a patient appointment, you should review the schedule carefully, evaluating the needs of each patient and considering the physician's preferences and availability of the office facilities (see next page).

Legal Tips

Appointment books are considered legal documents and could be subject to subpoena. Consequently, you must write or print clearly and make corrections neatly. Do not erase missed appointments or cancellations on the day of the appointment. Instead, put a mark through the patient's name (making sure the name is still readable). Then make a notation next to the patient's name indicating if the appointment was canceled, missed, or rescheduled.

Computerized Scheduling

A number of companies produce software designed to assist with such administrative functions as appointment scheduling. Some of the same principles used with an appointment book also apply when using computerized scheduling. However, computerized scheduling can often save time. For instance, you would still need to develop a matrix, but information that does not change (eg, hospital rounds from 7:30–8:30, lunch from 12:30–1:30) would need to be entered only once into the computer program. Computerized scheduling also offers a quick method for determining available appointment times. Typically, you would enter the desired date, and the computer would display the schedule for that day, showing which, if any, time slots were available. Depending on the specific software, you could also print numerous documents, such as the daily or weekly appointment schedule, appointment reminders, or billing slips.

Checkpoint Question
2. Before patient appointments are made, what task must be done?

➤ FACTORS THAT AFFECT SCHEDULING

Patients' Needs

People express their needs in varied ways. A patient might be experiencing several emotions including uncertainty, embarrassment, shyness, and fear. When these emotional states exist, it takes little in the way of real or

imagined miscommunication to create a negative response from the patient. Always be courteous and maintain your professionalism.

Before scheduling an appointment, you should determine:

- Why the patient wishes to see the physician
- How long the patient has had the symptoms
- If the problem is acute (abrupt onset) or chronic (long standing)
- The most convenient time for the patient to come in (eg, early morning or evenings)
- If the patient requires special transportation services (Community or hospital van services operate only during certain hours.)
- If the patient needs to see other office staff members

Control of the appointment schedule is your responsibility. Strive to accommodate a patient's requests whenever possible but not if it will overload the schedule. For example, if a patient requests a 2 PM appointment this Tuesday, and you already have patients in that time slot, politely explain that the request is not possible unless you have a cancellation. You might offer a later time on Tuesday or on another day at 2 PM. You can also ask if the patient wishes to be put on a "move-up" list to be notified if anything sooner opens up. In other words: You control the schedule, do not let it control you.

The Physician's Preferences and Needs

The management of the practice depends on the desires and requirements of the physician. Some physicians are always running behind schedule; others are extremely punctual. You will need to recognize your physician's habits and adjust the schedule accordingly. If a medical assistant is employed to assist the physician with clinical duties (eg, removing sutures, performing electrocardiograms, giving injections), the schedule can be adjusted to accommodate a larger number of patients, while still allowing the physician enough time to provide each patient with personal attention.

Keep in mind that the physician will need scheduled time to receive and return telephone calls, review laboratory and pathology reports, dictate chart notes or correspondence, and so on. If your physician is on the staff of a teaching hospital, you may also need to block off time for clinic conferences and other teaching duties.

The physician also will need time to meet with nonpatient or unscheduled office visitors. Such visitors might include other physicians or sales representatives from medical supply or pharmaceutical companies. You will need to determine in advance how the physician wants you to handle these visitors. For example, the physician may want to be notified immediately if another physician has come to the office. However, if the visitor is a salesperson or a pharmaceutical representative, the physician may have another staff member meet with the individual or may request that an appointment be scheduled for a more convenient time.

Physical Facilities

The physical facilities available in the medical office will have an impact on the management of the appointment schedule. Consider these points: How many physicians use the facility? How many examination rooms are there? Is it necessary to resterilize instruments between procedures or is more than one set of instruments available? You would not want to schedule two sigmoidoscopies at the same time, for example, if the office has only one appropriately equipped examination room. It is important to have a thorough understanding of the requirements for procedures to be performed in the office to schedule appointments wisely.

Checkpoint Question

3. What are three factors that can affect appointment scheduling?

➤ SCHEDULING GUIDELINES

Whether the patient is making an appointment by telephone or in person, you must be pleasant and maintain a helpful attitude. Always write each patient's telephone number on the schedule when making appointments. Emergencies and delays are unavoidable, and schedule corrections can be made quickly if the telephone number is handy.

It is also important for you to leave some time slots open during each day, perhaps 15 to 20 minutes in the morning and in the afternoon. Invariably, problems will arise (eg, late patients, emergencies) that can disrupt the regular appointment schedule. These open blocks can allow the schedule to "catch up." Also, patients calling for appointments will not appreciate being told that no time is available for 2 or 3 weeks. Open slots can be used to schedule brief appointments on an as-needed basis.

New Patients

Most appointments for new patients are made over the telephone (Fig. 8-3). When scheduling an appointment for a new patient, there are certain guidelines to follow. These are discussed in detail below and summarized in Box 8-1.

1. Allow an adequate amount of time for the appointment. To do so, obtain as much information as possible from the patient, such as:

   - Full name and correct spelling
   - Mailing address (not all offices require this)
   - Day and evening telephone numbers
   - Reason for the visit
   - Name of the referring physician or individual

2. Explain the payment policy of the practice. Most offices require full or partial payment at the time of an initial visit, and patients must understand this policy. Instruct patients to bring all pertinent insurance information.

3. Be sure patients know your office location; if needed, give them concise directions. You may also want to give patients an idea of how long they can expect to be at the office.

4. Some patients are sensitive about messages for them that are left on an answering machine or given to a coworker. To avoid violating patient confidentiality, ask the patient if it is permissible to call at home or at work.

5. Before ending the call, confirm the time and date of the appointment. You might say, "*Thank you for calling Mr. Brown. Your appointment is scheduled for Tuesday, December 10 at 2 PM.*" Always check your appointment book to be sure that you

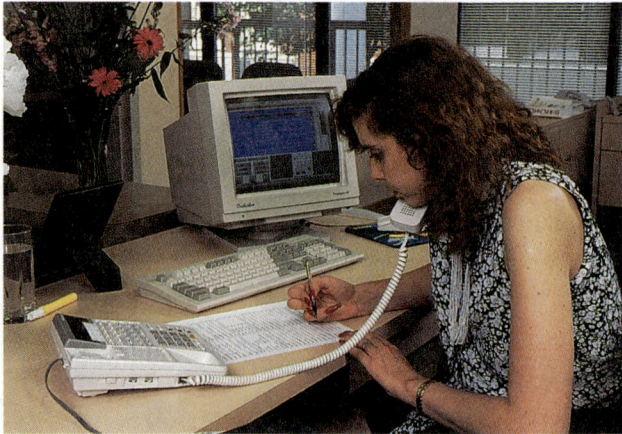

FIGURE 8-3
Be sure to obtain all pertinent information when a patient calls to schedule an office visit.

have placed the appointment on the correct day in the right time slot.

6. If the patient was referred by another physician, you may need to call that physician's office in advance of the appointment for copies of laboratory work, x-rays, pathology reports, and so on. *Remember*: The patient must give authorization to release medical documents (see Chap. 10, Medical Records and Records Management for more information). Give this information to the physician prior to the patient's appointment.

Double Bookings

Double booking means that more than one patient is scheduled for the same time slot. This can create negative feelings when patients discover that they were scheduled for the same appointment time. However, if you have three patients coming to the office and you know each will require only 5 minutes, it is permissible to have them all come in at 9 AM or 2 PM (or whenever your first morning or afternoon time slot may be) as long as you block off at least 15 minutes on the schedule. As the morning or afternoon progresses, you may find that this type of scheduling is not a good idea because delays or emergencies cannot be foreseen. Of course, double booking is not a problem if patients who are scheduled in the same time slot will be seeing different staff members (eg, medical assistant, x-ray technician) and not the same physician.

Double booking can also work when using **wave scheduling**, which has a couple of variations. With one variation, three or more patients may be scheduled for

a given hour. Each patient is instructed to arrive at the same time (eg, 11 AM), but patients are seen in the order of arrival. This approach helps prevent schedule delays due to lateness. With another variation, several patients may be scheduled for different times during the first half of the hour, while none are scheduled for the second half of the hour (eg, two patients may be scheduled at 11 AM, two at 11:15 AM, and one at 11:30 AM). By not booking appointments during the second half of the hour, the schedule can remain on time even if delays or other disruptions occur in the first half of the hour.

Return Appointments

Most return appointments are made while the patient is in the office. When doing so, follow these guidelines:

1. Carefully check your appointment book before offering an appointment. If a specific examination, test, or x-ray is to be performed on the return visit, you will want to avoid scheduling two patients for the same examination at the same time.
2. Offer the patient a specific time and date. For example, you might say, "*Mrs. Chang, I have next Tuesday, the 15th available at 3:30 PM.*" (Avoid asking the patient when he or she would like to return as this can cause indecision.) If the offered appointment is not convenient, offer another specific time and date.
3. Write the patient's name and telephone number in the appointment book.
4. Transfer the pertinent information to an appointment card and give it to the patient. Repeat aloud the appointment day, date, and time to the patient as you hand over the card (Fig. 8-4).

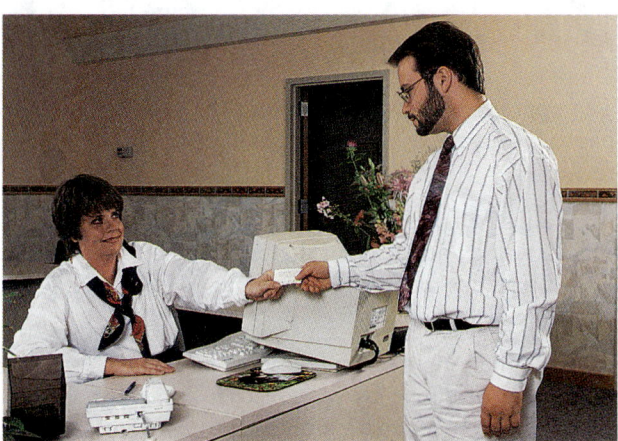

FIGURE 8-4
Use an appointment card to remind the patient of a return or follow-up visit.

5. Double check your book to be sure you have not made an error.
6. End your conversation with a pleasant word and a smile.

? Checkpoint Question
4. What method of scheduling is helpful with double bookings?

PREPARING A DAILY OR WEEKLY SCHEDULE

In most offices, the medical assistant is responsible for preparing a daily and weekly schedule of appointments. You should make a copy for the physician and other office staff members. When there are changes in the schedule, you need to ensure that corrections are made on all copies. Make sure the next day's schedule is placed on the physician's desk before he or she leaves for the day. Give the weekly schedule to the physician before he or she leaves on Friday. Schedules should not only include patient appointments, but also hospital rounds, surgeries, meetings, and any personal engagements you know about.

PATIENT REMINDERS

Various kinds of reminders can be used to tell a patient about an appointment that needs to be made or that an appointment has been made on a specific date and time. These reminders are the appointment card, the telephone call, and the mailed card.

Appointment Cards

The appointment card is given to the patient when he or she leaves the office. It should have the following information:

- Patient's name
- Day, date, and time of the return visit
- Physician's name and telephone number (Fig. 8-5)

If the patient requires a series of appointments, try to make them on the same day of the week and at the same time of day. This will make it easier for the patient to remember the appointments. However, unless your appointment card allows you to list the complete series of appointments, give the patient a card for the next appointment only and repeat the procedure after

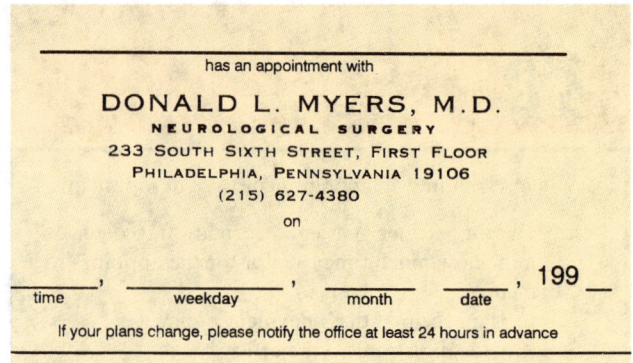

has an appointment with
DONALD L. MYERS, M.D.
NEUROLOGICAL SURGERY
233 SOUTH SIXTH STREET, FIRST FLOOR
PHILADELPHIA, PENNSYLVANIA 19106
(215) 627-4380
on

_____ , _____ , _____ , 199 __
time   weekday   month   date

If your plans change, please notify the office at least 24 hours in advance

FIGURE 8-5
Example of an appointment card.

each subsequent visit. When several cards have to be saved, they can easily be lost.

Telephone Reminders

All new patients and patients with advance bookings on your schedule should each receive a telephone reminder the day before the appointment. Remember: Do not call a patient at work unless you have been given permission to do so. Keep your telephone reminder simple. Identify your office, yourself, and state the date and time of the appointment. For example, you might say, *"This is Ms. Gonzales from Dr. Jordan's office. I'm calling to confirm your appointment for tomorrow, Thursday, February 10, at 3:30 PM."* Unless the patient has a question, say "thank you and good-bye." This reminder helps jog the patient's memory and if the appointment is canceled or rescheduled, you will have time to fill the slot from your move-up list. Make a notation on the appointment schedule, such as confirmed, left message, or no answer.

Mailed Reminder Cards

Reminder cards are usually sent to remind the patient that it is time to keep an upcoming scheduled appointment. These should be mailed at least a week before the date of the appointment. In addition, reminder cards are sent after a certain period of time has passed since a patient's last appointment. Reminder cards are often used to remind patients of annual examinations (eg, Pap smears, mammograms, prostate examinations).

To handle this kind of reminder, keep a supply of preprinted postcards in the office. The cards should

BOX 8-2 Tickler Files for Patient Reminders

A tickler file helps remind you to do something by a certain time in the future. It can be something as simple as a card file box (like a recipe box) or an accordion folder with insert guides in chronological order. The guides may be in weekly or monthly divisions. Put patient appointment reminder cards in the appropriate location in the file. Check the file each week or month, depending on the divisions, then mail the reminders.

have a simple one- or two-sentence message, such as: "According to our records, you are due for a follow-up visit. If you would kindly call the office, we will be glad to arrange an appointment for you." The physician's name, address, and telephone number should be printed on the card. Many physicians also include their specialty on the reminder card. However, because postcards can be read by anyone, this might not be a good idea if the physician is in a sensitive specialty such as plastic surgery or psychiatry. Place the card in a **tickler file** (Box 8-2) and mail it at the appropriate time (Fig. 8-6).

? Checkpoint Question
5. What are the three types of patient reminders?

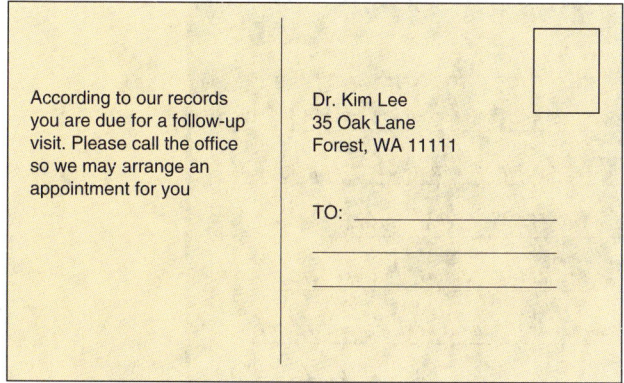

FIGURE 8-6
Reminder postcards are often used to remind patients to schedule annual examinations.

➤ ADAPTING THE SCHEDULE

Emergencies

When a patient calls with an emergency, your first responsibility is to determine if the problem can be treated in the office. The office should have a policy that you can follow to properly evaluate the situation. You also should have a list of appropriate questions to ask the patient (eg, "*Are you experiencing chest pain? Are you having difficulty breathing? How long have you had the symptoms?*") (See Chap. 28, Medical Office Emergencies for more detailed information.)

What If?
What if the patient who is calling is having chest pain? What should you do?

Follow your office policy. In general, any caller who appears to have an emergency (eg, chest pain, dyspnea) should be immediately referred to a physician or nurse. If the physician is not available, call your emergency service number (911 in most areas) while keeping the caller on the line and have the ambulance take the patient to the nearest hospital. It is not advisable to instruct patients with chest pain or dyspnea to drive themselves to the physician's office. Giving medical advice over the telephone is out of the scope of practice for medical assistants; you can be held legally accountable for practicing medicine without a license (see Chap. 3, Medicine and the Law).

Patients Who Are Acutely Ill

Patients who are acutely ill will usually have serious though not life-threatening conditions. These patients will need to be seen as soon as possible, but not necessarily on that same day. Obtain as much information about the patient's medical problem as you can so your message to the physician will allow him or her to decide how soon the patient should be seen.

Walk-in Patients

"Walk-in" patients are those who arrive at the office without a scheduled appointment and expect to see the physician that day. Typically, the physician will have told you how to handle such situations. In general, you must first determine the reason for the "walk in." Patients with medical emergencies will need to be seen immediately. Other patients can be asked to have a seat in the waiting room while you inform the physician of the patient's presence. The physician can then make the decision to see the patient or not.

If the patient is to be seen, explain that you will work him or her into the schedule as soon as possible for a brief examination. When the patient leaves the office, you might apologize for the delay, then ask the patient to schedule an appointment for the next visit.

If the physician decides not to see a walk-in patient, you will have to ask the patient to schedule an appointment and to return later.

Late Patients

Patients who are late inevitably cause problems in the schedule. Unfortunately, not only is the patient late, but he or she may also complain if there's a wait to be seen. You should gently but firmly apologize for the delay but tell the patient, "You were late and Dr. Steiner is seeing another patient now. The doctor should be able to see you in about 15 minutes." Patients who are routinely late should be advised in a polite manner that "according to our office policies patients who are more than 15 minutes late will have to be rescheduled." In addition, ask patients to call the office if they know they are going to be late.

Physician Delays

Of course, there will be times when the physician is delayed. If office hours have not yet begun, call the patients with appointments and give them the options of coming in later in the day or rescheduling the appointment for another day. If patients are waiting in the office, inform them immediately if the physician will be delayed. For example, you might say, "Dr. Samuel has been delayed and will probably be 20 to 30 minutes late. Would you like to wait, or would you prefer to reschedule for another time?" Always keep your patients informed; most people will understand if they know you have not ignored or forgotten them. If you reschedule an appointment, note in the patient's chart the reason for the cancellation or rescheduling.

Missed Appointments

A missed appointment or "no show" is when a patient neglects to keep an appointment and does not notify the office. When this happens, call the patient to try to determine why the appointment was missed and to reschedule for another time. If you are unable to reach the patient by telephone, send a card asking the patient to reschedule. Note in the patient's chart any missed appointment and that you have either rescheduled the appointment or mailed a card to schedule another appointment. If the patient habitually fails to keep appointments, you may want to call and remind the patient the day before the appointment.

Continued failure to keep appointments should be brought to the attention of the physician, who may want to either call the patient personally (particularly if the patient is seriously ill) or to send a letter expressing concern for the patient's welfare. Notations of all actions and copies of any letters sent to the patient

Charting Example

| 05/12/98 | 1530 Patient was called regarding missing scheduled appointment for today at 0930. Patient states that she "forgot" about the appointment. Appointment was rescheduled for 05/14/98 at 1000. Patient was advised of the need to have regular prenatal checkups. Patient verbalized understanding. Dr. Wong was notified that appointment was missed and rescheduled. ———————— Thomas Richards, RMA |

should become a permanent part of the individual's medical record.

➤ CANCELLATIONS

Cancellations by the Office

You may need to cancel a patient's appointment if the physician is ill, has an emergency, or has scheduled a short vacation. Patients who must be rescheduled need not be told the specific reason for the physician's absence. These cancellations should be noted in the patient's medical record.

When you have advance notice, write a letter to the patient indicating that the physician will be away from the office, but will return by a certain date. Patients should be alerted to cancellations a week before their appointments. Offer a specific date and time for a new appointment, or ask the patient to call the office to reschedule.

If you have to cancel on the day of the appointment, call the patient and explain. For example, you might say, *"Dr. Patel has been called out of town unexpectedly. Would it be convenient to reschedule your appointment for sometime next week?"* If the patient arrives at the office before you can contact him or her, apologize and politely explain the situation. Most patients will be understanding.

When a physician will be unavailable for an extended period, it is necessary to have another physician cover the practice or be "on call." Everyone in the office should have a list of names and addresses of "on call" physicians and you should give this information to your patients, according to your office policy.

Cancellations by the Patient

When a patient cancels an appointment, ask the reason for the cancellation and mark it on your appointment schedule and in the patient's chart. Offer to reschedule at another time. If the patient is being seen for a continuing problem, be sure he or she understands the necessity for reexamination. If the patient wants to call back for an appointment, make a note to yourself to check on the call back in a few days. If a patient cancels appointments frequently, you should bring it to the physician's attention.

If a patient cancels an appointment and you have a full schedule, nothing need be done. However, if your schedule is light, refer to your move-up list to try to fill the vacancy.

➤ MAKING APPOINTMENTS FOR PATIENTS IN OTHER FACILITIES

Referrals and Consultations

When calling another physician's office for an appointment for your patient, provide the following information:

- Physician's name and telephone number
- Patient's name, address, and telephone number
- Reason for the call
- Degree of urgency
- Whether the patient is being sent for consultation or referral

Record in the patient's chart the time, date of the call, and the person who received your call. Tell the person you are calling that you wish to be notified if your patient does not keep the appointment. If this occurs, be sure to tell your physician and enter this information in the patient's record.

Write the name, address, and telephone number of the doctor you are referring your patient to on your office stationery and include the date and time of the appointment. Give or mail this information to your patient. Occasionally, the patient may call the referring physician to make his or her own appointment. If this is the situation, ask the patient to call you with the appointment date, then document this in the chart.

Laboratory Tests or X-rays

These appointments are usually made while the patient is still in the office. Before scheduling, determine the exact test(s) the physician requires and how soon the results are needed. (Be sure to indicate to the facility if the results are needed immediately, or STAT.) Also, check with the patient for any time restrictions he or she may have. Give the facility the patient's name, address, telephone number, the exact test(s) required, and any other special instructions from the physician. Give the patient a laboratory or x-ray referral slip with the time and date of the appointment as well as the name, address, and telephone number of the outside facility.

Some laboratory studies or x-ray tests require advance preparation by the patient. Give your patient a written and verbal explanation of the required preparation, and be sure he or she understands the importance of following the instructions. On the patient's chart, note the name of the outside facility and the date and time of the appointment. Also place a reminder in your tickler file or on your appointment schedule to be sure the test results are received as requested.

Surgery

Before you can schedule a surgical procedure, you must know the exact procedure, the amount of time needed for the procedure, the urgency of the procedure, and the type of sedation or anesthesia required. Call the hospital operating room or outpatient surgical facility and specify the time and date the physician has requested. The operating facility will need to know the exact procedure, the amount of time needed, the type of anesthesia required, and any other special instructions your physician may have. The facility will also need the patient's name, age, address, telephone number, and insurance information.

If the hospital has supplied your office with preadmission forms, give a copy to the patient and make sure he or she understands the need to complete and return the form in a timely manner. Give the patient all preoperative instructions including the need for laboratory studies, x-ray testing, or autologous blood donation (donation of a person's own blood). Finally, note in the patient's record the name of the operating facility and the date and time the surgery is scheduled. You may also need to arrange for hospital admission.

➤ WHEN THE APPOINTMENT SCHEDULE DOES NOT WORK

No appointment schedule runs smoothly all the time, so an occasional glitch is to be expected. However, if you find that your schedule is chaotic nearly every day, you should determine the cause. To do so, evaluate the schedule over a period of time, generally 2 to 3 months. For example, make a list of all patients seen, their arrival times, the amount of time they spent with the physician, the time they left, and the amount of time needed to perform each examination or treatment.

Your evaluation may reveal that many of your patients are arriving late or that you have not allotted enough time for certain procedures. Sometimes, a habitually late physician is the problem. Or you may find that too many staff people are making appointments. If this is the case, you can assign only one staff person to handle all scheduling.

Some problems may never be completely solved. However, if they are identified, you can often make adjustments to avoid causing frustration for both patients and office personnel.

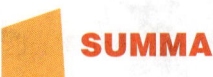

SUMMARY

Accurate appointment scheduling is essential for the success of any medical office setting. As a medical assistant, it is your responsibility to properly schedule patients, remind patients of their scheduled appointments, and to document any missed or rescheduled appointments.

CRITICAL THINKING CHALLENGES

1. Assume that you are the senior medical assistant in a physician's office. Create a policy and procedure for scheduling patients.
2. Reminder cards that are mailed can cause a breach in patient confidentiality. What other methods could you use that would limit the potential for invasion of patient privacy?
3. Review Chap. 4, Fundamental Communication Skills. What are some examples of kinesics and proxemics that would indicate to you that a patient is upset about delays in seeing the physician? What are some things that you can do to help this situation?
4. You notice that patients typically wait 30 to 45 minutes past their scheduled appointment times because of the physician. How would you approach a physician who chronically runs late?

ANSWERS TO CHECKPOINT QUESTIONS

1. The three systems that can be used for patient office visits include scheduled appointments, flexible hours, and open hours.
2. Before scheduling any appointments, you must create a matrix.
3. The three factors that can affect scheduling are patient needs, physician preferences, and the physical facilities.
4. Wave scheduling is helpful if your office does double bookings.
5. The three type of patient reminders are appointment cards, telephone reminders, and mailed reminder cards.

SUGGESTIONS FOR FURTHER READING

Andreas, A. (1996). *Saunders Manual of Medical Office Management*. Philadelphia: W. B. Saunders.

Johnson, J. M., & Johnson, M. W. (1994). *Computerized Medical Office Management*. Albany, NY: Delmar.

Written Communications

Chapter Outline

Letter Development
    Components of a Letter
    Letter Formats
    Writing a Business Letter
Memorandum Development
    Components of a Memorandum
Sending Written Communication
    Facsimile Machines
    Electronic Mail
    United States Postal Service
Receiving and Handling Incoming Mail
    Types of Incoming Mail

    Opening and Sorting Mail
    Annotation
Composing Agendas and Minutes
Transcription
    Transcription Machines
    The Dictating Process
Summary
Critical Thinking Challenges
Answers to Checkpoint Questions
Suggestions for Further Reading

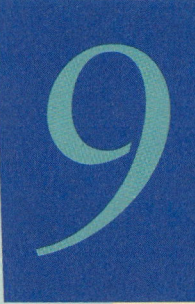

DACUM Components

1.3   Practice within the scope of education, training, and personal capabilities
1.4   Maintain confidentiality
2.7   Receive, organize, prioritize, and transmit information
2.10 Use medical terminology appropriately
2.11 Compose written communication using correct grammar, spelling, and format
3.1   Perform basic secretarial skills
3.5   Perform medical transcription

Chapter Competencies

Learning Objectives

Upon successfully completing this chapter, you will be able to:

1. Spell and define the Key Terms.
2. Describe the process of letter development.
3. Describe the process of memorandum development.
4. Discuss the various mailing options.
5. Identify the types of incoming written communication seen in a physician's office.
6. List the items that must be included in an agenda.
7. Identify the items that must be included in minutes.
8. Discuss the transcription process.

Performance Objectives

Upon successfully completing this chapter, you will be able to:

1. Create a business letter.
2. Create a memorandum.
3. Address and send written communication.
3. Open and sort mail.
4. Annotate a document.
5. Transcribe a document.

Key Terms

(See Glossary for definitions.)

annotation
block
closing
enclosure
full block
identification line
memorandum
proofreading
salutation
scanner
semiblock

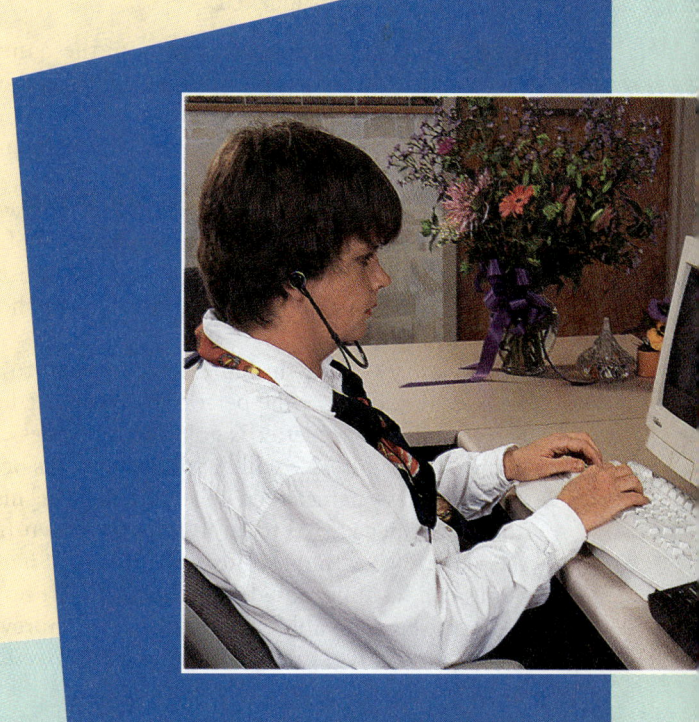

The ability to write well is an important skill for medical assistants. Your written communication must be clear, concise, and correct. Poorly written documents reflect negatively both on the physician's practice and on you. You will be responsible for creating and handling many types of written communication. This chapter discusses letter development, **memorandum** writing, sending written communication, handling incoming mail, composing agendas and minutes, and medical transcription.

➤ LETTER DEVELOPMENT

Writing effective business letters is a skill that requires practice and careful attention to detail. To write a professional business letter, you must:

- Understand the components of a letter
- Use the correct letter format
- Ensure the message is clear, concise, and accurate

Each of these areas is described in detail below.

Components of a Letter

A letter has 12 basic components. We will explore each one, beginning at the top of the page. For easy reference, Figure 9-1 displays a sample business letter with the various components marked.

1. *Letterhead*. The letterhead consists of the name of the practice or physician, address, and sometimes the company logo. The letterhead is often embossed in color and centered on the top of the page.
2. *Date*. The date includes the month, day, and year. It should be positioned two to four spaces below the letterhead or fifteen spaces below the top of the page if no letterhead is used. The date must be typed on only one line and no abbreviations should be used.
3. *Inside address*. The inside address refers to the name and address of the person to whom the letter is being sent. If the letter is going to a business, the name of the addressee will be followed by his or her title, business name, then the address. The inside address is placed two to twelve spaces down from the date. Never abbreviate city or town names. States can be abbreviated. (See Appendix III for list of approved state abbreviations.) Never abbreviate business titles (eg, President, Chief Executive Officer).
4. *Subject line*. The subject line, an optional component, is used to highlight the intent of a letter or to indicate about whom the letter is regarding. It is

placed two spaces below the inside address and is written as Re:_____ (an abbreviation for regarding).

5. *Salutation*. The **salutation** is the greeting of the letter. It is placed two spaces down from the inside address or the subject line. The first letter of each word is capitalized and the phrase is always followed by a colon. When writing to a physician, write out the word doctor. When writing to someone whose name you do not know, use either of the following salutations: To Whom It May Concern *or* Dear Sir or Madam.
6. *Body of the letter*. The body of the letter contains the message. It should be single spaced with double spaces between the paragraphs. Abbreviations should not be used unless they are widely accepted (eg, etc) or introduced in the letter.
7. **Closing**. The *closing* concludes the letter. Some common closings include: Sincerely, Yours truly, Regards, Respectfully, Cordially yours. Only the first word is capitalized and a comma follows the phrase. Closings are placed two spaces down from the end of the letter.
8. *Signature and typed name*. The name of the person sending the document is typed four spaces below the closing with the person's title typed directly below. The physician will read and sign the letter above the typed name. If you are instructed to sign the letter, sign the physician's name followed by a slash mark and your name.

   Example: Susan James, MD/Raymond Smith, RMA
9. *Identification line*. The **identification line**, an optional component, indicates who dictated the letter and who wrote it. It consists of abbreviations only. The initials of the person who dictated the letter are capitalized; the letter writer's initials are in lower case.
10. *Enclosure*. An **enclosure** is something that is included with a letter. It is abbreviated *Enc.* and is placed two spaces down from the identification line. The number of documents included is placed in parentheses; if only one document is included, just the abbreviation Enc. is used.
11. *Carbon copy*. The abbreviation *cc*, for carbon copy, is used to indicate that a duplicate letter has been sent. It is typed two spaces below the enclosure line. Usually, letters are copied to managers, supervisors, or to the physician who requested that the given information be dispersed.
12. *Margin*. The margin is the blank space around the letter. A 1-inch margin is used for both the left and right sides of the letter and the bottom. Margins are used to center the components of a letter in a standardized manner.

Vincent Delmar, M.D.   (1)
134 Morgan Street, Suite 313
Hartford, Connecticut 06157

May 17, 1998   (2)

Dr. Thomas Wilhelm   (3)
Medical Director
Family Practice Associates
134 N. Tater Drive
Hartford, Connecticut 06157

(12) Re: Mr. Mark Sieble   (4)

Dear Doctor Wilhelm: (5)

Thank you for asking me to evaluate Mr. Sieble. I agree with your diagnosis of rheumatoid arthritis. His prodromal symptoms include vague articular pain and stiffness, weight loss and general malaise. Mr. Sieble states that the joint discomfort is most prominent in the mornings, gradually improving throughout the day.

My physical examination shows a 45-year-old male patient in fair health. Heart sounds normal, no murmurs or gallops noted. Lung sounds clear. Enlarged lymph nodes were noted. Abdomen soft, bowel sounds present, and the spleen was not enlarged. Extremities showed subcutaneous nodules and flexion contractures on both hands.

Laboratory findings were indicative of rheumatoid arthritis. See attached laboratory data. I do not feel x-rays are warranted at this time.

My recommendations are to continue Mr. Sieble on salicylate therapy, rest and physical therapy. I suggest that you have Mr. Sieble attend physical therapy at the American Rehabilitation Center on Main Street.

Thank you for this interesting consultation.

Yours truly,   (7)

Vincent Delmar   (8)
Vincent Delmar, MD

VD/em   (9)

Enc. (2)   (10)

cc: Dr. Samuel Adams   (11)

FIGURE 9-1

Components of a business letter. This business letter, done in full block format, contains these components: (*1*) letterhead, (*2*) date, (*3*) inside address, (*4*) subject line, (*5*) salutation, (*6*) body, (*7*) closing, (*8*) signature and typed name, (*9*) identification line, (*10*) enclosure, (*11*) carbon copy. A one-inch margin is used (*12*).

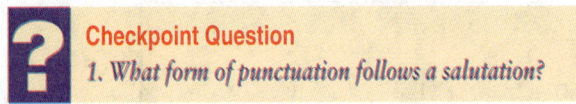

Checkpoint Question

1. What form of punctuation follows a salutation?

Checkpoint Question

2. What is the purpose of the identification line?

Letter Formats

There are three basic types of letter formats: **full block**, **semiblock**, and **block**. Office policy or physician preference dictates which format you will use.

Full Block

In this format, each line is justified to the left. Full block is the most formal format and is most commonly used for professional letters. (See Fig. 9-1 for an example of a letter done in full block format.)

Block

In the block format, the date, subject line, closing, and signatures are flush to the right margin. All other lines are justified to the left (Fig. 9-2).

Semiblock

The semiblock is the same as the block except the first sentence of each paragraph is indented five spaces (Fig. 9-3). Semiblock is also referred to as modified block.

William Erikson, MD
Storrs Family Practice
22 Maple Avenue
Storrs, Connecticut 06268

August 15, 1998

Ms. Karen Roberts
Office Manager
ABC Copier
Fifth Avenue
Storrs, Connecticut 06268

Dear Ms. Roberts:

We are pleased to announce that we have selected your firm to meet our copying needs for 1999.

Please forward a contract to us, including the stipulations that were previously discussed. After reviewing the contract, I will contact you to arrange for a date and time for a staff orientation session on using the new copier.

I look forward to working with you and ABC Copier.

Sincerely,

Jenny Jacobs, RMA

WE/jj

cc: William Erikson, M.D.

FIGURE 9-2
Sample letter in block format.

Elizabeth Jones, M.D.
750 East Street, Suite 205
Hialeah, Florida 33013

June 12, 1998

Margaret Trent
18 Cambridge Street
Hialeah, Florida 33013

Dear Ms. Trent:

As per our phone conversation, your blood glucose level remains elevated. It is essential that we stabilize your blood sugar level.

In order to achieve normal blood sugar levels, you must follow the enclosed diet. A meeting with a Registered Dietitian can be arranged for you to discuss any dietary concerns you may have.

I am also enclosing patient education instructions for the use of a glucometer. You must test your blood sugar every morning and keep a diary of your results. Glucometers can be purchased from any pharmacy. If you need assistance in using the glucometer, please contact Raymond Smith, CMA, at 555-6423.

Presently, I do not wish to prescribe any medications. If we are unable to get your blood sugar under control, I will prescribe an oral diabetic medication.

Please call my office and schedule an appointment for the week of June 20 for a blood draw and a follow-up visit.

Sincerely,

Elizabeth Jones, M.D.

EJ/rs

enc. (2)

FIGURE 9-3
Sample letter in semiblock format.

Checkpoint Question

3. What are the three formats in which letters can be written?

Writing a Business Letter

To create a professional business letter, follow these three steps: preparation, composition, and editing.

Preparation

Before you begin to type a letter, mentally prepare your message. You might start formulating the message by envisioning yourself talking to the person to whom you are sending the letter. Preparation offers three benefits:

1. It helps eliminate writer's block.
2. It gets you to focus on the message, not the mechanics (eg, spelling, grammar, punctuation).
3. It enhances your organization.

Box 9-1 discusses specific questions that you should ask yourself as you prepare your letter. Knowing the answers to these questions helps you target your message.

Composition

The goal of composition is to ensure that your message is transmitted clearly, concisely, and accurately to your reader. As you did during preparation, focus on the message, not on the mechanics.

A clear message ensures that your reader knows precisely what is expected; an unclear message leaves room for doubt. For example:

BOX 9-1 Letter Preparation: Questions to Ask Yourself

By determining the answers to these four questions, you can better prepare the message of your letter.

1. *Who is my reader?*
   It is very important that you use proper gender identification. Be especially careful with names that can be used for males or females (eg, Sam, Kelly, Ronnie, Alex, Tracy).
   Determine the reader's comprehension level. Letters to physicians will be more technical and will include the use of medical terminology. Letters to patients will be less technical and use medical terminology sparingly.
2. *What do I want my reader to do?*
   This is your call to action—make it **clear** and **specific.** For example, you might write: *Please complete the enclosed insurance form (2 pages). Be sure to include all necessary information and to sign your name. Place the form in the enclosed envelope and return it to our office by June 15, 1998.* Avoid the term "at your earliest convenience"—include a date for the required action. If possible, include a response mechanism, such as a self-addressed, stamped envelope.
3. *What do I want to say?*
   Briefly list the information that needs to be included. To help you remember all the necessary in-

formation, ask yourself: Who, what, where, when why, and how.

4. *How will I organize my message?*

Here are three basic formats that you can use to organize your message:

1. Chronologic: In this format, items are discussed in a sequential manner, beginning with the earliest date and proceeding to the most recent date. For example, when discussing the physician's career, you would list his or her earlier experiences before the most recent career achievements.
2. Problem-oriented: This format is used to let the reader know about a specific problem and to provide instructions on correcting the problem. For example, if a patient's blood work came back with abnormal results, a letter would be sent identifying the problem (low hematocrit) and advising the patient on the possible causes, treatments, and follow-up procedures.
3. Comparison: This format is used to evaluate the effectiveness of two or more items. For example, as an office manager, you may need to write to the physician comparing two different service contracts or two sample computer software packages.

Unclear: Please contact me.

Clear: Please contact me by Thursday, October 1.

Unclear: You need to make an appointment for blood work.

Clear: Call Temple Hospital laboratories (555-4010) and make an appointment for a blood glucose test on March 13.

A concise message is short and to the point. Extraneous phrases and adjectives should not be used. For example:

Not concise: Please enclose a check for the amount of $50.

Concise: Please enclose a $50 check.

Not concise: In the month of June, the practice saw 150 patients.

Concise: 150 patients were seen in June.

An accurate message includes the correct date, time, figures, and information. Inaccurate messages cause delays and confusion and can lead to poor public relations.

Checkpoint Question

4. What is the goal of composing?

Editing

After you have composed the letter, you need to edit it for both grammatical errors and factual information. Editing is a key step in making your letter a success. Editing involves two steps: **proofreading** and corrections.

PROOFREADING

Whenever possible, have a colleague proofread (read text and check for accuracy) your letter and provide constructive criticism (be sure to maintain confidentiality). If you are using a computer, consider printing out a hard copy of your document for proofreading; some individuals find it difficult to proofread a document on the computer screen. Check for the following items:

BOX 9-2 Basic Grammatical Tips

Capitalization

Always capitalize the first word in a sentence, proper nouns, the pronoun "I," book titles, and known geographical names. Names of persons, holidays, and trademark items should be capitalized. The expressions of time (AM and PM) are capitalized.

Punctuation

- Period (.)—Used at end of sentences and following abbreviations.
- Comma (,)—Used to separate words or phrases that are part of a series of three or more. The final comma before the "and" may be omitted. A comma can also be used after a long introductory clause or to separate independent clauses joined by and, but, yet, or, and nor.
- Semicolon (;)—Used to separate a long list of items in a series or to separate independent clauses not joined by a conjunction (eg, and, but, because).
- Colon (:)—Used to introduce a series of items, to follow formal salutations, or to separate the hours from minutes indicating time.
- Apostrophe (')—Used to denote omissions of letters and to denote the possessive cases of nouns.

- Quotation marks (")—Used to set off spoken dialogue, some titles (eg, journal articles, newspapers, or television and radio programs), and words used in a special way.
- Parentheses ()—Used to indicate a part of a sentence that is not part of the main sentence but is essential for the meaning of the sentence. Also used to enclose a number, for confirmation, that is spelled out in a sentence.

Abbreviations

Use these only when they are well known within a particular profession. The meanings of abbreviations may vary among medical offices (eg, BS can be used to abbreviate blood sugar, bowel sounds, or breath sounds). For this reason, a policy listing acceptable abbreviations for your office should be made.

Numbers

Write out numbers except when referring to particular laboratory data numbers, medication dosages, or specific medical number. Ordinal numbers are written out (eg, Fifth Avenue)—first through ninth; greater than ninth, use numerals.

BOX 9-3 Basic Spelling Tips

When in doubt about the spelling of a word, always use a dictionary or spell check (if you are using a computer) to confirm the spelling. Keep in mind that a computerized spell check will check for spelling but will not alert you to inappropriate word usage. Here is an example: "The expenses are listed on lie two." *Lie* is spelled correctly and will not be highlighted by a spell check; however, the writer intended to use the word *line*.

1. Remember this rhyme: *I* comes before *e*, except after *c*, or when sounded like *a* as in neighbor and weigh. Examples: achieve, receive. (The exceptions are either, neither, weird, leisure, and conscience.)
2. Words ending in *ie* drop the *e* and change the *i* to *y* before adding *ing*. Examples: die—dying, lie—lying.
3. Words ending in *o* that are preceded by a vowel are made plural by adding *s*. Example: studio—studios, trio—trios. Words ending in *o* that are preceded by a consonant form the plural by adding *es*. Examples: potato—potatoes, hero—heroes.

4. Words ending in *y* preceded by a vowel form the plural by adding *s*. Examples: attorney—attorneys, day—days. Words ending in *y* that are preceded by a consonant change the *y* to *i* and add *es*. Examples: berry—berries, lady—ladies.
5. The final consonant of a one-syllable word is doubled before adding a suffix beginning with a vowel. Examples: run—running, pin—pinning. If the final consonant is preceded by another consonant or by two vowels, do not double the consonant. Examples: look—looked, act—acting.
6. Words ending in a silent *e* generally drop the *e* before adding a suffix beginning with a vowel. Examples: ice—icing, judge—judging. The exceptions are dye, eye, shoe, and toe. However, the *e* is not dropped in suffixes beginning with a consonant unless another vowel precedes the final *e*. Examples: pale—paleness, argue—argument.
7. For all words ending in *c*, insert a *k* before adding a suffix beginning with *e, i,* or *y*. Examples: picnic—picknicking, traffic—trafficker.

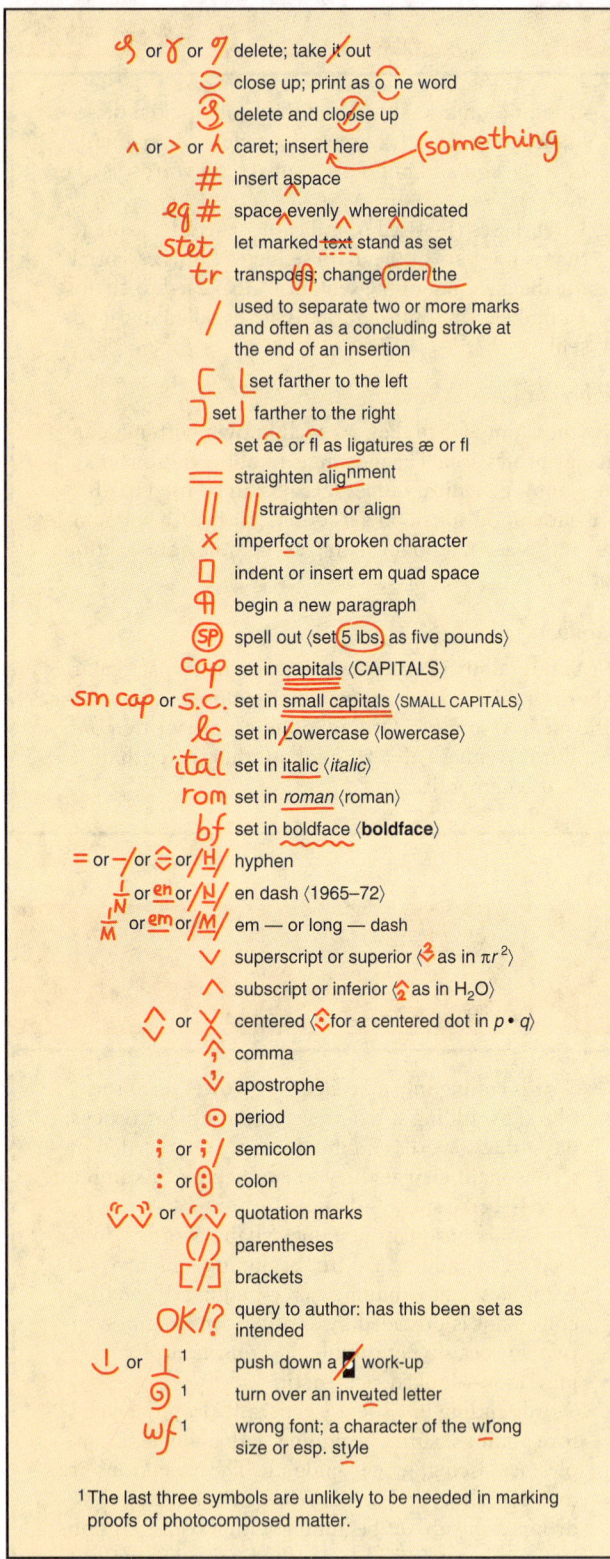

FIGURE 9-4
Standard proofreader's marks.

- Accuracy of all information
- Clarity and conciseness
- Clarity of the call to action (see Box 9-1)
- Grammar (Box 9-2)
- Spelling (Box 9-3)
- Punctuation
- Capitalization
- Logical organization

Use proofreader's marks (Fig. 9-4) to accelerate the editing process. These are standard marks used to indicate corrections. You should become familiar with the basic marks.

BOX 9-4   Writing A Business Letter

1. Prepare your message for the reader. Answer the four questions:
   - Who is my reader?
   - What do I want my reader to do?
   - What do I want to say?
   - How will I organize my message?
2. Begin composing your letter:
   - Select the type of letter format.
   - Insert the mandatory components (letterhead, date, inside address, body, closing, and signature line).
   - Insert optional components as needed (subject line, identification line, carbon copy, and enclosures.
3. Edit your message:
   - Print hard copy and proofread using proofreader's marks.
   - Make necessary corrections.
4. If your letter needs more than one page, use letterhead stationery for page one only. For the subsequent pages, the addressee's name and title, page number, date, and subject are typed on the seventh line from the top. The body of the letter is then started three lines down from the heading.
   Example: James Roberts, M.D. -3- May 24, 1999
   or
   James Roberts, M.D.
   Page two
   December 20, 1999
   Subject: Virginia Marshall
   Either style is considered acceptable.
5. Obtain the necessary signatures and prepare to send the letter. Always copy the letter before mailing it and file as per office policy.

After making corrections, print a final copy of the letter. It is important to note that computerized spell checks should be used with caution as they highlight misspelled words but not incorrectly used words.

Box 9-4 outlines the steps for writing a business letter.

➤ MEMORANDUM DEVELOPMENT

Memorandums (often called memos) are for interoffice communication only; they are never sent to patients. They are less formal then letters and generally are used for brief announcements.

Components of a Memorandum

A memorandum contains the standard elements listed below in bold. Follow the guidelines noted to properly complete each element.

Date: Use the same rules for letters when typing the date for memorandums.

To: List the names of all recipients, either in alphabetic or hierarchic order. If the memorandum is going to a particular group (eg, All Department Managers, All Employees), it can be addressed to the group.

From: List the name and title of the person sending the memorandum.

Subject: Insert a brief phrase describing the purpose of the memorandum.

Body: Write the message of the memorandum here.

Carbon copy (cc): Use the same rules as for letters when sending duplicate copies of memorandums.

Salutations and closings are not used in memorandums. All lines in a memorandum are justified left and 1-inch margins are used.

The Date, To, From, and Subject lines are double-spaced. The body is single-spaced with double spaces between paragraphs. Figure 9-5 shows a sample memorandum.

Writing a memorandum involves the same steps (preparation, composition, editing) as writing a business letter; however, instead of mailing the document, you will distribute it to the appropriate staff members. Be sure to keep a copy of the memorandum for your files.

➤ SENDING WRITTEN COMMUNICATION

After the document has been written, proofread, and signed, it is ready to be sent to its receiver. Written communications can be sent three ways: via facsimile machines, by electronic mail, or by postal service.

American Family Physician Practice
162 N. Plains Road
Boca Raton, Florida 33432

Date: August 16, 1998

To: All staff members

From: Ronald Jackson, Office Manager

Subject: Staff Meeting

The staff meeting scheduled for Thursday, August 18, has been changed to Tuesday, August 23, at 2 P.M. Please bring your productivity reports for July to the meeting.

Be prepared to discuss the advantages/disadvantages of purchasing a new automated office billing system.

Please call me at extension 4223 if you have any questions.

FIGURE 9-5
Sample memorandum.

Facsimile Machines

Facsimile machines, or fax machines, allow the medical office to send and receive printed material over a phone line. These machines offer a convenient and cost-effective way to transmit records, orders, prescriptions, test results, and other materials that require quick receipt. When you receive a fax, photocopy it if it is printed on thermal paper (text printed on thermal paper fades quickly), then forward it to the appropriate person.

Some fax machines have a function called a **scanner.** A scanner takes a picture of a written document and inserts the picture into the computer. (Scanners can also be independent pieces of equipment.)

Electronic Mail

Electronic mail, or E-Mail, allows computer-to-computer communication, whether within the same facility or anywhere throughout the world. The communication occurs through a modem. Each computer must be linked to an on-line service provider.

United States Postal Service (USPS)

Written communication is commonly sent via the United States Postal Service. Envelopes must be correctly prepared so that the optical scanners used by the postal service can sort the mail quickly and efficiently.

Addressing Envelopes

The standard business envelope is No. 10. USPS regulations state that the minimal size of an envelope is 3½ x 5 inches. It must be rectangular in shape and can be no less than 0.007 inches thick.

The return address is placed in the upper left hand corner. It should not exceed four lines. In most situations, the return address will be embossed.

The recipient's address is typed 12 spaces down from the top. **All words of the address should begin with a capital letter.** Only approved abbreviations for states should be used and you will note that no punctuation is used following the abbreviation (see Appendix III for a list of approved state abbreviations). All addresses must include the five-digit Zip Code; whenever possible, the four-digit expanded Zip Code should be used. The entire address should not exceed four lines.

Special notations such as "Confidential" or "Personal" are placed on the left hand side of the envelope two lines below the return address. Notations for "Hand Cancel" and "Special Delivery" are made in the upper right hand corner of the envelope below the postage. **Nothing should be printed on the right lower corner of the envelope because the USPS uses that space for its bar codes.** Figure 9-6 displays a properly addressed envelope. Box 9-5 describes the steps for properly addressing and sending written communication.

Checkpoint Question
5. Where would you type the notation "Personal" on an envelope?

Checkpoint Question
6. Where would you type the notation "Hand Cancel" on an envelope?

Affixing Postage

Proper postage must be affixed to the envelope either via a stamp or through the use of a postage meter machine (Fig. 9-7). Postage meter machines are inhouse

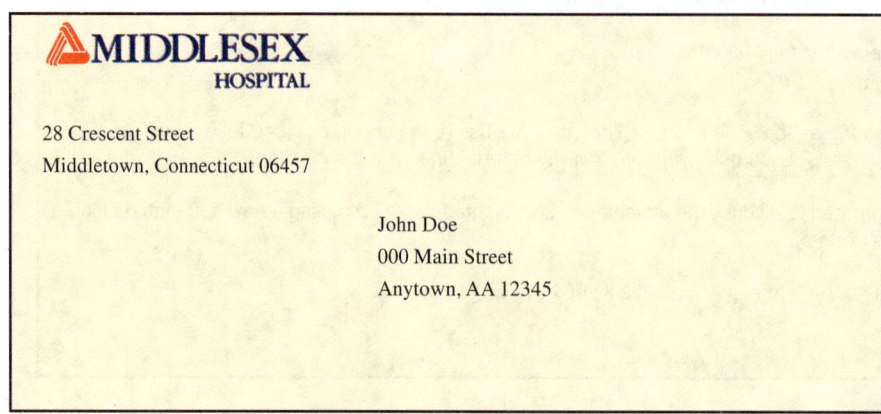

FIGURE 9-6
Properly addressed envelope.

BOX 9-5   Addressing and Sending Written Communication

1. Obtain a No. 10 envelope. If a return address is embossed, go to step number two. If there is no return address, type the return address in the upper left hand corner of the envelope.
2. Type the recipient's address twelve spaces from the top of the envelope.
3. Type any special notations. Personal and confidential should be typed two spaces below the return address. Special delivery or hand cancel notations should be typed below the postage.
4. Seal the envelope.
5. Select the type of mail service that is appropriate. Affix stamps and/or labels to the envelope.
6. Deposit the envelope in an appropriate postal service box.

machines that are regulated by the postal service. They contain a prepaid amount of postage and can either imprint the postage stamp directly on the envelope or onto an adhesive tape which is then applied to the envelope. Some machines also seal the envelope. The date on the postal machine must be changed daily and the ink roller must be kept full.

The advantage to using postage meter machines in the office setting is that they bypass the postal cancellation process, enhancing the speed at which the document reaches its final destination. They also help speed the mailing process when large numbers of documents need to be sent out.

Mailing Options

Mail can be sent in a variety of ways based on its urgency and value. The following is a brief description of the services offered by the USPS.

- *Express mail*, the fastest service, ensures delivery of your package by the next day (by noon in most areas). Express mail is delivered 7 days a week at no extra charge. The maximum weight for Express mail is 70 pounds; the combined length and girth must not exceed 108 inches.
- *Priority mail*, the second fastest service, offers 2-day delivery to most destinations. (Size requirements are the same as for express mail.)
- *First-class mail* is the service used for sending standard mail (letters and postcards) weighing up to 11 ounces.

P 011 437 846

Receipt for Certified Mail
No Insurance Coverage Provided
Do not use for International Mail
(See Reverse)
UNITED STATES POSTAL SERVICE

Sent to	
Street and No.	
P.O., State and ZIP Code	
Postage	$
Certified Fee	
Special Delivery Fee	
Restricted Delivery Fee	
Return Receipt Showing to Whom & Date Delivered	
Return Receipt Showing to Whom, Date, and Addressee's Address	
TOTAL Postage & Fees	$
Postmark or Date	

PS Form 3800, June 1991

Fold at line over top of envelope to the right of the return address

CERTIFIED

P 011 437 846

MAIL

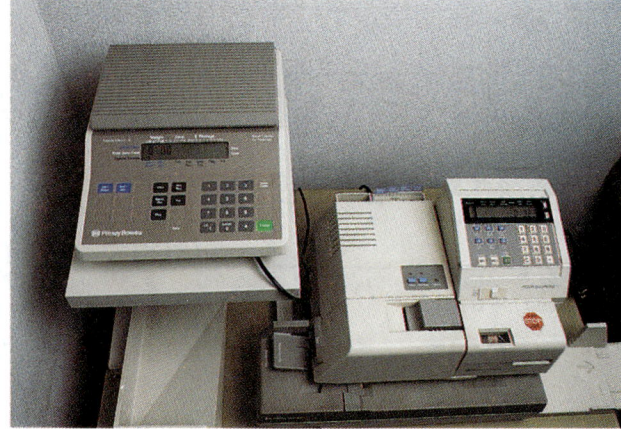

FIGURE 9-7
Postage meter machine.

FIGURE 9-8
Certified mail receipt.

- *Second-class mail* is used only by authorized publishers and registered news agencies.
- *Third-class mail* is used for mailing packages not exceeding 16 ounces. Bulk-mail rates (catalogs, circulars) also fall into this category.
- *Fourth-class mail*, also called parcel post, is used for packages weighing greater than 16 ounces and less than 70 pounds. The combined girth may not exceed 108 inches.

Because postal rates, fees, and services are subject to change, you must stay abreast of the latest information.

Special Services

A *certificate of mailing* is used to prove that a document was mailed. No record is kept at the post office.

Certified mail provides a mailing receipt and a record of the mailing at the local post office (Fig. 9-8). This service is available only for First-class and Priority mail. Return receipts can be purchased in conjunction with this.

Return receipts are used to prove that the recipient received the document (Fig. 9-9).

Insured mail allows you to insure packages (up to $600.00).

Collect on delivery (COD) allows the sender to receive payment for a given item and postage from the recipient for amounts not exceeding $600.00.

Registered mail provides the most protection for valuables. It is available only for Priority and First-class mail. The maximal insurance that can be obtained is $25,000.00. This service can be combined with return receipts and COD.

In addition to the regular postage for the document to be mailed, there is a fee for each of these special services.

International rates are available from your local post office. All international mail is treated with First-class service. Outgoing international mail should have the endorsement "Air Mail" or "Par Avion" printed on the envelope.

The United States Postal Service has a customer service line available to answer your questions: 1-800-222-1811. All offices should have a supply of Express and Priority mail envelopes along with a current fee schedule.

Other Delivery Options

There are many other companies that specialize in document and package delivery, particularly with next-day or second-day delivery services. Examples of these companies include Airborne Express, Federal Express, and United Parcel Service (UPS). Fees vary, so you need to contact each company for prices and available services.

RECEIVING AND HANDLING INCOMING MAIL

Part of the daily routine for a medical assistant is handling the incoming mail. To ensure efficient functioning of the medical office, incoming mail must be sorted correctly and promptly.

Is your RETURN ADDRESS completed on the reverse side?

SENDER:
- Complete items 1 and/or 2 for additional services.
- Complete items 3, 4a, and 4b.
- Print your name and address on the reverse of this form so that we can return this card to you.
- Attach this form to the front of the mailpiece, or on the back if space does not permit.
- Write *"Return Receipt Requested"* on the mailpiece below the article number.
- The Return Receipt will show to whom the article was delivered and the date delivered.

I also wish to receive the following services (for an extra fee):
1. ☐ Addressee's Address
2. ☐ Restricted Delivery

Consult postmaster for fee.

3. Article Addressed to:

4a. Article Number

4b. Service Type
☐ Registered ☐ Certified
☐ Express Mail ☐ Insured
☐ Return Receipt for Merchandise ☐ COD

7. Date of Delivery

5. Received By: *(Print Name)*

6. Signature: *(Addressee or Agent)*
X

8. Addressee's Address *(Only if requested and fee is paid)*

PS Form **3811,** December 1994 Domestic Return Receipt

Thank you for using Return Receipt Service.

FIGURE 9-9
Return mail receipt.

Types of Incoming Mail

Many types of mail are received daily in a physician's office. Examples include:

- Advertisements
- Bills for office services
- Consultation letters
- Hospital communications/newsletters
- Laboratory/radiographic reports
- Office supply magazines
- Patient correspondence
- Payments from insurance companies and patients
- Professional journals
- Literature from professional organizations
- Samples (drugs, laboratory test kits)
- Waiting room magazines

Opening and Sorting Mail

Each physician will have an individual policy on which mail should be opened and how it will be processed. Some physicians will have you sort, file, and respond to mail without their review. However, in some practices, all mail is placed in a special file folder and handled only by the physician or office manager. Box 9-6 lists general guidelines for opening and sorting the mail.

When the physician is away, the mail must be opened and handled appropriately. If the mail requires an urgent response, the covering physician should be contacted, unless otherwise directed. Mail should never be allowed to accumulate in outside mailboxes because patient information is confidential.

Annotation

Some physicians request that each letter be annotated. Annotation involves reading each document and highlighting the key points. If the letter is very detailed, a summary of the key points should be written in the margins. The summary should be factual and not editorialized.

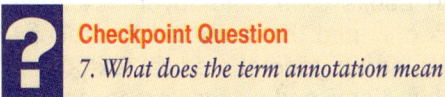
Checkpoint Question
7. *What does the term annotation mean?*

➤ COMPOSING AGENDAS AND MINUTES

Another type of written communication involves typing agendas and minutes. The purpose of an agenda is to outline briefly the topics to be discussed at a meet-

---

BOX 9-6 Opening and Sorting the Mail

1. Gather the necessary equipment: a letter opener, paper clips, and a date stamp.
2. Open all letters and check for enclosures; paper clip these to the letter. If the letter states that enclosures were sent but they are not in the envelope, contact the sender and request them. Indicate on the letter that the enclosures were missing and the name of the person you contacted.
3. Date stamp each item.
4. Sort the mail into categories and deal with it appropriately. Generally, you should handle the following types of mail as noted:
   - Use a paper clip to attach test results to the patient's chart; place the chart in a pile for the physician to review.
   - Record promptly all insurance payments and checks and deposit them according to office policy.
   - Account for all drug samples and appropriately log them into the sample book.
   - Dispose of miscellaneous advertisements, unless otherwise directed.
5. Distribute the mail to the appropriate staff members. For example, mail can be for the physician, nurse manager, office manager, billing clerk, or other personnel.

---

ing. It allows the meeting participants to prepare any necessary reports before the meeting and to anticipate questions. Agendas usually begin with a call to order, followed by a review of previous meeting minutes, old business updates, then new business. Adjournment is the last item on the agenda (Fig. 9-10).

Minutes of meetings should be typed as soon after the meeting as possible. The minutes of a meeting should include:

- List of members present
- List of members absent
- Date and time the meeting was called to order
- Statement regarding the acceptance of the previous minutes
- Brief description of discussions
- List of reports that were submitted
- Date and time of the next meeting
- Adjournment time
- Signature of the person who prepared the minutes and the chairperson's signature

```
              Quality Improvement Committee
                   February 15, 1998
                       Agenda

   I. Call to order
  II. Review and acceptance of the minutes from January
      15, 1998.
 III. Old business
      A. Copy machine updates
      B. Insurance updates for overdue accounts
  IV. New business
      A. New contract for laboratory supplies
      B. Scheduling guidelines for summer vacations
   V. Adjournment
```

FIGURE 9-10
Sample agenda.

➤ TRANSCRIPTION

Transcription is the process of typing a previously dictated message. The most common documents transcribed in a medical office are patient histories, progress notes, and physical examination reports. Other types of documents that you may transcribe are consultation reports, discharge summaries, minor surgical procedures, or general office correspondence.

To transcribe, the medical assistant must:

- Be an excellent typist
- Have a strong medical terminology vocabulary
- Have excellent listening skills
- Have good editing skills

Transcription Machines

Each transcription machine (Fig. 9-11) is slightly different; however, most have the basic parts described below.

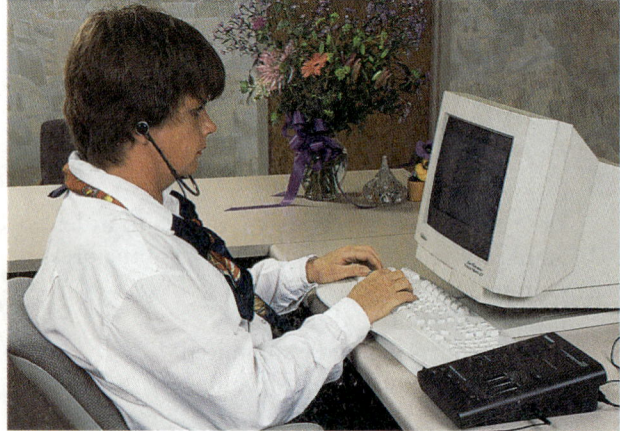

FIGURE 9-11
Transcription machine.

- The *foot pedal* is used to start, stop, fast forward, or rewind the tape.
- The *speed control* regulates the speed at which the tape is played. As a beginner, you want to keep the speed slow. As your listening and typing coordination improve, you will be able to increase the speed of the tape. When you become experienced with a particular physician's voice speed, you will be able automatically to set the speed control to match his or her voice speed and your typing speed.
- The *tone* dial can be adjusted to change the bass or treble of a dictator's voice.
- The *volume control* is used to adjust the sound level.
- The *headset* is used to eliminate distracting external noises. It is important to note that it is not a good habit to share headset ear plugs with fellow colleagues because ear infection transmissions can occur.

Because every transcription machine is slightly different, you should read the instruction manual before you begin working on a unfamiliar machine. All instruction manuals should be kept in one central location in the office for easy access.

What If?

What if you have trouble understanding a word or phrase on the tape? What should you do?

First, rewind the tape and listen again to the phrase. You can try to readjust the speed control to slow the pronunciation of the word. If you are still uncertain about the word or phrase, leave a blank space for that word and continue transcribing. Do not use reference materials until you have finished typing the whole document. Going back and forth between the dictionary and tape will cause you to lose speed and concentration. You should have a selection of reference materials available at your work station. Examples of useful reference books include a standard dictionary, a medical dictionary, both Physician Desk Reference (PDR) books (one is for over-the-counter medications only and the other is for prescribed medications), and a general medical textbook on anatomy, physiology, and disease processes.

The Dictating Process

The physician or health care provider will use a dictation machine to tape a message. After the message is taped, the tape will be removed and marked with some form of identification. In small medical offices, patient initials and/or dates are used. In large health care settings, codes are used to indicate the type of report and the level of urgency. In hospitals, dictation phones are on most patient care units and the tapes are centrally recorded in the medical records department. Box 9-7 describes the steps for transcribing a document.

Checkpoint Question

8. Which four reference books should you have available when you are transcribing?

BOX 9-7 Transcribing a Document

1. Gather the equipment: transcribing machine, head phones, transcription (dictation) tapes, computer or typewriter, and paper.
2. Select a transcription tape. All urgent codes must be typed first. If there are no urgent tapes, select the tape that has the oldest date.
3. Turn on the transcriber and insert the tape.
4. Put on the headset.
5. Position the foot pedal in a comfortable location.
6. Play a sampling of the tape. Adjust the volume, speed, and tone dials to your comfort level.
7. Set margins as appropriate for your computer or typewriter.
8. Rewind the tape to the beginning.
9. As a novice transcriptionist, you will need to play a segment of the tape, stop the tape, and type the message. As your speed and skills progress, you will not need to stop the tape.
10. If you come across an unfamiliar term, leave a blank space in the document and continue transcribing. After you have finished the document, contact the physician, colleague, or use a reference book to complete the blank.
11. Leave the document along with the tape in a designated area for review. After the dictator has reviewed and approved the document, erase the tape and return it to the dictation area. **Never erase a tape until the printed copy has been read and approved by the dictator.**
12. Turn off the power to the computer and transcription machine. Return all supplies. Leave the work area clean and free of trash.

SUMMARY

A medical assistant must have excellent written communication skills. You will use these skills to write letters, memorandums, and transcribe various reports. After writing these documents, you must be able to select the appropriate service for mailing them. Your primary goal with all written communication is to get your message across in a clear, concise, and accurate manner.

CRITICAL THINKING CHALLENGES

1. Create a business letter. Include all the components and use the full block format. Print your unedited copy and indicate your corrections using proofreader's marks. Make the corrections and reprint a final copy. Ask your instructor to review both copies.
2. Develop a one-page instruction sheet that can be posted in the workplace that describes the mailing options.
3. Make a copy of the full block letter example. Annotate the letter.
4. You are having trouble understanding a particular physician's dictation tapes because of his foreign dialect. How would you handle this situation?

ANSWERS TO CHECKPOINT QUESTIONS

1. A colon always follows a salutation.
2. The identification line indicates who dictated the document and who composed it.
3. The three letter formats are full block, semiblock, and block.
4. The goal of composing is to create a clear, concise, and accurate message for your reader.
5. The notation "Personal" is typed on the left side of envelope, two spaces below return address.
6. The notation "Hand Cancel" should be typed in the right-hand corner of envelope below the postage.
7. Annotation means to read, highlight, and summarize a document.
8. Four reference books that can help you in transcribing documents are the PDR, medical dictionary, English dictionary, and a general medical textbook.

SUGGESTIONS FOR FURTHER READING

Strunk, W., Jr and White E.B. (1979). *The Elements of Style*, 3rd ed. New York: Macmillian.

United States Postal Service.(1995). *Consumer's Guide to Postal Rates and Fees*. Publication 123.

Medical Records and Records Management

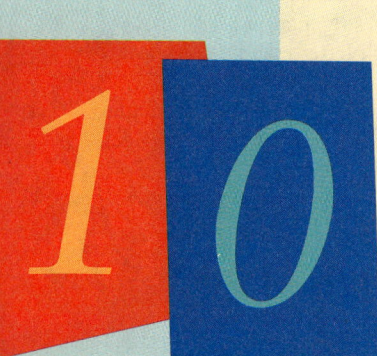

Chapter Outline

Standard Medical Records
  Contents of the Record
Medical Record Organization
  Source-Oriented Medical
    Record
  Problem-Oriented Medical Record
    (POMR)
Documentation Forms
  Progress Notes
  Flow Sheets
  Other Forms
The Medical History
Medical Record Entries
  Additions to Medical Records
Worker's Compensation Records
Filing Procedures

Procedure: Preparing a Medical Record
    File
Filing Systems
  Alphabetic Filing
  Numeric Filing
  Other Filing Systems
Classifying Medical Records
Storing Medical Records
  Statute of Limitations
Releasing Medical Records
  Releasing Records to Patients
Reporting Obligations
Summary
Critical Thinking Challenges
Answers to Checkpoint Questions
Suggestions for Further Reading

DACUM Components

1.2   Perform within ethical boundaries
1.3   Practice within the scope of education, training, and personal capabilities
1.4   Maintain confidentiality
2.7   Receive, organize, prioritize, and transmit information
2.10 Use medical terminology appropriately
3.1   Perform basic secretarial skills
3.3   Prepare and maintain medical records
3.4   Apply computer concepts for office procedures
5.1   Document accurately
5.3   Use appropriate guidelines when releasing records or information

Chapter Competencies

Learning Objectives

Upon successfully completing this chapter, you will be able to:

1. Spell and define the Key Terms.
2. Explain the process for releasing medical records to third-party payers and individual patients.
3. List the standard information included in medical records.
4. Identify and describe the types of formats used for documenting patient information.
5. Explain how to make an entry into a patient's medical record.
6. Identify the various ways medical records can be stored.
7. Compare and contrast the differences between alphabetic and numeric filing systems; give an example of each.

Performance Objective

Upon successfully completing this chapter, you will be able to:

1. Prepare a medical record file folder (Procedure 10-1).

Key Terms

(See Glossary for definitions.)
alphabetic filing
chronological order
cross-reference
demographic
filing system
microfiche
microfilm
numeric filing
statue of limitations
subject filing
tab
unit

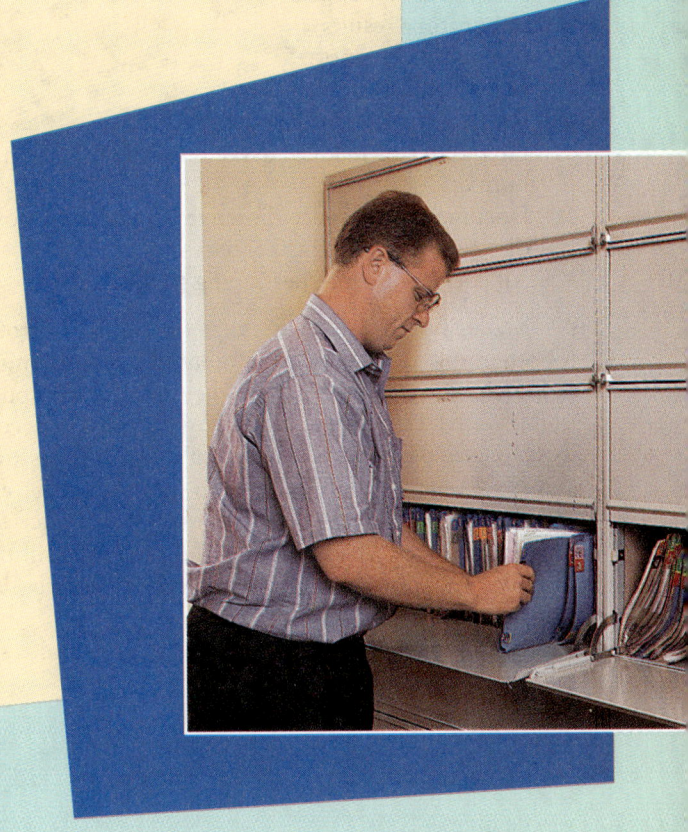

Medical records have a vital role in ensuring quality patient care. Proper medical records management requires adherence to certain legal, moral, and ethical standards. If these standards are disregarded, a breach of contract between patient and physician may occur, exposing the patient to potential embarrassment and making the physician vulnerable to lawsuits (see Chap. 3, Medicine and the Law). To avoid breach of contract, medical assistants must follow the guidelines discussed below when charting, filing, and releasing patients' medical records.

➤ STANDARD MEDICAL RECORDS

Contents of the Record

Typically, a patient's medical record—often called a chart or a file—contains the following information:

- History of present illness
- Past history
- Review of systems
- Chief complaint
- Progress notes
- Treatments
- Radiographic reports
- Laboratory results
- Consultation reports
- Medication administration
- Diagnosis or medical impression
- Physician's or medical assistant's identification (or both)
- Documented advance directives, living will, power of attorney for medical care
- All correspondence pertaining to the patient

Medical records can be kept on paper, **microfilm** (photographs of records in a reduced size), or **microfiche** (sheets of microfilm), or they may be computerized (Box 10-1). When deciding how to keep the records in your practice, consider the number of records to be stored, the type of information to be included in each record, and the accessibility of these records once they have been stored. Also keep in mind that you will need to make backup copies of computerized records daily and store them in a safe location.

No matter how the records are stored, make sure that the information is:

- Easily retrievable
- Kept in an orderly manner
- Complete
- Legible
- Accurate
- Brief

BOX 10-1 Safeguarding Computerized Patient Records

Use caution in storing patient medical histories on a computer. Evidence shows that persons with access to technology can invade patient records stored on computer data bases. This is a gross breach of confidentiality and is illegal. To maintain security, keep all computer disks in a safe location and periodically change log-in codes and passwords.

Keep in mind that, to be considered complete, all records should contain both subjective and objective information.

➤ MEDICAL RECORD ORGANIZATION

Information contained in the medical record is usually organized in a standard order and placed in a specially designed folder. The order in which documents are placed in the medical record will depend on the physician's preference. In general, the medical record will be organized in either a source-oriented or problem-oriented format.

Source-Oriented Medical Records

In source-oriented medical records, all similar categories or sources of information are grouped together. The typical groupings are:

- Billing/insurance information
- Physician orders
- Progress notes
- Laboratory results
- Radiographic results (magnetic resonance imaging, computed tomography scans, ultrasound)
- Patient education

All documentation in these categories is placed in reverse **chronological order**—that is, the most recent documents are placed on top of previous sheets.

Problem-Oriented Medical Records (POMR)

The problem-oriented medical record (POMR) lists each patient problem, usually at the beginning of the folder, and references each problem with a number throughout the folder. This method was developed by Dr. Lawrence Week and has become a common method of compiling information because of its logical flow and the ease with which information can be researched. For instance, if Mr. Jones has hypertension and hyperglycemia, each will be assigned a problem number as soon as the diagnosis is made:

2/4/9 #1. Hypertension
2/4/9 #2. Hyperglycemia

At each subsequent visit made by Mr. Jones, these problems will be referenced by these numbers. If a problem develops and is then resolved, the problem number will be terminated by a single strike-through with a date beside it or by adding an X to a heading that indicates resolution of problems. Chronic problems, such as hypertension and hyperglycemia, will be retained by their numbers for as long as the patient remains with the practice. These may be divided by headings of "acute" and "chronic" or "short-term" and "long-term" for convenience.

Problem-oriented medical records are divided into four components:

1. *Data Base*:
   - Chief complaint
   - Present illness
   - Patient profile
   - Review of systems
   - Physical examination
   - Laboratory reports
2. *Problem List*: Includes every problem the patient has that requires evaluation, including social, **demographic**, medical, and surgical problems. (Demographic problems relate to statistical characteristics of certain populations.)
3. *Treatment Plan*: Includes management, additional work-ups that may become necessary, and therapy.
4. *Progress Notes*: Structured notes corresponding to each problem; these are written using the SOAP method.

Checkpoint Question
1. What are the two ways in which the medical record can be organized?

➤ DOCUMENTATION FORMS

Whether the medical record is organized in the source-oriented or problem-oriented format, two documentation forms are commonly used. These are progress notes and flow sheets.

Progress Notes

Progress notes, or patient care notes, are written statements about various aspects of patient care. Typically, progress notes are placed on a lined piece of paper that has two columns. The left column is used to document the date and time, and the right column is used to write the note. The note can be written in four different formats:

1. Narrative
2. SOAP
3. PIE
4. Focus

Narrative

Narrative is the oldest documentation form and the least structured. It is simply a paragraph indicating what was wrong with the patient, what you did to help the patient, and whether the treatment worked. Figure 10-1 provides an example of a progress notes using the narrative format.

SOAP

SOAP (Subjective, Objective, Assessment, Plan) is one of the most common methods of documentation. The Subjective component is a statement depicting what the patient says. Whenever possible, you should use actual patient quotes. The Objective component is what you observed about the patient when you did your assessment. The Assessment portion is a phrase stating your impression of what is wrong; it is NOT a diagnosis. The Plan is a list of interventions that you have done. Figure 10-2 provides an example of a progress note using SOAP format.

Some facilities use variations of the SOAP format including SOAPIE, in which the "P" refers to what you plan to do, "I" refers to interventions that you have done, and the "E" pertains to evaluation of the interventions, and SOAPIER, in which the added "R" stands for revisions to the plan.

02/27/97	Patient arrived in the office complaining of a
1000	sore throat. Rapid strep test done—positive.
	Patient education brochure for strep throat
	was given to patient. Patient was discharged
	by physician. ————————
	———————————— Donna Chang, CMA

FIGURE 10-1
Example of progress note using narrative format.

10/15/98 1130	S	Patient states: "I hurt my left arm when I fell off my horse."
	O	Patient's left arm is edematous. Deformity noted. Left radial pulse present. Able to move fingers on left hand. Nailbeds on left hand pink and warm to touch.
	A	Left arm pain due to falling off horse.
	P	Left arm elevated on pillow. Ice applied to left arm. Left arm immobilized. Physician notified of patient's arrival. ————— ————————— Colleen O'Malley, RMA

FIGURE 10-2
Example of progress note using SOAP format.

Date/ Time	Focus	Patient Care Notes
07/19/98 1200	Soap in right eye	D: patient got laundry soap in right eye 45 minutes prior to her arrival. Eye appears red and teary.
		A: Right eye irrigated with normal saline through a morgan lens.
		R: Patient states eye feels better. Physician in to see patient. Bob Jones, CMA

FIGURE 10-4
Example of progress note using focus format.

PIE

PIE (Problem, Implementation, Evaluation) is another common charting form used in writing progress notes. The Problem is a brief phrase or statement explaining what the patient's problem is. Implementation refers to the list of interventions that were done. Evaluation is a statement reflecting how the implementation helped the patient. Figure 10-3 shows an example of a progress note using the PIE format.

Focus

Focus charting is a structured format using four elements: Focus, Data, Action, and Result. In this format the progress note page is divided into three columns: the date/time, focus, and the note. The focus depicts the patient problem in three or four words. The data, or "D," is the "O" in SOAP. The action, or "A," is the "P" in SOAP. The result, or "R," is the "E" in SOAPIER. Figure 10-4 is an example of a progress note using the focus format.

Flow Sheets

In addition to progress notes, the other common documentation form is flow sheets. A flow sheet is a preprinted checklist of the most commonly asked questions. Flow sheets are designed to limit the need for long handwritten patient care notes by allowing information to be recorded in either graphic or table form. They are usually customized to meet the needs of the individual practice. Generally, flow sheets are designed for a given task: vital signs documentation, patient assessment, patient education, or medication administration (Fig. 10-5).

No matter what form is used for documenting, you must always include the date, time the procedure was done, and your signature.

Other Forms

Two other documentation forms that you should be aware of are charting by exception (CBE) and computerized charting.

Charting by Exception

Charting by exception (CBE) represents a newer philosophy in charting. The foundation of CBE is that only the abnormal events are charted in narrative form; normal or expected findings are checked off in a flow sheet format. This method is used primarily in ambulatory care centers, intermediate care centers, and in hospitals.

Computerized Charting

Computerized charting is becoming more common in physician offices, hospitals, and in other health care facilities. This form has many advantages, including legibility, improved documentation, and easy storage and retrieval of information. Documentation is improved

11/26/98 1430	P	Abdominal pain in right lower quadrant for two days.
	I	Urine pregnancy test was done, negative. Urine dip was negative for blood and WBCs. pH 7.0. Urine was clear. Venipuncture was done on left forearm. Blood was sent to the laboratory for CBC and lytes. Vital signs: T-101.3 (R), P-94, R-16, BP-112/76. Tylenol 650 mg suppository given, as ordered, by Dr. Rogers.
	E	Patient states that she feels more comfortable now. Temperature 99.6 (R). ————— ————————— Lisa Fuentes, CMA

FIGURE 10-3
Example of progress note using PIE format.

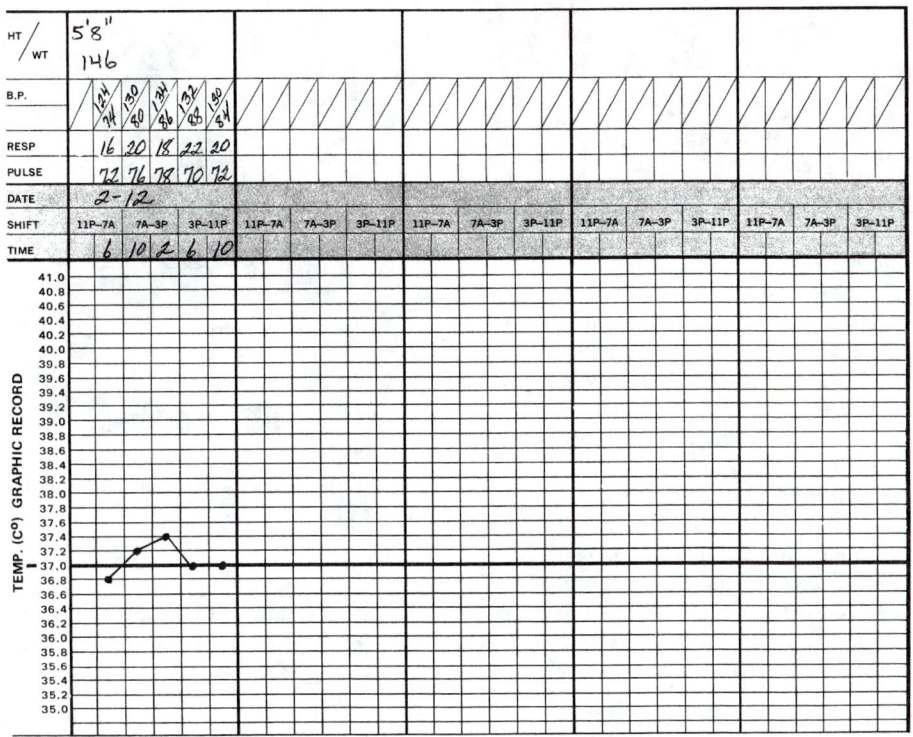

FIGURE 10-5
A graphic flow sheet is a preprinted checklist that is designed to document a specific task.

through computers because they will require that specific information be inserted. For example, when completing a patient history form, the computer will ask : "Is this patient a male or female?" The question must be answered to be able to move to the next screen, thus preventing missed documentation. Computerized charting takes less time than handwriting notes. However, computers do have some disadvantages, including downtime, cost, security issues, and the need for more in-depth staff training. Computerized charting can be done through bedside terminals (used in hospitals), microprocessors, or personal computers. In the medical office, the setup may consist of a mainframe with various terminals placed throughout the office.

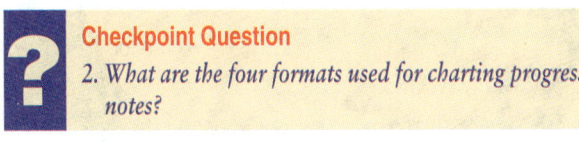

Checkpoint Question
2. What are the four formats used for charting progress notes?

➤ THE MEDICAL HISTORY

The patient's medical history reveals past and present medical treatments and diagnoses, family history, social history, and other pertinent medical information.

A medical history can be obtained by having the patient complete a standard form, or the physician or medical assistant can interview the patient. All information contained in the medical history is confidential and is not to be released to or shared with anyone without a consent form signed by the patient. Box 10-2 includes the kind of information obtained during a patient interview and provides a sample SOAP note. (See Chap. 20, Medical History and Patient Assessment, for more information about obtaining a medical history.)

➤ MEDICAL RECORD ENTRIES

Proper medical record entries are necessary for efficient communication and for legal considerations. The medical record allows health care practitioners to communicate among themselves and therefore provide the best care possible for the patient. Good communication fosters continuity of patient care.

The medical record also is a legal document that can be subpoenaed in a malpractice suit. If the documentation is accurate, timely, and legible it can help win a lawsuit—or prevent one altogether. However, if the documentation is messy, inaccurate, or improperly

BOX 10-2 Using the SOAP Method to Document Patient Information

Maria Moran states that her daughter Melissa has been vomiting all night. She also states that Melissa had diarrhea for 2 days before her appointment. Mrs. Moran states that Melissa has only eaten crackers and bananas since 6 PM last night. Dr. Daly's notes indicate that Melissa has lost 3 pounds since her last visit and that she appears pale, weak, and slightly dehydrated. He suspects a viral infection.

Dr. Daly ordered a stool culture along with a CBC with differential. He prescribed the BRAT diet and suggested that Mrs. Moran give Melissa Immodium D for the next 48 hours. He also told Mrs. Moran to call the office if Melissa's symptoms worsen and to bring her back for a recheck if the symptoms are not cleared up by the end of the week.

S: According to the patient's mother, the patient has been vomiting all night and has had diarrhea for the past 2 days. She has only eaten crackers and bananas since 6 PM the night before.

O: Patient appears pale, weak, and slightly dehydrated and has lost 3 pounds since her last visit.

A: Possible viral infection.

P: Stool culture, CBC with diff, BRAT diet, and Immodium for the next 48 hours. Call office if symptoms worsen; return to office if patient not well by the end of the week.

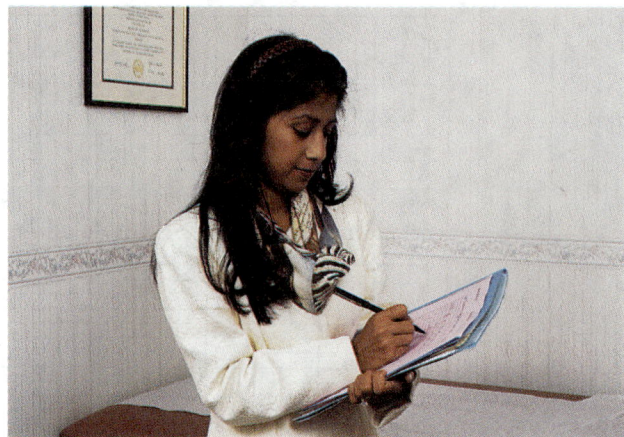

FIGURE 10-6
All communication with a patient must be documented in the patient's record

4. Always date and time all entries. Military time is preferred to limit any potential confusion between AM and PM (Fig. 10-7).
5. Write legibly.
6. Check the spelling of medical terms before entering them into the chart.
7. When using abbreviations, use only those that are accepted by your facility. Abbreviations can cause confusion and errors in patient care if they are overused, used incorrectly, or are open to interpretation. For instance, the abbreviation BS might

done, it can raise questions that might cause the practice to lose a malpractice suit.

The "golden rule" in documentation is: If it is not documented, it was not done. Therefore, all patient procedures, assessments, interventions, evaluations, teachings, and communications must be documented (Fig. 10-6).

Follow these guidelines for documenting in patients' medical records: ASAP.

1. Make sure you have the correct patient chart. If the patient's name is common, ask for a birth date or Social Security number as a double check.
2. Always document in ink. Generally, black or dark blue ink is preferred; other colors do not photocopy well.
3. Always sign your complete name and title.

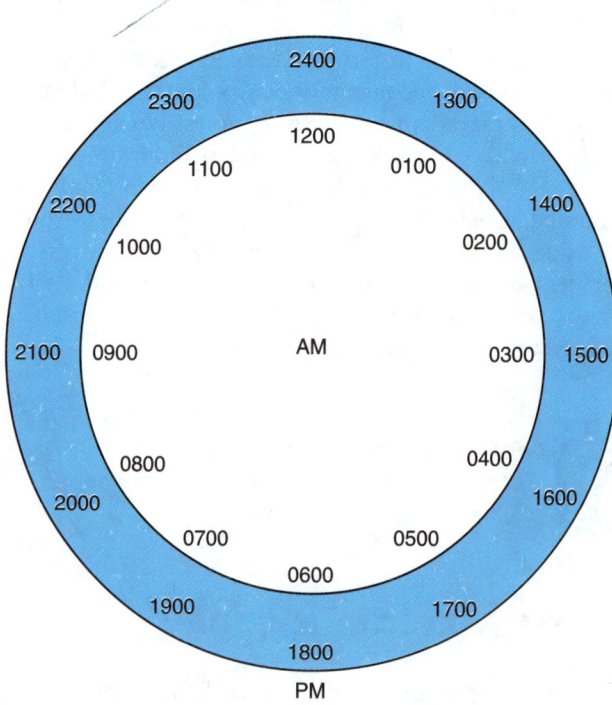

FIGURE 10-7
Military time is based on a 24-hour numbering system.

stand for bowel sounds, breath sounds, or blood sugar. (See Appendix IV for a list of commonly used abbreviations.)

8. When charting the patient's statements, use quotation marks to signify that these are the patient's own words.

9. Do not attribute any diagnosis. For example, if the patient states "My throat is sore," do not write that she has pharyngitis. It is not within the scope of training for medical assistants to diagnose.

10. Document as soon as possible after completing a task to promote accuracy.

11. Document missed appointments in the patient's chart. Chart your attempts to reach the patient to remind him or her of the appointment.

12. Document any telephone conversations in the chart.

13. Be honest. If you have given a wrong medication or done the wrong procedure, document it, then complete an incident report (see Chap. 12, Quality Improvement and Risk Management). State only the facts; do not draw any conclusions or place blame.

14. Never document for someone else, and never ask someone else to document for you.

15. Never document false information.

16. Never delete, erase, scribble over, or white-out information in the medical record because this can be construed as tampering with a legal document. If you do make an error, draw a single line through it, initial it, date it, and write "error." Then document the correct information (Fig. 10-8).

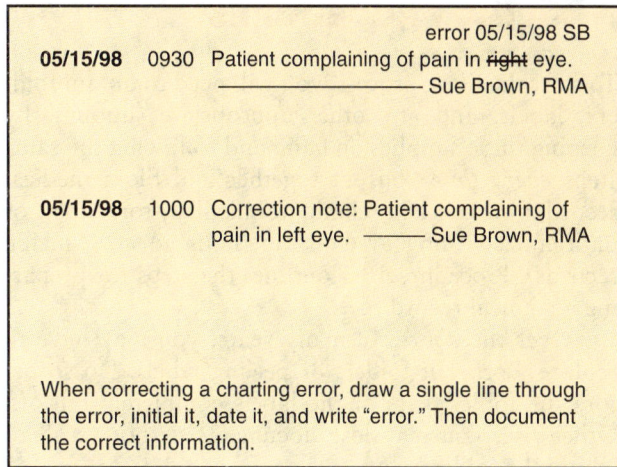

<table>
<tr><td></td><td></td><td>error 05/15/98 SB</td></tr>
<tr><td>05/15/98</td><td>0930</td><td>Patient complaining of pain in ~~right~~ eye.
————————— Sue Brown, RMA</td></tr>
<tr><td>05/15/98</td><td>1000</td><td>Correction note: Patient complaining of
pain in left eye. ——— Sue Brown, RMA</td></tr>
</table>

When correcting a charting error, draw a single line through the error, initial it, date it, and write "error." Then document the correct information.

FIGURE 10-8
Correcting a charting error.

Additions to Medical Records

Any additions to a medical record, such as laboratory results, should be transcribed onto a full sheet of paper or shingled and placed in the appropriate area of the chart. Most laboratory reports are computer generated and will come ready to insert into the chart. All additions to the medical record (eg, laboratory results, radiographic reports, consultation reports) should be initialed by the physician before they are inserted into the chart.

➤ WORKER'S COMPENSATION RECORDS

From time to time, a patient who is active within your practice may seek treatment as part of a worker's compensation claim. When this occurs, do not simply add the information to the patient's current medical record. Instead, start a new record. A worker's compensation medical record actually belongs to the employer, so the data in that record can be reviewed by the employer's insurance carrier. Consequently, any information about the patient's previous health or family history that is not pertinent to the workplace incident should not be made available to the insurance carrier.

Before treating a patient for a possible worker's compensation case, you must first obtain verification from the employer, unless the situation is life-threatening. Be sure to document the name of the person who authorizes treatment as well as any other information that becomes available during the verification process.

Worker's compensation cases are kept open for 2 years after the last date of treatment for any follow-up care that may be required. After that time, care may not be covered under the same case.

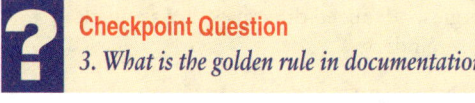

What If?

What if I tamper with a medical record? Can I get in trouble?

YES! It is against the law to falsify a medical record. If you or the physician is found guilty of tampering with medical records, you can face legal consequences and sanctions from professional organizations. These consequences may include fines, loss of licensure (for the physician), and either censure, suspension, or expulsion from professional organizations. Forensic specialists can detect handwriting changes or ink changes and can analyze typewriters to prove that tampering occurred.

Checkpoint Question
3. What is the golden rule in documentation?

➤ FILING PROCEDURES

To start the filing process, you will need to obtain folders, labels, and any other appropriate supplies. By keeping these supplies on hand and following the same steps *every time* you put together and file a medical record, you can help eliminate misfiled, torn, lost, or unorganized **filing systems** (methods for organizing records). Procedure 10-1 outlines the steps for preparing a medical record file.

Over the course of many years, you may have to replace worn out folders or peeling labels. Do so before the folder tears or the labels completely fall off. Otherwise, you may lose documents or not recall to whom the folder belongs.

To ensure efficient and speedy filing and document retrieval, consider the following factors:

- *Conditioning*—Gather all items together and prepare them by removing loose pieces of tape or paper clips and replacing with staples.
- *Indexing*—Separate business records from patient records.
- *Sorting*—Put each group of records in proper order to be filed onto shelves, either alphabetic or numeric. This makes actual filing time go much faster because you are not moving up and down and back and forth to find the proper letter area; you will just move down in order.
- *Storing*—Place each record in the proper storage area, as described below.

After preparing the folders, you may also want to prepare several outguides—plastic sheets with a **tab** (projection) and a pocket for index cards. Type "Out-

---

Procedure 10-1   Preparing a Medical Record File

Equipment/Supplies

- file folder
- title, year, and alphabetic or numeric labels
- special information labels (insurance information, drug allergies, advance directives)

Steps	Purpose
1. Decide the name of the file (either a patient's name, company name, or the name of the type of information to be stored within the record).	
2. Type a label with the selected title on it *in unit order* (eg, type: Lynn, Jessica A. *not* Jessica A. Lynn).	2. Typing the label in unit order helps avoid filing errors.
3. Place the label along the tabbed edge of the folder so that the title is extending out farther than the file folder itself. (Tabs can either be the length of the folder or tabbed in various positions such as left, center, and right.)	3. This ensures easy readability.
4. Place a year label along the top edge of the tab, before the label with the title. This will be changed each year that the patient has been seen. *Note:* Do not automatically replace these labels at the start of a new year; only remove the old year and replace with a new one when the patient comes in for the first visit of the new year.	4. Doing this makes the process of removing inactive files more time efficient. At the beginning of each new year, you can easily spot the records that are years beyond your storage time limit in the active file area. Doing this also can help you readily locate inactive files if patients return many years later. (By determining the last year the patient was seen, you can narrow your search to files with a matching year label.)
5. Place the appropriate alphabetic or numeric labels below the title.	5. This aids accurate filing and retrieval.
6. Apply any additional labels that your office may decide to use.	6. Labels noting special information (eg, insurance, drug allergies, advanced directives) act as quick and easy reminders.

guide" on the tabbed edge of the sheet. Then, when you need to remove a folder, write the title of the folder, your initials, and the date onto an index card. Place the card inside the outguide, and put the outguide in the spot where the folder was. An outguide indicates that the folder has been removed, so you will know that it is not lost or misfiled. The index card acts as a reference for anyone looking for the folder.

➤ FILING SYSTEMS

The two main filing systems are alphabetic and numeric. In some practices you may use both systems, each for different types of files.

Alphabetic Filing

As the name implies, alphabetic filing is a system involving the use of letters. Begin alphabetic filing by distinguishing the first, second, and third **unit** as described in Box 10-3. (A unit is each part of a name or title that is used in indexing.) Using the first letter of the first unit, place your records in small groups in order from A to Z. After that, take each small group and gradually work through the second and consecutive letters to put the small groups in order. Using this process allows you to work in a progressive order as you add records to the already existing files.

In cases in which the entire first unit is the same, move onto the second unit. If the second unit is still the same, move onto the third unit. Occasionally you will have records where units one, two, and three are identical. In such cases, it does not matter which one is filed first; however, use extreme caution when retrieving records with identical units to prevent errors. Using the patients' birth dates or mothers' maiden names can help avoid confusion.

With alphabetic filing, color coding may also be used. Specific letters are used on each folder, and a color-coded bar is placed next to the label with the patient's name on it. For example, names beginning with A to F would be blue; G to L, green; M to T, yellow; and U to Z, purple. Using this system, Michele Beals would have a blue color-coded strip, Geraldine Schmidt would have a yellow strip, Lauren Kayser's would be green, and Dana Warbeck would have purple.

Numeric Filing

Numeric filing involves the use of digits (usually six) to file records. The digits are typically grouped together, but read as three groups of two digits. For ex-

BOX 10-3 Indexing Rules for Alphabetic Filing

When filing records alphabetically, use the indexing rules below to help you decide the placement of each record. Indexing rules apply whether you use the title of the record's contents or a person's name.

- File records having a person's name according to last name, first name, middle initial, and *treat each letter in the name as a separate unit.* *Example:* Jamey L. Crowell should be filed as Crowell, Jamey L. and should be placed before Crowell, Jamie L.

- Make sure initials are placed after a full name. *Example:* John P. Bonnet, D.O. should be filed as Bonnet, John P., D.O.

- Treat hyphenated names as one unit. *Example:* Bernadette M. Ryan-Nardone should be filed as Ryan-Nardone, Bernadette M. *not* as Nardone, Bernadette M. Ryan.

- File abbreviated names as if they were spelled out. *Examples:* Finnigan, Wm. should be filed as Finnigan, William and St. James should be filed as Saint James.

- File Mac and Mc in regular order or grouped together, depending on your preference.

- File a married woman's record using her first name. *Example:* Helen Johnston should be filed as Johnston, Helen *not* as Johnston, Kevin Mrs.

- Disregard titles unless the complete name is not given. *Example:* Ignore the title Professor when filing Professor John Robinson (Robinson, John); however, use it for filing Professor Robinson (Robinson, Professor).

- Disregard Jr. and Sr., but use them in labeling the record.

- When names are identical, use the next unit such as birth dates or mothers' maiden name. *Example:* Use Durham, Rianna (2-4-94) and Durham, Rianna (4-5-45).

- Disregard apostrophes.

- Disregard *or, a, and, the,* or *of.* *Example:* File *The Cat in the Hat* under *Cat in Hat.*

- Treat letters in a company name as separate units. *Example:* For ASM, Inc., "A" is the first unit, "S" is the second unit, and "M" is the third unit.

ample, the record filed as 324478 would be read as 32, 44, 78. The commas would not be placed or any separation used when applying the labels to the tabbed edge of the file folder. The records would then be placed in numeric order without concern of duplication, which may sometimes happen with alphabetic. If you use this technique, it is called *straight digit filing* because you are reading the number straight out, from left to right.

Sometimes the file label will look the same as shown above, 324478, but will be read in the reverse order: 78, 44, 32. This technique is called *terminal digit filing*—that is, the groups of numbers are read from the end first, from right to left. You must beware to not mix the two filing systems together. If using both techniques within your office, be sure to keep them separate by means of changing the file folder color or some other means to prevent errors.

Regardless of which approach you choose, this type of filing plays an important role in the medical field. With tests for human immunodeficiency virus (HIV) and acquired immunodeficiency syndrome (AIDS) and their results being held in strict confidence,

the use of numeric filing is becoming even more popular. When this technique is used it is important to keep a **cross-reference** in a secure area listing the numeric code and the name of the patient. Such a reference is called a master patient index. This way, extremely limited numbers of people have knowledge of who the patient is, maintaining privacy. It is also important to keep any documents added into this record numerically coded and to avoid using the patient's name so that even when someone looks inside the record, patient identity is not revealed.

Boxes 10-4 and 10-5 provide examples of how to file patient records alphabetically or numerically.

BOX 10-4 Alphabetic Filing Examples

The following patient records are to be filed alphabetically:

Mary P. Martin
Floyd Pigg, Sr.
Automated Systems Management
AAMA (American Association of Medical
    Assistants)
Anita Putrosky
Macy's Furniture Outlet
Sister Mary Catherine
Cher
Stephen Dorsky, M.D.
Mrs. John Moser (Donna)

The proper order would be:

American Association of Medical Assistants
Automated Systems Management
Cher
Stephen Dorsky
Macy's Furniture Outlet
Mary P. Martin
Donna Moser
Floyd D. Pigg
Anita Putrosky
Sister Mary Catherine

BOX 10-5 Numeric Filing Examples

The following patient records are to be filed numerically:

Michelle Lanzarone	213456
Daniel Christopher	334387
Susan Coven	979779
Molly Pitcher	321138

In *straight digit filing*, the proper order would be:

213456
321138
334387
979779

In *terminal digit filing*, the proper order would be:

321138
213456
979779
334387

Sometimes, you may have files in which one or two groups of numbers are the same. In such situations, you would need to refer to the second or third groups or numbers.
Example: In *straight digit filing* (reading from left to right) the number 003491 would come before 004592. The first group of numbers ("00") is the same for both files, so you would determine the order of filing by the second group of numbers—in this case, 34 comes before 45.
Example: In *terminal digit filing* (reading from right to left), 456128 would come before 926128. The first two groups of numbers ("28" and "61") are the same for both files, so you would need to go to the third group of numbers—in this case, 45 comes before 92.

Other Filing Systems

Other filings systems include **subject filing**, in which documents are arranged alphabetically according to subject (eg, insurance, medications, referrals); geographic filing, in which documents are grouped alphabetically according to locations, such as state, county, or city; and chronological filing, in which documents are grouped in date order.

Checkpoint Question

4. What are the two main filing systems? Briefly describe each.

➤ CLASSIFYING MEDICAL RECORDS

Records are classified into three different categories: active, inactive, or closed.

Active records are those of patients who have been seen within the past few years. The exact amount of time is designated within each practice; it usually ranges from 1 to 5 years. Keep these records in the most accessible storage spot available because you will be using them regularly.

Inactive records are those of patients who have not been seen in more than the designated time set aside for active records. You will still keep these records within the office, but they do not need to be as accessible as the active files. Usually they are placed on bottom shelves to eliminate constant bending when reaching for active files, or they may be stored in another room within the office. "Inactive" patients have not formally terminated their contact with the physician, but they have either not needed the physician's services or have not contacted the office regarding a move, change in physician, or death.

Closed records are those of patients who have terminated their relationship with the physician. Reasons for such termination might include moving, problems with services or treatment, no further treatment necessary, or death. Store these records in the office in an out of the way area, such as a basement or attic. They may even be kept off site in the physician's home. This practice is permitted because the records legally belong to the physician, but it is not recommended because at any time the office staff may need access to these records.

➤ STORING MEDICAL RECORDS

Whether the records are active, inactive, or closed, you can choose from a variety of storage options.

Shelf files are stationary shelves made of either wood or metal. Rows are stacked on each other and units may be lined up alongside each other. These files may also be custom ordered to the width you need. Records are stored horizontally and labels read from the side.

Drawer files are a type of filing cabinet. The drawer pulls out for easy access and overview of all records (Fig. 10-9.) This type of filing system allows you easier access to all sides of files, which can help in trying to locate missing files that may have been pushed to the back or behind other files. Drawer files also allow easier filing because you can read from above the files, rather than squatting to read the labels from the sides as you work your way down to the lower shelves. A disadvantage is that these files take up a great deal of space.

Rotary circular or *lateral files* allow records to be stored in units that either spin in a circle or stack one behind the other, enabling you to rotate different units to the front. This system allows for maximum utilization of office space and is suggested for a medical office with large quantities of records to be stored. With shelf or drawer units, more wall space is needed to spread out each unit, but with rotary files, the amount of space is confined to one area (Fig. 10-9).

Automated files are increasingly being used as computer technology becomes an important part of the medical office. Computerized record keeping eliminates the need for conditioning, allows easy updating, provides a clearer understanding of record content, and speeds retrieval. Robotics in this type filing system is not commonly used within private practices but is more often used in hospitals or institutional settings because of the quantity of records maintained.

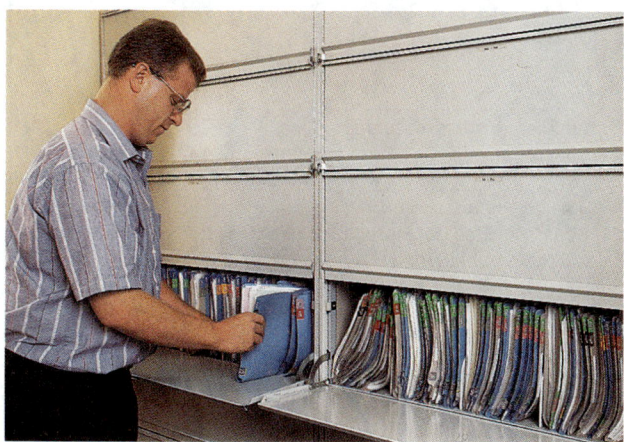

FIGURE 10-9
A drawer file storage system.

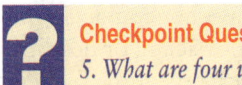

Checkpoint Question
5. What are four ways in which records can be stored?

Statute of Limitations

The **statute of limitations** (legal time limits) will vary from state to state. You will need to observe statutes of limitations in your particular state regarding the length of storage of medical and business records.

Legally, medical records should be stored for at least 7 years from the date of the last entry. However, it is recommended that medical records be stored permanently because any malpractice lawsuits can be filed within 2 years of the knowledge of malpractice—not 2 years from the date of the procedure (if the individual filing the suit was not immediately aware of the problem).

Tax records and liability plans, including old and new policies, should be permanently stored in a fireproof cabinet. Older liability plans may provide proof of coverage should a case of malpractice be filed during a time in which the current policy was not in effect.

Insurance policies (excluding liability policies) should be stored in a fireproof cabinet. You can keep the newest policy and discard the older one.

Canceled checks should be kept in fireproof storage for at least 3 years. After that, keep them indefinitely in regular storage.

Receipts for equipment should be kept until each item listed on the receipt is no longer of intrinsic value.

General correspondence should be kept as long as the information is pertinent. Periodically review the content of material, then discard anything that is unneeded.

➤ RELEASING MEDICAL RECORDS

Although the medical record legally belongs to the physician, any request for release of records must first be authorized by the patient or legal guardian. When releasing a medical record, provide a copy only. NEVER release the original medical record, except in limited circumstances.

Insurance companies, lawyers, other health care practitioners, and patients themselves may request copies of medical records. All requests should be made in writing stating the patient's name, address, and Social Security number and with patient's ORIGINAL signature authorizing the release of records. NEVER RELEASE INFORMATION OVER THE TELEPHONE. You will have no way of verifying that the person with

Legal Tips

The only time an original record should be released is when it is subpoenaed by a court of law. In such situations, the physician may wish to have the judge sign a document stating that he or she will temporarily take charge of the medical record. The signed document should be filed in the medical office until the record is returned. To further ensure the record's safety, a staff member can transport the original record to court on the day it is requested, then return the record at the end of the court session that day. When the court orders that a record be submitted to the court at a given date and time, the legal order is termed *subpoena duces tecum.*

whom you are speaking is the person who has authorization.

Unless the request is made by the patient, all other parties can be charged a fee for copying the medical record. The fee for reproduction of records should be no greater than $1 per page or $100 for the entire record, whichever is less. If the record is less than 10 pages the office may charge up to $10 to cover postage and miscellaneous costs associated with the retrieval process.

Certain guidelines must be followed even with a signed authorization release form (Fig. 10-10). Copies of all records *except* any documentation or references to mental health diagnosis or treatments, references to

---

Authorization for Release of Medical Record

I, _____, (patient or legal guardian) give permission to _____ (your organization's name) to release my medical records to _____ (other organization's name and address). I understand that my medical records include documentation about my health, laboratory and radiographic results, and various other forms.

Patient's signature   Date   Witness signature   Date

FIGURE 10-10

Sample authorization for release of medical records.

drug or alcohol abuse, references to HIV, AIDS, or any other sexually transmitted disease may be released. The above-mentioned information can only be released when asked for specifically on the signed authorization form. If it is not specifically requested when copying, place a piece of blank white paper over any such areas of information. Never white-out these areas on the original document or mention what these blank areas are.

Releasing Records to Patients

When patients request copies of their own records, be cautious in releasing any information that may be considered emotionally hazardous to their health, such as letters from family members regarding family medical history the patient is not aware of or diagnoses that the patient has not been made aware of.

Patients age 17 and under cannot get copies of their own medical records without a signed consent from either parent or legal guardian unless they are emancipated minors. However, they may obtain certain services independently (check your state's law regarding treatment of minors), and no contact to the parent or guardian can be made. Ironically, the parent or guardian may still be billed without the bill being itemized. The billing statement should include only the treatment date(s) and amount due. It should not note the diagnosis or specific services performed.

➤ REPORTING OBLIGATIONS

Although patients' records are confidential, certain situations require reporting to particular authorities. Requirements for reporting vary among states. Generally, the following types of items must be reported: vital statistics, communicable diseases, child and elderly abuse or maltreatment, and certain injuries. (Refer to Chap. 3, Medicine and the Law, for reporting obligations.)

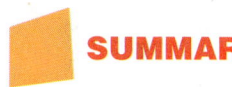

SUMMARY

Preparing and maintaining medical records is an important responsibility. To ensure efficient recording and retrieval, you must be familiar with the varied documentation forms as well as the different kinds of filing systems. In addition,

you must adhere to strict guidelines when releasing any information contained in patient medical records. Remember: Medical records are not only a means of communication among health care providers, but they also are legal documents depicting the quality of patient care.

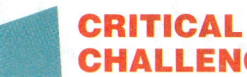

CRITICAL THINKING CHALLENGES

1. Interview a fellow student regarding a made-up injury. Document the incident and what treatments you did in narrative, SOAP, PIE, and focus formats.
2. Compare and contrast alphabetic filing with numeric filing. Which system do you think would work better? Justify your response.
3. Review the guidelines for documenting in the medical record. Create a policy that would educate new medical assistant employees on how to properly document in a medical record.

ANSWERS TO CHECKPOINT QUESTIONS

1. Medical records can be organized as either source-oriented or problem-oriented formats.
2. The four formats used for documenting progress notes are narrative, SOAP, PIE, and focus.
3. The golden rule in documenting is: "If it is not documented, it was not done."
4. The two main filing systems are alphabetic (using letters to file records) and numeric (using digits to file records).
5. The most common methods of storing records include shelf files, drawer files, rotary or circular files, and automated files.

SUGGESTIONS FOR FURTHER READING

Craven, R. F., & Hirnle, C. (1996). *Fundamentals of Nursing: Human Health and Function*, 2nd ed. Philadelphia: Lippincott-Raven.

Eggland, E. T., & Heinemann, D. S. (1994). *Nursing Documentation, Charting, Recording and Reporting.* Philadelphia: J. B. Lippincott.

Rosdahl, C. B. (1994). *Textbook of Basic Nursing*, 6th ed. Philadelphia: J. B. Lippincott.

Computers in the Medical Office

Chapter Outline

Computer Components
    Hardware
    Secondary Storage Systems
    Software
    Computer Accessories
Care and Maintenance of the System and Equipment
Operate a Computer
    Turning On a computer
    Turning Off a Computer
Training Options

Computer Applications
    Administrative Applications
    Clinical Applications
    Literature Searches
Automated Front Desk
Purchasing a Computer
Summary
Critical Thinking Challenges
Answers to Checkpoint Questions
Suggestions for Further Reading

DACUM Components

1.3 Practice within the scope of education, training, and personal capabilities
1.4 Maintain confidentiality
3.4 Apply computer concepts for office procedures

Chapter Competencies

Learning Objectives

Upon successfully completing this chapter, you will be able to:

1. Spell and define the Key Terms.
2. Identify basic computer components.
3. List five different maintenance regimens.
4. Describe three types of training options.
5. Discuss the types of administrative software that might be used in a physician's office.
6. Discuss the types of clinical software that might be used in a physician's office.
7. Discuss the advantages and disadvantages of an automated front office.
8. Describe the considerations involved in purchasing an office computer.

Performance Objectives

Upon successfully completing this chapter, you will be able to:

1. Turn on a computer.
2. Turn off a computer.

Key Terms

(See Glossary for definitions.)

back-up
boot
byte
CD-ROM
central processing
   unit (CPU)
crash
cursor
data
database
directory
disk drive

downtime
file
floppy disk
hard copy
hard drive
hardware
log-in
mainframe
megabyte
microprocessor
modem
monitor

motherboard
mouse
multimedia
on-line
operating system
printer
random access memory
   (RAM)
read only memory (ROM)
software
subdirectories

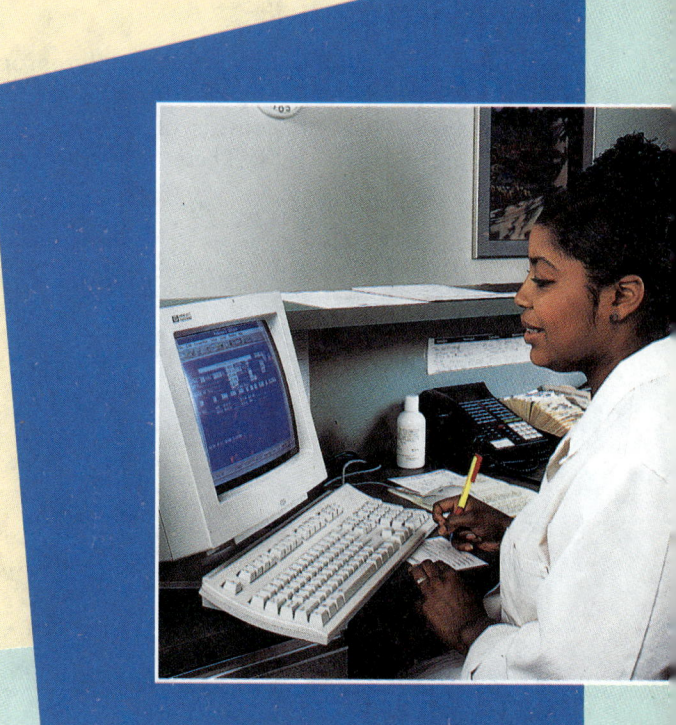

Computers play a major role in the physician's office. In the past, computers were often purchased solely to facilitate the billing process. Now computers can be used in a variety of ways to improve relations with patients, payers, and other physicians. In this chapter, you will learn basic computer concepts and care and maintenance of the system. You also will receive an overview of various computer applications.

➤ COMPUTER COMPONENTS

Computer components can be divided into four categories: **hardware**, secondary storage systems, **software** (application programs that direct the hardware to perform given tasks), and accessories.

Hardware

The computer hardware consists of the central processing unit (CPU), motherboard, keyboard, monitor, hard drive, disk drive, and the *printer* (Fig. 11-1). Hardware choice will be based primarily on the specific application software that the medical office needs. There should also be consideration as to the relative advantages and disadvantages of Macintosh versus IBM-type technology.

Central Processing Unit

The **central processing unit (CPU)** *or* **microprocessor** *is circuitry imprinted on a silicon chip that processes information.* The CPU consists of a variety of electronic and magnetic cells. These cells read, analyze,

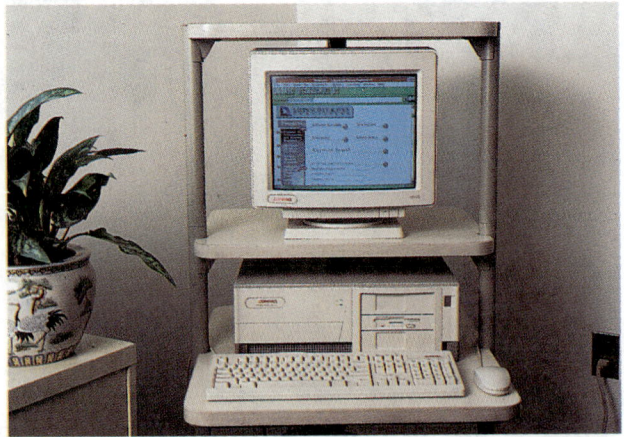

FIGURE 11-1
The computer hardware consists of the central processing unit, motherboard, keyboard, monitor, hard drive, disk drive, and the printer.

process, and instruct the computer on how to operate a given software program. All CPUs function basically the same way, but chips differ dramatically in capabilities and speeds. Software written for one kind of chip will not run on computers that use another kind of chip. To get around this barrier, many programs are written in two separate versions, one for each type of computer chip.

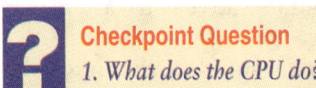

Checkpoint Question
1. What does the CPU do?

Motherboard

The **motherboard** *is a fiberglass board that contains the CPU, memory, expansion slots, and many other pieces of circuitry.* There are two types of memory chips within the computer, ROM and RAM. The **read only memory (ROM)** chip is the permanent memory inside the computer. Information cannot be entered into the ROM, it can only be accessed through the computer manufacturer or programmer.

The **random access memory (RAM)**, sometimes referred to as main memory, primary memory, or short-term memory, is contained in a set of silicon chips. It holds **data** (information) temporarily to allow the computer to communicate with software but does not retain the information when the computer is turned off. *The more RAM a computer has, the more data it can manipulate and the faster many programs will run.* With some application programs, the computer may actually slow to a halt if it does not have enough RAM.

Computer memory is measured in **megabytes (MB)**. This is simply the most convenient way to measure the quantity of computer information that a particular device can hold. Each character (eg, *A* or *3*) is called a **byte**. The prefix *mega* means million. Thus a megabyte is 1 million characters.

The amount of main memory installed in a computer or the storage capacity of a floppy disk or hard disk is measured by the number of characters it can hold. Most systems require a minimum of 4 MB to run reliably and quickly, but 8 MB is generally recommended. The larger your data and application files, the more you will benefit from extra RAM in your computer.

Keyboard

The keyboard is the primary means by which information is input (entered) into the computer. The keyboard is plugged into the computer and functions much like a typewriter. Besides the letter and number keys, there are additional keys—*special function keys*—that provide increased capabilities. Examples of special function keys are *Alt, Ctrl, Insert, Esc*. Each of these keys has a specific function for a given software package. These functions may include searching for and replacing words, moving blocks of text, indenting or centering text, and spell checking.

Monitor

The **monitor, or visual display terminal (VDT) as it is sometimes called, is a display unit that resembles a TV screen.** It shows the information that is being input via the keyboard. The point at which data will be entered on the monitor is marked by a flashing line called a **cursor**.

Monitors come in various sizes and qualities. The quality of the screen is based on the number of DPIs (dots per inch). The more DPIs, the clearer the picture. Monitors can display their information either in monochrome (a single foreground color like green or amber) or in color. Both types have adjustment dials for brightness and contrast.

Many people have come to prefer color monitors even though they are more expensive because the colors are less straining to the eyes and make it easier to distinguish different types of information on a crowded screen.

Checkpoint Question
2. *The quality of the monitor screen is based on what feature?*

Hard Drive

The **hard drive provides a place where the computer can store the programs and data files you use.** It is a sealed device that fits inside the computer or in a separate box alongside it. The capacity of a hard drive (ie, the quantity of program and data information it can hold) is measured in megabytes. Originally, hard drives could hold 5 MB (equivalent to about 2000 typed pages). But today, the most popular hard drives can hold as much as 1000 megabytes (also called a gigabyte) or more.

Because many of today's popular and important software applications occupy 10, 25, or even 40 MB of storage, it is common for computers in the medical office to contain hard drives rated at 600 MB or more. The actual amount of data storage your business requires is approximately the total of the following:

- The total amount of storage required by your computer's **operating system** (DOS) and an interface

such as Windows 95, can amount to as much as 50 MB.
- The total amount of storage required by all the application software you are likely to use, now and in the next few years.
- The total amount of data you are likely to store.
- The amount of room for expansion. (Buy at least twice as much disk capacity as you think you need.)

Disk Drive

The **disk drive is simply a device that gets the information on and off a floppy disk.** The information may consist of a software program or involve storing a document. Disk drives are often termed drives and labeled alphabetically (eg, Drive A, Drive B; the hard drive is Drive C). The number and size of the disk drives vary among computers.

Printer

The *printer* transfers computerized information onto paper (**hard copy**). Computer printers use various technologies, operate at different speeds, and print in black or in color. The printer allows you to generate bills, print letters, and produce a daily schedule. The three types of printers that will be discussed are: dot matrix, laser, or ink jet (Fig. 11-2).

Dot matrix printers, the least expensive models, imprint a series of dots on the paper in the form of characters. These printers are good for completing certain insurance forms and printing laboratory results. The disadvantage of dot matrix printers is the slow speed at which they print the information. Usually, they are not used for business letters because of their poor print quality. They should not be used to print patient discharge instructions unless the instructions can be clearly read.

Laser and ink jet printers provide the best quality, with lasers being the best. The main disadvantage to these printers in the medical office setting is the inability to print on carbon copy forms, such as insurance forms. These printers print data without mechanically touching the paper; therefore, duplicate forms print only on the top sheet.

Checkpoint Question
3. *What are three types of printers?*

Secondary Storage Systems

There are two types of secondary storage systems: floppy disks and cartridges.

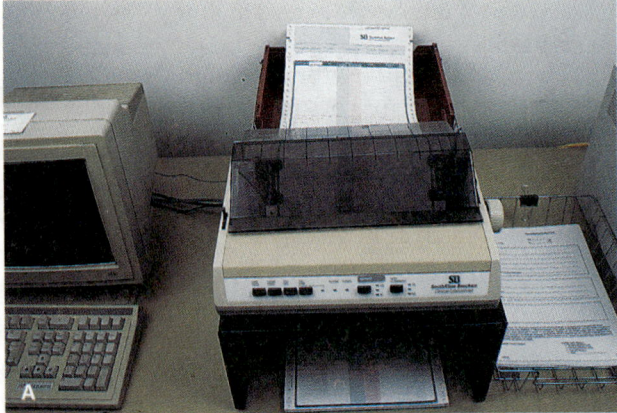

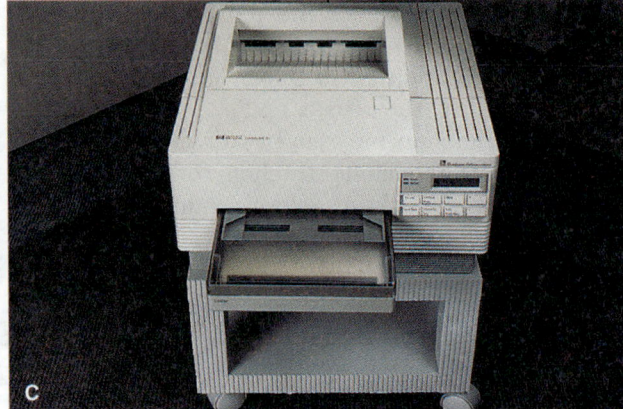

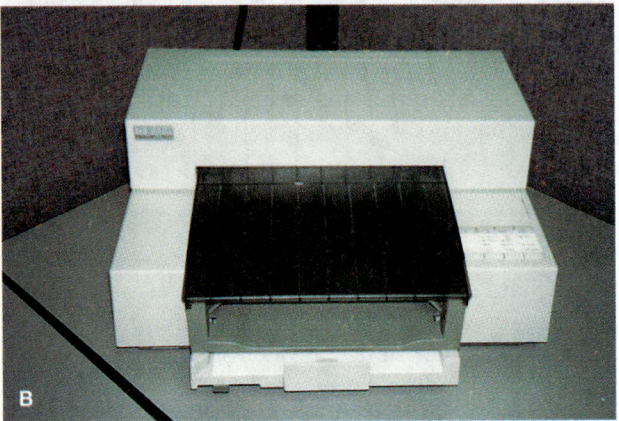

FIGURE 11-2
Types of printers (*A*) dot matrix, (*B*) ink jet, and (*C*) laser.

Floppy Disks

Data can be stored on diskettes (**floppy disks**) (Fig. 11-3), thin magnetic films that are inserted into the disk drives. Floppy disks come in a variety of sizes (eg, 3½ and 5¼ inches) and memory capacity. The size of the floppy disk you will use depends on your disk drive size. Each disk must be labeled to allow for identifica-

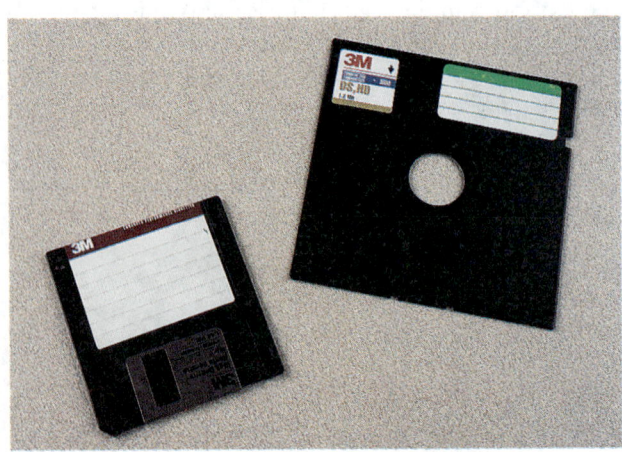

FIGURE 11-3
Floppy disks.

tion; some offices use color-coded labels for easier identification.

Information that is saved on a floppy disk is put in the form of a **file**, which should be named for easy retrieval. Files are created using applications. Some applications allow you to create file names using an unlimited number of characters; others have a maximum amount of characters that can be used.

Files on a related topic can be grouped into a **directory**, which is like the table of contents of a file system. A directory can be further broken down into **subdirectories**. For example, you might create a directory of diabetic patients cared for by the practice, with subdirectories for insulin-dependent and noninsulin-dependent patients. Files may be individually named using the patient's last name.

You should always make a **back-up** (duplicate) of your computerized files and store these in a secure location. That way, if the computer **crashes** (experiences a breakdown), you will be sure that all of your records are intact.

Checkpoint Question
4. How is information stored on a floppy disk?

Cartridges

Another type of secondary storage system, the data cartridge, is used to back-up the hard disk. Cartridges are primarily used in large office settings or in hospitals where individual computers are connected to **mainframe** computers. Mainframe computers contain large **databases** (collection of files) used by institutions; each department's computer is linked to the main system.

Software

A computer's memory capacity varies depending on the number of megabytes in the system. This is important when choosing the software components you wish to add to your system. In the physician's office, the types of software used will have either administrative or clinical applications.

Administrative applications are used for basic word processing, producing billing statements, processing insurance forms, maintaining patient files, printing mailing labels, and, in general, keeping a business ledger for the practice.

Clinical applications can provide patient discharge instructions, information on current disease pathologies and procedures, pharmacologic updates, and answers to a wide variety of clinical issues.

See the section "Computer Applications," below, for more information.

Checkpoint Question

5. What are the two types of software applications a physician's office may have?

Computer Accessories

Mouse

The **mouse** is a free-standing device that can be used to control the cursor on the display screen. Although you cannot type in characters using the mouse, you can move or delete individual characters, words, or entire blocks of text with it.

Multimedia Upgrades

Multimedia refers to computer capabilities that allow users to record and play back some combination of stereophonic sound, animation, full-motion video, photographs, and TV pictures. Because multimedia requires such massive amounts of data, information is generally stored on high-capacity disks that work with

the CD-ROM. A **CD-ROM** is a 5¼ disk that is inserted into a device similar to a disk drive. The CD-ROM allows video and sound reproduction. One CD-ROM disk can hold over 200,000 typewritten pages!

Battery Back-up

Battery back-up units allow the computer system to function in the event of a power failure. They come in various sizes depending on the size of your computer and the amount of work that needs to be accomplished during a power failure.

Modem

A **modem** is a communication device that connects your computer to the standard telephone system, allowing you to exchange information with other computers, including the Internet, on-line services, such as bulletin boards, and electronic mail systems. There are data modems that allow computers to exchange files and fax modems that allow computers to exchange information with standard facsimile machines. The device commonly called a *fax modem* actually contains both a data modem and a fax modem in one unit.

➤ CARE AND MAINTENANCE OF THE SYSTEM AND EQUIPMENT

As with any piece of equipment in the medical office, it is necessary to maintain your computer on a regular basis. Below are some general care guidelines:

- Place the monitor, keyboard, and printer in a cool dry area void of direct sunlight.
- Be aware that static electricity can cause memory loss, inaccurate data collection, and other adverse reactions. To control this problem, place the computer on an antistatic floor mat or carpet, or purchase a specific antistatic device. You can also use commercial sprays and dust covers to help eliminate the problem.
- Use available accessories to properly care for your system. For example, use dust covers for the keyboard and the monitor when they are not in use. Antistatic wipes are available to use on the screen and they should be used as an alternative to glass cleaners.
- When moving the computer, lock the hard drive to protect the CPU and disk drives.
- Keep keyboards free of debris and liquids, which can be hazardous to the keyboard as it is directly plugged into the computer. If the keyboard becomes wet, it may shock the user and cause memory loss in

BOX 11-1 Care of Floppy Disks

- Always handle the disk by the label or jacket.
- Store the disk in a cool dry place; avoid high moisture storage areas or areas with extreme temperature changes.
- Never spill liquids on the disk.
- Never store the disk near a magnetic field, such as a television, motors, or a cellular telephone.
- Store disks in the vertical position and in an appropriate disk file box.

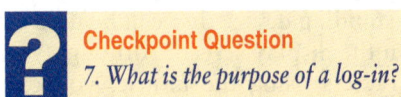

Richard Thompson, MD

Kansas City, MO

Log-in:

Password:

FIGURE 11-4
Log-in screen.

the hard drive. Vacuum the keyboard periodically to eliminate dust particles under the key pads.

- Be aware of any maintenance and warranty contracts for the computer system and do not hesitate to contact the service representative when needed. Some maintenance agreements require that a service representative clean and inspect the system on a regular basis for the warranty to be active.
- Handle floppy disks with special care. Box 11-1 provides some general guidelines to keep in mind.

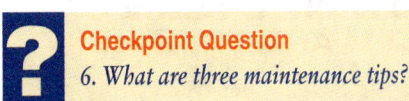

Checkpoint Question
6. What are three maintenance tips?

➤ OPERATE A COMPUTER

Turning on a Computer

The technical term for starting a computer is to **boot** it. Here are the basic steps to boot a computer.

1. Before turning on the computer, check to make sure that the disk drives are empty. No floppy disks can be in the drive when turning on the power. If you forget to remove a disk and start the computer, you will see a prompt: "Non-system disk or disk error; Replace disk and strike any key." If this happens, remove the disk and strike any key.
2. Turn on the power to the computer, monitor, and printer. Some offices have all of the electrical cords for these items plugged into a main console, making it easy to turn on the power. In other settings, you have to locate the power switch on the individual items.
3. Wait as the computer runs through a series of internal checks. It will count the memory and dis-

play it in the top left portion of the screen. Most computers scan for potential viruses at this point. After the memory check is clear and the viral check is negative, you will see a **log-in** screen (Fig. 11-4), which is designed to ensure security.

4. Type the log-in code in a precise manner and press enter. (A sample log-in may be your last name.) The cursor will go to the password. Type in your password and press enter. A password may be any combination of letters or numbers. In most situations, the actual letters or numbers will not be displayed on the monitor; this is for security purposes.
5. When the main menu appears on the screen (Fig. 11-5), use the cursor to highlight the desired selection or type the corresponding number at the C> prompt.

Sometimes a program error may require you to reboot your computer. Some programs will allow you to reboot your computer with the power on. In this case you would hold down the Ctrl and Alt keys simultaneously with one hand, then lightly press the Delete (Del) key with the other hand. The computer will then restart. If your computer does not allow this function, you will have to turn the power off then turn it on.

Checkpoint Question
7. What is the purpose of a log-in?

Turning Off a Computer

1. Make sure that you have saved all your data either on floppy disks, the main computer drive, or on cartridges.
2. Exit the program you are in. Most of the time, this command can be found on the category *file*.
3. When you have exited to the main menu, shut the power off. Never turn the power off if you have

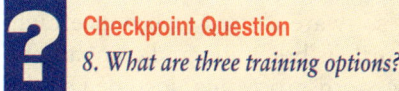

Family Practice Medical Associates
Middletown, CT

Main Menu

New patient entry

Display patient data

Procedural entry

Medical Record Reports

Insurance Billing

Micro-Medx

Word-Perfect

Highlight your selection

09/09/97

FIGURE 11-5
Sample main menu.

not properly exited a given software program as you may lose your data.
4. Place the floppy disks in a secure place.
5. Cover the computer, keyboard, and monitor with dust protectors.

What If?
What if the computer develops a virus?

A virus is a very serious problem capable of causing the entire system to crash. It can be caught by sharing floppy disks or bootlegged software or it can be generated from an on-line system. The symptoms include everything from self-changing data, blank screens, and inability to access or freezing of programs. Preventing a virus from entering your system is critical. Never share floppy disks with another system. If you use an on-line service, ascertain its internal prevention techniques for virus control. If your system develops viral symptoms, immediately notify your service representative. Wait for further instructions from a computer programmer before you do anything. Do not turn the computer off; this destroys data.

➤ TRAINING OPTIONS

To achieve the optimal benefit from any computer or software package, you must be trained in its use. There are a number of ways that this can be accomplished.

- The company from which the computer was purchased often provides personnel to train you and other staff members.
- A user's manual will come with your system. You can refer to it when troubleshooting system problems.
- Help screens installed with every software package allow the user to *self-teach*. The disadvantage of this method is that it is often time consuming.
- Some software packages come with a tutorial. This is an on-line short course on the use of the software.
- The computer manufacturer has a service called a help desk, which provides technical support. It is usually accessed by calling a toll-free number and is manned by computer professionals who can answer your questions concerning the system.

A combination of the above methods is the best approach to learning about your computer and software.

? Checkpoint Question
8. What are three training options?

➤ COMPUTER APPLICATIONS

Applications are relatively large and important programs that enable computers to do the kinds of work that small businesses require. Depending on the type of software selected for the system, the program capabilities are endless. The two broad groups of software packages that you will use in the medical office are administrative and clinical.

Administrative Applications

The tasks that administrative software can do are endless and are divided into the following groups.

Spreadsheets

Spreadsheets are used to calculate numbers entered into rows and columns. As a medical assistant, you may do spreadsheets for the physician showing the practice's revenue, financial accounts of patients, or insurance totals. Examples of some of the most commonly used spreadsheet programs are: LOTUS 1-2-3, EXCEL, and QUATRO-PRO.

Word Processing

Word processing software allows you to manipulate words to create documents such as letters, memorandums, and reports. As a medical assistant, you will use this software to write letters to patients, other physicians, or insurance companies. Some of the most commonly used word processing programs are WordPerfect and Microsoft Word.

Graphics

Graphics applications allow you to produce graphs, charts, symbols, and presentation materials. These packages also enable you to draw your own pictures on the screen. As a medical assistant, you may create graphs comparing previous year's data to current data or comparing the types of patients seen in a practice. Some of the most commonly used graphic programs are: Harvard Graphics, PC Paint, and Microsoft.

Desktop Publishing

Desktop publishing software is used to produce high-quality documents, such as brochures and company reports, by integrating word processing documents with graphics. It also is used for marketing a physician's practice. As a medical assistant, you may use this software to create patient education brochures or to promote the practice. Some of the most commonly used programs for desktop publishing are Pagemaker and Ventura.

Medical Office Management

This kind of software can be use for:

- Electronic claims submission. Payers like this because it saves them the expense of rekeyboarding data sent on paper claims.
- Patient scheduling. Electronic systems can make it easier to keep track of and remind patients of appointments.
- Tracking patients. A computer can prompt you or your staff to schedule follow-up visits, periodic screenings and vaccinations, or other long-range services patients may need.
- Patient record-keeping. More and more of a patient's record is computerized. Besides dates and test results, some systems allow progress notes and other text-based records.
- Referral letter preparation. Computers can help you track and follow-up on referrals. If you are us-

ing computerized patient records, relevant facts can easily be merged into referral letters.

- Marketing trends. Analysis of computer records can tell you where your patients are coming from and where you need to focus your efforts to expand the practice. Computer records also can be used to generate mailing lists for focused marketing efforts such as promotion of screening tests.
- Electronic billing for Medicare, Medicaid, and other commercial insurance companies using HCFA 1500 forms.
- Monthly and year-to-date billing statements
- Mailing labels
- Insurance forms
- Appointment scheduling
- Payroll
- Charge slips
- Monthly and yearly reports
- New patient entry and database creation

There are many programs that perform the tasks listed above. Some of those commonly used are: Medics II, MD Versa Form, Medicalis, PAS-3 Plus System III, Medx, Physician Choice System, Med-Ease, Econo-Med, and Genesis. It is important to note that the capabilities of each of these software programs to perform these tasks will vary. You must carefully investigate each system before it is purchased.

Checkpoint Question

9. What are five types of administrative software that may be used in the medical office?

Clinical Applications

Clinical application software programs help the health care practitioner in assessing, diagnosing, and implementing patient care. Several clinical applications are discussed below.

Drug Interactions

The practitioner can type in a variety of patient medications and the computer will cross reference them to determine how they will interact. Some medications when mixed with other medications can cause severe and even fatal results.

Disease Updates

This provides the practitioner with up-to-date information on hundreds of diseases. For example, if a patient arrives in a physician's office with Lyme disease, the practitioner can type in Lyme disease and find out what causes the disease, how it is transmitted, what diagnostic procedures to order, and what medications and treatments to initiate.

Toxicology

This assists the practitioner in determining how dangerous a particular substance is when it is ingested and how to treat the ingestion. For example, suppose a mother brings in a baby who just ingested Drano. The practitioner would type in "Drano" and the child's weight and age, and the computer will advise the physician about the complications of ingesting Drano and how to treat the child.

Discharge Instructions and Patient Education

This provides the practitioner with printed discharge instructions for patients (see Figure 4-2 for an example of computerized discharge instructions). In most programs, the instructions can be printed in both English and Spanish, and at various reading levels.

Emergency Care

This provides the practitioner with current medication doses, cardiopulmonary resuscitation (CPR) guidelines, and advance cardiac care instructions. For example, suppose an 8-year-old child suffers cardiac arrest while in the pediatrician's office. The physician can type in the age of the child and weight, and the computer will print out what medication and dose to give.

Examples of clinical application software include: Micro-Medx, Stat-Ref, Family Doc, Physicians on Line, Grateful Med.

Checkpoint Question

10. What type of clinical software would help a physician care for a patient who ingested a poisonous plant?

Literature Searches

Periodically, physicians need to obtain articles from professional journals regarding a specific disease entity. The most common software for literature searches is MEDLINE. MEDLINE has articles published from 1966 to the present. This software can be found in physician's offices, libraries, hospitals, and universities. MEDLINE allows you to search for a given topic or to search for a given author's publications.

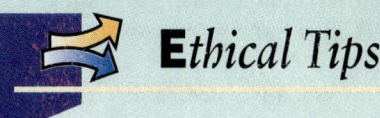

E*thical Tips*

You must remember that all patient data stored on computers is confidential. To ensure privacy:

- Always clear the screen of patient data before leaving the computer monitor.
- If your computer has fax capabilities, make sure that the intended receiver is at the receiving computer *before* you send the data.

➤ AUTOMATED FRONT DESK

Most physician offices have an automated front desk. However, some small physician offices are not automated. There are definitely pros and cons to having an automated front office, as noted below.

Advantages to automation:

- Accurate and faster completion of time-consuming tasks
- Easy accessibility to data
- Rapid generation of monthly billing statements
- Potential for lower labor costs (after initial training)
- Secure data; better patient confidentiality
- Neater work area
- Less chance of losing documents
- Helps organize the practice

Disadvantages to automation:

- Initial financial cost
- Initial data transfer can be long and tedious
- Requires total staff cooperation
- May increase labor hours initially
- Security risks
- **Downtime** (computer malfunction or time when the machine is not operational)

➤ PURCHASING A COMPUTER

Purchasing a new office computer system—or updating an existing one—is a very important business decision. All key members of the staff should be consulted *prior* to such a purchase and should be actively involved in selecting the hardware and software. Here are some general guidelines to follow when shopping for a computer and software:

- Determine your specific needs. For example, do you need both clinical and administrative applications?
- Visit different physician offices and clinics to see what other medical office staff members are using. Ask questions such as: *How user-friendly are the computer programs? How long did it take to educate the staff? What does the staff like and dislike about the programs?*
- Try out many software packages. Most software programs have demonstrator disks that can be used to evaluate the system.
- Interview and compare different computer vendors. Find out:

  1. How long they have been in service.
  2. How many service representatives they have and if they are available 24 hours a day.
  3. The specifics of their system.
  4. The specifics of any service and warranty contracts they provide.
  5. If they provide training; if so, whether there is an additional cost.
  6. How you can transfer your present data to a new system.
  7. How much the system costs.
  8. If the software can be customized; if so, the cost.
  9. Their response time for service or technical support calls.

Independent consultants can be hired to evaluate a particular office and make specific recommendations for that office. This option can be expensive and should be figured into the initial cost.

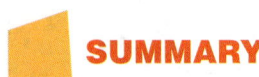

SUMMARY

As a medical assistant, you will be expected to have a basic understanding of computers and how they function. A medical assistant who can work in an automated office will have a hiring advantage and greater career mobility.

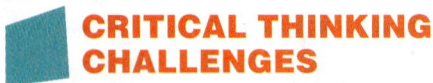

CRITICAL THINKING CHALLENGES

1. Write a policy on the care and maintenance of the office computer. Be sure to note who will be responsible for these duties.

2. You office has the software Micro-Medx. Tomorrow your computer will be on downtime for a good part of the day. What patient education instructions would you want to preprint today? Are there any other instructions or information that you would preprint? Explain your response.

3. Formulate a list of questions that you would ask a computer vendor if you were planning to purchase a computer. Then, look in your local phone book and prepare a list of vendors to contact.

ANSWERS TO CHECKPOINT QUESTIONS

1. The CPU reads, analyzes, processes, and instructs the computer on how to operate software.
2. The monitor's quality is based on the number of DPIs.
3. Types of printers are dot matrix, ink jet, and laser.
4. Information is stored on a floppy disk as files.
5. A physician's office may have software for administrative and clinical applications.
6. Answers vary but may include the following: Keep the computer away from sunlight and heat, avoid static electricity, use dust covers and antistatic wipes, lock the hard drive when moving the computer, keep keyboards clean, utilize service contracts, handle floppy disks carefully.
7. A log-in is a security password.
8. Answers vary but may include the following: Company-provided training, user manuals, help screens, tutorials, help desk.
9. Administrative software used in the medical office may include spreadsheets, word processing, graphics, desktop publishing, and medical office management applications.
10. A toxicology application can help the physician care for a patient who ingested a poisonous plant.

SUGGESTIONS FOR FURTHER READING

Johnson, J. M. and Johnson, M. W. (1994) *Computerized Medical Office Management.* Albany, NY: Delmar.

Connway, S. and Messerle, J. (1990) *Searching MEDLINE: Finding the Needles in the Medical Haystack.* Group Practice Journal 39(3): 26-34.

Arnold, J. M. and Pearson, G. A. (1992) *Computer Applications in Nursing Education and Practice.* National League of Nursing, New York, NY; Port City Press.

Quality Improvement and Risk Management

Chapter Outline

Quality Improvement Programs in the
Medical Office Setting
    Regulatory Agencies
Developing a Quality Improvement
Program
    Seven Steps for a Successful Program
Risk Management
    Incident Reports
    When to Complete an Incident
      Report

Information Included on an Inci-
dent Report
Guidelines for Completing an Inci-
dent Report
Trending Incident Reports
Putting It All Together: A Case Review
Summary
Critical Thinking Challenges
Answers to Checkpoint Questions
Suggestions for Further Reading

DACUM Components

1.3   Practice within the scope of education, training, and personal capabilities
1.5   Work as a team member
5.2   Determine needs for documentation and reporting
6.2   Operate and maintain facilities and equipment safely

12

Chapter Competencies

Learning Objectives

Upon successfully completing this chapter, you will be able to:

1. Spell and define the Key Terms.
2. List the three regulatory agencies that require medical office settings to have quality improvement programs.
3. Describe the accreditation process of the Joint Commission on Accreditation of Health Care Organizations (JCAHO).
4. Describe the steps to developing a quality improvement program.
5. List five guidelines for completing incident reports.
6. Explain how quality improvement programs and risk management work together in a medical office setting to improve overall patient care and employee needs.

Performance Objective

Upon successfully completing this chapter, you will be able to:

1. Complete an incident report.

Key Terms

(See Glossary for definitions.)

expected threshold

incident reports

Joint Commission on Accreditation
   of Health Care Organizations
   (JCAHO)

quality improvement (QI)

risk factors

task force

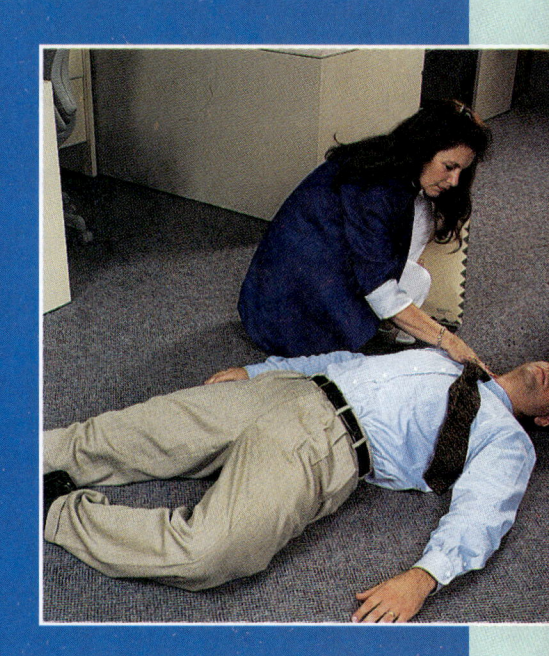

Quality improvement (QI) is the commitment and plan to improve every part of an organization. Its goal is both to meet and to exceed customer (patient) expectations and employee needs. Quality improvement plans examine the way care is delivered, analyze problems in the delivery system, and investigate methods to correct the problems.

In this chapter, we discuss why quality improvement programs exist in health care organizations, the process for developing and maintaining quality improvement plans in a medical office setting, and risk management.

➤ QUALITY IMPROVEMENT PROGRAMS IN THE MEDICAL OFFICE SETTING

Quality improvement programs allow an organization to scientifically measure the quality of its products and services. A health care organization's success depends on patient satisfaction. Patients select the health care organization that best meets their needs in terms of professional services and personal care.

Quality improvement programs have many other benefits for health care organizations. These include:

- Identification of delivery system failures
- Improvement of patient, family, and customer service
- Improvement of patient outcomes
- Improvement of employee efficiency and productivity
- Improvement of company morale
- Encouragement of teamwork within the institution or organization

Regulatory Agencies

Quality improvement programs exist in medical office settings both because of the benefits listed above and because of regulatory agency mandates. The three primary regulatory agencies that mandate QI programs are the **Joint Commission on Accreditation of Health Care Organizations (JCAHO)**, the Occupational Safety and Health Administration (OSHA), and the individual state health departments.

Joint Commission on Accreditation of Health Care Organizations (JCAHO)

JCAHO is a private agency that sets health care standards and evaluates an organization's implementation of these standards for health care settings. Prior to the mid 1990s, JCAHO's primary focus was on evaluating hospitals and in-patient care institutions such as nursing homes. In 1996, JCAHO expanded its jurisdiction to outpatient and ambulatory care settings. This change was in part owing to the shift of patient care from inpatient to outpatient services. JCAHO presently sets standards and evaluates the care in the following health care settings:

- Ambulatory care centers
- Birthing centers
- Chiropractic clinics
- Community health organizations
- Corporate health services
- County jail services
- Dental centers
- Dialysis centers
- Group practices
- Imaging centers
- Independent practitioner practices
- Lithotripsy centers
- Magnetic resonance imaging (MRI) centers (mobile and fixed)
- Oncology centers
- Ophthalmologic surgery centers
- Podiatry centers
- Rehabilitative centers
- Research centers
- Student health centers
- Womens' health centers

JCAHO surveys these centers and then assign them an accreditation title. Participation in JCAHO accreditation is voluntary for health care organizations; however, without a successful accreditation title, the health care organization may not be eligible to participate in particular federal and state funding programs, such as Medicare and Medicaid. In addition, accreditation indicates to the community that a particular organization has met basic practice standards, therefore improving its marketability.

ACQUIRING JCAHO ACCREDITATION

The process of acquiring JCAHO accreditation involves the following seven steps:

1. *The health care organization files a survey application with JCAHO.* The application, which is sent from JCAHO headquarters, consists of inquiries regarding:

    Ownership of the organization
    Demographics (eg, address, phone number)
    Types and volume of services provided

    Official records of operating licenses are also required. After the application is received, JCAHO will forward a set of its current standards for the organization to review.

2. *The health care organization prepares for the survey by reviewing each standard and assessing its compliance.* (Box 12-1 lists the various types of standards.) In addition, the organization reviews and updates all policy and procedure manuals. Personnel records are checked for accuracy and completion. In-house, mock JCAHO surveys are usually conducted.

3. *JCAHO informs the health care organization of the date and time of the survey.* The length of the survey depends on the size and complexity of the setting. Usually, first-time survey visits last 2 to 4 days. The survey is conducted by JCAHO surveyors who specialize in health care standards. The number of surveyors is based on the organization's needs.

4. *JCAHO conducts the survey, which consists of medical record reviews, patient and family interviews, and facility tours.* Employees will be interviewed to determine if they know where the policy and procedure manuals are located, what is in the manuals, and basic safety rules. An exit conference will be held between the surveyors and the administration (leadership) of the health care organization. Preliminary findings will be discussed.

5. JCAHO mails the accreditation decision to the health care organization within 60 days from survey completion. The five types of accreditation are explained in Table 12-1. Organizations can appeal to JCAHO for re-evaluation of the assigned title. The organization will receive a certificate indicating the level of accreditation which can be posted in the setting.

6. *If necessary, JCAHO will conduct a second survey.* A second survey, called a *focus survey*, may be required to prove that corrections have been made. This type of survey generally lasts 1 to 2 days.

7. *After 3 years (the time period for which JCAHO accreditation is valid), the health care organization submits a renewal application, resuming the cycle.*

JCAHO AND QUALITY IMPROVEMENT

The Joint Commission has termed its quality improvement standards as **Improving Organization Performance (IOP)**. The two primary focuses of IOP standards for the organization are to:

- Do the right thing.
- Do the right thing well.

Do the right thing. Does the organization demonstrate **efficacy** and **appropriateness** in caring for patients? Efficacy is determined by whether or not a given treatment is effective for the patient. For example, did giving an antibiotic to a patient with pneumonia cure the pneumonia? Appropriateness refers to whether or not correct tests and procedures were done according to standards of care. For example, was an x-ray study ordered and done for a patient with an injured leg?

Do the right thing well. Does the organization have the appropriate resources **available** and are they accessible in a **timely** fashion? Is there **continuity** of patient care? Is patient **safety** at risk? Is the care provided to the patient and family with **respect and dignity**?

BOX 12-1   Joint Commission on Accreditation of Health Care Organizations (JCAHO) Standards

Section I: Patient-Focused Functions
- Patient Rights and Organization's Ethics
- Assessment of Patients
- Care of Patients
- Education of Patients and Family
- Continuity of Care

Section II: Organization Functions
- Improving Organization Performance
- Leadership
- Management of the Environment of Care
- Management of Human Resources
- Management of Information
- Surveillance, Prevention, and Control of Infection

Table 12-1

Types of Accreditation Offered by the Joint Commission on Accreditation of Health Care Organizations (JCAHO)

Accreditation Title	Explanation
Accreditation with Commendation	This is the highest title that an organization can acquire. It indicates that the organization has demonstrated an exemplary performance.
Accreditation	This title indicates that the organization has met most of the standards. This title can come with or without type I recommendations. A type I recommendation is a specific failure to comply with a given standard. Type I recommendations must be corrected within a given time frame.
Conditional Accreditation	This title indicates that the organization is deficient in meeting various standards. A second survey will be conducted to ensure that corrections have been made.
Provisional Accreditation	This title is given to new organizations that have demonstrated basic compliance but have not been in operation long enough to demonstrate a proven track record. A second survey will be conducted.
Not Accredited	This title is used when the organization has been denied accreditation or its accreditation has been withdrawn by JCAHO.

Checkpoint Question

1. Why do health care organizations participate in JCAHO accreditation if it is voluntary?

Checkpoint Question

2. What are the two basic focuses of JCAHO IOP standards?

Occupational Safety and Health Administration (OSHA)

OSHA is a federal agency that regulates health care and other nonmedical companies (manufacturing plants, and so forth). OSHA requires that QI programs are in place to protect the health and welfare of patients and employees. A primary focus of OSHA is its attention to protecting health care workers from blood-borne pathogen exposures. Unlike JCAHO, OSHA compliance is not voluntary. Noncompliance with OSHA regulations can result in fines and closure of the organization's laboratory setting. The laboratory section of this

textbook discusses in detail Quality Improvement programs as they apply to laboratory settings.

State Health Departments

Each state has a specific agency that is designed to license and monitor health care organizations in the state. Each state has specific guidelines for required QI programs. Like OSHA, participation in state regulations is not optional.

➤ DEVELOPING A QUALITY IMPROVEMENT PROGRAM

The size and complexity of an organization's quality improvement program will vary based on the organization's particular needs. In large hospitals, there may be numerous committees assigned to monitor and implement these plans. (Examples of hospital QI committees may include critical care, patient education, and nursing services). Most hospitals have a specific person assigned to oversee all of these committees.

In the medical office and ambulatory care settings, QI programs tend to be less structured and more informal. Usually the office manager or senior physician is responsible for monitoring and implementing QI plans. However, as more outpatient centers become accredited by JCAHO, the QI programs will have to become more structured.

Seven Steps for a Successful Program

The following seven steps are essential for creating an effective quality improvement program.

1. *Identify the problem.* All organizations can improve their delivery of patient care. Suggestions for improving care can come from many resources, including:
   - Quality improvement managers
   - Office managers
   - Physicians (recommendations and complaints)
   - Other employees (eg, nurses and medical assistants)
   - Patients (interviews)
   - Postcare questionnaires
   - Incident report trending (see below)

   The person responsible for quality improvement in the medical office must review all recommendations for QI problems, then select which ones to address first. Problems given top priority are those that are high-risk (most likely to occur) and those that are most likely to cause injury to patients, family members, or employees.

   In the medical office setting, problems can be grouped into three areas: administrative, clinical,

and laboratory-related (Table 12-2). Problems in any of these areas can cause patient delays and poor patient care. They may also affect patient outcomes and eventually cause patient dissatisfaction.

2. *Form a* **task force**. A *task force* is a group of employees from different disciplines within the organization brought together to solve a given problem. In the medical office, the task force usually consists of the physician, nurse, medical assistant, and office manager. In large hospitals, various department managers will be involved.

3. *Assign an* **expected threshold**. The task force must establish the *expected threshold* (numerical goal) for the given problem. Thresholds must be realistic and achievable. Example: If the problem is patient falls, the expected threshold would be the number of falls that the task force feels is acceptable in a given period of time. For instance, the threshold may be three falls per month. It would not be realistic to say zero; this may be optimal but certainly not achievable.

4. *Explore the problem and propose solutions.* The task force investigates the problem thoroughly to determine all potential angles and solutions. After various solutions are discussed, a decision is made on what solution(s) to implement.

5. *Implement the solution.* The key to a successful implementation of the solution is staff education.

6. *Establish a QI monitoring plan.* After implementation, the solution must be evaluated to determine if it worked and how well it worked. QI monitoring plans have three elements:
   - Source of monitoring—where the numerical data will be obtained (eg, medical record re-

Table 12-2 *Problems Requiring Quality Improvement*	
Area	*Potential Problems*
Administrative	Patient complaints about: • Confusing billing systems • Insurance company delays in paying for care • Inability to access physicians after hours • Appointments delays Lack of collection of insurance co-payments
Clinical	Medication errors (eg, wrong medications given, wrong doses, wrong route) Patient falls Poor patient education Numerous needlesticks
Laboratory	Patients fainting with venipuncture Wrong tests done on wrong patients Inaccurate test results Long turnaround time for results

view, incident reports, laboratory reports, office logs)

- Frequency of monitoring—how often the data will be monitored and tallied (eg, once a week, once a month)
- Person responsible for monitoring—collects the data and depicts the results in graphic form, allowing for easy comparison of pre- and postsolution result

7. *Obtain feedback*. The members of the task force must review the graphs in relation to what their expected threshold was. Did they meet the threshold? If yes, the problem has been resolved. If no, the task force must determine if the expected threshold was unrealistic or if the solutions were inadequate. In either case, the problem has not been resolved; therefore, the task force must review each step and implement the necessary changes.

Checkpoint Question
3. What is an expected threshold?

Checkpoint Question
4. What are the seven steps for creating a quality improvement plan?

➤ RISK MANAGEMENT

Risk management is an internal process geared to decreasing the potential **risk factors** for patients and employees. These risk factors include safety and liability concerns. A risk factor is any issue that poses a safety or liability concern for a given practice. Examples of risk factors include patient falls, medication errors, employee needlesticks, or mistakes in therapeutic intervention. Risk factors for a particular health care organization are identified through the trending of incident reports (see below).

Incident Reports

Incident reports, sometimes referred to as occurrence reports, are written accounts of untoward patient, visitor, or staff events. Such events may be minor or life and limb threatening. Incident reports are often required by the insurance company that provides the institution's liability insurance.

An incident report is initiated by the staff member involved in or at the scene of the incident. The report is reviewed by a supervisor for completion and accuracy and is then sent to a central location. In a hospital, incident reports are sent to the risk manager. In the medical office, incident reports are usually kept on file by the office manager or the physician. Depending on the type of event and organizational policy, a physician may or may not document the event on the incident report. However, if an unusual event occurs to a patient, the physician should assess the patient and document the findings on the incident report.

When to Complete an Incident Report

Even in the most optimal settings, untoward patient events occur. These sometimes result from human error (eg, giving the wrong medication) or they may be idiopathic. Idiopathic means that something occurred for unknown reasons and was unavoidable (eg, an allergic reaction). Incident reports must be completed even if no injury resulted from an event. A few examples of situations requiring an incident report are:

- All medication errors
- All patient, visitor, and employee falls
- Drawing blood from a wrong patient
- Incorrect surgical instrument counts following surgery
- Employee needlesticks
- Workers' compensation injuries

The basic rule of thumb is, when in doubt complete an incident report. Many health care professionals are reluctant to complete incident reports owing to various myths, which are discussed and debunked in Box 12-2.

Checkpoint Question
5. What is the basic rule of thumb to follow regarding completing incident reports?

Information Included on an Incident Report

Although every agency has its own form, the following data should be included on an incident report (Fig. 12-1):

- Name, address, phone number of the injured party
- Date of birth and sex
- Date, time, and location of the incident
- Brief description of the incident and what was done to correct it
- Any diagnostic procedures or treatments that were needed
- Patient examination findings, if applicable

BOX 12-2   Debunking the Myths About Incident Reports

Myth: If I complete an incident report, it will hurt my defense in a malpractice lawsuit. Fact: Incident reports do not hurt you in a malpractice lawsuit and in some cases may actually help your organization's defense. Incident reports are confidential and are not usually available for prosecuting attorney review.

Myth: Incident reports are put in my personnel records. Fact: Incident reports do not go into your personnel file and are not "counted" against you in your performance evaluation. However, you may be educated regarding an error and the manager may choose to document the incident on a disciplinary action form for your personnel records.

Myth: If I complete an incident report, I am implying that I am at fault. Fact: Completing an incident report does not imply that you were at fault. It is just a statement of facts.

- Name and addresses of witnesses, if applicable
- Signature and title of person completing form
- Physician and supervisor signatures as per policy

Guidelines for Completing an Incident Report

When completing an incident report, follow these guidelines:

1. **State only the facts.** Do not draw conclusions or summarize the event. For example, if you walk into the reception room and find a patient on the floor, *do not* document *"Patient tripped and fell in reception area"*; that would be drawing a conclusion. Instead, document as follows: *"Patient found on the floor in the reception area. Patient states that he fell* (Fig. 12-2)."
2. Write legibly and sign your name legibly. Be sure to include your title.
3. **Complete the form in a timely fashion. In general, incident reports should be completed within 24 hours of the event.**
4. Do not leave any blank spaces on the form. If a particular area does not apply, write n/a (not applicable).
5. Never photocopy an incident report for your own records.
6. Never place the incident report in the patient's chart. Never document in the patient's chart that an incident report was completed. Only document the event. (By writing in the medical record that an incident report was completed, it opens the potential for discovery of the report should there be a malpractice lawsuit.)

What If?

What if you give the wrong medication and the patient has a bad reaction to it? Would you be better off not documenting the medication error?

NO! By not documenting the incident, you place yourself at more legal risk. These risks can include allegations of falsifying medical records, tampering with medical records, and failing to follow reporting policies and procedures. On the incident report, do not state "I gave the wrong medication"; just state the facts: "X medication was ordered. I gave Y medication." Then document who you told and when, what you were advised to do, and any other pertinent information. Your supervisor or the risk manager may call the medical office's insurance company to alert them to the incident. If the incident results in a malpractice lawsuit, an accurately completed incident report can prove helpful to your organization's attorney.

Trending Incident Reports

After incident reports are completed, they are reviewed and trended to highlight specific patterns. The statistical data obtained can then be used to identify problem areas, which can be corrected through quality improvement programs. Examples of statistical data that can be found in incident reports include:

- Particular days of the week when most untoward events happen. (If most events occur on Friday af-

text continues on page 178

INCIDENT REPORT FORM

PRIVILEGED & CONFIDENTIAL

Patient Stamp

☐ Inpatient ☐ Outpatient ☐ Visitor ☐ Volunteer ☐ Other   *NOT A PART OF THE MEDICAL RECORD–FORWARD TO RISK MANAGER WITHIN 72 HOURS*

Name		Age	Sex	Admit Date	Location of Incident	Room #
Diagnosis	Date of Incident	Time AM / PM	Date of Report	Person Reporting & Title (print)		

CONDITION BEFORE INCIDENT
☐ Alert   ☐ Disoriented   ☐ Unconscious   ☐ Agitated
☐ Confused   ☐ Sedated   ☐ Uncooperative   ☐ Other

Activity Orders
☐ Adlib   ☐ BRP   ☐ BRP c̄ help
☐ With assist   ☐ CBR
☐ Up in chair   ☐ BSC

Signature

INCIDENT (please check all items that apply)   FALLS

FALLS	PREFALL FACTORS	RESTRAINTS	RISK CONDITIONS	CURRENT MEDICATIONS
☐ Fall from Bed	☐ Bed Up	Restraints Ordered ☐ Y ☐ N	☐ Weakness ☐ Decreased Mobility	☐ None
☐ Fall from Chair	☐ Bed Down	Restraints in Use ☐ Y ☐ N	☐ Confusion	☐ NTG ☐ Diuretics
☐ Fall from Bedside Commode	☐ Brake On ☐ Y ☐ N	Type: ☐ Vest ☐ Wrist ☐ Ankle	☐ Neuro/ortho diagnosis	☐ Cathartic preps/enemas
☐ Fall from Stretcher	☐ Not working	☐ Secured Mittens	☐ Cardiovascular Diagnosis	☐ Antihypertensives
☐ Fall from Wheelchair	☐ Siderails Down	☐ Tied ☐ Untied by:	☐ Impaired Vision	☐ Antiseizure
☐ Fall from Toilet	____ 2 Up	____ Staff	☐ History of Syncope	☐ Antidepressants
☐ Fall while Ambulatory	____ 3 Up	____ Patient	☐ Poor Nutritional Status	☐ Antiemetics
☐ Other: _____	____ 4 Up	____ Family/S.O.	☐ Incontinence	☐ Antipsychotics
	____ Climbed Out	Call light in reach ☐ Y ☐ N	☐ History of fall last 6 months	☐ Analgesics/Hypnotics
		Fall follow-up program initiated	Safety Education given prior to fall:	☐ Narcotics
		prior to fall ☐ Y ☐ N	☐ None ☐ Patient ☐ Family/S.O.	☐ Cardiovascular

Environment: ☐ Floor wet ☐ Y ☐ N   ☐ Free from obstacles ☐ Y ☐ N   Describe: _____
☐ Night light on ☐ Y ☐ N ☐ N/A   ☐ Objects not in reach-searching for _____

MEDICATION VARIANCE, including IV & Blood Product(s)		PROCEDURE VARIANCE		MISCELLANEOUS
☐ Incorrect Pt Identification	☐ Incorrect IV Solution	☐ Record Error ☐ Transcription	☐ Documentation Error	☐ AMA/Elopement
☐ Incorrect Dosage	☐ Incorrect IV Rate	☐ Incorrect Pt Identification	☐ Consent Variance	☐ Admitted c̄ Pressure Sore
☐ Incorrect Route	☐ Incorrect Count/Missing Med	☐ Omitted Treatment	☐ Improper Prep of Pt	☐ Damaged/Lost Teeth/
☐ Incorrect Time	☐ Topical Substance Reaction,	☐ Delayed Treatment	☐ NPO Violated	Denture
☐ Incorrect Med Given	including Tape	☐ Omitted Diagnostic/Lab	☐ Radiation/Toxic Chemical Exposure	☐ Injury During Transport
☐ Incorrect Med Dispensed	☐ Allergy Not Documented	☐ Delayed Diagnostic/Lab	☐ X-ray Interpretation Discrepancy	☐ Self Inflicted Injury/Suicide
☐ Med Omitted	☐ Contrast Reaction/Complication	☐ Traumatic Venipuncture	☐ Airway/Intubation Problem	☐ Malpositioning/Incorrect
☐ Med Transcription Error	☐ Medication Past Due 1 hour	☐ Break in Sterile Technique	☐ Incorrect Level of Heat/Cold Applied	Body Alignment
☐ Incorrect Blood Given	or more	☐ Incorrect Surgical Count—Sponge	☐ Incorrect Procedure/Treatment	☐ Pt Self Extubation
☐ Pharmacy Notified	☐ Other: _____	☐ Incorrect Surgical Count—Needle	☐ Unordered Procedure/Treatment	☐ Tube/IV Catheter Out
☐ Infiltration		☐ Incorrect Surgical Count—Instrument	☐ Equip./Product Malfunction	☐ Accidental Striking Against
☐ Blood Reaction	☐ Given s̄ Order	☐ Retained Foreign Body	☐ User Error	an Object
☐ Med Reaction		☐ Other: _____	☐ Equipment Unavailable	☐ Fainted
		_____		☐ Pt Dissatisfied/Pt
		_____		Threatened Law Suit
				☐ Transfer to Critical Care
				p̄ incident
				☐ Behavior Out of Norm.
				☐ Other: _____

INJURY (please check all items that apply) All serious/significant injuries must be described on reverse side | PROCEDURE/LABOR & DELIVERY/NURSERY

SERIOUS	SIGNIFICANT	SUPERFICIAL	PROCEDURE/LABOR & DELIVERY/NURSERY
☐ None	☐ None	☐ None	☐ Newborn with apparent Cerebral dysfunction
☐ Spinal Cord Injury	☐ Major Infiltration	☐ Unknown	☐ Newborn with APGAR of four (4) or less at five (5) minutes
☐ Injury to Nerves	☐ Hospital Acquired Decubiti	☐ Abrasion	☐ Newborn with serious birth trauma
☐ Brain Injury	☐ Burn	☐ Bruising	☐ Precipitous Delivery
☐ Surgery to Wrong Pt	☐ Fracture	☐ Blister/Skin Tear	☐ Unattended Delivery
☐ Incorrect Surgical Procedure	☐ Sprain/Strain Joint/Muscle	☐ Skin Prick	**MEDICAL DEVICE/EQUIPMENT RELATED**
☐ Shock	☐ Injury to Blood Vessel	☐ Laceration	Equipment involved: _____
☐ Trauma Causing Internal Injury	☐ Dislocation of Joint	☐ Rash/Hives	Manufacturer: _____
☐ Hemorrhage	☐ Open Wound Needing Medical Care	☐ Other: _____	Serial #: _____
☐ Death	☐ Adverse Effect Due to Med/Anesthesia/Transfusion		Asset #: _____
☐ Unscheduled Return to OR	☐ Adverse Effect Due to Exposure to Toxic Chemical		Biomedical Dept. Notified: _____
☐ Other: _____	☐ Complication Due to Mechanical Device		Date
	☐ Prolongation of Hospital Stay		Tagged & Removed from Service: _____
	☐ Anoxia/Respiratory Distress		Date/Time
	☐ Cancellation of or after induction of anesthesia		**Maintain all components of device such as connectors, adaptors, tubings, etc. Document all readings/settings.**
			DO NOT ADJUST OR CLEAR ANY READINGS.

AMA FOLLOW-UP

Reason for leaving: _____
Patient admitted <24 hours   ☐ Yes   ☐ No
Patient/S.O. Teaching: ☐ Completed   ☐ Partial   ☐ None   ☐ Patient Uncooperative

FIGURE 12-1
Incident report form.

Description of event: _____
_____
_____
_____
_____
_____
_____
_____
_____
_____
_____
_____
_____
_____
_____
_____

Physician notified: ☐ Yes   ☐ No   Name of Physician (print): _____
Physician Remarks: _____
_____
_____
_____
_____
_____
_____
_____
_____
_____

_____   _____
Physician Signature   Date

Supervisor/Manager Investigation/Follow-Up Action: _____
_____
_____
_____
_____
_____

_____   _____
Supervisor/Manager Signature   Date

Witnesses: Name (print)	Department/Shift	Address	Phone

_____   _____
Risk Manager Signature   Date

FIGURE 12-1 Continued

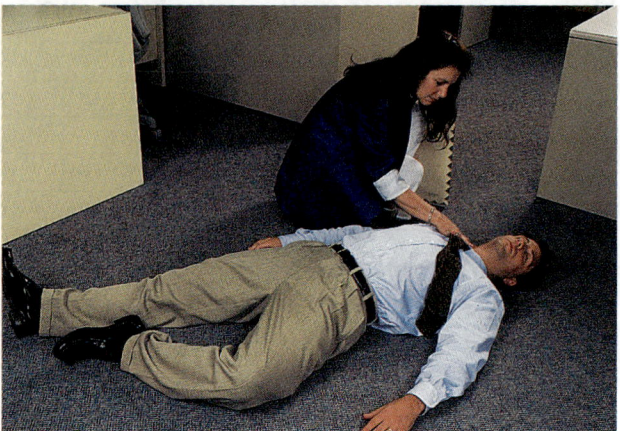

FIGURE 12-2
When completing an incident report form do not draw conclusions or summarize the event; state only the facts.

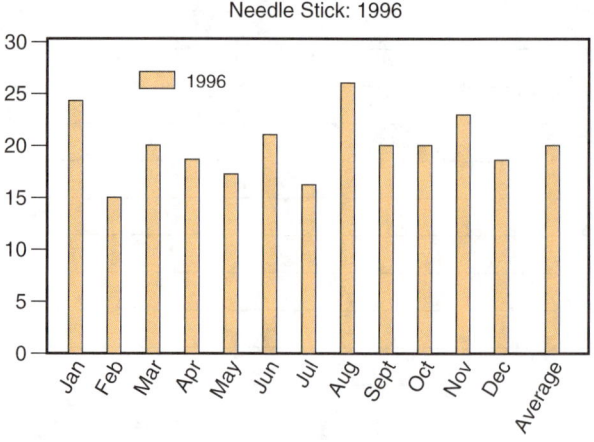

FIGURE 12-3
Graph depicting the number of needle sticks over a year period.

ternoon, perhaps staffing on Friday afternoon needs to be re-evaluated.)
- The most common area for patient falls. (If most falls happen in the lobby, a QI program may need to be established to assess why falls occur there.)
- Medication that is routinely given incorrectly. (This may be corrected by educating staff and using colored labels to highlight similar drug names.)
- The age group most likely to experience problems. (If most of your incident reports reflect problems in the geriatric population, a QI program focusing on geriatric care may need to be established.)

Incident reports should be kept in a special file in the manager's office. Some managers file these reports according to dates, whereas others file them according to the problem.

➤ PUTTING IT ALL TOGETHER: A CASE REVIEW

Below is a case study in which the elements of successful quality improvement and risk management programs are put into action.

Assume that you are working in a busy family practice setting. The average number of patients seen daily is 92. The physicians, nurses, and medical assistants are responsible for venipunctures. On the average, 40 venipunctures are done daily. Monthly needlesticks average 20.

The office manager brings a graph to a staff meeting depicting the number of needlesticks that occurred over a 12-month period (Fig. 12-3). She states that there are no specific trends indicating a difference between days of the week or times that needlesticks occur. It is decided that this is a significant employee safety problem and that a QI program needs to be de-

veloped to address the **identified problem of employee needlesticks**.

A task force is formed. It includes a physician, nurse, and medical assistant. The task force identifies the problem as a high-risk issue and **assigns the expected threshold** to be less than three needlesticks per month. The task force **identifies the factors related to the problem,** which includes lack of sufficient number of needle box holders, lack of a needleless system, and overall need for needlestick prevention education.

Solutions to these three problems are created. An additional needle box is placed in every patient room and two additional boxes are added in the laboratory area (Fig. 12-4). A needleless system is brought into the practice and **all employees receive inservice** training from the company representative. Finally, **inhouse education is conducted** to reinforce proper disposal of

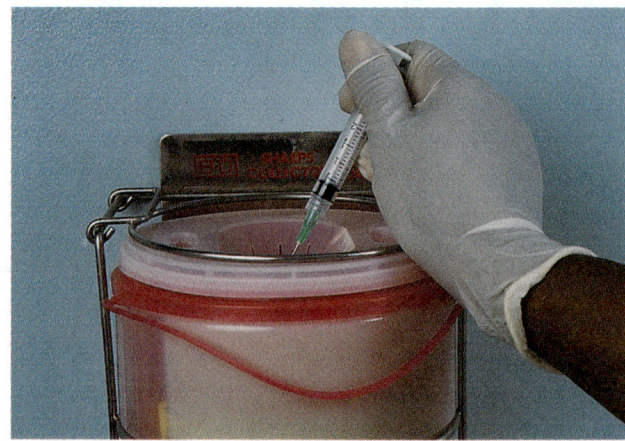

FIGURE 12-4
As part of the quality improvement program needle boxes were placed in every patient room.

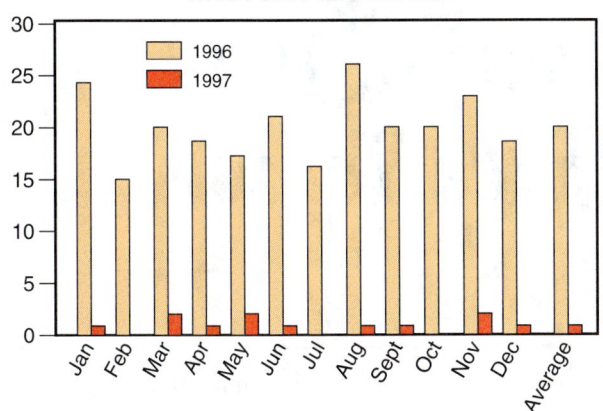

FIGURE 12-5
Graph depicting the number of needle sticks before the quality improvement program was enacted (1996) and after the quality improvement program was enacted (1997).

contaminated needles. A **QI monitoring plan is developed** to evaluate these changes:

1. The **source for monitoring** is the incident reports.
2. The **frequency of monitoring** is monthly, as incident reports became available.
3. The **person responsible** for monitoring is the medical assistant.

New graphs are developed showing the changes (Fig. 12-5). Because the threshold has been met and surpassed, the task force does not feel any changes are needed and therefore the **QI needlestick program is ended.**

SUMMARY

The use of quality improvement programs and risk management, serious problems can be identified and corrected. These two programs must work closely together to meet and exceed patients' expectations and staff members' needs.

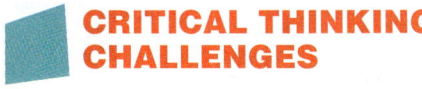

CRITICAL THINKING CHALLENGES

1. Create a list of potential patient-employee problems that would require a quality improvement program. Be sure to include some administrative, clinical, and laboratory examples. Then select three problems and develop a list of solutions for each problem.
2. Patient falls pose a serious problem for health care organizations. Review your clinical chapters on various body systems. Then make a list of diseases that would place a patient at high risk for falls. How could you help prevent patient falls? What groups of medications would increase the potential for patient falls?
3. How can you, as a medical assistant, help your employer with quality improvement and risk management?

ANSWERS TO CHECKPOINT QUESTIONS

1. The two reasons that health care organizations participate in JCAHO accreditation is that accreditation is needed to participate in federal programs and to improve their marketability.
2. The two basic focuses of JCAHO's IOP is to ensure that the health care organization does the right thing and does it well.
3. The expected threshold is a numeric goal.
4. The seven steps for creating a quality improvement program are to identify problem, form a task force, assign an expected threshold, explore the problem and propose solutions, implement the solutions, establish a QI monitoring plan, and obtain feedback.
5. Regarding incident reports, the rule of thumb is: When in doubt, complete an incident report.

SUGGESTIONS FOR FURTHER READING

1996 Accreditation Manual for Ambulatory Care, Vol. 1: Standards. (1996). Oakbrook, IL: Joint Commission on Accreditation for Health Care Organizations.

Craven, Ruth F., & Hirnle, Constance, J. (1996). *Fundamentals of Nursing, Human Health and Function*, 2nd ed. Philadelphia: Lippincott-Raven Publishers.

Eggland, Ellen T., and Heinemann, Denise S. (1994). *Nursing Documentation, Charting, Recording and Reporting.* Philadelphia: J.B. Lippincott.

Schroeder, Patricia. (1994). *Improving Quality and Performance: Concepts, Programs and Techniques.* St. Louis: Mosby-Year Book, Inc.

Management of the Medical Office Team

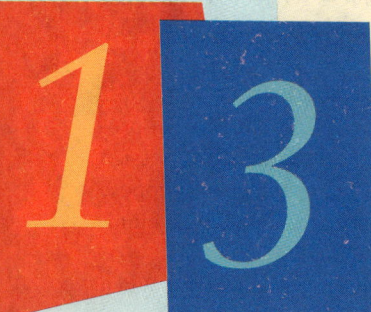

Chapter Outline

Overview of Medical Office Management
    Organizational Structure
    The Medical Office Manager
Responsibilities of the Medical Office Manager
    Communication
    Staffing Issues
    Policy and Procedure Manuals
    Developing Promotional Materials
    Financial Concerns
    Education

Legal Issues Regarding Office Management
    Americans with Disabilities Act
    Sexual Harassment
    Family and Medical Leave Act
    Other Legal Considerations
Summary
Critical Thinking Challenges
Answers to Checkpoint Questions
Suggestions for Further Reading

DACUM Components

1.1 Project a positive attitude
1.5 Work as a team member
1.6 Conduct one's self in a courteous and diplomatic manner
1.7 Adapt to change
1.8 Show initiative and responsibility
2.11 Compose written communication using correct grammar, spelling, and format
6.1 Maintain the physical plant
6.3 Inventory equipment and supplies
7.4 Orient and train personnel

Advanced-level skills:
Develop and maintain policy and procedure manuals
Supervise personnel
Develop educational materials

Chapter Competencies

Learning Objectives

Upon successfully completing this chapter, you will be able to:

1. Spell and define the Key Terms.
2. Describe what is meant by "organizational structure."
3. List seven responsibilities of the medical office manager.
4. Explain the five staffing issues that a medical office manager will be responsible for handling.
5. List the types of policies and procedures that should be included in a medical office's policy and procedure manual.
6. List five types of promotional materials that a medical office may distribute.
7. Discuss three financial concerns that the medical office manager must be capable of addressing.
8. Discuss four legal issues that affect medical office management.

Performance Objectives

Upon successfully completing this chapter, you will be able to:

1. Write a job description.
2. Create policy and procedure manuals.

Key Terms

(See Glossary for definitions.)
Americans with Disabilities Act
budget
Family and Medical Leave Act
job descriptions
mission statement
organizational chart
policy
procedure

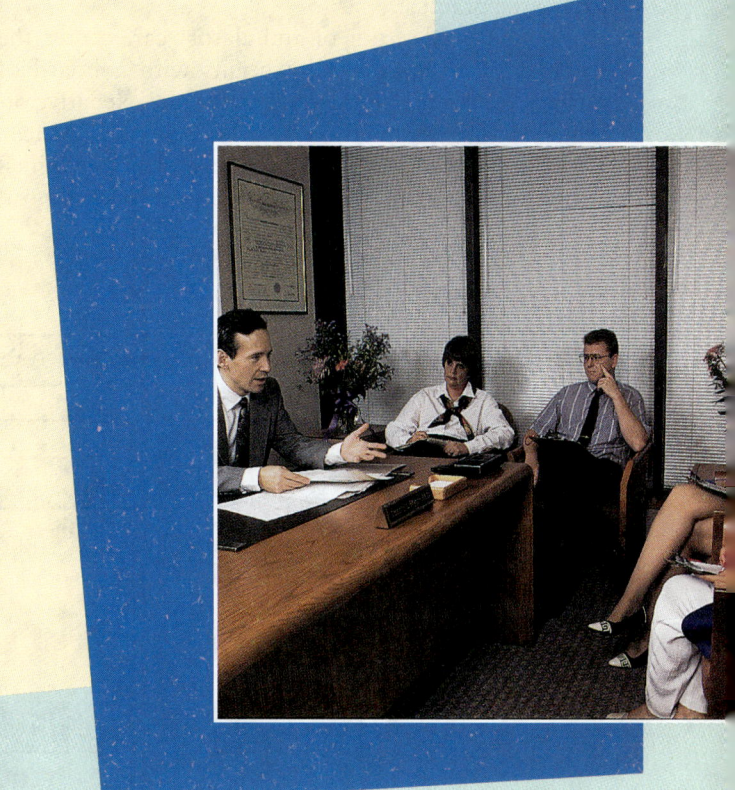

A successful medical practice needs an effective medical office management process. This process must be a team effort between the physicians, nurse managers, and the office manager. This chapter provides an overview of medical office management as well as a discussion of a medical office manager's specific responsibilities.

➤ OVERVIEW OF MEDICAL OFFICE MANAGEMENT

Each medical office is organized in a slightly different manner, depending on the size and complexity of the setting.

Organizational Structure

The medical office's organizational structure, or chain of command, is depicted in an **organizational chart, a flow sheet that allows the manager and employees to identify their team members and to see where they fit into the team.** Figure 13-1 displays a sample organizational chart for a physician's office in which there is a partnership between two physicians. In this example, it is assumed that both physicians have an equal partnership in the practice.

In a hospital setting or ambulatory care center, the organizational chart usually begins with a board of trustees. Below the board will be the chief executive officer, chief operating officer, and chief financial officer. Below these positions will be vice presidents, administrative directors, managers, and then the staff positions.

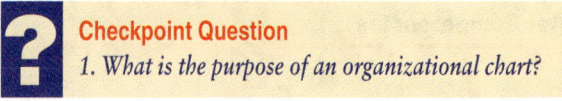

Checkpoint Question
1. What is the purpose of an organizational chart?

The Medical Office Manager

The medical office manager must be multiskilled, multitalented, and able to prioritize a variety of issues, juggle responsibilities, and communicate effectively with patients, staff, and physicians. In some settings, the medical office manager may be referred to as the "business manager". Managers may be nurses, medical assistants, or administrative support personnel. Although the qualifications and educational requirements for the position vary greatly among health care organizations, a successful medical office manager must be:

- Flexible
- A positive employee role model
- Honest and fair
- A good communicator
- A resource person for employees
- Supportive of all management decisions
- Well organized
- Able to focus on a given task
- Able to resolve conflicts
- Able to see the "big picture"

A medical office manager's responsibilities are varied and include such tasks as:

- Communicating with patients, physicians, and staff
- Handling staffing issues
- Writing and revising *policy* and *procedure* manuals
- Developing promotional materials
- Handling financial concerns

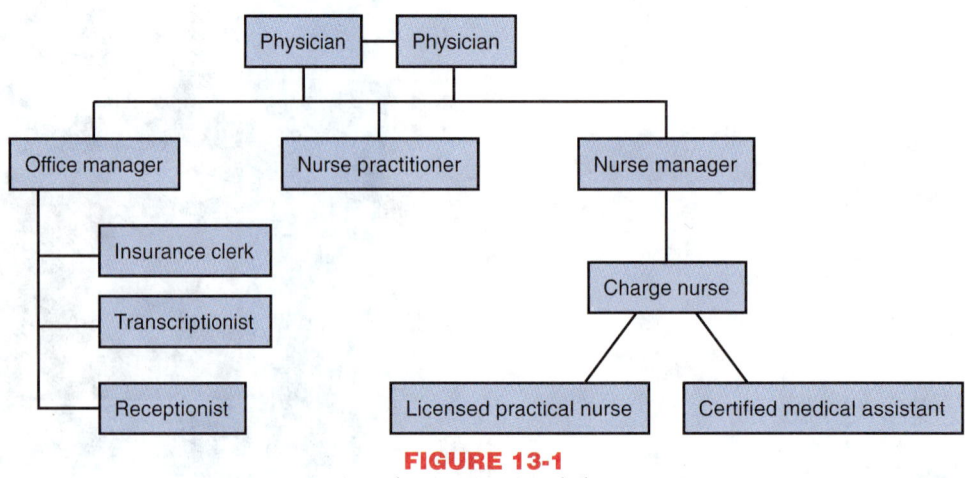

FIGURE 13-1
Sample organizational chart.

- Handling maintenance and inventory
- Ensuring the staff receives appropriate education

➤ RESPONSIBILITIES OF THE MEDICAL OFFICE MANAGER

Communication

Perhaps one of the hardest and yet most important aspects of being an effective manager is being able to communicate with fellow employees, colleagues, physicians, and patients. (The techniques for effective communication are discussed in Chapter 4, Fundamental Communication Skills.) You must be a good listener, have good interpersonal skills, and be aware of your own nonverbal language.

Communicating with Patients

Communication with patients on a management level can often be challenging. Patients come to you with a variety of complaints, such as incorrect billing, poor care, or long waits to see physicians. Of course, you must always be diplomatic. Your goal should be to correct the problem in a timely and professional manner and to alleviate any negative feelings the patient may have.

Communicating with Staff

Communication with staff members can be difficult depending on the number of employees, number and locations of satellite centers, and the variety of shifts that are in place. There are three ways to promote communication with staff members: staff meetings, bulletin boards, and communication notebooks.

Staff meetings. These meetings should be scheduled at a predictable frequency and time to allow the staff to plan (eg, they might be held the first Monday of every month at 8 AM and 3 PM. Meetings should never be canceled except in a true emergency. If the staff size is large (>20-25 employees), it is best to hold two separate meetings to allow all staff members the opportunity to attend.

Staff meetings must be well organized and should begin and end on time. Agendas should be created prior to the meeting and posted for staff review. (See Chap. 9, Written Communications, for information about agendas.) The agenda should be followed as closely as possible. Individual staff concerns or complaints should not be handled during a general staff meeting; the meeting should remain focused and constructive and not turn into a "battleground" for staff disagreements. Minutes should be taken and kept in a

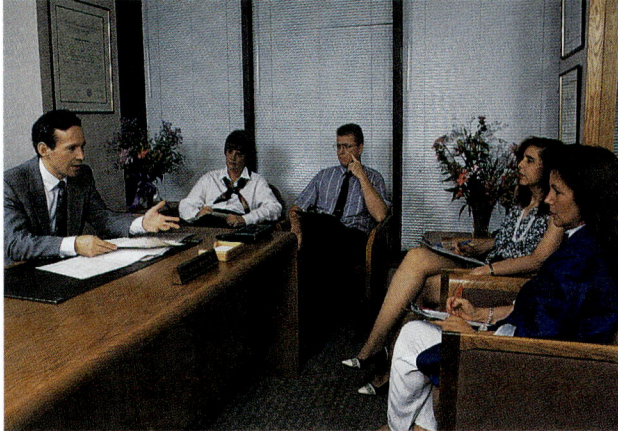

FIGURE 13-2
Conduct staff meetings in a private area.

notebook for staff to review as needed. (See Chap. 9, Written Communications, for information about minutes.)

Staff meetings should be conducted in a private area out of patient sight and hearing (Fig. 13-2). All interruptions, except for emergencies, should be avoided. The policy and procedure manual should clearly state the attendance policy for staff meetings. In addition, some offices include attendance as a "duty" in each employee's **job description** (statement of work-related responsibilities). To improve attendance at staff meetings, consider serving food or including an educational presentation.

Bulletin boards. Bulletin board postings allow employees to get a quick and easy look at **new** polices or procedures. To encourage staff members to read the postings, make sure the bulletin boards are attractive, well organized, and updated regularly. It is a good idea to have employees initial all messages on the bulletin board after reading them.

Communication notebooks. A simple notebook can serve as a two-way communication tool—you can write messages to employees and they can write back to you. Such a notebook is usually kept in the staff lounge. Again, staff members should initial any important messages after reading them. If the message is directed to you, be sure to respond as soon as possible.

Sometimes, the press of daily duties prevents managers from communicating with staff members on a personal level. To be an effective manager, you should not communicate only "bad" news to your employees but also positive messages. You can communicate positive messages through birthday and holiday cards and employee recognition awards. Bulletin boards can also be used to promote positive messages such as births, weddings, or engagement announcements.

Checkpoint Question
2. *What are three ways to promote communication with staff members?*

Staffing Issues

Staffing issues will occupy most of your time as an office manager. These concerns involve writing job descriptions, hiring new employees, evaluating present

---

Job Description

Title: Medical Assistant
Supervisor(s): Charge Nurse for Clinical Duties
Office Manager for Administrative Duties
Position summary: This is a 40 hour position that will require the employee to perform various duties including administrative, clinical and laboratory procedures. Scheduling will be variable to meet the needs of the office.
Hours: Hours will vary to meet the needs of the office. Hours will rotate from: 8 AM–4:30 PM and 10:00 AM–6:30 PM. You will be expected to work one Saturday per month.
Location: Our main office is located at 129 South Main Street. The satellite office is located at 56 West Road, Suite 102. This position will primarily require you to work at our main office. However, occasional days may be assigned at the satellite office.
Employment Requirements: The employee must have graduated from a medical assisting program. CMA or RMA is preferred. The employee must have a current CPR and First Aid card. One year of experience is preferred or completion of an externship.
• *Language skills:* The employee must be able to read and interpret documents and respond appropriately (verbally and/or in writing). Must be able to document in a professional manner.
• *Mathematical skills:* The employee must be able to add, subtract, multiply and divide whole numbers and fractions.
Physical requirements: The following are physical requirements for this job: Standing: 6–8 hours/day; Sitting: 6–8 hours/day; Lifting: 50 pounds; Twisting and rotating: 45 degrees; Squatting: As needed to assist patients or to perform office tasks.
Duties: You will be expected to perform the following duties after completing the orientation process. This is a partial list; and other duties can be added as necessary:
Administrative:

Scheduling appointments	Processing mail
Transcribing documents	Operating the telephone
Filing	Providing patient education
Completing insurance forms	

Clinical/Laboratory:

Operating centrifuge	Obtaining vital signs
Performing phlebotomy	Administering vaccines and other medications
Performing HCT/HGB/CBC	as ordered
Performing pregnancy and monospot tests	Providing patient education
Obtaining visual acuities	Assisting the physician as directed

Evaluation process: Three evaluations will be conducted in the first year. Thirty days from start date, ninety days from the start date, and then at the one-year anniversary date. Following the first year of employment, annual evaluations will be done.

I have read my job description and I understand what is expected of me. I am able to physically perform all the required duties.

Signature of employee: _____   Date: _____

Signature of supervisor: _____   Date: _____

Signature of supervisor: _____   Date: _____

Dates: original JD - 1977, revised March 1998.

FIGURE 13-3
Sample job description.

employees, taking disciplinary actions, handling terminations, and scheduling.

Writing Job Descriptions

Each job must have a description. The purpose of a job description is to inform the employee about the duties and expectations for a given position. Job descriptions also help you in interviewing applicants and evaluating existing employees.

Each employee should receive a copy of his or her job description at the time of hiring and after any revisions to the description are made. Some medical offices have a policy requiring the employee to read and sign the job description at the time of hiring.

Formats for writing job descriptions vary among offices. In general, the following elements are included: job title, supervisor, position summary, hours, location, employment requirements, physical requirements, duties, and the evaluation process (Fig. 13-3). The description should also include the date it was written and the date(s) it was revised.

If possible, involve staff members in writing and revising their job descriptions. Employee participation leads to greater cooperation.

Employee Evaluation Form

Employee: _____

Evaluation Date: _____

Job Title: _____

Ratings:

Traits	Score
Appearance	
Communication Skills	
Attendance	
Quality of work	
Reliability	
Initiative	
Other:	
Total Score:	

Rating scale:

5—excellent

4—above average

3—meets job expectations

2—below job expectations

1—does not meet job expectations

Supervisor comments:

_____

_____

Employee goals for the next year (to be completed by employee):

_____

_____

_____

Employee Comments:

_____

_____

_____

Supervisor signature: _____ Date:_____

Employee signature: _____ Date:_____

FIGURE 13-4

Sample employee evaluation form.

Hiring and Interviewing Employees

Only after creating or reviewing an existing job description can you begin the process of interviewing and hiring a new employee. Finding applicants for most medical office positions is not usually a problem. You can seek applicants through advertising in local newspaper classified sections, placement personnel at local schools that offer medical assisting programs, networking, and employment agencies.

All applicants should complete an application. State laws vary regarding the types of questions that can be asked on applications. In general, you must avoid any questions pertaining to an applicant's age, sex, race, religion, and physical or mental disabilities. Any employee application form should be reviewed by legal counsel prior to its use. It is always a good idea to request that the applicant bring a resume to the interview.

Before interviewing an applicant, prepare a list of questions. Again, use caution; you are not legally able to ask about the above-mentioned topics. During the interview, assess the applicant's ability to:

- Perform technical skills
- Treat patients in a caring manner
- Fit into your organization
- Communicate in a professional yet friendly manner
- Remain flexible

Evaluating Employees

All employees must be evaluated on an annual basis. The evaluation process should be a positive experience for the employee. Employee evaluations must be fair, accurate, and objective. Some type of written evaluation should be given to the employee to read, sign, and comment on. Most forms ask employees to list their objectives and goals for the coming year. (Fig. 13-4 displays a sample evaluation form.) Some organizations call evaluations "performance appraisals."

New employees should be evaluated 1 month after their start date, again in 90 days, and then at their 1-year anniversary date. This evaluation process helps new employees gain confidence and improve weaknesses.

Taking Disciplinary Action

Most offices have policies regarding documentation of disciplinary action. Disciplinary actions can be verbal or written. Verbal warnings are generally done for a

Discipline Record

Employee Name:_____ #:_____ Date of Warning:_____
Warning
Date of Violation:_____ Time:_____ Place: _____
Description of Violation:

_____
_____
_____
_____
_____
_____

_____ Verbal Warning   Action To Be Taken:
_____ Written Warning
_____ Probation—_____Days   _____
_____ Suspension—_____Days   _____
_____ Termination   _____
                                                    _____
                                                    _____
_____
Supervisor's Signature   Date

Employee's Remarks
Do you agree with the details above: Yes: _____ No: _____
Comments: _____
_____
_____

_____
Employee's Signature   Date

FIGURE 13-5
Sample disciplinary action form.

first-time minor occurrence (eg, not showing up for work and not calling in). A note should go into the employee's file stating that a verbal warning was given, the date, any actions that were taken, and any comments that the employee made.

Written notices are used for more serious problems (eg, breaching patient confidentiality, substance abuse) or recurrent minor ones. Employees should sign any written warning notices. These documents can be used as evidence in the event that there is a wrongful discharge lawsuit. Figure 13-5 shows a sample written disciplinary action form.

Terminating Employees

Having to terminate an employee is never an easy or pleasant task. It is essential that policies regarding termination be followed precisely. All disciplinary actions must be clearly and objectively stated. Terminating employees for unlawful reasons or failing to follow the organization's termination policy can result in lawsuits against you and the office. Reasons for terminations may include:

- Excessive tardiness or absenteeism
- Inappropriate dress or behavior
- Alcohol or drug use
- Lying or stealing
- Falsifying medical records
- Breaching patient confidentiality

What If?

What if you receive a call requesting a reference for an employee who was fired? What should you say?

Be careful! This situation can turn into a legal nightmare if not handled appropriately. If you give a wonderful report to the potential employer and say: "She was a great, never had any problems" you and the office might be sued by the former employee for wrongful discharge. In court, you would be asked: "If she was so wonderful, why did you fire her?" On the other hand, if you say, "She was a terrible employee and we fired her," you can be sued for defamation of character. Because of the legal concerns in providing employment references, most organizations have a policy stating that the only information to be released is verification of employment dates and job titles. When in doubt, give no information. Ask for the caller's name and phone number; discuss the issue with the physician in charge, then return the phone call.

Scheduling

The primary goal of scheduling is to meet the needs of the office. The secondary goal is to meet the requests of your employees. You must be fair in scheduling and always follow your organization's policies for weekend and holiday or personal day requests. Depending on the number of employees that you need to schedule and the complexity of the hours or shifts, you can either schedule by hand or through computerized programs. Most office managers schedule by hand. If your organization is small and cohesive, you may want to assign a senior staff member to do the scheduling or you might allow the employees to self-schedule. No matter what scheduling format is used, you are ultimately responsible for ensuring that the appropriate number and type of employees needed are scheduled.

Requests for time off should be put in writing. Depending on the size of the organization, such requests may have to be received by a given date or time. For example: "A request for a day off in May may need to be received by April 15. Any requests for time off filed after the cutoff date will be approved whenever possible." This eliminates your having to repeatedly adjust the staffing schedule.

Checkpoint Question

3. What is the medical office manager's primary goal in scheduling?

Policy and Procedure Manuals

Policy and Procedure manuals contain written guidelines to inform the employee about various issues. A policy is a statement regarding the organization's rules on a given topic. A procedure is a series of steps required to perform a given task. Policies and procedures must be written in a clear, concise and understandable format. To make the process easier, follow these tips:

1. Contact local organizations, medical offices, or ambulatory care centers and ask how they perform a given task. Ask for copies of their policies.
2. If you are writing a procedure on using a new piece of equipment, ask the sales representative for educational pamphlets. Some companies have pre-printed sample procedures.
3. Form a policy and procedure committee. If staff members help develop the policies, they are more likely to follow them.
4. Create a sample master sheet with all the required elements. This makes it faster and easier to com-

plete the task. Each policy and procedure should have the following elements:

- Name: This should be in a logical, easily identifiable format. Example: Infection Control Procedure—Handwashing.
- Purpose: This should be a sentence or two (at most) explaining the intent of the policy or procedure.
- Necessary equipment or forms: This is a comprehensive list of all the items needed to complete the task. Also indicate if no special equipment or forms are necessary.
- Steps to complete task or policy explanation: The steps must be complete and in a logical order. It should never be assumed that the reader knows how to perform a given step (eg, handwashing). If there are no specific steps, the policy is written out in paragraph form.
- Signatures: All policies and procedures must be signed. Clinical procedures will usually be signed by the nurse manager and a physician. Policies regarding medical office management will be signed by the physician and medical office manager.
- Date that the policy was written and revised: All policies and procedures should be reviewed annually to assess for currentness and accuracy. If changes are needed, the policy or procedure is rewritten, signed, and dated with the new revision dates. The previous dates are generally listed as well.
- Numbering system: All policies and procedures should be numbered to allow for easy access and identification. Example: "HR #14" means human resource section, policy number 14.

? Checkpoint Question

4. Which seven elements must be included when writing a policy or procedure?

Types of Policies and Procedures

There are many types of policies and procedures. In general, the following areas are included in a policy and procedure manual:

Section 1: Mission Statement
Section 2: Organizational Structure
Section 3: Human Resources/Personnel
Section 4: Quality Improvement/Risk Management
Section 5: Clinical Procedures
Section 6: Administrative
Section 7: Infection Control

North Shore Family Practice is a group practice dedicated to providing quality care through compassion, innovation, performance and education. It is our goal to provide medical care to the community of Rochester, New York. The physicians, nurse practitioners and all staff members are committed to working together as a team to provide the patient with the best care possible.

FIGURE 13-6
Sample mission statement.

Section 1: Mission Statement. A **mission statement** describes the goals of the practice and who it serves. Often a mission statement provides a philosophic look at an organization. It is generally one to two paragraphs long (Fig. 13-6).

The mission statement should not only be included only in the policy and procedure manual; it should also be available to patients. Often it is framed and placed in the waiting room or printed in the patient instruction booklet.

Section 2: Organizational Structure. The organizational chart is included in this section as well as policies regarding:

- Chain of command
- How and when to contact various members of the team
- Coverage for managers
- Physician on-call policies

Section 3: Human Resources/Personnel. This section consists of policies relating to staff responsibilities, benefits, and employee rules and regulations. Box 13-1 lists the kinds of policies found in this section of the manual. A sample human resources policy is displayed in Figure 13-7.

Section 4: Quality Improvement/Risk Management. This section includes policies outlining who is in charge of quality improvement, the steps for developing a quality improvement plan, and explanations of incident reporting. (See Chapter 12, Quality Improvement and Risk Management, for more information.)

Section 5: Clinical Procedures. Any task that requires patient intervention should be listed in this section. (Some offices separate laboratory procedures into a different section for convenience.) In addition, clinical procedures should include specific infection control guidelines for the particular procedure, patient education guidelines, and instructions for documentation. Sample documentation forms should be included in this section. It is a good idea to complete the sample form correctly so that it can serve as a model. Throughout this textbook, sample clinical procedures are in-

---

Benjamin William, MD
2295 Matthews Drive
Boca Raton, Florida 33432
POLICY AND PROCEDURE MANUAL

Policy title: Human Resources; Call offs
Purpose: The purpose of this policy is to advise all employees of the policy for call offs and to prewarn employees regarding the disciplinary steps that will be taken as a result of not complying with this policy.
Equipment/Forms necessary: No equipment or forms are required.
Explanation:
- If you are going to call in sick, you must call in two hours prior to your assigned time. Messages should be left with the answering service if the office is not open.
- If you have personal days accrued, you can use them for compensation.
- If you are going to be out sick for more than three consecutive working days, you will need to obtain a physician's note to document the illness.
- Employees are allowed six (6) call offs per year without disciplinary action. Seven (7) call offs will result in a verbal warning regarding attendance. Eight (8) call offs will result in a written warning. Nine (9) call offs will result in termination. Exceptions to disciplinary action will be reviewed on an individual basis and are at the joint discretion of the office manager and physician.

_____   _____
Susan Rogers, RMA   Benjamin William, MD
Office Manager

date: original policy - 06/96, revised 07/98
HR: 14

FIGURE 13-7
Sample human resources policy.

cluded. In the medical office setting, these procedures may vary slightly to meet the needs of the office, physician requests, or manufacturer guidelines.

Section 6: Administrative. This section includes a policy or procedure on all tasks that the administrative office staff must perform. Sample forms should also be included and updated as necessary. Examples of administrative tasks include:

- Accounting/bookkeeping
- Appointment scheduling
- Collections
- Computer care and operations
- Insurance filings
- Medical records management
- Mail and postal machines operations

Section 7: Infection Control. Depending on the length of this section, some offices opt for a separate manual dedicated to infection control and prevention. Examples of these policies include:

Types of personal protection equipment available
Biohazardous waste disposal
Handling of various disease identities
Handling of employee exposures or needle sticks
Documentation required by OSHA
Employee education for infection control

Developing Promotional Materials

The medical office manager is often responsible for developing and distributing promotional literature for the practice. Depending on the budgetary allowance, promotional materials can be created and produced at commercial printing shops or done in the office with desktop publishing computer software programs. Examples of promotional materials include:

- Patient education booklets
- Patient handbooks
- Newsletters
- Holiday cards
- Birthday cards (usually used by pediatricians)
- Newspaper articles
- Yellow pages
- Direct mail
- Business cards

Follow these guidelines when creating promotional materials:

Double check all spelling and grammar.
Ensure accuracy.
Use clear and specific language.
Avoid abbreviations and complex medical terms.
Use brightly colored materials.

BOX 13-1 Types of Human Resources/Personnel Policies

Absentee policies	Office hours
Cafeteria plans	Orientation process
Confidentiality policy	Overtime reports
Continuing education requirements	Parking
Disciplinary action procedures	Payroll
Emergency procedures	Personal phone calls
Employee benefits (health and dental insurance)	Resignations
	Sexual harassment
Evaluation process and performance appraisals	Sick leave and family leave
	Staff meetings
Grievance procedures	Tardiness
Grooming and uniforms/appearance	Termination process
Holiday coverage and compensation for holidays	Time recording
	Vacation days
Jury duty	

If you are using a commercial printer, be sure to carefully review the proofs before the final printing.

Financial Concerns

Budgets

A budget is a financial planning tool that helps an organization estimate its anticipated expenditures and revenues. Budgeting has many purposes for an organization. For example, it:

- Forces the manager and physician to plan
- Causes managers and staff to become cost conscious
- Promotes communication among staff and managers
- Helps the organization achieve a financial goal

The medical office generally has both an operating and a capital budget. Operating budgets consist of all costs to run the office. These include, but are not limited to, payroll, office and medical supplies, education, promotional materials, and electricity and telephone services. Capital budgets consist of large outlays of money. These usually include large purchases (usually over $500), building maintenance, property management, and equipment.

Developing and writing a budget takes practice and instructions from the financial officer or physician. In general, the previous year's expense report is reviewed, revenues are projected for the following year, then figures are assigned to ensure that income balances with the outgoing expenses.

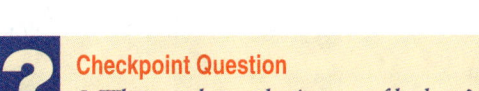

Checkpoint Question

5. What are the two basic types of budgets?

Payroll

Another financial concern for the manager is payroll. All employees expect to receive the correct amount of pay on time, and those expectations must be met. Payroll is a complex task that involves both state and federal laws regarding deductions for Social Security and other taxes. Some offices outsource this service owing to its complexity and to time consuming issues. (See Chap. 16, Accounts Payable and Payroll, for more information.)

Petty Cash

Most offices keep a small amount of cash in the office. Petty cash is used to purchase small items (eg, postage, emergency office supplies) or to reimburse employees for small items. It is essential that the office manager keep close tallies on the petty cash fund. Most offices have some form of a petty cash receipt. Petty cash must be kept in a separate drawer from the change box. (See Chap. 15, Bookkeeping and Banking, for more information.)

Maintenance and Inventory of Supplies

One of the medical office manager's key responsibilities is to keep the office neat, clean, and organized. Most offices have an outside cleaning agency to maintain the lobby, patient rooms, and offices. Special attention to waiting room toys is necessary because they can pose a safety threat to children (see Chap. 49, Pediatric Patients). Staff should be encouraged to periodically check the lobby for neatness and assist in routine cleaning and straightening.

Service Contracts

The medical office manager is responsible for keeping track of all service contracts. A service contract is an agreement between the medical organization and a service company in which the company agrees to perform regular inspections of and care for a specific piece of equipment. Service contracts are usually obtained for copiers, computers, fax machines, and other large and expensive pieces of equipment.

Inventory

Extensive amounts of supplies are needed to run a medical office. As a medical office manager, you must develop a logical system to keep track of them. There should be a policy outlining who is responsible for ordering supplies and the procedure for ordering. There also must be some process to check that deliveries of supplies are complete and accurate.

Education

Staff Education

The medical office manager must keep the staff up to date on current trends regarding new medical procedures, new drugs and vaccines, new insurance coding and billing regulations, and any other topics that promote good patient care. In addition to these topics, annual education is usually conducted on cardiopulmonary resuscitation (CPR), infection control, and fire and electrical safety.

PLANNING EDUCATION EVENTS.

As the medical office manager, you should select an educational topic for each month. In some offices, the educational topic is covered during the monthly staff meetings, whereas other offices have separate educational programs. After choosing the monthly topic, select an appropriate presenter. Suggestions for presenters include colleagues, physicians, sales representatives, local hospital staff development coordinators, or specialists in a given area. Presenters for CPR classes must be CPR instructors who are approved by either the American Red Cross or the American Heart Association. To promote attendance, create informative flyers and distribute them to all staff members. Keep attendance records for all classes given.

In addition to formal educational programs, there are other ways to keep your staff up to date. For instance, educational videos can be rented or purchased for staff viewing; consider developing a posttest to assess for comprehension. Also, many professional magazines have continuing education articles on various topics, usually accompanied by a posttest. Finally, staff members should be sent to one to two seminars a year. Outside seminars help increase employee productivity, self-esteem, and retention.

Patient Education

Patient education must occur on a daily basis by all members of the health care team. As a manager, you may not provide patient education directly, but you are responsible for assisting the staff in performing this task. You can help the staff by creating patient education booklets, developing patient education posters, and by teaching your staff how, when, and what to teach patients and families.

Patient education brochures should be colorful and easy to read. Close attention to spelling, grammar, punctuation, and accuracy is essential. All patient education brochures should be reviewed by a physician. Depending on your office's clientele, the brochures should be printed in various languages. Refer to Chapter 5, Patient Education, for more details on creating patient education brochures.

Manager Education

Managers should attend workshops and conferences and read appropriate printed materials to enhance their knowledge and skills in managing a medical office. All new managers can benefit from courses on time management, stress management, solving personnel conflicts, and budget preparation. Memberships in professional organizations can also assist the new office manager. Two such organizations are:

Medical Office Management Association
1355 South Colorado Boulevard, Suite 900
Denver, CO 80222-3331
Professional Association of Health Care
    Office Managers
Suite 102
2929 Langley Avenue
Pensacola, FL 32504-7355

➤ LEGAL ISSUES REGARDING OFFICE MANAGEMENT

Americans with Disabilities Act (ADA)

Formerly called the Rehabilitation Act, the **Americans with Disabilities Act** was expanded in 1994. All companies with more than 15 employees must comply with regulations designed to meet the needs of people with physical and mental disabilities. This act requires that all buildings be accessible to physically challenged people. Following is a partial list of ways the medical office can comply with this act:

- Entrance ramps
- Widened rest rooms to be wheelchair accessible
- Elevated toilet bowls for easier transferring from wheel chairs
- Easy-to-reach elevator buttons
- Braille signs
- Access to special telephone services to communicate with hearing-impaired patients

Sexual Harassment

It is illegal for any employee or patient to be sexually harassed. Sexual harassment can come in many forms. As a medical office manager, it is your responsibility to be alert for signs of harassment and to have in place a policy for handling complaints regarding this.

Family and Medical Leave Act

The Family and Medical Leave Act, approved in 1993, allows an employee to leave his or her job for up to 12 weeks (unpaid) to meet family needs (eg, the birth or adoption of a child; serious illness of a child, parent, spouse, or self). Employers must hold the employee's job position or offer the employee a position of similar nature upon return.

Other Legal Considerations

The Clinical Laboratory Improvement Amendments (CLIA) of 1988 contain specific rules and regulations regarding laboratory safety. These issues are discussed in Unit 7, Performing Laboratory Procedures.

The Occupational Safety and Health Administration (OSHA) is a federal agency that sets standards for employee safety. OSHA regulations are also discussed in Unit 7.

The Joint Commission on Accreditation of Health Care Organizations (JCAHO) is a private organization

Legal Tips

There are many acts and regulations that affect health care organizations and their operations. As a medical office manager, you must keep current on all legal updates. Most states publish a monthly bulletin that reports on newly passed legislation; read these on a regular basis. Each office should have legal counsel who can assist in interpreting legal issues. It is important for a new manager to meet with the medical office's attorney to discuss legal concerns for the practice.

that sets standards for health care administration. JCAHO is discussed in Chapter 12, Quality Improvement and Risk Management.

Each state also has specific laws regarding patient care, insurance billing, payroll management, and so forth that a medical office manager must understand.

Checkpoint Question
6. What are some legal issues of concern to the medical office manager?

SUMMARY

Effective management of the medical office is essential for a health care organization to succeed in the competitive marketplace. A good manager must be able to perform a variety of tasks in an organized and efficient manner. These tasks include communicating with patients and staff, handling staffing issues, developing policy and procedure manuals, creating promotional materials, preparing budgets, and overseeing educational programs. In addition, the medical office manager must keep current on legal requirements related to office operations.

CRITICAL THINKING CHALLENGES

1. Review the list of qualities that a manager should have. Which ones do you have? How would you acquire the others? Are there any other qualities that should be listed?
2. Review the the types of sections that are often included in policy and procedure manuals. Now assume that you are to help a physician set up a practice. How would you

organize your policy and procedure manual? Create one sample sheet for each section of your manual. Be sure to include all necessary elements when you write your policies and procedures.

3. Create a description for your ideal job. How would you go about finding this position?

ANSWERS TO CHECKPOINT QUESTIONS

1. An organizational chart is a flow sheet that allows the manager and employees to identify their team members and to see where they fit into the team.

2. Three ways to communicate with staff members are through bulletin boards, staff meetings, and communication notebooks.

3. The primary goal of scheduling is to ensure that the needs of the office are met.

4. The elements that must be in a policy or procedure are: document name, purpose, equipment or forms needed, steps or explanations, signatures, numbering system, and dates.

5. The two basic types of budgets are operating and capital.

6. Some of the legal issues are the Americans with Disabilities Act, Sexual Harassment laws, Family and Medical Leave Act, CLIA, and OSHA.

SUGGESTIONS FOR FURTHER READING

Andress, Alice A. (1996). *Saunders Manual of Medical Office Management*. Philadelphia: W.B. Saunders.

Johnson, Joan M., & Johnson, Marc, W. (1994). *Computerized Medical Office Management*. Albany, NY: Delmar Publishers.

Unit 4

Managing Finances in the Practice

The medical practice must operate in a financially sound manner to continue to serve the patient's needs. Knowledge of health insurance and reimbursement policies for medical services will ensure that the business of medicine is self-supporting and available to all patients.

Credit and Collections

Chapter Outline

Fees
    Setting Fees
    Discussing Fees in Advance
    Forms of Payment
    Payment by Insurance Companies
    Adjusting Fees

Credit
    Extending Credit
    Legal Considerations

Collections
    Legal Considerations
    Collecting a Debt
    Collection Alternatives

Summary

Critical Thinking Challenges

Answers to Checkpoint Questions

Suggestions for Further Reading

DACUM Components

1.2   Perform within ethical boundaries
1.6   Conduct oneself in a courteous and diplomatic manner
1.8   Show initiative and responsibility
8.4   Manage accounts receivable
8.6   Maintain records for accounting and banking purposes

14

Chapter Competencies

Learning Objectives

Upon successfully completing this chapter, you will be able to:

1. Spell and define the Key Terms.
2. Explain how a physician sets fees.
3. Discuss forms of payment.
4. Explain the legal considerations in extending credit.
5. Discuss the legal implications of credit collection.
6. Describe three methods of debt collection.

Performance Objectives

Upon successfully completing this chapter, you will be able to:

1. Use an aging schedule.
2. Write a collection letter.

Key Terms

(See Glossary for definitions.)
adjustments
aging schedule
collection
credit
professional courtesy
write off

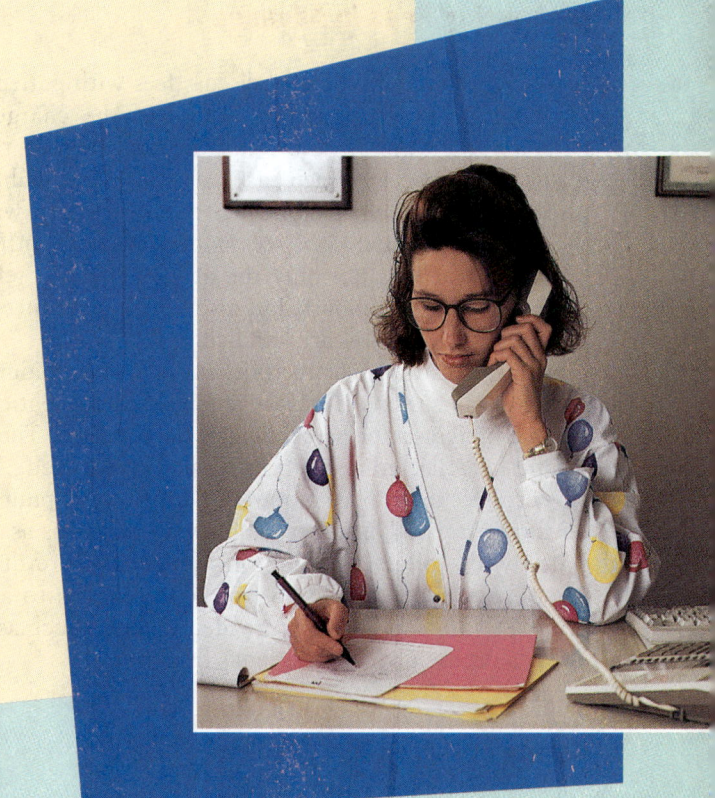

The medical office runs on the fees generated by patient visits, laboratory work, and in-office procedures. Without these fees, the medical office would be unable to pay for staff, office space, and supplies. Therefore, collecting fees—whether paid by the patient, an insurer, or a third party—is essential for the medical practice to succeed.

➤ FEES

Setting Fees

Generally, the physician sets the fees for office visits, laboratory work, and in-office procedures based on the UCR concept: (1) *U* (usual)—fair value of the service; (2) *C* (customary)—competitive rates charged by other physicians; and (3) *R* (reasonable)—that which meets the other two criteria. Fee setting also considers the Resource-Based Relative Value Scale (RBRVS), by which fees are determined based on the relative value of a particular service and adjusted for geographical differences. (See Chap. 17, Diagnostic and Procedural Coding, for more information about RBRVS and Chap. 18, Health Insurance, for more information about UCR fees.)

Discussing Fees in Advance

It is always a good policy to discuss fees with patients in advance, so that they are aware of the charges. Patients will want to know in advance whether the medical office accepts their insurance or if they will be responsible for paying the fee. A good and easy way to initiate a discussion of fees is by having an office brochure that lists not only the office's address, telephone number, and hours, but also which insurance is accepted and how fees are handled.

Many insurance companies and health maintenance organizations (HMOs) require that the patient pay a co-payment or percentage of the total fee. These should be collected at the time service is rendered. Always collect the entire amount due from a new patient on the first visit. The great majority of problems associated with **collection** (acquiring funds that are due) come from patients who go from one practice to another. Be sure you get a picture identification such as a driver's license on a new patient's first visit.

Forms of Payment

Depending on the medical office's policies, the patient can usually pay for services in one of two ways: with cash or by personal check. If a new patient is paying by check, get two forms of identification. Many larger practices accept credit card (Visa, Mastercard, Discover) payments as well. By agreeing to accept a credit card payment, the medical office also agrees to pay the credit card company a percentage of the total charge (usually 1.8%). Although this may seem costly, it is sometimes more cost effective to receive payment by credit card rather than to receive it in installments—or not at all—from the patient.

Payment by Insurance Companies

By far the largest proportions of fees are paid by insurance companies and HMOs. Therefore, it is imperative that patient insurance information be kept current. Most medical practices require that a patient submit a medical insurance card for each visit; this way, changes in insurance can quickly and easily be noted. Always make a copy of the patient's insurance card and staple in the appropriate section of the chart for billing reference.

Adjusting Fees

Sometimes, **adjustments** (changes in a posted account) must be made to a standard fee, as when the medical office accepts a set insurance rate for a service that is lower than the practice's rate. You must charge the patient the normal fee for the service; however, when the insurance carrier sends payment, the explanation of benefits (EOB) will show how much you may collect for the service. The difference between the physician's normal fee and the insurance carrier's allowed fee will be adjusted in the credit adjustment column on the patient's account.

Other fee adjustments include **professional courtesy** fees, in which other health care professionals are charged a reduced rate. The physician may even choose not to charge a fee at all; this too is considered a professional courtesy and should not be confused with writing off a fee. (A **write off** refers to the cancellation of an unpaid debt; these generally can be claimed on the practice's federal taxes.) Again, you would charge the normal fee and then adjust the designated amount in the adjustment column with "professional courtesy" in the description column.

? Checkpoint Question

1. To avoid collection problems, what should you get from a new patient on the first visit?

➤ CREDIT

Extending Credit

It is not always possible for patients to pay their entire bills at the time when such costs are incurred. Depending on the medical office's policy, **credit** may be extended to patients on an installment plan. The extension of credit to a patient is a decision that is often made solely by the physician.

Legal Considerations

When a medical practice extends credit to a patient, it may charge interest on the patient's unpaid balance. If this is the case, the medical office is legally required to disclose this information to the patient, along with any other fees or charges incurred by the patient's acceptance of credit. This legal documentation is called a "truth-in-lending statement" and must be filed in the patient's medical chart.

Different states have different laws concerning the extension of credit. Generally, credit cannot be denied based on age, gender, race, marital status, religion, national origin, or source of income (ie, if a patient receives public assistance). If your facility has given credit to one patient, you typically may not refuse the same arrangements for another patient. Some states have laws limiting the amount of interest that can be charged. The practice's accountant should be able to provide the information required for the state and municipality in which the practice is located.

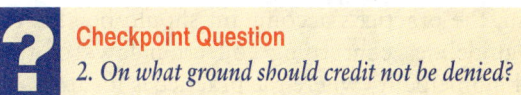

Checkpoint Question
2. On what ground should credit not be denied?

➤ COLLECTIONS

When a patient has an unpaid bill or has not paid an installment per a credit agreement, those funds must be collected. Collecting fees can be time consuming and is regulated by a variety of consumer protection laws.

Legal Considerations

When attempting to collect a bill, certain procedures should be followed. A debt collector—in this case, the administrative medical assistant or billing clerk—must exercise reasonable restraint when contacting a patient about a bill. For instance, a debt collector **may not:**

1. Contact the patient at his or her place of employment if the employer objects
2. Contact a third party about payment of a debt without court authorization
3. Contact the patient except between the hours of 8:00 AM and 9:00 PM
4. Contact the patient at all if the patient has filed bankruptcy
5. Harass or intimidate the patient, that is, use abusive language, provide false or misleading information, or pose as someone other than a debt collector

---

BOX 14-1 Collecting Debts From a Patient's Estate

When a patient dies, the family needs time to grieve and accept the death. Collecting debts from an estate requires professionalism and tact. Never contact the family regarding a debt immediately after a patient's death. Most offices have a policy stating that family members of deceased patients will not be contacted until a week after the funeral date. At the appropriate time, call the next of kin listed in the patient's chart. Offer your sympathy and ask for the name of the patient's executor, the individual responsible for handling the patient's affairs after death. The executor may be an attorney, spouse, friend, or other relative. Call the executor and introduce yourself. Obtain the executor's address and send a final billing notice. It is important that all claims for a patient's estate be made promptly. In case the estate does not have enough funds to meet all of its debts, the local probate court will decide the priority list for debt collection.

Again, the practice's accountant should be able to provide guidelines concerning collection laws of the state and municipality where the practice is located.

Attempting to collect a debt from a patient's estate requires particular diplomacy. Box 14-1 offers some guidelines to follow in such a situation.

Collecting a Debt

Monthly Billings

The easiest way to collect a debt or an installment is by monthly billing. Once a month, the medical office sends bills to its patients who have unpaid balances. Larger offices set up a billing cycle and divide the alphabet, sending statements once a week to each selected group. For example, patients with names beginning with the letters A to G might be billed on the 1st of the month, H to N on the 8th, O to S on the 15th, and T to Z on the 22nd. If your facility changes a billing cycle, you are legally required to notify patients of the change 3 months prior to the change taking effect.

The noncomputerized office will normally just copy the ledger cards of the patients who owe balances; the computerized office can easily send statements. If the account is on an installment plan, the patient receives a bill that lists the amount due for that month as well as the total amount due. This way, the patient has the option of paying more than is due for that particular month (and thereby reducing the amount of interest paid) and is aware of the current balance.

Aging Accounts

Unpaid accounts must be monitored to determine how overdue or in arrears they are. For this purpose, the medical office keeps an **aging schedule** (Fig. 14-1) that lists the patient's name, balance, any payments, and comments such as reminders or second notices sent. Such a schedule can be kept on a large sheet of paper or by a comprehensive computer billing program.

Aging of an account is calculated from the first date of billing, not by the procedure date. For example,

FIGURE 14-1
Sample aging of accounts receivable report.

Aging of Accounts Report: April 30, 2000			
Patient Name	**Account Number**	**Due Date**	**Amount**
Accounts 30 Days Past Due:			
Doe, John C.	000-00-0000	3/6/00	625.00
Graham, Paula R.	000-00-0000	3/29/00	450.00
O'Toole, William Q.	000-00-0000	3/13/00	25.00
Parker, Mary W.	000-00-0000	3/25/00	299.00
Reeves, Chris A.	000-00-0000	3/11/00	58.00
South, Cheryl C.	000-00-0000	3/8/00	385.00
Yarkony, Ralph M.	000-00-0000	3/11/00	108.00
Accounts 60 Days Past Due:			
Forest, Patricia L.	000-00-0000	2/19/00	476.00
Heany, Beverly O.	000-00-0000	2/12/00	57.00
Thomas, Walter T.	000-00-0000	2/27/00	185.00
Accounts 90 Days Past Due:			
Glick, Rhonda K.	000-00-0000	1/4/00	28.00
Payne, Robert A.	000-00-0000	1/25/00	456.00
Accounts 120 Days or More Past Due:			
Baird, Jane C.	000-00-0000	10/3/99	45.00
Wallace, Michael S.	000-00-0000	12/15/99	349.00
Total Overdue Accounts Receivable			**$3,546.00**

a patient has an office visit on January 5, and the first statement is sent on February 1. The account will not be past due until March 1.

Aging of accounts is a measure of the practice's ability to collect its fees. The vast majority (80%) of fees should be collected within 30 days. If the aging shows a high percentage (50%) of fees being collected 30 days or more after billing, the practice's billing and collection procedures may need to be reviewed.

Collecting Overdue Accounts

The three most common ways of collecting an overdue account are sending an overdue notice to the patient, telephoning the patient to let him or her know the account is overdue, and informing the patient at the next office visit.

OVERDUE NOTICES

Overdue notices (Fig. 14-2) are fairly simple to prepare. Often, they consist of a copy of the patient's monthly billing with the words "overdue" or "second notice" stamped on it in red. Alternatively, a form letter with spaces for the patient's particulars may be sent. If a computer billing program is used, the computer often can automatically generate overdue notices.

TELEPHONING THE PATIENT

If written notices bring no response, you may need to telephone the patient to inquire about an overdue account. Always ask when payment might be forthcoming and document this on the patient's account. If payment is not received as promised, contact the patient again.

IN-OFFICE REMINDERS

A patient can be reminded of an overdue balance when he or she comes to the office to see the physician. To handle this situation discreetly, simply give the patient a copy of the most recent overdue notice. Once again, ask when payment might be forthcoming and follow through.

Family Practice Associates
2345 Oak Street
Forest, OR 77777
(234) 567-8900

June 23, 1999

Mary W. Parker
300 Red Bird Lane
Lake, OR 77771

Dear Ms. Parker:

It has recently come to our attention that your account with our office is slightly overdue. Your balance of $299.00 is over 30 days past due. Please pay this amount as soon as possible. If you are having trouble paying this amount, please call our office and make arrangements to pay your balance.

If you have recently paid this amount and your payment is on the way to us in the mail, please disregard this letter. If you have any questions or concerns, feel free to contact me at the phone number above.

Sincerely,

Kathy Porter
Accounting Manager

FIGURE 14-2
Sample overdue notice.

What If?

What if a patient who has an overdue account wants to schedule an appointment?

As a medical assistant, you are not responsible for deciding whether a patient who has an outstanding balance gets to be seen by the physician. Schedule the appointment, then discuss the issue privately with the physician. Ethically, the physician may opt to care for the patient until the disorder is resolved. Legally, the physician is obligated to care for this patient until the physician-patient relationship is terminated (see Chap. 3, Medicine and the Law).

Checkpoint Question

3. What are three ways of collecting overdue accounts?

Collection Alternatives

Sometimes it is more cost effective for collections to be handled outside the medical office. Three common alternatives include collection agencies, small claims court, and credit bureaus. Collection agencies specialize in collecting debts. For either a fee or a percentage of the debt, the collection agency attempts to collect the monies due by the methods listed above. In addition, the collection agency can represent the medical practice in a small claims court suit and can have the bad debt listed with credit reporting agencies.

The medical practice can, of course, sue patients in small claims court or list patients with credit reporting bureaus itself, but it is often more time and cost effective to hire an outside agency.

SUMMARY

The success of a medical office is based on the ability of the staff to collect physician fees. This must be done in a professional manner and in accordance with state and federal laws.

Legal Tips

The Fair Debt Collection Act is a federal law that states how and when a collector can attempt to collect a debt. It is a violation of the law to threaten to send a patient to a collection agency if you do not intend to do so. Unlawful threats can result in a lawsuit for harassment against the caller.

CRITICAL THINKING CHALLENGES

1. Under what sorts of circumstances might a patient need credit?
2. A patient has an overdue account balance. What steps would you take to collect the debt? Create a collection letter for a patient account that is 60 days overdue.

ANSWERS TO CHECKPOINT QUESTIONS

1. On a new patient's first visit, collect the entire amount due and get a picture identification.
2. Credit cannot be denied based on age, gender, race, marital status, religion, national origin, or source of income.
3. Overdue accounts can be collected by sending overdue notices, telephoning patients, and informing patients at the next office visit.

SUGGESTIONS FOR FURTHER READING

Andress, A. A. (1996). *Saunders Manual of Medical Office Management*. Philadelphia: W. B. Saunders.
Becklin, K. J., & Sunnaborg, E. M. (1992). *Medical Office Procedures*. 3rd Ed. New York: Glencoe/McGraw-Hill.
Humphrey, D. D. (1990). *Contemporary Medical Office Procedures*. Cincinatti: South Western Publishing.

Bookkeeping and Banking

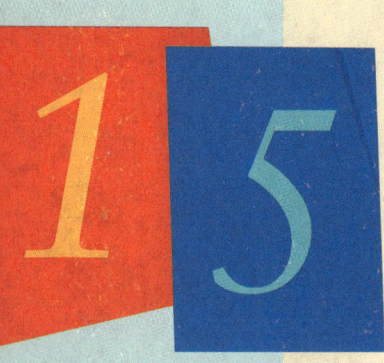

Chapter Outline

Bookkeeping Systems
   Pegboard Bookkeeping System
   Posting a Charge
   Posting a Payment
   Posting a Credit
   Posting a Credit Adjustment
   Posting a Debit Adjustment
   Posting to Cash Paid Out Section of
      Day Sheet
   Computerized Bookkeeping Systems

Banking
   Choosing a Bank
   Receiving Checks and Making
      Deposits
   Bank Statements
Petty Cash
Summary
Critical Thinking Challenges
Answers to Checkpoint Questions
Suggestions for Further Reading

DACUM Components

1.2   Perform within ethical boundaries
1.8   Show initiative and responsibility
8.1   Use manual bookkeeping systems
8.4   Manage accounts receivable
8.6   Maintain records for accounting and banking purposes

Chapter Competencies

Learning Objectives

Upon successfully completing this chapter, you will be able to:

1. Spell and define the Key Terms.
2. Explain the concept of the pegboard bookkeeping system.
3. Describe the components of the pegboard system.
4. Identify and discuss the special features of the pegboard day sheet.
5. Discuss how to balance a day sheet.
6. Compare pegboard and computer bookkeeping systems.
7. Explain how to balance a monthly bank statement.

Performance Objectives

Upon successfully completing this chapter, you will be able to:

1. Record financial transactions, such as charges, payments, credits, and adjustments to patient ledger cards.
2. Complete a bank deposit slip and make a deposit.
3. Maintain a petty cash account.

Key Terms

(See Glossary for definitions.)

accounts payable	ledger
accounts receivable	ledger card
balance	overdraft protection
credit	posting
daily journal	returned check fee
day sheet	service charge
debit	superbill
endorse	

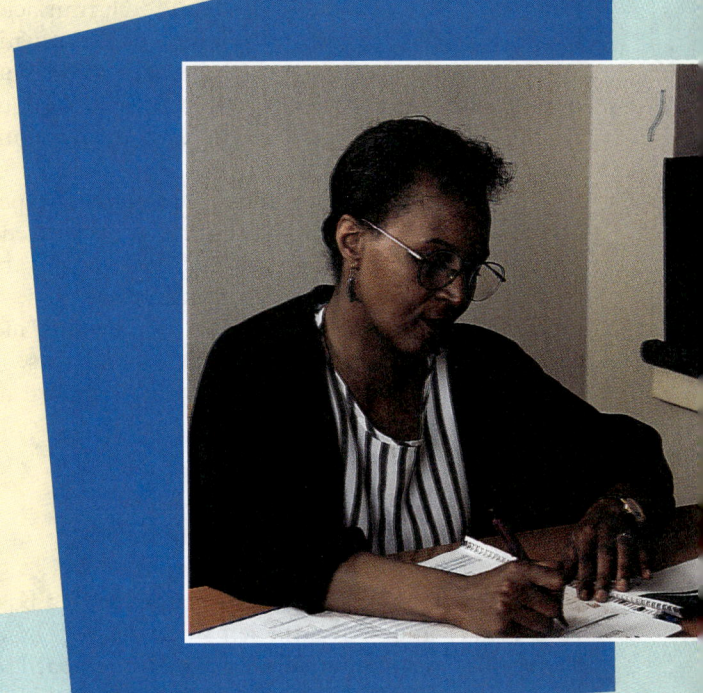

Bookkeeping and banking are important facets of medical office management. In most medical practices, bookkeeping and banking include maintaining both patient and office account records, including petty cash, **accounts receivable** (money owed to the practice), and **accounts payable** (money owed by the practice).

➤ BOOKKEEPING SYSTEMS

There are two basic types of bookkeeping systems used by most medical practices: single entry and double entry.

In a single-entry system, the bookkeeper—in this instance, the administrative medical assistant—records a financial transaction such as a payment into the bookkeeping system only once; hence the term single entry.

In a double-entry system, the bookkeeper records the transaction in two different places; thus the term double entry. The foundation of the double-entry system is the accounting equation:

$$Assets = Liabilities + Equity$$

Assets are all things of value relating to the practice. *Liabilities* are monies owed. *Equity* refers to the amount of capital the physician has invested in the practice. Because the two sides of the accounting equation must always **balance** (be equal), each transaction requires a **debit** (charge) on one side of the equation and a **credit** (payment) on the other side of the equation; the amount of the debit and credit must be equal. Double-entry systems are usually used by accounting firms and corporations.

Most medical facilities use the "cash basis" type of accounting, which means that income is considered as income only when the money is collected and payables (money owed) are considered expenses when paid.

Single-entry systems, which are used by most medical practices, are available in a variety of formats. The most popular of these formats are the pegboard and computerized single-entry systems.

Pegboard Bookkeeping System

The pegboard bookkeeping system starts with a board with pegs running down the left side. The pegs hold a **day sheet**, or **daily journal**, in place on the board. All transactions for the day will be recorded on this day sheet. Each patient has a **ledger card** (record of the patient's financial activities), which will fit into a given

pegboard. Whenever a patient transaction occurs, the bookkeeper places the ledger card over the day sheet with the **superbill** (preprinted patient bill) or encounter form charge slip over the ledger card, on the next available entry line, and makes the appropriate entry on the ledger card (Fig. 15-1).

Ledger cards have carbon paper or noncarbon (NCR) backings; thus, the entry recorded on the ledger card even when a superbill is not used is also recorded on the day sheet. As the day progresses, each patient's ledger card is placed on the next available line on the day sheet, so that the day's entries appear consecutively. At the end of the day, all of the transactions are added.

The various components required in the pegboard system and the specific steps for recording patient transactions are discussed in greater detail below.

Day Sheet

The day sheet keeps track of daily patient transactions, such as charges for services to patients, payments from patients and insurance carriers, and adjustments to patient accounts. A day sheet should be kept for each day that the physician sees patients; on busy days or for practices with more than one physician, more than one day sheet may be required.

The day sheet has several sections: a deposit slip, distribution columns, a section for payments, a section for adjustments, and a section for **posting** proofs (listing financial transactions in a ledger).

The deposit slip is a detachable portion of the day sheet. All payments received are noted on the deposit slip, and at the end of the day it is torn from the day sheet and deposited with that day's payments.

The distribution columns are used to assign charges for various services. How these columns are

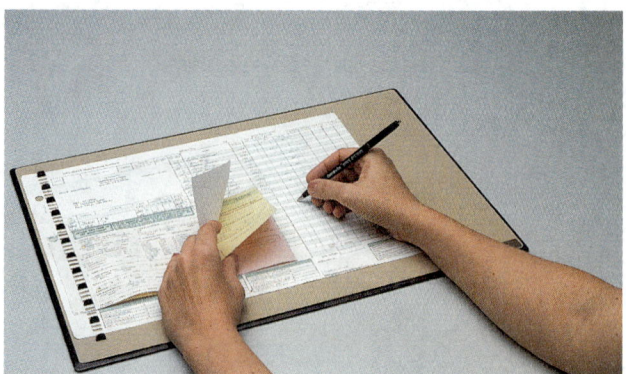

FIGURE 15-1
Sample day sheet with ledger card and superbill. (Courtesy of Control-o-fax, Waterloo, IA)

used depends on the needs of the individual practice. In a group practice, each practitioner may be assigned his or her own column. Some practices may assign columns to the various insurance plans they accept. Finally, these columns can be used to provide information on quality improvement issues (see Chap. 12, Quality Improvement and Risk Management). **The distribution columns, regardless of how they are assigned, provide the physician with important information about how the practice earns its income.**

The adjustments section allows for the adjustment in an office fee, as with professional courtesy discounts and insurance disallowances (see Chap. 14, Credit and Collections). The adjustments section also allows for crediting an account for uncollectible monies without using the payment column. It can also be used to add charges back to an account in cases where the patient's payment has been returned by the bank for insufficient funds.

The posting proofs section is where the day's totals are entered and the day sheet is balanced, much as one would balance a checkbook. Once the day sheet is complete, each column or section is totaled individually. It is best to total each column twice to make sure that no mathematical errors have been made. After all the columns have been totaled, the posting proofs section is filled out.

If the posting proofs do not balance, an error has been made on the day sheet. To locate the error, go over each transaction one by one. Add the previous balance to the fee or subtract the payment from the previous balance to check if the new balance listed is correct. If the posted charges are correct, total each column again. **Errors should not be erased or whited-out; instead, a line should be drawn through the erroneous entry and the transaction entered on a new line** (Box 15-1). When a transaction must be reentered on the day sheet, the ledger card must be pulled and used again as well.

The day sheet is important because it keeps track of ongoing accounts receivable. The accounts receivable total changes every time a charge, payment, or ad-

BOX 15-1 Basic Bookkeeping Tips

- Always use black ink; do not use pencil.
- Write legibly.
- Never erase or white-out errors.
- Always double check each entry.

What If?
What if you cannot balance the day sheet?

First, take a short break. Then return to the day sheet and double check each entry and all arithmetic. (A common error is transposing numbers, such as entering 69 instead of 96.) If you are still unable to find the error, ask a colleague to check the day sheet. After all attempts to balance the sheet have been exhausted, notify the physician.

justment is made to an account. You should add all the totals of the outstanding balances on the ledger cards at the end of every month to ensure that they equal your accounts receivable.

Completed day sheets are filed chronologically in a **ledger** (a book of accounts) with the most recent day sheet on top. **Completed day sheets are important legal documents and must be kept for at least 7 years for tax purposes.** They should be stored in a safe, dark area to avoid loss or fading.

Checkpoint Question
1. What are five sections of a pegboard day sheet?

Ledger Cards

The ledger card is a record of the patient's financial activities as they pertain to the medical practice. Most ledger cards include areas for the responsible person's name, address, telephone number, and insurance information (Fig. 15-2). Other information that may appear on the ledger card includes employment information and primary and secondary insurance information. Patient information appears on the top portion of the ledger card; the bottom portion is used to record the patient's financial activities.

Many practices use photocopies of an individual's ledger card as a bill, mailing the photocopy to the patient each month for payment. If you use a copy of the ledger card for the monthly statement, you must ensure that no information is visible outside the window envelope other than the billing name and address. Allowing other information to be visible is a breach of privacy.

The ledger card is a legal document and should be kept for the same length of time as the patient's medical record. Ledger cards are filed alphabetically in a

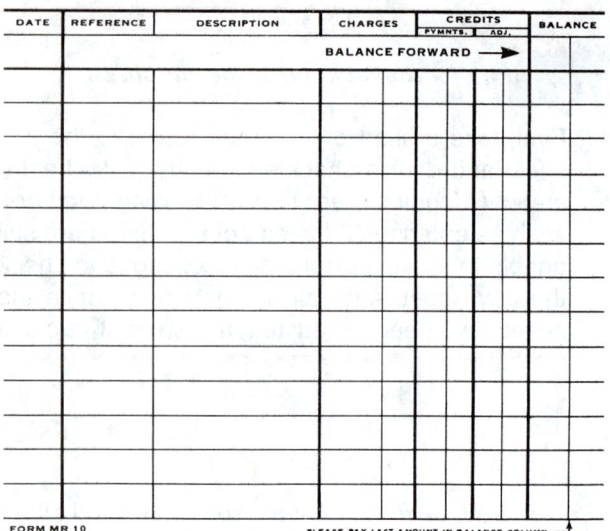

THIS IS A COPY OF YOUR ACCOUNT AS IT APPEARS ON OUR RECORDS

FIGURE 15-2
Sample ledger card.

ledger tray . A medical practice may require more than one ledger tray. Ledger cards with outstanding balances are kept separate from paid ledger cards; this makes it easier to photocopy the monthly bills or find a ledger card when a patient calls about an outstanding bill. If the office uses only one ledger tray, the ledger cards with outstanding balances are filed alphabetically in the front of the ledger tray, with the paid ledger cards filed alphabetically in the back of the tray.

Superbills

Superbills are preprinted patient statements that list codes for basic office charges and have sections for the patient's current balance and next appointment. Most superbills have three-part copies:

1. The first copy is kept by the facility for auditing purposes (all are numbered).
2. The second copy is given to the patient for insurance filing.
3. The third copy, which has a carbon line at the top to match your ledgers and day sheets, is given to the patient as a receipt of services.

Superbills are designed to be used in conjunction with ledger cards. They often have differently colored NCR copies. (Fig. 15-3).

Some offices use the encounter form in place of the superbill. An encounter form includes the same general information as the superbill and is a three-part form, but it is computer-generated.

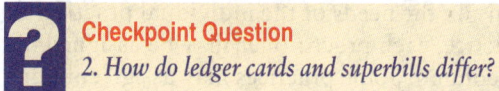

Checkpoint Question
2. How do ledger cards and superbills differ?

Posting a Charge

The charge column of the day sheet is for original charges incurred for services received by the patient from the physician or staff on a specific date. Examples include office visits, electrocardiogram, blood work, hospital visits, consultations, and fees for returned checks.

To post a charge, follow these steps:

1. Place a fresh day sheet on the pegboard and enter the date. Align the patient's ledger card on top of the sheet. If the patient was seen in the office, a superbill can also be used. Place it appropriately on top of the ledger card.
2. Record the patient's name and previous balance (last balance showing on the patient's ledger card) in the appropriate columns. If the patient does not have a previous balance, enter 0. If a superbill is also being used, place the number of the superbill in the appropriate receipt number column.
3. Record the date of posting in the date column. If the date of posting and the procedure date are different (as in posting charges incurred by this patient on a previous day), you will show the procedure date in the description column. A date must be entered for every transaction recorded.
4. Enter the appropriate procedure code in the description column. Enter the total charges for that procedure in the fee column. Add the previous balance to the new fee and record the new balance in the balance column. If the distribution columns are used, enter the fee or appropriate information in the appropriate columns.
5. Return the patient's ledger card to the ledger file.

Posting a Payment

Payments received by the practice may include insurance checks received in the mail, money orders, credit card payments, or cash received from patients.

To post a payment, follow these steps:

1. Align the patient's ledger card on the day sheet. If the patient is paying for services received by the physician today, a superbill should also be in place that shows today's total charges.
2. Enter the patient's name and previous balance in the appropriate columns. If using a superbill, make sure you place the superbill number in the receipt

Patient Name: _____

Patient ID #: _____ DOB: _____ Sex: _____

PCP: _____

SSN: _____ Financial Class: _____

Phone: _____ (home) _____ (work)

Medical Record #: _____ Date of Service: _____

Benefit Pkg: _____ Copay $ _____

Encounter #: _____

Service Provider: _____

Appt. Status: ☐ Scheduled   ☐ Same Day   ☐ Walk-in

Check-in Time: _____   Check-out Time: _____
Escorted to Exam Room: _____   Time Patient Seen: _____
Appointment Time: _____

Is Patient Being Seen in Relation to:
☐ Motor Vehicle Accident   ☐ Workman's Compensation

Appointment Failure Reason:
☐ Patient Cancel   ☐ No Show   ☐ Walk Out   ☐ PHA Cancel

TYPE OF VISIT

✓	CODE	DESCRIPTION	FEE	✓	CODE	DESCRIPTION	FEE	✓	CODE	DESCRIPTION	FEE	✓	CODE	DESCRIPTION	FEE
		OFFICE VISITS-EST.				**OFFICE VISITS-NEW CONT.**				**PREVENTATIVE, NEW**				**COUNSELING**	
	99211	Minimal			99204	Compreh.			99385	E&M 18-39			99401	15 Min.	
	99212	Focused			99205	Comp. & Complex			99386	E&M 40-64			99402	30 Min.	
	99213	Expanded				**NURSE VISIT**			99387	E&M 65 & over			99403	45 Min.	
	99214	Detailed			99211	Minimal				**CONSULTATION**			99404	60 Min.	
	99215	Compreh.				**PREVENTATIVE, EST.**			99241	Focused					
		OFFICE VISITS-NEW			99395	E&M 18-39			99242	Pre-Op Consult					
	99201	Focused			99396	E&M 40-64			99244	2nd Opinion					
	99202	Expanded			99397	E&M 65 & over									
	99203	Detailed													

PROCEDURES

✓	CODE	DESCRIPTION	FEE	✓	CODE	DESCRIPTION	FEE	✓	CODE	DESCRIPTION	FEE	✓	CODE	DESCRIPTION	FEE
	88170	Aspiration - Cyst			11200	Skin Tag Removal				**IMMUNIZATIONS/INJECTIONS**				**IMMUNIZATIONS/INJECTIONS CONT.**	
	20600	Aspiration - Joint (Small)			20550	Trigger point/Tendon Inj.			G0009	Administration Fee - Pneumovax			J2203	Triamcinolone Inj.	
	20605	Aspiration - Joint (Interm.)							G0010	Administration Fee - Hepatitis B			J3420	Vitamin B$_{12}$	
	20610	Aspiration - Joint (Large)				**SPECIALTY SERVICES**			95115	Allergy Injection Single				**IN-HOUSE LABORATORY**	
	16020	Burn Dressing			99070	Ace Bandage			95117	Allergy Injection Multiple			89050	Cell Count, except blood	
	69210	Ear Irrigation			E0110	Crutches			90788	Antibiotic IM			89060	Crystalanalysis	
	10120	Foreign Body Removal, Skin			29130	Finger Splint			J2910	Aurothioglucose			82948	Glucose	
	10060	I&D Abscess, simple			29125	Wrist Splint			G0008	Flu Vaccine			85013	HCT	
	90780	IV Infusion Therapy			99080	Form Completion			J1600	Gold Injection			85018	Hemoglobin Screen	
	12001	Laceration Repair, Simple				**TESTING/SCREENING**			90731	Hepatitis B			81025	Pregnancy	
	13160	Laceration Repair, Extens.			95004	Allergy - Skin Test			90741	Immune Globulin			81002	Urinalysis, Dipstick	
	64450	Medial Nerve Infiltration			92557	Audiometry			90724	Influenza			81000	Urinalysis, Full	
	17110	Molluscum/Wart Rmvl			93000	EKG			J9217	Lupron 3.75 mg			G0001	Venipuncture	
	94640	Nebulizer			92506	Hearing Screen			J9217	Lupron 7.5 mg				**OTHER PROCEDURES**	
	82270	Stool for Blood (Hemocult)			86580	PPD			J9250	Methotrexate 2-5 mg					
	12001	Suturing, Superficial			94010	Pulmonary Function			90732	Pneumovax					
	13100	Suturing, Complex			94760	Pulse Oximetry, Single			90718	Td					
	11050	Skin Les./Wart Cautery			45330	Sigmoidoscopy, Flexible			90782	Therapeutic SQ or IM					

P = PRIMARY   S = SECONDARY   S1-S9 = NUMBERED SECONDARY

DIAGNOSIS

✓	CODE	DESCRIPTION	✓	CODE	DESCRIPTION	✓	CODE	DESCRIPTION
	789.0	Abdominal Pain		780.6	Fever		462	Pharyngitis (sore throat)
	879.8	Abrasion/Laceration		704.8	Folliculitis		486	Pneumonia
	995.3	Allergic Reaction		535.5	Gastritis		V70.3	Pre-Marital Testing
	477.9	Allergic Rhinitis		558.9	Gastroenteritis		V72.81	Pre-op Cardiac Exam
	285.9	Anemia		274.9	Gout		V72.83	Pre-op Exam, Other
	413.9	Angina		V72.3	Gyn Exam		601.0	Prostatitis
	300.00	Anxiety		784.0	Headache		600	Prostatism
	716.90	Arthritis		389.9	Hearing Loss		782.1	Rash
	427.9	Arrhythmia		536.8	Heartburn/Indigestion		569.3	Rectal Bleeding
	493.90	Asthma		573.3	Hepatitis		530.81	Reflux
	611.72	Breast Lump		455.6	Hemorrhoids		V81.2	Screening for Cardiac Condition
	490	Bronchitis		553.9	Hernia		780.3	Seizure Disorder
	727.3	Bursitis		401.9	Hypertension (NOS)		473.9	Sinusitis
	354.0	Carpal Tunnel Syndrome		272.4	Hyperlipidemia		848.9	Strain/Sprain
	682.9	Cellulitis		242.00	Hyperthyroidism		438	Stroke
	786.50	Chest Pain		251.2	Hypoglycemia		305.90	Substance Abuse
	575.1	Cholecystitis		380.4	Impacted Cerumen		099.9	STD
	372.3	Conjunctivitis		780.52	Insomnia		727.00	Tenosynovitis, Tendonitis
	496	COPD		564.1	Irritable Bowel Syndrome		451.9	Thrombophlebitis
	414.9	Coronary Artery Disease		719.40	Joint Pain		246.9	Thyroid Disease
	290.9	Dementia		592.0	Kidney Stones		435.9	TIA
	311	Depression		464.0	Laryngitis		463	Tonsillitis
	692.9	Dermatitis		724.2	Low Back Pain		011.90	Tuberculosis
	250.01	Diabetes, IDDM		710.0	Lupus		465.9	Upper Respiratory Infection
	250.00	Diabetes, NIDDM		V70.0	Medical Exam/Physical		599.0	Urinary Tract Infection
	558.9	Diarrhea		346.9	Migraine		V04.8	Vaccination, Flu
	562.10	Diverticular Disease		278.0	Obesity		V03.9	Vaccination, Pneumovax
	780.4	Dizziness		382.9	Otitis Media		616.10	Vaginitis
	995.2	Drug Reaction		614.9	Pelvic Inflammatory Disease		424.9	Valvular Heart Disease
	782.3	Edema		533.9	Peptic Ulcer Disease		079.9	Viral Syndrome
	780.7	Fatigue/Tiredness/Malaise		443.9	Perpheral Vascular Disease			

Comments:

PREVIOUS BALANCE $

TODAY'S CHARGES $

PAYMENT $

BALANCE $

RETURN APPOINTMENT:
_____ Days _____ Weeks _____ Months
APPT. LENGTH: _____ PROVIDER: _____

APPT. REASON:

PROVIDER SIGNATURE:

Adult

Philadelphia
Health Associates
Tax ID #23-2350500
PHA Group # PH75923

☐ 3550 Market Street
Philadelphia, PA 19104
(215) 823-8660

☐ The Bourse Building
111 S. Independence Mall
East • 7th Floor
Philadelphia, PA 19106
(215) 625-9100

OTHER DIAGNOSIS

✓	CODE	DESCRIPTION	✓	CODE	DESCRIPTION

PHA-019 (6/95)

FIGURE 15-3
Sample superbill.

number column. Enter the posting date in the date column.

3. Enter the type of payment being made in the description column, whether personal check (pers. ck.), money order (mo), MasterCard (MC), or insurance check (ins. ck.). Enter the amount of payment in the payment column and also on the deposit section of the day sheet in the cash or checks column.

4. Subtract the payment amount from the previous balance and record the new balance in the new balance column. If only a payment is being posted, no entry is made in the fee area. If an entry has been made in the fee area, you will start with the previous balance, add the charges, and then subtract the payment and put the new balance in the balance column.

Posting a Credit

There are times when an account is overpaid either by the patient or the insurance company. Such an overpayment is termed a credit (money owed to the patient or insurance carrier by the facility). This will show on the patient's ledger card as the last balance with brackets [ ] indicating a credit, for example, [25.00]. Brackets are used to show the opposite of the column's normal meaning. In this case, the balance column is normally a debit to the patient, meaning that the patient owes the doctor money. Brackets around an amount indicate that the doctor owes the patient money.

Checkpoint Question

3. What do brackets around an amount listed in a column indicate?

Credits are handled in one of two ways: (1) the credit is left on the account and subtracted from the charges on the patient's next visit, or (2) the patient is mailed a refund for the amount of the overpayment. The way in which an overpayment is handled depends on office policy and the amount of the overpayment. Generally, overpayments under $5.00 are left on account as a credit, whereas overpayments over $5.00 are refunded.

To post a credit, follow these steps:

1. Align the patient's ledger card on the day sheet. Enter the patient's name, previous balance, and the date in the appropriate columns.

2. Enter the bank identification number in the appropriate area of the deposit slip and amount of the payment in the payment section and on the deposit slip. Starting with the previous balance, subtract the payment from the previous balance. The result will be a negative number, that is, a number preceded by a minus (-) sign.

3. Enter the negative amount in the new balance column in brackets, for example, [4.00].

Posting a Credit Adjustment

The adjustments section is used for adjusting office fees and for crediting an account for uncollectible monies. Below are three specific situations that would require a credit adjustment.

Example 1. The physician wishes to give a registered nurse a 25% professional discount on charges incurred today for an office visit. Legally, the physician must charge everyone the same fee for the same procedure. Therefore, you would enter the normal fee in the charge column, show in the description column an office visit with a professional discount of 25%, and put the 25% in the adjustment column. Assume that an office visit was $40.00. You would put $40.00 in the charge column and $10.00 (25% of $40.00) in the adjustment column. The patient would owe your facility $30.00 for this visit.

Example 2. Most medical offices belong to insurance groups, which means that the physician has signed an agreement with the insurance carrier to accept the fee for services set by that carrier instead of the physician's normal fee. Again, you must charge the same fee for the same procedure. However, when payment is received, the explanation of benefits from that carrier will show the agreed-on amount for that procedure. You will post the payment in the normal way, but you must write off the difference between what the physician actually charged the patient for this procedure and the agree-on amount. Assume that the doctor charged $40.00 for an office visit and the insurance carrier's agreed-on amount was $35.00. You would post the payment in the payment column and $5.00 in the adjustment column to arrive at the agreed-on amount.

Example 3. Most facilities request that you write off the balance of an account when you turn it over to a collection agency to keep better control on the accounts receivable. Therefore, if the patient's balance is $1200.00, you would show "Collection Agency" in the description column of the ledger and put the $1200.00 in the adjustment column, which would bring the balance to 0.

To post a credit adjustment, follow these steps:

1. Align the patient's ledger card on the day sheet.
2. Record the patient's name, previous balance, and the date in the appropriate columns.

3. Record the amount of the adjustment in the adjustment column of the ledger card. Enter a description of the adjustment in the professional service column, that is, insurance adjustment or correction adjustment.
4. Subtract the amount of the adjustment from the previous balance and record the new balance in the balance column.

Note: Payments and adjustments can be posted at the same time. The payment is recorded in the payment column and the adjustment is entered in the adjustment column. Both are subtracted from the previous balance and the new balance is recorded in the new balance column.

Posting a Debit Adjustment

Generally, a credit adjustment reduces the patient's account balance, whereas a debit adjustment increases or adds to the patient's account balance. Below are three specific situations that would require a debit adjustment.

Checkpoint Question

4. How does a credit adjustment differ from a debit adjustment?

Example 1. You receive an nonsufficient funds (NSF) check back from the bank today from a payment made earlier by a patient and posted as such to his account. The previous payment is no longer valid. Therefore, you must eliminate that payment because the patient now owes it again. Because this is not an original charge, you may not use the charge column for this entry. To post this debit adjustment to the patient's account, you will show NSF in the description column and the amount of the NSF check in the adjustment column with brackets.

Example 2. Assume that you have turned over an account to a collection agency and the patient comes in later to pay the amount owed. You must first put the money back on the account or you will create a credit balance. Place the ledger card on the day sheet and in the description column write "Reverse Collection." Again, this is not an original or new charge, so you may not use the charge column. Show the amount in the adjustment column in brackets because you are "adding" the amount back to the patient's balance. You may now show the payment in the payment column.

Example 3. Your office requires that you refund all money over $5.00 to the patient or insurance car-

rier. You must also post this to eliminate the credit balance on the account. Place the ledger card on the day sheet and in the description column show "Refund to Patient" (or insurance carrier). To eliminate a credit balance, you must debit the account. You will put the amount of the refund in the adjustment column in brackets indicating it is a debit, not a credit adjustment.

To post a debit adjustment, follow these steps:

1. Align the patient's ledger card on the day sheet.
2. Record the patient's name, previous balance, and the date in the appropriate columns.
3. Record the amount of the debit adjustment in the adjustment column of the ledger card. Because this is the opposite of what that column normally means, you will post a debit adjustment on the ledger card with brackets [ ] around the amount.
4. Starting with the previous balance, you will add a debit adjustment to this and record the total in the balance column.

Posting to Cash Paid Out Section of Day Sheet

Sometimes, the physician may need to take out cash from the day's receipts. When this happens, your bank deposit for that day will be short by the amount taken out. The best way to account for this is to have the physician sign in the cash paid out section of the day sheet for the amount. This documents the transaction and prevents anybody else from being able to do this.

Some insurance carriers keep money overpaid to your facility out of money they are paying your facility for other patients. Because you will be posting the correct amounts in the payment column for each patient,

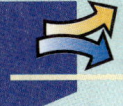

Ethical Tips

Overpayment of an account is more common than you might realize, especially when multiple insurance companies are billed along with the patient. If your office receives an overpayment by an insurance company, notify the company and send the overpayment back. Be sure to discuss this with the physician first. Ethically (and legally), it is wrong to keep overpayments.

your check amount from the insurance carrier will be "short" the refund or kept out money. You will show this in the cash paid out section of the day sheet with an explanation of "insurance refund on account of (patient's name)." It is also a good idea to make a copy of the explanation of benefits and staple it to the back of your day sheet for future reference.

Computerized Bookkeeping Systems

Computer programs are available that fulfill many of the same functions as a pegboard system, but do so much faster. Instead of recording entries on a day sheet, entries are keyed into a computer program. The administrative medical assistant can then print out invoices and receipts for patients and insurance companies. Depending on the individual computer program, you can easily generate daily, monthly, and yearly reports or reports for the transactions for an individual physician in a group practice.

Computer bookkeeping programs have a variety of advantages over pegboard bookkeeping. Computer programs frequently work as expanded calculators and will perform the mathematical functions, such as balancing individual accounts and the day's totals. Many bookkeeping programs also have check writing capabilities. Programs are available that permit electronic banking to occur between the office and computer and the bank's computer system. Furthermore, an individual computer can run programs for bookkeeping, for making appointments, and for generating other office reports, such as forms for insurance reimbursement.

Until recently, cost was considered a disadvantage to a computer system, but personal computers have become so inexpensive and efficient that, in the long run, the savings in time and money is substantial. Most bookkeeping programs on the market today are easy to use and require a minimum of computer skills. It is essential that data stored on computer be downloaded to magnetic tape or floppy disk, so that backup copies of the data are available in case the computer "crashes."

➤ BANKING

Choosing a Bank

Existing medical practices already have established checking accounts, but opening or changing a business checking account is a simple procedure. This should by done by the owner of the practice. When opening a new business checking account, choose a bank that is either close to the office or otherwise easily accessible because you will be making daily deposits.

Banks require signature cards for each person authorized to sign checks. In most cases, this is limited to the physician(s). At the time that a new checking account is opened, the actual checks must be ordered with a check order form. The administrative medical assistant must continually maintain the checkbook and ensure that checks are available by reordering checks as needed.

Besides physical location, several other factors should be considered when choosing a bank for the office business account. These factors include the monthly service fees, **overdraft protection** programs (protection against bouncing checks), interest-bearing accounts, and returned check fees.

Banks have different policies concerning monthly service charges. A **service charge** is a fee charged monthly for using an account. The charge can be a fixed amount or may be an individual charge for each check written on the account. Some banks do not levy a service charge if a specific minimum balance is maintained for the account; other banks offer interest on checking accounts that maintain a specific minimum balance.

Overdraft protection guarantees that checks written against the account will be paid even when there is not enough money in the account at the time. Usually, the bank pays the checks and retrieves the money owed to it when the account balance is restored. Many banks offer overdraft protection only up to a certain dollar amount.

Some banks charge a **returned check fee**, which is a fee charged for any check that is deposited into the checking account but that is later returned to the bank because the account it was issued from had insufficient funds with which to pay the check. Such a check is often referred to as a "bounced" check. Most facilities charge this amount back to the patient. Because this is an original charge, this bad check fee would be listed in the charge column of the patient ledger and day sheet with the amount of the check being recorded as a debit adjustment.

Checkpoint Question

5. What are several factors to consider when choosing a bank for a business account?

Receiving Checks and Making Deposits

When checks are received in the office, the first thing that should be done is to **endorse** them. To endorse a check requires writing (or rubber stamping) the name

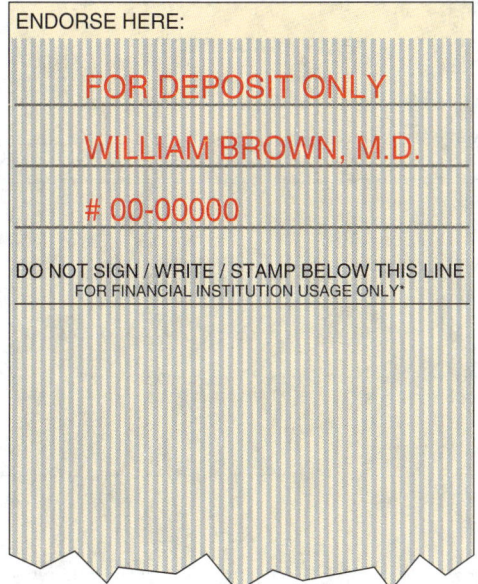

FIGURE 15-4
An endorsed check.

and account number of the account into which it will be deposited on the back of the check (Fig. 15-4). This way, if the payments are lost or stolen, no one will be able to cash them. It also ensures that the bank will deposit the payments to the correct account. An endorsement stamp can be purchased from your bank.

After the payments have been posted, total all the checks for the day and all the cash received for the day. This total should match the totals of the payments column on your day sheet. Detach the deposit sheet from the day sheet and stamp the back with the endorsement check. If a computer program is used, print out a deposit slip. Wrap the deposit slip around the checks and complete a bank deposit slip for the account the deposit will be placed in. The deposit can be hand delivered or mailed to the bank.

If the deposit is hand delivered, it may be taken to a teller, who will issue a deposit receipt, or it may be dropped in a depository. If the deposit is mailed, make sure that sufficient postage has been affixed to the envelope. Never include cash payments in a deposit that is mailed or placed in a depository. Cash deposits

---

1. Subtract any fees or charges that appear on this statement from your checkbook balance.
2. Add any interest paid on your checking account to your checkbook balance.
3. List the checks you have written that have not been paid (these checks did not yet appear on your bank statement). You can also include in this list any withdrawals you have made since the ending date of the banking statement that do not appear on the statement:

Check Number	Amount
_____	_____
_____	_____
_____	_____
Total	_____

4. If you have entered deposits or other additions to your checkbook that do not appear on the statement, list them here:

Date	Amount
_____	_____
_____	_____
Total	_____

5. Enter the ending balance from your statement here: _____
   Add the total deposits from Step 4: + _____
   Subtract the total from Step 3: − _____
   Total (this should equal your checkbook balance): _____

If these balances do not equal your checkbook balance:
- Check the addition and subtraction in your checkbook
- Check the amount of each transaction in your checkbook with the amount shown on your statement
- Check to see that all transactions from your previous statement have been accounted for
- Call your bank manager for assistance

FIGURE 15-5
Bank statement reconciling worksheet.

should always be hand delivered and a teller's receipt should always be obtained.

Bank Statements

All banks mail monthly statements to account holders listing all transactions that have occurred since the last closing date. It is important that the bank statement is reconciled each month.

The statement consists of one or more pages that numerically lists all checks written and their amounts, all deposits made and their amounts, any electronic transactions, and any service charges. Verify that all checks and deposits are listed correctly. Make a check mark on the checkbook stub of each check that has been paid by the bank. On the back of the statement is a worksheet that explains how to balance the account (Fig. 15-5). By following the steps listed on the worksheet, balancing the account is a fairly easy procedure.

➤ PETTY CASH

A petty cash account is a cash fund kept in the office specifically for small purchases, such as buying postage stamps or office supplies. It is an impress account, which means that the value of the account always remains the same. A petty cash fund is always a designated sum of money. When money is taken from the fund, a voucher (Fig. 15-6) or receipt is placed in the fund to verify the purchase. The remaining cash and the sum of the vouchers should always equal the designated sum; for example, a petty cash fund of $40.00 with $13.00 in actual cash should have receipts that amount to $27.00.

Petty cash funds should be kept separate from patient cash payments. All cash should be kept in a secure, locked area. One person should be designated to maintain the petty cash fund and issue vouchers. A voucher with an attached receipt should always be placed back into the petty cash fund both to provide proof of the purchase and to keep the account balanced. The petty cash fund normally is replenished once a month. To replenish the fund, a check is cashed for the exact amount as the vouchers. The money is placed in the fund and the vouchers are removed for filing.

Some offices keep a petty cash expense record. This record is similar to a checkbook that keeps track of the account balance as checks are written, such as personal checkbook. This expense record also categorizes the purchases so that they can be included with the monthly office expenses. Purchases such as stamps and office and medical supplies can be deducted as office expenses and added to the accounts payable expense record.

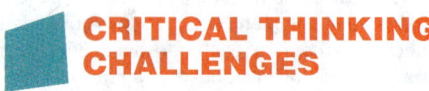

PETTY CASH RECEIPT

.... 19 ....

To Office Manager:
   Please furnish for..

Supplies:

Postage:

Travel Expenses:

Other:

Approved

TOTAL

Received Above Amount

FIGURE 15-6
A petty cash voucher.

Checkpoint Question
6. *What is an impress account?*

SUMMARY

Whether a medical practice uses a manual bookkeeping system, such as the pegboard system, or a computerized system, you will be responsible for keeping records of accounts payable, accounts receivable, and petty cash. You also will be responsible for banking functions, such as receiving checks, making deposits, and reconciling monthly bank statements. To carry out these responsibilities effectively, you must record all transactions accurately and promptly.

CRITICAL THINKING CHALLENGES

1. Your day sheet deposit slip and your posting proofs do not agree. How would you find the error?
2. Last year a patient moved to another state and changed physicians. How long should you keep his ledger card?

3. Your office is considering going from a pegboard system to a computerized bookkeeping system. What features would you look for when considering computer bookkeeping programs?

ANSWERS TO CHECKPOINT QUESTIONS

1. Five sections of a pegboard day sheet include the distribution columns, the adjustment column, the deposit slip, the payments section, and the posting proofs section.

2. A superbill is a receipt that may double as an appointment card; it still requires the use of a ledger card.

3. Brackets indicate the opposite of the normal meaning of that column.

4. Generally, a credit adjustment reduces the patient's account balance, whereas a debit adjustment increases the patient's account balance.

5. Factors to consider when choosing a bank are location, service fees, overdraft protection, interest-bearing accounts, and returned check fees.

6. An impress account means that the value of the account always remains the same.

SUGGESTIONS FOR FURTHER READING

Andress, A. A. (1996). *Saunders Manual of Medical Office Management*. Philidelphia: W. B. Saunders.

Becklin, K. T., & Sunnaborg, E. M. (1992). *Medical Office Procedures*. 3rd ed. New York: Glencoe/Mcgraw-Hill.

Accounts Payable and Payroll

Chapter Outline

Accounting Cycle
Record-Keeping Components
Accounts Payable
    Ordering Goods or Services
    Receiving Supplies
    Paying Invoices
Payroll
    Types of Payroll Systems

Employee Records
    Tax Withholdings
Preparation of Reports
Assisting With Audits
Summary
Critical Thinking Challenges
Answers to Checkpoint Questions

1 6

DACUM Components

8.5   Manage accounts payable
8.6   Maintain records for accounting and banking purposes
8.7   Process employee payroll

Chapter Competencies

Learning Objectives

Upon successfully completing this chapter, you will be able to:

1. Spell and define the Key Terms.
2. Describe the accounting cycle.
3. Describe the components of a record-keeping system.
4. Explain the process of ordering supplies and paying invoices.
5. Discuss the types of payroll records.
6. Explain which taxes are withheld from paychecks.

Performance Objectives

Upon successfully completing this chapter, you will be able to:

1. Issue a payroll check using the pegboard system.
2. Calculate the amount of an employee's payroll check for a given pay period.

Key Terms

(See Glossary for definitions.)

audit
check register
check stub
gross income
Internal Revenue Service (IRS)
net pay
packing slip
payroll
payroll journal
purchase order
tax withholding
federal unemployment tax

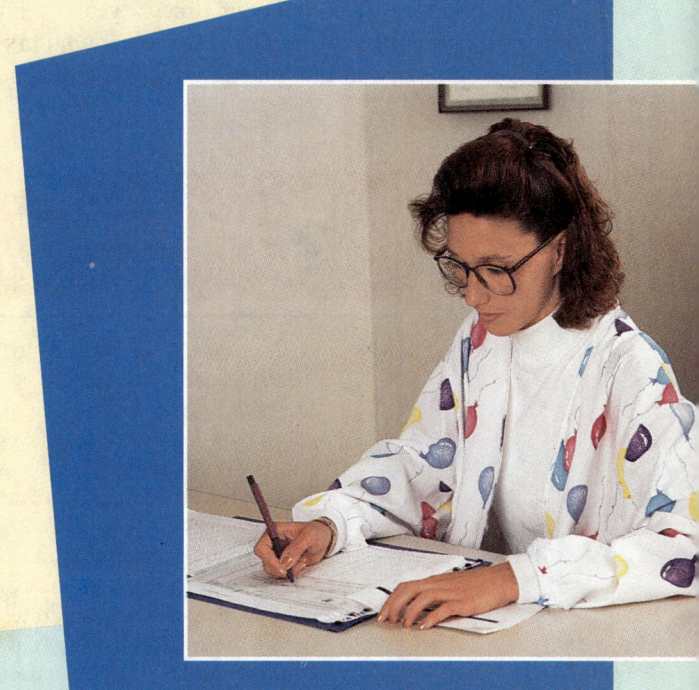

Accounting is the compilation of a business's financial records. It provides an assessment of the practice's financial history, which in turn serves as the basis for sound future financial management. The medical office, like other businesses, requires strict adherence to sound record-keeping practices. Records must be maintained in an orderly fashion to facilitate the examination of office financial records at any time and to present an organized picture of the business's finances. A system of checks and balances is an integral part of record management. Generally, the check-and-balance status of accounts is examined monthly by the administrative medical assistant; the practice's accountant also will closely scrutinize these records at scheduled intervals for tax reporting purposes.

ACCOUNTING CYCLE

Medical practices operate in one of two 12-month intervals or durations. The office accounting records will follow either the fiscal year (a consecutive 12-month period starting with a specified month) or a calendar year (January through December). The yearly interval used depends on the way the practice's accountant has structured the business of the practice. (For example, the medical practice can exist as a sole proprietorship or as a professional corporation.)

The **Internal Revenue Service (IRS)** examines a business's income statements for the amount of profit and the resulting owed tax four times a year by quarterly estimated tax returns. The practice's annual tax return is a summary of the quarterly returns and reports the final, year-end profit or loss (income minus expenses equals profit or loss) for the fiscal or calendar reporting period. If financial records are scrupulously maintained all year, the preparation of the annual income tax return for the practice should merely be a summation of existing accounting facts. Well maintained office records not only facilitate IRS returns, but also provide data that define the practice's business picture.

There are many reasons why a physician along with an accountant may need to review financial data on a regular basis. Financial records reflect growing expenditures and growth in the business. Conclusions can be drawn from financial data that will affect future financial decisions. Tax records need to be available in case of IRS inquiries or **audits** (reviews of accounts). Records such as receipts should be retained for 7 years, but records such as banking statements, canceled checks, and IRS tax returns should be kept for the duration of the business.

RECORD-KEEPING COMPONENTS

The practice's financial records should include a running record of the practice's income, total expenditures including **payroll** (employee salaries), cash on hand, and liabilities that are due. Expenditures can be broken down into categories (Box 16-1). This is important because it enables the record keeper to track the practice's expenses and provide the physician and accountant with a cohesive picture of the practice's expenses at tax time.

Categories can be accommodated by several types of bookkeeping systems; a simple business checkbook does

---

BOX 16-1 Categories of Expenditures

- *Office supplies*—items used by the facility's employees (paper, pencils, day sheets, ledger cards, etc)
- *Medical supplies*—items used for patients (examination gowns, electrocardiograph paper, syringes, tongue depressors, etc)
- *Drugs*—drug purchases, such as injectables; some facilities keep a separate column for these purchases and others put this amount in the medical supplies category
- *Payroll*—gross amount paid to employees
- *Taxes*—taxes paid, such as FICA, Medicare, federal withholding, state withholding, etc; list these separately
- *Rent*—the amount paid to rent the facility
- *Utilities*—utilities (gas, electric, telephone) paid by the facility
- *Maintenance*—routine care of the facility such as cleaning personnel
- *Travel*—physician's car lease payment, gas mileage if paid to employees, etc
- *Personal*—any money used personally by the physician

not allow this. Pegboard systems are available that allow the bookkeeper to write the check once over the **check register** (a place to record checks) or the ledger sheet and then have multiple pages with columns to distribute an expense into categories, including a back sheet for payroll. These columns are totaled and balanced at the completion of each check register sheet and can be subtotaled monthly, quarterly, and annually. (See "Pegboard Payment," p. 220, for more detailed information.) By keeping a monthly accounts payable disbursement sheet, the administrative medical assistant can compare past years' monthly expenses for the same time period more easily.

Computer software packages offer the most sophisticated way to maintain financial records, not just for the categorization of expenses, but also for the rapid formation of financial reports. Automating accounts payable does, however, require a personal computer (PC) and software and the training to use it.

There are advantages and disadvantages to both automating and maintaining paper records. Each practice should make this decision based on its particular volume and needs. Either system (pegboard or computer) can provide the practice and its accountant with the ability to pay and track expenses and to furnish the financial data necessary to create reports.

Multiple summation reports—such as the payroll report, itemized category report, account balances, and the profit-loss statement—need to be prepared for the practice's accountant. If financial data are entered diligently into the bookkeeping system, monthly, quarterly, or yearly, preparing reports should not be a daunting task. Income tax accounting cycles are divided into quarters: January through March, April through June, July through September, and October through December. Payroll reports are necessary based on the amount of taxes being withheld and made monthly, quarterly, or annually. Normally the practice's accountant will send you necessary reports and have you mail the checks.

➤ ACCOUNTS PAYABLE

Ordering Goods or Services

There are many ways to purchase office supplies or equipment economically. For instance, purchasing cooperatives (co-ops) offer bulk-rate discounts by allowing physicians to order in a pool with other purchasers. Vendors may offer discounts for buying in volume or for paying promptly. Large, warehouse-type merchandisers and companies with discount catalogs also offer competitive prices. Researching and cost comparing office products and medical supplies can be time consuming, but it is worth the effort, especially for items used frequently. Merchandise prices should be compared by comparing past invoices with prices in new catalogs.

Besides cost, other considerations come to bear when purchasing office supplies. For example, office supply companies often provide free delivery, but office warehouse chains may charge a fee or require a minimum order to receive free delivery. Quality also plays a role. Supplies should be standard quality as well as economical. It is common to use several different office supply vendors based on quality or pricing of goods.

Office supplies or equipment can be ordered in a number of ways. Once an account is set up, offices can place orders by telephone, fax, mail, or e-mail. These orders can be paid monthly by check or by credit card. It is preferable to pay for supplies by check or credit card rather than by cash, but when cash purchases are necessary, retain a detailed receipt for tax purposes. Credit card purchases can be made over the telephone or through mail order, but for security reasons, credit card account numbers should not be faxed.

When placing orders for supplies, give the office's account number to the vendor or write it on the order form. It is a good idea to use a **purchase order** that lists the supplies ordered and their order numbers, so that order numbers for frequently ordered items can be pulled from the previous purchase order; this saves time with subsequent orders. Be sure to record the charges for your order and verify them against the bill later. It is also handy to keep a list of all vendors, telephone numbers, and account numbers.

Checkpoint Question
1. When purchasing office supplies, what other factors besides costs should you consider?

Receiving Supplies

When goods are delivered to the office, a receipt or **packing slip** listing the enclosed items should always accompany the order. The office staff member who receives the supplies must check the packing slip against the actual contents to ensure that all supplies are accounted for. The person should initial the packing slip, which shows the administrative medical assistant that all goods were received. When it is time to issue checks for payables, the assistant can then pay the invoice. These receipts or packing slips should be placed in a "bills pending" file, so that they may be compared to the bill when it arrives. If the bill has already been paid by check or credit card, then the invoice should be placed in the appropriate paid accounts payable file; there should be such a file for each fiscal or calendar year.

Paying Invoices

Invoices for supplies and other types of bills payable by the practice should be kept together in a bills pending file to avoid loss or misplacement of a bill. Bills can be paid on a daily, weekly, biweekly, or monthly basis.

Manual Payment

The manual payment of bills requires a checkbook and checks. The practice's accountant may recommend the purchase of a log or record book into which is entered information about each check, such as payroll taxes or the breakdown of expenses for a monthly credit card bill. The large checks and checkbooks available from banks and business printers offer more space for writing memos or itemizing of a check. Each check, once written, is detached from a **check stub**, which remains in the checkbook. If you make a mistake while writing a check, void the check and stub and staple the voided check to the stub. Never make corrections on the facility's checks. Checkbook stubs should be filed with other fiscal or calendar year records and kept for the life of the practice.

The information recorded on the checkbook stub includes the check number, the date the check was issued, the payee (the party to whom the check was written), and the full amount of the check. Notes should be written on both the memo section of the check and on the check stub; for example, "payee: Office Communications Co." or "new beeper for Dr. Smith." The check is then attached to the bill or invoice and signed by an authorized individual.

Memos or notations on check stubs can be referenced later in the event that a question arises concerning payment by a particular check. A log or record book enables the bookkeeper to make entries for each expense, categorize expenses, and maintain detailed payroll records. It should be kept in mind that, unlike one-write (pegboard) or computer systems, multiple entries must be made by hand to track office bill paying. This can seem laborious when compared to other bookkeeping systems, but it may be ideal for smaller practices.

Pegboard Payment

The same pegboard system that is used for accounts receivable (see Chap. 15, Bookkeeping and Banking) may be used for bill paying and has several advantages over the ordinary manual method of paying bills. Instead of using a day sheet, a check register page is used to record the checks that have been written. The check is then aligned on the pegboard over

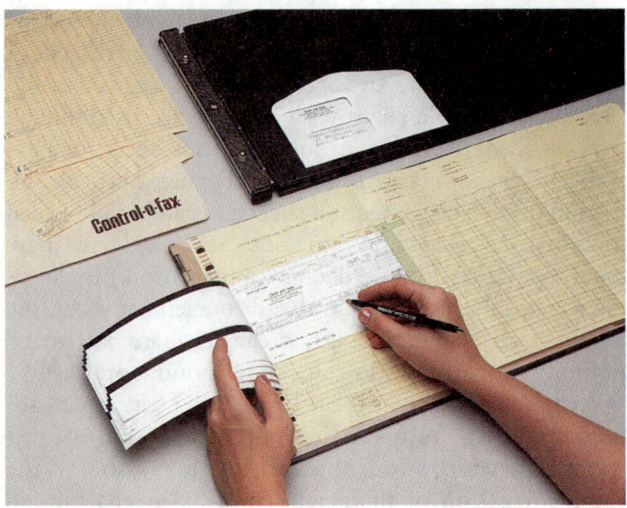

FIGURE 16-1

Sample pegboard check and check register. (Courtesy of Control-o-fax, Waterloo, IA.)

the register page and is filled out as with any other check (Fig. 16-1). Pegboard checks, however, have a carbon or transfer strip, and on this strip is written the date, the payee, the check number, and the amount. The information that was written on the strip is recorded automatically on the check register. These check-writing systems are referred to as "one-write" systems for this reason. The check can then be addressed directly beneath the payee line and mailed in a window envelope, which saves time by not having to address a separate envelope.

The pegboard check register has approximately 20 columns that can be used to categorize expenses, such as rent, insurance, office supplies, utilities, service contracts, postage, or any other applicable categories. All entries on the check register are totaled when the register is completed; these totals are carried forward to the new register page. Each fiscal or calendar year begins with a new first page (page 1), and the last check register page will have totals for the entire year. The check register provides a system of checks and balances even before the bank statement arrives because the check register must be balanced, similar to reconciling a bank statement.

The check register also allows for entries for bank deposits, and the back page of the register is used for payroll record keeping. As with pegboard accounts receivable, completed pegboard check registers are filed in a separate binder in chronological order, with the most recent register on top.

Computer Payment

A computer accounts payable system has all the advantages that a pegboard system offers: access at a glance to check registers, itemized categories and their totals, payroll records, and entries for bank deposits. To use such a system, you must have a personal computer (PC), accounts payable program software, a computer printer, and bank checks that are compatible with the software and printer. The initial expense with a computer system is considerable when compared to manual or pegboard systems. Office personnel will need some computer training to use the program. It is also obvious that a computer requires electricity and may be inoperational during power failures. However, a good computer accounting program will provide functions for both accounts receivable and accounts payable. Financial data should be recorded in three forms: on the computer's hard drive, on a magnetic tape or floppy disk, and in print-out form ("hard copy").

Although inputting data onto the computer may at first be time consuming, this is less of a concern when the bookkeeper becomes experienced in using the computer program. Furthermore, financial reports can be compiled and printed in a fraction of the time required with manual or pegboard systems. The computer program can also perform the record-keeping arithmetic; as a result, mathematical errors are practically nonexistent.

Paying bills by computer requires using the software program to open the file in which the check-writing account is located. Checks are presented on the computer screen in the same way that a paper check would normally appear (Fig. 16-2), and the information that is required to appear on the check is input on the computer keyboard. The information is then stored and the check printed out; the computer program automatically subtracts the amount of the check from the account's balance. The bookkeeper can print one check at a time or a batch of checks together.

Checks can be "memorized" by the computer so that the information on them can be recalled and reprinted without re-inputting; this is especially helpful with payroll checks. A good accounting program also allows for bill reminders and disk or magnetic tape back-up reminders. Of course, it is essential to back up financial data on magnetic tapes or floppy disks in case of computer problems.

Checkpoint Question

2. *Whether using a manual, pegboard, or computer accounts payable system, two steps must always occur when ordering and receiving supplies. What are they?*

➤ PAYROLL

Types of Payroll Systems

The medical office will have payroll obligations to its staff and payroll taxes due according to federal, state, and city guidelines for its employees. The administrative medical assistant may issue payroll checks for the practice's entire staff, including the physician, or just for the office staff. Or an outside payroll service may

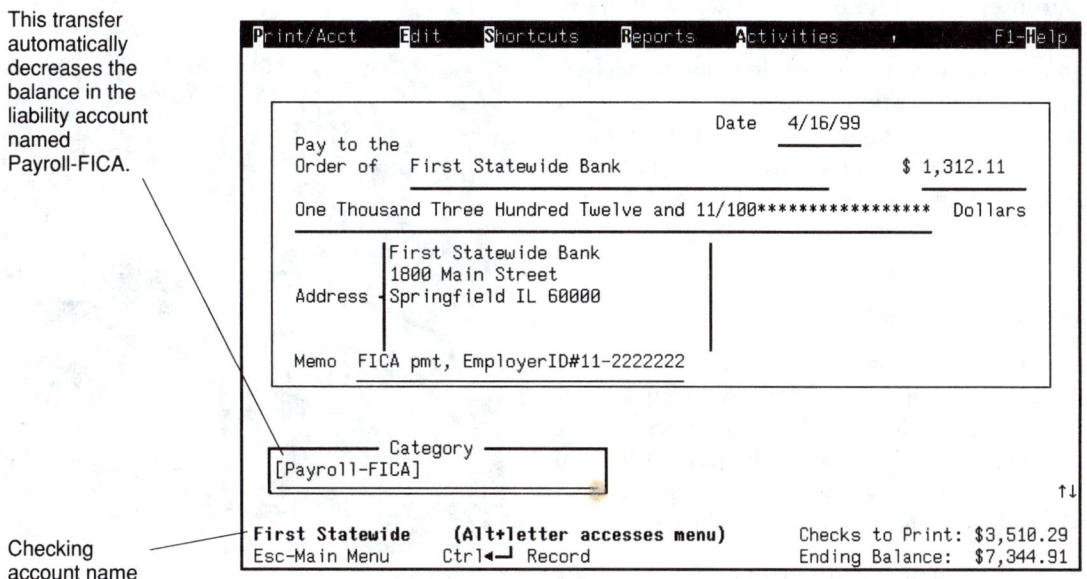

This transfer automatically decreases the balance in the liability account named Payroll-FICA.

Checking account name

FIGURE 16-2

Computer screen showing a check for payroll taxes.

BOX 16-2 Outside Payroll Services

Payroll services can be provided by outside accounting firms that specialize in computing, withholding, and paying taxes and payroll for small businesses. Such a firm can provide all of these services for considerably less than it would cost for office time and personnel or for an accountant. The larger the practice's staff, the more economical a payroll service becomes. Firms that provide payroll services are especially cost effective in that they are highly accurate, aware of changes in tax laws, and legally liable.

be retained to issue payroll checks and provide payroll record keeping (Box 16-2). Generally, payroll checks for the medical office will be issued at one of the following intervals:

- Weekly (52 pay periods/year)
- Biweekly (26 pay periods/year)
- Monthly (12 pay periods/year)

The pay period is set up by your employer and is the same for all employees.

There are different ways to record payroll expenditures, depending on what type of bookkeeping system is used by the office.

Manual Payroll Systems

When payroll checks are issued manually without a pegboard system, separate records must be kept for payroll purposes. The checkbook stub will indicate to whom the check was issued, in what amount, and on what date. A separate record or log book must be maintained to keep track of gross income and tax withholdings for each employee. These withholdings should be totaled monthly, quarterly, and annually; for this reason it is advisable to maintain payroll records in a timely manner throughout the year.

Pegboard Payroll Systems

The pegboard system allows for payroll entries as well as the accumulation of payroll data by using an employee payroll record form and the correlating back page of each check register, called the **payroll journal** (Fig. 16-3). To issue a payroll check using the pegboard system, follow these general guidelines:

1. Align the carbon or transfer strip at the top of the check on the employee's payroll record, then align both on the payroll journal.

2. Enter the employee's name first, followed by the check number, the payroll period, and the **gross income** (the amount of money an employee earned before taxes are withheld) plus any additional earnings.

3. From the gross income, subtract federal, state, and local taxes and Social Security; this is called **tax withholding**, and is described in detail on p. 226.

4. Enter the **net pay** (amount of money an employee is paid after taxes are withheld) on the detachable payroll slip. Fold this slip behind the check when it is placed in the envelope to protect the employee's privacy.

The payroll journal is totaled when each page is completed; total amounts of income and tax withholdings should be accrued for each quarter for tax reporting purposes.

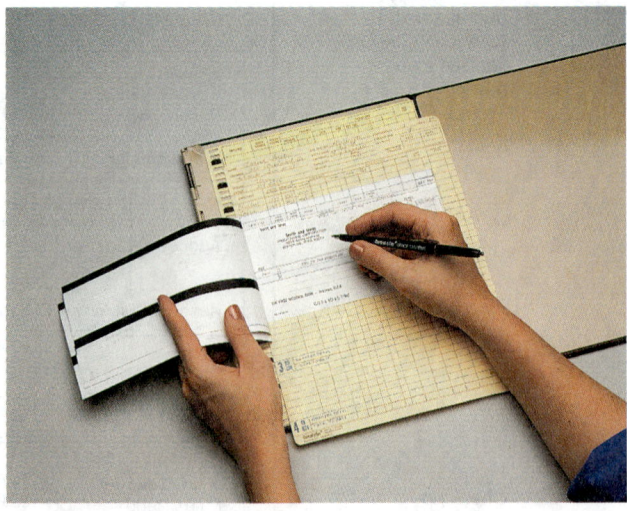

FIGURE 16-3

Sample pegboard payroll journal. (Courtesy of Contol-o-fax, Waterloo, IA.)

Box 16-3 provides a detailed example of how to calculate the amount of an employee's paycheck.

Computer Payroll Systems

Payroll records can be maintained with various computer software packages; many such packages integrate payroll with other accounting functions, such as accounts receivable and accounts payable. Computer payroll programs can calculate tax withholdings automatically as well as record payroll data and print payroll checks. In most cases, a computer program provides substantial time savings over manual and pegboard payroll systems.

Employee Records

Regardless of the payroll system used, it is necessary to maintain an individual personnel file for each employee that contains pertinent employment information. The employee personnel file should include the following information:

- Employee's original resume or completed job application
- Job references
- Hourly rate or salary at the time of hire
- Dates and amounts of pay raises
- Job evaluations

BOX 16-3 Calculating Employee Earnings

To calculate the amount of an employee's payroll check, begin by calculating the employee's annual gross wage using the following formula:

Hourly Wage × Number of Hours Worked per Week × 52
(number of weeks in a year) = Gross Annual Wage

Assume an employee earns $7.00 per hour and works 40 hours per week:

$7.00 × 40 × 52 = $14,560 annual gross wage

If the pay period for your facility is biweekly or monthly, you would then divide this sum by 26 or 12, respectively, to calculate this pay period's gross wages.

What if the employee missed a day during the pay period and you must deduct this? Always start with the normal gross wage (actual earned amount), then deduct a day's pay. To do this, go back to the year's gross amount, divide by 52 weeks in a year and then divide by 5 (work days in a week) to get the amount of a day's pay. Deduct this amount from the gross wage to get the adjusted gross wage from which you will withhold taxes. Using the example above, the calculation would be as follows:

($14,560 ÷ 52) ÷ 5   = Day's pay
$280 ÷ 5   = $56
$280 − $56 = $224 (Adjusted Gross Wage)

If you always go to the yearly gross wage when figuring deductions or increases to gross wages, you will get the exact amount.

Increases to gross wages might be overtime worked. Overtime is defined as hours worked over the normal for the pay period. Overtime is calculated by paying 1½ times the normal hourly wage. If the employee earns $7.00 per hour, overtime pay would be calculated by dividing $7.00 in half ($3.50) and adding that amount to the hourly wage: the hourly pay rate for overtime would be $10.50.

Once you have calculated the employee's gross wages, refer to the appropriate tax tables for the deductions for taxes (eg, federal, FICA/Medicare, state taxes). Subtract the taxes from the gross or adjusted gross wages to obtain net pay. This is the amount for which you would write the payroll check.

- All employee withholding authorization forms, such as W-4 forms (see below)
- Pension plan or health or life insurance paperwork
- Vital facts about the employee (eg, date of birth, name of spouse, Social Security number, current address and telephone number, name and daytime phone number of emergency contact person, etc)

Tax Withholdings

Federal, state, and possibly city or local taxes must be withheld from employees' paychecks; for this reason, each employee must complete a W-4 form (Fig. 16-4) on the first day of hire. This form needs to be completed by the employee before the first pay period; otherwise, you are required to withhold taxes at the highest rate, which is classified as single with no dependents. The W-4 form lists the employee's name, Social Security number, current address, marital status, and the number of exemptions to be used in the calculation of tax withholding. If any of the information contained on an employee's W-4 form changes, the employee must fill out a new form, which is then placed in the personnel file.

The federally mandated taxes are Social Security (FICA), Medicare, and federal income tax. Each of these taxes is based on a percentage of total gross income; the federal income tax also factors in marital status and the number of withholding exemptions claimed on the W-4 form.

The employer must match the amount withheld from each employee's paycheck for Social Security and Medicare taxes. For example, if $150 was withheld from an employee's paycheck for Medicare and Social Security taxes, then the employer must pay $300 to the IRS ($150 withheld from the employee plus $150 matching amount). The employer does not match federal, state, or local taxes. The practice's accountant should advise the office bookkeeper on current tax rates and withholdings. Usually each pay period or at least monthly, you will deposit the federal taxes withheld from all employees plus FICA doubled in an account at a federal depository (normally the facility's bank). Your accountant normally will send you the estimated federal depository slips for this purpose.

The employer must also pay a **federal unemployment tax** (FUTA) for each employee based on that employee's gross income. The amount of this tax is calculated by the practice's accountant and paid either quarterly or annually. Individual states may levy their own unemployment tax; this tax should also be calculated by the practice's accountant.

Other withholdings from an employee's paycheck might include health, life, or disability premiums; pen-

sion plan contributions; or court-ordered garnishment of wages owed to a third party.

Checkpoint Question

3. What taxes must be withheld from an employee's paycheck?

Payment of Taxes

Payroll taxes are paid according to different schedules as determined by the IRS and the state and local tax authorities. Federal taxes such as Social Security, Medicare, and federal wage tax must be paid monthly, bimonthly, or more frequently depending on the size of the gross payroll. Always remember to match the Medicare and Social Security payments withheld from the employee's check (the amount withheld × 2). These payments are made on IRS Form 941 for deposit requirements; the IRS furnishes these forms free of charge.

Currently, if the total federal taxes due are more than $3000, these payroll taxes must be paid within 3 calendar days from the time the payroll check was issued. State taxes that are withheld from the employee's pay check are usually paid by mail and must be paid and mailed before the tax due date to avoid penalties.

The IRS also requires the employer to file quarterly returns for all federal taxes withheld; these returns are due by April 30, July 31, October 31, and January 31 each year. This quarterly return is a summary of the Social Security, Medicare, and federal wage taxes paid. State quarterly returns have the same due dates and are usually paid by mail. Your accountant will keep you informed of taxes due.

What If?

What if the practice does not pay its payroll taxes?

The Internal Revenue Service (IRS) charges penalties and interest on all unpaid taxes. The IRS can attach the business and its assets and close the business.

W-2 forms

At the end of the calendar year, all pertinent payroll information should be summarized for each employee and made available to the practice's accountant. The

text continues on page 227

Form W-4 (1995)

Want More Money In Your Paycheck?
If you expect to be able to take the earned income credit for 1995 and a child lives with you, you may be able to have part of the credit added to your take-home pay. For details, get Form W-5 from your employer.

Purpose. Complete Form W-4 so that your employer can withhold the correct amount of Federal income tax from your pay.

Exemption From Withholding. Read line 7 of the certificate below to see if you can claim exempt status. *If exempt, complete line 7; but do not complete lines 5 and 6.* No Federal income tax will be withheld from your pay. Your exemption is good for 1 year only. It expires February 15, 1996.

Note: *You cannot claim exemption from withholding if (1) your income exceeds $650 and includes unearned income (e.g., interest*

and dividends) and (2) another person can claim you as a dependent on their tax return.

Basic Instructions. Employees who are not exempt should complete the Personal Allowances Worksheet. Additional worksheets are provided on page 2 for employees to adjust their withholding allowances based on itemized deductions, adjustments to income, or two-earner/two-job situations. Complete all worksheets that apply to your situation. The worksheets will help you figure the number of withholding allowances you are entitled to claim. However, you may claim fewer allowances than this.

Head of Household. Generally, you may claim head of household filing status on your tax return only if you are unmarried and pay more than 50% of the costs of keeping up a home for yourself and your dependent(s) or other qualifying individuals.

Nonwage Income. If you have a large amount of nonwage income, such as interest or dividends, you should consider making

estimated tax payments using Form 1040-ES. Otherwise, you may find that you owe additional tax at the end of the year.

Two Earners/Two Jobs. If you have a working spouse or more than one job, figure the total number of allowances you are entitled to claim on all jobs using worksheets from only one Form W-4. This total should be divided among all jobs. Your withholding will usually be most accurate when all allowances are claimed on the W-4 filed for the highest paying job and zero allowances are claimed for the others.

Check Your Withholding. After your W-4 takes effect, you can use Pub. 919, Is My Withholding Correct for 1995?, to see how the dollar amount you are having withheld compares to your estimated total annual tax. We recommend you get Pub. 919 especially if you used the Two Earner/Two Job Worksheet and your earnings exceed $150,000 (Single) or $200,000 (Married). Call 1-800-829-3676 to order Pub. 919. Check your telephone directory for the IRS assistance number for further help.

Personal Allowances Worksheet

A	Enter "1" for **yourself** if no one else can claim you as a dependent	A _____
B	Enter "1" if: { • You are single and have only one job; or • You are married, have only one job, and your spouse does not work; or • Your wages from a second job or your spouse's wages (or the total of both) are $1,000 or less. } . .	B _____
C	Enter "1" for your **spouse.** But, you may choose to enter -0- if you are married and have either a working spouse or more than one job (this may help you avoid having too little tax withheld)	C _____
D	Enter number of **dependents** (other than your spouse or yourself) you will claim on your tax return	D _____
E	Enter "1" if you will file as **head of household** on your tax return (see conditions under **Head of Household** above) .	E _____
F	Enter "1" if you have at least $1,500 of **child or dependent care expenses** for which you plan to claim a credit . .	F _____
G	Add lines A through F and enter total here. **Note:** This amount may be different from the number of exemptions you claim on your return ▶	G _____

For accuracy, do all worksheets that apply.
- If you plan to **itemize or claim adjustments to income** and want to reduce your withholding, see the Deductions and Adjustments Worksheet on page 2.
- If you are **single** and have **more than one job** and your combined earnings from all jobs exceed $30,000 OR if you are **married** and have a **working spouse or more than one job,** and the combined earnings from all jobs exceed $50,000, see the Two-Earner/Two-Job Worksheet on page 2 if you want to avoid having too little tax withheld.
- If **neither** of the above situations applies, **stop here** and enter the number from line G on line 5 of Form W-4 below.

-------- **Cut here and give the certificate to your employer. Keep the top portion for your records.** --------

Form **W-4** Department of the Treasury Internal Revenue Service	**Employee's Withholding Allowance Certificate** ▶ **For Privacy Act and Paperwork Reduction Act Notice, see reverse.**	OMB No. 1545-0010 19**95**

1	Type or print your first name and middle initial	Last name	2	Your social security number

	Home address (number and street or rural route)	3	☐ Single ☐ Married ☐ Married, but withhold at higher Single rate. **Note:** *If married, but legally separated, or spouse is a nonresident alien, check the Single box.*

	City or town, state, and ZIP code	4	If your last name differs from that on your social security card, check here and call 1-800-772-1213 for a new card . . . . . ▶ ☐

5	Total number of allowances you are claiming (from line G above or from the worksheets on page 2 if they apply) .	**5**
6	Additional amount, if any, you want withheld from each paycheck	**6** $
7	I claim exemption from withholding for 1995 and I certify that I meet **BOTH** of the following conditions for exemption: • Last year I had a right to a refund of **ALL** Federal income tax withheld because I had **NO** tax liability; **AND** • This year I expect a refund of **ALL** Federal income tax withheld because I expect to have **NO** tax liability. If you meet both conditions, enter "EXEMPT" here . . . . ▶	**7**

Under penalties of perjury, I certify that I am entitled to the number of withholding allowances claimed on this certificate or entitled to claim exempt status.

Employee's signature ▶		Date ▶	, 19

8	Employer's name and address (Employer: Complete 8 and 10 only if sending to the IRS)	9	Office code (optional)	10	Employer identification number

Cat. No. 10220Q

FIGURE 16-4
Sample W-4 form.

Deductions and Adjustments Worksheet

Note: *Use this worksheet only if you plan to itemize deductions or claim adjustments to income on your 1995 tax return.*

1   Enter an estimate of your 1995 itemized deductions. These include qualifying home mortgage interest, charitable contributions, state and local taxes (but not sales taxes), medical expenses in excess of 7.5% of your income, and miscellaneous deductions. (For 1995, you may have to reduce your itemized deductions if your income is over $114,700 ($57,350 if married filing separately). Get Pub. 919 for details.)   **1** $ _____

2   Enter: { $6,550 if married filing jointly or qualifying widow(er) / $5,750 if head of household / $3,900 if single / $3,275 if married filing separately }   . . . .   **2** $ _____

3   **Subtract** line 2 from line 1. If line 2 is greater than line 1, enter -0- . . . .   **3** $ _____

4   Enter an estimate of your 1995 adjustments to income. These include alimony paid and deductible IRA contributions   **4** $ _____

5   **Add** lines 3 and 4 and enter the total . . . .   **5** $ _____

6   Enter an estimate of your 1995 nonwage income (such as dividends or interest) . . . .   **6** $ _____

7   **Subtract** line 6 from line 5. Enter the result, but not less than -0- . . . .   **7** $ _____

8   **Divide** the amount on line 7 by $2,500 and enter the result here. Drop any fraction . . . . .   **8**   _____

9   Enter the number from Personal Allowances Worksheet, line G, on page 1 . . . .   **9**   _____

10   **Add** lines 8 and 9 and enter the total here. If you plan to use the Two-Earner/Two-Job Worksheet, also enter this total on line 1 below. Otherwise, **stop here** and enter this total on Form W-4, line 5, on page 1 . . . . .   **10**   _____

Two-Earner/Two-Job Worksheet

Note: *Use this worksheet only if the instructions for line G on page 1 direct you here.*

1   Enter the number from line G on page 1 (or from line 10 above if you used the Deductions and Adjustments Worksheet)   **1**   _____

2   Find the number in **Table 1** below that applies to the **LOWEST** paying job and enter it here . . . .   **2**   _____

3   If line 1 is **GREATER THAN OR EQUAL TO** line 2, subtract line 2 from line 1. Enter the result here (if zero, enter -0-) and on Form W-4, line 5, on page 1. **DO NOT** use the rest of this worksheet . . . .   **3**   _____

Note: *If line 1 is **LESS THAN** line 2, enter -0- on Form W-4, line 5, on page 1. Complete lines 4–9 to calculate the additional withholding amount necessary to avoid a year end tax bill.*

4   Enter the number from line 2 of this worksheet . . . .   **4**   _____

5   Enter the number from line 1 of this worksheet . . . .   **5**   _____

6   **Subtract** line 5 from line 4 . . . .   **6**   _____

7   Find the amount in **Table 2** below that applies to the **HIGHEST** paying job and enter it here . . . .   **7** $ _____

8   **Multiply** line 7 by line 6 and enter the result here. This is the additional annual withholding amount needed   **8** $ _____

9   Divide line 8 by the number of pay periods remaining in 1995. (For example, divide by 26 if you are paid every other week and you complete this form in December 1994.) Enter the result here and on Form W-4, line 6, page 1. This is the additional amount to be withheld from each paycheck . . . .   **9** $ _____

Table 1: Two-Earner/Two-Job Worksheet

Married Filing Jointly				All Others	
If wages from **LOWEST** paying job are—	Enter on line 2 above	If wages from **LOWEST** paying job are—	Enter on line 2 above	If wages from **LOWEST** paying job are—	Enter on line 2 above
0 - $3,000	0	39,001 - 50,000	9	0 - $4,000	0
3,001 - 6,000	1	50,001 - 55,000	10	4,001 - 10,000	1
6,001 - 11,000	2	55,001 - 60,000	11	10,001 - 14,000	2
11,001 - 16,000	3	60,001 - 70,000	12	14,001 - 19,000	3
16,001 - 21,000	4	70,001 - 80,000	13	19,001 - 23,000	4
21,001 - 27,000	5	80,001 - 90,000	14	23,001 - 45,000	5
27,001 - 31,000	6	90,001 and over	15	45,001 - 60,000	6
31,001 - 34,000	7			60,001 - 70,000	7
34,001 - 39,000	8			70,001 and over	8

Table 2: Two-Earner/Two-Job Worksheet

Married Filing Jointly		All Others	
If wages from **HIGHEST** paying job are—	Enter on line 7 above	If wages from **HIGHEST** paying job are—	Enter on line 7 above
0 - $50,000	$380	0 - $30,000	$380
50,001 - 100,000	700	30,001 - 60,000	700
100,001 - 130,000	780	60,001 - 110,000	780
130,001 - 230,000	900	110,001 - 230,000	900
230,001 and over	990	230,001 and over	990

FIGURE 16-4 Continued

W-2 statement provided to the employee at the year's end should list the following information:

- Total gross income
- Total federal, state, and local taxes withheld
- Any taxable fringe benefits
- The employee's total net income

Checkpoint Question

4. What information does the employee list on the W-4 form? What happens if this information changes?

➤ PREPARATION OF REPORTS

The bookkeeper must also prepare reports for the practice's accountant or the IRS based on financial data stored in the office's bookkeeping system. For this reason, care should always be taken when recording financial data.

The manual system, when assisted by the use of a log or record book, should be able to provide monthly, quarterly, and annual summaries for income, expenditures, and payroll. It is advisable to have subtotals and totals for these periods for tax payment purposes.

The pegboard system is also practical for providing summaries of income, expenses, and payroll and can be totaled monthly, quarterly, and yearly. Each day sheet, check register, and payroll journal is individually totaled with all balances forwarded to the next page. These records are stored in binders and kept for future reference.

The computer system of accounting offers all of the previously mentioned reports, as well as other, more complicated reports that would generally require more advanced accounting skills. The great advantage with report generating by computer is that the computer will perform all of the mathematical calculations for the time frame requested.

➤ ASSISTING WITH AUDITS

Audits may be informal (in-house) and used to assist the practice's accountant with tax preparation, or they may be formal audits held by the IRS. If meticulous attention has been paid throughout the year to record keeping, the preparation time needed for such an audit should be minimal. It is important to save all banking statements, copies of annual and quarterly tax returns, and all receipts for expenditures. Can-

celed checks and payroll records should be readily available.

Manual and pegboard systems can provide spending category and payroll summaries in addition to the examination of the actual entries for the period being audited. A computerized accounting system can provide all of the above plus reports such as profit-loss statements, which normally would be compiled by an accountant.

SUMMARY

Accounting is a complex process involving many legal issues. As a medical assistant, your responsibility is to keep all accounting records in a neat and organized manner. You also will be expected to understand how to order goods and services efficiently and economically, and the methods of paying invoices. In addition, you must understand the process for handling employee payroll.

CRITICAL THINKING CHALLENGES

1. Explain the advantages of manual, pegboard, and computer accounting systems.
2. What factors influence choosing one office supply vendor over another?
3. An employee gets divorced. Does she need to file a new W-4 form? Why?
4. What reports does the practice's accountant need at the end of the year?

ANSWERS TO CHECKPOINT QUESTIONS

1. Besides cost, consider delivery charges and product quality when purchasing office supplies.
2. The bookkeeper must write out a purchase order and compare the packing slip and final invoice to the purchase order.
3. Social Security, Medicare, and federal, state, and local wage taxes must be withheld from an employee's paycheck.
4. The employee provides his or her name, Social Security number, marital status, current address, and number of withholding exemptions. If any of this information changes, the employee must complete a new W-4 form for the employer.

Diagnostic and Procedural Coding

Chapter Outline

Diagnostic Coding
> International Classification of Diseases, 9th Revision, Clinical Modification (ICD-9-CM)

Procedural Coding
> Physician's Current Procedural Terminology (CPT)
> HCFA's Common Procedure Coding System (HCPCS)

Reimbursement
> Diagnostic Related Groups (DRGs)
> Resource-Based Relative Value Scale (RBRVS)

Fraud and Coding

Summary

Critical Thinking Challenges

Answers to Checkpoint Questions

Suggestions for Further Reading

DACUM Components

1.2   Perform within ethical boundaries
2.10   Use medical terminology appropriately
8.2   Implement current procedural terminology and ICD-9 coding

17

Chapter Competencies

Learning Objectives

Upon successfully completing this chapter, you will be able to:

1. Spell and define the key terms.
2. Name two coding systems used to describe diseases, injuries, and procedures and explain the differences between each.
3. Give four examples of how diagnostic and procedural coding is used.
4. Discuss the goals of resource-based relative value system (RBRVS).
5. Explain what diagnostic related groups (DRGs) are and how they are used to determine Medicare payments.
6. Explain the format of Current Procedural Terminology (CPT-4) and its use.
7. Explain HCFA's Common Procedure Coding System (HCPCS) and level 2 and 3 codes.
8. Describe the relationship between coding and reimbursement.

Key Terms

(See Glossary for definitions.)

category codes
Current Procedural Terminology (CPT)
Diagnostic Related Group (DRG)
HCFA's Common Procedure Coding System (HCPCS)
Health Care Financing Administration (HCFA)
International Classification of Diseases (ICD)
nonessential modifiers
outlier
Resource-Based Relative Value Scale (RBRVS)
subcategory codes
upcoding

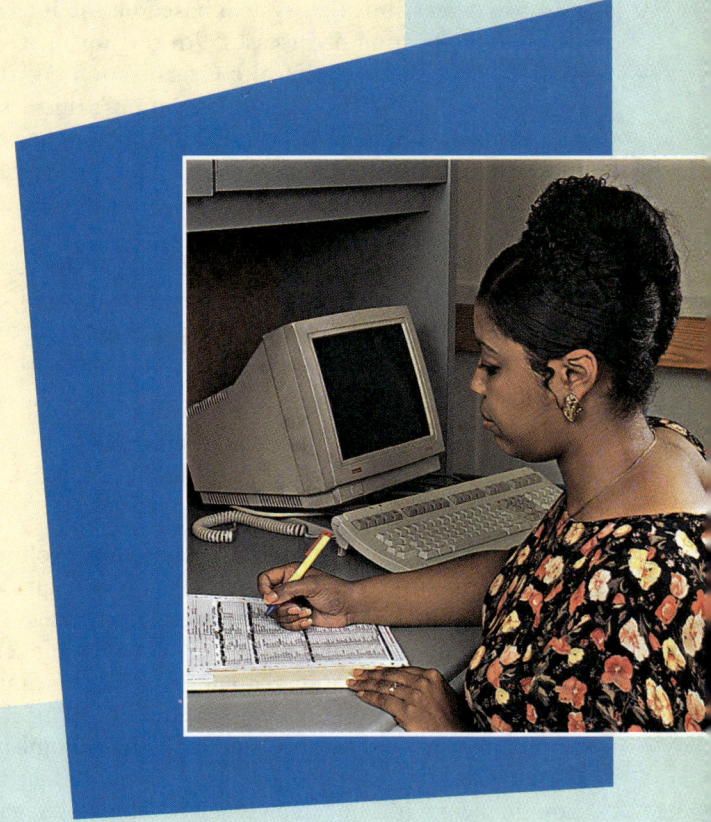

The simplest definition of coding is that it is the assignment of a number to a verbal statement or description. However, medical coding is anything but simple. Two of the most common coding systems used to describe diseases, injuries, and procedures are ICD-9-CM (International Classification of Diseases, 9th revision, Clinical Modification) and CPT-4 (Physician's Current Procedural Terminology).

Coding is a way to standardize medical information for purposes such as collecting health care statistics, performing a medical care review, and indexing medical records. It also is used for health insurance claims processing (see Chap. 18, Health Insurance, for more information). Because coding is linked to reimbursement, it is imperative that you code accurately and precisely. Incorrect, insufficient, or incomplete coding on claims forms can lead to improper reimbursement for the hospital or individual physician as well as an inaccurate database.

➤ DIAGNOSTIC CODING

International Classification of Diseases, 9th Revision, Clinical Modification (ICD-9-CM)

International Classification of Diseases (ICD)-9-CM is a statistical classification system based on the International Classification of Diseases, 9th revision (ICD-9), developed by the World Health Organization (WHO). The CM stands for "clinical modification"; this designation appears because ICD-9 was modified to be used more effectively to help health professionals collect basic health statistics, perform medical care reviews, and index medical records.

ICD-9-CM represents the most current and comprehensive statistical classification of its kind. Containing more than 10,000 diagnostic codes and over 1000 procedure codes, it consists of three volumes:

- Volume 1: Tabular List of Diseases
- Volume 2: Alphabetic Index of Diseases
- Volume 3: Tabular List and Alphabetic Index of Procedures

Depending on the publisher, these three volumes may be under one cover. In the typical physician's office, only volumes 1 and 2 are used regularly.

The diagnostic classification (Volumes 1 and 2) is maintained by the National Center for Health Statistics (NCHS); the procedure classification (Volume 3) is maintained by the **Health Care Financing Administration (HCFA)**, a federal agency that regulates health care financing. It is updated regularly, with codes being added, revised, and sometimes deleted. Changes in ICD-9-CM are published by NCHS and HCFA with the

approval of the World Health Organization (WHO.) Both the American Health Information Management Association and the American Hospital Association advise and assist in keeping the classification system current.

To ensure accurate coding, update your ICD-9-CM coding books and software (encoders) as needed. (Updates and addenda can be purchased from the particular publisher of your coding book.) You must update codes on **superbills** (preprinted bills listing a variety of procedures) or any other forms you use. It is important also to watch for the dates that new codes are accepted by insurance companies or Medicare/Medicaid.

Checkpoint Question
1. *What are the three volumes in the ICD-9-CM coding book?*

Checkpoint Question
2. *What organization must approve any changes to the disease classification system?*

ICD-9-CM, Volume 1

Volume 1 contains the classification of diseases (conditions) and injuries by code numbers. These 17 chapters cover groupings of diseases and injuries by etiology (eg, infectious diseases) and by anatomic system (eg, digestive, respiratory). Each chapter has a heading or title. Following the title in parenthesis is the range of three-digit categories included in it. Within each chapter you will find subtitles in large type followed by a range of three-digit categories in parentheses. These are called *sections*. Three-digit codes with titles are referred to as **category codes** (eg, 037 is Tetanus).

In many instances, a fourth digit has been added to a category to provide more information or specificity. These codes are referred to as **subcategory codes**. Some codes have a fifth digit added because of the need to code along a different axis from that at the fourth digit level. For example, the diabetes mellitus category is 250. It is necessary to use one of the fourth digit subcategories to indicate the specific complications that may accompany the diabetes and then add a fifth digit to indicate whether the diabetes is insulin-dependent or noninsulin-dependent. Incomplete coding here impacts on reimbursement and causes data errors.

Supplementary classifications in Volume 1 include "V" and "E" codes. V-codes, which range from V01-

V82, provide a means of indexing the reason for hospital or physician office care for other than current or genuine illness, such as a history of an illness, immunizations, or live born infants according to type of birth. An example of a V-code would be V10.04, which would be used for a person with a personal history of a malignant neoplasm of the stomach.

E-codes, which range from E800 to E999, are used to classify external causes of injuries and poisoning. Specificity is limited to the fourth digit level. E-codes are used in conjunction with codes in chapters 1-17. They help to provide information of interest to industrial medicine, insurance underwriters, national safety programs, public health agencies, and others concerned with causes of injuries (eg, auto accidents, accidents caused by heavy industrial machinery).

There is a separate index to access E-codes that can be found in Section 3 of Volume 2. It is called the "Alphabetic Index to External Causes of Injury and Poisoning."

Volume 1 also has five appendices:

APPENDIX A: Morphology of Neoplasms
This appendix can be used in conjunction with chapter 2 in ICD-9-CM when coding neoplasms. It lists the five-digit alpha-numeric codes used to identify the morphology of a neoplasm. For example, in the morphology code M8070/3, the 8070 indicates the morphology type is squamous cell carcinoma. The /3 indicates that it is the primary site.
APPENDIX B: Glossary of Mental Disorders
Alphabetical list of mental disorders, which includes detailed descriptions of each disease.
APPENDIX C: Classification of Drugs by American Hospital Formulary Service (AHFS) List Number and the ICD-9-CM Equivalents
This appendix lists the AHFS list number (eg, 24:04 for cardiac drugs) and the ICD9-CM code number for each one (eg, 24.04 cardiac drugs would be equivalent to category 972.9, the ICD9-CM category titled "Other and unspecified agents primarily affecting the cardiovascular system").
APPENDIX D: Classification of Industrial Accidents by Agency
This includes codes that can be used as a supplement to describe types of equipment or materials that may be responsible for an industrial accident or illness.
APPENDIX E: List of Three-Digit Categories
This is simply a list of all the three-digit categories that appear in ICD9-CM.

Checkpoint Question
3. How many digits will a subcategory code have?

Checkpoint Question
4. Which appendix would most likely help you when coding a chart in a psychiatric facility?

ICD-9-CM, Volume 2

Volume 2, the Alphabetic Index of Diseases, contains many diagnostic terms that do not appear in Volume 1. (That is because the diagnostic terms in Volume 2 are examples of only disease categories). The index is arranged by *condition*. Always check all indentations in the index under the condition to ensure that you have the one most appropriate to the diagnosis you intend to code. Often, a diagnosis may be an eponym (eg, Meniere's Disease or Syndrome). These terms can be found in the index under the eponym or under the main entry "disease" or "syndrome."

Following the main entry is a code number, which refers you to the tabular listing (Volume 1). You must not accept this number as the correct code without checking the tabular list. NEVER CODE DIRECTLY FROM THE ALPHABETIC INDEX! This could result in an incorrect coding assignment.

The Alphabetic Index has three sections:

- *Section 1, Alphabetic Index to Diseases and Injuries*, is organized by main terms printed in boldface type. When trying to locate a diagnosis in this index, look under the condition. However, keep in mind the following exceptions to this rule:
  1. Obstetric conditions may be found under the main terms delivery, pregnancy, and puerperal.
  2. Complication of medical (or surgical) procedures can be found under "complication."
  3. Late effects are found under "late effect."
  4. V-codes are found under main entries such as Admissions, Examination, History of Observation, Problem (with), Status, Vaccination, Encounter for, and Follow-up.
- **Nonessential modifiers** are terms that appear in parentheses after a main term in the index. Their presence or absence in the diagnosis has no effect on the selection of the code numbers. For instance, the code for acute appendicitis is 540.9; the code for acute inflammatory, retrocecal appendicitis also is 540.9. Despite the fact that the modifiers "inflammatory" and "retrocecal" have been added, the code is the same.
- *Section 2, Table of Drugs and Chemicals*, includes an extensive listing of drugs, chemical substances, and toxic agents. It also shows E-codes and AHFS List Numbers. The AHFS List Numbers are located in the table under the main term "drug."

• Section 3, *Alphabetic Index to External Cases of Injuries and Poisonings*, leads you to codes that describe circumstances of injuries, accidents, or violence. These codes are not used for coding medical diagnoses. Main entries in this section usually represent a type of accident or violence (eg, assault, fall, collision). These codes can supplement the diagnostic code, but they should never be used alone or as principal diagnosis codes.

For example, a person who had fractured a tibia in a fall off a sidewalk curb would be given a code from chapter 17 in ICD9-CM for the injury (eg, "Fracture of Tibia, closed" is 823.80) an additional code, E880.0, would indicate the accident was a fall off a sidewalk curb.

ICD-9-CM, Volume 3

Volume 3, the Tabular List and Alphabetic Index of Procedures, is based on anatomy—not surgical specialty. There are no alphabetic characters in these procedure codes. The codes are based on two-digit categories with a maximum of two decimal digits where necessary. The majority of codes refer to surgical procedures, the rest cover miscellaneous diagnostic and therapeutic procedures. An example of a procedure code would be 31.61, larynx laceration suture.

➤ PROCEDURAL CODING

Physician's Current Procedural Terminology (CPT)

Physician's *Current Procedural Terminology* (CPT) is a comprehensive listing of medical terms and codes for the uniform coding of procedures and services provided by physicians. First published in 1966 by the American Medical Association (AMA), CPT focused mainly on surgical procedures with a limited number of other codes to describe medical, radiology, laboratory, and pathology procedures. It was revised in 1970, 1973, and for the fourth time in 1977. The 4th edition, CPT-4, contains more than 7000 codes and is updated annually. The new CPT-4 book is available in December of each year.

CPT-4 contains a listing of all current and Food and Drug Administration-approved physicians' procedures and services. It was developed in collaboration with the AMA and various other health organizations. In the early 1980s, Congress decided to use CPT-4 to code all physicians' procedures and services for Medicare patients. The aim of CPT-4 was to establish a way in which interested parties could get an idea of what procedures and services had been provided to the patient without reading a lengthy report. For example, the CPT-4 allows insurance companies to:

• Communicate easily with one another
• Compare reimbursable amounts for procedures
• Speed claims processing

CPT-4 is a system of five-digit numeric codes and corresponding meanings, as illustrated by the following example: 99201—Office or other outpatient visit for the evaluation and management of a new patient, which requires the following three key components:

1. Problem-focused history
2. Problem-focused examination
3. Straightforward medical decision-making

Every code means something different and is used only once to describe a specific procedure, service, or medical supplies provided by physicians to their patients. Codes and descriptions are regularly updated, revised, or changed. If your physician's office uses a superbill or preprinted routing slip that lists the procedures performed, it is imperative that you update this form yearly.

The CPT-4 book is divided into six major sections:

1. Evaluation and Management (E/M)
2. Anesthesia
3. Surgery
4. Radiology
5. Pathology and Laboratory
6. Medicine

Each section begins with its own specific guidelines and a listing of specific procedures and services applicable to the particular field. The guidelines contain: definitions, explanatory notes, a listing of the previously unlisted procedures found in that particular section, how to file a special report, modifiers for use in that particular section, and definitions to assist the coder.

Checkpoint Question
5. How often are CPT-4 codes updated?

Evaluation and Management (E/M) Codes

E/M codes are five-digit numbers that begin with the number 9. These are the most frequently used codes. E/M codes describe various histories, examinations, and decisions physicians must make in evaluating and treating patients in various settings (eg, office, outpatient, hospital). In essence, the E/M codes address what the physician does when interacting with the patient. For this reason it is important that the physician becomes involved in deciding which code to use for a specific patient-physician encounter.

To code the services described in the E/M section, you must be sure that two or three of the "key components" are present (depending on the category of the service). These components are the elements that make up the visit. All E/M codes contain the following components:

- History
- Physical Examination
- Medical Decision-Making
- Counseling
- Coordination of Care
- Nature of Presenting Problem
- Time

However, not all of these are *key* components for a visit. The key components for a visit listed in CPT-4 are:

- History
- Physical Examination
- Medical Decision-Making

There are four kinds of *Histories* and *Physical Examinations* described in CPT-4. These include:

- Problem-focused
- Expanded problem-focused
- Detailed
- Comprehensive

Table 17-1 describes these in greater detail. When coding, you must pick one of these based on information *provided by the physician.*

The third key component, *Medical Decision-Making,* is defined in CPT-4 as either:

- Straightforward
- Low Complexity
- Moderate Complexity
- High Complexity

Medical decision-making refers to the kinds of things the physician must do to establish a diagnosis for the patient (eg, determine the management options available, the amount and complexity of the data to be reviewed, the risk of complications, or other problems [ie, worsening of the illness or death]). To qualify for a particular decision-making level, you need to be sure the physician meets or exceeds two of the three elements.

Time spent with a patient (eg, conducting counseling or coordinating patient care) can *sometimes* be a factor when choosing E/M codes. When time spent with the patient is greater than 50% of the total time for the visit, then time becomes the deciding factor in choosing an E/M code. For example, if a physician

spends an additional 15 minutes counseling a patient in what would normally be only a 10-minute expanded, problem-focused history and physical examination, the counseling was more than 50% of the usual 10-minute face-to-face time. You would then choose an E/M code with a 25-minute time frame (10 minutes and an extra 15 minutes counseling).

Special considerations regarding E/M codes: Initial Hospital Care codes can be used only by the admitting physician. All other physicians must use Consultation codes or subsequent Hospital Care codes. Emergency Department Service codes are to be used only when the service is rendered in a 24-hour hospital-based facility that specializes in providing treatment of unscheduled events.

Checkpoint Question

? 6. To code for a service in the E/M section, two of the three key elements must be present. What are the three key elements?

Anesthesia Codes

Anesthesia codes are five-digit codes that begin with 0. Anesthesia codes are divided by anatomic site and by specific type of procedure (eg, head, neck, thorax are anatomic sites and the codes in each section represent the specific procedure, such as plastic repair of cleft lip).

There are two types of modifiers used in the anesthesia section. One type is the standard modifier that is found in all the other sections of CPT. The other type is the physical status modifier, which is a two-digit code beginning with the letter "P" and ending in a number from 1-6. These physical status modifiers indicate the patient's condition at the time of anesthesia and the corresponding complexity of services (eg, "P" indicates a normal, healthy patient and "P_5" indicates a patient in a dying state who is not expected to survive without the procedure).

Surgery Codes

Surgery codes begin with the numbers 1 through 6. You need to be aware of the following elements, which are discussed in the guidelines of the surgery section.

Nonstarred codes. The CPT-4 codes in this section that **do not have a star** (*) refer to codes that include a "surgical package." The code that follows identifies the surgical package and would include normal, uncomplicated follow-up care. The surgical package means that local infiltration, digital block or topical

Table 17-1
History and Physical Examinations

The physician will assist you in selecting which history and physical examination code to use. However, you should have a basic understanding of each category. It is important to note that there are separate codes for each category and separate codes for both new and established patients.

Type of history and physical examination	Patient problems and physician time required	Examples
Problem focused	Patient problems are self-limited and minor. Physician time: usually 10 minutes.	• 9-month-old patient with diaper rash • 40-year-old patient with sunburn • 18-year-old patient with poison ivy • 60-year-old patient with a routine blood pressure check
Expanded problem focused	Patient problems are mild to moderate. Physician time: between 15–20 minutes.	• 55-year-old patient with recurrent urinary tract infections • 16-year-old patient with chronic asthma presents with a cold • 76-year-old patient with osteoarthritis • 56-year-old patient with a stomach ulcer
Detailed	Patient problems are moderate to severe. Physician time: usually 30 minutes.	• 18-year-old patient with first Pap smear and contraceptive education • 67-year-old patient with new onset of dysuria • 18-month-old patient with delayed motor skill development. • 34-year-old patient with diabetes requiring insulin dose changes
Comprehensive	Patient problems are moderate to severe. Physician time: usually 45 minutes.	• 36-year-old patient with infertility • 8-year-old patient with new onset of diabetes • 65-year-old patient with history of left-sided weakness and confusion

anesthesia, the operation itself, and normal uncomplicated follow-up care are included in the code that covers the operation itself.

Health Care Financing Administration (HCFA) has defined the surgical package for Medicare recipients somewhat differently. According to CPT-4, any complications or problems related to the surgery are not included in the surgical package. If additional procedures are performed to correct or alleviate these problems, they should be coded separately. However, according to HCFA and Medicare, complications that do not require a revisit to the operating room are included in the price of surgery.

Some insurance carriers have a set number of follow-up days that is consistent for all nonstarred surgical services. Check with your carrier to learn what these are so you can bill for the additional office, outpatient, or hospital visits made.

Starred codes. Codes with a star (*) are for the surgical service itself. The surgical package does not apply. You should code any preoperative anesthesia and postoperative components *separately*.

If there is no star next to the code, it means that you cannot bill separately for preoperative and postoperative components.

Example: Repair—Simple superficial wounds of scalp, neck, axilla, external genitalia, and so forth.

12001*—2.5 cm or less
12002*—2.6 cm to 7.5 cm
12004*—7.6 cm to 12.5 cm
12005—12.6 cm to 20.10 cm (notice no star)

If a patient came in for routine follow-up care of a scalp wound that had been coded 12001, 12002, or 12004, the coder could also code for both office visits (99212). There is a corresponding fee for this service. If, however, the patient was returning for routine follow-up care for a wound repair that had originally been coded 12005, the code 99024 (postoperative follow-up visit) could be used but there is *no* charge for this because the service was included in the surgical package. Remember, 12005 was not a starred procedure. Third-party payers have different rules about what constitutes a surgery package, so the coder needs to check with the third-party payers in their area.

Integumentary system. In this section, there are codes for which a measurement is necessary. It is important that the size of both the defect and the size of the specimen are measured before they are sent to the laboratory. All excisions listed in the Integumentary section *include* simple closure.

Repairs. There are three types of repairs defined in CPT-4: simple, intermediate, and complex. Repairs should be measured and recorded in centimeters to be coded appropriately.

Cast re-application (replacement). You cannot assign the same code for cast replacement as you did for the original cast application because the code for replacement does not include the "treatment" of the fracture, as the original cast application code did; it therefore carries a lower reimbursement rate.

Multiple procedures furnished on the same day. Unless these are part of the overall global service, they should be coded separately and placed on the claims form in order from major to minor.

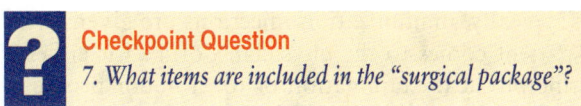

Checkpoint Question
7. What items are included in the "surgical package"?

Radiology Codes

This section of CPT-4 is divided into the four subsections listed below:

- Diagnostic Radiology/Diagnostic Imaging
- Diagnostic Ultrasound
- Radiation Oncology
- Nuclear Medicine

All Radiology codes are five-digit numbers that begin with the number 7 that generally are arranged by anatomic site, from the top of the body to the bottom. If a physician performs the procedure as well as supervises and interprets a procedure (eg, injecting a contrast medium and supervising and interpreting the procedure), two codes should be used. The code for the procedure is usually found in the Surgery section and the code for supervision/interpretation is usually found in the Radiology section.

Pathology and Laboratory Codes

All codes in this section are five-digit numbers that begin with the number 8. A subsection, Automated Multichannel Tests, deserves a special note. When coding, check that the tests performed are included in the lists under this subsection. For example, the physician may perform the following three tests for a patient: bilirubin, direct; cholesterol; and blood urea nitrogen (BUN). When coding, you would assign the code 80003, three clinical chemistry tests, because all of these tests are listed under the Automated Multichannel Test subsection. However, if the tests performed were bilirubin, direct; cholesterol; and blood acetaldehyde, you would need to code 80002, two clinical chemistry tests, and 82000, blood acetaldehyde. That is because blood acetaldehyde was not on the list of clinical chemistry tests in the Automated Multichannel Test subsections.

Medicine Codes

Like the E/M codes, Medicine codes are five-digit numbers that begin with the number 9. As with the other five sections of the CPT-4, this section includes guidelines for appropriate coding. You may want to pay particular attention to the information related to the Immunization Injections subsection, which includes codes from 90701-90749.

Typically, immunization injections are given when the patient comes to the physician's office for either a routine physical examination or for a minor problem, such as a sore throat. When the injection is given at the same time as such a visit, use two codes: one for the service (usually an E/M code) and one for the immunization injection. For example, an established patient may come into the physician's office for a brief examination for a minor problem. The patient may be examined briefly and may also be given an immunization for poliomyelitis. The coding for this would be:

1. **99211** Office and other outpatient visit for the evaluation and management of an established patient, which may not require the presence of a physician. Usually the presenting problems are minimal. Typically, 5 minutes are spent performing or supervising services.
2. **90713** Poliomyelitis vaccine.

The Immunization Injections subsection of the Medicine section is the only one that advises and allows the coder to bill for an E/M service even when an injection is the only service provided. For therapeutic or diagnostic injections (codes 90782–90799), you need *to specify* what was injected. Examine the code: **90782** Therapeutic injection of medication (specify); subcutaneous or intramuscular?

As you can see, the code would be the same for a number of injectable therapeutic substances. However, you need to find a way to distinguish among the various kinds of injectable substances to protect the physician's profile. (A profile is defined as a fixed dollar amount per code that the computer expects to see after a particular CPT-4 code.)

For coding Medicare claims, the cost of administering injections will be included in the price of office/outpatient visits or other procedures furnished on the same day. However, supplying the drug is a separate billable service and can be assigned to HCPCS National Code. (This may not be true of other carriers, however, so you need to check with them.)

Using the most specific codes for different injectable substances and supplies protects the physician's profile and locks in a specific dollar amount for a particular code.

Checkpoint Question

8. A patient comes to the office for a tetanus booster, and the physician gives the booster plus completes a routine physical examination. How many codes would you use for this visit?

CPT-4 Modifiers

CPT-4 provides a way to give additional information about a procedure through the use of additional numbers called **modifiers.**

There are several ways to write modifiers. For example, you can:

BOX 17-1   Examples of CPT-4 Modifiers

Here are just a few examples of CPT-4 modifiers. A complete list can be found in Appendix A of CPT-4.

–20 microsurgery

This modifier signifies that the surgeon used an operating microscope to perform a procedure.

–23 unusual anesthesia

This modifier signifies that anesthesia was used in a procedure that normally would not require it.

–26 professional component

This modifier signifies that there are two components to the procedure, a professional and a technical one. For example, when a physician requests an x-ray, the radiologic technologist takes the x-ray and the physician reads it. This modifier lets the insurance carrier know that both service components were not provided by the physician.

- Write the five-digit code with a dash followed by the two-digit modifier (eg, 28702-22).
- Write the code without a dash separating it from the modifier (eg, 2870222).
- Write the five-digit code with the modifier listed directly beneath it as a five-digit code beginning with the number 099:
  - 28702
  - 09922 (modifier)

Of course, the modifier can never appear on the claim form by itself because it refers to the procedure and must be directly below it on the claim form (Fig.17-1).

Box 17-1 provides a few examples of modifiers. A separate listing of available modifiers can be found in Appendix A of CPT-4. This saves you from having to go to each section to find the modifiers. However, only the modifiers listed in the guidelines of each section

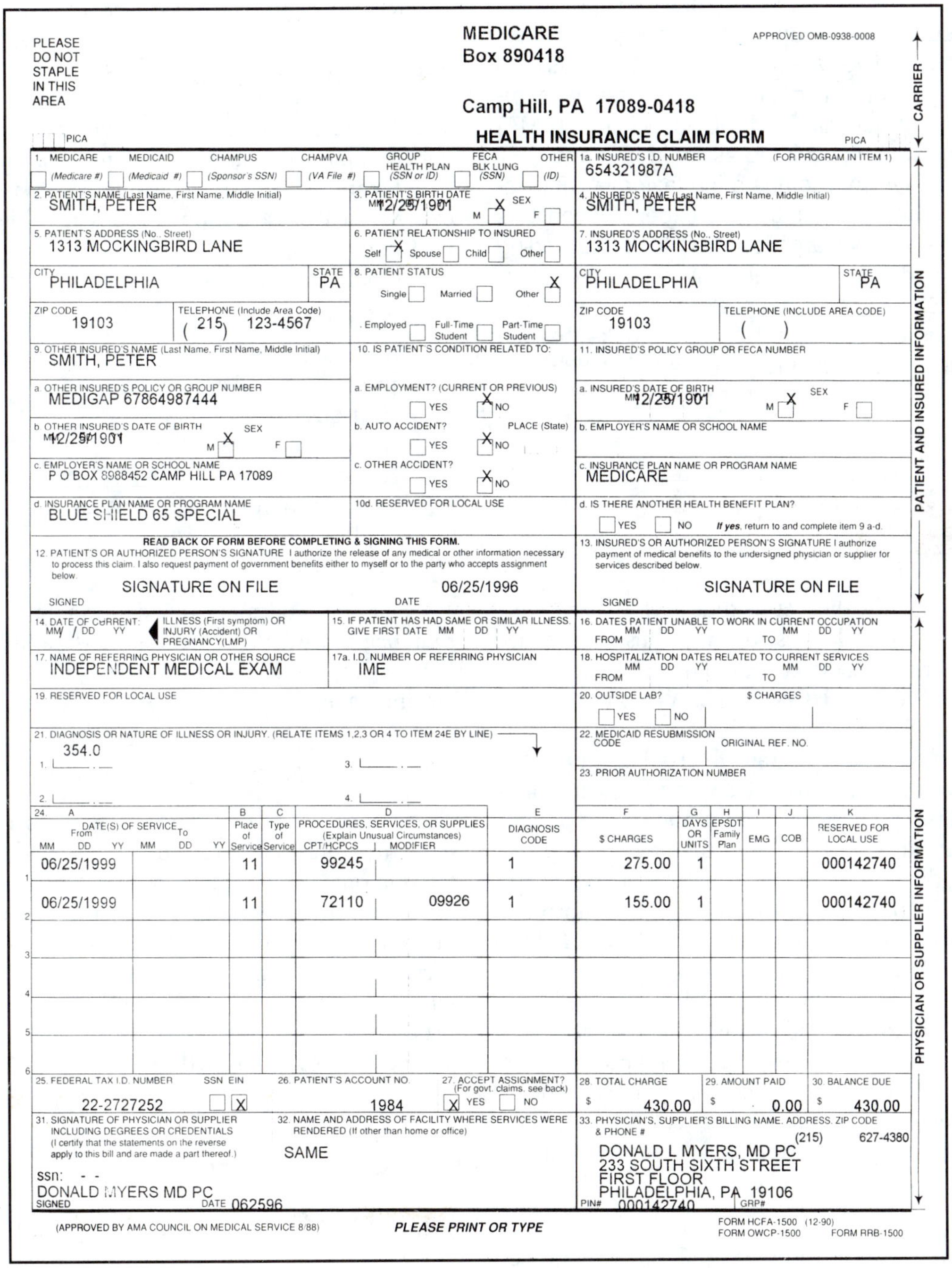

PLEASE DO NOT STAPLE IN THIS AREA

MEDICARE
Box 890418

Camp Hill, PA 17089-0418

APPROVED OMB-0938-0008

CARRIER

PICA

HEALTH INSURANCE CLAIM FORM

PICA

1. MEDICARE (Medicare #) MEDICAID (Medicaid #) CHAMPUS (Sponsor's SSN) CHAMPVA (VA File #) GROUP HEALTH PLAN (SSN or ID) FECA BLK LUNG (SSN) OTHER (ID)

1a. INSURED'S I.D. NUMBER (FOR PROGRAM IN ITEM 1): 654321987A

2. PATIENT'S NAME (Last Name, First Name, Middle Initial): SMITH, PETER

3. PATIENT'S BIRTH DATE: 12/25/1901 SEX M X F

4. INSURED'S NAME (Last Name, First Name, Middle Initial): SMITH, PETER

5. PATIENT'S ADDRESS (No., Street): 1313 MOCKINGBIRD LANE

6. PATIENT RELATIONSHIP TO INSURED: Self X Spouse Child Other

7. INSURED'S ADDRESS (No., Street): 1313 MOCKINGBIRD LANE

CITY: PHILADELPHIA STATE: PA

8. PATIENT STATUS: Single Married Other X; Employed Full-Time Student Part-Time Student

CITY: PHILADELPHIA STATE: PA

ZIP CODE: 19103 TELEPHONE (Include Area Code): (215) 123-4567

ZIP CODE: 19103 TELEPHONE (INCLUDE AREA CODE): ( )

9. OTHER INSURED'S NAME (Last Name, First Name, Middle Initial): SMITH, PETER

10. IS PATIENT'S CONDITION RELATED TO:

11. INSURED'S POLICY GROUP OR FECA NUMBER

a. OTHER INSURED'S POLICY OR GROUP NUMBER: MEDIGAP 67864987444

a. EMPLOYMENT? (CURRENT OR PREVIOUS) YES NO X

a. INSURED'S DATE OF BIRTH: 12/25/1901 SEX M X F

b. OTHER INSURED'S DATE OF BIRTH: 12/25/1901 SEX M X F

b. AUTO ACCIDENT? PLACE (State) YES NO X

b. EMPLOYER'S NAME OR SCHOOL NAME

c. EMPLOYER'S NAME OR SCHOOL NAME: P O BOX 8988452 CAMP HILL PA 17089

c. OTHER ACCIDENT? YES NO X

c. INSURANCE PLAN NAME OR PROGRAM NAME: MEDICARE

d. INSURANCE PLAN NAME OR PROGRAM NAME: BLUE SHIELD 65 SPECIAL

10d. RESERVED FOR LOCAL USE

d. IS THERE ANOTHER HEALTH BENEFIT PLAN? YES NO *If yes,* return to and complete item 9 a-d.

READ BACK OF FORM BEFORE COMPLETING & SIGNING THIS FORM.

12. PATIENT'S OR AUTHORIZED PERSON'S SIGNATURE I authorize the release of any medical or other information necessary to process this claim. I also request payment of government benefits either to myself or to the party who accepts assignment below.

SIGNED: SIGNATURE ON FILE DATE: 06/25/1996

13. INSURED'S OR AUTHORIZED PERSON'S SIGNATURE I authorize payment of medical benefits to the undersigned physician or supplier for services described below.

SIGNED: SIGNATURE ON FILE

PATIENT AND INSURED INFORMATION

14. DATE OF CURRENT: MM / DD YY ILLNESS (First symptom) OR INJURY (Accident) OR PREGNANCY(LMP)

15. IF PATIENT HAS HAD SAME OR SIMILAR ILLNESS. GIVE FIRST DATE MM DD YY

16. DATES PATIENT UNABLE TO WORK IN CURRENT OCCUPATION FROM MM DD YY TO MM DD YY

17. NAME OF REFERRING PHYSICIAN OR OTHER SOURCE: INDEPENDENT MEDICAL EXAM

17a. I.D. NUMBER OF REFERRING PHYSICIAN: IME

18. HOSPITALIZATION DATES RELATED TO CURRENT SERVICES FROM MM DD YY TO MM DD YY

19. RESERVED FOR LOCAL USE

20. OUTSIDE LAB? YES NO $ CHARGES

21. DIAGNOSIS OR NATURE OF ILLNESS OR INJURY. (RELATE ITEMS 1,2,3 OR 4 TO ITEM 24E BY LINE)

1. 354.0
2.
3.
4.

22. MEDICAID RESUBMISSION CODE ORIGINAL REF. NO.

23. PRIOR AUTHORIZATION NUMBER

24. A DATE(S) OF SERVICE From MM DD YY To MM DD YY	B Place of Service	C Type of Service	D PROCEDURES, SERVICES, OR SUPPLIES (Explain Unusual Circumstances) CPT/HCPCS	MODIFIER	E DIAGNOSIS CODE	F $ CHARGES	G DAYS OR UNITS	H EPSDT Family Plan	I EMG	J COB	K RESERVED FOR LOCAL USE
1 06/25/1999	11		99245		1	275.00	1				000142740
2 06/25/1999	11		72110	09926	1	155.00	1				000142740
3											
4											
5											
6											

25. FEDERAL TAX I.D. NUMBER: 22-2727252 SSN EIN X

26. PATIENT'S ACCOUNT NO.: 1984

27. ACCEPT ASSIGNMENT? (For govt. claims, see back) YES X NO

28. TOTAL CHARGE: $ 430.00

29. AMOUNT PAID: $ 0.00

30. BALANCE DUE: $ 430.00

31. SIGNATURE OF PHYSICIAN OR SUPPLIER INCLUDING DEGREES OR CREDENTIALS (I certify that the statements on the reverse apply to this bill and are made a part thereof.)

ssn: - -
DONALD MYERS MD PC
SIGNED DATE 062596

32. NAME AND ADDRESS OF FACILITY WHERE SERVICES WERE RENDERED (If other than home or office): SAME

33. PHYSICIAN'S, SUPPLIER'S BILLING NAME, ADDRESS, ZIP CODE & PHONE #: (215) 627-4380
DONALD L MYERS, MD PC
233 SOUTH SIXTH STREET
FIRST FLOOR
PHILADELPHIA, PA 19106
PIN# 000142740 GRP#

PHYSICIAN OR SUPPLIER INFORMATION

(APPROVED BY AMA COUNCIL ON MEDICAL SERVICE 8/88)

PLEASE PRINT OR TYPE

FORM HCFA-1500 (12-90)
FORM OWCP-1500 FORM RRB-1500

FIGURE 17-1
Sample insurance claim form for consultation and chest x-ray.

can be used with codes in that particular section. Failure to use an appropriate modifier causes database and billing errors.

If you have a question about coding, **never** guess; find the correct answer. For example, you can ask colleagues, office managers, or even the physician. Insurance companies may have a "help line" to assist you. If you are a member of a professional health care organization, network with fellow members. The American Medical Association (AMA) publishes various books to assist in ICD and CPT coding. The AMA also has a magazine—"CPT Assistant"—that is written by CPT experts. It contains many articles that are designed to make coding easier. In addition, this magazine will keep you current with updates and changes. For further information on the CPT Assistant or other books that the AMA publishes on coding, call 1-800-621-8335.

HCFA's Common Procedure Coding System (HCPCS)

Because CPT-4 codes did not include such items as ambulance service, wheelchairs, or injections, HCFA designed another coding system based on the CPT-4. This system is referred to as **HCPCS** (HCFA's Common Procedure Coding System).

HCPCS uses codes contained in CPT-4 plus expanded codes developed by HCFA and fiscal intermediaries to classify physician and nonphysician patient care services. Since 1985, physicians have had to use HCPCS to bill for services provided to Medicare patients either in the medical office or in the hospital. Since October 1986, physicians also have used HCPCS to bill for services provided to Medicaid patients.

Beginning July 1, 1987, federal law required hospitals to use HCPCS to report outpatient surgery services to patients receiving health benefits sponsored by the federal government. By October 1, 1987, federal law had extended ambulatory surgical center (ASC) prospective payment methodology to hospital outpatient surgical payments. The purpose of this was twofold:

- To permit identification of ASC surgery procedures so a blended payment rate could be applied to ambulatory surgery performed in the hospital outpatient department

- To provide a database for future prospective payment amounts for all hospital outpatient services

HCPCS includes three levels of codes, which are discussed below.

HCPCS Level 1 Codes

Level 1 codes are in CPT-4. This is a listing of terms and codes that provide a means to report physician's procedures and services under both private and government-sponsored health insurance programs.

HCPCS Level 2 Codes: National Codes

This listing comes out once a year in a National Coding Manual. The National Coding Manual can be ordered from the American Hospital Association, American Medical Association, or other publishers of the CPT coding book.

It includes codes for:

- Chemotherapeutic drugs
- Dental services
- Durable medical equipment
- Injections
- Ophthalmologic services
- Orthotics
- Some pathology and laboratory and rehabilitation supplies
- Vision care

National codes are five-digit alpha-numeric codes that begin with the letters A-V. (Example: L8100 is Elastic support, Elastic Stocking, Below knee, Medium weight, each).

HCPCS Level 3 Codes: Local Codes

These codes were developed to address regional coding—the ability to code something performed or offered in one state that may or may not be performed or offered in another state. These codes, which are produced and made available through your state Medicare carrier, may vary from state to state. Local codes begin with letters W-Z. HCFA takes full responsibility for the codes that go in the National Coding Manual, leaving local codes up to Medicare carriers in each state.

➤ REIMBURSEMENT

Diagnostic Related Groups (DRGs)

Diagnostic related groups (DRGs) are categories into which patients are placed according to the similarity of their diagnoses, treatment, and length of stay. Initially, these categories were developed by Yale University researchers in the mid 1970s to aid the process of utilization review. Some 13,000 codes were run through a computer and grouped according to their clinical similarities (including similarities in resources used). Today, DRGs are used to determine reimbursement for Medicare patients' inpatient services. The fee attached to each DRG is based on the national average of all Medicare discharges and is adjusted for regional differences in hospital wages and updates. Hospitals are paid a set amount for each DRG—regardless of actual costs for treating the patient. For example, if a hospital uses fewer resources to care for a patient and discharges that patient in less time, it may keep the difference between its actual cost and the DRG payment. Conversely, if the patient stays longer than usual and requires more services, the hospital absorbs the loss. A patient who has an unusually long stay or a complicated case is considered an outlier, and the hospital may be paid more than the standard DRG rate if the added expenses can be justified.

Assigning the correct ICD-9-CM code will influence the DRG to which the patient will be assigned. Selecting the proper DRG is based on:

- Principal diagnosis
- Surgeries
- Complications and comorbid conditions

Physicians can help with coding by:

- Recording the appropriate documentation to identify each patient's problems, complaints, or other reasons for the encounter or visit.
- Working with the medical records or the office coding and billing staffs to determine the proper diagnosis to code, using terminology that includes specific diagnoses as well as symptoms, problems, or reasons for the encounter (ICD-9-CM codes describe all of these)

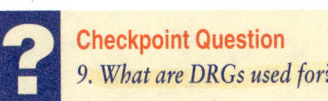

Checkpoint Question

9. What are DRGs used for?

Resource-Based Relative Value Scale (RBRVS)

As part of the 1989 Omnibus Budget Reconciliation Act (OBRA), Congress stipulated that reimbursement to physicians for Medicare services is based on a fee schedule. This fee schedule sets a maximal fee for each service based on the **resource-based relative value scale (RBRVS)**. The goal of RBRVS is to reduce

Medicare Part B costs and to establish national standard for coding and payment. The system requires the use of the Evaluation and Management codes in CPT-4.

A fee is calculated based on the following factors:

- Intensity of the service
- Time required
- Skills needed
- Overhead expenses
- Malpractice premiums

The particular fee is adjusted by a geographical practice cost index (GPCI), which reflects the difference in health care costs in different parts of the country. Finally, a conversion factor (CF) is applied.

➤ FRAUD AND CODING

Even though the physician you work for may have already been paid for a claim submitted, the medical office still may be audited. As a federal program, Medicare has the same authority as the Internal Revenue Service to audit claims and may do so retroactively. This means that an audit can occur even a couple of years after payment has been received for claims. If the medical practice is found to be in error, the physician may be required to repay an amount owed plus interest. Even worse, such errors can jeopardize the physician's ability to participate in Medicare funded programs.

To avoid costly errors, be certain that you can justify your coding. To do this, make sure that you:

- Keep adequate, accurate, and complete documentation

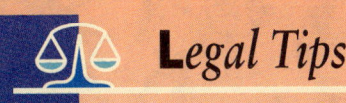

Legal Tips

When submitting Medicare or other insurance claims, **do not** bill for services the physician has not performed, and **do not** bill more for a service than it is worth by upcoding.

Millions of dollars have been budgeted to investigate fraud and abuse. Fiscal intermediaries randomly review and compare the documentation in the record and report their findings to the particular providers. Peer review organizations (PROs) have been authorized by HCFA to obtain medical records of Medicare beneficiaries for review. There also is a legislative mandate for Health Care Financing Administration (HCFA) to develop a method of reviewing records in the office setting.

- Use the proper tools to code
- Follow the coding rules by becoming familiar with new rules and keeping up to date on any changes to existing ones

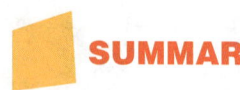

SUMMARY

Medical coding involves the use of numbers to describe diseases, injuries, and procedures. It has several purposes, including indexing medical records, performing medical care reviews, deriving health statistics, and reimbursing physicians and hospitals for services provided. Two main coding systems are used for claims reimbursement: ICD-9-CM and CPT-4. Each system is organized differently. As a medical assistant, you are responsible for knowing the format and usage of each one. Accurate and thorough coding is essential to ensure appropriate reimbursement. Because learning to code is an ongoing process, continuing education is vital. This can be accomplished by attending workshops in your geographic area or by joining a local association of coders, which may also sponsor coding problem clinics.

CRITICAL THINKING CHALLENGES

1. How would you handle a physician who you feel "over-bills" for procedures? To whom would you report this? How might you collect documentation of fraud?
2. Create a reminder card that could be used when you are to assist with coding.
3. Assume that you are working for a family practice physician. Identify three patient problems that you might encounter. Then use the CPT and ICD-9-CM coding books at your school library or the local hospital library to find the correct codes.

ANSWERS TO CHECKPOINT QUESTIONS

1. The three volumes in the ICD-9-CM coding book are the tabular list of diseases, the alphabetic index of diseases, and the alphabetic list and tabular list of procedures.
2. The World Health Organization must approve any disease classification changes.
3. Subcategory codes have four digits.
4. Appendix B covers psychiatric disorders.
5. CPT codes are updated annually.
6. The three key elements are history, physical examination, and medical decision-making.
7. The surgical package consists of local infiltration, digital blocks, topical anesthesia, the operation, and normal uncomplicated follow-up care.
8. There would be two codes: one for the service and one for the immunization.
9. DRGs are used to determine the reimbursement for Medicare patients' inpatient services.

SUGGESTIONS FOR FURTHER READING

Adams, W. L. (1995). *Adam's Guide to Coding and Reimbursement.* St. Louis: Mosby Lifeline.
Buck, C. J. (1996). *Step by Step Medical Coding.* Philadelphia: WB Saunders.

Health Insurance

Chapter Outline

Health Benefits Plans
    Group Health Benefits
    Individual Health Benefits
    Government-Sponsored (Public)
       Health Benefits
Filing Claims
    Electronic Claims Submission
    Explanation of Benefits
Managed Care
    Health Maintenance Organizations
      (HMOs)

Preferred Provider Organizations
    (PPOs)
Physician Hospital Organizations
Other Managed Care Programs
Policies in the Practice
Summary
Critical Thinking Challenges
Answers to Checkpoint Questions
Suggestions for Further Reading

18

DACUM Components

1.4   Maintain confidentiality
5.3   Use appropriate guidelines when releasing records or information
8.3   Analyze and use current third-party guidelines for reimbursement

Chapter Competencies

Learning Objectives

Upon successfully completing this chapter, you will be able to:

1. Spell and define the Key Terms.
2. Describe group, individual, and government-sponsored (public) health benefits and explain the differences between them.
3. Explain the differences between Medicare and Medicaid.
4. List the information required on a medical claim form and explain why each piece of information is needed.
5. Name two legal issues affecting claims submissions.
6. Explain how managed care programs work.
7. Explain the differences between health maintenance organizations (HMOs), preferred provider organizations (PPOs), and physician hospital organizations.

Performance Objectives

Upon successfully completing this chapter, you will be able to:

1. Fill out a HCFA 1500 claim form.

Key Terms

(See Glossary and Box 18-1 for definitions.)

assignment of
  benefits
balance billing
birthday rule
capitation
carrier
claim
claims
  administrator
coinsurance
coordination of
  benefits
co-payment
crossover claim
deductible

dependent
disability
eligibility
employee
explanation of
  benefits (EOB)
fee-for-service
fee schedule
group member
health maintenance
  organization
  (HMO)
independent practice
  association (IPA)
insurance

insured
managed care
peer review
  organization
physician hospital
  organization
plan maximums
pre-existing condition
preferred provider
  organization (PPO)
third-party
  administrator (TPA)
usual, customary, and
  reasonable
utilization review

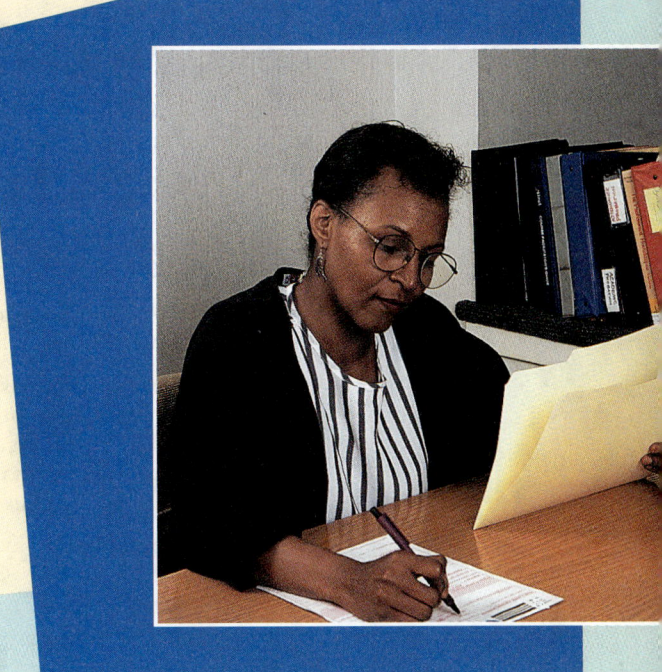

Health benefits plans were initially offered to Americans in the 1930s. Blue Cross plans, the first available, were offered by hospitals to cover the costs of hospitalization. Health benefits were originally intended to protect families from catastrophic financial burdens in the event of a serious illness or accident. A few years later, however, Blue Shield plans were introduced to pay for the portion of medical fees charged by physicians. Blue Shield plans were developed by medical societies and operate as nonprofit entities, as allowed by state regulations.

Today, virtually every state has a Blue Cross and a Blue Shield plan. Health benefits also are provided by insurance companies, self-funded group plans, and government plans such as Medicare and Medicaid. The benefits available vary with each plan and from state to state.

Approximately 80% of Americans are enrolled in health benefits plans. Consequently, most of the patients you will encounter in the physician's office will have some type of health insurance. As a medical assistant, you will need to understand the differences in health benefits plans and the requirements of each so that you can complete and file **claim** forms appropriately. You will also need to learn the special terminology associated with health insurance claims (Box 18-1). In addition, you may need to instruct patients about filling out claim forms.

BOX 18-1 Important Health Insurance Terms and Concepts

Assignment of Benefits: The patient gives written authorization for the claims administrator to reimburse the physician for billed charges. An assignment of benefits is necessary if the physician agrees not to collect fees from the patient but to wait for payment from the claims administrator.

Balance Billing: If the patient is billed the difference between what the claims administrator paid and what the physician's charges actually were, the patient is balance billed. Most managed care contracts prohibit the physician from balance billing the patient.

Birthday Rule: If a dependent child is covered by the benefit plans of both parents, the plan of the parent whose birthday falls earliest in the calendar year (*not* the oldest parent) is primary. The birthday rule is used by benefit plans and claims administrators to coordinate the benefits of dependent children covered by two plans.

Capitation: A capitated plan is one that pays the provider a flat amount per covered member, regardless of services provided, rather than on a fee-for-service basis. Health Maintenance Organizations are often capitated.

Carrier: An insurance company that insures a medical benefit plan is often referred to as the carrier.

Claim: A written and documented request for reimbursement of an eligible expense under a plan. Making a claim for benefits payable.

Claims Administrator: This may be an insurance company, a third-party administrator (see p. 246), or other entity responsible for the examination and processing of claims. The adjudication of a claim is at the discretion of the claims administrator in accordance with the provisions of the benefit plan. Claims are submitted to the claims administrator by the provider or patient.

Coinsurance: A benefit plan pays a percentage of the eligible benefits after the deductible has been paid. The percentage not paid by the plan is the coinsurance portion for which the patient is responsible.

Coordination of Benefits: If a patient has benefits under more than one plan, the benefits are coordinated to determine how much each plan pays.

(continued)

BOX 18-1   Important Health Insurance Terms and Concepts *(Continued)*

Co-payment (or co-pay): An amount specified by the plan that the patient pays for a service before the plan pays. Commonly used in managed care plans, a small co-pay for each office visit is paid by the patient.

Crossover Claim: When a patient is eligible for both Medicare and Medicaid, the claim is referred to as a crossover claim.

Deductible: The amount of eligible charges each patient must pay each calendar year before the plan begins to pay benefits. For example, if the plan deductible is $200 per calendar year, the first $200 of eligible expenses incurred by the patient is the responsibility of that patient. Eligible charges beyond the $200 are then paid according to plan provisions.

Dependent: A person who is covered by a benefit plan by virtue of their relationship to the employee, member, or insured. A spouse or child may be covered dependents. Dependents must meet specific eligibility requirements as set forth in the plan.

Disability: An illness or injury that prevents a person from performing routine tasks and therefore requires an absence from employment.
Disability benefits require ongoing verification by the physician.

Eligibility: Criteria defined by each plan that determine who may receive benefits under the plan.

Employee: In group health plans, the employee is a person who, by virtue of employment, may participate and receive benefits from the group health plan. In group health plans, the term employee has the same meaning as member.

Explanation of Benefits (EOB): The claims administrator prepares and issues an EOB explaining how the claim was settled, indicating deductible, coinsurance, and ineligible information.

Fee-for-service: A common term describing physician reimbursement based on the services provided, in contrast to a capitated or prepaid plan.

Fee Schedule: A schedule of the amount that will be paid by the plan for each procedure or service. This fee schedule is determined by the claims administrator and applied to claims that are subject to the fee schedule by virtue of the provider's managed care contract.

Group Member: A person covered by a health benefits plan, usually referring to the primary person covered (not to covered dependents of the member).

Health Maintenance Organization (HMO): A group of physicians and other health care providers who have a contractual arrangement to provide services to subscribers (participating patients) on a capitated or negotiated fee-for-service basis.

Independent Practice Association (IPA): In the narrowest sense, several independently practicing physicians contracted with an HMO to provide services to HMO members.

Insurance: The term insurance is widely used to refer to a health benefits plan, whether the plan is insured or self-funded. Technically, the term insurance refers to health benefits plans that are funded by an insurance contract.

Insured: A person who is covered by a health benefits plan.

(continued)

BOX 18-1 Important Health Insurance Terms and Concepts *(Continued)*

Managed Care: A term used to describe a feature of many health benefits plans that requires such things as precertification of hospitalizations, documented and approved referrals for specialist care, benefits payments in accordance with a fee schedule, and other requirements for claims payment. Managed care contracts with physicians require the physician to provide specified services.

Peer Review Organization: Also referred to as the Professional Review Standards Organization (PRSO). This is a group of physicians who review cases for appropriateness and hospitalizations and discharges.

Physician Hospital Organization: An entity owned and managed by a hospital and physicians to deliver a managed care product.

Plan Maximum: Benefit plans may restrict or limit the amount of benefit payable for a certain benefit to an annual maximum or a lifetime benefit.

Pre-existing Condition: Plans may exclude coverage for a specified period of time for a condition that existed prior to the patient joining the health plan. The condition is referred to as pre-existing.

Preferred Provider Organization (PPO): An organization sponsored by a hospital or group of physicians or owned and marketed by an insurance company or other entity. A physician who is contracted with a PPO is considered a participating provider.

Third-Party Administrator (TPA): A claims administrator who provides claims processing services for the sponsor of a self-funded benefit plan. The plan sponsor (usually an employer) contracts with the TPA to process claims and provide other administrative services to the health plan.

Usual, Customary, and Reasonable: A data base of charges for each procedure indicating the charge of the majority of physicians in a geographic area. Plans that are not subject to a fee schedule are administered by UCR. If the physician's charges exceed the UCR limit, any amount over that limit will be considered ineligible and not considered for payment.

Utilization Review (or Utilization Management): A term used to describe plan requirements to obtain prior approval for certain services, most often inpatient hospitalizations.

➤ HEALTH BENEFITS PLANS

Group Health Benefits

Group health benefits are sponsored by an organization such as an employer, a union, or an association. A person covered by group health benefits is either an **employee** or a **group member**, who, by virtue of employment or membership in an organization, may participate in and receive benefits from a health plan.

Benefits may be either **insured** or *self-funded*. Commonly, health benefits are referred to as **insurance**. However, it is important to distinguish between the actual benefits and the vehicle used to fund and provide them.

With *insured benefits*, a monthly premium is paid by the employer or organization to an insurance company. The insurance company, in turn, is obligated to pay for any eligible health benefits. In contrast, *self-funded benefits* are provided to eligible employees or members by their employer or organization. Claims are processed by a professional **claims administrator**, such as a **third-party administrator (TPA)**. The claims are paid from the sponsor's funds. Many employers now choose to self-fund their group benefit plans rather than insure them.

You will need to be aware of these funding differences as they relate to state and federal regulations. For instance, insured benefit plans are subject to state regulations. Many states mandate that certain types of benefits be included in any insurance plan. These mandated benefits vary from state to state but often include such medical services as childhood immunizations, routine diagnostic care, and treatment for substance abuse.

Self-funded benefit plans are not subject to these state-mandated benefits. However, they must comply with federal regulations issued in 1974 as the Employee Retirement Income Security Act, often referred to as ERISA. Although this law does not mandate specific benefits, it contains complex rules regarding the individual rights of employees and the funding of claims.

Checkpoint Question

1. What is the difference between an insured benefits plan and one that is self-funded?

You also need to understand that although a plan designed and funded by insurance companies has the same benefits for all employers or organizations that buy that particular plan, every self-funded benefit plan is different. Each sponsor develops and designs the benefit provisions for their self-funded plan, so these kinds of plans can vary dramatically from one organization to another.

For the group benefit plan to cover (pay for) eligible expenses, the patient must meet several criteria, called **eligibility** requirements. These are defined in the policy or plan document and may include a minimum number of hours worked per week and a waiting period from the date of employment until benefits are effective.

Eligibility is based on criteria to be met by the employee or member. The eligibility of **dependents** (spouse and children) is based on the employee's eligibility. Certain eligibility limitations apply to dependent children. For example, children are eligible until they reach the limiting age as defined by the plan. The age limitation is usually extended if the child is a full-time student. Most plans also require that children be the unmarried natural or adopted children of the employee, unmarried stepchildren, or children for whom the employee has legal guardianship.

To confirm a patient's eligibility, call the claims administrator for the health benefits plan. A provider inquiry telephone number is commonly included on the patient's identification (ID) card (Fig. 18-1).

Individual Health Benefits

Individual health benefits policies are purchased by an individual from an insurance company. The premiums are submitted by the individual directly to the insurance company, and the company then reimburses the covered individual for eligible medical expenses.

Individual health policies are underwritten; that is, the applicant must disclose any health-related matters and health history. Only applicants who are determined by the insurance company not to be at a high health risk are insured.

For patients with individual health benefits, the criteria for completing and filing claims is the same as for patients with group health benefits. However, individual health policies commonly have less generous coverage than group health plans. An individual policy may also have a rider that limits or eliminates benefits for certain illnesses or injuries, based on the determination of the underwriter at the time the policy was issued.

Government-Sponsored (Public) Health Benefits

Government sponsored benefit programs are funded and regulated by the federal or state governments. Government programs have been developed over the years to assist persons who do not otherwise have health benefits, such as the elderly, the indigent, and others unable to obtain benefits. Government programs include Medicare, Medicaid, CHAMPUS/CHAMPVA, and Workers' Compensation.

Medicare

Initially, Medicare was designed to provide medical care and benefits for the elderly population. Medicare has since been expanded to provide benefits for persons of any age with end-stage renal disease (ESRD) as well as for blind or disabled persons. The medical costs of organ donors and recipients are now also covered by Medicare benefits. The Medicare patients you will probably encounter most often are the elderly.

Patients may have part A or parts A and B of Medicare. Persons who are entitled to Social Security are automatically enrolled in Medicare part A, which covers hospital services and expenses only, after an annual **deductible**. Medicare part B covers the physician's charges for inpatient or outpatient care as well as diagnostic services, after an annual deductible (which increases each year). Part B does not cover routine examinations, well care, routine immunizations, or cosmetic surgery. Eligible persons electing to participate in the Medicare part B program must pay a monthly premium for these benefits.

A patient with Medicare coverage who is actively employed and covered by the employer's plan will have secondary Medicare benefits. A retired person age 65 or over who has retirement or private supple-

(Front)

(Back)

ABC Insurance Company

1-800-555-5555
Provider Inquiry: 1-555-555-5555

Employee: Jane Doe

Employer: XYZ Company

SSN: 555-55-5555

Pre-certification Requirements: You must call ABC
Company for authorization prior to any hospital
admission. For emergency admissions, you must call
within 48 hours of admission . Failure to comply will
result in a reduction of benefits.

Submit all claims to: ABC Company
555 Fifth Avenue
New York, NY

(Front)

(Back)

ABC Insurance Company - Managed Network

1-800-555-5555
Provider Inquiry: 1-555-555-5555

Employee: Jane Doe

Employer: XYZ Company

SSN: 555-55-5555

Coverage: Family

All non-emergency medical care must be provided by
your Primary Care Physician. Office visit charges of
your Primary Care Physician are subject to a $10.00
co-pay.
You or your physician must pre-certify any non-emergency hospital admission; failure to do so will result in a
reduction of benefits. In the event of emergency, you or
your physician must certify your hospitalization within
48 hours of admission to avoid a reduction in benefits.

FIGURE 18-1

ID card samples. (*A*) Identification card for a plan requiring pre-certification or hospitalizations. (*B*) Identification card for a managed care plan.

mental benefits will have primary Medicare benefits.
Physicians are required to submit claims to Medicare
on behalf of Medicare patients. These claims must be
filed within 1 year of the time the service is incurred.
(See section "Filing Claims," p. 250, for more information.)

After the deductible has been met, Medicare reimburses to the physician 80% of the Medicare-
approved charges. The patient is then responsible for
the remaining 20% of the Medicare-approved fee. The
patient may not be subject to **balance billing** for the
difference between the physician's charges and the
Medicare-approved charges. If patients are financially
unable to pay the 20%, they may also be eligible for
Medicaid. This is referred to as a **crossover claim** because the patient is eligible under both Medicare and
Medicaid and the claim crosses over from one cover-

age to the other. In this situation, Medicare is primary
and Medicaid is secondary. Medicare will accept original claims (no copies) filed on HCFA 1500 claim
forms only.

The Health Care Financial Administration (known
as HCFA) is a government agency that oversees the financial aspects of health care in the United States.
HCFA has adopted a revised Current Procedural Terminology (CPT) coding system, which must be used
for Medicare claims. Medicare B claims use the standard CPT codes. For services not listed in the CPT code,
HCFA has established Health Care Procedural Coding
System (HCPCS) codes. (See Chap. 17, Diagnostic and
Procedural Coding, for more information.)

It is important to inquire of the patient regarding
supplemental or Medigap coverage. Some Medicare patients purchase a policy to cover those charges not cov-

ered by Medicare. In this case, a second claim filing becomes necessary.

Medicaid

This government-sponsored program provides health benefits to low-income or indigent persons. Often, eligibility for Medicaid is based on a patient's eligibility for other state programs, such as welfare assistance. The federal government provides funds to each state for Medicaid costs; each state is then required to provide a Medicaid program. Although the federal government stipulates the minimum coverage, states can provide coverage beyond the federally required minimums. Therefore, Medicaid eligibility and benefits vary from state to state. At a minimum, Medicaid provides coverage for:

- Inpatient hospital care
- Outpatient treatment and services
- Diagnostic services
- Family planning services
- Skilled nursing facilities
- Diagnostic screenings for children

Medicaid patients receive a new ID card each month. Make a photocopy of the card for the patient's file on the first visit of each month. Most states require prior authorization before any services are rendered. Not all physicians accept Medicaid patients; they are not required to do so. However, if Medicaid patients are accepted, certain important regulations must be followed. Because requirements vary from state to state, you need to be familiar with Medicaid as administered in your state.

CHAMPUS/CHAMPVA

The Civilian Health and Medical Program of the Uniformed Services (CHAMPUS) is a part of the U.S. Department of Defense and provides supplemental medical coverage for dependents of active service personnel, dependents of service personnel who died dur- ing active duty, and retired service personnel. If a patient lives within 40 miles of a uniformed services hospital, a statement of nonavailability is required for treatment by a physician's office or civilian hospital. This statement means that the local uniformed services hospital is unable to provide the required care. Patients who live more than 40 miles from a uniformed services hospital do not need this statement to receive care.

The *Civilian Health and Medical Program of the Veterans Administration* (CHAMPVA) covers dependents of veterans who have total and permanent service-connected disabilities. The CHAMPVA program is administered by the area Veterans Administration hospital. Once admitted to the CHAMPVA program, patients select their own physician.

Workers' Compensation

Employees in every state are covered by a Workers' Compensation program administered by the state. Workers' Compensation benefits were developed to cover the expenses resulting from a work-related illness or injury. In the event of a work-related illness or injury, claims submitted to the group or individual health benefits plan will be returned with direction to file with the Workers' Compensation administrator, who determines the validity of the claim and reimburses accordingly. For this reason, it is important to determine at the time services are rendered if the illness or injury is work-related and, if so, to separately account and file for those services.

You are responsible for knowing your state's Workers' Compensation regulations and procedures. Consult your state's office for Workers' Compensation or your state's designated claims administrator of the Workers' Compensation program for specific information.

Focus on the Patient: Ensuring Fair Treatment

All patients must be treated equally and fairly. Financial issues regarding the patient's type of insurance or lack of insurance should have no bearing on the care you provide. As a medical assistant, you must avoid stereotyping and care for the patient in an objective, professional manner.

➤ FILING CLAIMS

If the provider requires patients to make full payment on examination, the physician *may* still submit a claim on the patient's behalf; however, the patient may need to submit claims to the claims administrator for reimbursement. However, most providers will accept **assignment of benefits**. To do this, the patient must give written authorization for the claims administrator to reimburse the physician for billed charges. The medical assistant is responsible for obtaining all necessary claims information from the provider and the patient, then submitting a claim for payment to the claims administrator.

The patient's ID card is one source of information necessary for complete and accurate claims submission. Keep a copy of this card in the patient's file and be sure to update it regularly because the patient's employment and eligibility may change.

In addition, a patient may be covered by more than one group plan. For example, a patient may be covered as an employee on the employer's group plan and as a dependent on the spouse's group plan. The primary plan—the one that pays first—is the plan provided by the patient's employer. Any unpaid amount is then considered for payment by the spouse's group plan, which is considered secondary. This is called **co-ordination of benefits**.

Dependent children may be covered under only one parent's plan or under each parent's plan. Unless the plans state otherwise, the plan of the parent whose birthday occurs first each calendar year (not necessarily the oldest parent) is the primary plan. This is known as the **birthday rule**. This rule is commonly used by benefit plans and claims administrators to coordinate the benefits of dependent children covered by two plans. However, if the parents are legally separated or divorced, the primary plan is the plan of the parent who has custody or, in some instances, is subject to a court order or divorce decree.

After establishing the primary plan and the claims submission destination, the medical assistant prepares the claim for filing. The HCFA 1500 was developed by the American Medical Association to standardize an acceptable claim form for different plans and different claims administrators. It is the most widely used method of filing a health claim (Fig. 18-2). The HCFA 1500 is accepted by most claims administrators, including Blue Shield, Medicare, Medicaid, and CHAMPUS/CHAMPVA.

Most plans include a clause that excludes coverage for a stated period of time (usually 12 months) for a condition that existed before the plan's effective date (a **pre-existing condition**). For example, a patient with a diagnosis of depression before the effective date of his or her plan would be covered for all other conditions from the effective date forward, but would not be covered for services related to the diagnosis or treatment of depression for the pre-existing exclusion period (in this example, 12 months).

Many pieces of information are necessary for timely and efficient claims processing (Box 18-2). Claims with incomplete or inaccurate information cannot be processed and will be returned to the provider for completion, correction, and resubmission. This lengthens the time the provider must wait for reimbursement, making accurate claims submission a critical aspect of a medical assistant's responsibilities.

Ethical Tips

The following scenario might occur in a medical office:

While you are filing an insurance claim, the physician tells you to "readjust" the laceration length from 4 cm to 9 cm. (The physician can bill more for a 9-cm laceration.) When you question him about this, he says, "Don't worry. The patient isn't paying the difference, the insurance company is—and they have plenty of money." How should you handle this situation?

Ethically and legally, you cannot change the length of a laceration on the medical record or the bill. This is fraud. You need to explain to the physician that you are uncomfortable with this request and that you are ethically and legally bound to truthful billing.

A physician who operates in an unethical manner should be reported. If he is a partner in a practice, alert the other physicians about his actions. You can also contact your state medical association, the American Medical Association, or the institutional review board at the hospital where your physician is affiliated.

What If?

What if the reason for a rejection or denial of a claim is not clear?

If the reasons for denial of the claim are not clear, a telephone call to the claims administrator should provide the necessary information. Following is a list of the most frequent causes for denial of a claim and the corrective actions that you can take.

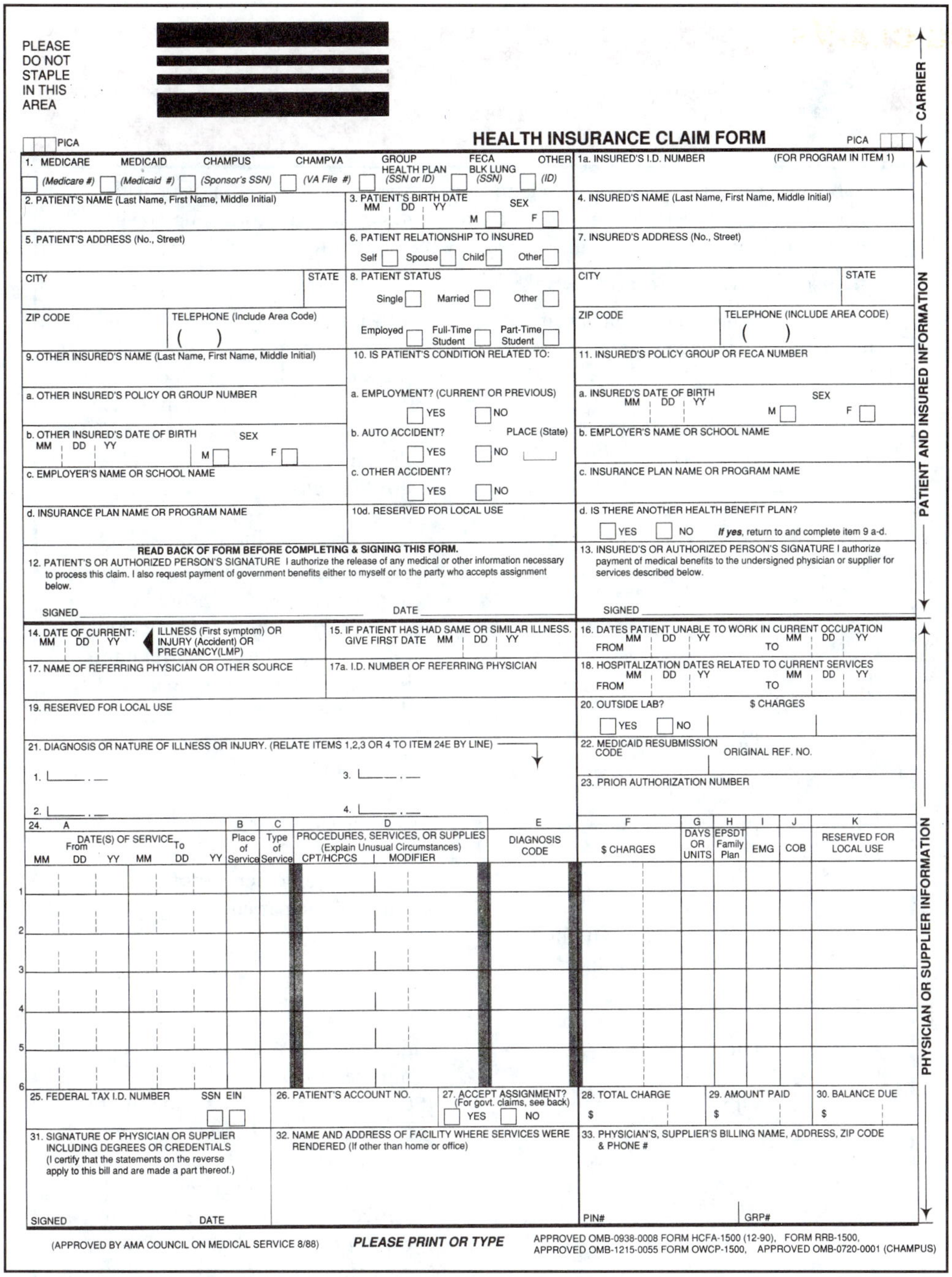
PLEASE DO NOT STAPLE IN THIS AREA

CARRIER

PICA

HEALTH INSURANCE CLAIM FORM

PICA

1. MEDICARE (Medicare #) MEDICAID (Medicaid #) CHAMPUS (Sponsor's SSN) CHAMPVA (VA File #) GROUP HEALTH PLAN (SSN or ID) FECA BLK LUNG (SSN) OTHER (ID)

1a. INSURED'S I.D. NUMBER (FOR PROGRAM IN ITEM 1)

2. PATIENT'S NAME (Last Name, First Name, Middle Initial)

3. PATIENT'S BIRTH DATE MM DD YY SEX M F

4. INSURED'S NAME (Last Name, First Name, Middle Initial)

5. PATIENT'S ADDRESS (No., Street)

6. PATIENT RELATIONSHIP TO INSURED Self Spouse Child Other

7. INSURED'S ADDRESS (No., Street)

CITY STATE

8. PATIENT STATUS Single Married Other

CITY STATE

ZIP CODE TELEPHONE (Include Area Code) ( )

Employed Full-Time Student Part-Time Student

ZIP CODE TELEPHONE (INCLUDE AREA CODE) ( )

9. OTHER INSURED'S NAME (Last Name, First Name, Middle Initial)

10. IS PATIENT'S CONDITION RELATED TO:

11. INSURED'S POLICY GROUP OR FECA NUMBER

a. OTHER INSURED'S POLICY OR GROUP NUMBER

a. EMPLOYMENT? (CURRENT OR PREVIOUS) YES NO

a. INSURED'S DATE OF BIRTH MM DD YY SEX M F

b. OTHER INSURED'S DATE OF BIRTH MM DD YY SEX M F

b. AUTO ACCIDENT? PLACE (State) YES NO

b. EMPLOYER'S NAME OR SCHOOL NAME

c. EMPLOYER'S NAME OR SCHOOL NAME

c. OTHER ACCIDENT? YES NO

c. INSURANCE PLAN NAME OR PROGRAM NAME

d. INSURANCE PLAN NAME OR PROGRAM NAME

10d. RESERVED FOR LOCAL USE

d. IS THERE ANOTHER HEALTH BENEFIT PLAN? YES NO *If yes*, return to and complete item 9 a-d.

READ BACK OF FORM BEFORE COMPLETING & SIGNING THIS FORM.

12. PATIENT'S OR AUTHORIZED PERSON'S SIGNATURE I authorize the release of any medical or other information necessary to process this claim. I also request payment of government benefits either to myself or to the party who accepts assignment below.

SIGNED DATE

13. INSURED'S OR AUTHORIZED PERSON'S SIGNATURE I authorize payment of medical benefits to the undersigned physician or supplier for services described below.

SIGNED

PATIENT AND INSURED INFORMATION

14. DATE OF CURRENT: MM DD YY ILLNESS (First symptom) OR INJURY (Accident) OR PREGNANCY(LMP)

15. IF PATIENT HAS HAD SAME OR SIMILAR ILLNESS. GIVE FIRST DATE MM DD YY

16. DATES PATIENT UNABLE TO WORK IN CURRENT OCCUPATION FROM MM DD YY TO MM DD YY

17. NAME OF REFERRING PHYSICIAN OR OTHER SOURCE

17a. I.D. NUMBER OF REFERRING PHYSICIAN

18. HOSPITALIZATION DATES RELATED TO CURRENT SERVICES FROM MM DD YY TO MM DD YY

19. RESERVED FOR LOCAL USE

20. OUTSIDE LAB? YES NO $ CHARGES

21. DIAGNOSIS OR NATURE OF ILLNESS OR INJURY. (RELATE ITEMS 1,2,3 OR 4 TO ITEM 24E BY LINE)

1. 2. 3. 4.

22. MEDICAID RESUBMISSION CODE ORIGINAL REF. NO.

23. PRIOR AUTHORIZATION NUMBER

24. A DATE(S) OF SERVICE From MM DD YY To MM DD YY; B Place of Service; C Type of Service; D PROCEDURES, SERVICES, OR SUPPLIES (Explain Unusual Circumstances) CPT/HCPCS MODIFIER; E DIAGNOSIS CODE; F $ CHARGES; G DAYS OR UNITS; H EPSDT Family Plan; I EMG; J COB; K RESERVED FOR LOCAL USE

1 2 3 4 5 6

PHYSICIAN OR SUPPLIER INFORMATION

25. FEDERAL TAX I.D. NUMBER SSN EIN

26. PATIENT'S ACCOUNT NO.

27. ACCEPT ASSIGNMENT? (For govt. claims, see back) YES NO

28. TOTAL CHARGE $

29. AMOUNT PAID $

30. BALANCE DUE $

31. SIGNATURE OF PHYSICIAN OR SUPPLIER INCLUDING DEGREES OR CREDENTIALS (I certify that the statements on the reverse apply to this bill and are made a part thereof.)

SIGNED DATE

32. NAME AND ADDRESS OF FACILITY WHERE SERVICES WERE RENDERED (If other than home or office)

33. PHYSICIAN'S, SUPPLIER'S BILLING NAME, ADDRESS, ZIP CODE & PHONE #

PIN# GRP#

(APPROVED BY AMA COUNCIL ON MEDICAL SERVICE 8/88) PLEASE PRINT OR TYPE APPROVED OMB-0938-0008 FORM HCFA-1500 (12-90), FORM RRB-1500, APPROVED OMB-1215-0055 FORM OWCP-1500, APPROVED OMB-0720-0001 (CHAMPUS)

FIGURE 18-2
HCFA 1500 form.

1. *The patient cannot be identified as a covered person*: Confirm that coverage information on file is current, including insurance company and group number and that the Social Security number is accurate.
2. *Coding is deemed inappropriate for services provided*: Review provided services and recode, as necessary.
3. *The patient is no longer covered by the plan*: Bill the patient for the charges. The patient may provide confirmation on new coverage.
4. *The data are incomplete*: Complete the required data and resubmit the claim.
5. *Services are not covered by the plan*: Bill the patient for the charges, unless there is a basis for an appeal.

Electronic Claims Submission

Although many practices continue to submit claims on paper through the mail, and most claims administrators continue to accept this practice, the use of electronic claims filing is growing rapidly. The physician's office computer software will include the HCFA 1500 format

text continues on page 254

BOX 18-2 Important Information Required on a Medical Claim

Because the HCFA 1500 is the claim form most frequently used, it is provided here as the example for completing a claim form. Other claim forms may be in different formats but will require essentially the same information.

Box #	Information to be Entered	Comments
1	Where the claim is being submitted	Confirm the patient's coverage and accuracy of your file information. A change in the patient's coverage will change how the claim is filed.
1a	The *insured*'s ID number	**Important:** It is the ID number of the "Insured" (or "Employee")—*not the patient*—that is required here. This is a frequent filing error and will result in the rejection of the claim. The insured's ID number is often the insured's Social Security number (SSN); check the ID card—the correct ID number required by the company may differ from the SSN.
2	Patient's name	The correct order is important (last, first, middle initial)
3	Patient's birthday	
4	Insured's name	Again, be sure that it is the name of the "insured" (or "employee") that is entered here—not the name of the patient.
5	Address of the patient	
6	Patient relationship to the insured	
7	Address of the insured	Check and update regularly.
8	Patient status	This will need to be checked and updated frequently.
9	Other insured's name	If the patient is covered under more than one plan, the second plan should be entered here. For example, if Jane's claim is being submitted to the insurance company for her employer but she is also covered under her husband Joe's plan, Joe's name would be listed here.
9a	Other insured's policy or group number	Joe's policy number would be entered here.
9b	Other insured's date of birth	Joe's date of birth and sex
9c	Employer's name or school name	The name of Joe's employer
9d	Insurance plan name or program name	The name of Joe's insurance company
10	Patient's condition	
10a	Patient's condition related to employment?	If yes, the claim should be submitted to the Worker's Compensation carrier.

(continued)

BOX 18-2   Important Information Required on a Medical Claim (Continued)

Box #	Information to be Entered	Comments
10b	Related to an auto accident?	If yes, the claim will not be processed unless a police report is attached.
10c	Other accident?	If yes, details of that accident must be attached for the claim to be processed.
11	Insured's policy group or Federal Employee Compensation Act (FECA) number	**Very important**—some payers will automatically return the claim if the group number is not indicated here. The group number will be on the patient's ID card.
11a	Insured's date of birth	Again note—this is the *insured*—not the patient
11b	Employer's name	The *insured*'s employer or school name
11c	Insurance plan name or pro-gram name	
11d	Is there another health plan?	If the patient is covered under more than one plan, check yes. If yes, the coverage will be coordinated between the plans covering the patient.
12	Patient's or authorized per-son's signature	This signature authorizes the release of information necessary to process the claim. If a "Signa-ture on File" has been signed and is in the patient file, then "Signa-ture on File" may be entered here.
13	Insured's signature	The signature of the insured
14	Date of current	This is not the date of service, but is the date the illness began, accident occurred
15	If patient has had same or similar illness	Has the patient had this illness in the past. If so, enter the date the patient first had this illness.
16	Is patient unable to work	This information is required for the patient to receive *disability* pay-ments.
17	Name of referring physician	If this patient was referred by another physician, enter that physician's name here.
17a	ID number of referring physician	Enter the Employer ID Number (EIN) of the physician who referred the patient
18	Hospitalization dates	If the patient has been hospitalized due to this illness or the reason for this visit, enter the dates of the hospitalization here

(continued)

BOX 18-2 Important Information Required on a Medical Claim *(Continued)*

Box #	Information to be Entered	Comments
20	Outside lab	If lab charges were incurred related to this visit and were provided by an outside lab, check yes and enter amount of charges. If not, simply check no.
21-24	Codes	The accuracy of the information entered in these sections determines the accuracy of the reimbursement received by the physician. A thorough understanding of coding is essential in completing this section. Please refer to Chap. 17.
25	Federal tax ID number	Enter the EIN of the physician
26	Patient's account number	If you have an account number assigned to the patient, enter that number here
27	Accept assignment?	If you will accept assignment of the benefits, check yes. If not, check no
28	Total charge	Enter the total amount of charges for this visit or service
29	Amount paid	Enter here any amount paid by the patient
30	Balance due	Subtract any amount paid from the total charge and enter that amount here
31	Signature of physician	
32	Name and address of facility where services were rendered	If the service was rendered outside of the physician's office, enter that address here
33	Physician's billing name, addresss, zip code and phone	This is the information that will be used to mail reimbursement. Be sure it is current. Note that the physician's billing name is required—this may be a practice or corporate name. If so, be sure to enter that billing name here.

for convenient and automated claims filing. With a computer and a modem, health claims can be filed immediately, reducing the time for the reimbursement cycle.

Several regional and national clearinghouses receive health benefits claims and electronically direct them to the appropriate claims administrators. This system allows you to file all electronic claims through one clearinghouse, rather than filing separately to hundreds of claims administrators.

The system requires that all fields on the electronic claim form are completed and in the required format. If the claim is incomplete or inaccurate, the system will interrupt the electronic transmission. You can make the completion or correction on-line, and the transmission can continue.

Claims submitted electronically that do not meet the criteria will be rejected by the clearinghouse and must be submitted by mail. In addition, claims that are

Legal Tips

Keeping patient information *confidential* is a primary concern in the medical practice. You should not release any information about the patient to any party, including the claims administrator, without the written authorization of the patient or the patient's guardian. Obtain a written authorization to release information from each patient on his or her first visit to the practice. Keep this information in the individual patient's file. Any claims submitted to the claims administrator by the physician's office must have "signature on file" on the claim form. With written authorization for the release of information, only such information as is pertinent to the claim and necessary for the processing of that claim should be released. Releasing any patient information without written consent is a breach of confidentiality.

Another legal issue sometimes encountered by the medical assistant is a request to misrepresent diagnoses or services rendered on the claim form or to alter the date the services were incurred. To do so would be considered *fraud*. Any requests to alter or misrepresent the medical records or claims of a patient must be firmly denied.

It is also fraudulent to misrepresent or expand the services rendered on the coding of a claim so as to receive additional reimbursement. "Unbundling" procedures so as to receive a greater reimbursement is also fraudulent. "Unbundling" refers to the practice of submitting a claim with several separate procedure codes rather than the single code that represents the services performed. Most payers now have software that will detect such practices and reject the claim.

particularly complicated or cumbersome, have attachments, or are otherwise unsuitable for electronic submission should be filed on paper with the claims administrator.

Explanation of Benefits

When the claims administrator settles a claim, that is, makes a payment, an **explanation of benefits** (EOB) statement is issued to both the provider and the patient (Fig. 18-3). The EOB statement tells how the payment was made, including deductible and **coinsurance** information. Some EOB statements include information for several claims that may have been processed during a particular time period. You will be responsible for checking the EOB to be sure that all payments made to the physician are for the appropriate procedures and in the correct amounts.

➤ MANAGED CARE

Throughout the 1970s and 1980s and into the 1990s health care costs in the United States grew at about twice the general rate of inflation. As a result, the United States now spends more for health care services than any other industrialized nation, both as a percentage of gross national product and on a per person basis. At the same time, a smaller percentage of our population has health insurance coverage than is true for other advanced nations.

In the United States, most people obtain health coverage through their employer. The exceptions are Medicare and CHAMPUS for the elderly and military dependents, the Medicaid programs for low-income Americans, and those who do not have access to group coverage and buy coverage directly from insurers. In total, these programs cover fewer people than employer-paid health plans.

The rapid rate of health care inflation affected the premiums paid by employers. Health premiums grew so quickly that they began to reduce the profitability of companies that offered health benefits to their employees and the amount these companies could afford to pay their employees. In response, employers began to offer **managed care** programs, which were less costly than traditional insurance coverage systems. Managed care programs vary greatly from one another but all involve a different relationship between the insurer, health care provider, and the covered individual. To understand this difference, we will first discuss the traditional insurance system.

In traditional insurance systems, the covered person (patient) may seek care from any provider. Normally the patient and physician decide what care is needed. Then services are rendered and the insurer pays a portion of the provider's bills (after deductibles and coinsurance). The insurer has no relationship with the provider.

In managed care systems, the insurer has a contractual relationship with the provider. The contract usually establishes what prices will be charged for each service and the conditions under which a service would be covered. Most managed care programs contain the following elements:

- *Precertification of hospital admissions (often also called utilization management or* **utilization re-**

Explanation of Benefits

Employee Name: Joe Doe   Date of Service: 6-15-96

SSN: 555-55-5555   ①   Provider: Dr. Jekyll

Group No. 55555   Provider TIN: 35-5555555

Patient Name: Joe Doe

Date of Service ②	Comment Code ③	Amount of Charge ④	Amount Allowed ⑤	At ⑥	Amount Paid ⑦
6-15-96	57	87.00	82.00	80%	65.60

Total ⑧	65.60
Less Deductible ⑨	25.00
Amount Paid ⑩	40.60

Payable to: Dr. Jekyll
                 Address

Comment Code:
57 - The amount charged exceeds Usual and Customary

Reading the EOB (Explanation of Benefits)

After the claim has been processed, an EOB will be issued. Although each payer has his or her own EOB format, this sample EOB illustrates the key points included in an EOB. The terms used may differ, and the formats will differ widely.

① The top section typically includes the name of the employee and the Social Security number (SSN) or other identifying number, as well as the name of the patient, the group number, the date of service and provider name and employer identification number (EIN) (Federal identification number assigned to the physician).

② The date of service is included and is shown as the date the service is actually rendered, not the date that it was posted or billed.

③ The Comment Code is a tool used on many EOBs to indicate a coded comment that is either printed on the back or explained at the bottom. In this case, the Code 57 is explained on the bottom as exceeding "Usual and Customary." In this situation, the claim will be processed on the Usual and Customary amount. The difference between the amount charged ($87.00) and the amount allowed ($82.00) is $5.00. Unless the physician is contractually bound by an agreement with a managed care plan that forbids the practice of balance billing, that difference of $5.00 may be billed to the patient.

④ Amount of Charge shows the amount that the physician's office billed for the service.

⑤ Amount Allowed shows the amount of charge upon which the claim processing will be based (in this example, it is the amount of Usual and Customary).

⑥ This indicates the percentage of co-insurance payable by the plan.

⑦ Amount Paid shows the amount payable by the plan after co-insurance has been applied, but is not necessarily the amount that is actually paid (see #10).

⑧ The Total shows the total submitted and payable after the claim has been processed.

⑨ After all processing on the claim has been completed, any deductible is applied. In this example, Joe still had $25.00 to be applied to his annual deductible. Therefore, $25.00 is deducted from the amount paid and the actual reimbursement to the physician is $40.60. The amount applied to the deductible should be billed to the patient.

⑩ The amount actually reimbursed.

FIGURE 18-3
Explanation of benefits (EOB) statement.

view—UM or UR). A patient can be admitted to a hospital for certain conditions only if that admission has been certified (approved) by the insurer. The goal of this requirement is to ensure that a patient's care is provided in the most cost-effective setting. For example, many surgical procedures that used to require an inpatient hospital stay can now be performed in an outpatient setting if proper education and support are available to the patient. Conflict between a UR guideline and the physician's requirements for the patient can be sent to an impartial **peer review organization** comprised of physicians and specialists who will review the case and make the final recommendation.

- *Approved referrals.* In many managed care plans a specialty physician can provide services to a managed care patient only on referral from the patient's primary care physician. The purpose is to ensure that the services provided by the specialist are medically necessary and, again, provided in the most cost-effective setting.

- *Network.* A network consists of those providers (physicians, hospitals, pharmacies, and other providers and suppliers) who have signed contracts with the insurer or health maintenance organization (HMO) to provide services to covered persons in individual, group, or public health plans. A patient is normally required to use network providers to receive full coverage. The financial penalties (lost coverage) are often very high if a patient does not use these providers.

- *Assignment of benefits.* The network provider cannot bill the patient for any amounts not paid by the insurer (no balance billing) except for **co-payments**, coinsurance, and deductibles. If payment for a service provided by a network physician or hospital is denied by the insurer because it was not properly authorized, the provider cannot bill the patient for these services. This puts teeth into the control features of the managed care program.

Most physicians have contracts with more than one managed care program and each of these programs will have different requirements and different reimbursement schedules. To provide the health care services needed by the patient while ensuring that the physician is paid for his or her services, you should understand the requirements of each patient's program. From this perspective, the UM or precertification requirements are extremely important. Check the patient's ID card for details. UM requirements may only apply to inpatient services but many apply to a variety of outpatient and doctor office services. Until you are very familiar with the requirements of each of your patient's managed care programs, you

should call the number on the ID card before a patient is admitted to a hospital (on a nonemergency basis), referred to another physician, or scheduled for a significant laboratory, radiologic, or other test or evaluation. For inpatient admissions, the UM firm may ask for diagnosis, procedure(s) to be performed, and other related information before approving the admission and, once approved, may only approve a specified length of stay in the hospital. Failure to comply with precertification requirements results in a financial penalty for the patient and may result in financial penalties for your physician and the hospital as well.

The next most important feature, from the patient's perspective, is the network. The physician, hospital, laboratory, or other provider you normally refer a patient to may not be in the network. By calling the UM number, you can avoid penalties and improve the satisfaction of the patient with your services.

Checkpoint Question
4. *What are the four elements of a managed care program?*

Health Maintenance Organizations (HMOs)

It is easiest to understand how a **health maintenance organization (HMO)** functions if we contrast it with a traditional health insurance program. In the traditional insurance system, the relationship between the covered individual and the insurer (or self-insurer) is purely financial. The insurer promises to reimburse (indemnify) the individual if he or she incurs certain types of covered medical expense. There are often limits to coverage (exclusions and limitations) and normally the coverage has a deductible (amounts below which are not reimbursable by the insurer) and coinsurance (the patient pays a percentage of the medical expense after the deductible is satisfied).

The covered individual seeks medical services and, thereby, incurs an expense. The individual, not the insurer, is responsible for this expense. If the medical treatment is covered as defined in the insurance policy, the company will reimburse the patient a portion of the amount incurred (after deductibles and coinsurance).

In contrast to the traditional insurance system, an HMO promises to provide covered services rather than pay for them. In this respect, the HMO acts both as an insurer and a provider of service. HMO policies are written differently from insurance policies. The HMO policy lists the medical services the member is entitled to receive and the physicians and hospitals that will provide these services. The HMO has a contract with both the patient and provider. It must provide covered services to the member either directly with its own physician staff and hospitals or indirectly by contracting with physicians and hospitals and obligating them to provide the services promised to the member. The HMO, rather than the patient, is responsible for the costs of medical services and providers bill the HMO rather than the patient if a reimbursable service has been rendered to an HMO member.

This is one reason why HMOs do not normally use deductibles and coinsurance, which are standard features of health insurance programs. A patient does not receive a provider's bill, so deductibles and coinsurance cannot apply. Instead, HMOs will use dollar denominated co-payments (eg, $10 per physician office visit) to reduce premium prices.

Health maintenance organizations come in many forms. Kaiser Permanente Health Plan is generally recognized as the nation's first HMO (there were earlier organizational forms but none that lasted into the modern era). In the early 1930s Kaiser Industries needed to provide physician services for its employees in remote areas. No physicians were available. Kaiser sought the services of a physician to build a medical group that would provide the necessary services. Rather than paying for these services on a **fee-for-service** basis, the company paid the physicians on a per employee basis (as the company did for other Workers' Compensation coverage).

Over time the physician group grew and became the Permanente Medical Group. Coverage was expanded first to include non–work-related illness and injury for employees and then services for the dependents and spouses of employees. Finally, the program was expanded to allow other employers to purchase care for their employees from the Permanente Medical Group and the organization was restructured into three mutually dependent entities: Kaiser Permanente Health Plan, Permanente Medical Group (a very large multispecialty group practice), and Kaiser Foundation Hospitals. This company is the best example of the group model HMO and serves over 6 million members. The health plan (HMO) contracts with employers to cover their employees. The medical group and hospitals contract with the health plan to provide the services required in the health plan's contract with employers.

Consistent with its history, the health plan does not pay the medical group a fee for each service provided. Instead, it pays each party based on the number of members enrolled in the health plan. This is often called **capitation** because there is one payment per capita. Capitation payments are also used by other types of HMOs.

As group model HMOs developed (they were called prepaid group practices until 1973 federal legislation changed their names), nongroup physicians organized into an entity called an **independent practice association (IPA)**. The early IPA HMOs were often sponsored by a local medical society and were developed to allow independent physicians to compete with prepaid group practices.

The IPA HMOs contract with employers in the same manner as do group model HMOs and their members are required to receive covered services from IPA physicians. However, the HMO's contracts with physicians are different because these physicians are not organized into a single multispecialty group practice. IPA physicians are paid in a number of ways. Some are paid on a capitation basis, or some may be paid on a fee-for-service basis using a **fee schedule** established by the HMO. Often a portion of any reimbursement is withheld by the HMO and returned only if the HMO's total medical expense is within budget.

In some of these HMOs, the IPA is a separate corporation, often owned by physicians. With this structure (still called an IPA HMO) the IPA contracts with physicians and the HMO contracts with the IPA instead of directly with each physician.

Over the years, HMOs have evolved and many are now a mixture of the models discussed above. For a medical assistant, this means that you must know what type of relationship the practice has with the HMO before you can determine how it will be reimbursed. Most HMOs will require that claims be submitted even if payment is a capitation rather than fee for service. And many HMOs also require the collection and transmission of other patient information, which is not required in the traditional insurance industry.

Checkpoint Question

5. How does an HMO differ from a traditional health insurance program?

Preferred Provider Organizations (PPOs)

Whereas HMOs promise to provide services and have a financial risk in their relationships with subscribers, a preferred provider organization (PPO) is an organization whose purpose is simply to contract with providers, then lease this network of contracted providers to health care plans. The PPO network is not risk bearing—it does have any financial involvement in the health plan. PPOs are typically developed by hospitals and physicians as a vehicle to attract patients, although some are developed and managed by insurance **carriers**.

The PPOs contract with participating providers (including hospitals and physicians). These contracts allow the PPO to contract with insurers and other purchasers of health care services on behalf of the participating providers, who typically accept less than their normal charges and agree to follow the utilization management and other administrative protocols as specified by the PPO.

Typically, a health plan with a PPO offers benefits at two different levels, commonly referred to as in network or out of network. Unlike an HMO, patients may visit any provider they wish for services. If the provider is in network (a participating provider), the levels of benefits for the patient are greater than if the patient receives services from an out-of-network (nonparticipating) provider.

A typical health plan with a PPO could look like this:

As you can see from the example, each time the patient sees an in-network provider, he or she receives significantly better benefits. A primary difference between an HMO and PPO, therefore, is that patients can see any physician of their choice and receive benefits; they simply have an incentive in the form of higher benefits when they see an in-network provider.

As part of your responsibilities, you should identify the PPOs with which the physician has contracted and determine the administrative requirements set forth by each PPO in the contract. To understand the administrative services agreed to by the physician, review all managed care contracts carefully. Additionally, be aware that most PPOs have a provider relations representative who works with the contracted providers (physicians) to answer questions and clarify procedures. The PPO is typically operated by a group of hospitals or physicians or by an insurance company or independent organization. Physicians agree to participate in PPOs to serve their existing patients who now have PPO plans and sometimes to gain additional patients who will often seek the services of a PPO physician.

Participating physicians have agreed to perform certain administrative services for PPO patients. Commonly, the physician's office must accept assignment of benefits and provide claims filing services for the patient. The physician agrees to accept the reimbursement by the claims administrator as payment in full and agrees not to balance bill the patient for any difference between the physician's usual charge and the PPO-negotiated charge for the service. The participating physician is responsible for collecting any co-pay amount at the time of service. The physician also agrees to comply with any precertification requirements stipulated by the plan.

Checkpoint Question

6. *What is the primary difference between an HMO and PPO?*

Physician Hospital Organizations

Physicians and hospitals have become more active in developing managed care alternatives. **Physician hospital organizations (PHOs) are a coalition of physicians and a hospital contracting with large employers, carriers, and other benefits groups to provide discounted health services.** There are numerous variations of PHOs. A PHO may look much like a PPO with no risk-bearing elements, in which case the network of providers constituting the PHO are under no financial obligation to subscribers. A PHO may look more like an HMO, wherein the participating providers in the PHO do have a risk-bearing contract and assume responsibility for the overall medical budget of subscribing units. Physician organizations (POs) are such groups consisting of physicians only. As with any managed care program, it is important to know and understand the particulars of each managed care contract and requirements of the provider and obligations to patients and the managed care entity.

Health Plan With a PPO

Benefit	In-network	Out-of-network
Deductible	$100	$300
Coinsurance	90%	70%
Routine care	$200 per calendar year	-0-
Mental health	80%	50%
Office visit	$10 co-pay; no deductible	70%

Other Managed Care Programs

Although HMOs, PPOs and, increasingly, PHOs are the most common managed care programs, there are many others covering patients today and still more being developed.

Although requirements vary, a *gatekeeper* provision is commonly included. A gatekeeper is a primary care physician. Participants are required to see a primary care physician for all nonemergency services.

BOX 18-3 The Future of Managed Care

At the time of this writing, approximately 73% of covered employees nationally are in HMOs or PPOs. Growth of managed care has been rapid and the pace of change has increased in the 1990s. In 1995 alone, enrollment in HMOs increased by 20%. By the end of 1995, over 33% of Medicaid recipients and over 10% of Medicare participants were enrolled in HMOs. This represents an increase in excess of 25% in just a year. The rise in Medicare managed care is particularly significant as these seniors represent only 13% of the nation's population, but almost 40% of the nation's total personal health care expenditures.

Managed care is strongest in urban areas and less in rural areas and stronger on the West Coast than the East Coast, but it is growing in all parts of the country. Unless the regulatory climate changes abruptly, managed care in one variety or another is expected to replace traditional indemnity coverage in all markets.

Managed care is also changing the organizational structures of medicine. To form risk-bearing organizations, physicians and hospitals are combining into new relationships with one another. Hospitals are buying physician practices and small group or solo practice physicians are combining into larger group practices. Some of these are forming public companies and raising investment capital to foster even more rapid growth in size and geographic scope. The size of medical practice is increasing and is expected to continue to increase in the foreseeable future.

The role of primary care physicians is changing relative to subspecialty physicians. In many managed care programs, primary care physicians act as patient care managers. Services authorized by these gatekeepers are covered, whereas those not authorized by the patient's primary physician may be denied or paid at a lower rate. Patients often join managed care organizations only if their primary care physician is a participant in a particular plan.

As coverage changes from an insured/fee-for-service system to a managed care system with incentives to decrease the cost of patient care, employers and other purchasers have become much more interested in measuring the quality of care provided by different managed care organizations. The very largest employers worked with leading HMOs to develop a report called HEDIS (Healthplan Employer Data Information Set). This uniform data set (reporting many indicators of health care quality such as immunization rates, cesarean section rates, etc.) is now required of any HMO that wishes to serve the largest employers in the nation. HEDIS is upgraded continuously and is being adopted by governmental organizations and many smaller employers as a prerequisite for an HMO to cover employees and governmental populations. This is only a start. Demands for increasingly sophisticated medical information will intensify.

The new demands on the medical care system, to reduce the cost of care while measuring quality and improving it over time, have led many organizations to develop increasingly sophisticated patient care protocols. These require documentation of efficacy and quality, information contained in patient medical records. These demands are leading to the automation of medical records. With automated medical records, a patient's medical history can be instantaneously available to any provider in virtually any location. Not only will it be easier to document quality and measure improvement over time, a complete medical record that is available to any provider (with the patient's permission) will improve coordination among physicians and reduce iatrogenic illness. This alone could lead to substantial improvement in the quality of care provided to patients.

(continued)

That physician will either treat the patient or, if necessary, refer the patient to a specialist. The physician must complete and submit a referral form or call the claims administrator for approval of the referral.

The gatekeeper provision seeks to reduce the plan cost of specialists. For example, without such a provision, a patient might see a specialist first at a more costly fee, even though the condition may have been adequately treated by a less costly primary care physician. The gatekeeper approach also encourages patients to establish a relationship with a primary care physician, who is then in a position to manage the patient's care.

The continuing progress of managed care and its impact on medical care is discussed further in Box 18-3.

➤ POLICIES IN THE PRACTICE

In an era of managed care contracts and negotiated services, many practice policies are affected. Medical assistants must be knowledgeable and precise in administering practice policies, especially with regard to assignment of benefits and balance billing.

Assignment of benefits is a patient service that may be provided by the practice. If assignment of benefits is accepted, the patient's signature must be on file authorizing the claims administrator to reimburse the physician. Managed care plans require physicians to accept assignment; however, many physicians do not accept assignment for nonmanaged care patients. If assignment is not accepted, the patient is responsible for paying all charges and then filing a claim with the claims administrator for reimbursement directly to the patient.

Balance billing is a practice prohibited by most managed care contracts. The physician cannot charge the patient the difference between the physician's usual charge and the allowable charge specified by the contract. For plans without managed care contracts, balance billing is not subject to any restrictions and the practice may balance bill the patient any difference between the physician's charged fee and the amount allowable by the plan according to **usual, customary, and reasonable** (UCR) tables.

A few national firms provide UCR data to claims administrators who use that data to determine the maximum amount payable for any given service (the **plan maximum**). UCR data are calculated from surveys of the amount physicians charge for each service or procedure. That amount is calculated on a geographic (zip code) basis to reflect regional variations in health care costs. Nonmanaged care plan physician reimbursements are based on a maximum allowable charge as specified in the UCR data. The physician may choose to bill the patient for the difference between the amount charged and the UCR amount.

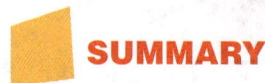

SUMMARY

Most patients you will encounter in the physician's office will have some type of health care plan. Types of plans include group, individual, and government-sponsored health benefits such as Medicare or Medicaid. Many physicians have contracts with managed care plans such as HMOs and PPOs. Each type of plan has certain requirements regarding eligibility and claims submission, and you must be knowledgeable about those requirements. In particular, one of your primary duties is to file claims in a timely and accurate manner to ensure appropriate reimbursement for the physician. When filing claims, you must be careful to maintain patient confidentiality and to avoid fraud.

CRITICAL THINKING CHALLENGES

1. Jane and Joe are married and each are employed and cover themselves and their two children on their health plans. Jane's birthday is July 23 and Joe's birthday is August 9. Joe is 2 years older than Jane. When claims are submitted for their two children, which spouse's plan is primary? Fill in the spaces below, noting which plan is primary and secondary for each family member.
2. The requirements for Medicaid vary from state to state. How would you determine the Medicaid requirements for your particular state? Locate the name, address, and telephone number of your state's resource.

Coordination of Benefits

Family Member	Jane's Plan Birthday: July 23	Joe's Plan Birthday: August 9
Jane		
Joe		
Child		
Child		

ANSWERS TO CHECKPOINT QUESTIONS

1. With insured benefits, a monthly premium is paid by the employer or organization to an insurance company. The insurance company, in turn, is obligated to pay for any eligible health benefits. In contrast, self-funded benefits are provided to eligible employees or members by their employer or organization. Claims are processed by a professional claims administrator, such as a third-party administrator.
2. Persons who are entitled to Social Security are automatically enrolled in Medicare part A, which covers hospital services and expenses only, after an annual deductible. Medicare part B covers the physician's charges for inpatient or outpatient care as well as diagnostic services, after an annual deductible (which increases each year). Part B does not cover routine examinations, well care, routine immunizations, or cosmetic surgery.
3. Medicaid patients receive a new ID card each month.
4. The four elements of managed care programs are precertification of hospital admissions (often also called utilization management or utilization review—UM or UR), approved referrals, network, and assignment of benefits.
5. In a traditional insurance system, the individual, not the insurer, seeks medical services and, thereby, incurs the expense. An HMO promises to provide covered services rather than pay for them.
6. A primary difference between an HMO and a PPO is that patients can see any physician of their choice and receive benefits; they simply have an incentive in the form of higher benefits when they see an in-network provider.

SUGGESTIONS FOR FURTHER READING

Beard, P. C. (1993). What the Medicare fraud squad looks for in claims. *Medical Economics*, 42–46.

Buck, C. J. (1996). *Step by Step Medical Coding*. Philadelphia: W. B. Saunders.

White, O. (1993). Seven ways to make insurers pay you quicker. *Medical Economics*, 39–41.

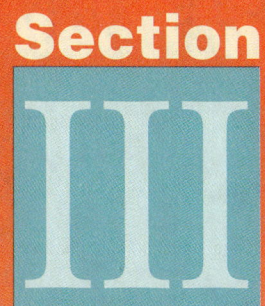

Section

III

The Clinical Medical Assistant

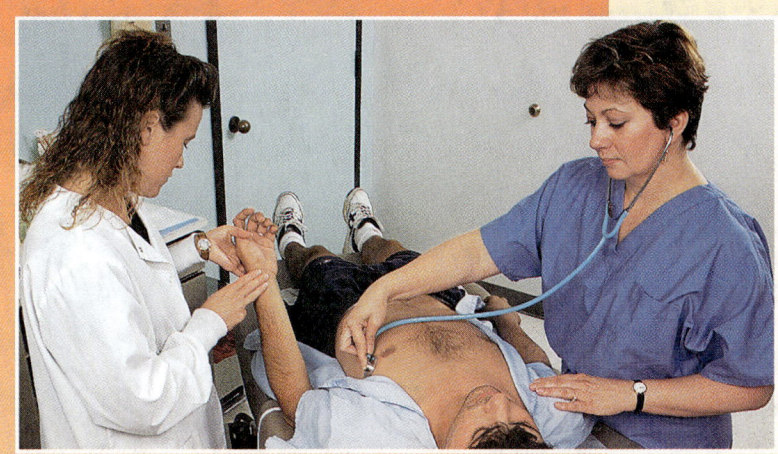

Unit 5

Performing Clinical Duties

In the clinical area of the medical office, we begin the process of gathering together the pieces of patient information that provide clues about the patient's illness. Following standard protocol for the protection of the health care worker and patient will help to ensure that the procedures and treatments prescribed by the physician are safely and properly performed to assist in the patient's return to health.

Asepsis and Infection Control

Chapter Outline

Microorganisms and Normal Flora
Conditions That Favor the Growth of Pathogens
The Infection Cycle
Modes of Transmission
  Direct Transmission
  Indirect Transmission
  Sources
Medical Asepsis
Maintaining Medical Asepsis
Procedure: Handwashing for Medical Asepsis
Isolation Precautions
Surgical Asepsis
Surgical Scrub
Procedure: Performing a Surgical Scrub
Procedure: Sterile Gloving

Procedure: Removing Gloves After a Procedure
Infection Control
  Levels of Infection Control
  Handling Environmental Contamination
  Cleaning and Decontaminating Spills of Blood or Body Fluids
  Handling Soiled Linens
  Decontaminating and Laundering Protective Clothing
  Disposing of Infectious Waste
Summary
Critical Thinking Challenges
Answers to Checkpoint Questions
Suggestions for Further Reading

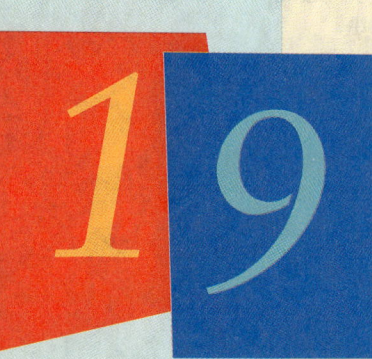

DACUM Components

1.3 Practice within the scope of education, training, and personal capabilities
4.1 Apply principles of aseptic technique and infection control
7.3 Teach patients methods of health promotion and disease prevention

Chapter Competencies

Learning Objectives

Upon successfully completing this chapter, you will be able to:

1. Spell and define the Key Terms.
2. Identify and describe conditions that promote the growth of pathogens.
3. Define the chain of infection.
4. Describe how microorganisms are transmitted.
5. Distinguish between medical and surgical asepsis.
6. Explain the difference between medical aseptic handwashing and surgical scrubbing.
7. Explain the purpose of following Standard Precautions with all patients.
8. Identify and describe the levels of infection control.

Performance Objectives

Upon successfully completing this chapter, you will be able to:

1. Perform a medical aseptic handwashing (Procedure 19-1).
2. Perform a surgical scrub (Procedure 19-2).
3. Put on sterile gloves (Procedure 19-3).
4. Remove gloves after a procedure (Procedure 19-4).
5. Clean and decontaminate spills of blood or body fluids.

Key Terms

(See Glossary for definitions.)

asepsis	exogenous	phagocytized
carrier	medical asepsis	surgical asepsis
centigrade (c),	microorganisms	transient flora
Celsius (C)	normal flora	vector
disease	pathogens	virulent

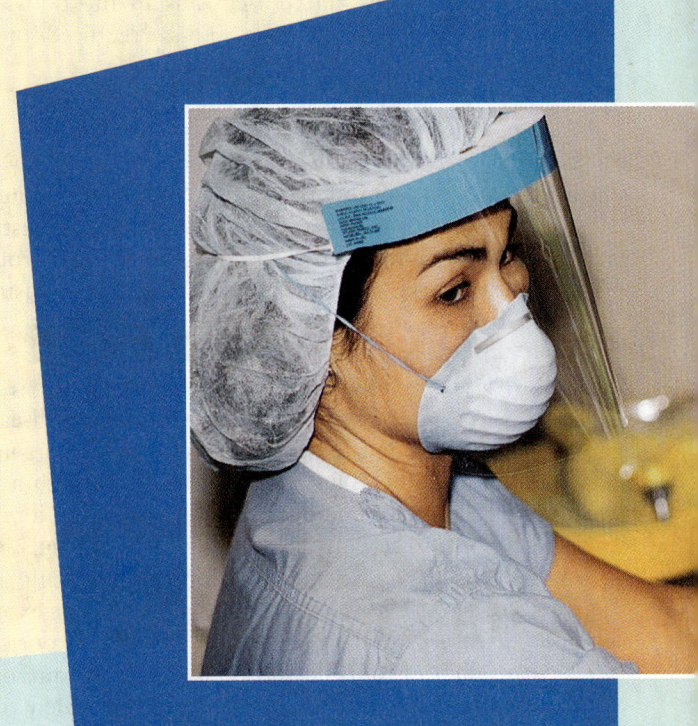

To prevent the spread of **disease** (illness), aseptic technique must be used in every aspect of work in the medical office. **Asepsis** means free from infection or a condition in which pathogenic organisms are absent. The medical aseptic handwash is the most important factor in the prevention of disease transmission. As a medical assistant, you must adhere to strict aseptic procedures, and you must also encourage patients and their families to practice good handwashing and medical aseptic technique in the home. In addition, you must recognize the importance of using standard precautions—the new guideline for isolation precautions issued by the Centers for Disease Control and Prevention (CDC)—for all patients. Finally, you must be aware of the various levels of infection control that can be used in the medical office.

MICROORGANISMS AND NORMAL FLORA

Microorganisms—microscopic living organisms—are all around us and all through our bodies. They can be classified as bacteria, fungi, viruses, protozoa, and metazoa (see Chap. 43, Microbiology, for a more detailed discussion). They are abundant on the skin, throughout the gastrointestinal and genitourinary tracts, and in the respiratory system. They are even found in parts of the body not connected to the outside environment. Most microorganisms in the body are normal flora (or resident flora) and are required for the normal functioning of the various systems.

When microorganisms produce disease, they are called pathogens. Pathogens are easily spread from one person to another either directly or indirectly by inhalation (from contaminated air droplets from coughs and sneezes from a contaminated person), ingestion (from eating contaminated foods), or injection (through a break in sterile procedure). See "Modes of Transmission," below.

Persons who are infected with transmissible diseases but who are asymptomatic may be carriers, or reservoirs, of disease. They can still transmit those diseases simply by coming in contact with a susceptible person.

Many beneficial microorganisms reside within the body. Each type of microorganism is specific to its special section of the body. The presence of normal flora in that section triggers the immune system to build and release antibodies that protect the body from **exogenous** disease-producing microorganisms (microorganisms originating outside the body) or from microorganisms that are normal in the body but alien to a specific system. For instance, *Escherichia coli* is normal for the lower gastrointestinal tract but is pathogenic in the urinary system. When a chemical imbalance is created in the body through chemotherapy or antibiotic drugs, an imbalance may exist in the normal flora, decreasing the protection they offer and allowing pathogens to grow.

The body is protected by many nonspecific defenses against disease. If the barriers are overpowered or breached, other backup systems are in place to protect us from the multitude of microorganisms that surround us.

- **Skin**. Normal flora on the skin consists mainly of *Staphylococcus aureus*. As long as the skin is kept clean and intact, the bacteria are not considered dangerous. Frequent washing of the skin flushes the bacteria away. Keeping the skin intact prevents a portal of entry.
- **Eyes**. Tears flush potentially dangerous bacteria from the eyes and contain a bacteria-destroying enzyme called lysozyme.
- **Mouth**. The greatest variety of microorganisms found in the body are in the oral cavity, which is itself the ideal host for pathogens to thrive. Good oral hygiene removes the pathogens or prevents their growth. Saliva is slightly bactericidal.
- **Gastrointestinal tract**. Normal hydrochloric acid in the stomach destroys many disease-producing pathogens. The normal flora of the colon and small intestines, which are vital for digestion of nutrients, are usually not disease-causing microbes as long as they remain within the gastrointestinal tract.
- **Respiratory tract**. Nostril hair and cilia are early defenses against airborne bacteria. If these barriers are insufficient, mucus from the membranes lining the respiratory tract constantly waves along the cilia, trapping and transporting microorganisms to the pharynx for swallowing. Digestive enzymes usually neutralize airborne microorganisms. Those that make it to the lung fields are usually **phagocytized** (engulfed and digested) by macrophages in the alveoli and interstitial spaces.
- **Genitourinary tract**. The reproductive tracts and the urinary system are slightly acidic to provide a less hospitable environment for microorganisms. Frequent flushing by the urinary tract with urination removes many transient pathogens.

All of these systems may be overpowered by a particularly **virulent** (highly pathogenic) organism or they may be overcome if the barriers and resistance are depressed, as in old age, existing pathology, or unusual stress. **Transient flora**—organisms that do not normally reside in a particular area—are not usually pathogenic. They are not as well adapted to the body as the normal flora and will only become pathogenic if the disease resistance of the host is decreased for some reason.

➤ CONDITIONS THAT FAVOR THE GROWTH OF PATHOGENS

As living organisms, the pathogens found in the clinical setting need certain conditions for optimum growth and reproduction. As a medical assistant, you are responsible for reducing pathogens in the clinical setting by eliminating as many of their life requirements as possible. These requirements include:

- *Moisture.* Few microbes survive well in dry places. Those that form spores may remain dormant until moisture is available.
- *Nutrients.* Microorganisms depend on their environment for sustenance; a nutrient-rich environment fosters growth.
- *Temperature.* Although microorganisms may survive in freezing or boiling environments, those that thrive at body temperature—98.6° Fahrenheit or 37° **centigrade**—are more likely to be pathogenic to humans. (Centigrade, or Celsius, is a temperature scale on which 0° is the freezing point and 100° is the boiling point of water at sea level.)
- *Darkness.* Virtually no bacteria pathogenic to humans will thrive in sunlight or bright light.
- *Neutral to slightly alkaline pH environment.* The pH of the blood at 7.35 to 7.45 is preferred by those microorganisms that prefer the human body.
- *Oxygen.* Most pathogens require free air; those that do are called aerobes. A few, however, do not live well in an oxygen-rich environment; these are called anaerobes (eg, tetanus, botulism).

If any one of these conditions is changed in any way, the result can be a change in the growth and replication of the pathogen.

➤ THE INFECTION CYCLE

The infection cycle is often referred to as links of a chain around a causative agent, which is the invading microorganism (Fig. 19-1). The first link in the infection cycle is a reservoir host. If the microorganism cannot find a host on which it can feed, it will die. This reservoir host provides nutrients and an incubation site for the pathogen. The pathogen may cause disease symptoms in the reservoir host, or it may asymptomatically incubate new generations there and then leave the first host to search for a second host.

The second link in the infection cycle is the means of exit, sometimes referred to as the portal of exit. This refers to the manner by which the pathogen leaves the host—for example, by coughing, sneezing, direct contact by shaking hands, or through an open wound as exudate.

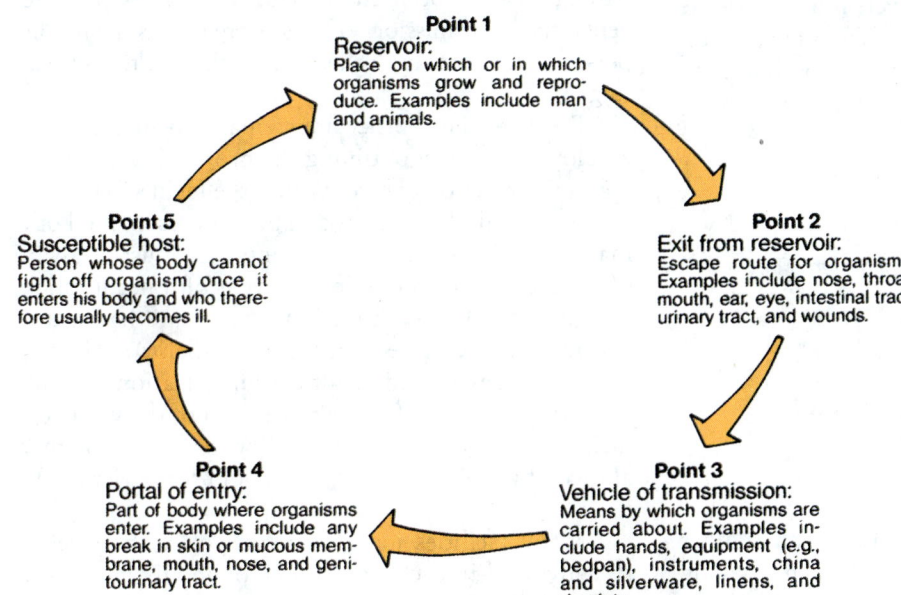

Point 1
Reservoir:
Place on which or in which organisms grow and reproduce. Examples include man and animals.

Point 2
Exit from reservoir:
Escape route for organisms. Examples include nose, throat, mouth, ear, eye, intestinal tract, urinary tract, and wounds.

Point 3
Vehicle of transmission:
Means by which organisms are carried about. Examples include hands, equipment (e.g., bedpan), instruments, china and silverware, linens, and droplets.

Point 4
Portal of entry:
Part of body where organisms enter. Examples include any break in skin or mucous membrane, mouth, nose, and genitourinary tract.

Point 5
Susceptible host:
Person whose body cannot fight off organism once it enters his body and who therefore usually becomes ill.

FIGURE 19-1
This sketch illustrates the infectious process cycle. Infections and infectious diseases are spread by starting from the reservoir (*Point 1*), and moving full circle to a susceptible host (*Point 5*). Microorganisms can be controlled by using methods that interfere at any point within the cycle.

BOX 19-1   The Susceptible Host

The susceptible host is unable to resist the invading pathogen for a variety of reasons:

- *Age.* As the body ages, defense mechanisms begin to lose their effectiveness. The immune system is no longer as active or as efficient. In the very young, the immune system may not be fully functional.
- *Existing pathology.* Stress of an existing illness will occupy or deplete the immune system to leave the way clear for an additional illness.
- *Poor nutrition.* A nutritionally deficient diet will not allow cells to repair and reproduce as they are weakened by disease.
- *Poor hygiene.* Although multitudes of microbes exist on our skin, keeping the numbers down will allow normal flora to maintain a proper balance with pathogens.

The third link in the infection cycle is the means, or vehicle, of transmission. This includes contaminated air droplets from coughing and sneezing, pathogens on a unclean hand passing on to another by direct contact, or contact with wound drainage.

The fourth link in the infection cycle is a means of entrance, or portal of entry. This could occur by breathing in contaminated airborne droplets or ingesting contaminated food or drink. Any break in the skin or mucous membrane is a portal of entry for a pathogen. Any break of sterile procedure is a means of entrance for a pathogen.

The fifth link in the infection cycle is a susceptible host (Box 19-1). A host that permits easy entrance similar to the means of exit and allows the pathogen to grow and multiply then becomes a new reservoir host, causing the chain to repeat the cycle.

Checkpoint Question

3. How are the first and fifth links of the infection cycle related?

➤ MODES OF TRANSMISSION

Direct Transmission

Direct transmission requires direct contact with another person. Direct transmission occurs through shaking hands, sexual contact, direct contact with blood or body fluids, inhaling contaminated air droplets, or kissing.

Indirect Transmission

Indirect transmission occurs through contact by a vehicle, either biologic or mechanical, called a vector. Examples include food, milk, water, disease-carrying insects (eg, mosquitoes, ticks, lice, or fleas) or an inanimate object (eg, air, soil, instruments, wound exudate, drinking glasses).

Sources

Most reservoir hosts are humans, animals, and insects. Human hosts include people who are ill with an infectious disease, people who are carriers of an infectious disease, and people who are in the incubation or ambulatory stage of a infectious disease. With the exception of flies and roaches, which carry many diseases, most of the insect sources are those that draw blood from an infected reservoir, such as ticks and mosquitoes, and pass the disease to their next victim. The animal sources are less abundant but include infected animals such as those that transmit anthrax or rabies.

Table 19-1 provides some examples of common diseases and their methods of transmission.

➤ MEDICAL ASEPSIS

Medical asepsis, commonly referred to as "clean technique," means an object or area is free from infection. It requires destroying organisms after they have left the body. There will still be nonpathogens present on a clean or medically aseptic substance or surface, but all pathogens have been eliminated. Medical asepsis prevents the transmission of microorganisms from one person or area to any other within the health care setting.

Every medical office must make available to its employees a policy outlining the protocol to follow to maintain infection control within the facility. This may be bound with the policies and procedures manual or it may be kept separately. Every employee must be aware of procedures to follow in the event of a needle stick, for instance, or how infectious wastes are handled in this facility (see "Infection Control," below). The Occupational Safety and Health Administration (OSHA) has strict guidelines for the protection of the worker; a facility may adopt a stronger policy for protection than allowed by law, but it may not adopt less strict guidelines.

Many facilities include in the policy the level of risk involved in each procedure commonly performed on site, with clear instructions for avoiding or reducing danger to the worker. For example, any procedure that

Table 19-1
Common Communicable Diseases

Disease	Method of Transmission
AIDS (acquired immunodeficiency syndrome)	Direct contact with body fluids, sexual contact, contact with contaminated needles
Bacillary dysentery	Fecal/oral route (spread by vectors such as flies and contaminated food)
Cholera	Ingestion of contaminated food or water
Diphtheria	Airborne droplets, carriers
German measles (rubella)	Airborne droplets
Influenza	Direct contact, contaminated articles, airborne droplets
Measles (rubeola)	Airborne droplets
Mononucleosis	Airborne droplets, contamination by infected saliva
Mumps	Direct contact with materials contaminated with infected saliva, airborne droplets
Pneumonia	Airborne droplets, direct contact
Rabies	Saliva of infected animal (bites)
Tetanus	Spores or animal feces transmitted by direct contact

involves blood or body fluid (eg, phlebotomy) is high risk for contamination, whereas taking vital signs is considered low risk. Job descriptions may also list risk categories; for instance, a receptionist is not usually at risk for exposure, but the clinical assistant is frequently in high-risk situations.

MAINTAINING MEDICAL ASEPSIS

Handwashing is the MOST IMPORTANT medical aseptic practice and is crucial in preventing microorganism transmission in the medical office. Hands must be washed frequently using proper technique (Procedure 19-1). For example, handwashing must be performed:

- Before and after patient contact
- Before putting on gloves
- After removing gloves
- After contact with any blood or body fluid
- After contact with contaminated material
- After handling specimens
- After coughing, sneezing, or blowing the nose
- After using the restroom

It is your responsibility to practice medical aseptic techniques in the office (Box 19-2). Patients and their families must be taught the proper medical aseptic techniques to use in the home, such as proper handwashing and proper disposal of contaminated articles or dressings. Patient education will frequently be your responsibility, so you will need to instruct and observe the patient or caregiver in proper procedures to reduce the transmission of disease.

ISOLATION PRECAUTIONS

In January 1996, the Centers for Disease Control and Prevention (CDC) and the Hospital Infection Control Practices Advisory Committee (HICPAC) issued revised

BOX 19-2 Guidelines for Maintaining Medical Asepsis

1. Avoid touching clothing with soiled linen or instruments. Both should be held above waist level and away from the body. Roll used linen or table paper inward with the clean surface outward. Do not allow used supplies or equipment to touch clothing.
2. Always consider the floor to be contaminated. Any item dropped must be discarded or re-cleaned to its former level of asepsis.
3. Clean immediately. Areas kept clean are less likely to harbor microorganisms or encourage their growth.
4. Always presume that blood and body fluids are contaminated. Follow guidelines published by OSHA and CDC to protect yourself and to prevent transmission of disease.

Procedure 19-1   Handwashing for Medical Asepsis

Steps	Purpose
1. Remove all rings and wrist watch (or move watch above the wrist several inches).	1. Rings may harbor pathogens that may not be washed away. Raising the watch protects it from water damage.
2. Stand close to but not touching the sink.	2. Standing close makes it easier to perform a proper hand wash without splashing, but the sink is considered contaminated and standing too close may contaminate your clothing.
3. Turn on the faucet using a paper towel. Discard the towel. *Note:* Some facilities have faucets with knee controls, rather than hand controls. Water force is controlled by a back and forth motion and water temperature is controlled by an up and down motion. Knee controls are preferred over hand controls for surgical scrubs but may not be available in many office settings.	3. The faucets are considered to be contaminated and the towel cannot be used again.
4. Wet hands and wrists under running warm water and apply liquid antibacterial soap. Scrub wrists.	4. Water too warm or too cool will cause the hands to chap and crack, providing a break in the protective barriers of the hands. Antibacterial soaps help lower the number of pathogens.
5. Work soap into a lather by rubbing the palms of the hands together, then intertwine the fingers of both hands and rub the soap between the fingers at least 10 times.	5. This motion dislodges microorganisms from between the fingers.

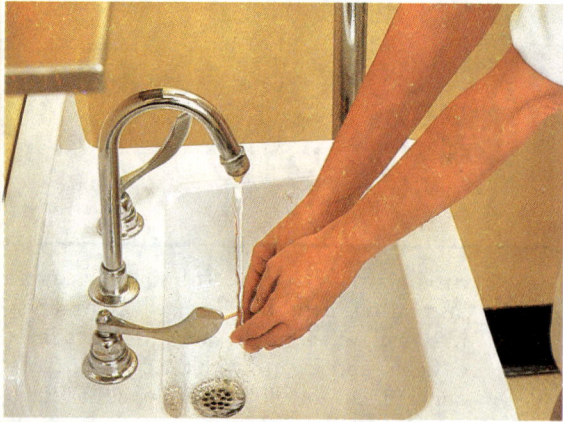

Step 4. Wet hands and wrists.

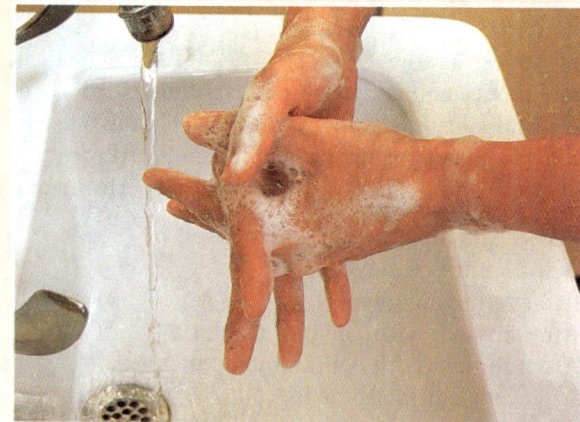

Step 5: Wash hands and wrists with firm rubbing and circular motions.

6. Scrub the palm of one hand with the fingertips of the other hand to work the soap under the nails of that hand then reverse the procedure and scrub the other hand.	6. Friction helps remove microorganisms.

(continued)

Procedure 19-1

Handwashing for Medical Asepsis *(continued)*

Steps	Purpose
7. Use an orangewood stick under the nails.	7. Nails may harbor microorganisms. Metal files or pointed instruments may break the skin and cause an opening for bacteria.
8. Holding the hands in a downward position, rinse the soap from both hands allowing the water to drip off the fingertips. Rinse well.	8. Hands held lower will allow microorganisms to flow off the hands and fingers rather than back up the arms.
9. If hands are grossly contaminated, repeat the procedure. (See note regarding knee controls.)	
10. Dry the hands gently with a paper towel and discard the towel.	10. Hands must be dried completely to prevent drying and cracking. The paper is wet now and may wick contaminants back onto the clean hands.

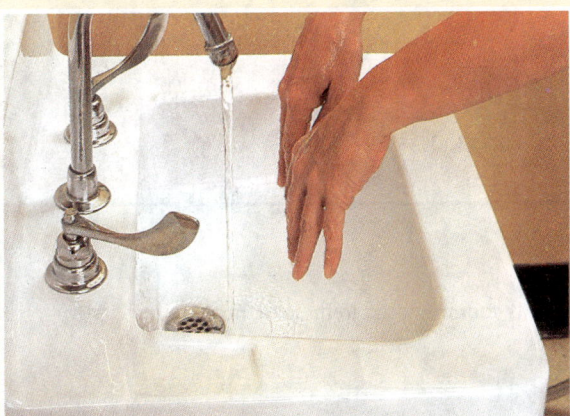

Step 8: Rinse hands thoroughly.

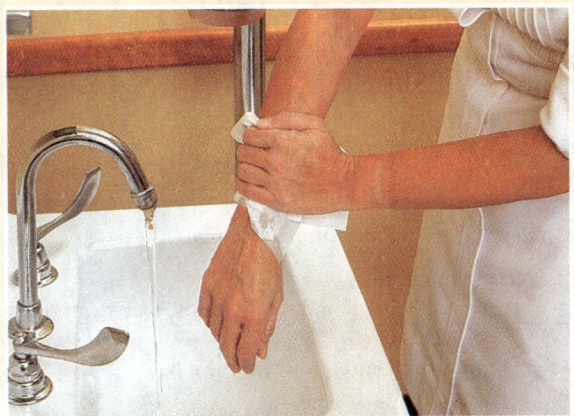

Step 10: Dry hands with a paper towel.

11. Use a dry paper towel to turn off the faucets and discard the towel.	11. Hands are now clean and should not touch the contaminated handles.
12. If the sink is splattered, wipe with a clean dry paper towel to reduce available moisture for pathogens and to remove as many as possible. Discard the paper towel.	

Note: This procedure should take 1–2 minutes.

guidelines for isolation precautions. These guidelines supersede previous CDC recommendations. Under the new system, two tiers of precautions are recognized:

1. *Standard Precautions* are to be used for all patients, regardless of their known (or suspected) infection status. Standard Precautions synthesize the major features of two isolation systems: universal precautions (designed to reduce the risk of transmission of blood-borne pathogens [eg, human immunodeficiency virus and hepatitis B virus]) and body substance isolation (designed to reduce the risk of transmission of pathogens from moist body substances). Box 19-3 describes Standard Precautions in greater detail.

2. *Transmission-based precautions* are to be used for patients known (or suspected) to be infected with

Patient Education: Basic Aseptic Technique

While performing procedures, take the opportunity to instruct your patients in basic aseptic techniques they can use at home.

- *Handwashing.* Performing this routine as part of daily hygiene is particularly important for patients who are immunosuppressed, very young or old, steroid dependent, or required to perform at-home dressing changes. Instruct patients that hands should be washed before and after eating meals; after sneezing, coughing, or nose blowing; after using the bathroom; before and after changing wound dressings; and before and after changing a child's diaper.

- *Tissue use.* Explain to patients with respiratory symptoms that using a disposable tissue to cover the mouth and nose when coughing or sneezing decreases the potential of transmitting the illness throughout the household.

- *Dressing changes.* Instruct patients regarding the differences between sterile dressings and clean bandages. Demonstrate the procedure and have patients return the demonstration to ensure comprehension.

- *Sanitation.* Explain to your patients the proper techniques for disposing of waste from members of the household with communicable diseases.

BOX 19-3 Standard Precautions

Under Standard Precautions, you must:

- Wash your hands:
    - after touching blood, body fluids, secretions, excretions, and contaminated items whether you have worn gloves or not
    - immediately after you remove gloves
    - between patient contacts
    - when necessary to prevent transfer of microorganisms
- Use plain soap for routine handwashing and an antimicrobial or antiseptic agent for specified situations.
- Wear clean, nonsterile gloves when touching blood, body fluids, secretions, excretions, mucous membranes, non-intact skin, and contaminated items.
- Change gloves between procedures on the same patient after exposure to potentially infective material.
- Remove gloves immediately after patient contact and wash your hands.
- Wear protective barrier equipment (eg, mask, goggles, face shield, gown) to protect the mucous membranes of your eyes, nose, and mouth and to avoid soiling your clothing when performing procedures that may generate splashes or sprays of blood, body fluids, secretions, or excretions.
- Care for equipment and linens that are contaminated with blood, body fluids, secretions, or excretions in a way that avoids skin and mucous membrane exposures, clothing contamination, and microorganism transfer to other patients and environments. Dispose of single-use items appropriately.
- Take precautions to avoid injuries before, during, and after any procedures using needles, scalpels, or other sharp instruments.
- Ensure that used needles are not recapped, purposely bent, broken, removed from disposable syringes, or otherwise manipulated by hand. Never direct the point of a needle toward any part of your body; instead use a one-handed "scoop" technique or a device designed for holding the needle sheath.
- Place used disposable syringes and needles, scalpel blades, and all other used sharps in a puncture-resistant container that is located as close to the area of use as possible.
- Use barrier devices (eg, mouthpieces, resuscitation bags) as alternatives to mouth-to-mouth resuscitation.

(Based on information from "Guidelines for Isolation Precaution in Hospitals" developed by the Centers for Disease Control and Prevention [CDC] and the Hospital Infection Control Practices Advisory Committee [HICPAC], January 1996.)

Table 19-2

Transmission-Based Precautions
In addition to Standard Precautions, the following types of transmission-based precautions are to be used in specified situations.

Type	Precautions	Indications and Illnesses
Airborne precautions	• Place patient in a private room with negative airflow and appropriate ventilation. • Wear a mask when entering patient's room. • Have patient wear a mask during transport.	Use for infections that can be transmitted by airborne droplet nuclei (small particles) Examples: measles, varicella, tuberculosis
Droplet precautions	• Place patient in a private room or with another patient who has the same infection. • Wear a mask when working within 3 feet of patient. • Have patient wear mask during transport.	Use for infections that can be transmitted by droplets (large particles) during coughing, sneezing, or talking. Examples: *Haemophilus influenzae* disease, *Neisseria meningitidis* disease, streptococcal pharyngitis, mumps, rubella
Contact precautions	• Place patient in a private room or with another patient who has the same infection. • Wear gloves when entering patient's room and while providing care; change gloves after contact with infectious material. • Wear gown if clothing may have contact with patient or with infectious material.	Use for infections that can be transmitted by contact directly with patient or patient's items. Examples: multidrug-resistant infections, *Clostridium difficile, Shigella,* herpes simplex virus, impetigo, pediculosis, scabies

(Based on information from "Guideline for Isolation Precautions in Hospitals" developed by the Centers for Disease Control and Prevention [CDC] and the Hospital Infection Control Practices Advisory Committee HICPAC], January 1996.)

highly transmissible or epidemiologically important pathogens that can be transmitted by the airborne, droplet, or direct-contact routes. Transmission-based precautions are to be used in addition to Standard Precautions for specified patients. Table 19-2 describes transmission-based precautions in greater detail.

Standard Precautions are to be used for all patients in all situations and apply to:

- Blood
- All body fluids, secretions, and excretions *except sweat* regardless of whether or not they contain visible blood
- Nonintact skin
- Mucous membranes

Figure 19-2 shows a medical assistant wearing personal protective equipment (PPE).

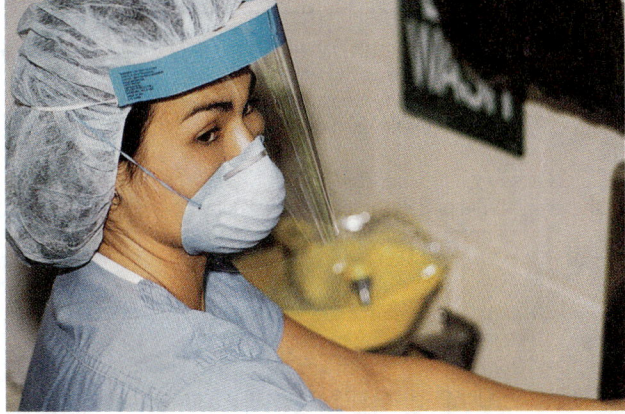

FIGURE 19-2
Personal protective equipment (PPE) includes a face shield and mask in situations that may result in splashes and splatters of blood or body fluids. An impervious gown will also be worn.

What If?
What if your patient is offended that you are wearing gloves when drawing his blood?

Sometimes patients will become defensive and make statements to the effect that they are "disease free." If this happens, reassure the patient that wearing gloves is standard practice for all patient procedures in which there may be exposure to blood, body fluids, secretions, or excretions. Then explain that gloves are worn for the protection of the patient also. Use the occasion to educate the patient about Standard Precautions and the importance of following these guidelines.

SURGICAL ASEPSIS

The principle of **surgical asepsis** is to free an item or area from all microorganisms, both pathogens and nonpathogens (Table 19-3). The practice of surgical asepsis, also known as "sterile technique," should be used when entering any part of the body that is normally sterile. Examples of this would include maintaining a sterile field for office surgery, handling sterile instruments to be used for incisions and excisions, or changing dressings over surgical or accidental wounds. (See Chap. 24, Assisting With Minor Office Surgery, for more information.)

Surgical asepsis prevents microorganisms from entering the patient's environment as opposed to medical asepsis, which prevents them from leaving the patient to spread to others.

You should use the principles of sterile technique when preparing for, setting up, and assisting with any surgical procedure in the medical office. This includes anything as simple and quick as ear piercing to a more lengthy and complex removal of a lesion.

The physician trusts you to use sterile technique when you set up a sterile field. It must be quickly acknowledged if that sterile field has been contaminated by contact with an unsterile object so that steps can be taken to restore sterility. The physician also expects you to be knowledgeable of sterile technique and to be able to maintain sterility throughout the procedure. Any break in sterile technique, no matter how small, can lead to infections the body cannot fight. Even mild infections delay recovery and are physically, mentally, and financially costly to the patient.

Checkpoint Question
4. What is surgical asepsis and when should you use it?

SURGICAL SCRUB

If you are required to assist the physician in the performance of a procedure, it will be necessary to scrub before putting on sterile gloves (Procedures 19-2 and 19-3). It is not possible to sterilize the hands, but washing in the appropriate manner will eliminate the greatest number of pathogens possible.

After assisting with a procedure that involves blood and body fluid, as all surgical procedures will, your gloves will be more contaminated than your hands. Care must be taken to avoid contaminating the hands when removing the gloves (Procedure 19-4).

INFECTION CONTROL

Maintaining effective infection control in the medical office will require knowledge of varying levels of sanitation and disinfection. Not all equipment needs to be

text continues on page 284

Table 19-3 *Comparing Medical and Surgical Asepsis*		
	Medical Asepsis	*Surgical Asepsis*
Definition	Destroys microorganisms after they leave the body	Destroys microorganisms before they enter the body
Purpose	Prevents the transmission of microorganisms from one person to another	Maintains sterility when entering a normally sterile part of the body
When used	Used when coming in contact with a body part that is not normally sterile (eg, when performing an enema)	Used when entering a normally sterile part of the body (eg, when performing urinary catheterization)
Differences in hand-washing technique	Hands and wrists are washed for 1–2 minutes; brush is not necessary. Hands are held down to rinse so water runs off fingertips. Paper towel is used for drying.	Hands and forearms are washed for 5–10 minutes; brush is used for hands, arms, and nails. Hands are held up to rinse so water runs off elbows. Sterile towel is used for drying.

Procedure 19-2 Performing a Surgical Scrub

Steps

1. Remove all jewelry.

2. Stand close to but not touching the sink.

3. Turn on the faucet using a paper towel. Discard the paper towel. *Note:* Some facilities have sinks equipped with knee controls rather than hand controls. Water force is controlled by a back and forth movement, temperature is controlled by an up and down movement. Knee controls are preferred for surgical scrubs but may not be available in many office settings.

4. Wet hands by allowing warm water to flow over them to wet completely. Keep hands above waist level.

5. Apply liquid bactericidal soap and work up a lather; intertwine the fingers and work the soap between the fingers and around the nails.

Purpose

1. Jewelry may harbor microorganisms and is never worn during a sterile procedure.

2. Standing close makes it easier to perform a proper hand wash without splashing, but the sink is considered contaminated and standing too close may contaminate your clothing.

3. The faucets are considered to be contaminated and the towel cannot be used again.

4. Warm water removes more microorganisms than cold but will not chap and crack hands as hot water will do. Hands should not be allowed to drop below waist level during a surgical scrub.

5. Intertwining cleans surfaces between the fingers; soaping the nails dislodges particles.

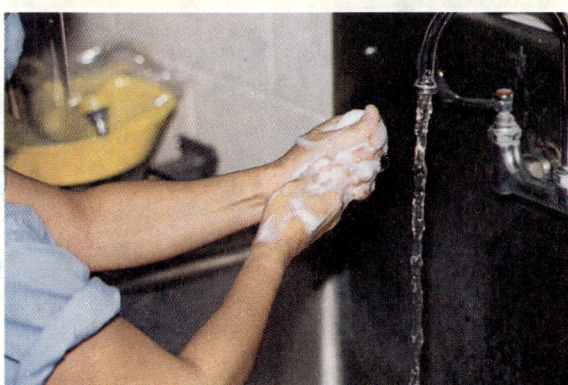

Step 5: Lather hands well.

(continued)

Procedure 19-2   Performing a Surgical Scrub *(continued)*

Steps

6. Using a brush, scrub the nails, backs, and palms of the hands and wrists and forearms.

7. Using an orangewood stick or nail instrument, clean under each nail.

Purpose

6. A brush helps dislodge and remove the maximum number of microorganisms.

7. Nails harbor microorganisms that must be removed by an instrument that is not likely to injure the integumentary system.

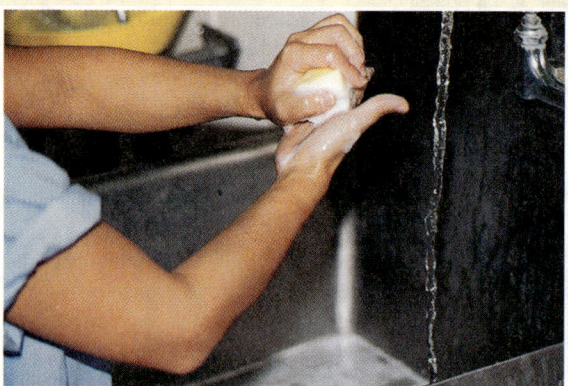

Step 6: Using the surgical scrub brush, scrub all surfaces of both hands and the forearms.

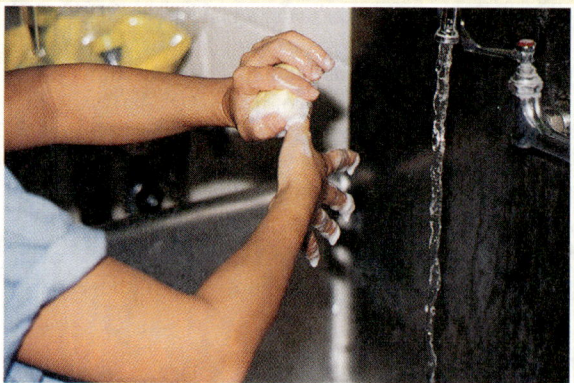

Step 6: Continued

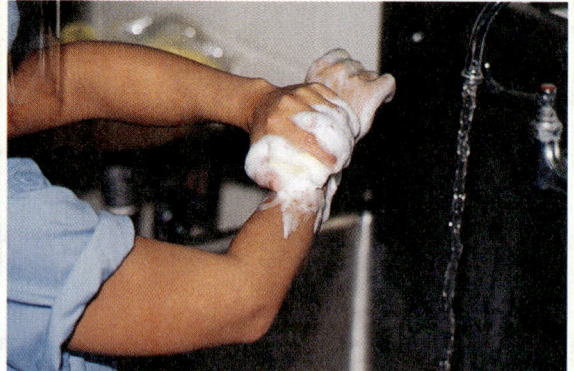

Step 6: Continued

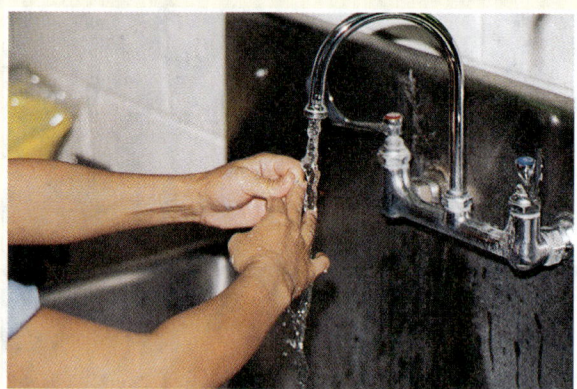

Step 7: Using a nail instrument, clean under each nail.

(continued)

Procedure 19-2

Performing a Surgical Scrub (continued)

Steps	**Purpose**

8. Rinse thoroughly.
    a. Rinse from the fingertips to the forearms.
    b. Keep the hands higher than the elbows so that water runs down the arms rather than off of the fingertips.
	8. Water running back over the hands will return microorganisms to the cleaned hands.

9. Dry from the hands to the forearms with a sterile towel.	9. Drying in this fashion prevents returning microorganisms to the cleaned hands.

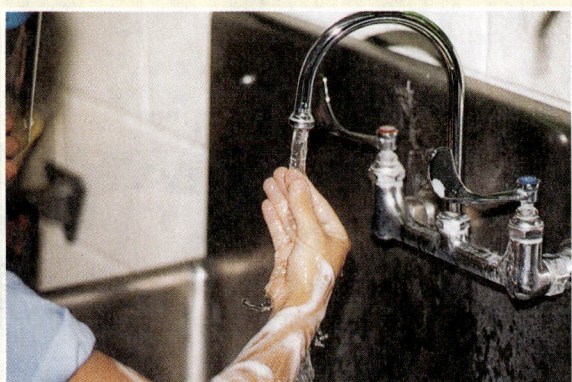

Step 8A: Rinse from the fingertips to the forearm.

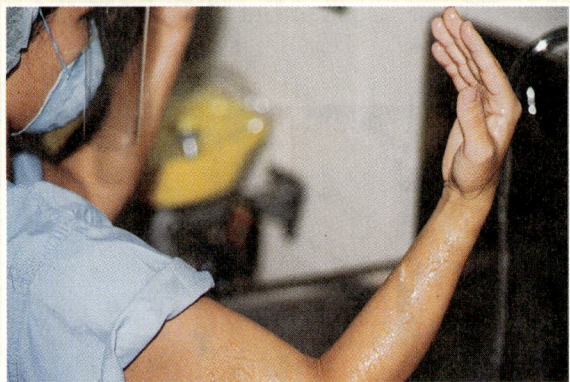

Step 8B: Hold the hands higher than the elbows.

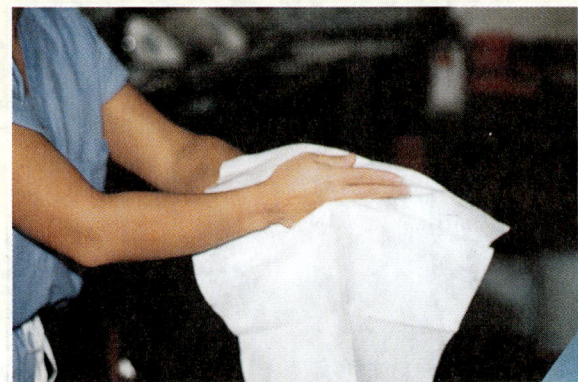

Step 9: Dry with a sterile towel from the fingertips to the forearms.

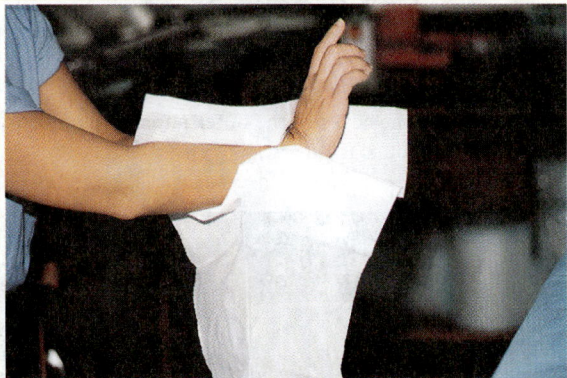

Step 9: Continued

10. Turn off the faucet with the knee controls or with the forearm, or by using a dry, sterile towel.	10. The contaminated faucets are not to be touched by the clean hands.

Note: This procedure should take 5–10 minutes.

Procedure 19-3 Sterile Gloving

Steps	Purpose
1. Remove rings and other jewelry.	1. Rings may pierce the gloves and contaminate the procedure.
2. Wash hands using the surgical aseptic technique (see Procedure 19-2).	2. Gloving is not a substitute for handwashing but must be done in addition to handwashing.
3. Place the prepackaged gloves on a clean, dry, flat surface with the cuffed end toward you. 　a. Pull the outer wrapping apart to expose the sterile inner wrap. 　b. With the cuffs toward you, fold back the inner wrap to expose the gloves.	3. Gloves are packaged for ease of application in this fashion.

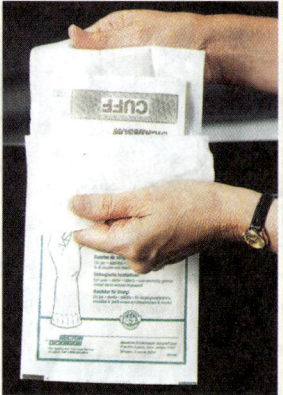

Step 3A: Pull the outer wrapping apart to expose the sterile inner wrap.

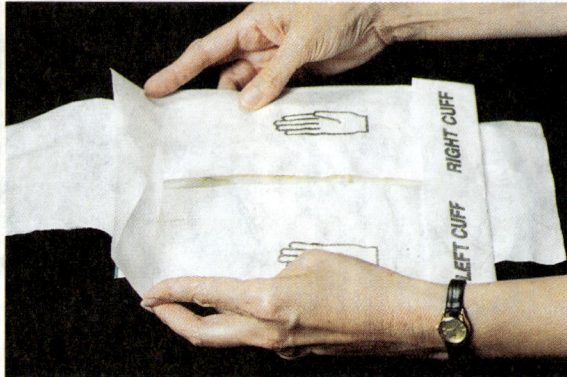

Step 3B: With the cuffs toward you, fold back the inner wrap.

4. Grasping the edges of the outer paper, open the package out to its fullest.	4. The inner surface of the package is a sterile field.

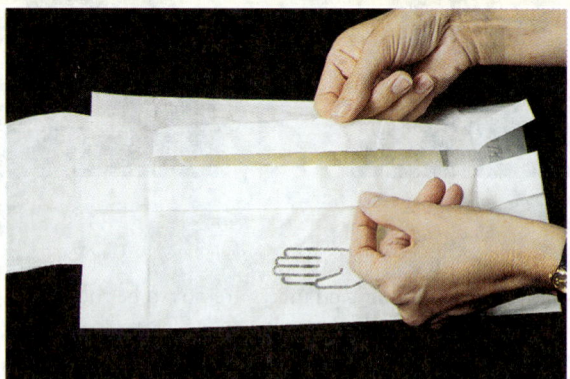

Step 4: Grasp the edges and open the package.

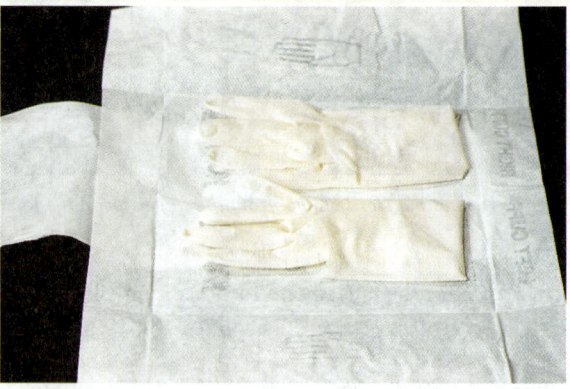

Step 4: Continued

(continued)

Procedure 19-3   Sterile Gloving *(continued)*

Steps	Purpose
5. Using your nondominant hand, pick up the dominant hand glove by grasping the folded edge of the cuff, lifting it up and away from the paper. The folded edge of the cuff is contaminated as soon as it is touched with the ungloved hand. Be very careful not to touch the outside surface of the sterile glove with your ungloved hand.	5. Lift it up and away to avoid letting the fingers of the glove brush an unsterile surface.

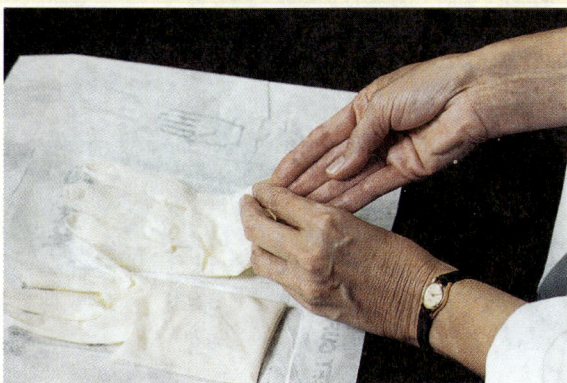

Step 5: Using the nondominant hand, lift the cuff of the glove for the dominant hand, touching only the inner surface of the cuff. Curl the thumb inward as the hand is inserted.

Steps	Purpose
6. Curl the fingers and thumb together to insert them into the glove. Then straighten the fingers and pull the glove on with the nondominant hand still grasping the cuff.	6. This prevents accidental touching of the outside surface of the glove.
7. Unfold the cuff by pinching the inside surface that will be against the wrist and pulling it toward the wrist.	7. This ensures that only the unsterile portions are touched by the hands.

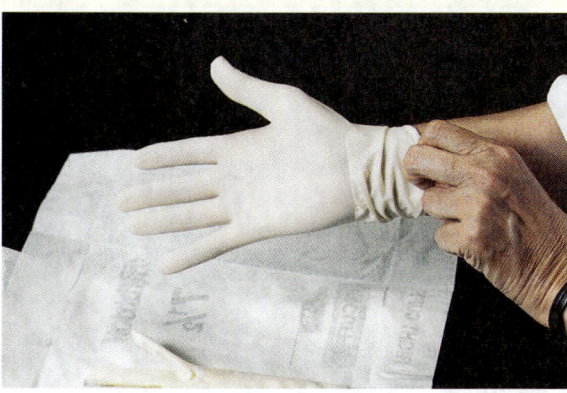

Step 7: Pull the glove snugly into place by using just the inside surface of the cuff.

(continued)

Procedure 19-3   **Sterile Gloving** *(continued)*

Steps	Purpose
8. Place the fingers of the gloved hand under the cuff of the remaining glove, lift the glove up and away from the wrapper, and slide the ungloved hand carefully into the glove with the fingers and thumb curled together.	8. This avoids letting the sterile glove accidentally touch an unsterile surface and ensures that the fingers will not brush the sterile surface of the glove.
9. Straighten the fingers and pull the glove up and over the wrist by carefully unfolding the cuff.	9. At all times, sterile must touch sterile only. Folding the cuffs out to their fullest allows the greatest area of sterility.
10. Settle the gloves comfortably onto the fingers by lacing the fingers together and adjusting the tension over the hands.	10. The gloves should fit snugly without wrinkles or areas that bind the fingers.

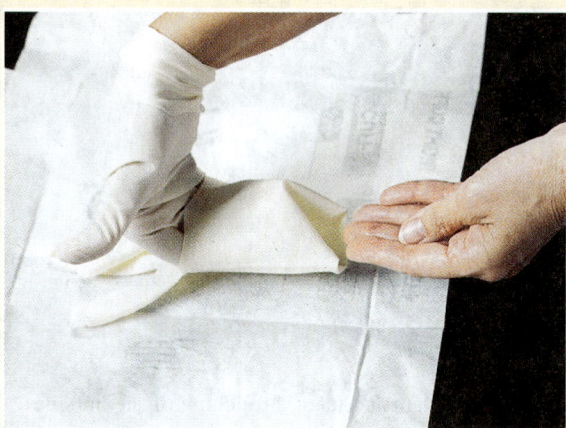

Step 8: With the thumb curled, slip the gloved dominant hand into the cuff of the remaining glove.

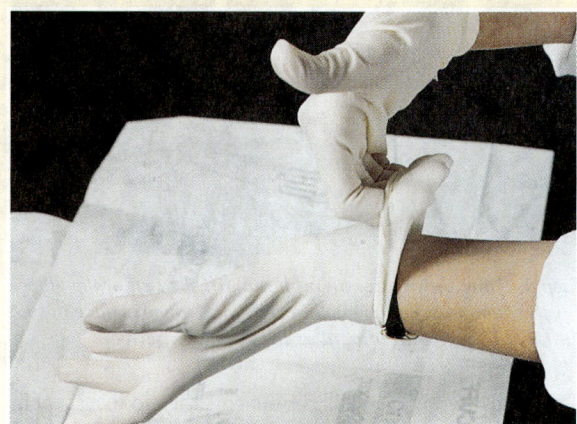

Step 9: Unfold the cuff and pull the glove on snugly.

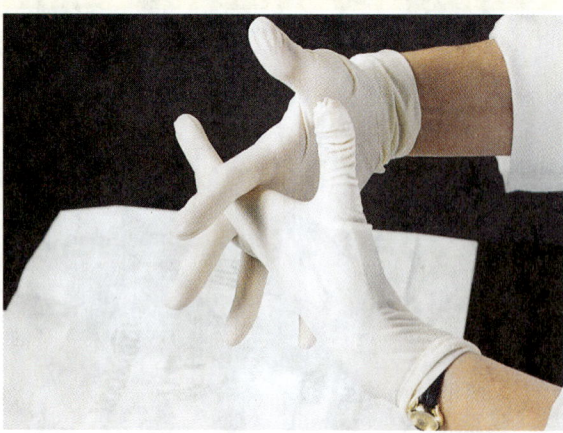

Step 10: Adjust the fingers for a comfortable fit.

Procedure 19-4   Removing Gloves After a Procedure

Steps

1. With the gloved dominant hand, grasp the area of glove over the wrist or at the palm of the nondominant hand and pull it away from the hand.

2. Stretch this soiled glove down over the fingers by pulling it away with the gloved hand.

3. As you pull the glove from the hand, ball it into the palm of the still gloved hand.

Purpose

1. This avoids touching soiled glove to clean hand.

2. This frees the hand without touching the soiled surface.

3. Balling it into a small area prevents the fingers of the glove from accidentally brushing a clean area.

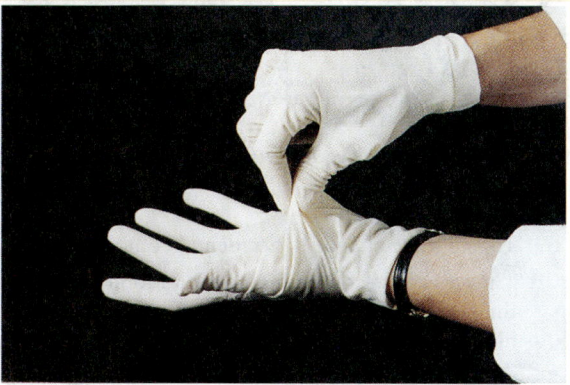

Step 1: Grasp the palm of the nondominant gloved hand.

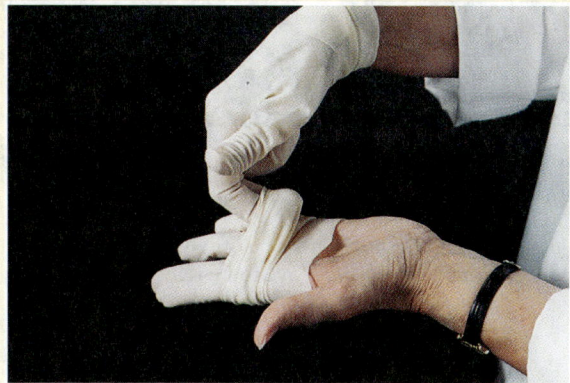

Step 2: Carefully remove the glove. Avoid contaminating your bare skin.

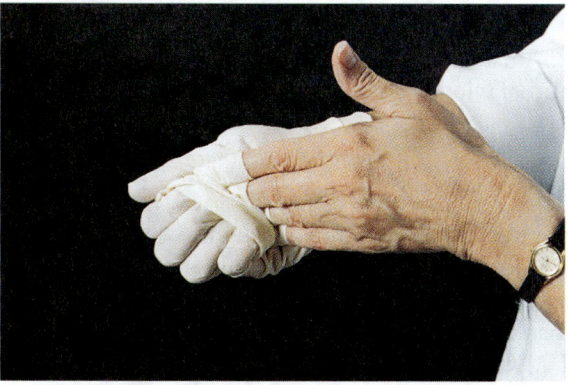

Step 3: Grasp the soiled glove with the gloved dominant hand.

4. Holding the soiled glove in the palm of the gloved hand, slip the ungloved fingers under the cuff of the gloved hand against the skin, being careful not to touch the soiled outside of the glove.

5. Stretch the glove up and away from the hand and turn it inside out as it is pulled off over the first glove.

4. This ensures skin touches skin, with no opportunity to touch the soiled area of the glove.

5. Turning it inside out exposes only clean surfaces. Soiled surfaces will be enclosed within.

(continued)

Steps	**Purpose**

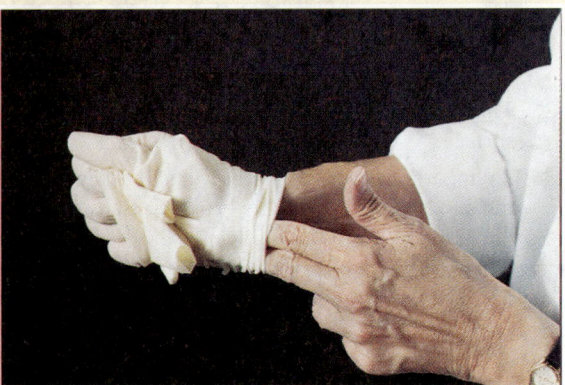

Step 4: Slip the free hand under the cuff of the remaining glove.

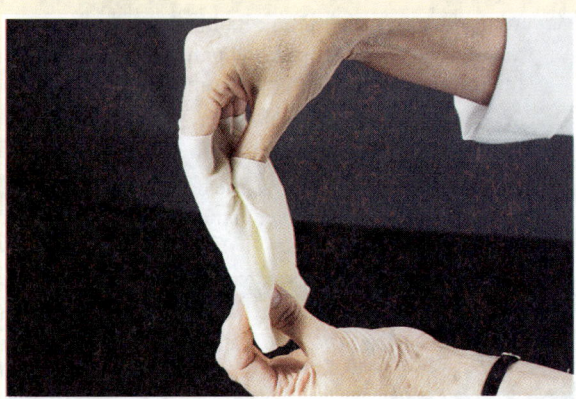

Step 5: Remove the glove by turning it inside out over the previously removed glove.

6. Both gloves should now be off with the first inside the palm of the last glove to be removed and the last glove should be inside out.	6. To avoid the chance of accidental contamination.
7. Discard in a biohazard waste receptacle.	7. The gloves are contaminated with blood and body fluid and are a potential source of infection by blood-borne pathogens.
8. Wash the hands well.	8. Gloving is not a substitute for handwashing.

Note: This procedure is also used for removing nonsterile treatment gloves.

sterile, but all equipment must be clean to a certain degree. To ensure the effectiveness of any sterilization or disinfection process, equipment and instruments must first be thoroughly cleaned or sanitized of all visible soil.

Levels of Infection Control

Sterilization

Sterilization is the highest level of infection control and destroys all forms of microorganisms including most forms of bacterial spores. Sterilization methods include steam under pressure (autoclave), gas (ethylene oxide), dry heat, or immersion in an Environmental Protection Agency (EPA)-approved chemical sterilant for a prescribed period of time. Sterilization is used for instruments or devices that penetrate the skin or contact normally sterile areas of the body (eg, scalpels, needles, catheters). Disposable invasive equipment eliminates the need to reprocess these types of items. (See Chap.

23, Instruments and Equipment, for the procedure for autoclaving.)

High-Level Disinfection

High-level disinfection is slightly less effective than sterilization, destroying all forms of bacterial life except high numbers of spores. Methods of high-level disinfection are hot water pasteurization using 80° to 100°C for 30 minutes, or exposure to an EPA-approved disinfecting chemical for a shorter exposure time, such as 10 to 45 minutes. High-level disinfection is required for reusable instruments that come in contact with mucous membranes (eg, laryngoscopes or endotracheal tubes).

Intermediate-Level Disinfection

Although intermediate-level disinfection destroys *Mycobacterium tuberculosis*, vegetative bacteria, most viruses, and most fungi, it does not kill bacterial spores.

Methods of intermediate-level disinfection are EPA-approved chemical germicides with tuberculocidal properties or hard-surface germicides or solutions containing a 1:10 dilution of common household bleach, or approximately ¼ cup of bleach per quart of tap water. Intermediate-level disinfection is used for surfaces that come in contact only with intact skin (eg, stethoscopes, blood pressure cuffs, splints) and have been visibly contaminated with blood or body fluids. Surfaces must be precleaned to remove contaminants before the germicidal chemical is applied for disinfection.

Low-Level Disinfection

Most bacteria and some viruses and fungi are destroyed by low-level disinfection, but *M. tuberculosis* or bacterial spores are not. Methods of low-level disinfection are EPA-approved disinfectants with no tuberculocidal properties. Low-level disinfection is used for routine cleaning or removing surface debris in the absence of visible blood or body fluid contamination.

Checkpoint Question

5. How does high-level disinfection differ from low-level disinfection?

Handling Environmental Contamination

Clean and disinfect environmental surfaces that have become soiled, using any cleaner or disinfectant agent intended for environmental use. These surfaces include floors, woodwork, countertops, and so on.

Cleaning and Decontaminating Spills of Blood or Body Fluids

All spills of blood and blood-contaminated fluids should be promptly cleaned using an EPA-approved germicide or a 1:10 solution of household bleach in the appropriate manner.

1. Put on gloves. Wear protective eyewear and an impervious apron or gown if you anticipate that splashing may occur.
2. Remove visible material with disposable towels or other means that will prevent contact with the fluid.
3. Dispose of the material in a biohazard container.
4. Decontaminate the area with an appropriate germicide and discard the material used for wiping up the area in an appropriate biohazard container.

5. Wash your hands after removing and discarding the gloves.
6. Place soiled items in the biohazard container and dispose of them according to facility policy. Plastic bags should be available for removal of contaminated items from the site of the spill.

Note: Your shoes can become contaminated with blood as well. Where there is massive blood contamination on floors, the use of disposable impervious shoe coverings should be considered. Protective gloves should be worn to remove contaminated shoe coverings. The coverings and gloves should be disposed of in the biohazard containers.

Handling Soiled Linens

Although soiled linen may be contaminated with pathogenic microorganisms, the risk of actual disease transmission is small. Rather than use rigid procedures and specifications, hygienic storage and processing of clean and soiled linen are recommended. Handle soiled linen as little as possible and with minimum agitation to prevent contamination of the air and the persons handling the linen. All soiled linen should be bagged at the location where it was used. Linen soiled with blood should be placed and transported in impervious bags. Normal laundry cycles should be used according to the washer and detergent's recommendations.

Decontaminating and Laundering Protective Clothing

Protective clothing contaminated with blood or body fluids to which standard precautions apply should be placed and transported in impervious bags. Anyone involved in bagging, transporting, and laundering contaminated clothing should wear gloves.

Disposing of Infectious Waste

Procedures for disposal of infectious waste are selected by determining the relative risk of disease transmission and by applying local regulations (which vary widely). In all cases, local regulations should be consulted and followed before disposal.

Generally, infectious wastes should either be incinerated or decontaminated before disposal in a sanitary landfill. Bulk blood, suctioned fluids, excretions, and secretions may be carefully poured down a drain connected to a sanitary sewer, where local regulations permit. Sanitary sewers may also be used to dispose of

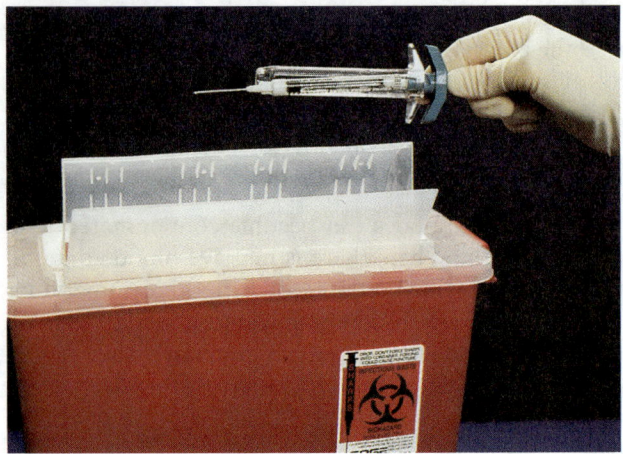

FIGURE 19-3
Disposal container for contaminated sharps.

other infectious wastes capable of being ground and flushed into the sewer, where permitted. Sharp items should be placed in puncture-proof containers (Fig. 19-3) and blood-contaminated items should be placed in leakproof plastic bags for transport to an appropriate disposal location.

Checkpoint Question
6. *What should you use to clean spills of blood or blood-contaminated body fluids?*

SUMMARY

Following the principles of medical and surgical asepsis and infection control will ensure a safe environment for patients and colleagues in the medical office. If you fail to follow these principles meticulously, you will place yourself and others at risk for infection that could impair patient recovery or affect health care worker performance in your medical setting. <u>Remember:</u> *Handwashing is the single most effective measure to prevent the spread of infection.*

CRITICAL THINKING CHALLENGES

1. Review Table 19-1 on common communicable diseases. Compare the various modes of transmission, then create a patient education booklet that focuses on preventing the spread of these diseases.
2. Identify the conditions that favor the growth of pathogens, then formulate a list of ways to control each of these factors.

3. Your patient has a leg wound that must be cared for at home. He says he knows what to do, but you suspect that he may be confused. How would you handle this situation? What other health caregivers may be able to assist your patient at home? How would you contact them?
4. Determine which of the following procedures would require medical asepsis and which would require surgical asepsis:
   • Rectal temperature
   • Excision of cyst
   • Catheterization
   • Injection
   • Throat culture
   • Cystoscopy

ANSWERS TO CHECKPOINT QUESTIONS

1. Normal flora are organisms normally found in a particular area of the body. Their presence triggers the immune system to build and release antibodies to defend against pathogens.
2. The six conditions that favor the growth of pathogens include moisture, nutrients, temperature, darkness, neutral to slightly alkaline pH, and oxygen.
3. The first link in the infection cycle, the reservoir host, provides nutrients and an incubation site for the pathogen. The fifth link, the susceptible host, allows the pathogen easy entrance and permits it to grow and multiply and thus becomes a new reservoir host, repeating the cycle.
4. Surgical asepsis, also known as sterile technique, means that an item or area is free from both pathogens and nonpathogens. It is used whenever entering any part of the body that is normally sterile.
5. High-level disinfection destroys all forms of bacterial life except high numbers of spores. Low-level disinfection destroys most bacteria and only some viruses and fungi.
6. Use an EPA-approved germicide or a 1:10 solution of household bleach to promptly clean all spills of blood or blood-contaminated body fluids.

SUGGESTIONS FOR FURTHER READING

Blood Borne Pathogens Regulations, OSHA Instructions 29CFR 1910.1030.
Burton, G. R. W. (1992). *Microbiology for the Health Sciences*, 4th ed. Philadelphia: J. B. Lippincott.
Centers for Disease Control. (1988). Recommendations for prevention of HIV transmission in the health care setting. *MMWR*, 37(24).
Ernest, V. V. (1992). *Clinical Skills in Nursing Practice*, 2nd ed. Philadelphia: J.B. Lippincott.

Haman, B. (1994). *Disease: Identification, Prevention and Control*. St. Louis: Mosby-Yearbook.

Lewis, L., & Timby, B. (1992). *Fundamental Skills and Concepts in Nursing Care*, 5th ed. Philadelphia: J. B. Lippincott.

Smeltzer, S. C., & Bare, B. C. (1996). *Brunner and Suddarth's Textbook of Medical-Surgical Nursing*, 8th ed. Philadelphia: Lippincott-Raven.

Staines, N., Brostoff, J., & James, K. (1993). *Introducing Immunology*. London: C. V. Mosby.

Taylor, C., Lillis, C., LeMone, P. (1993). *Fundamentals of Nursing: The Art and Science of Nursing Care*, 2nd ed., Philadelphia: J.B. Lippincott.

Volk, W. A., et al. (1995). *Essentials of Medical Microbiology*, 5th ed., Philadelphia: J.B. Lippincott.

Medical History and Patient Assessment

Chapter Outline

The Medical History
    Methods of Collecting
        Information
    Elements of the Medical
        History
Conducting the Patient Interview
    Preparing for the Interview
    Introducing Yourself
    Barriers to Communication

Assessing the Patient
    Signs and Symptoms
    Chief Complaint and Present Illness
Procedure: Interviewing the Patient to
        Obtain a Medical History
Summary
Critical Thinking Challenges
Answers to Checkpoint Questions
Suggestions for Further Reading

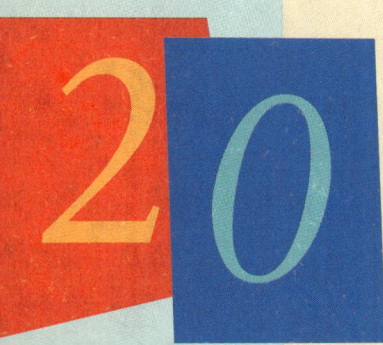

20

DACUM Components

1.4   Maintain confidentiality
1.5   Work as a team member
2.1   Listen and observe
2.5   Serve as liaison between physician and others
2.9   Interview effectively
3.3   Prepare and maintain medical records
4.6   Interview and take patient history
5.1   Document accurately

Chapter Competencies

Learning Objectives

Upon successfully completing this chapter, you will be able to:

1. Spell and define the Key Terms.
2. List the different sections of the medical history and give examples of the type of information included in each.
3. Explain why certain information is included in the various sections.
4. List guidelines for conducting a patient interview.
5. Explain the difference between a sign and a symptom and give examples of each.
6. Explain chief complaint and present illness.

Performance Objective

Upon successfully completing this chapter, you will be able to:

1. Interview a patient and correctly complete appropriate sections of the medical history form (Procedure 20-1).

Key Terms

(See Glossary for definitions.)

assessment
chief complaint
familial
hereditary
medical history
over-the-counter
signs
symptoms

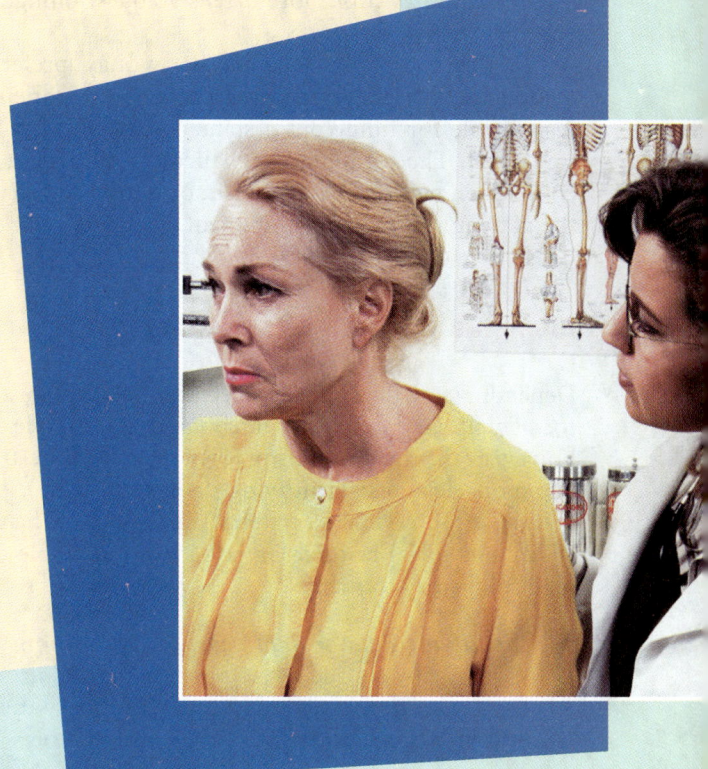

Diagnosing a patient's present illness requires that the physician have access to the patient's past and current health status. The medical assistant is responsible for eliciting this information as part of the **medical history** and patient **assessment**. The medical history is a record containing information about a patient's past and present health status. Assessment is the process of gathering information to determine the patient's problem or reason for seeking medical treatment. To ensure consistent care, you will ask standard questions and obtain specific information about each patient. Responses are usually documented on preprinted forms or in a manner decided by the physician (see Chap. 10, Medical Records and Records Management, for information on documentation).

➤ THE MEDICAL HISTORY

Methods of Collecting Information

In many practices, the medical assistant and the physician work cooperatively to obtain the patient's complete medical history. The medical assistant gathers initial patient information by obtaining answers to a printed list of questions and conducting a patient interview. The physician then reviews that information, using it as the basis for more extensive questioning and data gathering.

In other practices, the physician may prefer to complete the medical history. In others, the patient is responsible for filling out a standardized medical history form. The form may be mailed to the patient for completion before the initial visit, or it may be given to the patient at the first appointment.

Elements of the Medical History

Depending on the practice specialty, medical history forms will vary somewhat in content and complexity; however, the medical history is composed of these common elements: identifying data (data base), past history (PH), review of systems (ROS), family history (FH), and social history. Fig. 20-1 is an example of a medical history form.

- *Identifying data or data base.* Information in this section always includes the patient's name and date of birth and will usually include the patient's address, home and work telephone numbers, insurance carrier and policy number, social security number, gender, and race. This information is required for administrative purposes.

Legal Tips

You are responsible for ensuring that information obtained as part of the patient's medical history is kept confidential. Legally and ethically, the patient has a right to privacy concerning his or her medical records, which should be kept in a secure place. Only those health care providers directly involved in the patient's care should be allowed access to the records.

- *Past history (PH).* This is a summary of the patient's prior health status. It can include allergies, immunizations, childhood diseases, current and past medications, previous illnesses, traumatic injuries, surgeries, and hospitalizations. Knowing this information can help the physician plan appropriate care for the patient's present illness.
- *Review of systems (ROS).* A thorough review of each body system elicits information that the patient may have forgotten to mention or may have felt was irrelevant. Careful questioning can uncover potential areas of concern for the physician to explore further.
- *Family history (FH).* The health status of the patient's parents, siblings, and grandparents is summarized, including any specific diseases or disorders that any immediate family member may have. This information is important because certain diseases have **familial** or **hereditary** tendencies. Familial diseases tend to occur more often in a particular family. Hereditary diseases are transmitted from parent to offspring. If any of the patient's family members are deceased, you should obtain information about the cause of death.
- *Social history.* Included in this information is the patient's life-style, such as marital status, occupation, education, and hobbies. It may also include questions about the use of alcohol and tobacco and a sexual history. Knowing this information aids the physician in understanding how the patient's present illness, and any planned treatment, may affect the individual's life-style.

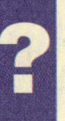

Checkpoint Questions

1. *What are the common elements of a medical history?*
2. *What is the difference between the past history and family history?*

text continues on page 293

Professional Medical Associates – History Form

NAME: _____ DATE OF BIRTH: _____

What is the main reason for your visit to the doctor? _____

_____

Were you referred? _____ if so, by whom? _____

PAST MEDICAL HISTORY:

Are you allergic to any medication? _____

If so, list medications: _____

List current medications, dosage, and how many times you take them a day:

Medication   **Dose**   **Times A Day**

_____

_____

Alcohol Consumption: What type? _____ Amount _____ How Often? _____

                        History of Alcoholism? _____

When was your last TB or Tine test? _____

Have you ever had a positive test for tuberculosis? _____

When was your last Tetanus shot? _____

List all surgeries you have had in the past:

Date   **Type of Surgery**

_____

_____

List all past hospitalizations (not involving surgeries above):

Date   **Reason For Hospital Stay**

_____

_____

List all past problems with trauma (broken bones, lacerations, etc.):

_____

REVIEW OF SYSTEMS, PAST MEDICAL PROBLEMS:

If you have been told you have any of the problems listed below, or are having any of the problems listed below, please CIRCLE:

1. <u>GENERAL:</u> Weight loss, weight gain, fever, chills, night sweats, hot flashes, tire easily, problems with sleep, crying spells, history of cancer.

2. <u>SKIN:</u> Rash, sores that won't heal, moles that are new or changing, history of skin problems.

3. <u>HEENT:</u> Headache, eye problems, hearing problems, sinus problems, hay fever, dizziness, hoarseness, sores in your mouth that won't heal, dental problems.

   Do you chew tobacco or dip snuff? _____

4. <u>METABOLIC/ENDOCRINE:</u> Thyroid problems, diabetes or sugar problems, high cholesterol.

FIGURE 20-1

A sample medical history form.

5. RESPIRATORY: Cough, wheezing, breathing problems, history of asthma, history of lung problems.

Do you smoke cigarettes or pipe? _____

How much? _____ For how long? _____

6. BREAST (WOMEN): Breast lumps, changes in nipples, nipple discharge, breast problems, family history of breast cancer. When was your last mammogram? _____

7. CARDIOVASCULAR: Heart murmur, rheumatic fever, high blood pressure, angina, heart problems, heart attack, abnormal heart rhythm, chest pain, palpitations, leg swelling, history of phlebitis or blood clots.

8. GI: Problems with appetite, swallowing, heartburn, nausea, vomiting, pain in the abdomen, constipation, diarrhea, blood in stool, history of ulcers, liver problems, hepatitis, jaundice, pancreas problems, gallbladder problems, or colon problems.

9. REPRODUCTIVE (WOMEN): Problems with irregular menstrual cycles, abnormal vaginal bleeding or discharge, history of venereal diseases, sexual problems.

AGE OF FIRST MENSES (PERIOD) _____ AGE OF MENOPAUSE _____

LAST PAP SMEAR _____ METHOD OF CONTRACEPTION _____

Obstetric History (Women)

NUMBER OF PREGNANCIES _____ PLEASE LIST AS FOLLOWS:

Delivery Date	Pregnancy Complications	Type Delivery	Body Weight

MEN: Problems with genital discharge, history of venereal diseases, sexual problems, prostate problems.

METHOD OF CONTRACEPTION _____

10. UROLOGIC: Problems with painful urination, urinary frequency, blood in urine, weak urinary stream, history of bladder or kidney infections, or kidney stones.

11. MUSCULOSKELETAL: Arthritis, back pain, cramps in legs.

12. NEUROLOGIC: Seizures, stroke, arm or leg weakness or numbness, black-out spells, memory or thinking problems, depression, anxiety, psychiatric problems.

13. HEMATOLOGIC: Anemia, bleeding problems, enlarged lymph nodes.

HAVE YOU EVER HAD A BLOOD TRANSFUSION? _____ DATE _____

FAMILY HISTORY:

List any medical problems that run in your family and which family members have these problems.

_____

_____

SOCIAL HISTORY:

MARITAL STATUS: _____

OCCUPATION: _____

EDUCATION: _____

HOBBIES: _____

WHAT DO YOU DO FOR ENJOYMENT? _____

FIGURE 20-1 Continued.

➤ CONDUCTING THE PATIENT INTERVIEW

Preparing for the Interview

An interview involves reviewing past or current medical history. As a medical assistant, your primary goal during the patient interview is to obtain accurate and pertinent information. To do this, you will need to understand the basic components of communication and to use active listening skills. You also will need to use a variety of interviewing techniques, including reflecting, paraphrasing, asking for examples, asking questions, summarizing, and allowing silence. (See Chap. 4, Fundamental Communication Skills, for specific information on these techniques.) Procedure 20-1 outlines the process for conducting a successful patient interview.

Be sure you are familiar with the medical history forms and questions before you start interviewing. Shuffling papers while the patient is talking or backtracking in your line of questioning distracts the patient and disrupts the flow of the interview. Know the order of the questions and the type of information the physician is trying to elicit. If the patient is new to the practice, review his or her new patient questionnaire before beginning. If the patient is an established one, review his or her chart.

To enhance the potential for open communication—and to safeguard patient confidentiality—find a private and comfortable place, such as an office or conference room, in which to conduct the interview. Avoid areas where distractions are likely, such as the reception area. Interview the patient alone, unless he or she wishes to have family members or significant others present (Fig. 20-2).

Introducing Yourself

For both new and established patients, begin by identifying yourself and stating the purpose of the interview. For example, you might say, "Good morning, Mr. Frank. My name is Angela and I'm Dr. Martin's medical assistant. I want to ask a few questions that will help the doctor plan appropriate care for you. Please be assured that your responses will be kept strictly confidential."

The initial impression you make on the patient will be a lasting one. So be sure your demeanor and words communicate genuine respect and concern. By developing a professional rapport, you will gain the patient's confidence and trust.

Barriers to Communication

As you begin speaking with the patient, assess any barriers to communication. Determine the patient's level of understanding and adjust your questioning accordingly—for instance, avoid using highly technical terms. Also note if the patient is hearing or visually impaired or has trouble understanding or speaking English. Again, adjust your interviewing techniques to best fit the patient's needs. (See Chap. 4, Fundamental Communication Skills, for more information.)

text continues on page 295

 **F**ocus on the Patient: Helping Patients Feel at Ease

Over time, many medical procedures will become routine for you. But for many patients, these "routine" procedures are cause for fear and intimidation during a visit to the physician's office. To help put patients at ease, follow these tips:

Treat each patient as an individual with unique needs. Help elderly or disabled patients onto the examining table. If they are unsteady, keep them seated in a regular chair.
When weighing patients, do not announce their weight verbally because this may be embarrassing. Instead, ask them in the privacy of the examining room if they want to know their weight.

Always offer a sheet or blanket to a patient who is changing into an examining gown.
When preparing a woman for a gynecologic examination, have her sit on the examining table until the physician is ready. Then assist her into the stirrups.
If the physician is delayed, let the patient know. Explain that an emergency has occurred, and let the patient know the approximate length of the delay. You can further help the situation by offering the patient a magazine or a glass of water. Also invite the patient to use the telephone to alert family, friends, or employers about the delay.

Procedure 20-1 — Interviewing the Patient to Obtain a Medical History

Equipment/Supplies

- medical history form or questionnaire
- pen

Steps	Purpose
1. Gather the supplies.	1. This ensures you have everything you need before you start.
2. Review the medical history form.	2. It is important that you become familiar with the order of the questions and the type of information required.
3. Find a private and comfortable place.	3. A quiet place avoids distractions and ensures patient confidentiality.
4. Sit across from the patient at eye level and maintain frequent eye contact.	4. Standing above the patient may be perceived as threatening and may result in poor communication.
5. Introduce yourself and explain the purpose of the interview.	5. This helps you establish a professional rapport with the patient.
6. Using language the patient can understand, ask the appropriate questions and document the patient's responses. Be sure to determine the patient's chief complaint (CC) and present illness (PI).	6. You must obtain accurate and complete data.
7. Listen actively, stop writing from time to time, and look at the patient while he or she is speaking.	7. Patients can sense when the interviewer is not listening, so be sure you show interest in what the patient is saying.
8. Regardless of the confidences shared by the patient, avoid projecting a judgmental attitude by your words or your actions.	8. You must maintain your professionalism and ensure the patient's trust in you.
9. If appropriate, explain to the patient what to expect during any examinations or procedures that may be scheduled for the day.	9. Keeping the patient properly informed about his or her care is vital.
10. Thank the patient for cooperating during the interview and offer to answer any questions.	10. Courtesy encourages the patient to have a positive attitude about the physician's office.

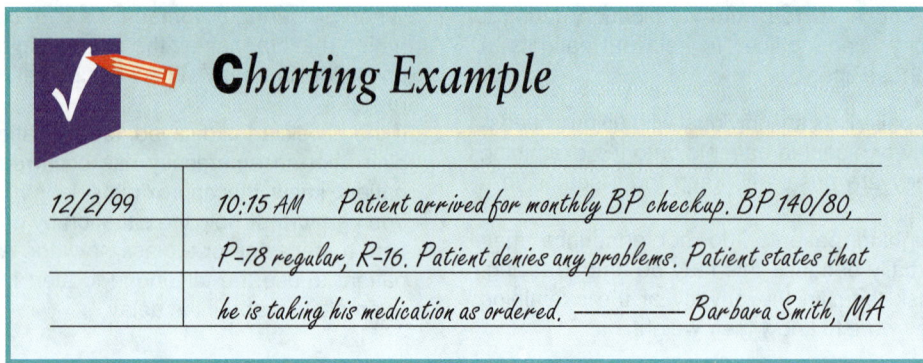

Charting Example

12/2/99	10:15 AM Patient arrived for monthly BP checkup. BP 140/80,
	P-78 regular, R-16. Patient denies any problems. Patient states that
	he is taking his medication as ordered. ———— Barbara Smith, MA

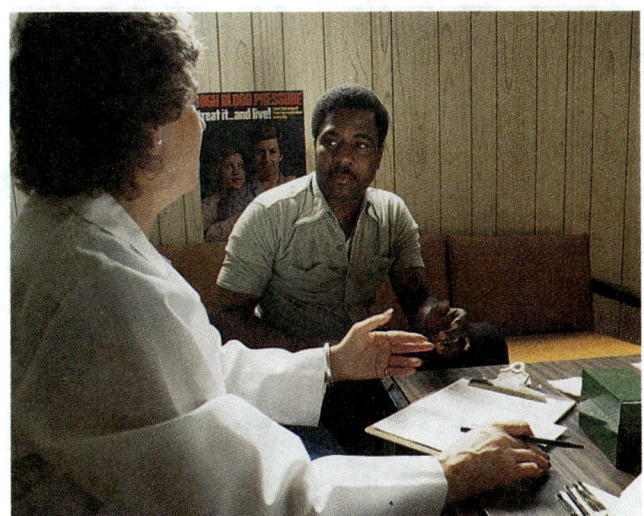

FIGURE 20-2
Conduct the patient interview in a private and comfortable place.

Checkpoint Question
3. *What should you do before beginning a patient interview?*

What If?
What if the patient is highly anxious about the interview? For example, when you ask a question, the patient speaks so quickly you have trouble understanding the answer. The patient also seems unable to focus on one topic at a time and often rambles.

Speak slowly and softly. Reassure the patient that people commonly feel nervous when talking about their health. Let the patient know that there is no rush and that you can take as much time as needed to complete the interview.

➤ ASSESSING THE PATIENT

Signs and Symptoms

You must listen carefully as the patient describes current medical problems to identify **signs** and **symptoms.** These are also referred to as subjective and objective information. Symptoms are subjective indications of disease or changes in the body as sensed by the patient; they are not discernible by anyone else. Examples of symptoms a patient may describe include "leg pain," "headache," or "nausea." Signs are objective indica-

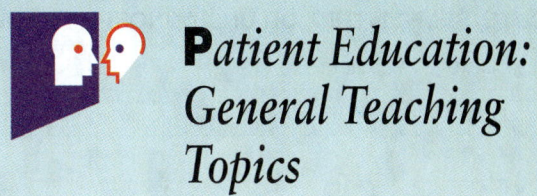

Patient Education: General Teaching Topics

While performing a patient assessment, you can initiate patient education. The teaching may consist of information about a specific disease or general care. For example, a diabetic patient may need instruction on glucose testing or diet control. General topics for *all* patients can include:

- blood pressure management
- stress management techniques
- diet or weight control tips
- the importance of exercise and sample exercises
- the effects of alcohol and the need to limit alcohol consumption
- instructions for conducting breast or testicular self-examination
- proper immunizations
- cancer prevention tips

tions of disease or bodily dysfunction that can be perceived by others, such as vital signs or findings made by the physician. Signs include a rash, bleeding, cough, discharge, or blood pressure readings.

Chief Complaint and Present Illness

After recording the patient's medical history and reviewing the information for accuracy and clarity, you must find out exactly why the patient has come to see the physician. To do this, ask an open-ended question—a question that allows a broad response—to encourage the patient to describe the chain of events leading to this appointment. For example, you might ask, "What can we do to help you?" or "What is the reason for your appointment today?" or "Can you describe what has been going on?"

The patient's answer will reveal the **chief complaint** (CC). The CC is a description of the symptom(s) that led the patient to seek the physician's care. Examples might include "I've had a headache for the last 3 days" or "Yesterday I lifted a heavy crate and strained my back." Document the CC in the patient's record using the patient's own words. Fig. 20-3 is an example of a form used to document a patient's CC.

text continues on page 298

ACUTE, SELF-LIMITED, OR UNDIAGNOSED PROBLEMS

	Date	Problem
A		
B		
C		
D		
E		
F		
G		
H		
I		
J		
K		
L		

PROFESSIONAL
MEDICAL ASSOCIATES, P.A.

CUMULATIVE PROBLEM LIST

	Date	Problem Title
1		
2		
3		
4		
5		
6		
7		
8		
9		
10		
11		
12		
13		
14		
15		
16		
17		

FIGURE 20-3
A cumulative problem list used to document a patient's chief complaint.

MEDICATION RECORD

Drug Intolerances:

Drug	Reaction	Date

LONG-TERM MEDICATIONS

Date	Problem	Medication

FIGURE 20-3 Continued.

Continue to probe for more details to define the patient's present illness (PI)—a more specific account of the CC. The PI includes a chronologic order of events including dates of onset, home remedies used by the patient, and over-the-counter medications taken by the patient. Over-the-counter medications are those that are available without prescriptions. Questions to ask might include:

- "How did this first begin?"
- "Can you describe the pain?"
- "What medications have you taken for the pain?"

Avoid suggesting answers, such as, "Is the pain sharp?" or "Is the pain worse when you walk?" Many patients will agree or answer positively because they think this must be the expected answer. Anything the patient has felt or has done up to this time should be noted on the initial interview.

After asking several open-ended questions, go to closed-ended questions to obtain specific data. For example, you might ask the patient, "How long have you had this pain?" This kind of question requires only a short answer, not a lengthy description.

Both the CC and the PI include subjective and objective information. The medical assistant must carefully describe and correctly designate each as either subjective or objective findings.

Of course, not all patients visit the doctor because they are ill. Some patient appointments are for routine examinations or tests. You must document the reasons for these visits in the patient record as well.

her clothes do not match. Is this worth noting on her chart?

2. Mrs. Brown speaks English as a second language. You need to ask her about her urinary symptoms. Compare the following phrases. Which one should you use? Why?
   - "Do you have trouble voiding?" "Do you have trouble passing your water?"

3. Review the following items. Determine in which section of the medical history each should be included and explain why. Identify any items that are irrelevant.
   - Sister died of breast cancer.
   - Son had chickenpox last year.
   - Patient has many allergies.
   - Father died of heart disease.
   - Mother living and well.
   - Brother works in real estate.
   - Patient smokes three packs of cigarettes a day.
   - Patient works in cotton mill.
   - Patient is a runner and teaches aerobics.
   - Patient has recently lost 60 pounds.
   - Patient had angioplasty last year.

4. Determine which of the following are signs and which are symptoms.
   nausea
   vomiting
   itching
   rash
   dizziness
   abdominal pain
   pallor
   tingling toes
   fever
   edema

Checkpoint Question

4. What is the difference between a sign and a symptom? Give an example of each.

SUMMARY

Every medical practice will obtain a history from each patient. As a medical assistant, you are responsible for knowing the components of a standard medical history and for obtaining the patient's medical history if appropriate. You may also conduct an interview to elicit the patient's chief complaint and present illness. The physician relies on the information you gather in diagnosing and treating patients, so it is essential that you question the patient carefully and document accurately.

CRITICAL THINKING CHALLENGES

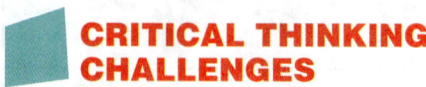

1. Mrs. Jones has always been impeccably groomed. Today her hair is not combed, she has on no makeup, and

ANSWERS TO CHECKPOINT QUESTIONS

1. The common elements of a medical history include identifying data, past history (PH), review of systems (ROS), family history (FH), and social history.

2. The past history summarizes the patient's prior health status; the family history summarizes the health status of the patient's parents, siblings, and grandparents.

3. Before beginning a patient interview, you should:
   - Review the patient's past and current medical history.
   - Familiarize yourself with the medical history form and questions.
   - Choose a private and comfortable place to conduct the interview.
   - Introduce yourself and explain the purpose for the interview.

4. A sign is an objective indication of disease or bodily dysfunction that can be perceived by others; examples include rash, bleeding, or discharge. A symptom is a subjective indication of disease or changes in the body that can be perceived only by the patient; examples include leg pain, headache, or nausea.

SUGGESTIONS FOR FURTHER READING

Bates, B., Buckley, L. S., Hockleman, R. A. (1995). *A Guide to Physical Examination and History Taking*, 6th ed. Philadelphia: J.B. Lippincott.

Craven, R. F., Hirnle, C. J. (1992). *Fundamentals of Nursing*, Philadelphia: J.B. Lippincott.

Kerschner, V. (1992). *Health Unit Coordinating, Principles and Practices*. Albany, NY: Delmar.

Kozier, B., & Erb, G. (1993). *Techniques of Clinical Nursing*, 4th ed. Addison and Wesley, Redwood City, CA.

Smeltzer, S., & Bare, B. (1996). *Brunner and Suddarth's Textbook of Medical-Surgical Nursing,* 8th ed. Philadelphia: Lippincott-Raven.

Timby, B., & Lewis, L. (1992). *Fundamental Skills and Concepts in Patient Care,* 5th ed. Philadelphia: J. B. Lippincott.

Anthropometric Measurements and Vital Signs

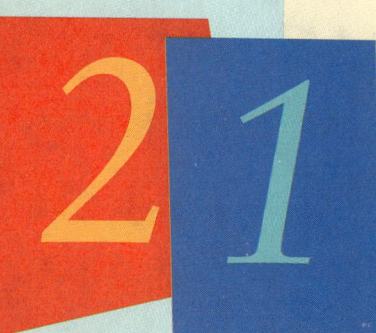

21

Chapter Outline

Weight
Procedure: Measuring Weight
Height
Procedure: Measuring Height
Temperature (T)
Fever Processes
Stages of Fever
Types of Thermometers
Oral Temperature
Procedure: Measuring Oral Temperature
Using a Glass Mercury Ther-
mometer
Rectal Temperature
Procedure: Measuring Rectal Temperature
Using a Glass Mercury Ther-
mometer
Axillary Temperature
Procedure: Measuring Axillary Tempera-
ture Using a Glass Mercury
Thermometer
Procedure: Measuring Temperature Using
an Electronic Thermometer
Tympanic Temperature
Procedure: Measuring Temperature
Using a Tympanic
Thermometer

Cleaning Thermometers
Procedure: Disinfecting a Glass
Thermometer
Pulse (P)
Characteristics
Averages and Ranges
Factors Affecting Pulse Rates
Procedure: Measuring the Radial Pulse
Procedure: Measuring the Apical Pulse
Respiration (R)
Characteristics
Averages and Ranges
Procedure: Counting Respirations
Blood Pressure (BP)
Korotkoff Sounds and the Five
Phases of Blood Pressure
Pulse Pressure
Auscultatory Gap
Factors Influencing Blood Pressure
Choosing the Correct Cuff Size
Procedure: Measuring Blood Pressure
Charting Vital Signs in the Hospital Setting
Summary
Critical Thinking Challenges
Answers to Checkpoint Questions
Suggestions for Further Reading

DACUM Components

1.3 Practice within the scope of education, training, and personal capabilities
1.6 Conduct oneself in a courteous and diplomatic manner
2.2 Treat all patients with empathy and impartiality
4.1 Apply principles of aseptic technique and infection control
4.2 Take vital signs
5.1 Document accurately
7.3 Teach patients methods of health promotion and disease prevention

Chapter Competencies

Learning Objectives

Upon successfully completing this chapter, you will be able to:

1. Spell and define the Key Terms.
2. Explain the procedures for measuring a patient's height and weight.
3. Identify and describe the different types of thermometers.
4. Explain the procedure for measuring a patient's temperature using the oral, rectal, axillary, or tympanic methods.
5. Explain the procedure for measuring a patient's pulse rate.
6. Explain the procedure for counting a patient's respirations.
7. Describe Korotkoff sounds and the five phases of blood pressure.
8. Explain the procedure for measuring a patient's blood pressure.
9. State normal values and value ranges for temperature, pulse, respirations, and blood pressure in a variety of patients.

Performance Objectives

Upon successfully completing this chapter, you will be able to:

1. Measure and record a patient's weight (Procedure 21-1).
2. Measure and record a patient's height (Procedure 21-2).
3. Measure and record a patient's oral temperature using a glass mercury thermometer (Procedure 21-3).
4. Measure and record a patient's rectal temperature using a glass mercury thermometer (Procedure 21-4).
5. Measure and record a patient's axillary temperature using a glass mercury thermometer (Procedure 21-5).
6. Measure and record a patient's temperature using an electronic thermometer (Procedure 21-6).
7. Measure and record a patient's temperature using a tympanic thermometer (Procedure 21-7).
8. Disinfect a glass thermometer (Procedure 21-8).
9. Measure and record a patient's radial pulse (Procedure 21-9).
10. Measure and record a patient's apical pulse (Procedure 21-10).
11. Count a patient's respirations (Procedure 21-11).
12. Measure a patient's blood pressure (Procedure 21-12).
13. Auscultate a patient's pedal pulse using a Doppler unit.

Key Terms

(See Glossary for definitions.)

anthropometric	cardinal signs	intermittent
baseline	diastole	postural hypotension
calibrated	diaphoresis	remittent
cardiac cycle	febrile	systole
cardiac output	hypertension	

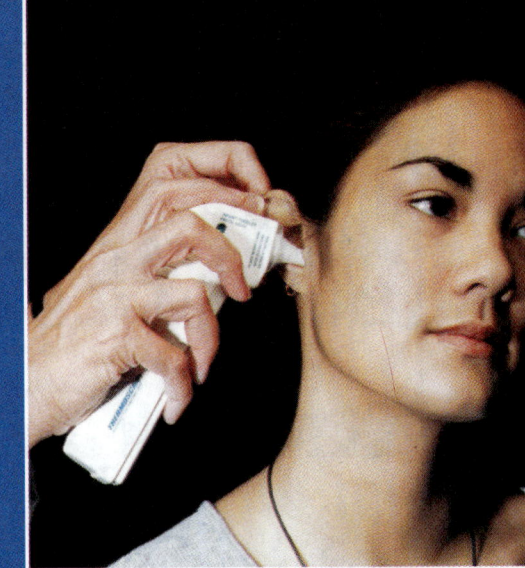

Vital signs, also called **cardinal signs**, are measurements of the functions essential to sustaining life. These include temperature (T), pulse (P), respiration (R), and blood pressure (BP). These signs are recorded at almost every visit made to the medical office.

Height and weight measurements, called **anthropometric** measurements, usually are acquired as the patient is escorted to the examining room. Height and weight are considered to be as important as any of the measurements required for diagnosis and treatment.

At the first visit, anthropometric measurements and vital signs are recorded as **baseline** data, or reference points, for comparison during all subsequent visits. These measurements are the most frequently performed procedures in the medical assistant's daily schedule.

➤ WEIGHT

Weights are always required for prenatal patients, infants, children, and the elderly. In addition, constant weight monitoring may be required if the patient is prescribed medications that must be carefully calculated by body weight. When the physician is following a patient who is attempting to gain or lose weight, the ideal is compared to the weights in an adult desirable weight chart.

The placement of the scales in the office should be carefully considered. Many patients will be uncomfortable if weight is measured in a place that is not private. The type of scales used to measure weight include balance beam scales (Fig. 21-1), digital scales, or dial scales. Weight may be measured in pounds (lb) or kilograms (kg). (See Appendix V for information about metric and U.S. equivalents for weight, length, and volume.) Procedure 21-1 describes how to measure weight.

➤ HEIGHT

Height may be measured using the movable ruler on the back of most scales (Procedure 21-2), or it may be measured against a graph mounted on a wall. A most accurate measure will be made by any device with a parallel bar that can be moved against the patient's head. Height can be measured in inches or centimeters, depending on the physician's preference.

➤ TEMPERATURE (T)

Temperature is defined as the balance between heat produced and heat lost by the body (Fig. 21-2). All human beings have a temperature that is produced by the energy generated during the physical and chemical changes called metabolism and lost through respiration, elimination, and conduction through the skin. Table 21-1 describes and illustrates processes by which heat is transferred.

Metabolism is the process of breaking down and burning energy sources by the cells for life mainte-

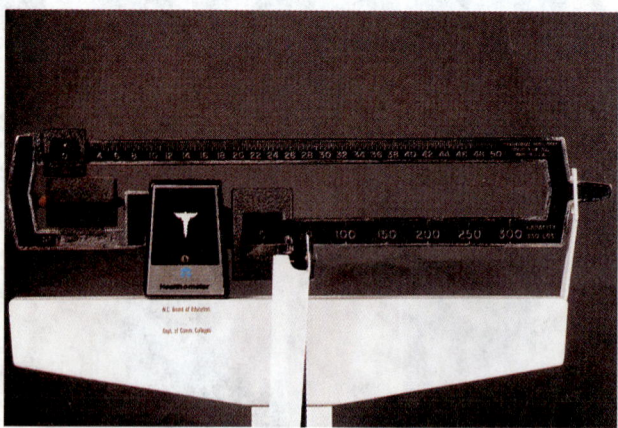

FIGURE 21-1

A balance beam scale. The large weight indicator is the bottom bar; measurements are in 50-pound increments. The small weight indicator is the top bar; measurements are in ¼-pound increments. On the small weight indicator bar, the even number pounds are numbered (eg, 0, 2, 4, 6) while the odd number pounds are each represented by a long line. Between the numbers and the long lines are smaller lines that represent ¼-pound measurements. A very slightly longer line is at ½-pound increments.

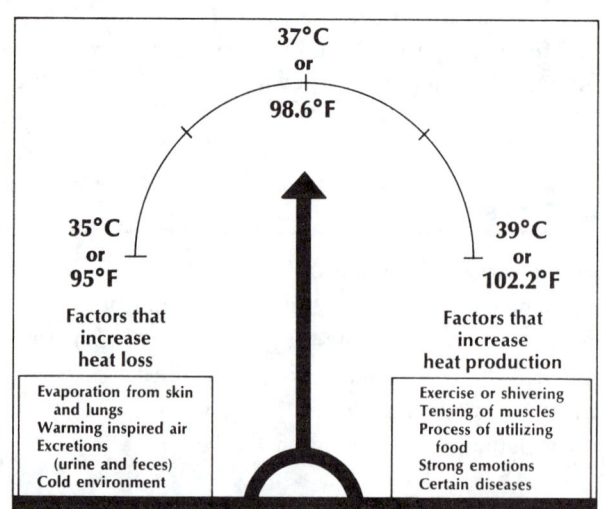

FIGURE 21-2

Factors affecting temperature balance. The illustration shows the balance between factors that increase heat loss and factors that increase heat production.

nance. This activity can be measured in four different ways using thermometers designed for each method: oral, rectal, axillary, and tympanic. The two scales used to measure temperature are Fahrenheit and centigrade (Celsius). Because thermometers may be **calibrated** (marked) in either scale (Fig. 21-3), you should be able to convert from one scale to another (see Appendix VI).

Each temperature is fairly constant in relation to the others. The oral temperature is the most common with all other temperatures relating to its average of 98.6° Fahrenheit or 37.0° centigrade. Rectal temperatures are generally 1° higher than oral due to the vascularity and tightly closed environment of the rectum. Axillary temperatures are usually 1° lower due to the lower vascularity in the area and the difficulty in keeping the axilla tightly closed. Tympanic membrane temperatures are taken with tympanic thermometers, which have been designed to produce a reading that is comparable to the oral temperature.

A patient whose temperature is above normal is referred to as **febrile**, and one whose temperature is normal is said to be afebrile. Pyrexia refers to fevers of 102°F or higher rectally or 101°F or higher orally. An extremely high temperature, at the danger level of 105° to 106°F, may be referred to as hyperpyrexia.

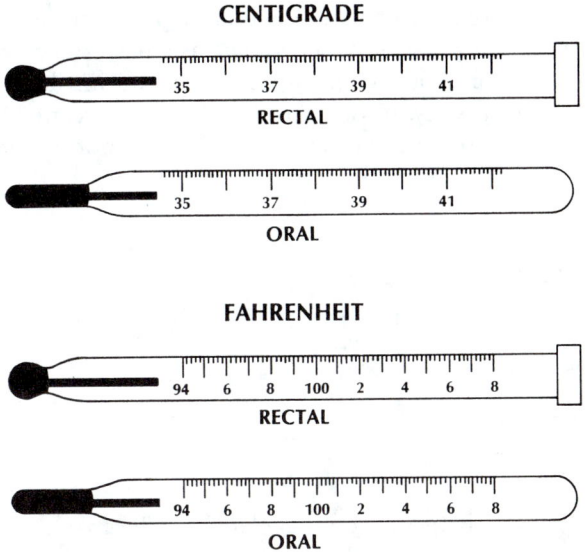

FIGURE 21-3
The two glass thermometers on the top use the centigrade scale to measure temperature; the two on the bottom use the Fahrenheit scale. Note the blunt bulbs on the rectal thermometers and the long thin bulb on the oral thermometers.

Table 21-1 Mechanisms of Heat Transfer			
Radiation	*Convection*	*Evaporation*	*Conduction*
Definition			
The diffusion or dissemination of heat by electromagnetic waves	The dissemination of heat by motion between areas of unequal density	The conversion of a liquid to a vapor	The transfer of heat to another object during direct contact
Example			
The body gives off waves of heat from uncovered surfaces.	An oscillating fan blows currents of cool air across the surface of a warm body.	Body fluid in the form of perspiration and insensible loss is vaporized from the skin.	The body transfers heat to an ice pack, causing the ice to melt.
Illustration			

From Taylor, C., Lillis, C., & Le Mone, P. (1993). Fundamentals of Nursing, *2nd ed., p. 388.* Philadelphia: J. B. Lippincott.

Abnormal temperature is usually produced by the presence of a disease process, such as a bacterial or viral infection. Body temperature may rise during intense exercise, anxiety, passion, or dehydration unrelated to a disease process, but these elevations are not considered fevers.

Checkpoint Question

1. How does an oral temperature differ from a rectal temperature? Why?

Fever Processes

The body temperature is regulated by the hypothalamus. When the hypothalamus senses that the body is too warm, it initiates peripheral vasodilation to carry core heat to the body surface and increases perspiration to cool the body by evaporation. If the temperature registers as too low, vasoconstriction and shivering will usually maintain a fairly normal core temperature. Temperature elevations and variations are a *sign* of disease and are not a disease in themselves (Box 21-1).

Temperatures that vary from the normal are caused by:

Age—Children usually have a higher metabolism and therefore a higher body temperature than adults. The elderly, with slower metabolism, usually have lower readings than younger adults. Temperatures for both the very young and the very old are easily affected by the environment.

Gender or hormones—Women usually have a slightly higher temperature than men, especially at the time of ovulation.

Exercise—Activity raises the need for cellular metabolism, causing the body to respond by raising the temperature to burn more calories for energy.

Time of day or diurnal influences—The body temperature is usually lowest in the early morning before activity has begun.

Emotions—Temperature tends to be higher during times of stress and lower with depression.

Illness—Most variations in temperature, either higher or lower, are an indication of a disease process.

Stages of Fever

Fever has several clearly defined stages, as described below.

1. The *onset* may be abrupt or gradual.
2. The *course* or *stadium* will range from a day or so to several weeks. Fever may be *sustained* (constant), **remittent** (fluctuating), or **intermittent** (occurring at intervals). Table 21-2 describes and graphically illustrates these courses of fever. Fever may also be *relapsing* (return after an extended period of normal readings).
3. The *resolution*, or return to normal, may occur as either a crisis (abrupt return) or lysis (gradual return).

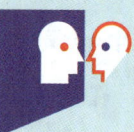

Patient Education: Fever

When instructing patients about fever, explain that current theories suggest that temperature elevations are a natural response to disease and that efforts to bring the temperature back to normal are counterproductive. However, if the patient is uncomfortable, or the temperature is abnormally high, it should be brought down to about 101°F. At 101°F, the body's natural defenses may still be able to destroy the pathogen without extreme discomfort to the patient.

After consulting with the physician, instruct all patients regarding the following comfort measures:

- Consume clear fluids as tolerated to rehydrate the tissues, if nausea and vomiting are present.
- Keep clothing and bedding clean and dry, especially after **diaphoresis** (sweating).
- Avoid chilling. Chills bring on shivering, which raises the temperature to compensate.
- Rest and eat a light diet as tolerated.
- Use antipyretics to keep comfortable, but **do not** give aspirin to children younger than 18 years with viral fevers. Aspirin has been associated with Reye's syndrome, a potentially fatal disorder, following cases of varicella zoster (chickenpox) and viral illnesses.

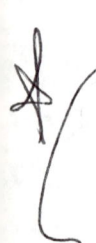

BOX 21-1 Temperature Comparisons

	Fahrenheit	*Centigrade*
Oral	98.6°	37.0°
Rectal	99.6°R	37.6°
Axillary	97.6°A	36.4°
Tympanic	98.6°T	37.0°

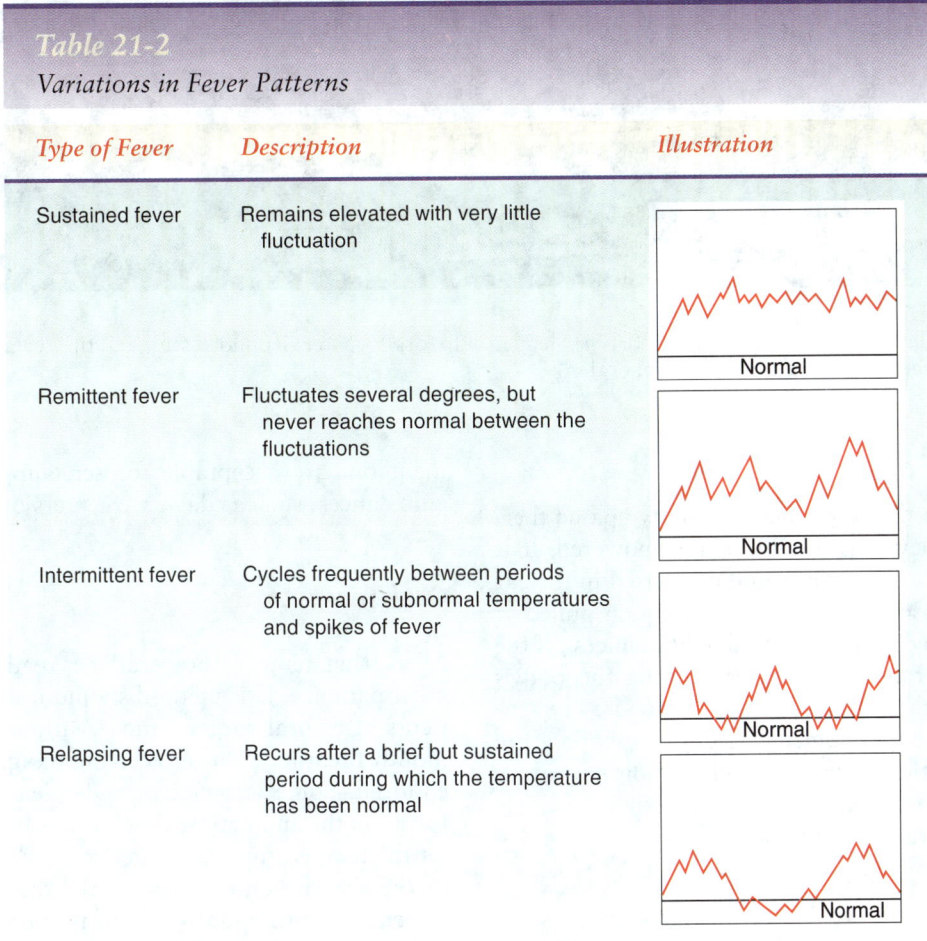

Table 21-2		
Variations in Fever Patterns		
Type of Fever	**Description**	**Illustration**
Sustained fever	Remains elevated with very little fluctuation	
Remittent fever	Fluctuates several degrees, but never reaches normal between the fluctuations	
Intermittent fever	Cycles frequently between periods of normal or subnormal temperatures and spikes of fever	
Relapsing fever	Recurs after a brief but sustained period during which the temperature has been normal	

From Timby, B. K. (1996). *Fundamental Skills and Concepts in Patient Care*, *6th ed.*, p. 147. Philadelphia: Lippincott-Raven Publishers.

Checkpoint Question

2. How does a child's normal body temperature differ from an adult's? Why?

Types of Thermometers

Glass Mercury Thermometers

Oral, rectal, and axillary temperatures have traditionally been measured by the glass mercury thermometer. This thermometer is a glass tube divided into two major parts. The bulb end is filled with mercury and shaped in a long slender form for oral use, and a rounded stub form for rectal use. Heat expands the mercury, which rises up the glass column to measure degrees of temperature.

The major portion or glass stem of the Fahrenheit thermometer is calibrated with lines designating temperature in even degrees—94°, 96°, 98°, 100°, and so on. Uneven numbers are marked only with a longer line. Between these longer lines are four smaller lines designating temperature in 0.2°F increments. Therefore a large line marked 100 with the mercury falling on the second smaller line after it would read 100.4°F.

Some glass thermometers are color coded, with blue tips meaning oral use and red tips meaning rectal use. Some thermometers will have "rectal" or "oral" written on them or etched into the glass. Rectal and oral thermometers are never used interchangeably. Figure 21-4 shows oral and rectal thermometers.

Electronic Thermometers

Electronic thermometers use portable battery-operated units with sheath-covered probes (Fig. 21-5). The temperature is sensed and a digital read-out is given in the window of the hand-held base. Electronic thermometers are kept in a charging unit when not in use to ensure that the batteries are operative at all times. Most units can be used for either oral or rectal measurement but will have clearly marked probes to avoid errors.

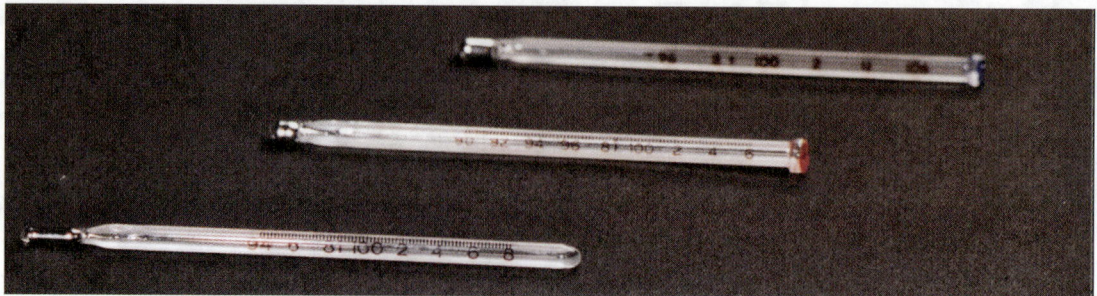

FIGURE 21-4
Glass mercury thermometers. (*front*) Slender bulb, oral. (*center*) Rounded stub, red tip, rectal. (*back*) Rounded stub, blue tip, oral.

Tympanic Thermometers

The newest type of thermometer is the tympanic thermometer. This device is usually battery powered. It is fitted with a disposable cover and is inserted in the ear much like an otoscope (Fig. 21-6). A trigger is pulled or a button is pressed and an infrared light bounces off the tympanic membrane (eardrum), recording the body's temperature on the digital screen in 2 seconds. The sensor in a tympanic thermometer checks the temperature of the blood in the tympanic membrane on its way to the hypothalamus; this is considered a highly reliable form of temperature measurement.

Disposable Thermometers

Disposable, single-use thermometers register quickly with color changes on a strip (Fig. 21-7). Although many disposable thermometers are fairly accurate, they are not considered as reliable as either electronic or glass thermometers. Single-use patches or tapes are applied to the forehead or chest and register by changing colors on dots or stripes or by displaying an array of colors. They are not reliable for definitive measure-

ment but are acceptable for screening in special circumstances, such as day-care centers or schools.

Oral Temperature

Measuring temperature orally is readily accepted by most patients. This method should not be used for patients after oral surgery, those with seizure disorders, mouth breathers, those receiving oxygen, or for small children. Some agencies provide clear plastic sheaths for glass thermometers; these are to be disposed of after the temperature has been taken. Check for integrity of the sheath before inserting the thermometer in the patient's mouth and dispose of properly after the procedure. Sheath designs vary somewhat; follow the manufacturer's directions for applying the sheath available at your facility (Fig. 21-8). Procedure 21-3 describes the steps for measuring oral temperature using a glass mercury thermometer. See Procedure 21-6 for taking an oral temperature electronically.

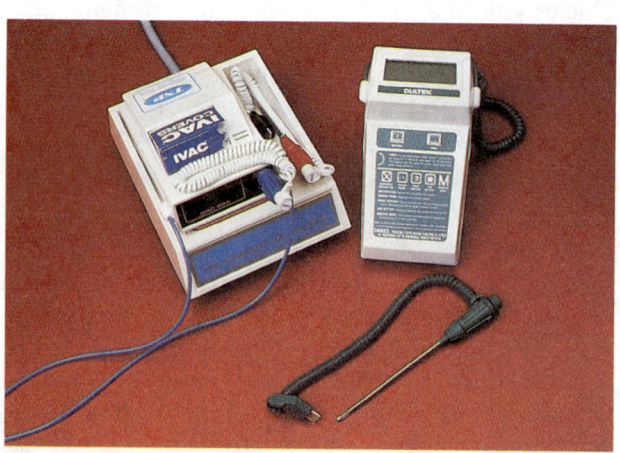

FIGURE 21-5
Two types of electronic performometers cland probes.

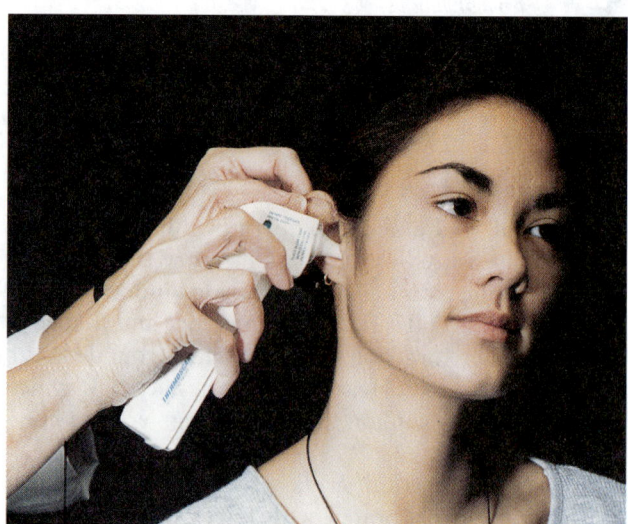

FIGURE 21-6
The tympanic thermometer in use.

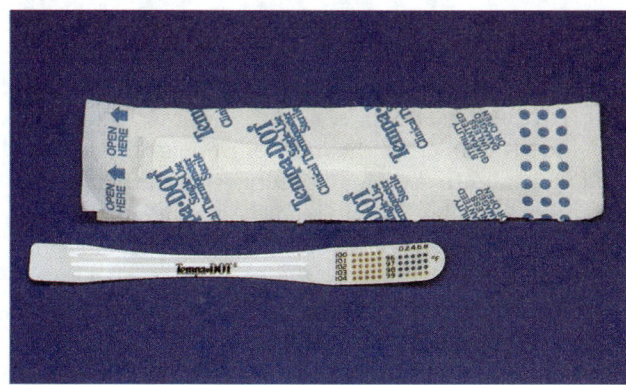

FIGURE 21-7
Disposable paper thermometer. The dots change color to indicate temperature.

Rectal Temperature

The rectal temperature is thought to be more accurate than the oral temperature because of the closed, highly vascular environment of the rectal canal. This is the least acceptable method for patients and is not considered to be accurate if stool is present in the rectum. This method may never be used for patients closely following rectal surgery and is discouraged for patients with seizure disorders or cardiac disorders. Unless properly performed, there is the danger of anal perforation. Procedure 21-4 outlines the steps for measuring rectal temperature using a glass mercury thermometer. See Procedure 21-6 for taking a rectal temperature electronically.

Axillary Temperature

If performed properly, axillary measurements are considered to be very accurate. This method of measurement is becoming more acceptable to the medical profession and

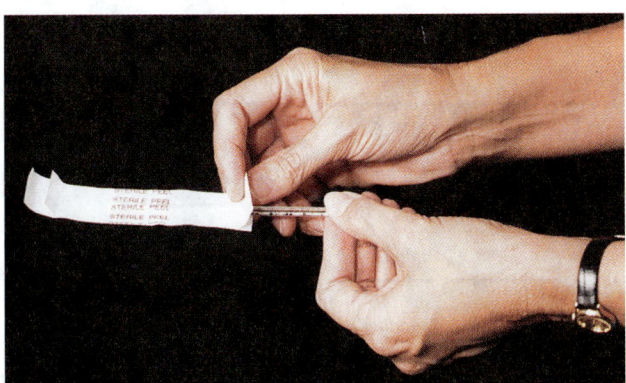

FIGURE 21-8
Standard thermometer sheaths are applied by inserting the bulb end into the indicated opening and removing the paper cover as directed.

> ## Charting Example
>
> | 03/09/99 | 8:30 AM | Mother arrived carrying baby in her arms. According to the mother, the baby has been pulling on his ears for 2 days and has had a fever. Rectal temp-100.3° F, P-140, R-28. Mother instructed on procedure for taking rectal temps. Mother verbalized understanding. |
> | --- | --- | --- |
> | | | —— Jack Kimble, CMA |

always has been preferred by patients who were unable to use the oral site. It is safe and there is less chance of the transfer of microorganisms. It may be used for children, mouth breathers, patients receiving oxygen, postoperatively for patients who have undergone oral surgery, or in any instance where the oral route is contraindicated. Procedure 21-5 explains how to measure axillary temperature using a glass mercury thermometer. See Procedure 21-6 for measuring axillary temperature electronically.

Tympanic Temperature

Temperatures taken via the tympanic route are noninvasive and are readily acceptable to patients. In addition, the site is easily accessible. For these reasons, this route is rapidly becoming the route of choice. Procedure 21-7 outlines the steps for assessing temperature using a tympanic thermometer.

Checkpoint Question
3. Why would a tympanic membrane temperature be more accurate than an axillary?

Cleaning Thermometers

After use, thermometers must be sanitized and disinfected for the next patient. Electronic units and tympanic thermometers only need to be wiped down with disinfectant during environmental cleaning. Glass thermometers must be thoroughly disinfected (Procedure 21-8). During the disinfecting process, check all equipment for safety and function. Check the glass thermometer for chips or cracks, for example. Check the electronic base for malfunction.

In addition to cleaning thermometers, medical assistants are often responsible for disinfecting the instrument trays used for storing thermometers or the special thermometer containers. These must be washed with hot soapy water and dried thoroughly. Some facilities will recommend daily autoclaving. The containers are then refilled with the proper freshly prepared solution. It is customary to place a gauze sponge in the bottom of instrument trays to avoid damage to the glass instruments.

➤ PULSE (P)

As the heart beats, it forces blood into the arteries causing them to expand. As the heart relaxes, the arteries relax. Each heart beat is counted at the point of expansion of the artery.

Although every artery in the body has a pulse, the pulse usually is measured only at a point where an artery may be pressed against a bone or other underlying firm surface. These are called pulse points.

There are several pulse points at which the heart beat can be palpated (felt) or auscultated (heard). From head to foot, these are: temporal, facial, carotid, apical, brachial, radial, femoral, popliteal, posterior tibialis, and dorsalis pedis. Figure 21-9 shows some of these pulse sites. The apical pulse usually cannot be palpated unless the patient has a circulatory abnormality, but it is easily auscultated and is considered the most accurate measurement. All of the others listed usually are palpated or may be auscultated with a Doppler unit.

Palpation of the pulse is performed by placing the index and middle finger, the middle finger and ring finger, or all three fingers, over a pulse point (Fig. 21-10). Auscultation usually requires a stethoscope to hear the pulse or a Doppler unit to broadcast the sound. For apical auscultation, the bell of the stethoscope is placed over the apex of the heart and the beats are counted for 1 minute.

Characteristics

Although you will know the terms that apply to the measurements of the pulse, it is not within the scope of practice for medical assistants to diagnose the readings. Observations will be made about the characteristics of the pulse. However, the rate should never be listed as bradycardia, a pulse of less than 60 beats per minute (bpm or beats/min), or tachycardia (an adult

pulse of more than 100 bpm). Only the number should be listed with observations regarding the characteristics. The characteristics of the pulse to be assessed are rate, rhythm, and volume.

Rate is defined as the number of heartbeats occurring in 1 minute. You may observe that the rate is fast (rapid) or slow but should record only the number and let the physician diagnose beyond that point.

Rhythm is defined as the time interval between each heartbeat or the pattern of the beats. In the normal heartbeat, this pattern will be regular. A regular heartbeat will be recorded as such; an irregular beat will be recorded as arrhythmic or irregular.

Volume is defined as the strength or force of the heartbeat and can be described as soft, bounding, weak, thready, feeble, strong, or full.

Averages and Ranges

In the healthy adult, the average pulse rate is 70 to 80 beats per minute (bpm). With other ages, there is a large variance of pulse rates as shown in Table 21-3.

Factors Affecting Pulse Rates

Many factors affect the force, speed, and rhythm of the heart. As noted on Table 21-3, young children and infants normally have a much faster heart rate than adults. It is not unusual for a conditioned athlete to present with a normal heart rate below 60 bpm. Older adults may very well exhibit an increased heart rate as the myocardium begins to compensate for decreased efficiency. Other factors that affect pulse rates are listed in Table 21-4.

The pulse is counted most often at the radial point for convenience and because most patients prefer this site (Procedure 21-9). If the radial pulse is irregular or hard to count or if cardiac disease is present, the apical

Table 21-3
Variations in Pulse Rates by Age

Age	Beats per Minute
Birth to 1 y	110–170
1–10 y	90–110
10–16 y	80–95
16 y to midlife	70–80
Elderly adult	55–70

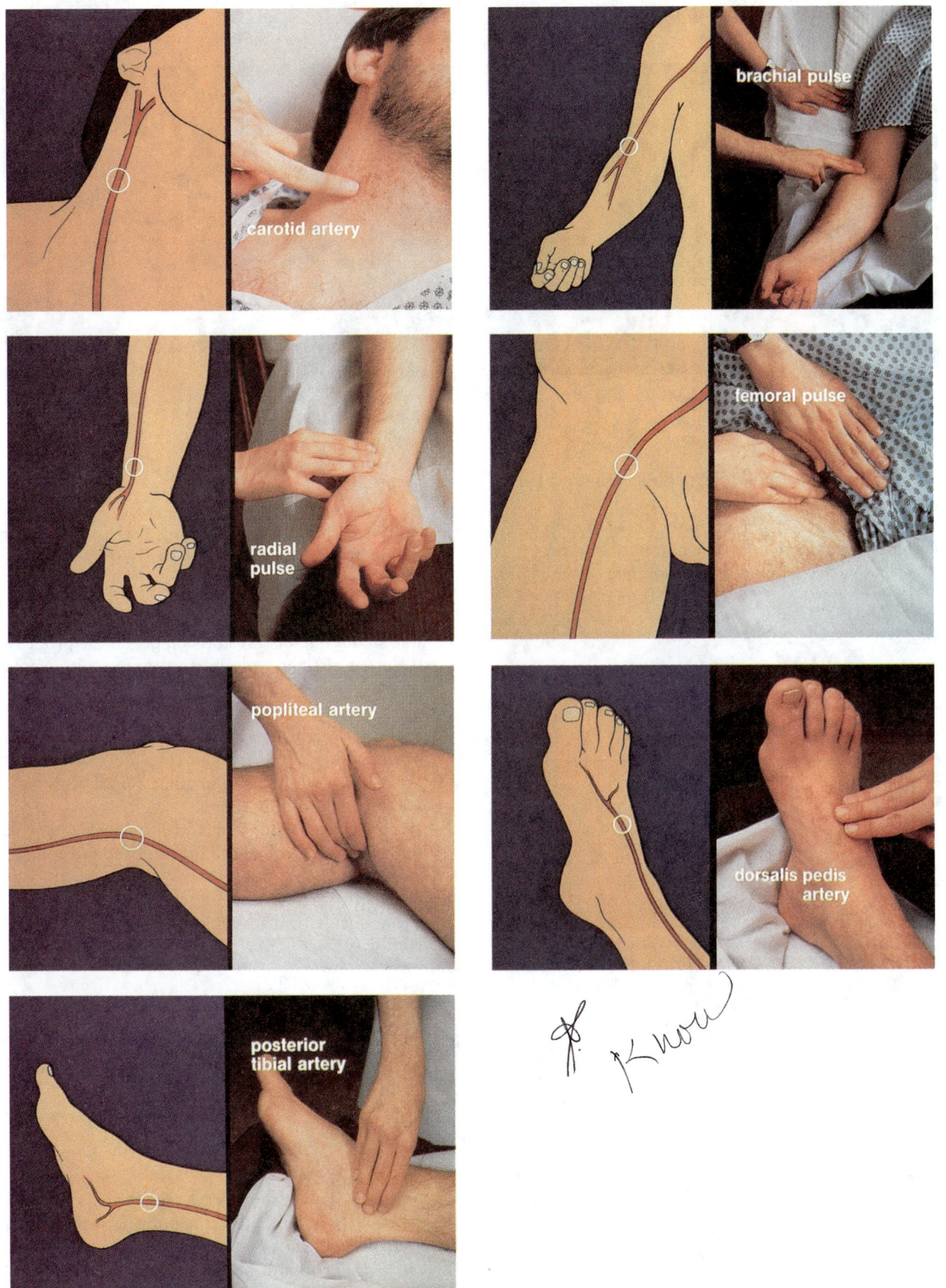

FIGURE 21-9
Sites for palpation of peripheral pulses. (Lippincott Learning Systems.)

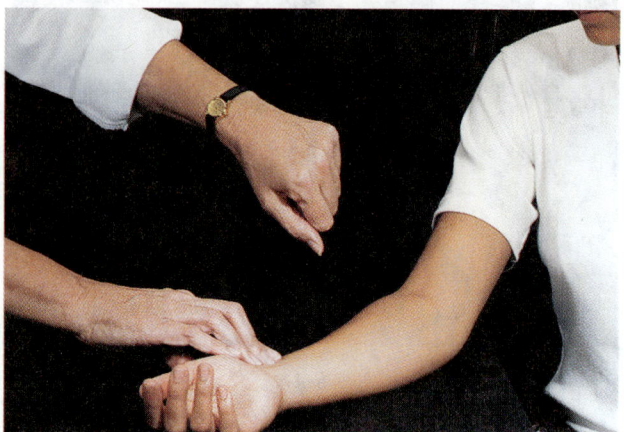

FIGURE 21-10
Measuring a radial pulse.

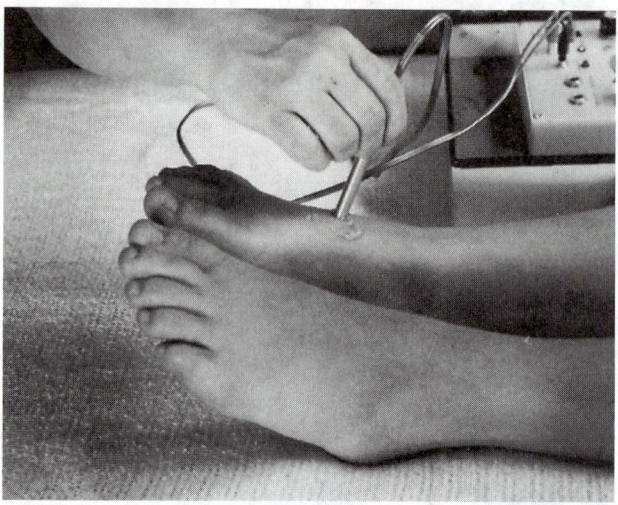

FIGURE 21-11
Auscultation of the pedal pulse using a Doppler unit.

pulse is the site of choice for pulse measurement (Procedure 21-10).

Note: Some peripheral pulses are counted using a Doppler ultrasound unit. The unit may be attached to earpieces such as found on stethoscopes so that only you can hear the pulse, or it may be set to broadcast the sound for counting purposes. These devices are battery powered. Follow these steps to use a Doppler unit:

1. Use a coupling or transmission gel on the probe to make an airtight seal and to promote ultrasound transmission.
2. With the machine "on," hold the probe at a 45° angle with light pressure to ensure contact but to avoid obliterating the pulse (Fig. 21-11). Arteries are usually loud with a pumping sound; veins have a lighter, whooshing sound.
3. If the vein sound interferes with the measurement, reposition the probe until the artery sound is dominant.
4. Assess the rate, rhythm, and volume and record.
5. Clean the patient's skin and the machine probe with warm water to remove the coupling gel.

Checkpoint Question
4. *When measuring a patient's pulse, what characteristics are to be assessed? Briefly explain each.*

RESPIRATION (R)

Respiration is defined as the exchange of gases between the atmosphere and blood of the body. External respiration involves the intake of air through the respiratory tract to the alveoli and bloodstream; internal respiration refers to the exchange of gases between the bloodstream and the tissue cells. The major gases exchanged are carbon dioxide (CO_2) and oxygen (O_2). Respiration is controlled by the respiratory center in the brain stem

---

Table 21-4
Factors Affecting Pulse Rates

Factor	Affect
Time of day	The pulse is usually lower early in the morning than later in the day.
Gender	Women have a slightly higher pulse rate than men.
Body type and size	Tall, thin people usually have a lower pulse rate than shorter, stockier people.
Exercise	The heart rate increases with the need for increased **cardiac output** (amount of blood ejected from either ventricle per minute).
Stress or emotions	Anger, fear, excitement, and stress will raise the pulse; depression will lower it.
Fever	The increased need for cell metabolism in the presence of fever raises the cardiac output to supply oxygen and nutrients; the pulse may rise as much as 10 beats/min per degree of fever.
Medications	Many medications raise or lower the pulse as a desired effect or an undesirable side effect.
Blood volume	Hemorrhage or loss of blood volume as in dehydration or loss of tissue fluid will increase the need for cellular metabolism and will increase the cardiac output to supply the need.

(primarily in the medulla oblongata), and by feedback from the chemosensors in the carotid that check for an increase in the CO_2 content of the blood.

As the body breathes, it brings into the lungs O_2 from the atmosphere by inspiration or inhalation. It forces out CO_2 and other wastes by expiration or exhalation. Inspiration and expiration are accomplished by the mechanical muscular action of the diaphragm and ribs. When you inhale, the diaphragm contracts and flattens as the rib cage lifts and expands, creating a negative pressure within the chest cavity that must be filled by the intake of air. When you exhale, the diaphragm relaxes and moves upward in a dome shape; the rib cage falls and compresses the pleura and the air is pressed out. Each respiration is counted as one full inspiration and one full expiration.

Observing the rise (inspiration) and fall (expiration) of the chest to count respirations is usually performed as a part of the pulse measurement to obtain an accurate reading. Patients can and usually do change the voluntary action of breathing if they are aware that they are being watched; therefore, it is generally considered best not to announce that you will now count the respirations. However, when appropriate, you may need to use a stethoscope to auscultate the respirations.

Characteristics

The characteristics of respiration are rate, rhythm, and depth. *Rate* is defined as the number of respirations occurring in 1 minute; the written descriptions medical assistants should use are normal, rapid, or slow. The physician may diagnose and record these as eupnea (easy, normal respirations), tachypnea (fast respirations), or bradypnea (slow respirations); this is not the responsibility of the medical assistant. (See Chap. 37, Caring for Patients With Respiratory Disorders, for more information about abnormal breathing patterns.)

When measuring respirations by auscultation and using a stethoscope, the count is performed for 1 minute and may be recorded as an odd number. When measuring respirations by observation in a patient without respiratory or cardiac symptoms, it is equally proper to count the respirations for 15 seconds and then multiply by four or for 30 seconds and multiply by two. This type of measurement is always recorded in even numbers.

Rhythm is defined as the period of time (spacing) between each respiration to determine a pattern. This interval or pattern will be equal in normal respirations and is written as regular. Any abnormal rhythm is described by what is detected and is written as irregular.

Depth is defined as the volume of air being inhaled and exhaled. When a person is at rest, the depth should be regular and consistent. There should be no notice-able sounds other than the regular exchange of air, and the written description should be either deep or shallow. If sounds are present, it is usually a sign of a disease process. Such sounds are referred to with specific descriptions, such as crackles, gurgles, stertorous, wheeze, and so on. (See Chap. 37, Caring for Patients With Respiratory Disorders, for more information about abnormal breath sounds.)

Averages and Ranges

In the healthy adult the average respiratory rate is 14 to 20 breaths per minute. With other ages there is a large variance of respiratory rates, as Table 21-5 shows. In fever states, as the pulse rises to satisfy the increased cellular needs, the respiratory rates will increase as well to bring in more oxygen. It is generally noted that each degree of temperature rise will increase the pulse by as many as 10 bpm; the respiratory rate will follow by increasing one respiration for each four to five beats per minute of the pulse.

A respiration rate that is significantly slower than the average is called bradypnea. A respiration rate that is much faster than the average is called tachypnea. Further descriptions that can be given are:

- Dyspnea—difficult or labored breathing
- Apnea—no respirations
- Hyperpnea—abnormally deep, gasping breaths
- Hyperventilation—a respiratory rate that greatly exceeds the oxygen demand
- Hypopnea—shallow respirations
- Orthopnea—inability to breathe or difficulty breathing in a supine or prone position; the patient usually has to sit upright to breathe.

The Cheyne-Stokes breathing pattern is a noticeable pattern that usually begins with slow shallow breathing, escalates to deep rapid breathing, then decreases to slow shallow breathing again. This pattern is followed by a period of apnea. The pattern continues until the apnea is permanent and death occurs. Cheyne-Stokes breathing sometimes precedes the

Table 21-5	
Variations in Respiration Ranges by Age	
Age	**Respirations per Minute**
Infant	20 +
Child	18–20
Adult	14–20

"death rattle," which is caused by mucus accumulating in the throat as the cough reflex diminishes and the patient can no longer swallow this accumulation.

Procedure 21-11 lists the steps for counting respirations.

Checkpoint Question

5. What happens within the chest cavity when the diaphragm contracts?

➤ BLOOD PRESSURE (BP)

Blood pressure is the pressure of the blood as it is forced against the arterial walls. The heart contracts and ejects the blood within it during a phase called **systole**. As the heart pauses briefly to rest and refill, the arterial pressure drops; this phase is called **diastole**.

Pressure is measured in both the contraction and relaxation phases. As the heart contracts, the highest pressure level is recorded as systolic pressure. When the heart relaxes, the lowest pressure level is recorded as diastolic pressure.

Systolic and diastolic pressure are the two parts of the **cardiac cycle**, the period from the beginning of one heartbeat to the beginning of the next. The average adult blood pressure is 120/80 with a normal range between 100 and 140 systolic and 60 to 90 diastolic. Pressures of greater than 140/90 are considered hypertensive; pressures of less than 100/60 are considered hypotensive. A lower pressure may be normal for athletes with exceptionally well conditioned cardiovascular systems. A pressure that drops suddenly when the patient stands is referred to as **postural hypotension** or orthostatic hypotension. These patients will experience vertigo and may actually faint.

Diastolic and systolic pressures are measured by using a stethoscope and an instrument called a sphygmomanometer (Procedure 21-12). There are two basic types of sphygmomanometers: the aneroid, which has a dial for the readings, and the mercury, which has a calibrated, mercury-filled glass tube for the readings (Fig. 21-12). The mercury is considered to be the more accurate. Each type measures blood pressure in millimeters of mercury, which is abbreviated "mm Hg." Both are attached to a cuff by a rubber tube. A second rubber tube is attached to a pump with a screw valve used to blow up the rubber bladder held within the cuff. This arrangement of tubes and bladder presses the artery and records the pressure exerted by the blood as it flows through the vessel.

Electronic sphygmomanometers work well at home and either broadcast the sound or display a digital read-

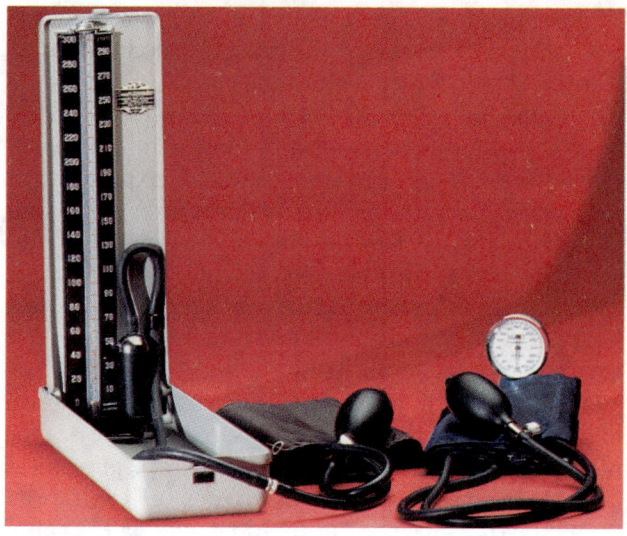

FIGURE 21-12
The mercury column sphygmomanometer and the aneroid sphygmomanometer.

out. Most offices currently prefer the more traditional and reliable aneroid or mercury equipment. As technology improves the electronic instruments, their use in the medical office will increase.

A stethoscope is needed for you to hear the pressure sounds with the standard methods of measurement (Fig. 21-13). Some offices may use a Doppler type of pressure measurement that will broadcast the sound of the systolic pressure without the use of a stethoscope.

A pressure of 120/80 indicates the force needed to raise a column of mercury to the 120 mark on the glass tube during systole and 80 during diastole. The pressure indicates the elasticity of the arteries, the strength of the heart muscle, and the quantity or viscosity (thickness) of the blood in the circulatory system.

The results of a blood pressure measurement are recorded as a fraction, with the systolic as the numerator and the diastolic as the denominator (eg, 120/80).

Checkpoint Question

6. What is happening in the heart during systole? During diastole?

Korotkoff Sounds and the Five Phases of Blood Pressure

Korotkoff sounds are those sounds heard through the stethoscope during the measurement of blood pressure. These sounds consist of two basic types: the first sound producing a "lubb" reflects the systolic period of the

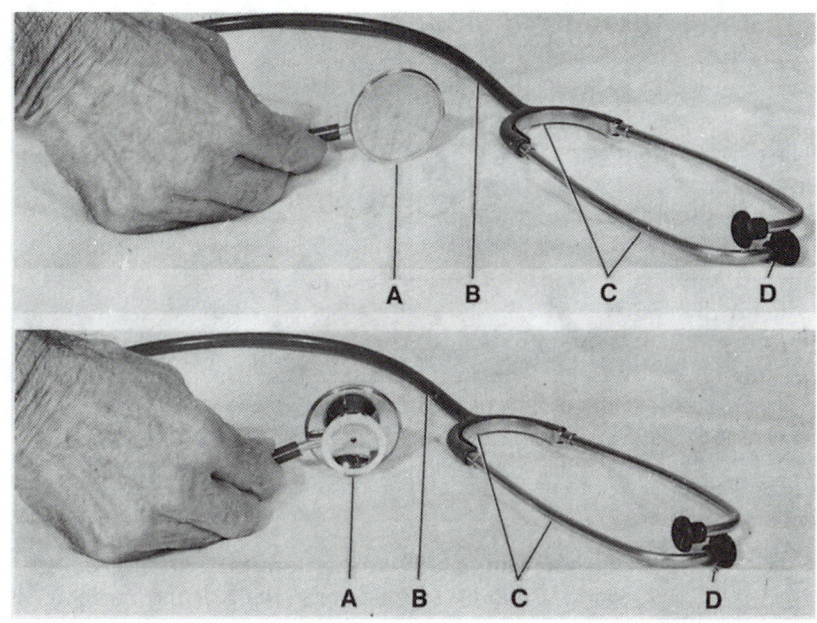

FIGURE 21-13

(*A*) The chest piece on this stethoscope contains both a diaphragm (top) and a bell (bottom). The diaphragm is used for listening to high-pitched sounds. The bell is better for detecting low-pitched sounds; it is used when obtaining the blood pressure. (*B*) The tubing may be rubber or plastic. Unnecessarily long tubing decreases good sound conduction. A length of about 50 cm (20 in) seems best. (*C*) The brace and binaurals are the metal portions connecting the tubing and the chest piece. The binaurals should clear the examiner's face. The brace prevents the tubing from kinking. (*D*) The eartips are rubber or plastic and should fit snugly but comfortably into the ears. They should be placed so that they are directed downward and forward. If the eartips are not properly positioned in the ear canal, sound quality will be poor, and, in measuring blood pressure, a falsely low systolic and falsely high diastolic pressure are likely to be obtained.

cardiac cycle and the second sound producing a softer "dubb" reflects the diastolic period of the cardiac cycle. Thus one heartbeat consists of the "lubb-dubb" sound and reflects one cardiac cycle of contraction and relaxation. The Russian neurologist Nicolai Korotkoff classified these sounds into five phases as described in Table 21-6.

Pulse Pressure

Pulse pressure is the difference between systolic and diastolic readings. For example, the difference in the normal adult average blood pressure of 120/80 is 40. The range for pulse pressure normal values is 30 to 50 mm Hg and a general rule is that the difference should be no more than one-third of the systolic reading.

Auscultatory Gap

An auscultatory gap may be observed in patients who have a history of **hypertension** (elevated blood pressure) and occurs in phase II of the cardiac cycle. An auscultatory gap is the loss of sounds for as many as 30 mm Hg or more during the fall of the needle or mercury. The beat is then heard again and continues to fade away. If this is not properly measured, the blood pressure may be tragically undermeasured. The recording of an auscultatory gap should be written as the first sound heard/the second sound heard (after the gap)/the last sound heard (eg, 210/130/120).

Table 21-6
Five Phases of Blood Pressure

Phase	Sounds
I	Faint tapping sounds heard as the cuff deflates (systolic)
II	Soft swishing sounds
III	Rhythmic, sharp, distinct tapping sounds
IV	Soft tapping sounds that become faint
V	No sounds (diastolic)

Charting Example

| 07/12/99 | 1400 | Patient arrived complaining of a headache. BP 180/120. Dr. Rodriguez was notified immediately. |
| | | — Susan Gomez, RMA |

Factors Influencing Blood Pressure

Atherosclerosis and arteriosclerosis are two factors that greatly influence blood pressure. These diseases affect the size of the vessel lumen and the elasticity of the vessels. The general health of the patient is also a major factor and includes dietary habits, alcohol and tobacco use, the amount and type of exercise, previous heart conditions or myocardial infarctions, and family history for cardiac dysfunction or coronary heart disease.

Other factors affecting blood pressure include:

Age—As the body ages, vessels begin to lose elasticity and will require more force for expansion. The build up of atherosclerotic patches will also increase the force needed for blood flow.
- *Activity*—Exercise raises the pressure; depression will lower it.
- *Stress*—The sympathetic nervous system raises the pressure in response to the flight-fright-fight syndrome.
- *Position*—Pressure is usually lower in the supine position.
- *Medications*—Some medications will lower and other will raise the pressure.

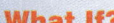

What If?

What if a patient has a dialysis shunt (a surgically made venous access port allowing the patient to be connected to a dialysis machine) in his left arm? Could you use that arm to take his blood pressure?

NO! By taking blood pressure in that arm, you could cause the shunt to be permanently damaged. The patient's chart should clearly indicate the shunt's location. Also, most dialysis patients are keenly aware of their conditions and will alert you to the location of their shunts. Additionally, you should not draw blood from the affected arm.

Choosing the Correct Cuff Size

Choose the correct size of cuff before beginning to measure blood pressure. The blood pressure measurement may be inaccurate by as much as +/− 30 mm Hg if the cuff size is incorrect. The width of the cuff should be 40% to 50% of the circumference of the arm. To determine the correct size, hold the narrow edge of the cuff at the midpoint of the upper arm. Wrap the width, not the length, around the arm. The cuff width should

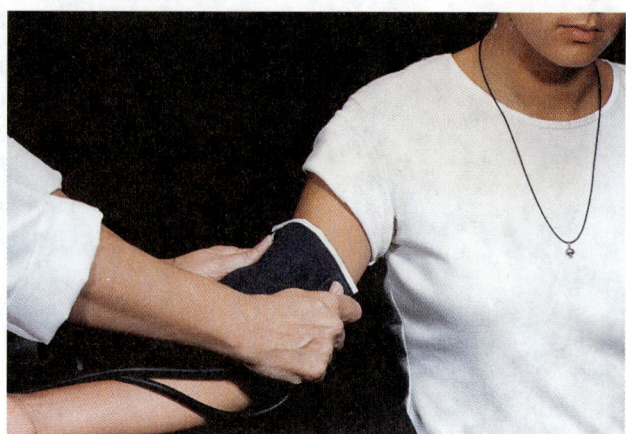

FIGURE 21-14
Choosing the right blood pressure cuff.

reach not quite half way around the arm (Fig. 21-14). Varying widths of cuffs are available, from about 1 inch for infants to 8 inches for obese adults (Fig. 21-15). It is your responsibility to carefully choose the size most appropriate for the patient.

Errors in blood pressure readings may not only be caused by using the wrong cuff size, but also by other factors. Box 21-2 lists additional causes of errors in blood pressure readings.

► CHARTING VITAL SIGNS IN THE HOSPITAL SETTING

Medical assistants who are employed as unit clerks in the hospital setting usually will not perform vital sign assessments but will record on graphic sheets the readings brought to them by the nurses on the unit. The vital signs are recorded in the TPR form, with temperature first, pulse second, and respiration third, (eg, 98.6–80 –18) and *never* in any other order.

The medical assistant records the data on special graphic forms with areas for the temperature, pulse,

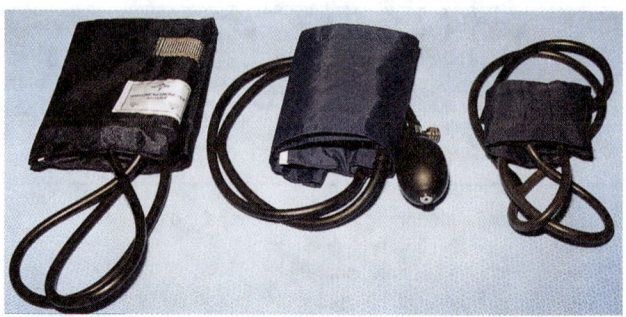

FIGURE 21-15
Three sizes of blood pressure cuffs (from left): a large cuff for the obese adult, a normal cuff, and a pediatric cuff.

BOX 21-2 Causes of Errors in Blood Pressure Readings

- Wrapping the cuff improperly
- Failing to keep the patient's arm at heart level
- Failing to support the patient's arm on a stable surface
- Recording auscultatory gap for diastolic pressure
- Failing to maintain the gauge at eye level
- Pulling the patient's sleeve up tightly above the cuff
- Listening through clothing
- Allowing the cuff to deflate too rapidly or too slowly
- Failing to wait 1–2 minutes before rechecking

respiration, blood pressure, height, and weight on admission and as needed through the hospital stay (Fig. 21-16). Most forms also include an area for bowel elimination and intake and output. There will be dates across the top with space for the day of the hospital stay, postoperative day, or postpartum day. The first day in the hospital will be listed as ADM (day of admission), the second day will be listed as Day 1. If surgery is performed or if this is a maternity patient, the first full day after noting PO (postoperative) or PP (postpartum) will be listed as Day 1 in the spaces below the listing for the hospital stay.

The graphic record gives an instant picture of the vital sign fluctuations during the hospital stay. The graph usually has heavy lines for full numbers or degrees and lighter lines for fractions of degrees of temperature, multiples of five for pulse (50, 55, 60, 65, 70, 75, etc.), and whole number multiples of 10 for respirations. The forms will vary by the facility and the variety of information required and the structure for recording is infinite.

In all cases, the medical assistant will enter dots on the perpendicular hour line and the horizontal reading line. Line the dot under the time and across from the reading. A straight edge corner aligned with the reading and moved across the page to the time column will help avoid errors. Make a dot at this point and connect it to the dot for the previous reading. If the temperature is axillary or rectal, note an A or an R beside the dot; if the pulse is apical, note this also. The lines are small and errors are easy to make, even using a straight edge guide. If an error is made, mark X through the dot, initial the space and make the correction.

Some facilities use military time for graphic sheets and for charting. The day starts at 1 minute past midnight as 0001. One AM is recorded as 0100; 10 minutes past 2:00 AM is recorded as 0210. Noon is 1200 and midnight is 2400.

Many hospitals and clinics now use computers for recording the vital sign data. You will need to familiarize yourself with the system used by the facility in which you work.

text continues on page 333

Charting Example

04/15/99	1300
	S: "This is my first visit at this office."
	O: 42-year-old man. Baseline data obtained: Ht: 65 1/2 inches;
	Wt: 138 lb. T-98.2 tympanic. Apical pulse-92 regular, R-14,
	BP 122/76.
	A: New patient—baseline appointment.
	P: 1. Educated pt. on office policies.
	2. Pt. completed medical history form.
	3. Dr. Goldstein in to see pt. ———— Yolanda Torres, CMA

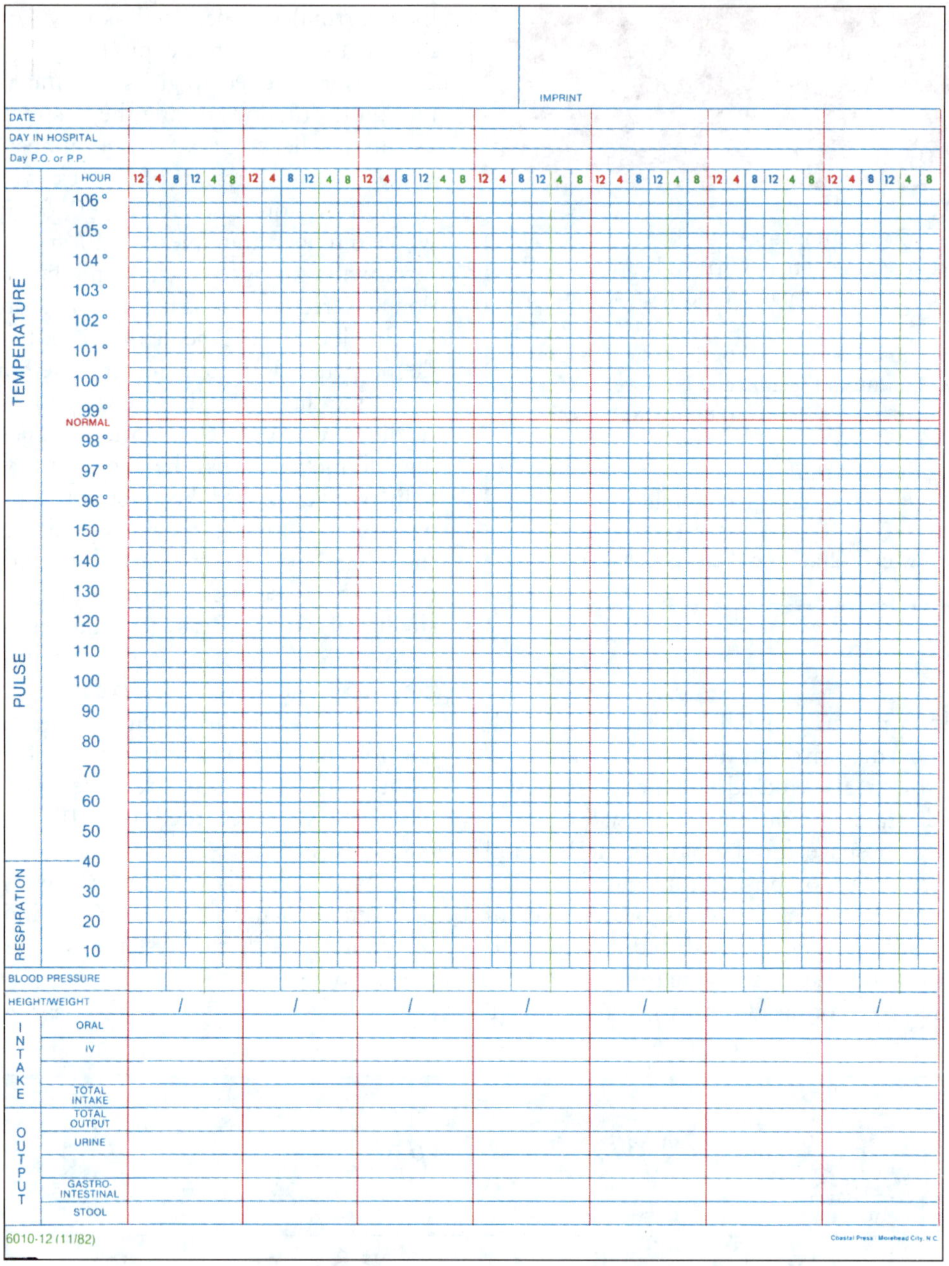
IMPRINT
DATE
DAY IN HOSPITAL
Day P.O. or P.P.
HOUR 12 4 8 12 4 8 12 4 8 12 4 8 12 4 8 12 4 8 12 4 8 12 4 8 12 4 8 12 4 8 12 4 8 12 4 8 12 4 8 12 4 8
TEMPERATURE 106° 105° 104° 103° 102° 101° 100° 99° NORMAL 98° 97° 96°
PULSE 150 140 130 120 110 100 90 80 70 60 50
RESPIRATION 40 30 20 10
BLOOD PRESSURE
HEIGHT/WEIGHT
INTAKE ORAL IV TOTAL INTAKE
OUTPUT TOTAL OUTPUT URINE GASTRO-INTESTINAL STOOL
6010-12 (11/82)
Coastal Press · Morehead City, N.C.

FIGURE 21-16
A graphic sheet for recording vital signs.

Procedure 21-1   Measuring Weight

Equipment/Supplies
- calibrated scale
- paper towel

Steps	Purpose
1. Wash your hands.	1. Handwashing aids infection control.
2. Ensure the scale is properly calibrated.	2. This avoids error in measurement.
3. Greet and identify the patient. Explain the procedure.	3. Identifying the patient prevents errors. Explaining the procedure helps ensure cooperation.
4. Escort the patient to the scale. Place a paper towel on the scale.	4. The patient will be standing barefooted or in socks or stocking feet; the paper towel helps minimize microorganism transmission.
5. Make sure the scale is balanced at zero. (A balance beam scale should always be returned to zero after each use.)	5. A scale is a delicate instrument and may easily become inaccurate. Ensuring that it registers zero will eliminate one source of error.
6. Have the patient remove shoes, heavy coats or jackets, put down the purse, and step up onto the scale. *Note:* Certain circumstances require that the patient be weighed wearing only a gown. In this situation, ensure patient privacy by moving the scale to the examining room, where the gowned patient will be waiting.	6. Unnecessary items must be removed for an accurate weight.
7. Assist the patient onto the scale. Have the patient stand steady without touching anything; watch closely for a loss of balance.	7. Some patients may lose balance and fall. Some may feel unsteady as the plate of the scale settles momentarily.
8. Weigh the patient.	
a. *On a balance beam scale:* Slide counterweights on the bottom and top bars from zero to the approximate weight. Each counterweight should rest securely in the notch, with the indicator mark at the proper calibration. To obtain the measurement, the balance bar must hang freely at the exact midpoint. To calculate the weight, add the top reading to the bottom reading (Example: If the bottom counterweight reads 100 and the top one reads 16 plus three small lines, the weight is 116¾ lb.)	
b. *On a digital scale:* Read the weight, which will automatically be displayed on the digital screen.	
c. *On a dial scale:* The indicator arrow will rest at the proper weight. Read this number from directly above the dial.	c. Reading at an angle will result in an incorrect measurement.

Note: *If the physician prefers pounds to kilograms or vice versa, the preferred scale will usually be provided. If it is necessary to convert pounds to kilograms or vice versa, remember that 1 k = 2.2 lb.*

To change pounds to kilograms: Divide the number of pounds by 2.2.

To change kilograms to pounds: Multiply the number of kilograms by 2.2.

Procedure 21-2   Measuring Height

Equipment/Supplies

* scale with ruler

Steps	Purpose
1. Have the patient stand straight and erect on the scale, heels together, eyes straight ahead. (The patient may be measured on the scale facing the ruler, but a better measurement will be made with the patient's back to the ruler.)	1. The posture must be erect for an accurate measurement.
2. With the measuring bar perpendicular to the ruler, slowly lower it until it firmly touches the patient's head. Press lightly if the hair is full and high.	2. Height is being measured, not hair.
3. Read the measurement at the point of movement on the ruler. If the measurements are in inches	

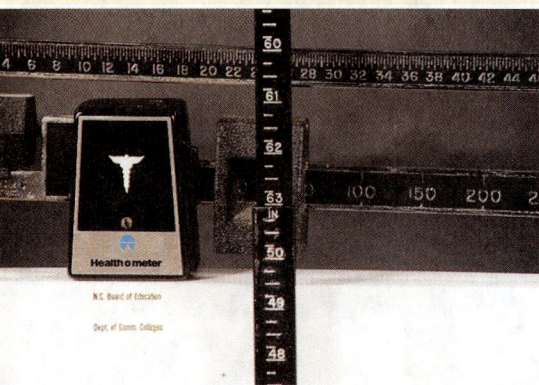

Step 3: Measure at the point of movement. (This measure reads 63 inches or 5 feet 3 inches.)

(with smaller marks for ¼, ½, and ¾), convert the inches to feet and inches. (Example: If the point of movement reads 65 plus two smaller lines, read it as 65½. Remember that 12 inches equal 1 foot; therefore, the patient is 5 feet 5½ inches tall.)	
4. At the completion of the procedure, assist the patient from the scale.	
5. Record the weight and height measurements. If these measurements are to be recorded on a graph, carefully align the points to accurately reflect the patient's measurements.	5. Procedures are considered not to have been done if they are not recorded.
6. Return the balance bar on the scale to zero and return the measuring bar to a safe position for the next procedure.	

Note: *If the physician prefers inches to centimeters or vice versa, the ruler will usually be in the preferred measurement. If it is necessary to convert from inches to centimeters or vice versa, remember that 1 inch = 2.5 cm.*

To convert inches to centimeters: Multiply the number of inches by 2.5.

To convert centimeters to inches: Divide the number of centimeters by 2.5.

Procedure 21-3

Measuring Oral Temperature Using a Glass Mercury Thermometer

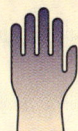

Equipment/Supplies

- glass mercury thermometer designed for oral use
- tissues or cotton balls
- disposable plastic sheath (if used)
- gloves

Steps	Purpose
1. Wash your hands.	1. Handwashing aids infection control.
2. Assemble the equipment and supplies. Check the thermometer for chips or cracks.	2. This ensures that everything you need is available. A safety check prevents patient injury.
3. Greet and identify the patient. Explain the procedure. Check for recent eating, drinking, gum chewing, or smoking.	3. Identifying the patient prevents errors in treatment. Explaining the procedure helps ease anxiety and ensure compliance. Recent eating, drinking, gum chewing, or smoking may alter the reading for oral temperature.
4. Rinse and dry the thermometer if it has been stored in solution. Wipe it from bulb to stem.	4. Chemical disinfectants can be irritating to the oral mucosa. Wipe always from the cleanest to the less clean area.
5. Read the thermometer by holding it by the stem horizontal to the face and turning it slowly to see the mercury column.	5. It will be easier to see the column in this position. The thermometer should not be held by the bulb, which will be inserted in the patient's mouth.
6. If the mercury registers above 94°F, grasp the thermometer by the stem with the thumb and forefinger and snap the wrist quickly several times to shake the mercury down to about 94°F. Avoid hitting the thermometer against anything.	6. The mercury must be below the lowest mark to register correctly. Glass thermometers are fragile and break easily.
7. If using a clear plastic sheath, cover the thermometer now.	7. Sheaths reduce the number of microorganisms on the thermometer. Follow package instructions for application.
8. Put on gloves.	8. Standard Precautions must be followed when there is potential exposure to body fluids.
9. Place the thermometer under the tongue to either side of the frenulum.	9. This is the area of the highest vascularity and will give the most accurate reading.

Step 9: Place the thermometer at either side of the frenulum.

(continued)

Steps

Purpose

10. Tell the patient to keep the mouth closed but caution against biting down on the glass column.

11. Leave the thermometer in place for 3–5 minutes. *Note:* The pulse and respirations may be taken at this time. (See Procedure 21–9, Procedure 21–10, and Procedure 21–11)

12. Remove the thermometer after the prescribed time. Remove and discard the sheath (if used) in an appropriate container or wipe the thermometer with a clean tissue or cotton ball from stem to bulb.

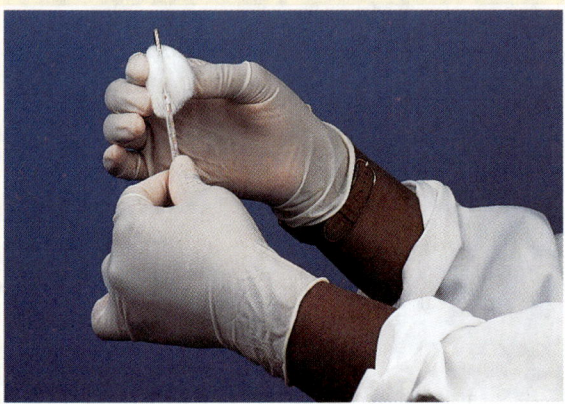

Step 12: Wipe the thermoneter from stem to bulb. (© B. Proud).

13. Hold the thermometer as before and note the reading.

14. Thank the patient and provide appropriate instructions.

15. Disinfect the thermometer according to the facility's policy. Remove gloves. Wash your hands.

16. Record the reading.

10. The reading will be inaccurate if air is entering the mouth. Biting down on the thermometer may cause it to break.

11. The thermometer may be left in place for 3 minutes if there is no evidence of fever and the patient is compliant. It should be left in for 5 minutes if the patient is febrile or noncompliant.

12. If the sheath remains on or if mucus is present, either may obscure the column. Wipe from clean to dirty.

14. Courtesy encourages the patient to have a positive attitude about the physician's office.

15. This prevents the spread of microorganisms.

16. Procedures are considered not to have been done if they are not recorded.

Procedure 21-4   Measuring Rectal Temperature Using a Glass Mercury Thermometer

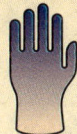

Equipment/Supplies

- glass mercury thermometer designed for rectal use
- surgical lubricant
- tissues
- disposable plastic sheath (if used)
- gloves

Steps	Purpose
1–7. Follow steps 1–7 as described in Procedure 21–3.	
8. Spread lubricant onto a tissue, then from the tissue to the thermometer. Put on gloves.	8. Never lubricate directly from the tube to avoid the spread of pathogens that might be present on the thermometer. Lubricants must be used for rectal insertion to avoid patient discomfort. Gloves are required under Standard Precautions when there is potential exposure to body fluids or excretions.
9. Ensure privacy. Place the patient in a side-lying position facing toward the examination room door. Drape appropriately.	9. This procedure may embarrass the patient. If the door is opened inadvertently, it will be less embarrassing if the patient is facing the door with less chance of exposure. The patient must be side-lying to expose the anus.
10. Expose only the buttock area. With the nondominant hand, lift the topmost buttock. Visualize the anus.	10. Never expose the patient unnecessarily. Never insert the thermometer without a clear view of the anus.
11. Touch the thermometer to the anus lightly. The anus will usually reflexively tighten against the intrusion. When the anus relaxes, insert the thermometer gently past the sphincter. Have the patient breathe deeply with the mouth opened.	11. Never force the thermometer; forcing may perforate the anal canal. Breathing through the mouth will relax the patient.
12. Insert the thermometer about 1½ inches for an adult, 1 inch for a child, and ½ inch for an infant.	12. These depths make it less likely that the anal canal will be perforated.
13. Release the upper buttock and drape the sheet back over the patent. Hold the thermometer in place for 3 minutes.	13. The patient must be covered for privacy. The thermometer will not stay in place if not held.
14. At the end of 3 minutes, remove the thermometer. Offer the patient a tissue for cleaning or assist as needed. Wipe the thermometer from stem to bulb,	14. The patient may be uncomfortable with extra lubricant around the anal area. Lubricant or the sheath will obscure the mercury column. Turning

(continued)

Procedure 21-4   Measuring Rectal Temperature Using a Glass Mercury Thermometer (continued)

Steps	Purpose
or remove the sheath (if used) by turning it inside out as it is pulled from the thermometer. Discard sheath in appropriate container.	the sheath inside out will reduce the transmission of pathogens.

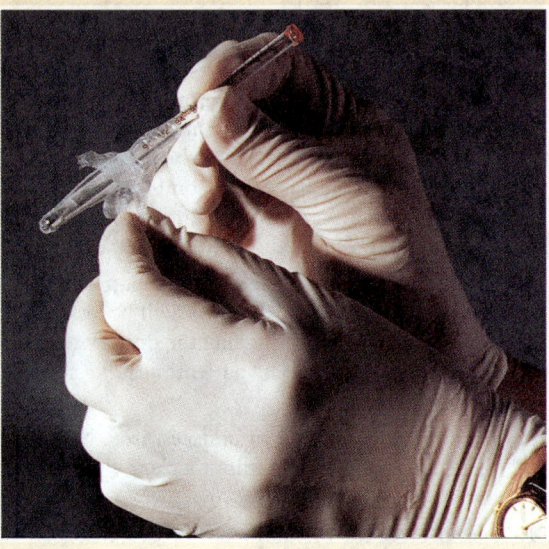

Step 14: Remove the sheath by grasping the end nearest the tip and inverting the plastic toward the bulb. The soiled area should now be inside the sheath.

Steps	Purpose
15. Note the reading. Remove and dispose of gloves.	
16. Thank the patient and provide appropriate instructions.	16. Courtesy encourages the patient to have a positive attitude about the physician's office.
17. Disinfect thermometer according to the facility's policy. Wash your hands.	17. This prevents the spread of microorganisms.
18. Record the reading, marking an R next to it to indicate rectal.	18. Procedures are considered not to have been done if they are not recorded. Temperatures are presumed to be oral unless otherwise noted.

Note: *Infants and very small children may be held in the lap or over the knees for this procedure or may remain on the examining table with the parent close by. Hold the thermometer and the buttocks with the dominant hand while securing the child with the nondominant hand. If the child moves with the thermometer in place, the thermometer and the hand will move together and avoid perforating the anal canal.*

Procedure 21-5	Measuring Axillary Temperature Using a Glass Mercury Thermometer

Equipment/Supplies

- glass mercury thermometer (either oral or rectal, according to facility's policy)
- tissues or cotton balls

Steps	Purpose
1–7. Follow steps 1–7 as described in Procedure 21–3.	
8. Expose the axillary area. Do not expose more of the patient's chest or upper body than is necessary to ensure the proper placement of the thermometer.	8. The patient's privacy must be observed.
9. Dry the axilla with patting motions.	9. Friction will increase the surface temperature. The axilla should be dry to remove perspiration, which may cause the thermometer to slip.
10. Place the bulb of the thermometer well into the axilla. Close the arm down over the axilla and cross the forearm over the chest. Drape the clothes or gown over the patient for privacy.	10. This position offers the best exposure to the mercury column and maintains a closed environment.
11. Leave the thermometer in place for 10 minutes. Stay with the patient.	11. Axillary temperatures take longer than oral or rectal. Staying with the patient ensures compliance.
12. Remove the thermometer after the prescribed time. Remove the sheath. Clean from stem to bulb. Note the reading.	12. Clean the thermometer of any surface dirt or perspiration before reading. Clean from the cleanest area to the least clean.
13. Thank the patient and provide appropriate instructions.	13. Courtesy encourages the patient to have a positive attitude about the physician's office.
14. Disinfect the thermometer according to the facility's policy. Wash your hands.	14. This prevents the spread of microorganisms.
15. Record the reading, marking an A next to it to indicate axillary.	15. Procedures are considered not to have been done if they are not recorded. Temperatures are presumed to be oral unless otherwise noted.

Note: *This is an excellent method for assessing a child's temperature but is time consuming and requires that the child remain still. Have the parent hold the child with the arm holding the thermometer against the parent's body to keep the thermometer in place. The parent may read to the child during this time or may give the child a bottle if appropriate.*

Procedure 21-6   Measuring Temperature Using an Electronic Thermometer

Equipment/Supplies

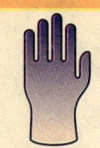

- battery-powered unit with probes and covers
- gloves
- lubricant (for rectal temperature)

Steps	Purpose
1. Wash your hands.	1. Handwashing aids infection control.
2. Assemble the equipment and supplies.	2. This ensures that everything you need is available.
3. Greet and identify the patient. Explain the procedure.	3. Identifying the patient prevents errors. Explaining the procedure helps ease anxiety and ensure compliance.
4. Choose the method most appropriate for the particular patient (eg, oral, rectal, axillary) and cover the probe to be used. Almost all units have a probe for oral and one for rectal. Covers are carried with the unit in a specially fitted box attached to the back of the unit. Put on gloves.	4. Comply with the facility's policy for the appropriate method for each patient. Standard Precautions must be observed when there is potential exposure to body fluids.
5. Place the thermometer as described for measuring an oral temperature (Procedure 21–3), rectal temperature (Procedure 21–4), or axillary temperature (Procedure 21–5).	
6. If taking an oral temperature, help the patient hold the probe. If taking a rectal temperature, you must hold the probe.	6. The electronic probe is heavier than the glass thermometer and is harder for patients to hold in place.
7. Note that the electronic unit will emit a beep when the temperature shows no signs of rising beyond this point. This will usually be within 20–60 seconds.	
8. Remove the probe. Note the reading; most will retain the reading until the probe is reinserted into the unit.	
9. Discard the probe cover in a waste receptacle. If this was a rectal temperature, help the patient to clean away any remaining lubricant. Remove gloves. Wash your hands.	9. The probe cover will be contaminated and must be disposed of properly.
10. Thank the patient and provide appropriate instructions.	10. Courtesy encourages the patient to have a positive attitude about the physician's office.
11. Record the temperature and the route. Return the unit to the charging base.	11. Procedures are considered not to have been done if they are not recorded. The route used must be specified. The unit must be kept charged and ready for use.

Note: *Electronic thermometers do not require the time limits set for glass thermometers. Most will provide a reading in well under 60 seconds.*

Procedure 21-7

Measuring Temperature Using a Tympanic Thermometer

Equipment/Supplies

- tympanic thermometer
- disposable probe covers

Steps	Purpose
1. Wash your hands.	1. Handwashing aids infection control.
2. Assemble the equipment and supplies.	2. This ensures that everything you need is available.
3. Greet and identify the patient. Explain the procedure.	3. Identifying the patient prevents errors. Explain the procedure to ease anxiety and ensure compliance.
4. Remove the tympanic thermometer from the base and put the disposable cover on the probe.	
5. Insert the probe, sealing the opening of the ear canal. Press the button to take the temperature, which will be displayed on the digital screen in about 2 seconds.	
6. Remove the probe and note the reading. Discard the probe cover in a waste receptacle.	6. The probe cover will be contaminated and must be disposed of properly.
7. Thank the patient and provide appropriate instructions.	7. Courtesy encourages the patient to have a positive attitude about the physician's office.
8. Record the temperature and the route. Return the unit to the base.	8. Procedures are considered not to have been done if not recorded. The route used must be specified. The unit must be kept charged and ready for use.

Procedure 21-8

Disinfecting a Glass Thermometer

Equipment/Supplies

- thermometer to be disinfected
- soft tissue or cotton ball
- soap
- gloves

Steps	Purpose
1. Put on gloves.	1. Gloves will prevent the spread of infection.
2. Wipe the thermometer with a soft tissue or cotton ball from stem to bulb with a rotating friction.	2. A soft material will remove more surface substances than a firmer material such as a paper towel. Friction will dislodge most substances. Wipe all surfaces from the cleanest area to the less clean.
3. Rub the thermometer briskly with cool or tepid soapy water.	3. Water too warm causes mercury to rise too quickly and may damage the thermometer. Water that is too cool is not as effective as tepid water. Soap dissolves fats and oils that remain on the surface.
4. Rinse with cool water.	4. The soap residue must be removed before placing in a soaking solution.
5. Dry well.	5. Moisture left on the thermometer will dilute the soaking solution and render it ineffective.
6. Place in the disinfectant soaking solution of choice, such as 70% alcohol.	6. Heat disinfection can not be used with thermometers.

(continued)

Steps

Purpose

7. After the prescribed period of time for the soaking solution of choice, remove the thermometers, rinse and store dry.

7. Chemicals left on thermometers may irritate the patient's mucosa. Instructions will be provided with the solution stating the time for disinfection to occur; these times must be carefully observed.

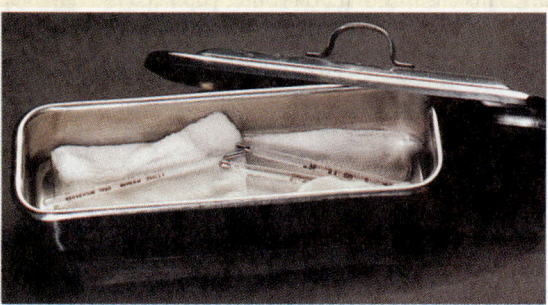

Step 7: Store clean thermometers in a covered instrument tray padded with gauze to prevent chipping.

Procedure 21-9

Measuring the Radial Pulse

Equipment/Supplies
- watch with sweep second hand

Steps

Purpose

1. Wash your hands.
2. Assemble the equipment.
3. Greet and identify the patient. Explain the procedure.
4. Place the patient with the arm relaxed and supported.
5. With the index, middle, and ring fingers of the dominant hand, use the fingertips to press firmly enough to feel the pulse, but gently enough not to obliterate it.

6. If the pulse is regular, count for 30 seconds and multiply by two. If this is a baseline pulse or if it is irregular, count for a full 60 seconds.
7. Record rate, rhythm, and volume, using terms described above. Record other data used to assess the cardiovascular system when appropriate. Observations about skin color (cyanosis, pallor, flushing) or temperature (cool and pale or hot and dry) may be required.

1. Handwashing aids infection control.
2. This ensures that everything you need is available.
3. Identifying the patient prevents errors. Explain the procedure to ease anxiety and ensure compliance.
4. If the arm is not supported and relaxed, or patient is uncomfortable, the pulse count may be affected.
5. The fingertips have greater sensitivity than other portions of the fingers. Using more than one finger increases the chance of finding the pulse. Avoid using the thumb; it has a slight pulse of its own and may be confused with the patient's. The thumb may be used on the opposite side of the patient's hand to steady the patient's hand and yours.
6. Counting an irregular pulse for less than 60 seconds will give an accurate measurement. You may check at other sites if unsure of the reading.
7. Procedures are considered not to have been done if they are not recorded.

Procedure 21-10 Measuring the Apical Pulse

Equipment/Supplies

- stethoscope
- watch with sweep second hand

Steps	Purpose
1. Wash your hands.	1. Handwashing aids infection control.
2. Assemble the equipment. Ensure that the stethoscope has clean earpieces.	2. This ensures that everything you need is available. Dirty earpieces may spread disease.
3. Greet and identify the patient. Explain the procedure.	3. Identifying the patient prevents errors. Explaining the procedure helps ease anxiety and ensure compliance.
4. Place the patient in a comfortable sitting or supine position. Remove the upper clothing or open it sufficiently to allow access to the chest wall. Drape for privacy with a gown or sheet.	4. If the patient is uncomfortable, the pulse rate may be affected. If clothing interferes with sound transmission or placement of the stethoscope, an inaccurate reading may result. Privacy for the patient must be ensured.
5. Locate the apex of the heart by palpating to the fifth intercostal space, between the fifth and sixth ribs. Move laterally to the left along the intercostal space to the nipple line or the midclavicular line.	5. This will locate the cardiac apex where the sound will be the loudest.

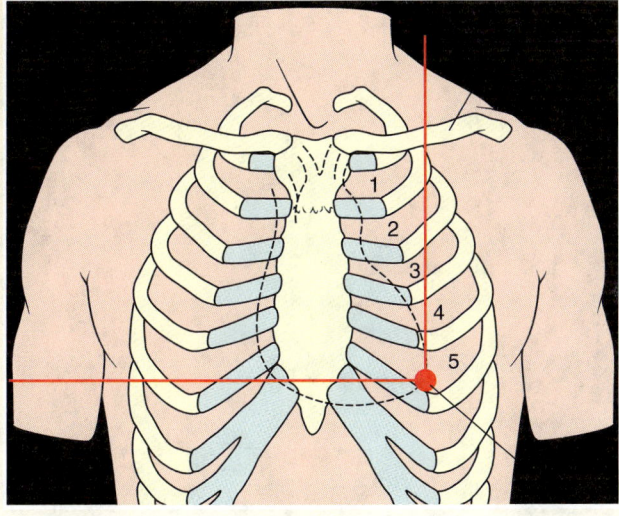

Step 5: Finding the apical pulse site.

6. Clean the stethoscope diaphragm with alcohol and warm it in the palm of the hand.	6. The stethoscope head should be cleaned between patients to avoid the spread of microorganisms. A cold stethoscope may cause the patient to be uncomfortable and may cause the heart rate to speed.
7. Insert the earpieces into the ear canals with the openings pointing slightly forward. A Doppler unit may also be used as noted above.	7. The ear canal in adults angles slightly forward. Inserting the earpieces to follow the line of the canal will make it easier to hear.

(continued)

Steps	Purpose
8. Listen for the S_1 and S_2 (sinus) sounds that will sound like "lubb, dubb." Together, they count as one beat.	8. The "lubb" sound is made when the atrioventricular valves close; the "dubb" sound is made when the semilunar valves close.
9. Count for one full minute.	9. If the heart rate must be counted by the apical pulse, it usually means that there is cardiovascular pathology present and a full minute will be needed to assess the count properly.
10. Assess the rate, rhythm and volume and record as an apical pulse.	10. Procedures are considered not to have been done if they are not recorded. If it is not otherwise noted, most pulses are presumed to be radial.

Note: If cardiovascular disease is present, it may be necessary to compare the radial pulse with the apical pulse to evaluate the *pulse deficit.* This is the difference between the sounds heard at the apex and the pulse felt at the radius. If there is a difference, the apex will always be the higher number. Generally it works best to have two people take the opposite

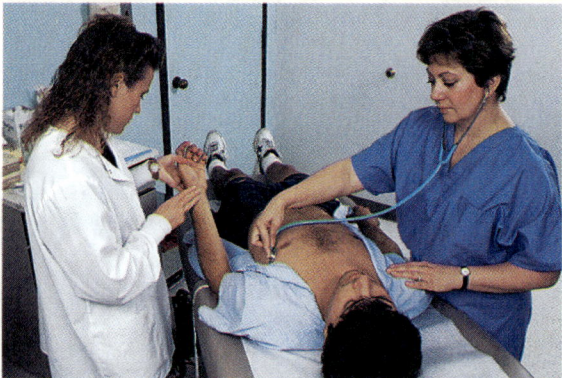

Two healthcare workers taking the apical and radial pulses to determine the pulse deficit.

pulses simultaneously, one at the apex, the other at the radius. With the watch at a point that both may see the sweep second hand, the apical recorder will call "start," usually as the hand reaches 12, 3, 6, or 9, to make it easier to keep track. The assistant who called "start" will call "stop" at the appropriate time and the numbers will be compared and recorded. If two workers are not available, one worker may perform the procedure by counting first one pulse for 60 seconds, then counting the other. Pulses performed in this manner will be recorded as "Apical/Radial" or "A/R."

Procedure 21-11: Counting Respirations

Steps	Purpose
1. With patient already in position and sweep second hand in view, count a complete rise and fall of the chest as one respiration. *Note:* Some patients breathe at rest using the abdominal muscles more than the chest muscles. Observe carefully for the easiest area to assess for the most accurate reading.	1. One complete cycle is counted as a respiration.
2. If pattern is regular, count respirations for 30 seconds and multiply by two, or count for 15 seconds and multiply by four. If pattern is irregular, count respirations for a full minute.	2. A full 60 seconds will be necessary for accuracy if the rate is not regular.
3. Record on the patient's chart with observations regarding the rate, rhythm, sounds, and effort. Record physical observations appropriate to assessment of the respiratory system, such as cyanosis, complaints of shortness of breath.	3. Procedures are considered not to have been done if they are not recorded. Simply recording a number may not provide sufficient information, especially if other observations are made.

Respirations are usually counted just after measuring the radial pulse, with your hand still on the patient's wrist. If patients are aware that breaths are being counted, it is not unusual for them to alter the pattern.

Procedure 21-12: Measuring Blood Pressure

Equipment/Supplies

- sphygmomanometer • alcohol wipe
- stethoscope

Steps	Purpose
1. Wash your hands.	1. Handwashing aids infection control.
2. Assemble the equipment and supplies.	2. This ensures that everything you need is available.
3. Identify the patient and explain the procedure. Ask the patient about recent smoking, caffeine, exercise, or emotional upset.	3. Identifying the patient prevents errors. Explain the procedure to ease anxiety and ensure compliance. The listed factors affect pressure levels.
4. Position the patient. Have the patient's arm supported and slightly flexed with the palm upward. The upper arm should be level with the heart. The patient's legs should not be crossed and the feet should be flat on the floor.	4. Patients are usually sitting unless the physician specifies a standing or lying pressure. (Always record the position if it is other than sitting.) Positioning the arm with the palm upward makes it easier to palpate the brachial artery. If the upper arm is higher than heart level, the pressure will be inaccurate. If the legs are crossed, the pressure may be higher than normal.
5. Expose the area. Remove the garment if the sleeve is too tight to raise above the area.	5. Tight clothing may act as a tourniquet and decrease the flow of blood. If clothing remains over the area, the sounds may be obscured.

(continued)

Equipment/Supplies

- sphygmomanometer
- alcohol wipe
- stethoscope

Steps	**Purpose**
6. Center deflated cuff over the brachial artery on the medial aspect of the upper arm. To assess the center of the cuff, fold the bladder in half; place the midpoint just above the brachial artery. The lower edge of the cuff should be 1–2 inches above the antecubital area.	6. Pressure must be applied over the artery for the correct reading. If the cuff is too low on the arm, it may interfere with the stethoscope placement and increase the environmental noises to obscure the pressure sounds.
7. Wrap the cuff smoothly. It should fit snugly against the arm without being too tight. (Cuffs vary. Some fasten with Velcro, some fasten with hooks, and others with long cloth tails.)	7. The cuff must be wrapped smoothly and snugly to ensure an accurate reading.
8. If using a mercury manometer, keep it vertical and at eye level. An aneroid must register with the needle at zero before beginning.	8. If the meniscus of the mercury is read at other than eye level, reading may be falsely high or low. If the aneroid needle doesn't register zero, it shouldn't be used until professionally calibrated.
9. Palpate the brachial pulse with the fingertips of the nondominant hand in the antecubital area.	9. It will be easier to hear the pulse sounds if the stethoscope is directly over the artery.
10. With air pump in the dominant hand and valve between the thumb and forefinger, turn the screw clockwise (right to tighten). Do not tighten it to the point that it will be difficult to turn back.	10. The cuff will not fill with the valve open. If the valve is too tight, it will be difficult to loosen with one hand.

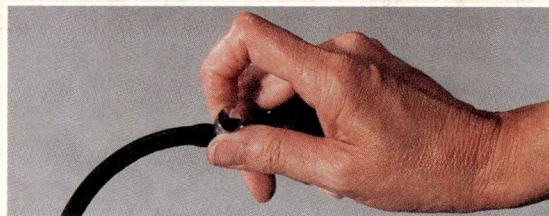

Step 10: Holding the bulb and screw valve properly will allow you to inflate and deflate the cuff easily.

11. With the fingers of the nondominant hand still at the pulse, inflate the cuff and note the point at which the brachial pulse is no longer felt. This number will be slightly below the first Korotkoff sound heard on auscultation.	11. Noting this point will give you a reference for assessing the pressure and a goal for re-inflating the cuff.

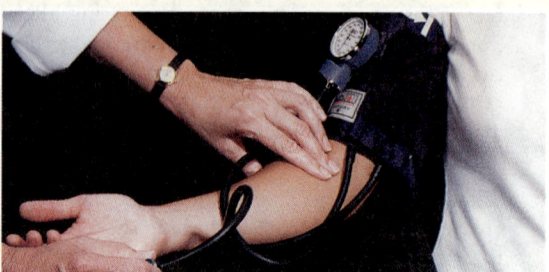

Step 11: Palpate brachial pulse before auscultating pressure.

(continued)

Procedure 21-12   Measuring Blood Pressure *(continued)*

Steps	Purpose
12. Deflate the cuff by turning the knob counterclockwise (left to loosen). Wait at least 30 seconds before re-inflating the cuff.	12. This interval allows the circulation to return to normal. The patient may raise or flex the arm and hand briefly to restore full circulation.
13. Clean the stethoscope diaphragm with alcohol. Place the stethoscope earpieces in the ear canal with the openings pointing slightly forward. Stand about 3 feet from the manometer, with the gauge at eye level. The stethoscope tubing should hang freely and should not rub against anything.	13. A clean bell prevents cross contamination. With earpieces pointing forward, the openings will follow the line of the ear canal. With manometer at eye level, there is less chance of error. If stethoscope rubs against objects, extraneous environmental noises may obscure the sound of the pulse.
14. Place the bell against the brachial artery but do not press hard. Hold with the nondominant hand.	14. The bell magnifies low-pitched sounds better than the diaphragm. The diaphragm covers more area, which may assist with finding the pulse if the brachial has been hard to palpate. If not pressed firmly enough, the sounds may not be heard; if pressed too firmly, the pulse may be obliterated.

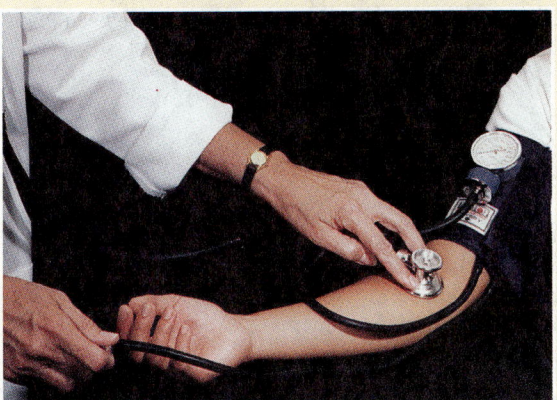

Step 14: Hold the stethoscope bell against the brachial artery.

15. With the valve in the dominant hand, thumb and forefinger on the valve screw, turn the screw just tightly enough to inflate the cuff. Pump the valve to about 30 mm Hg above the number felt on palpation.	15. If the screw is tightened too much, it will be difficult to release. Inflating above the 30 mm Hg point is uncomfortable for the patient and is unnecessary; inflating less than 30 mm Hg may cause the highest systolic reading to be missed.
16. With the thumb and forefinger remaining on the screw, slowly release the air at about 2–4 mm Hg per second.	16. Releasing too fast will cause missed beats; too slow will interfere with circulation.
17. Listening carefully, note the point on the gauge at which the first clear tapping sound is heard. This is the first systolic sound or Korotkoff I.	
18. Read at the top level of the meniscus (curved surface) of the mercury or at the number indicated by an arrow on the aneroid. Aneroid and mercury measurements are usually recorded as even numbers.	18. Reading at an angle will give an inaccurate measurement.
19. Maintaining control of the valve screw, continue to deflate at about 2–4 mm Hg a second and identify each of the Korotkoff sounds.	19. Many physicians will require that all sounds be recorded rather than the traditional systolic/diastolic.

(continued)

Procedure 21-12   Measuring Blood Pressure (continued)

Steps	Purpose
20. When the last sound is heard, note the reading and quickly deflate the cuff. *Note:* Never immediately re-inflate the cuff if you are unsure of the reading. Totally deflate the cuff and wait at least 1 minute before repeating the procedure. Have the patient raise the arm and flex the fingers of that hand to restore circulation and relieve vasocongestion if the pressure must be reassessed.	20. This will be the diastolic or Korotkoff V sound.
21. Remove cuff and press the air from the bladder.	
22. If this is the first recording or the first patient visit, the physician may want a reading in the opposite arm or in a position other than sitting.	22. Pressures will vary from arm to arm or according to position.
23. Record the result with the systolic over the diastolic, and any other sounds that might have been heard (eg, 160/110/80, if an auscultatory gap was heard). Record the patient's position if other than sitting, and the arm if other than the right arm.	23. Procedures are considered not to have been done if they are not recorded.
24. Clean and store the equipment. Wash your hands.	

Note: The palpatory method may be used if the Korotkoff sounds cannot be heard. Using the properly placed cuff, pump 30 mm Hg above the last felt pulse. Watching the mercury column or the aneroid needle as they drop, record the number at which the systolic pulse is felt at the radius. The diastolic cannot be assessed in this manner.

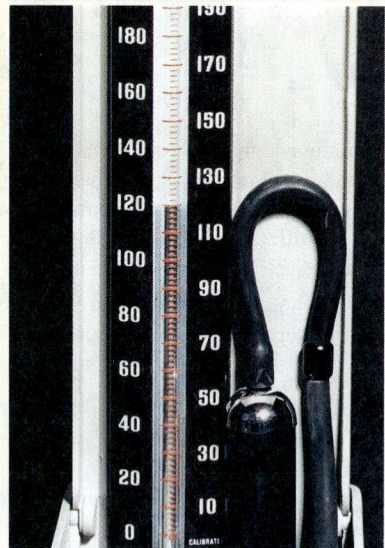

The meniscus reads 120 mm Hg.

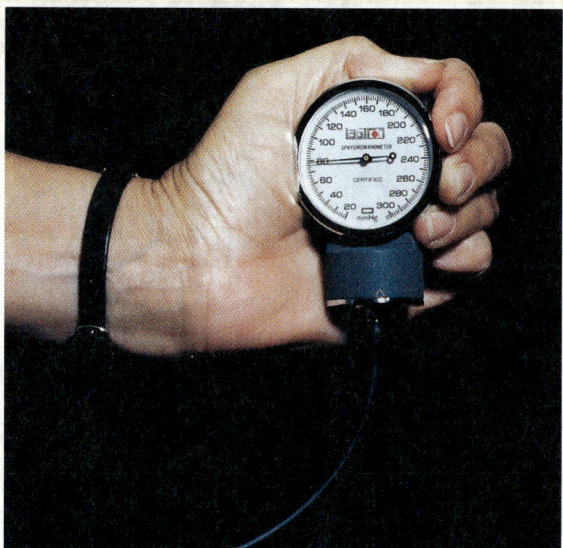

The gauge reads 120 mm Hg.

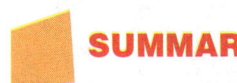

SUMMARY

Anthropometric measurements include height and weight. Vital signs include temperature (T), pulse (P), respiration (R), and blood pressure (BP). When a patient first visits the medical office, these measurements are recorded as baseline data. The physician then compares the baseline with measurements taken during all subsequent visits. Because anthropometric measurements and vital signs provide important data for the physician to use in diagnosing and treating illnesses, they are among the most frequently performed procedures in the medical assistant's daily schedule.

CRITICAL THINKING CHALLENGES

1. You are asked to teach a patient, Mr. Stone, how to take his blood pressure at home. Create a patient education brochure that explains the procedure in understandable terms and that includes normal blood pressure values. In addition, the physician wants Mr. Stone to record his blood pressure readings for 1 month. Design a sheet that Mr. Stone can easily use to record these readings.
2. Ms. Black has had a bad morning. She had car trouble on the way to the office. She could not find a parking place in the office lot. She was late for her appointment and had to be worked in. How would you expect this to affect her vital signs? Explain your response.
3. Mrs. Cooper is an elderly female with very little muscle mass. She weighs 90 lb. Which type of sphygmomanometer cuff will she likely need? Why?

ANSWERS TO CHECKPOINT QUESTIONS

1. Rectal temperatures are usually 1° higher than oral temperatures because of the rectum's vascularity and tightly closed environment.

2. A child's body temperature is usually higher than an adult's because of the child's higher metabolism.
3. Temperature taken by the tympanic route measures the temperature of the blood in the tympanic membrane on its way to the hypothalamus. The ear canal is a closed environment with the probe in place, resulting in a rapid, noninvasive, and accurate reading.
4. Measuring a patient's pulse involves assessing the rate (number of heartbeats in 1 minute), rhythm (time between each heartbeat), and volume (strength of the heartbeat).
5. When the diaphragm contracts, a negative pressure results and must be filled with inhaled air.
6. During systole, the heart contracts and forces out the blood. During diastole, the heart relaxes and fills with blood.

SUGGESTIONS FOR FURTHER READING

Earnest, V. V. (1992). *Clinical Skills in Nursing Practice*, 2nd ed. Philadelphia Lippincott-Raven.

Kerschner, V. L. (1992). *Health Unit Coordinating, Principles and Practices*. Albany NY: Delmar Publishers.

Kozier, B., & Erb, G. (1993). *Techniques of Clinical Nursing*, 4th ed. Redwood City, California: Addison-Wesley.

Memmler, R. L., Cohen, B. J., & Wood, D. L. (1992). *Structure and Function of the Human Body*, 5th ed. Philadelphia: Lippencott-Raven Publishers.

Rosdahl, C. B. (1995). *Textbook of Basic Nursing*, 6th ed. Philadelphia: Lippencott-Raven Publishers.

Smeltzer, S. C., & Bare, B. G. (1996). *Brunner and Suddarth's Textbook of Medical-Surgical Nursing*, 8th ed. Philadelphia: Lippincott-Raven Publishers.

Taylor, C., Lillis, C., & LeMone, P. (1993). *Fundamentals of Nursing: The Art and Science of Nursing Care*, 2nd ed. Philadelphia: Lippincott-Raven Publishers.

Timby, B. K. (1996). *Fundamental Skills and Concepts in Patient Care*, 6th ed. Philadelphia: J. B. Lippincott.

Physical Examination

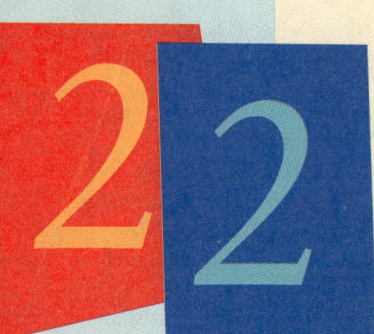

22

Chapter Outline

Components of the Physical Examination
Basic Instruments and Supplies
    Percussion Hammer
    Tuning Fork
    Nasal Speculum
    Otoscope
    Ophthalmoscope
    Audioscope
    Examination Light
    Gooseneck Lamp
    Tape Measure
    Gloves
    Stethoscope
    Tongue Depressor
    Penlight and Flashlight
Special Instruments and Supplies
    Headlight or Head Mirror
    Laryngeal Mirror
    Laryngoscope
    Vaginal Speculum
    Ayre Spatula or Histobrush
    Cotton-tipped Applicators
    Fixative
    Slides, Slide Covers, and Laboratory Request Forms
    Lubricant
    Anoscope
    Proctoscope
    Sigmoidoscope
Examination Techniques
    Inspection
    Palpation

    Percussion
    Auscultation
    Mensuration
    Manipulation
Responsibilities of the Medical Assistant
    Room Preparation
    Patient Preparation
    Assisting the Physician
    Postexamination Duties
Procedure: Assisting With the Physical Examination
Physical Examination Format
    Head
    Neck
    Eyes
    Ears
    Nose and Sinuses
    Mouth and Throat
    Chest
    Reflexes
    Breasts
    Abdomen
    Genitalia and Rectum
    Legs
    Posture, Gait, Coordination, Balance, and Strength
General Health Guidelines and Checkups
Summary
Critical Thinking Challenges
Answers to Checkpoint Questions
Suggestions for Further Reading

DACUM Components

1.3   Practice within the scope of education, training, and personal capabilities
1.5   Work as a team member
1.6   Conduct oneself in a courteous and diplomatic manner
4.1   Apply principles of aseptic technique and infection control
4.2   Take vital signs
4.5   Prepare and maintain examination and treatment area
4.7   Prepare patients for procedures
4.8   Assist physician with examinations and treatments

Chapter Competencies

Learning Objectives

Upon successfully completing this chapter, you will be able to:

1. Spell and define the Key Terms.
2. Identify and state the function of the instruments and supplies used for the physical examination.
3. Describe six methods used to examine the patient.
4. List the basic sequence of the physical examination.
5. State the responsibilities of the medical assistant before the examination.
6. Summarize the assisting duties of the medical assistant during the physical examination.

Performance Objectives

Upon successfully completing this chapter, you will be able to:

1. Assist the physician in all aspects of the physical examination (Procedure 22-1).

Key Terms

(See Glossary for definitions.)

applicator	gait	percussion
asymmetry	hernia	peripheral
auscultation	inguinal	PERRLA
baseline	inspection	range of motion
bimanual	lubricant	rectovaginal
bruit	manipulation	sclera
cerumen	mensuration	speculum
diagnosis	nasal septum	symmetry
digital	occult	transillumination
extraocular	palpation	tympanic membrane
fixative	Papanicolaou	

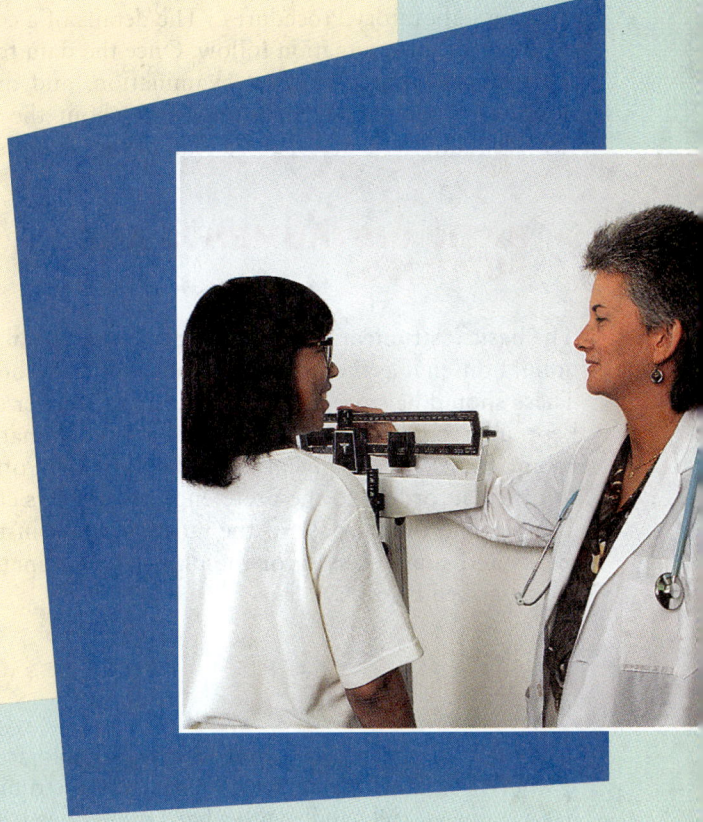

The purpose of the complete physical examination is to assess the patient's general state of health by examining each body system. Early signs and symptoms of disease may be detected during this procedure. All new patients usually receive a complete physical examination, which gives the physician **baseline** information about the patient. Baseline information is valuable for future comparison; it can aid the physician in **diagnosis** (identifying a disease or condition). Routine examinations are then performed at regular intervals to maintain health and prevent disease. As a medical assistant, you will be responsible for assisting the physician in the performance of routine physical examinations.

► COMPONENTS OF THE PHYSICAL EXAMINATION

The three components to the complete physical examination are: medical history, actual physical examination, and laboratory and diagnostic tests.

The specific procedures for obtaining a medical history and performing routine diagnostic and laboratory tests are described elsewhere in this text. (See pertinent chapters in Unit 5: Performing Clinical Duties; Unit 6: Assisting With Diagnostic Tests and Therapeutic Procedures for Common Disorders; and Unit 7: Performing Laboratory Procedures.) The details of a complete physical examination follow. Once the data from the medical history, physical examination, and diagnostic tests are evaluated, a judgment about the patient's conditions is made, and a plan of care is devised.

► BASIC INSTRUMENTS AND SUPPLIES

The basic instruments used for the general physical examination enable the physician to examine the body. These should be stored in a special tray or drawer and kept in a convenient location in each examination room. The exact equipment used will vary from office to office according to the preference of the physician. The use and the purpose of the most common instruments and supplies used for the physical examination are described below.

Percussion Hammer

The percussion hammer is used to test neurologic reflexes. Also called the reflex hammer, this instrument has a stainless steel handle with a hard rubber head. The head is used to test reflexes by striking the tendons of the ankle, knee, wrist, and elbow. The tip of the handle is used to stroke the sole of the foot. Some hammers are equipped with a brush and needle in their handles for testing sensory perception (Fig. 22-1).

Tuning Fork

The tuning fork is used to test hearing. It is a stainless steel instrument consisting of a handle and two prongs. The examiner strikes the prongs against his or her hand, which causes them to vibrate and produce a humming sound (Fig. 22-2).

Nasal Speculum

The nasal **speculum** is a stainless steel instrument that is inserted into the nose for visual **inspection** (examination) of the lining of the nose, nasal membranes, and septum. By squeezing the handles, the tips open to dilate the nostrils for visualization (Fig. 22-3). Nasal specula are available in a disposable form also. In addition, an otoscope with a special attachment may be used.

Otoscope

The otoscope permits visualization of the ear canal and **tympanic membrane**—a thin membrane in the middle ear that transmits sound vibrations (also called

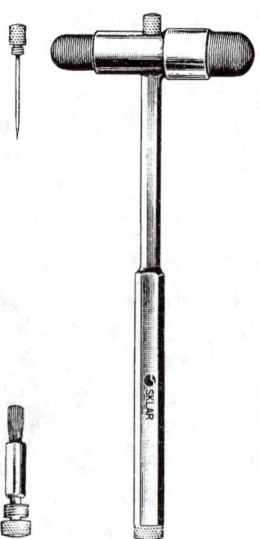

FIGURE 22-1

The Buck neurologic hammer. Note the pin and brush that fit within the frame of the hammer and are used to assess sensation. (Courtesy of Sklar Instruments, Westchester, PA)

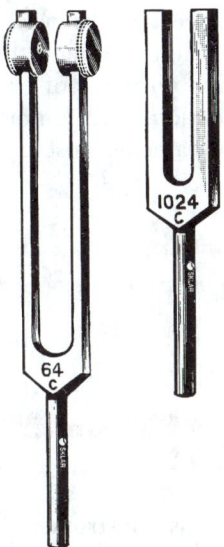

FIGURE 22-2
Tuning forks. (Courtesy of Sklar Instruments, Westchester, PA)

the eardrum). It has a stainless steel handle containing batteries and a head with a light, a magnifying lens, and a cone-shaped hollow tipped speculum that is placed into the ear. The interchangeable specula come in a variety widths and are numbered according to size. They must be thoroughly cleaned with a disinfectant, such as alcohol, after each use. Most offices use disposable covers so the tip does not directly contact the patient. Disposable specula are also available. The nose may also be examined with the otoscope by attaching specialized nasal specula tips.

Ophthalmoscope

The ophthalmoscope is used to examine the interior structures of the eye. It has a stainless steel handle containing batteries and a head with a light, magnifying lenses, and an opening through which to view the eye.

The examination of the eye, ear, and nose can be accomplished by using a common handle or base unit and changing only the head (or tip) for each part of the examination.

The otoscope and the ophthalmoscope operate on batteries located in the handle. A unit with rechargeable batteries must be placed in a charger when not in use. Some offices are equipped with wall-mounted electrical units to which the scopes are attached. Batteries are not necessary with these units (Fig. 22-4).

Audioscope

The audioscope is used to screen patients for hearing loss. It looks like an otoscope. The examiner places the tip into the patient's ear, and the instrument produces a variety of tones. The patient is asked to respond as each tone is heard.

Examination Light

Some offices are equipped with an adjustable overhead examination light. As a medical assistant, you have the responsibility to see that light is directed toward the area of the patient's body that the doctor is examining.

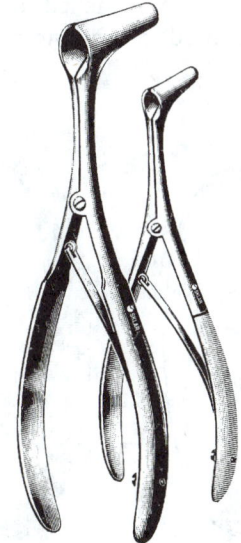

FIGURE 22-3
Nasal specula. (Courtesy of Sklar Instruments, Westchester, PA)

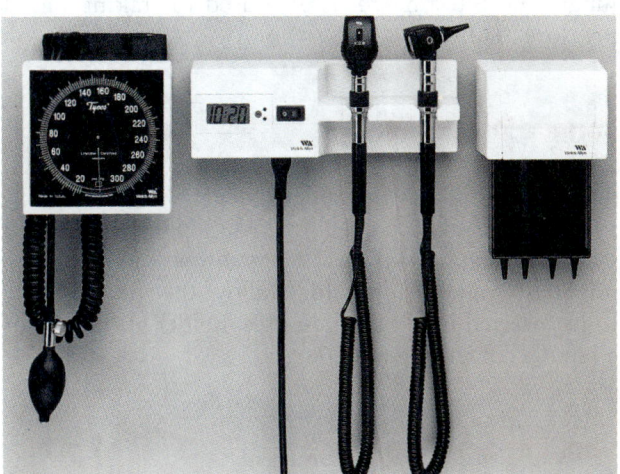

FIGURE 22-4
Wall-mounted examining instruments. From left: sphygmomanometer with cuff, ophthalmoscope, otoscope, and dispenser for disposable otoscope covers. (Courtesy of Welch Allyn, Skaneatels Falls, NY)

Gooseneck Lamp

The gooseneck lamp is a flexible floorlamp on a movable stand. It is capable of movement in a variety of directions to provide good visibility. Again, you have the responsibility to see that light is directed toward the area of the patient's body that the doctor is examining.

Tape Measure

The tape measure is a flexible ruler that is measured in inches and feet or centimeters and meters. It is used to measure head circumference and height in the infant, height of the uterus (fundus) during pregnancy, and the size of the body parts and abnormalities.

Gloves

Disposable examination gloves are used when the mouth, vagina, and rectum are examined to protect the patient and physician from microorganisms. Under Standard Precautions, gloves should be worn when touching blood, body fluids, secretions, excretions, mucous membranes, nonintact skin, and contaminated items.

Stethoscope

The stethoscope is used for listening to body sounds. At its end is a diaphragm or bell that is placed on the patient's body. This is connected to two earpieces by flexible rubber or vinyl tubing. The examiner uses the stethoscope to auscultate the sounds of the heart, lungs, and intestines. It is also used for taking blood pressure readings.

Tongue Depressor

The tongue depressor (tongue blade) is a thin, flat, smooth piece of wood about 6 inches long used to hold down the tongue to inspect the mouth and throat. Illuminated tongue blade holders allow the tongue blade to be inserted into a stainless steel holder at the end of a handle containing batteries.

Penlight and Flashlight

The penlight or flashlight are used to provide light during the examination. The penlight is the shape and size of a ballpoint pen. It is battery operated and has a clip on its side that is pressed to produce light. It is

usually used for inspecting the eyes, nose, and throat. Other uses include shining a light through the sinuses and scrotum for the purposes of examination; this is called **transillumination**. The common flashlight may also be used for the same purposes.

Checkpoint Question

1. Which instruments are used to test hearing and how do they work?

➤ SPECIAL INSTRUMENTS AND SUPPLIES

In addition to the basic instruments and supplies described above, other specialized equipment may be used for the physical examination.

Headlight or Head Mirror

An ear, nose, and throat specialist (otorhinolaryngologist) may wear a headlight or head mirror for the examination. This consists of a light or mirror attached to a headband that fits over the head (Fig. 22-5). Because the examiner needs a light source to examine the ear, nose, and throat, this provides illumination for these areas either directly or reflected from the examining light.

Laryngeal Mirror

The laryngeal mirror is a stainless steel instrument with a long, thin handle. Attached to its end is a small round mirror. It is used to examine the throat and larynx (Fig. 22-6).

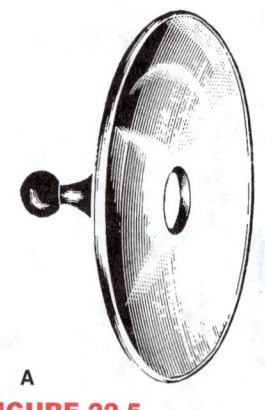
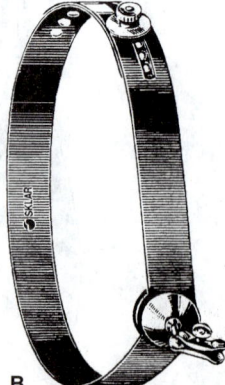

A   B

FIGURE 22-5
A head mirror (**A**) and head band (**B**). (Courtesy of Sklar Instruments, Westchester, PA)

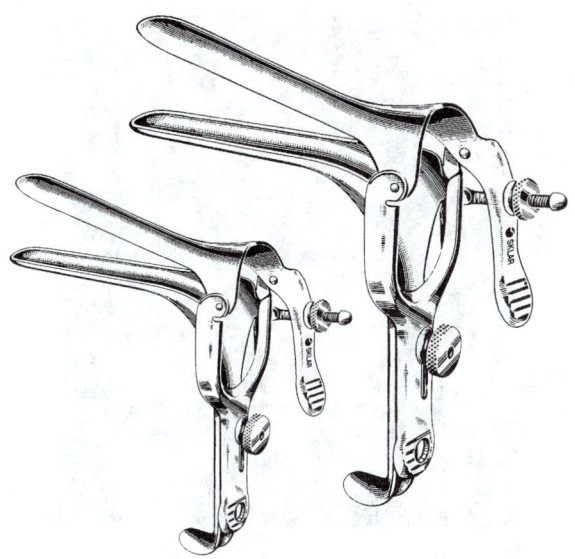

FIGURE 22-7
Two sizes of vaginal specula. (Courtesy of Sklar Instruments, Westchester, PA)

It is made of reusable stainless steel or a disposable plastic.

Ayre Spatula or Histobrush

The Ayre spatula, or cervix scraper, is a thin, flat, smooth piece of wood about 6 inches long. One tip has an irregular shape that is placed in the cervical opening and rotated to collect the specimen for a Pap smear. The other end is rounded and is used to collect cells from the vaginal cul-de-sac.

The histobrush is about six inches long, made of nylon or plastic, and tipped with soft bristles in a spiral that can be rotated in the cervical os to remove cells for a Pap smear if the physician prefers this instrument (Fig. 22-8).

Cotton-tipped Applicators

Cotton-tipped **applicators** are bits of cotton attached to a slender wooden or plastic stick. They may be small for specimen collection or may be large for medication application or for removing excess secretions that may interfere with treatment or visualization (see Fig. 22-8).

Fixative

A **fixative** is a chemical spray made of 50% alcohol and 50% ether or 95% ethyl alcohol. It "fixes" the Pap smear specimen on the slide and preserves it for cytology testing. Hair spray is sometimes used for this purpose.

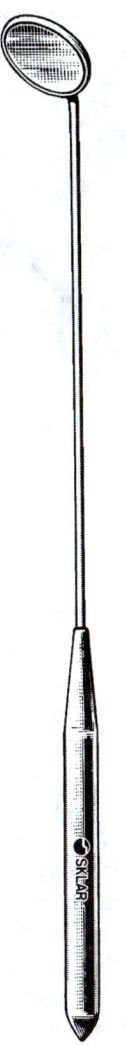

FIGURE 22-6
A laryngeal mirror. (Courtesy of Sklar Instruments, Westchester, PA)

Laryngoscope

The laryngoscope is an instrument with lights and mirror used to visualize the larynx.

Vaginal Speculum

The general physical examination for the female may include a pelvic examination and **Papanicolaou** (Pap) smear, a simple smear method of examining tissue cells for cancer (especially of the cervix). The vaginal speculum is a broad-billed bivalved instrument that is inserted into the vagina to expand the vaginal opening (Fig. 22-7). It permits the physician to visualize the cervix and vaginal walls and to obtain specimens.

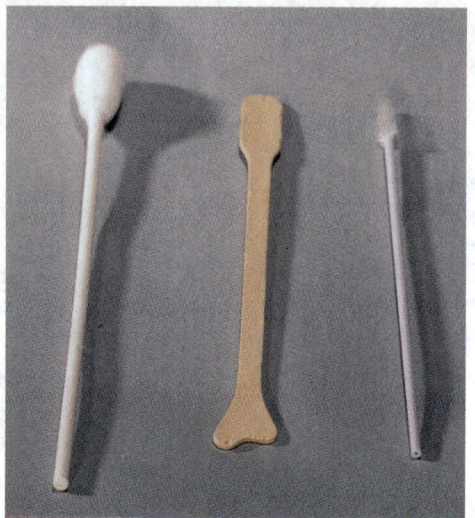

FIGURE 22-8
Cotton-tipped applicator (**left**), Ayre spatula (**center**), and histobrush (**right**). Cotton-tipped applicators of this size are frequently used to remove excess vaginal secretions or to apply medications during the gynecologic examination.

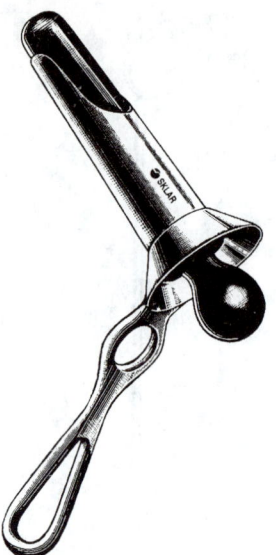

FIGURE 22-9
Anoscope. (Courtesy of Sklar Instruments, Westchester, PA)

Slides, Slide Covers, and Laboratory Request Forms

Glass microscope slides are used for specimens. Slides are placed into covers to preserve and protect them for transportation to the laboratory for analysis. Laboratory request forms are necessary to identify the patient and to provide patient data.

Lubricant

A lubricant is a gel used to reduce friction and provide for easy insertion. It may be used to facilitate speculum insertion or the **bimanual** (two hand) examination after the Pap smear is completed. It may also be used for the rectal examination.

Anoscope

The anoscope is a stainless steel speculum that is inserted into the rectum to inspect the anal canal. An obturator with a rounded tip extends beyond the anoscope to guide it into the rectum. After the instrument is inserted the obturator is removed for visualization. Some anoscopes have a knob that rotates the inserted end without having to turn the handle (Fig. 22-9).

Proctoscope

The proctoscope is a speculum used to visualize the rectum and anus. It consists of a straight tube with an obturator inside of it with a rounded tip that extends beyond the tube to direct or guide it along the canal. After the instrument is inserted, the obturator is removed and a fiberoptic light handle and magnifying lens are attached so that the physician can see through the tube. The tube is marked in centimeters so that any abnormalities noted may be located according to their depth in the canal. The proctoscope is longer than the anoscope and shorter than the sigmoidoscope.

Sigmoidoscope

The sigmoidoscope is an instrument used to visually inspect the rectum and sigmoid colon. It consists of a tube with an obturator, fiberoptic light handle, and magnifying lens. A suction machine, cotton-tipped applicators, glass microscope slides, slides covers, and laboratory request slips should be available when any rectal procedures are done. Tissue or stool specimens may be obtained.

In many offices, the larger, inflexible scopes have been replaced with flexible fiberoptic instruments that are smaller in diameter and are more comfortable for the patient. These newer instruments also allow for greater depth of examination and better visualization of the intestinal mucosa.

➤ EXAMINATION TECHNIQUES

The physician uses six basic techniques to gather information during the physical examination.

Inspection

Inspection involves looking at areas of the body to observe physical features. The examiner inspects the patient's general appearance, movements, coloring, contours, **symmetry** (equality in size or shape) or **asymmetry** (inequality in size or shape), deformities, injuries, and skin condition. Inspection may be done with the naked eye, with instruments, or with a light source.

Palpation

Palpation involves touching the body with the fingers or hands. The examiner palpates the body to determine pulse rate, the size, shape, and location of organs, the presence of masses, and the existence of swelling, tenderness, or pain. Skin temperature, moisture, texture, and elasticity may also be assessed. Palpation may be performed with both hands (bimanual), the full length of the fingers (**digital**), one hand, the fingertips, or the palm of the hand.

Percussion

Percussion involves tapping or striking the body with the hand or an instrument to produce sounds. Direct percussion is performed by directly striking the body with a finger. Indirect percussion is done by placing a finger on the area and then striking it with a finger of the other hand. In both methods, the examiner listens to the sounds and feels for vibrations produced to determine the position, size, and density of body organs and cavities. Percussion may be done with the finger, knuckles, or side of the hand. A percussion hammer is used to test reflexes.

Auscultation

Auscultation involves listening to the sounds of the body. The examiner uses a stethoscope to hear heart sounds (such as the heart beat and murmurs), lung sounds (such as respirations and signs of infection), blood vessel sounds (such as the movement of blood through the vessels), and abdominal sounds (such as the movement of gases and fluids). Direct auscultation may be done by placing the ear directly on the patient's body.

The above methods are usually performed in the order given for each area of the body as it is examined. For the abdominal examination, auscultation is performed before palpation and percussion because doing these first may alter the normal bowel sounds.

Mensuration

Mensuration refers to the measurement of height, weight, length, diameter, flexion, extension, hearing, vision, and pressure.

Manipulation

Manipulation is the passive movement of the joints of the body to determine extent of movement, or range of motion. The examiner moves the joints of the head, arms, hands, legs, and feet.

➤ RESPONSIBILITIES OF THE MEDICAL ASSISTANT

Room Preparation

As a medical assistant, you are responsible for seeing that the room is prepared for the examination. The examination room should be clean, well lighted and ventilated, and at a comfortable temperature for the patient. The examining table should be covered with clean paper and all evidence of previous patients removed.

Patient Preparation

Once the examining room is ready, call the patient by name from the waiting room and escort him or her to the examining room. It is important that you develop rapport with your patients and practice good interpersonal skills. This will help to put patients at ease and will increase their confidence in you. Your goal is to create a positive, supportive, caring, and friendly atmosphere. Assess the patient's facial expression and level of anxiety by noting verbal and nonverbal behavior. Treat the patient as an individual and speak clearly with a confident tone of voice as you explain the procedure.

Take and record the patient's history and chief complaint if this is your responsibility. Take and record the vital signs and the results of the visual acuity and blood tests. Explain how to obtain a urine specimen and direct the patient to the bathroom. Label the specimen and see that it arrives in the laboratory. Return the patient to the examining room and give instructions for disrobing and gowning. Some physicians have preferences for the gown opening in the front or the back. Leave the room while the patient undresses unless your assistance is needed. When the patient is ready, obtain an electrocardiogram if one is ordered. Then, have the patient sit on the edge of the examination table and cover the legs with a drape sheet. Place the chart outside the door of the examining room and notify the physician that the patient is ready.

Assisting the Physician

During the process of the physical examination, for legal reasons you must remain in the room when a male physician examines a female patient. In every examination, your responsibility is to assist the physician by handing the instruments and supplies needed and directing the light appropriately.

You must also assist the patient in assuming appropriate positions (Fig. 22-10) as the doctor proceeds, making sure to adjust the drapes to expose only those body parts being examined. Patient support and reassurance are also vital assisting duties during the examination. Table 22-1 lists the various examination positions, the body parts usually examined in the positions, and the instruments needed by the physician.

Postexamination Duties

At the completion of the physical examination, you are expected to perform follow-up treatments and procedures if necessary. Direct the patient to dress, and leave the room unless your assistance is required. Return to the examining room and ask if the patient has any questions. Reinforce any instructions that have been given and provide patient education. Escort the patient to the front office, where any future appointment may be scheduled and billing questions clarified.

Return to the examining room and clean all used instruments and equipment and dispose of used supplies. Clean the examining table and counter surfaces with disinfectant. (See Chap. 19, Asepsis and Infection

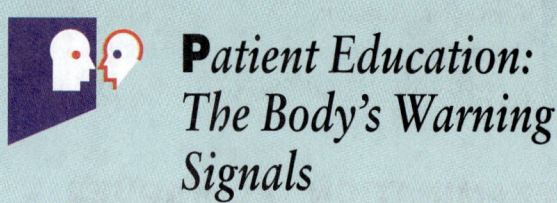

Patient Education: The Body's Warning Signals

Teach patients to recognize the following early warning signs of cancer:

C—change in bowel or bladder habits
A—a sore that does not heal
U—unusual bleeding or discharge
T—thickening, lump, or change in shape of the breasts or testes
I—indigestion or difficult swallowing
O—obvious change in a wart or mole; bleeding, enlargement, or itching
N—nagging cough or hoarseness

Frequent severe headaches and persistent abdominal pain are other signals that should not be ignored.

Instruct parents not to overlook the following signs in their children:

- continual crying for no obvious reason
- unexplained nausea and vomiting
- general failure to thrive
- spontaneous bleeding or bleeding that does not stop in the normal amount of time
- bumps, lumps, masses, or swelling anywhere on the body
- frequent stumbling for no apparent reason

Control.) Cover the examination table with clean paper and prepare the room for the next patient. Check the patient's medical record to be sure that all data have been accurately documented.

Procedure 22-1 describes the steps for assisting the physician with the physical examination.

Checkpoint Question

4. What are the four basic responsibilities of the medical assistant in the performance of the physical examination?

➤ PHYSICAL EXAMINATION FORMAT

The physical examination of the patient by the physician begins with the patient seated on the examining table with a drape sheet over the lap and covering the

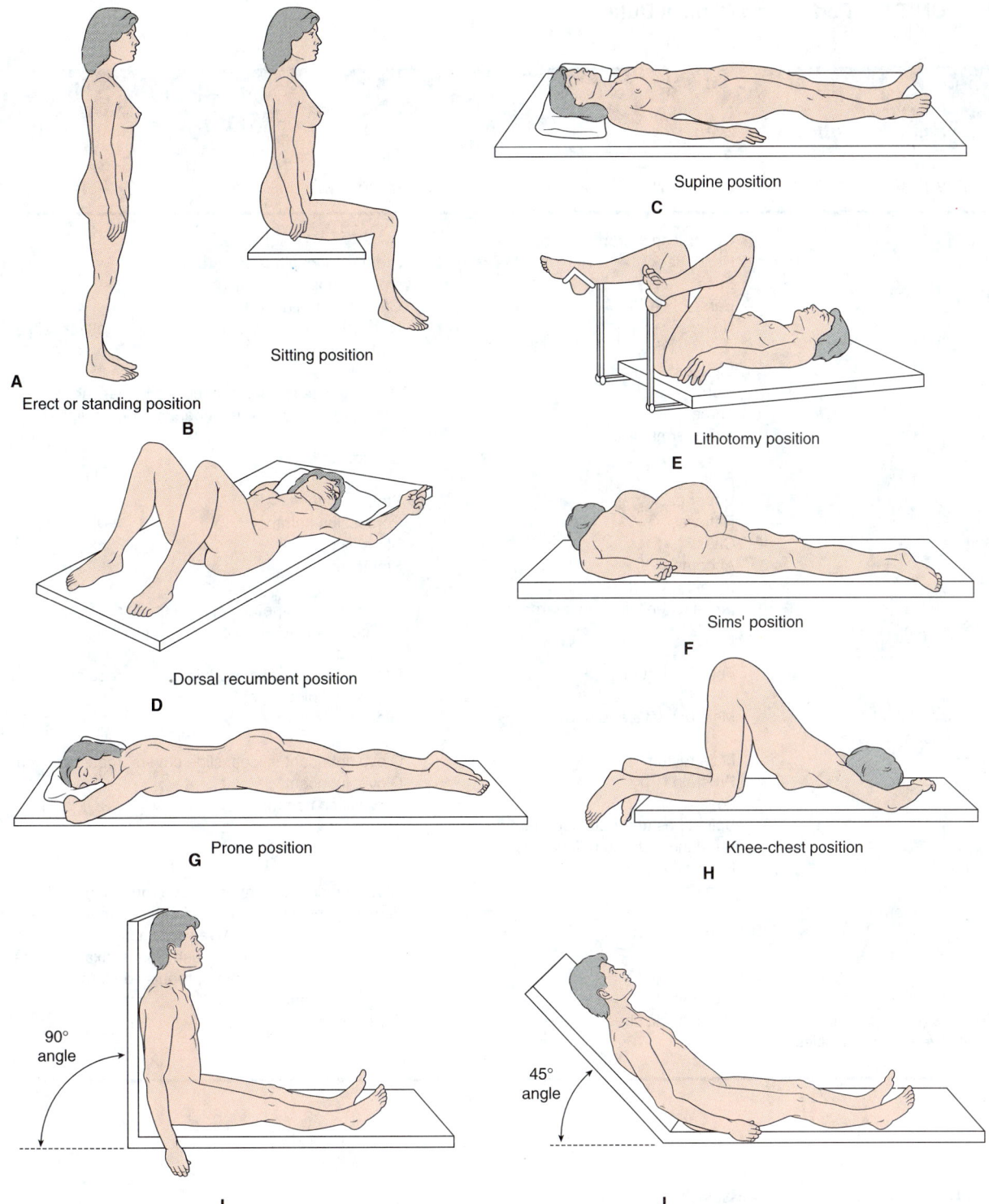

FIGURE 22-10

Patient examination positions. (**A**) Sitting position. The patient sits erect at the end of the examining table with the feet supported. (**B**) Standing position. The patient's body is erect and facing forward with the arms down at the sides. (**C**) Supine position. The patient lies on the back with arms at the sides. A pillow is usually placed under the head for comfort. (**D**) Dorsal recumbent position. The patient is in the supine position with the legs separated, knees bent, and feet flat on the table. (**E**) Lithotomy position. This position is similar to the dorsal recumbent position, but the patient's feet are placed in stirrups rather than flat on the table. The stirrups should be level with each other and about 1 foot from the edge of the table. The patient's feet should be moved into or out of the stirrups simultaneously to prevent back strain. (**F**) Sims' position. The patient lies on the left side with the left arm and shoulder behind the body, the right leg and arm sharply flexed on the table, and the left knee slightly flexed. (**G**) Prone position. The patient lies on the abdomen with the head supported and turned to one side. The arms may be placed under the head or by the sides, whichever is more comfortable. (**H**) Knee-chest position. The patient kneels on the table with the arms and chest on the table, hips in the air, and back straight. (**I**) Fowler's position. The patient is in a semi-sitting position with the head of the bed elevated 80°–90°. (**J**) Semi-Fowler's position. The patient is in a semi-sitting position with the head of the bed elevated 30 °–45° and knees slightly bent.

Table 22-1

Examination Positions and Their Uses

Patient Position	Body Part(s) Examined	Instruments Needed
Sitting	General appearance	
	Head, neck	Stethoscope, glass of water
	Eyes	Ophthalmoscope, penlight
	Ears	Otoscope, tuning fork
	Nose	Nasal speculum, penlight, substances to test sense of smell
	Sinuses	Penlight
	Mouth	Glove, gauze square, tongue blade, penlight
	Throat	Glove, tongue blade, laryngeal mirror, penlight
	Axilla, arms	
	Chest	Stethoscope
	Breasts	
	Upper back	Stethoscope
	Reflexes	Percussion hammer
Supine	Chest	Stethoscope
	Abdomen	Stethoscope
	Breasts	
Lithotomy, dorsal recumbent, or Sims'	Female genitalia and internal organs	Glove, vaginal speculum, Ayre spatula, histobrush, slides, fixative, slide covers, requisition form, lubricant
	Female rectum	Glove, lubricant, slides, slide covers, requisition form or occult blood test
Standing, dorsal recumbent, or Sims'	Male genitalia and hernia	Glove
	Male rectum	Glove, lubricant, slides, slide covers, requisition form
	Prostate	Glove, lubricant
	Legs	Percussion hammer
	Spine, posture, gait, coordination, balance, strength, flexibility	
Prone	Back, spine, legs	
Knee-chest (genupectoral)	Rectum	Glove, lubricant, sigmoidoscope (optional)
	Female genitalia	Glove, lubricant, vaginal speculum, Ayre spatula, histobrush, slides, fixative, slide covers, requisition form
	Prostate	Glove, lubricant
Fowler's (used for patients with breathing difficulties)	Head, neck, chest	Stethoscope

legs. The doctor usually progresses through the examination in orderly and methodical sequences. The patient's general appearance, behavior, speech, posture, nutritional status, hair distribution, and skin are observed throughout the examination.

Head

The patient's skull, scalp, hair, and face are inspected and palpated for size, shape, and symmetry. The examiner is looking for nodules, masses, or local trauma.

Neck

The patient may be asked to roll the head around in all directions to assess for range of motion and to check for any limitations of movement. The lymph nodes are located in the neck and are palpated. The trachea is inspected and palpated. The thyroid gland is inspected and palpated for size and symmetry.

The patient may be asked to swallow several times and small sips of water may be offered so the physician may palpate the thyroid gland. However, this is not always necessary because just the normal act of swallowing produces the same result. The carotid arteries are

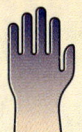

Procedure 22-1	Assisting With the Physical Examination

Equipment/Supplies

- appropriate instruments may include: stethoscope, ophthalmoscope, penlight, otoscope, tuning fork, nasal speculum, tongue blade, laryngeal mirror, percussion hammer, speculum
- glass of water (optional)
- substances for testing sense of smell (optional)
- gloves
- gauze squares
- lubricant
- vaginal spatula/histobrush
- slides, slide covers, and fixative
- requisition slips as appropriate
- tissues
- specimen container
- gown
- drape
- electrocardiograph

Steps	Purpose
1. Wash your hands.	1. Handwashing aids infection control.
2. Prepare the examining room.	2. A clean room that is free from contamination prevents transfer of microorganisms.
3. Assemble the equipment.	3. This ensures that all supplies are available.
4. Greet the patient by name and escort to the examining room.	4. Identifying the patient by name acknowledges the patient as a person and prevents errors.
5. Explain the procedures.	5. Explaining the procedure helps ease anxiety and ensure compliance.
6. Obtain and record the medical history and chief complaint if that is your responsibility.	6. A medical history gives the physician important background information about the patient's health and symptoms.
7. Take and record the patient's temperature, pulse, respirations, blood pressure, height, weight, and visual acuity. Draw blood if necessary.	7. The vital signs and diagnostic tests give the physician an overall picture of the patient's health.
8. Instruct the patient in obtaining a urine specimen and escort to the bathroom.	8. The urinalysis provides data on the patient's general health. An empty bladder facilitates the palpation of the abdomen.
9. See that the specimen is properly labeled and received in the laboratory.	9. Proper labeling of specimens helps to prevent errors.
10. Escort the patient back to the examining room. Instruct patient to disrobe completely and put on a full gown opening down the back or front as directed by the physician. Leave the room unless the patient needs assistance.	10. The gown must open in the direction that provides accessibility for the examination. Patients often prefer to disrobe in private; elderly and disabled patients may need assistance in disrobing and gowning.
11. Perform an electrocardiogram if ordered.	11. The electrocardiogram gives the physician information about the heart's conduction system.
12. Assist the patient into a sitting position on the edge of the examination table. Cover the lap and legs with a drape sheet.	12. Greeting the physician in a sitting position is psychologically beneficial to the patient and it is the position in which the physician begins the examination. A drape sheet provides privacy by covering those body parts not being examined.
13. Place the patient's chart outside the examination room door and notify the physician that the patient is ready.	13. Good communication between office personnel helps to prevent delays.

(continued)

Procedure 22-1   Assisting With the Physical Examination *(continued)*

Steps	Purpose

14. Assist the physician during the examination by handing the instruments needed for examination of each body area and ensuring proper patient positioning.

    a. Begin by handing the physician the instruments necessary for examining the:
- head and neck—stethoscope and glass of water
- eyes—ophthalmoscope, penlight
- ears—otoscope, tuning fork
- nose—nasal speculum, penlight, substances for testing sense of smell
- sinuses—penlight
- mouth—glove, gauze square, tongue blade, penlight. *Note:* Hand the tongue blade to the physician by holding it in the middle. When it is returned to you after use, grasp it in the middle again so that you do not touch the end that was in the patient's mouth.
- throat—glove, tongue blade, laryngeal mirror, penlight. *Note:* Warm the laryngeal mirror by placing it in warm water before handing it to the physician.

    b. Assist the patient in removing the gown to the waist so the physician can examine the chest and upper back. Hand the physician the stethoscope.

    c. Assist the patient in putting on the gown and remove the drape sheet from the legs so the physician may test the reflexes. Hand the physician the reflex hammer.

    d. Assist the patient to a supine position, opening the gown at the top to expose the chest once again. Place the drape sheet from the waist down to the toes. Hand the physician the stethoscope.

    e. Cover the patient's chest and lower the drape sheet to the pubic area to expose the abdomen. The physician will use the stethoscope.

    f. Assist with genital and rectal examinations. Hand the patient tissues following these examinations.

    For females:
- Assist the patient into the lithotomy position and drape appropriately.
- For examination of the genitalia and internal reproductive organs, provide a glove, lubricant, speculum, spatula or brush,

---

Purpose

14. Anticipating the physician's needs promotes efficiency and saves time.

    a. Holding the tongue blade in the center allows the physician to grasp one end of it so that the clean end may be placed in the patient's mouth. Warming the laryngeal mirror prevents fogging.

    b. Only those parts being examined are exposed; the rest of the body remains covered.

    f. Tissues may be used to wipe off excess lubricant used.

(continued)

Steps	**Purpose**

slides, fixative, slide covers, and requisition slip.
- For rectal examination, provide a glove, lubricant, slides, slide covers, and requisition slip.
- Assist the patient to a standing position.

For males:
- Assist the patient to a standing position. In this position, the physician can check for a hernia; by having him bend over the table, the physician can perform a rectal and prostate examination.
- For hernia examination, provide a glove.
- For rectal examination, provide a glove, lubricant, slides, slide covers, requisition slip.
- For prostate examination, provide a glove and lubricant.

e. With the patient in the standing position, hand the physician the reflex hammer to assist with examination of the legs and gait, coordination, and balance.

15. Help the patient to return to a sitting position at the edge of the examining table.

16. Perform any follow-up procedures or treatments.

17. Leave the room while the patient dresses unless needed for assistance with clothing.

18. Return to the room to answer questions, reinforce instructions, and provide patient education.

19. Escort the patient to the front office.

20. Properly clean or dispose of all used equipment. Clean the room with disinfectant and prepare for the next patient.

21. Wash your hands.

22. Record the procedures.

Purpose column:

15. The physician often discusses the findings with the patient at this time and provides instruction.

17. This provides privacy.

18. Patient compliance depends on full understanding of the treatment plan. Patient education is the responsibility of all health care workers.

19. You can help clarify appointment scheduling or billing questions, if any.

20. All instruments, supplies, and equipment that come into direct contact with patients must be appropriately decontaminated or disposed of.

22. Procedures are considered not to have been done if they are not recorded.

palpated and auscultated on both sides to check for any **bruits** (abnormal sounds) caused by possible blockage.

Eyes

The visual acuity test is usually performed by the medical assistant before the doctor's examination. (See Chap. 33, Caring for Patients with Sensory Disorders, for the procedure for visual acuity testing.) The physician inspects the **sclera**, the fibrous tissue covering the eye, for normal color (white in Caucasians and lightly yellow in African Americans). The pupils are inspected with a light to see if they are equal in size and round, and their reaction to light and accommodation is evaluated. Normal pupil reaction is indicated as **PERRLA** (pupils equal round reactive to light and accommodation). Eye movement is assessed by having the patient follow the examiner's fingers. If this is normal, it is abbreviated EOM intact, for **extraocular** (outside the eye) movement intact. **Peripheral** vision (side vision) is also assessed to test the horizontal and vertical fields of vision.

Using the ophthalmoscope, the physician is able to visualize the interior of the eye. The condition of the retina can be assessed. Pathology of the intraocular vessels will also be evaluated.

Ears

The ears are inspected and palpated for size, symmetry, lesions, and nodules. The otoscope is used to examine the interior of the ear canal. The examiner is able to visualize the ear canal noting the presence of **cerumen** (ear wax). The tympanic membrane can also be checked for coloration and scarring and to see if it is intact. Normally, the tympanic membrane is pearly gray and concave in appearance, but infection may cause discoloration and fluids from infection behind the eardrum may cause the membrane to bulge. Auditory acuity is tested with the tuning fork.

Nose and Sinuses

The external nose is inspected and palpated for abnormalities. The interior of the nose is examined using a nasal speculum and light. The position of the **nasal septum** is noted for deviation to the right or left. The nasal septum divides the nostrils. Each nostril is inspected for coloration of the mucosa, discharge, lesions, obstruction, polyps, swelling, or tenderness. The sense of smell may be assessed by having the patient close the eyes and identify a common substance such as alcohol, lemon, strawberry, or peppermint.

The paranasal sinuses are inspected and palpated. The technique of transillumination may be used to visualize the sinuses by darkening the room and placing a penlight in the patient's mouth or against the upper cheek or periorbital ridge.

Mouth and Throat

The physician inspects the mucous membranes, gums, tongue, teeth, tonsils, and throat using clean gloves, a light source, and a tongue blade. A laryngeal mirror may be used to inspect the throat. The mucous membranes and tongue may be palpated using a gauze square. The examiner is assessing general dental hygiene and salivary gland function and is looking for abnormalities in color, ulcerations, and nodules.

Checkpoint Question

5. What is the tympanic membrane and how does the presence of infection affect it?

Chest

The anterior chest is examined with the gown removed to the waist. The physician inspects the anterior chest and breasts observing the general appearance, symmetry, respiratory rate and pattern, and obvious masses or swelling. Palpation is then performed and includes the axillary (underarm) lymph nodes and the area over the heart. Percussion of the underlying structures follows. Using a stethoscope, the examiner auscultates the lungs for abnormal sounds and the patient may be asked to take deep breaths. The heart sounds and apical pulse are also assessed.

The posterior areas of the chest are inspected. Palpation includes assessment of the respiratory pattern and the muscles of the back and the spine. This is followed by percussion of the back to assess lung fields. Then, using a stethoscope, the examiner listens to the lung sounds and the patient is asked to take deep breaths.

Reflexes

The examiner uses the percussion hammer to strike the biceps, triceps, patellar, Achilles, and plantar tendons looking for a response. The physician may prefer to test the plantar reflexes in the supine position.

The patient is then assisted to a supine position with the anterior chest exposed and a drape sheet from the waist down. The heart may be reexamined in this position using inspection for visible external movements and an auscultation of the heart sounds. The patient may be asked to turn briefly onto his left side while the examiner listens to the heart sounds with the stethoscope.

Breasts

The breasts may be palpated in both the male and female. The supine position is preferred for palpation of the breasts because the breast tissue flattens out so that abnormalities, if present, are more easily felt.

Abdomen

To examine the abdomen, the drape sheet is lowered to the pubic area. A drape is placed across the chest or the gown is replaced and raised to just beneath the breasts. The abdomen is inspected for contour, symmetry, and pulsations. Auscultation follows. The examiner uses the stethoscope to listen to the bowel sounds and abdominal blood vessels. Percussion determines the outlines of the abdominal organs and palpation evaluates for enlargement, masses, pain, or tenderness.

The groin area is palpated for enlargement of **inguinal** lymph nodes or the presence of a **hernia**. A hernia is the protrusion of an organ through the muscle wall of the cavity that normally surrounds it. The femoral blood vessels may also be palpated and auscultated.

Checkpoint Question

6. *Why is the patient asked to assume the supine position for palpation of the breasts?*

Genitalia and Rectum

The physician wears clean gloves to examine the external male genitalia and rectum. Inspection is done to note symmetry, lesions, swelling, masses, and hair distribution. The scrotal contents may be visualized using transillumination in a darkened room. In addition, the scrotum is palpated for testicular size, contour, and consistency. The patient is then asked to stand and bear down while the examiner places a gloved index finger upward along the side of the scrotum into the inguinal ring to assess for a hernia. The patient is then asked to bend over the examination table. The examiner inspects the anus for lesions or hemorrhoids and then places a lubricated and gloved index finger into the rectum to palpate the rectal sphincter muscle tone and the prostate for

size, consistency, or masses. An **occult** (hidden) blood test is obtained from stool on the gloved finger.

The female genitalia and rectum are examined with the patient in the lithotomy position and draped appropriately. The examiner wears a clean latex glove on the dominant hand. The gooseneck lamp is adjusted to direct light on the vaginal area. The external genitalia are inspected for lesions, edema, cysts, discharge, and hair distribution. The vaginal speculum in inserted to inspect the condition of the cervix and vaginal mucosa. A Pap smear is obtained and possibly a sample of the secretions in the vagina. After the speculum is removed, a bimanual examination is done to palpate the internal reproductive organs for size, contour, and masses. Two fingers of the gloved hand are inserted into the vagina while the ungloved hand is placed on the lower abdomen to compress the internal organs. Sometimes a **rectovaginal** examination is necessary to palpate the posterior uterus and vaginal wall. The examiner places a gloved index finger in the vagina and the middle finger in the rectum at the same time.

The rectum is inspected and palpated for lesions, hemorrhoids, and sphincter tone. A stool specimen is obtained for occult blood.

What If?

The physician will be performing a genital examination on an disabled female patient. What if she is unable to assume the lithotomy position?

Both the genital and rectal examinations may be performed in the dorsal recumbent or Sims' position for those patients (such as the elderly or those with disabilities) who cannot assume the more uncomfortable positions such as the lithotomy position.

Legs

The legs are inspected and peripheral pulse sites are palpated in the supine position. The patient is then assisted to the standing position where the peripheral pulse sites may be palpated again and the legs observed for varicose veins.

Posture, Gait, Coordination, Balance, and Strength

The spine may be inspected and palpated and general posture assessed in the standing position. In addition, the patient may be asked to walk and perform other movements so that **gait** and coordination may be observed. A balance test may be done by having the patient stand with feet together and eyes closed. Range of motion and muscle strength are assessed on both the arms and the legs.

Each physician has an established pattern for performing physical examinations. The sequence may vary or certain aspects may be added or deleted based on the findings for each patient.

Checkpoint Question
7. What is the purpose of the rectovaginal examination?

➤ GENERAL HEALTH GUIDELINES AND CHECKUPS

Physicians vary as to how often they recommend a complete physical examination for their patients. For patients aged 20 to 40, physical examinations are scheduled about every 1 to 3 years. Annual examinations are typical for patients over age 40, unless an existing medical condition requires more frequent visits.

For women, the first Pap smear is recommended between ages 18 and 20 and then annually thereafter. A breast examination by a doctor is recommended every 3 years from ages 20 to 40 and annually after that. Breast self-examination should be performed monthly. A baseline mammogram is recommended between ages 35 and 40, every 2 years during the forties, and then annually after 50 years of age. If the patient is at risk for breast cancer, the doctor may recommend mammograms earlier and more often.

All patients should have a baseline electrocardiogram at age 40 and follow-up only as necessary. A rectal examination and stool for occult blood are recommended annually beginning at age 40. At ages 50 and 51 a proctoscopic examination is recommended and then every 3 to 5 years after that if the initial tests are negative.

Adult immunizations are recommended according to the following guidelines:

- Tetanus booster every 10 years or if the patient sustains a severe injury
- One injection of pneumonia vaccine (Pneumovax) between 60 and 65 years of age
- After age 65, annual flu shot (influenza A and B)
- Some doctors also recommend a series of three hepatitis B injections for their adult patients.

Patients should be instructed regarding signs and symptoms that may signal health problems and when to call the physician.

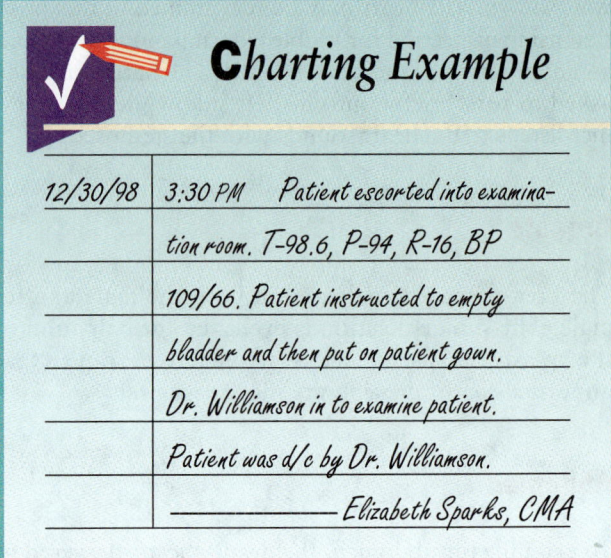

Charting Example

12/30/98	3:30 PM	Patient escorted into examination room. T-98.6, P-94, R-16, BP 109/66. Patient instructed to empty bladder and then put on patient gown. Dr. Williamson in to examine patient. Patient was d/c by Dr. Williamson.

— Elizabeth Sparks, CMA

SUMMARY

Clinically, your role as a medical assistant during the physical examination is to assist both the physician and the patient. Efficiency, accuracy, and attention to detail cannot be overemphasized in performing your duties as a helper to the physician and in anticipating what is needed. Assessing patient needs, developing good interpersonal relationships, and providing support to patients are important skills that help the patient to experience a more pleasant office visit.

CRITICAL THINKING CHALLENGES

1. During the physical examination, the physician asks the patient to walk across the room. What can be determined about the patient's health from observing the patient's way of walking?
2. After the physical examination, the patient asks you: "Why did the physician strike my chest and listen?" How would you explain this?
3. Why is it possible for the physician to assess vascular health by checking the eyegrounds?

ANSWERS TO CHECKPOINT QUESTIONS

1. The tuning fork and the audioscope are used to test hearing. To use the tuning fork, the examiner strikes its prongs against the hand, causing them to vibrate and produce a humming sound. To use the audioscope, the examiner places the tip into the patient's ear; as the instrument produces various tones, the patient responds when each tone is heard.

2. The anoscope is used to inspect the anal canal. The proctoscope is used to visualize the rectum and anus. The sigmoidoscope is used to visually inspect the rectum and sigmoid colon.

3. Auscultation involves listening to body sounds. Palpation stimulates bowel sounds, so if it is performed before auscultation, it may alter the normal bowel sounds.

4. As a medical assistant, you are responsible for preparing the examination room, preparing the patient, assisting the physician during the examination, and cleaning the room and equipment afterward.

5. The tympanic membrane, also called the eardrum, is a thin membrane in the middle ear that transmits sound vibrations. Normally, it is pearly gray and concave in appearance. However, in the presence of infection, it may become discolored. Also, infected fluids behind the eardrum may cause the membrane to bulge.

6. When the patient is in the supine position, the breast tissue flattens out. This makes it easier for the physician to feel any abnormalities, if present.

7. The rectovaginal examination is done to palpate the posterior uterus and vaginal wall.

SUGGESTIONS FOR FURTHER READING

Bates, B., Buckley, L. S., Hoekelman, R. A. (1995). *A Guide to Physical Examination and History Taking,* 6th ed. Philadelphia: Lippincott-Raven.

Rosdahl, C. B. (1995). *Textbook of Basic Nursing,* 6th ed., Philadelphia: J. B. Lippincott.

Smeltzer, S. C., & Bare, B. G. (1996). *Brunner and Suddarth's Textbook of Medical-Surgical Nursing.* 8th ed. Philadelphia: Lippincott-Raven.

Taylor, C., Lillis, C., & Lemone, P. (1993). *Fundamentals of Nursing,* 2nd ed. Philadelphia: J. B. Lippincott.

Timby, B. K., & Lewis, L. W. (1992). *Fundamental Skills and Concepts in Patient Care,* 5th ed. Philadelphia: J. B. Lippincott.

Instruments and Equipment

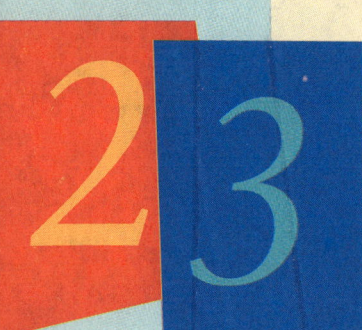

Chapter Outline

Instruments
   Forceps
   Scissors
   Scalpels and Blades
   Towel Clamps
   Probes and Directors
   Retractors
Instruments and Equipment Used by
   Specialists
Care and Handling of Instruments
Principles and Practices of Asepsis
Sanitation
Procedure: Sanitizing Equipment for
   Sterilization or Disinfection
Disinfection

Sterilization
   Sterilization Equipment
   Autoclave
   Sterilization Indicators
   Loading the Autoclave
   Operating the Autoclave
Procedure: Operating an Autoclave
Boiling
Storage and Recordkeeping
Maintaining Surgical Supplies
Summary
Critical Thinking Challenges
Answers to Checkpoint Questions
Suggestions for Further Reading

DACUM Components

1.3   Practice within the scope of education, training, and personal capabilities
4.1   Apply principles of aseptic technique and infection control
6.2   Operate and maintain facilities and equipment safely
6.3   Inventory equipment and supplies

Chapter Competencies

Learning Objectives

Upon successfully completing this chapter, you will be able to:

1. Spell and define the Key Terms.
2. Identify an instrument by its characteristics.
3. Categorize instruments based on use.
4. State the difference between reusable and disposable instruments.
5. Define sanitation.
6. Distinguish between the need for disinfection and sterilization.
7. Name several types of methods used for sterilization.
8. Identify instruments specific to designated specialties.
9. Maintain adequate maintenance checkups and servicing of equipment.
10. Keep adequate supplies (light bulb, lens, and so on) on hand for equipment needs.
11. Identify the need for special storage of supplies (ie, disinfectants and sterilants), instruments, and equipment.
12. Maintain adequate documents and records of maintenance or sterilization for instruments and equipment.

Performance Objectives

Upon successfully completing this chapter, you will be able to:

1. Sanitize equipment for disinfection or sterilization (Procedure 23-1).
2. Properly wrap equipment in preparation for sterilization in an autoclave.
3. Operate an autoclave observing protocol for pressure, time, and temperature appropriate for the material to be sterilized (Procedure 23-2).

Key Terms

(See Glossary for definitions.)

autoclave	OSHA
disinfectant	ratchets
disinfection	sanitation
ethylene oxide	sanitizing
forceps	scalpel
germicide	scissors
hemostat	serrations
instrument	sterile field
needle holder	sterilization
obturator	

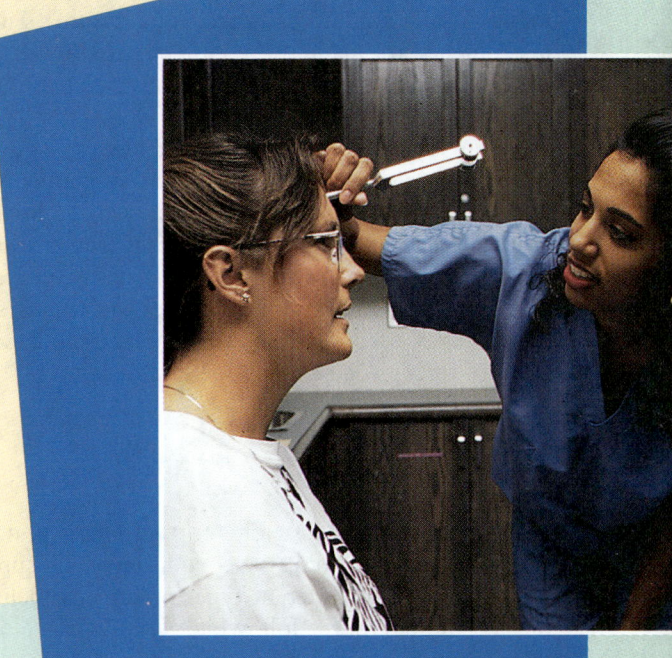

As a medical assistant, you will be responsible for assisting with minor surgical procedures in an office or clinical setting. To effectively manage this responsibility, you must:

- Become familiar with many types of surgical instruments
- Understand the principles and practices of asepsis
- Have a working knowledge of disinfection and sterilization techniques
- Be able to use equipment designed for sterilization, treatment, and diagnostic purposes

You must also be competent in maintaining accurate records of the purchases and maintenance performed on office equipment, performing routine equipment maintenance, and maintaining inventory to ensure adequate supplies are available for sterilization procedures, medical or surgical treatment, and diagnostic testing.

➤ INSTRUMENTS

In an office or clinical setting, you must be able to identify surgical **instruments** by their design and function. A surgical instrument is a tool or device designed to perform a specific function, such as cutting, dissecting, grasping, holding, retracting, or suturing. Surgical instruments are designed to perform specific tasks based on their shape; they may be curved, straight, sharp, blunt, serrated, toothed, or smooth. Many are made of steel and are designed to be durable. Surgical instruments are made to be either reused or disposed of, depending on the instrument's use and the manufacturer's recommendations.

You should be able to name or identify and know the proper use and care of the surgical instruments used for clinic or office procedures. Most can be identified for use by carefully examining the instrument and its parts; instruments are so specifically designed that the configurations will usually give clues to their uses. The most widely used surgical instruments include several types of forceps, scissors, scalpels, and clamps.

Forceps

Forceps are surgical instruments used to grasp, handle, compress, pull, or join tissue, equipment, or supplies. There are several different types of forceps including, but not limited to, the following:

- **hemostat** *clamp*—a surgical instrument with slender jaws used for grasping blood vessels and establishing hemostasis

- *Kelly clamp*—a curved or straight forceps or hemostat; those with long handles widely used in gynecologic procedures
- *sterilizer forceps*—used to transfer sterilizer supplies, equipment, and other surgical instruments
- *needle holder*—used to hold and pass a suturing needle through tissue
- *spring or thumb forceps*—usually consist of a spring handle and a serrated or toothed point used for grasping tissue for dissecting or suturing; examples: tissue forceps and splinter forceps

Figure 23-1 shows various types of forceps.

All forceps are available in a multitude of sizes, with or without **serrations** or teeth, with curved or straight blades, with ring tips, blunt tips, or sharp tips. Many have **ratchets** in the handles to hold the tips tightly together. These are notched mechanisms that click into position to maintain tension. Some have spring handles that are compressed to grasp objects.

Each physician will use a variety of forceps for procedures performed in the office. You must spend time studying the names and purposes of each to assist the physician when a specific instrument is requested.

Scissors

Scissors are sharp instruments composed of two opposing cutting blades, held together by a central pin on which the blades pivot. Scissors are used for dissecting superficial, deep, or delicate tissues and for cutting sutures and dressing. Scissors have blade points that are blunt or sharp or a combination of both, depending on the use of the instrument. The several types of scissors include:

- *straight scissors*—used during operations or procedures to cut deep or delicate tissue and for cutting sutures
- *curved scissors*—used for dissecting superficial and delicate tissues
- *suture scissors*—used to cut sutures; made with a straight top blade and a "curved-out" or hooked, blunt-shaped bottom blade to fit under, lift, and grasp sutures for snipping
- *bandage scissors*—have a flattened blunt tip on the bottom longer blade for fitting under bandages safely. These are usually angled to maneuver more easily under bandages. The most common type is the Lister bandage scissors.

Figure 23-2 shows various types of scissors.

text continues on page 357

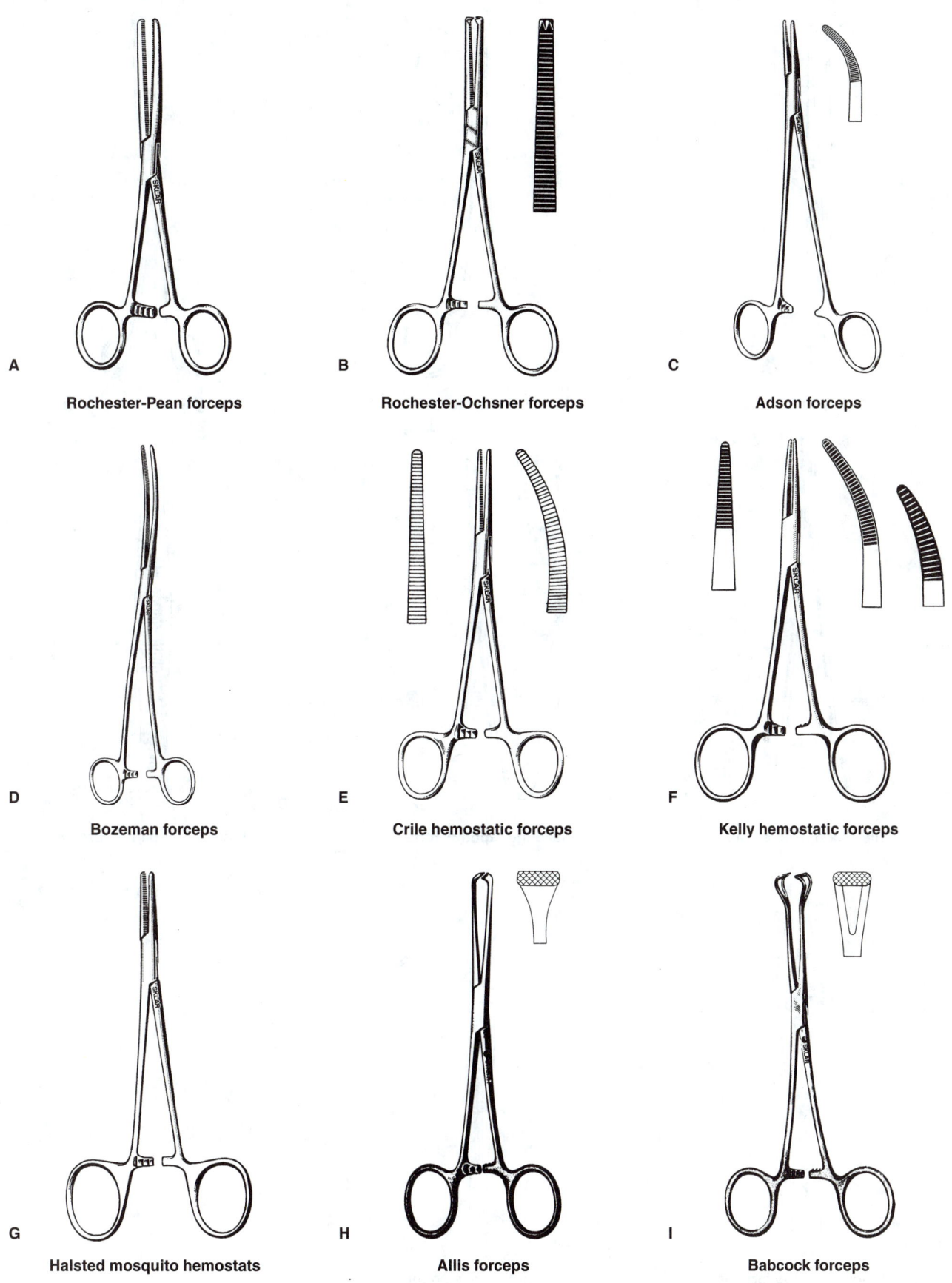

A   Rochester-Pean forceps

B   Rochester-Ochsner forceps

C   Adson forceps

D   Bozeman forceps

E   Crile hemostatic forceps

F   Kelly hemostatic forceps

G   Halsted mosquito hemostats

H   Allis forceps

I   Babcock forceps

FIGURE 23-1
Types of forceps. (Sklar Instruments, Westchester, PA)

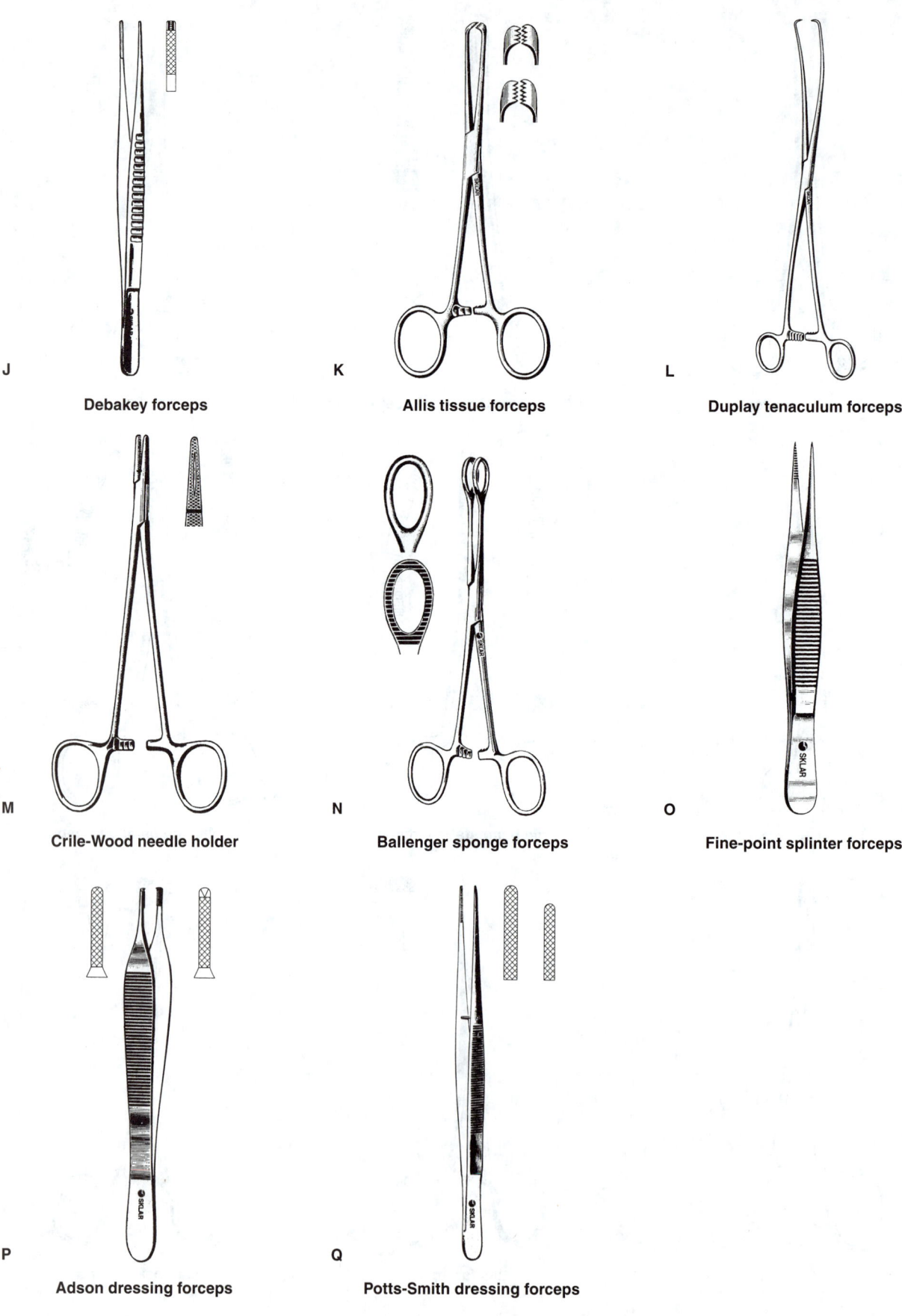

J   Debakey forceps

K   Allis tissue forceps

L   Duplay tenaculum forceps

M   Crile-Wood needle holder

N   Ballenger sponge forceps

O   Fine-point splinter forceps

P   Adson dressing forceps

Q   Potts-Smith dressing forceps

FIGURE 23-1 (continued)

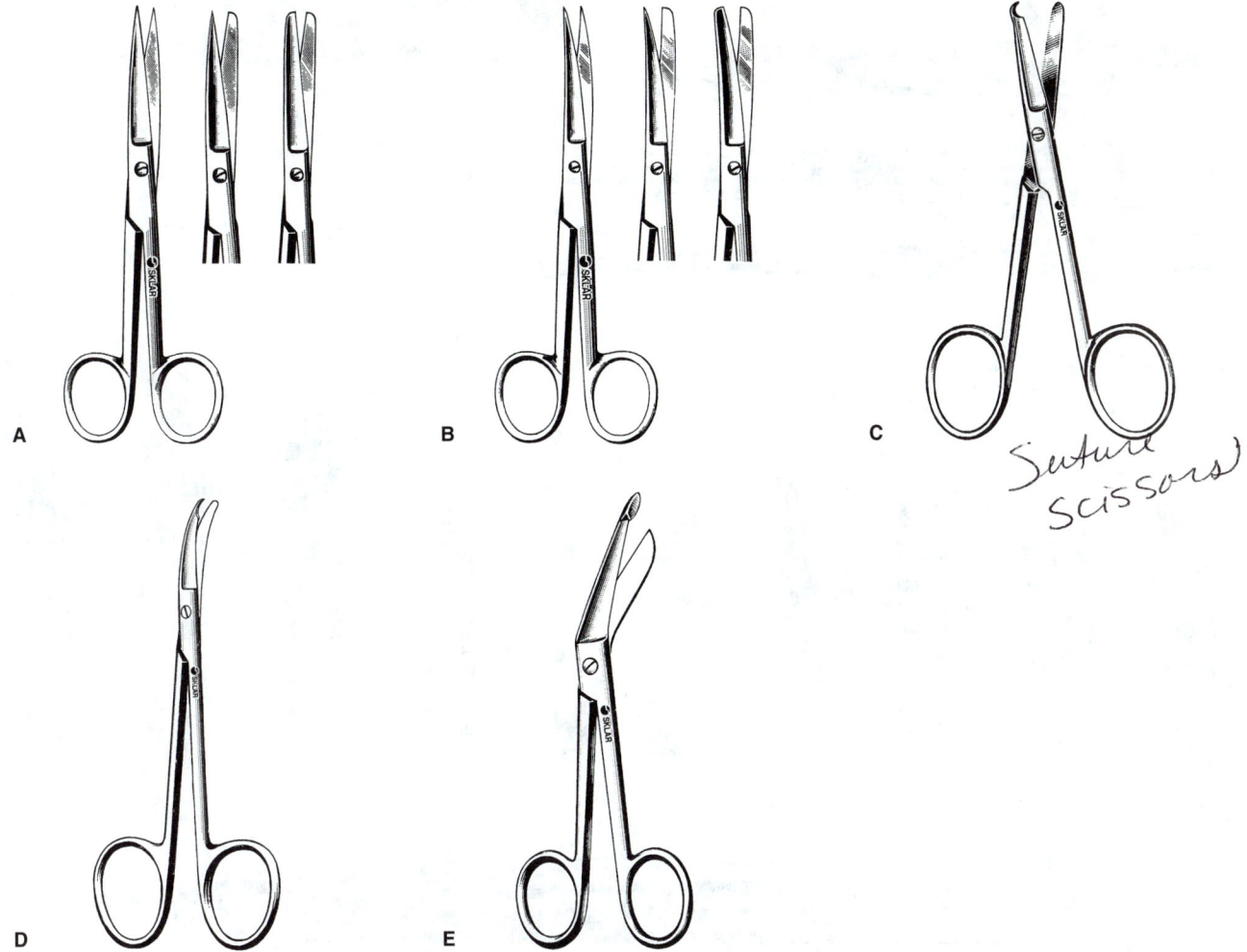

Suture Scissors) [handwritten annotation]

FIGURE 23-2

Types of scissors. (**A**) Straight-blade operating scissors, *left to right:* sharp/sharp (S/S), sharp/blunt (S/B), blunt/blunt (B/B). (**B**) Curved-blade operating scissors, *left to right:* sharp/sharp (S/S), sharp/blunt (S/B), blunt/blunt (B/B). (**C**) Spencer stitch scissors. (**D**) Suture scissors. (**E**) Lister bandage scissors. (Sklar Instruments, Westchester, PA)

Scalpels and Blades

A **scalpel** is a small surgical knife with a straight handle and a sharp convex blade edge. The scalpel handle can use interchangeable blades, based on the type of surgical procedure to be performed. Straight or pointed blades are used for incision and drainage purposes; curved blades are used to excise tissue. If a reusable handle is used, the blade will always be disposable. Many offices use disposable handles and blades. Figure 23-3 shows various scalpels and blades.

Towel Clamps

Towel clamps are used to maintain the integrity of the sterile field by holding the sterile drapes in place, allowing exposure of the operative site (Fig. 23-4). A sterile field is a specific area that is considered free of microorganisms.

Probes and Directors

Before entering a cavity or site for a procedure, the physician may first probe the depths and direction of the operative area. The probe will show the angle and depth of the operative area, and the director will guide the knife or instrument once the procedure has begun (Fig. 23-5).

Retractors

Retractors hold open layers of tissue, exposing the areas underneath to view. They may be plain or toothed; the toothed retractor may be sharp or blunt. Retrac-

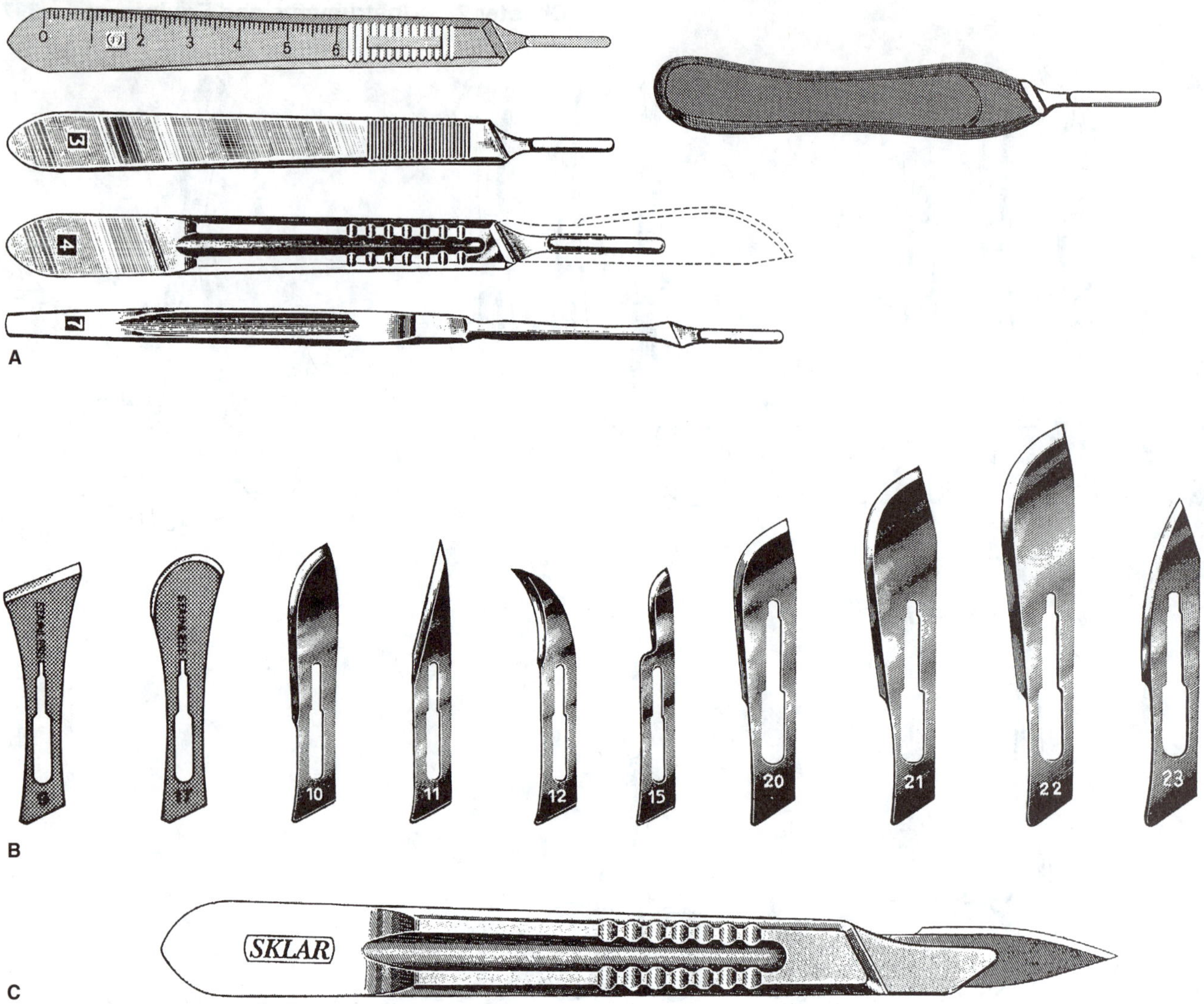

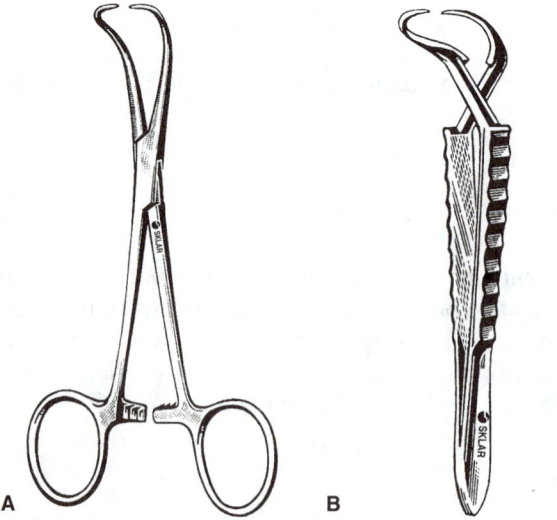

FIGURE 23-3
(**A**) Scalpel handles. (**B**) Surgical blades. (**C**) Sterile disposable scalpel-complete. (Sklar Instruments, Westchester, PA)

FIGURE 23-4
(**A**) Backhaus towel clamp. (**B**) Jones cross-action towel clamp. (Sklar Instruments, Westchester, PA)

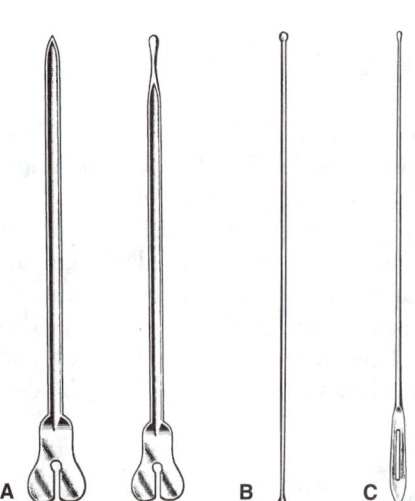

FIGURE 23-5
(**A**) Director and tongue tie. (**B**) Double-ended probe. (C) Probe with eye. (Sklar Instruments, Westchester, PA)

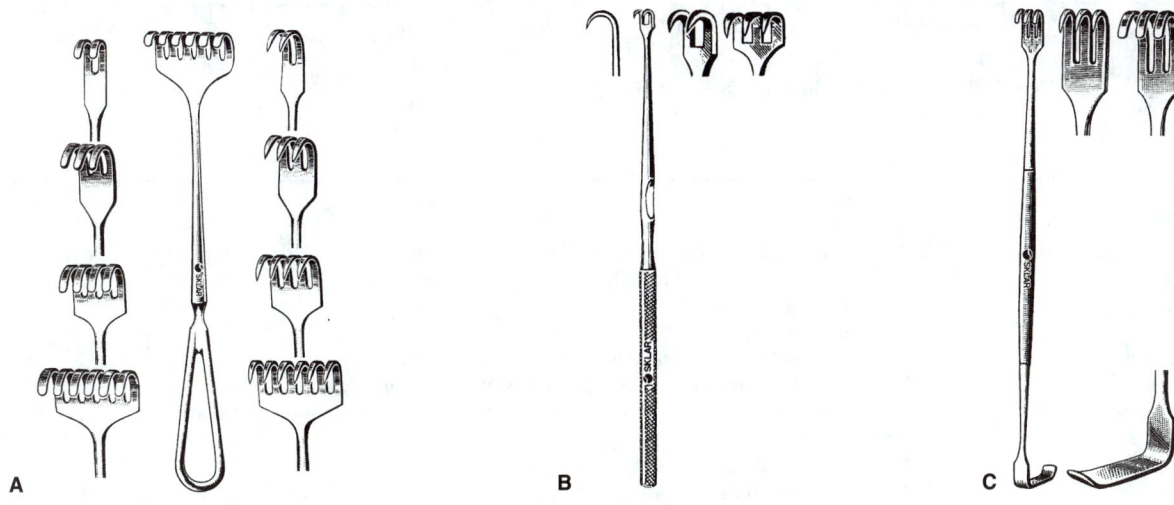

FIGURE 23-6
(**A**) Volkman retractor. (**B**) Lahey retractor. (**C**) Senn retractor. (Sklar Instruments, Westchester, PA)

tors may be designed to be either held by an assistant or screwed open to be self-retaining. Figure 23-6 shows several types of retractors.

Checkpoint Question
1. What are forceps, scissors, scalpels, and towel clamps used for?

▶ INSTRUMENTS AND EQUIPMENT USED BY SPECIALISTS

Physicians have preferences for certain types of instruments specific to their practices. An obstetrician will not usually have equipment normally used only by orthopedists, such as cast cutters and splints. Nor would the orthopedist have equipment usually used by an otologist, such as Buck's ear curet or otic lavage equipment.

As a medical assistant, you will not be required to identify a large assortment of instruments or equipment, but you must know the names, uses, and care of the equipment, instruments, and supplies used by the specific practice in which you work. Table 23-1 shows, by specialty, the most commonly used instruments and equipment.

Many of the instruments listed in Table 23-1 and in the section on instruments (above) may be reused. However, many are manufactured for "single-use only" and must be disposed of properly. Disposable instruments should not be reprocessed. Reusable items should be processed according to the designated use of the instrument or based on the manufacturer's recommendations.

In selecting the method of cleaning, disinfecting, or sterilizing, you must consider the uses for the instrument (medical asepsis versus surgical asepsis) and know any effects that certain chemicals may have on the equipment (ie, etching of glass or metal by solvents).

▶ CARE AND HANDLING OF INSTRUMENTS

To ensure that surgical instruments always function properly, follow these guidelines:

1. Avoid dropping or tossing instruments into basins or sinks. Surgical instruments are delicate and may have sharp blades or pointed tips easily damaged by improper handling. Should an instrument be dropped accidentally, it should be carefully inspected to identify damage. Damaged instruments can usually be repaired and should not be discarded unless repair is not feasible.
2. Avoid stacking instruments into a pile. They may become tangled and be damaged when separated.
3. Sharp instruments should always be stored separately to prevent dulling or damaging the sharp edges, as well as to prevent accidental injury. Disposable scalpel blades should be removed from reusable handles and placed in puncture-proof sharps containers; if the handle is also disposable, the whole unit is discarded in the container. Sy-

text continues on page 363

Table 23-1

Commonly Used Instruments and Equipment, by Specialty

Instruments	Use

Obstetrics and Gynecology

Speculum (pl. specula)	Opening the vagina for viewing the vaginal walls and cervical os and to perform procedures; are sized and may be reusable metal or disposable plastic
Fetal monitor	Assessing the health of the fetus
Ultrasound	Visualizing the fetus
Vaginal swabs	Applying or removing substances from the vagina or cervix
Tenaculum	Grasping and holding a part with hooklike tips and clasps tightly with ratchets
Uterine sounds	Assessing the depth of the uterus or location of the fundus; are graduated in inches or centimeters
Uterine dilators	Widening the cervical os; usually sized 3–18 mm
Curet	Scraping the endometrium; may be blunt or sharp
Dressing forceps	Sponging the area clean or applying treatments; may be ring forceps or Kelly forceps
Biopsy forceps or curet	Securing bits of tissue for microscopic study

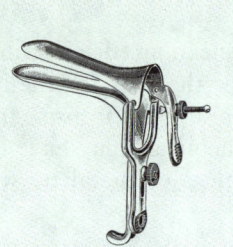
Graves vaginal speculum

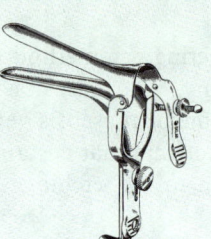
Pederson vaginal speculum

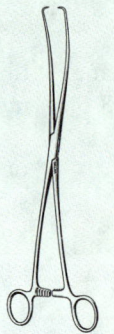
Duplay tenaculum forceps

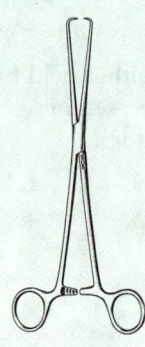
Schroeder tenaculum forceps

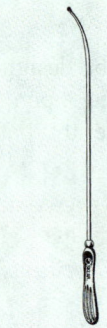
Sims uterine sound

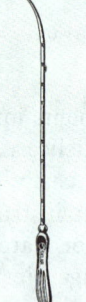
Simpson uterine sound-malleable

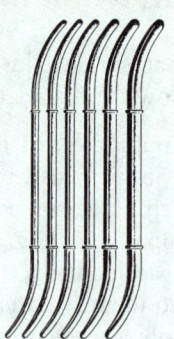
Hank uterine dilator

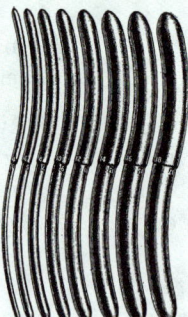
Hegar uterine dilator

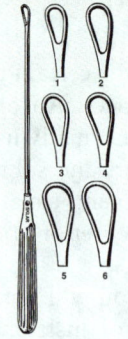
Thomas uterine curets

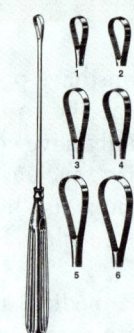
Sims uterine curets

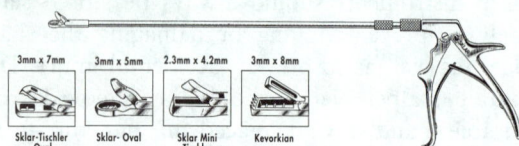
Universal style biopsy instruments

(continued)

Instruments	Use
Orthopedics	
Splints, braces, straps, supports, and immobilizers	Securing a part to prevent movement during healing
Cast saw or cutters and spreaders	Removing the cast at the completion of treatment
Dust collector or suction	Minimizing the debris of cast removal
Goniometer	Measuring range of motion and joint function
Rachiometer	Measuring spinal curvature

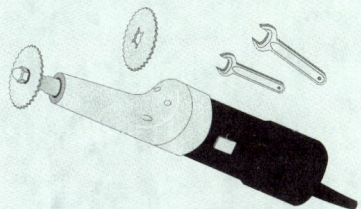

Oscillating plaster saw

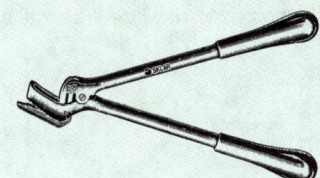

Stille plaster shears

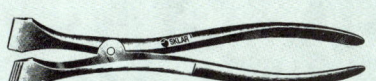

Hennig plaster spreader

Instruments	Use
Urology	
Cystoscope	Viewing the interior of the bladder
Catheter kits	Emptying the bladder for procedures or for securing a sterile specimen for diagnostic procedures; may be straight for one use, or may be Foley to remain in the bladder for a period of time
Prostate biopsy instruments	Removing bits of tissue for further microscopic study
Urethral sounds	Exploring the bladder depth and direction and for meatal dilation in cases of urethral stenosis; sized Fr 8–26
Microscopes, culture media, strip testing supplies	Diagnosing disorders

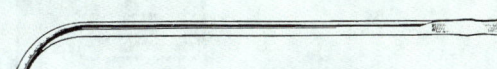

Otis/Dittel urethral sound

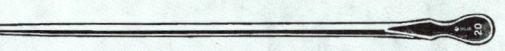

Dittel urethral sound

Instruments	Use
Proctology	
Anoscopes, sigmoidoscopes, proctoscopes	Visualizing the interior of the lower intestinal tract; are usually lighted and primarily flexible fiberoptic with a power source. Most will have an **obturator** for ease of insertion and patient comfort. Some will be equipped with suction devices.
Anal specula	Opening the anal walls for visualization
Biopsy instruments (punch or alligator)	Removing tissue (punch biopsy involves removing a small piece of tissue by making a small circular hole; alligator biopsies use an instrument with jaws that grasp and excise tissue)
Hemorrhoidal ligator	Applying a band to the base of the hemorrhoid to cause it to necrose and slough off

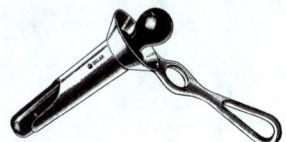

Ives rectal speculum (Fansler)

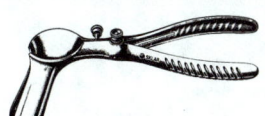

Pratt rectal speculum

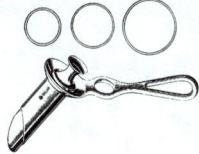

Hirschman anoscope

(continued)

Table 23-1

Commonly Used Instruments and Equipment, by Specialty (Continued)

Instruments	Use

Otology and Rhinology

Instruments	Use
Audioscope	Viewing the tympanic membrane and screening for decibel level losses
Tympanometer	Detecting otitis media and other middle ear pathologies; equipped with a printer for hard copy to assess the status of tympanic membrane pressure
Nasal or ear forceps	Visualizing the site of concern
Curets	Removing cerumen or scraping the nasal passages
Syringes	Washing out the ear canal; may be either bulb or plunger type
Nasal speculae	Extending the nostrils to visualize the nasal passages

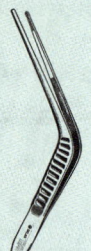

Wilde ear forceps

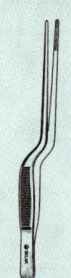

Lucae bayonet forceps

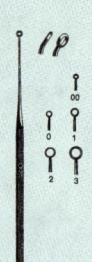

Buck ear curet

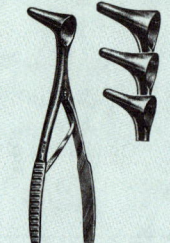

Vienna nasal speculum

Ophthalmology

Instruments	Use
Iris and strabismus scissors	Performing surgery
Eye loop and lid retractor	Assisting with finding and removing foreign bodies
Tonometer	Measuring the intraocular pressure to diagnose glaucoma

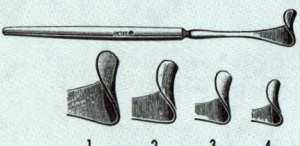

Desmarres lid retractor

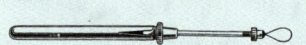

Bailey foreign body remover

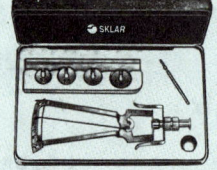

Schiotz tonometer

Dermatology

Instruments	Use
Punch biopsy	Removing small circular sections of skin for microscopic studies; sized 2–8 mm, either disposable or reusable
Comedone extractors	Removing blackheads and opening pustules

Keyes cutaneous punch

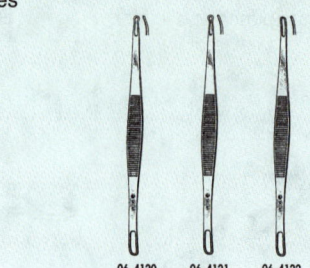

06-4120   06-4121   06-4122

Schamberg comedone extractor

Instruments courtesy of Sklar Instruments, Westchester, PA

ringes with needles attached and suture needles are placed in an approved sharps containers and never placed in the trash or with other instruments for processing. Delicate instruments, such as those with lenses, delicate scissors, or tissue forceps, are kept separate so they may be processed appropriately.

4. Keep ratcheted instruments in an open position when not in use to avoid damage to the rachet mechanism.

5. Rinse gross contamination from instruments as quickly as possible to prevent drying and hardening, which makes the cleaning process more difficult.

6. Check instruments before sterilization to ensure that they are in good working order; this allows you to identify instruments in need of repair.
   a. Blades or points should be free of bends and nicks.
   b. Tips should close evenly and tightly.
   c. Instruments with box locks should move freely but should not be too loose.
   d. Instruments with spring handles should have enough tension to grasp objects tightly.
   e. Scissors should close in a smooth, even manner with no nicks or snags. (Scissors may be checked by cutting through gauze or cotton to be sure there are no rough areas.)
   f. Screws should be flush with the instrument surface. They should be freely workable but not loose.

7. Use instruments only for the purpose for which they were designed. For instance, surgical scissors should never be used to cut paper or open packages because this may damage the cutting edges.

8. Sanitize instruments before they are sterilized so that sterilization procedures will work effectively.

Checkpoint Question
2. Why should you avoid dropping surgical instruments, and what should you do if one drops accidentally?

▶ PRINCIPLES AND PRACTICES OF ASEPSIS

As a medical assistant, you are responsible for minimizing the onset and spread of infection based on the principles and practices of asepsis as it relates to instruments, equipment, and supplies. Asepsis is the absence of microorganisms, infection, or infectious material. Asepsis is classified as either medical asepsis or surgical asepsis.

Medical asepsis (clean technique) is the removal or destruction of disease organisms or infected material.

Surgical asepsis (sterile technique) refers to practices designed to render and maintain objects and areas maximally free from microorganisms. (See Chap. 19, Asepsis and Infection Control, for a detailed discussion of medical and surgical asepsis and handwashing.)

You must be able to distinguish between the need for disinfection versus the need for sterilization. By becoming familiar with the manufacturer's recommendations for processing instruments and equipment based on the purposes for which the items will be used, you will be able to determine the level of asepsis appropriate in each instance. The method of sterilization to be used in any procedure depends on the nature of the material to be sterilized and the type of bacteria to be destroyed. It is recommended that procedures of sterilization be assigned to one or two workers in the facility. The occasional worker may not have the experience or knowledge to ensure that true sterilization will be accomplished.

▶ SANITATION

Surgical instruments and equipment have to be cared for and cleaned according to the recommendation of the manufacturer and with their eventual uses in mind. All instruments and equipment must be sanitized, which means they will be cleaned with warm soapy water and mechanical action to remove all organic matter and other residue.

Sanitation is the science of maintaining a healthful, disease-free and hazard-free environment. Sanitation results in the reduction of the microbial population on an inanimate object to a safe or relatively safe level. Cleaning or sanitizing must precede disinfection and sterilization procedures (Procedure 23-1). Disinfection destroys most pathogenic organisms; sterilization destroys all microorganisms.

▶ DISINFECTION

Disinfection describes a process that eliminates many or all pathogenic microorganisms on inanimate objects, with the exception of bacterial spores. The process kills pathogenic organisms or renders them inert.

In the health care setting, disinfection is generally accomplished by the use of liquid chemicals or wet pasteurization (Table 23-2). Disinfectants are chemicals that can be applied to instruments and equipment to destroy microorganisms. Disinfection is affected by a number of factors, any of which may limit the effectiveness of the process. These include:

- Prior cleaning of the object
- The amount of organic material on the object

Procedure 23-1   Sanitizing Equipment for Sterilization or Disinfection

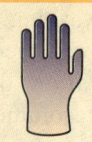

Equipment/Supplies

- equipment to be sanitized
- gloves
- impervious gown
- eye protection (goggles, face shield)

Steps	Purpose
1. Put on gloves, gown, and eye protection.	1. These devices protect against splattering and prevent contamination of your clothes.
2. Take apart pieces that require assembly. If cleaning is not possible immediately, disassemble the pieces and soak the sections to avoid having them stick together.	
3. Check for the operation and integrity of the equipment. If the equipment is defective, it should be repaired or discarded.	
4. Rinse with cool water.	4. Hot water "cooks" proteins onto the equipment.
5. After the initial rinsing, force streams of soapy water through any tubular or grooved instruments to clean the inside as well as the outside.	
6. After the cool rinse, use a hot soapy soak to dissolve fats or lubricants left on the surface. Use the soaking solution of choice for the facility.	
7. Use friction with a soft brush or gauze to loosen transient microorganisms. Abrasive materials should not be used on delicate instruments and equipment. Brushes work well on grooves and joints. Open and close the jaws of scissors or forceps several times to ensure that all material has been removed.	
8. Rinse well.	8. Proper rinsing removes soap or detergent residues and any remaining microorganisms.
9. Dry well before autoclaving or soaking.	9. Excess moisture will cause super wet steam and decrease the effectiveness of the autoclave process by delaying drying; it may also wick microorganisms into the damp packs. Moisture will dilute the soaking solution.
10. Be aware that any items used in the sanitation process are considered grossly contaminated and must be properly sanitized or discarded.	

- The type and level of microbial contamination
- The concentration of the **germicide** (chemical that kills pathogens)
- The length of exposure to the germicide
- The shape or complexity of the object
- The temperature of the disinfection process

Categories of disinfection include:

- High level—destroys all microorganisms, with the exception of bacterial spores.

- Intermediate—inactivates mycobacterium, tuberculosis, vegetative bacteria, most viruses, and some fungi, but does not necessarily kill bacterial spores
- Low level—can kill most bacteria, some viruses, and some fungi, but cannot be relied on to kill resistant microorganisms such as tubercle bacilli or bacterial spores

(See Chap. 19, Asepsis and Infection Control, for a more complete description of these categories.)

Table 23-2 Disinfection Methods	
Method	**Uses and Precautions**
Alcohol (70% isopropyl alcohol or ethyl alcohol)	Used for noncritical items (countertops, oral thermometers, stethoscopes) Flammable Damages some rubber, plastic, and lensed equipment
Chlorine (sodium hypochlorite or bleach)	Dilute to 1:10 (1 part bleach to 10 parts water) Used for a broad spectrum of antimicrobial activity Inexpensive and fast acting Corrosive, inactivated by organic matter, relatively unstable
Iodine or iodophores	Bacteriostatic agent used for skin surfaces Not to be used on instruments May cause staining
Phenols (tuberculocidal)	Used for environmental items and equipment Requires gloves and eye protection Can cause skin irritation and burns
Formaldehyde	Disinfectant and sterilant Regulated by OSHA Presence must be marked on all containers and storage areas
Hydrogen peroxide	Stable and effective when used on inanimate objects Attacks membrane lipids, DNA, and other essential cell components Can damage plastic, rubber, and some metals
Glutaraldehyde	Alkaline or acid based Effective against bacteria, viruses, fungi, and some spores OSHA regulated; requires adequate ventilation, covered pans, gloves, and masks Must display biohazard or chemical label

DNA, deoxyribonucleic acid; OSHA, Occupational Safety and Health Administration.

Disinfectants or germicides inactivate virtually all recognized pathogenic microorganisms but not necessarily all microbial forms, such as spores, on inanimate objects.

➤ STERILIZATION

Disinfection practices are not sufficient to process instruments and equipment for sterile technique; objects requiring surgical asepsis must be sterilized. Sterilization is the complete elimination or destruction of all forms of microbial life including spore forms. It is accomplished by either physical or chemical processes. Steam under pressure, dry heat, **ethylene oxide** (a gas), and liquid chemicals are principle sterilizing agents.

Critical medical devices or patient care equipment that enter normally sterile tissue or the vascular system, or through which blood flows, should be sterilized before each use.

Two types of bacteria are major concerns in sterilization: spore formers and nonspore formers. Spores are extremely resistant to heat. They can be destroyed most effectively by steam under pressure in an **autoclave**, an appliance used to sterilize medical instruments. Nonspore formers vary widely in their reaction to heat, but most of them are destroyed by boiling water, chemical agents, or gases. The method of sterilization to be used in any procedure depends on the nature of the material to be sterilized and the type of bacteria to be destroyed.

The most frequently used sterilant in the clinic or office setting is the autoclave, which uses steam under pressure. Other types of sterilants include liquid chemicals (glutaraldehyde or formaldehyde) and gas solvents (ethylene oxide). The liquid chemical form is the second most frequently used sterilant for instruments with successful sterilization after 10 hours of total submersion in the chemical liquid agent. Ethylene gas is rarely used in clinics or offices because of the dangers associated with its use. The Occupational Safety and Health Administration (OSHA) has issued stringent guidelines for its use and workers must be specially trained in safety measures.

Table 23-3 describes various methods of sterilization.

What If?

What if, while pouring glutaraldehyde into a container, the chemical spills?

OSHA and state regulations have defined a specific law to protect you from hazardous materials. The law is termed "The Right to Know" and requires that all companies using hazardous materials have Material Safety Data Sheets (MSDS) available to their employees. MSDS forms are prepared by the chemical manufacturer and clearly state how to handle and dispose of the chemical. These forms also include a list of potential health hazards to workers and identify the safety equipment needed when using the chemical. Never handle any type of chemical spill without first reading the MSDS form.

Checkpoint Question

3. What are the differences between sanitation, disinfection, and sterilization?

Sterilization Equipment

Several different types of sterilization equipment are necessary in the clinic or office setting. As a medical assistant, it is your responsibility to:

- Become familiar with the uses and operation of each piece of equipment
- Schedule periodic preventive maintenance or servicing of the equipment
- Maintain adequate supplies for general operational needs

Table 23-3
Sterilization Methods

Method	Concentration or Levels
Heat	
Moist heat (steam under pressure)	250°F or 121°C for 30 min
Boiling	100°C or 212°F at least 30 min
Dry heat	171°C for 1 h
	160°C for 2 h
Liquids	
Glutaraldehyde	Follow manufacturer's recommendation
Formaldehyde	or OSHA requirements and guidelines
Gas	
Ethylene oxide	450–500 mg/L 50°C

OSHA, Occupational Safety and Health Administration

Autoclave

The most frequently used piece of equipment for sterilizing instruments today is the autoclave (Fig. 23-7). The autoclave consists of two chambers, an outer unit where pressure builds and an inner chamber where the actual sterilization occurs. Water is added to a reservoir where it is converted to steam as the preset temperature is reached. The steam is forced into the inner chamber, increasing the pressure, which raises the temperature of the steam to a higher degree than that of boiling water (212°F or 100°C). (The pressure has no effect on sterilization; its purpose is to increase the temperature of the steam. The higher the pressure, the higher the temperature of the steam, which allows for more rapid destruction of most spores and viruses.)

An air vent exhaust at the bottom of the autoclave allows the air present in the chamber to be pushed out and replaced by the pressurized steam. When no more air is present, the chamber seals and the temperature gauge begins to rise. Newer automatic autoclaves can be set to vent, time, turn off, and exhaust at preset times and levels. Older models may require that the steps be advanced manually. All manufacturers provide instructions for operating the machine and recommendations for times necessary to sterilize different types of loads. These instructions should be posted in a prominent place near the machine.

Remember: Sterilization is required for surgical instruments and equipment that will come in contact

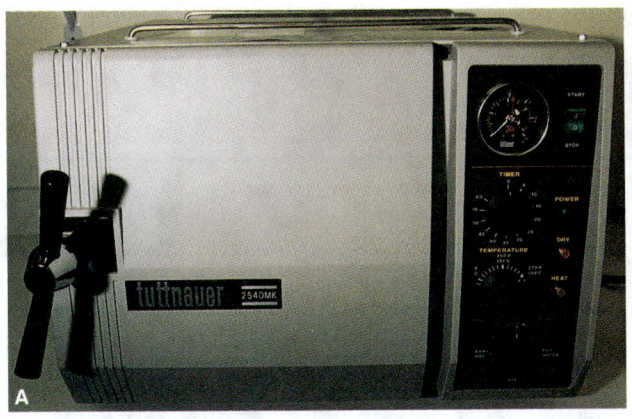
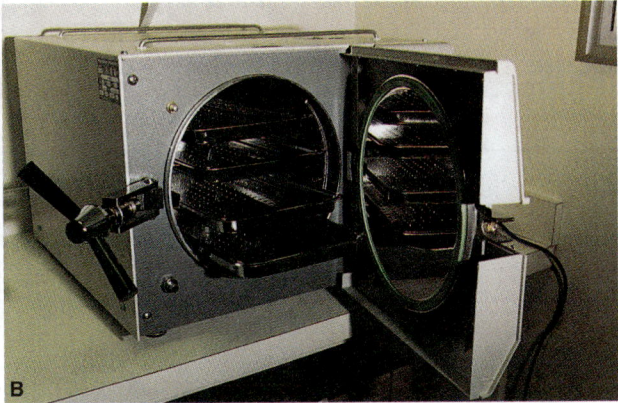

FIGURE 23-7
(**A**) An office-sized autoclave; note the clearly marked dials and gauges.
(**B**) The interior of the autoclave.

with internal body tissues or cavities that are considered sterile. The autoclave is commonly used to sterilize minor surgical instruments, surgical storage trays and containers, and some surgical equipment such as cystoscopes (lighted instruments guided through the urethra to visualize the bladder) and proctoscopes (lighted instruments guided through the anus to visualize the lower colon). Autoclaving is not recommended for many types of scopes; follow the manufacturer's recommendations.

You must be knowledgeable not only about the use of, the need for, and the care of the autoclave, but you also must know how to operate the equipment properly and how to prepare the items for sterilization. No matter how well the equipment is operated, if the items are not properly prepared for the autoclaving process, the sterility of the items cannot be ensured (Box 23-1).

 Checkpoint Question
4. What is an autoclave and how does it work?

Sterilization Indicators

Tapes applied to the outside of the packets will indicate that the items have been exposed to heat and pressure but will not ensure sterility of the contents (Box 23-2). Sterilization indicators placed in the packs will register that the proper pressure and temperature were present for the required time to allow steam to penetrate to the inner parts of the pack (Fig.

23-10). Improper wrapping, loading, or operation of the autoclave will prevent the indicator from registering properly.

Forms of indicators include those that change colors as higher temperatures are reached. If the required temperature is reached, it will register within the safe zone on the indicator. Specially designed tubes containing wax pellets are also used to indicate by the melted wax that the required temperature was reached.

Although most types of sterilization indicators work well, the best method of determining the effectiveness of sterilization is the culture test. Strips impregnated with heat-resistant spores are wrapped and placed in the center of the autoclave between the packages in a specific load. The strips are removed from their packets and placed in a broth culture to be incubated according to the instructions of the manufacturer. At the end of the incubation period, the culture is compared to a control to determine that all spores have been killed. If sterilization was incomplete, the entire load processed with the indicators must be reprocessed.

 **Checkpoint Question**
5. What is a sterilization indicator and what can prevent it from registering that sterilization has occurred?

Loading the Autoclave

Load loosely to allow steam to circulate throughout the items. If too many items are packed in, steam will not penetrate to those items in the center.

BOX 23-1 Wrapping Equipment for Sterilization

After sanitizing and checking the equipment, dry it well and prepare it to be wrapped. The wrapping material must have certain properties. It must:

- Be permeable to steam but not contaminants
- Resist tearing and puncturing during normal handling
- Allow easy opening to prevent contamination of the contents
- Maintain sterility of the item during storage

The wrap may be double layers of cotton muslin, special paper, or appropriately sized instrument pouches (Fig. 23-8). The pouches are gaining wide acceptance because of their convenience. They are sized for a small, single instrument or for an entire tray or setup and all sizes in between. They are transparent on one side so that the contents can be checked before opening. They offer good protection from contamination, are easy to use, take up little space, and, when opened properly, form a sterile field from which to work. They are somewhat stiff to work with and, if a large sterile field must be set up, an additional barrier drape must be wrapped within the package to form the table drape.

To ensure effective wrapping, follow these guidelines:

1. Package hinged instruments in an open position to allow steam to reach all surfaces.
2. If trays are packaged with the suitable instruments for a specific procedure, place a cloth or a barrier drape in the bottom of the tray to absorb condensation and to protect the instruments from damage.
3. Prevent sharp instruments from piercing their wraps by placing a cotton ball or gauze between the tips before wrapping.
4. When using pouches or bags, insert the instruments in such a way that when the package is opened the instruments will be removed in their functional position.
5. Make up lists of items to include in packages; pull the card and assemble the equipment to ensure that each package is complete.

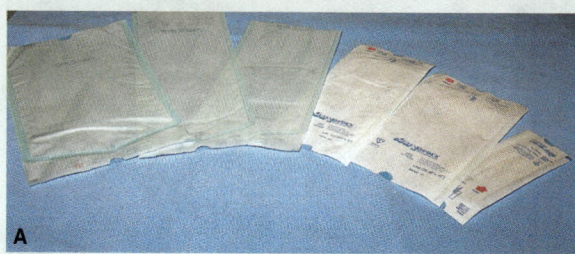
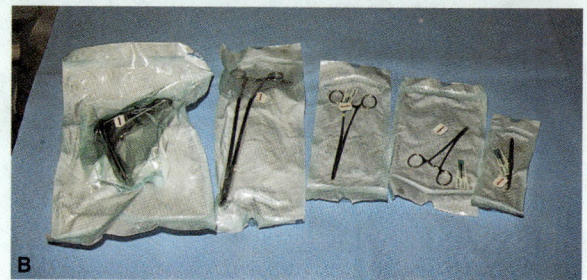

FIGURE 23-8
(**A**) Instrument pouches in a variety of sizes and (**B**) after autoclaving.

6. When wrapping trays, instruments, or fields in barrier wraps, place the item on a diagonal and fold one corner over with a tab folded back, fold in the left corner, fold in the right corner, each with a tab folded back, then fold over the last corner. If the pack is to be double wrapped, follow the same order and fold the last corner under the previous folds. Seal with labeled sterilization indicator tape (Fig. 23-9). Indicate on the tape the enclosed item or type of set up, the date of processing, and your initials.
7. If wrapping many items together for a field, place the larger, heavier items on the bottom.
8. Place in each pack the sterilization indicator of choice for the facility.
9. Wrap or place dressings on the tray in multiples of five or ten.

(continued)

Place containers on their sides with lids off. If containers are placed in the autoclave in an upright position, air, which is heavier than steam, will settle into the interior of the container and keep steam from circulating to the inner surfaces.

Place all packs vertically (on their sides) to allow for the maximum steam circulation and penetration. Like materials should be autoclaved together—soft with soft, metal with metal—as much as possible.

Items should be packed on a perforated tray for steam circulation.

Figure 23-11 shows a properly loaded hospital autoclave.

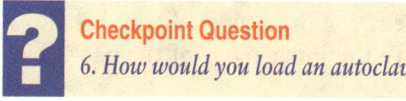

?   Checkpoint Question
6. How would you load an autoclave?

BOX 23-1
Wrapping Equipment for Sterilization (Continued)

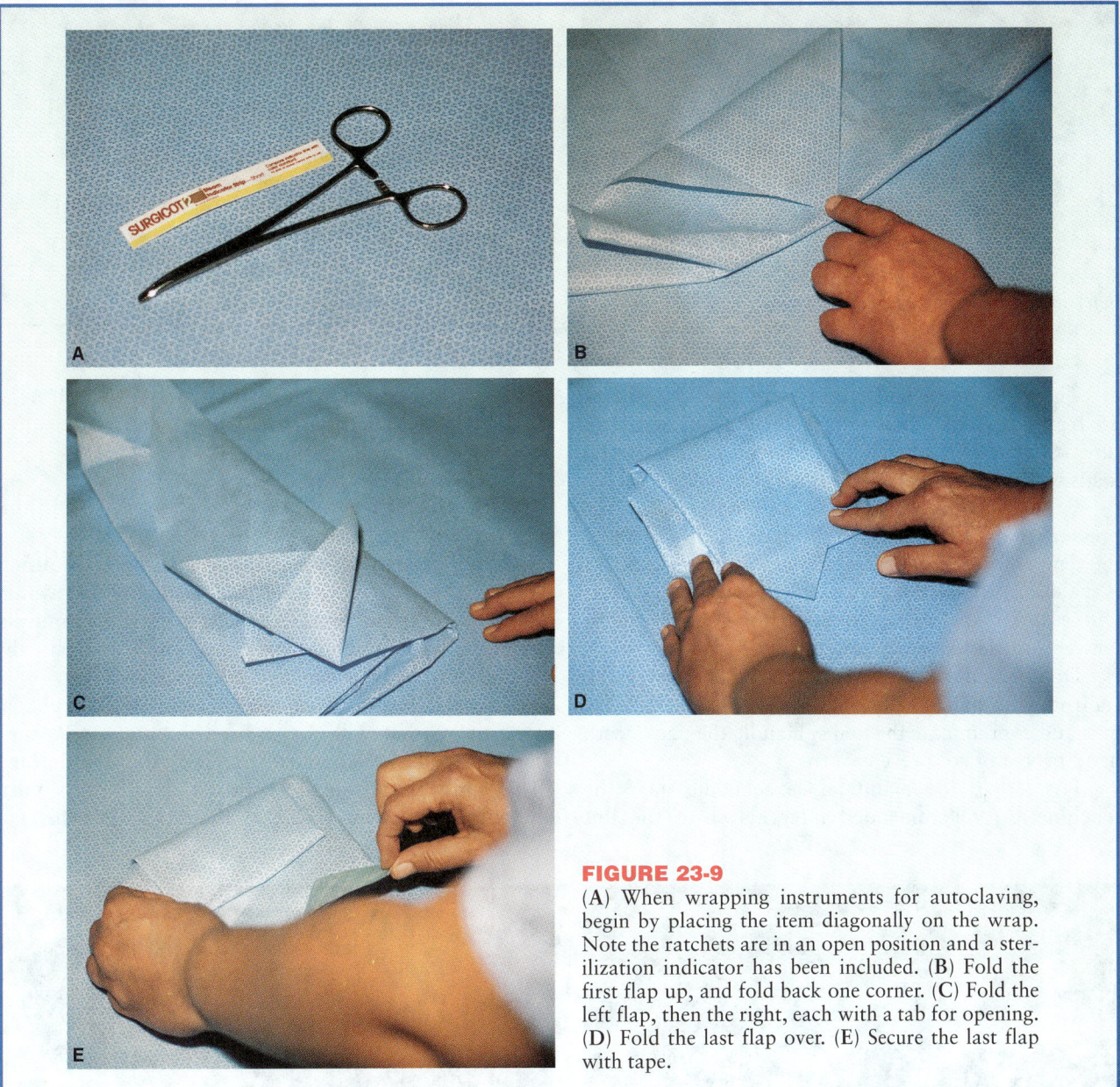

FIGURE 23-9

(**A**) When wrapping instruments for autoclaving, begin by placing the item diagonally on the wrap. Note the ratchets are in an open position and a sterilization indicator has been included. (**B**) Fold the first flap up, and fold back one corner. (**C**) Fold the left flap, then the right, each with a tab for opening. (**D**) Fold the last flap over. (**E**) Secure the last flap with tape.

Operating the Autoclave

All components of the autoclaving process—temperature, pressure, steam and time—must be in place for the items to reach a state of sterility. Follow the instruction manual carefully. All machines use the same principles, but operation may vary. Become familiar with the function of the machine in your facility. Instructions may be covered in plastic or laminated and posted beside the machine for easy reference. Procedure 23-2 outlines the general steps for operating an autoclave.

Use distilled water only. Tap water contains chemicals that will coat the interior, clog the exhaust valves, and hinder operation. Fill the reservoir only to the fill line. Too much water will cause saturated steam and will not be as efficient; too little water will not produce the required amount of steam.

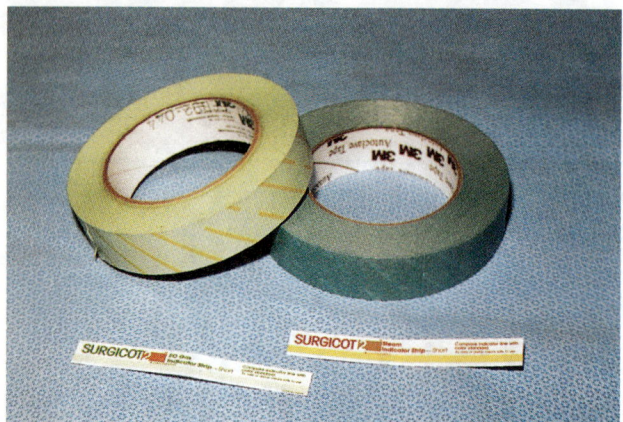

FIGURE 23-10

Sterilization indicators and tape. Gas indicator and tape (*left*) and steam indicator and tape (*right*).

The temperature and pressure are usually 250°F at 15 lb pressure for 20 to 30 minutes. Follow the manufacturer's instructions for the load content. Solid or metal loads will take slightly less time than soft, bulky loads.

Be sure to vent when the timer sounds to allow the pressure to drop safely. Open the door slightly to allow the temperature to drop and the load to cool and dry. If the door is opened more than ¼ to ½ inch, colder air will rush in and cause condensation on the items. Newer autoclaves vent automatically.

Do not remove the items until they are dry. Bacteria from your hands will wick through the moist coverings and contaminate the items. Handle the packs with hand protectors to prevent burns.

Post a routine maintenance schedule near the machine. At recommended intervals clean the lint trap, wash out the interior with a cloth or soft brush, and check the function of all components.

➤ BOILING

Boiling kills many of the pathogens found in an office but will not kill spores and the hepatitis virus. Water will boil to a temperature of 212°F or 100°C and no higher. Rapidly boiling water is no hotter than slowly bubbling water; it is simply evaporating faster.

Items to be boiled are usually metal or firm rubber. Only items that will not be used to enter sterile surfaces are to be boiled; most specula fit this description. They must be thoroughly sanitized and all parts must be under the boiling water. Set the timer when the wa-

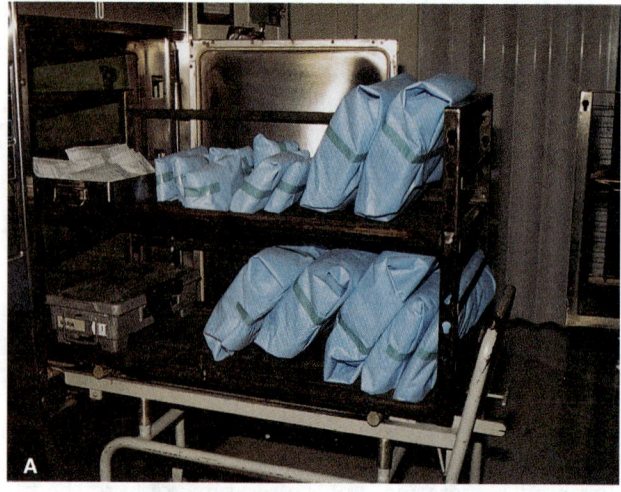
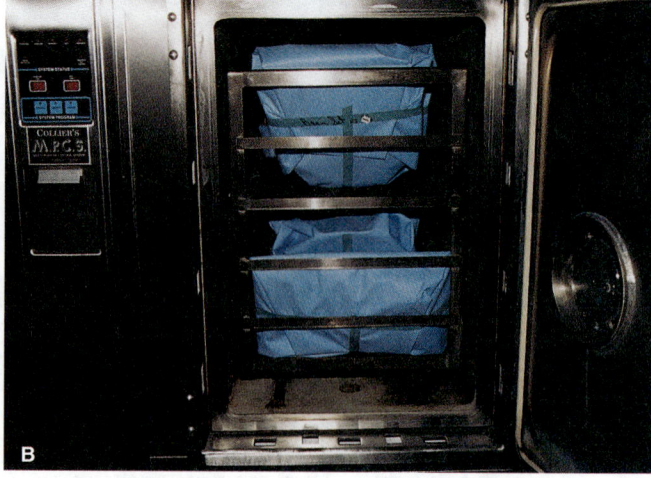

FIGURE 23-11

(**A**) A properly loaded hospital autoclave. Note the arrangement of the packs. Small packs are placed in a perforated tray to allow steam to circulate. (**B**) There is room on all sides for steam circulation.

Operating an Autoclave

Equipment/Supplies

- sanitized, wrapped articles sealed with indicator tape
- distilled water
- autoclave operating manual

Steps	Purpose
1. Assemble the equipment. An indicator should be wrapped within the pack. An indicator may also be included and wrapped separately to check the efficiency of the process without disturbing the wrapped packages.	1. Doing this ensures that all supplies are available. Including a wrapped indicator separately will allow you to check that the procedure was performed properly.
2. Check the water level and add more if needed, just to the fill line.	2. Too little water causes too little steam, too much water causes saturated steam that will extend the drying time and may wick microorganisms into the damp packs.
3. Load the autoclave:	3.
a. Place trays and packs on their sides, from one to three inches from each other and from the sides of the autoclave.	a. Air circulation is not possible if items are tightly packed. Placing items vertically allows heavier air to be forced out rather than pooling in the containers.
b. Put containers on their sides with the lids ajar.	b. Containers on their sides with lids ajar allow air to circulate within.
c. In mixed loads, place hard objects on the bottom shelf and softer packs on the top racks.	c. Harder objects may form condensation that will drip onto softer items and cause them to be wet.
d. Pack an indicator in the middle of the load.	
4. Read the instructions that should be available close to the machine. Almost all machines follow the same protocol:	
a. Close the door and secure it.	
b. Switch on the machine.	
c. When the temperature gauge reaches the temperature required for the contents of the load (usually 250° F or 121° C), set the timer. Many autoclaves can be preprogrammed for the required time.	
d. When the timer indicates that the cycle is over, vent the chamber. (Most autoclaves do this automatically.)	
e. Most loads dry in 5–20 minutes. Hard items dry faster than soft items.	
5. When the load has cooled, remove the items. Wear thermal gloves to prevent burns.	
6. Check the separately wrapped indicator for proper sterilization.	6. If the indicator registers that the load was properly processed, the items should be sterile; if the indicator has not registered, the load will need to be reprocessed.
7. Store the items appropriately in a clean, dry, dust-free area. Site-prepared packs are considered sterile for 30 days.	
8. Clean the autoclave by manufacturer's suggestions, which usually involve scrubbing with a mild detergent and a soft brush. Attention to the exhaust valve will prevent lint from occluding the outlet. Rinse the machine thoroughly and allow it to dry.	

ter reaches a full boil. Time is usually set for at least 20 minutes. Efficiency is increased with the addition of a 2% solution of sodium carbonate.

Boiling is rarely used in medical offices today. It is not considered a safe method of sterilization. More efficient methods of eliminating microorganisms have replaced the office boiler.

➤ STORAGE AND RECORDKEEPING

When using and maintaining sterilization and treatment equipment, the facility and staff are responsible for providing appropriate storage of these items, for keeping accurate records of warranties and maintenance agreements, and for keeping reordering information on hand.

Familiarize yourself with the manufacturer's recommendation for proper storage of instruments and equipment. Does this equipment need to be sterilized and stored wrapped in barrier protection? Or can it be stored in a clean area with a dustcloth or dustcover, such as electrocardiograph machines and ultrasound equipment? Is this an article of supply that warrants the need for special storage? Should the item be labeled and displayed so that employees are aware of potential hazards?

Most facilities have specific storage or supply rooms for housing sterile and nonsterile instruments and equipment. This area should be kept clean and dust free; it is usually located close to the area of need. Clean and sterile supplies and equipment must be separated from soiled items and waste.

In addition to providing proper storage for instruments and equipment, medical assistants are also responsible for keeping accurate records of sterilized items and equipment. Information that must be recorded includes maintenance records and "load" or sterilization records. Load or sterilization records should include:

- Date and time of the cycle
- General description of the contents of the load
- Exposure time and temperature
- Name or initials of the operator
- Results of the sterilization indicator
- Expiration date of the load (usually 30 days)

The maintenance records will include service by the manufacturer's representative as well as daily maintenance or maintenance as recommended to keep the equipment in optimum working condition.

Checkpoint Question

7. What six items should be included on a sterilization record?

➤ MAINTAINING SURGICAL SUPPLIES

As a medical assistant, you should keep an up-to-date master list of all supplies with all purchases and replacements. It is best to have one person responsible for maintaining the inventory, for keeping maintenance schedules, and for placing orders. If too many workers are involved, the care and handling of the facility equipment may either be overlooked or efforts may be duplicated.

Instruction manuals for all equipment should be kept on file and used when ordering supplies for replacement or maintenance. Equipment records for each item should include:

- Date of purchase
- Model number and serial number of the equipment
- Time period that service is recommended
- Date that service was requested
- Name of the individual requesting the service
- Reason for the service request
- Description of the service performed and any parts replaced
- Name of the person performing the service and the date the work was completed
- Signature and title of the person who acknowledged completion of the work

Warranties and guarantees should be kept with the equipment records. It is helpful also to have the name of the manufacturer's contact person attached to the records.

A tickler file should be kept to remind the staff of the need for manufacturer service maintenance as well as concurrent or periodic maintenance to be performed by the facility personnel.

Parts and supplies for items that are vital to the operation of the facility should always be kept on hand. The shelf life of the item, the storage space available, and the time required to order and receive an item should be considered in maintaining an inventory. If the piece of equipment cannot function without all of its components—and if some of those components have a short life span—replacements must be readily available. For example, an ophthalmoscope without a light is virtually useless.

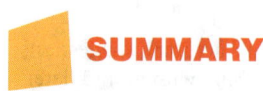

SUMMARY

As a medical assistant, you have to be reliable, responsible, and conscientious. You will be responsible for becoming familiar with several types of surgical instruments, understanding the principles and practices of asepsis, knowing disinfection and sterilization techniques, using equipment for sterilization and treatment purposes, and keeping accurate records and adequate supplies on hand for all sterilization and treatment equipment.

CRITICAL THINKING CHALLENGES

1. You are the senior medical assistant at Dr. Will's office. She instructs you to orient new employees on various aspects of the practice and requests that you develop an orientation booklet for all staff members. Design a booklet that contains the following information:
   - basic explanations of the instruments commonly used in the practice
   - procedures for sanitizing, disinfecting, and sterilizing the instruments
   - operating instructions for the autoclave
2. Create a record that can be used to document sterilization.
3. Develop a system for maintaining the office's surgical supplies.

ANSWERS TO CHECKPOINT QUESTIONS

1. Forceps are used to grasp, handle, compress, pull, or join tissue, equipment, or supplies. Scissors are used for dissecting superficial, deep, or delicate tissues and for cutting sutures and dressings. Scalpels are small knives used for surgery. Towel clamps are used to maintain the integrity of the sterile field by holding sterile drapes in place, allowing exposure of the operative site.

2. Because surgical instruments are delicate, improper handling may easily damage sharp blades or pointed tips. If you do drop an instrument, check it carefully to identify any damage. Note that damaged instruments can usually be repaired.

3. Sanitation is the science of maintaining a healthful, disease-free, and hazard-free environment. Disinfection is a process the destroys pathogenic organisms. Sterilization is a process that destroys all microorganisms.

4. An autoclave is an appliance for sterilizing medical instruments using steam under pressure. It consists of two chambers, an outer unit where pressure builds and an inner chamber where the actual sterilization occurs. Water is added to a reservoir, where it is converted to steam. This steam is then forced into the inner chamber, thereby increasing the pressure, which in turn raises the temperature of the steam. The higher the steam temperature, the more rapid is destruction of microorganisms.

5. A sterilization indicator, which is placed inside a pack to be autoclaved, registers the effectiveness of the sterilization process. Improper wrapping of packages, loading, or operation of the autoclave can prevent the indicator from registering correctly.

6. Load the autoclave loosely; do not try to pack in too many items because the steam cannot penetrate to those in the center. Place containers on their sides with the lids off. Place all packs on their sides to allow for maximum steam circulation and penetration.

7. The six items to include on a sterilization record are date and time of the cycle, general description of the load contents, exposure time and temperature, name or initials of the operator, results of the sterilization indicator, and load expiration date.

SUGGESTIONS FOR FURTHER READING

APIC. (1990). *APIC Guidelines for Selection and Use of Disinfectants and Sterilants.*

Caldwell, E., & Hegner, B. (1991). *The Nursing Assistant: A Nursing Process Approach,* 6th ed. Albany, NY: Delmar.

Donowitz, L. (1994). *Infection Control for the Health Care Worker.* Chicago: Mosby-Yearbook.

Preventing Disease Transmission in Personal Service Worker Occupations. (1994). Rockville, MD: U.S. Department of Health and Human Services, Public Health Service.

Assisting With Minor Office Surgery

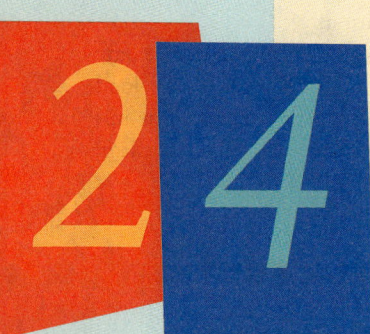

Chapter Outline

Preparing and Maintaining a Sterile Field
Sterile Surgical Packs
Procedure: Opening Sterile Surgical Packs
Ensuring Package Sterility
Sterile Transfer Forceps
Procedure: Using Sterile Transfer Forceps
Pouring a Sterile Solution
Procedure: Adding Sterile Solution to the Field
Adding Sterile Items from Peel-Back Packages
Preparing the Patient for Minor Office Surgery
Patient Instructions and Consent
Positioning and Draping
Preparing the Patient's Skin
Procedure: Performing Skin Preparation and Hair Removal
Local Anesthetics
Scalpels and Blades
Attaching a Scalpel Blade
Discarding Sharps
Wound Closure
Needles
Sutures
Assisting with Wound Closure
Steri-strips
Assisting with Suture Removal
Procedure: Removing Sutures
Assisting with Staple Removal

Procedure: Removing Staples
Sterile Dressings
Procedure: Applying a Sterile Dressing
Procedure: Changing an Existing Sterile Dressing
Bandaging
Types of Bandages
Bandage Application Guidelines
Montgomery Straps
Procedure: Applying Tubular Gauze Bandage
Commonly Performed Office Surgical Procedures
Excision of a Lesion
Procedure: Assisting with Excisional Surgery
Incision and Drainage
Procedure: Assisting with Incision and Drainage
Electrosurgery
Safety Measures
Care of Equipment
Laser Surgery
Specimen Collection During Office Surgery
Postsurgical Procedures
Cleaning the Examination Table
Cleaning the Operative Area
Summary
Critical Thinking Challenges
Answers to Checkpoint Questions
Suggestions for Further Reading

DACUM COMPONENTS

1.3 Practice within the scope of education, training, and personal capabilities
1.5 Work as a team member
4.1 Apply principles of aseptic technique and infection control
4.5 Prepare and maintain examination and treatment areas
4.7 Prepare patients for procedures
4.8 Assist physician with examinations and treatments
5.1 Document accurately
7.2 Instruct patients with special needs

Chapter Competencies

Learning Objectives

Upon successfully completing this chapter, you will be able to:

1. Spell and define the Key Terms.
2. List your responsibilities in the performance of minor office surgery.
3. List the guidelines and procedures for preparing and maintaining sterility of the field and the surgical equipment.
4. Explain the difference between dressings and bandages and give the purposes for both.
5. Describe the guidelines for the application of dressings and bandages.
6. State your responsibility in relation to informed consents and patient preparation.
7. Identify types and sizes of sutures and needles and give reasons for the selections of each.
8. Explain the purpose of local anesthetics and list three commonly used in the medical office.
9. Describe two methods of skin closure performed in the medical office.
10. Describe the procedure for attaching a scalpel blade to a reusable handle.
11. State your responsibility during surgical specimen collection.
12. List the types of laser and electrosurgery in the medical office and explain procedures and precautions for each.
13. Practice environmental disinfection to prevent cross contamination between patients and personnel.

Performance Objectives

Upon successfully completing this chapter, you will be able to:

1. Open sterile surgical packs (Procedure 24-1).
2. Use sterile transfer forceps (Procedure 24-2).
3. Add sterile solution to a sterile field (Procedure 24-3).
4. Open sterile packets.
5. Add the contents of peel-back packets to the sterile field.
6. Perform hair removal and skin preparation (Procedure 24-4).
7. Attach a surgical blade to a scalpel handle.
8. Remove sutures (Procedure 24-5).
9. Remove staples (Procedure 24-6).
10. Apply a sterile dressing (Procedure 24-7).
11. Change an existing sterile dressing (Procedure 24-8).
12. Wrap roller bandages using various techniques.
13. Apply tubular gauze bandage (Procedure 24-9).
14. Assist with excisional surgery (Procedure 24-10).
15. Assist with incision and drainage (Procedure 24-11).

Key Terms

(See Glossary for definitions.)

approximate	electrode
atraumatic	preservative
bandage	ratchets
cautery	swaged needle
coagulate	traumatic
dressing	

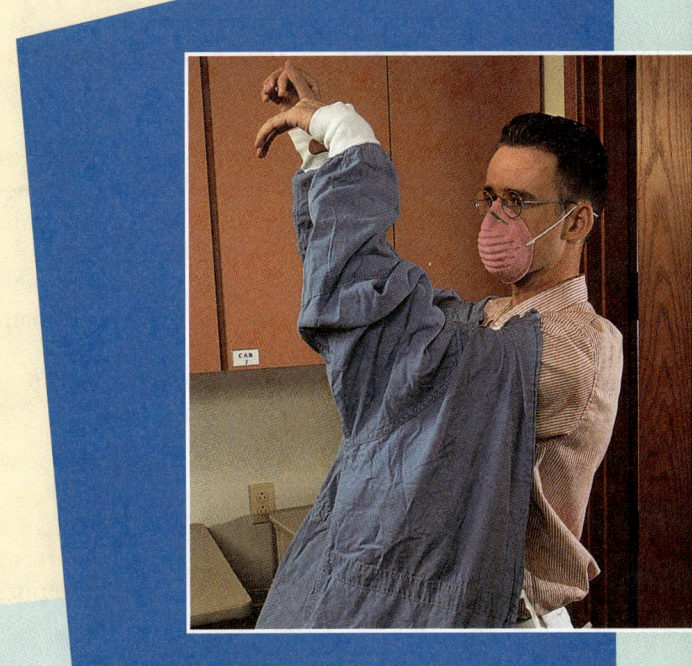

As a medical assistant, you will have many responsibilities when minor surgery is performed in the physician's office. These include:

1. Reinforcing the physician's instructions regarding preparation for surgery, including at-home skin preparation, fasting, bowel preparations, and so on.
2. Identifying the patient and the procedure before the physician arrives in order to gather the proper equipment and supplies.
3. Preparing the treatment room, instruments, supplies, and equipment.
4. Assisting the physician during the procedure.
5. Applying the **dressing** (wound covering).
6. Instructing the patient in postoperative wound care (eg, frequency of dressing changes, application of topical medication, observation of the wound for changes indicating healing or infection).
7. Assisting the patient as needed before, during, and after the procedure.
8. Assisting with postoperative instructions, prescriptions, medications; scheduling return visits.
9. Removing and caring for instruments, equipment, and supplies, including disposable items, "sharps," and contaminated and unused instruments.
10. Preparing the room for the next patient.

In addition, frequently you will be asked by the physician to witness the patient signing the informed consent document.

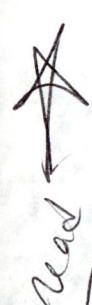

➤ PREPARING AND MAINTAINING A STERILE FIELD

Minor office surgery involves procedures that penetrate the body's normally intact surface. Whenever there is an open wound, surgical asepsis must be maintained (see Chap. 19, Asepsis and Infection Control). Because hands can never be sterilized, sterile transfer forceps or sterile gloved hands must be used to handle sterile objects during a sterile procedure.

Follow the guidelines below during a sterile procedure:

1. Do not let sterile packages become damp or wet. Microorganisms can be drawn into the package by a wicking action. If a package sterilized in the medical office becomes moist, it must be repackaged in a clean, dry wrapper and resterilized. Damp or wet disposable packages must be discarded.
2. Always face a sterile field. If you must leave the area or work with your back to the sterile field, the field must be covered with a sterile drape using sterile technique.

3. Hold all sterile items above waist level. When sterile items are not in the field of vision, they may become contaminated without your knowledge.
4. Place sterile items in the middle of the sterile field. A 1-inch border around the field is considered contaminated.
5. Do not spill any liquids, even sterile liquids, onto the sterile field. Remember, the surface below the field is not sterile and moisture will allow microorganisms to wick up to the surgical field.
6. Do not cough, sneeze, or talk over the sterile field. Microorganisms from the respiratory tract can contaminate the sterile field.
7. Never reach over the sterile field. Dust or lint from clothing can contaminate the sterile field.
8. Be aware that soiled supplies, such as gauze or instruments, should not be passed over or placed on the sterile field.
9. If you know or suspect that the sterile field has been contaminated, alert the physician. Sterility must be re-established before the procedure can continue.

Sterile Surgical Packs

Many medical offices keep a box with index cards or a loose-leaf binder listing surgical procedures that are commonly performed in the office and the items needed for setup. Some medical offices prepackage sterile setups in a suitable wrapper and prepare them in the office by autoclave sterilization (see Chap. 23, Instruments and Equipment, for autoclaving procedure). These setups are labeled according to the type of procedure (eg, lesion removal, suture setup) and contain the general instruments for these procedures. Some basic supplies (eg, gauze sponges, cotton balls, and towels) may also be included before autoclaving.

Because of the time and effort involved in the strict quality control that must be maintained to ensure that items autoclaved on site are sterile after processing, many offices use commercially packaged, disposable surgical packs. Disposal surgical packs have become increasingly popular because they are convenient and come in an almost infinite variety of forms with a wide assortment of contents. They may contain one sterile article (such as a 4 x 4 sterile dressing) or a complete sterile surgical setup.

Many of the supplies will be packaged in peel-apart wrappers with two loose flaps to be pulled apart and the sterile item dropped carefully onto the operative field. The insides of the wrappers may be opened out and used as sterile fields. If the sides of the packages are pulled completely apart, items left within the wrapper may be set out to the side of the procedural setup for use as needed. Some of the packages are enclosed in plastic and wrapped inside a barrier material that can be used as a sterile field.

Directions for opening are clearly marked on the outside of the pack and should be read and understood. If the surgical pack is opened improperly, the contents will be contaminated and cannot be used. Commercially prepared sterile packs are generally more expensive than medical practice site-prepared packs; therefore, care must be taken to avoid waste. Large surgical packs contain items specific for various types of surgery; the contents of the pack will be noted on the label. Commercially prepared packs list the contents item by item; site-prepared packs usually only state the type of setup. Procedure 24-1 describes the steps for opening sterile surgical packs.

Ensuring Package Sterility

There should be a sterilization indicator inside each surgical package to show that it has been properly sterilized. Tapes, strips, and packaging with indicator stripes or dots on the outside of the packs are not 100% accurate and do not guarantee sterility. These devices are designed to change color when exposed to high temperatures, as in an autoclave. Indicator strips, tapes, and packages should never be stored near the autoclave or in other unusually warm areas as the indicators may change colors as if the package had gone through a sterilization cycle.

In the autoclave, sterility is achieved only by the right combination of temperature, pressure, steam, and time. All four elements must be present at the proper levels in the autoclave cycle to ensure sterility. In addition, an improperly packed autoclave can impede steam penetration to the articles, which will prevent sterilization but will allow the package indicator to change colors. Therefore, sterilization indicators should be packaged within each pack and must be checked before beginning the surgical procedure. (See autoclaving procedures in Chap. 23, Instruments and Equipment.) When opening a package of sterile objects, the procedure is the same whether the items are site-prepared reusables or commercially prepared disposables. For all sterile packs or supplies, keep in mind that:

1. The unsterile area is the outside surface of the outside wrapper.
2. The sterile area includes the inside surface of the outside wrapper, the inside wrapper (if included), and the contents of the package.
3. Items are considered contaminated and should be repackaged and resterilized:
   a. When moisture is present
   b. When they have been dropped from the sterile field

   c. If they are out of date (on-site prepared packages expire 30 days from preparation; commercial packs have a posted expiration date)
   d. If the sterilization indicator has not turned color
   e. If the wrapper is torn or damaged
   f. When any area is known or thought to have been touched by an unsterile item

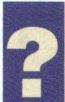

Checkpoint Question

1. What are nine guidelines that must be followed to maintain a sterile field?

Sterile Transfer Forceps

Sterile transfer forceps can be used to move sterile articles from one sterile area to another sterile area. The forceps' tips and the sterile articles being transferred must both remain sterile. The handles of the forceps are considered medically aseptic and are not considered sterile because these are touched by bare hands (Fig. 24-1).

Sterile transfer forceps are stored either in a dry sterile container, in a wrapped sterile package, or in a sterile solution in a closed container system, such as Bard Parker, which helps protect the forceps from contamination and slows evaporation of the soaking solution. In a closed dry container system, the forceps and container must be sanitized and autoclaved daily. In a closed sterile solution system, the forceps and the container are resterilized at least every day, or more often if needed, and fresh solution is added daily. Only one forceps should be stored per container because separate containers decrease the chance of contamination when removing forceps and avoid damage caused by tangling.

Proper use of sterile transfer forceps requires that certain guidelines be followed (Procedure 24-2).

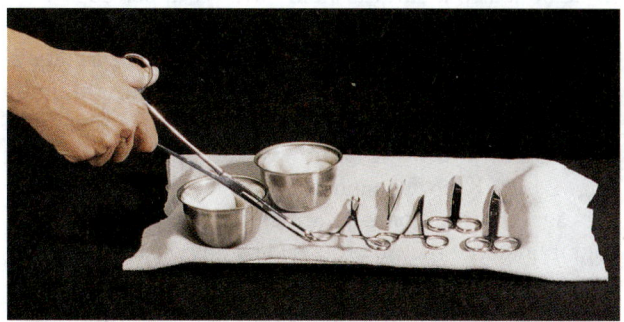

FIGURE 24-1
Sterile transfer forceps may be used to move items on the sterile field.

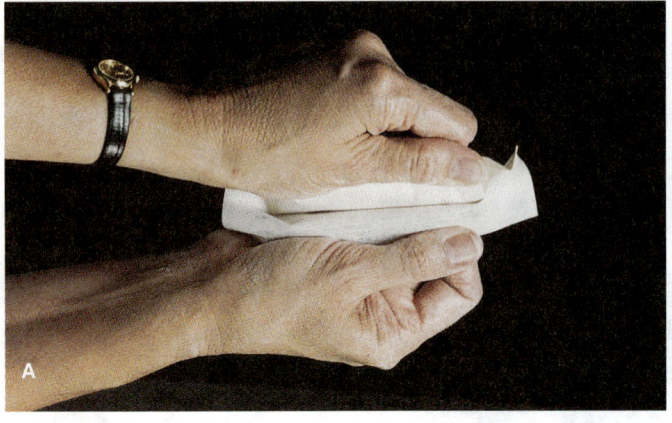

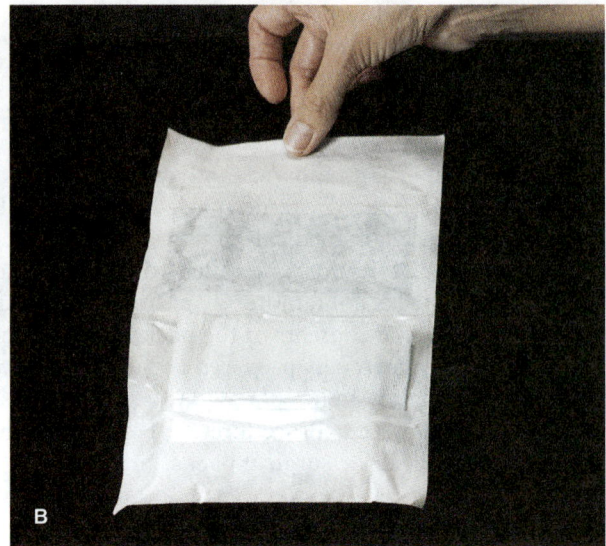

FIGURE 24-2
Sterile packets. (*A*) Open sterile packets by grasping the edges and rolling the thumbs outward. (*B*) Opening the packet properly forms a sterile field.

Pouring a Sterile Solution

Whether site-prepared or commercially prepared, trays are not processed or stored with liquids in open containers. Solutions must be added as needed at the time of setup. Some procedures require sterile water or saline, others may require an antiseptic solution. These will be poured into containers already arranged into position by using transfer forceps (Procedure 24-3).

Adding Sterile Items from Peel-Back Packages

Procedure packages are frequently prepared with supplies (eg, cotton balls, gauze squares, and so forth) to eliminate the need to add more at the time of setup. However, patient assessment at the time of surgery may suggest the need for additional items. These small supplies are usually provided commercially in peel-apart packages.

Peel-apart packages containing small or single items to be added to a surgical field have an upper edge with two flaps that are used to open the package in a manner that maintains the sterility of the contents. The package is properly opened by using both hands. With the thumbs just inside the tops of the edges, the flaps are separated using a slow, outward motion of the thumbs and flaps (Fig. 24-2). Keep in mind that the inside of the sealed package and the contents are sterile; they will become contaminated if they are touched by any unsterile object.

There are three ways in which the contents of peel-back packages can be added to the sterile field:

1. *By using sterile transfer forceps*. Peel the edges apart with a rolling motion as described above.

With the two edges held down, the contents may be lifted up and away with forceps. (Fig. 24-3)
2. *By using the sterile gloved hand*. This method requires two persons, usually the medical assistant who will open the package and the physician who will remove the contents with sterile gloved hands. You must carefully hold the edges to avoid contaminating the physician's gloves (Fig. 24-4).
3. *By flipping the contents onto a sterile field*. To do this, you must step back from the sterile field to prevent the hands and the unsterile outer wrapper of the pack from crossing over the sterile field. The edges are pulled down and away from the package contents and the item is carefully tossed or flipped onto the field without crossing the sterile area.

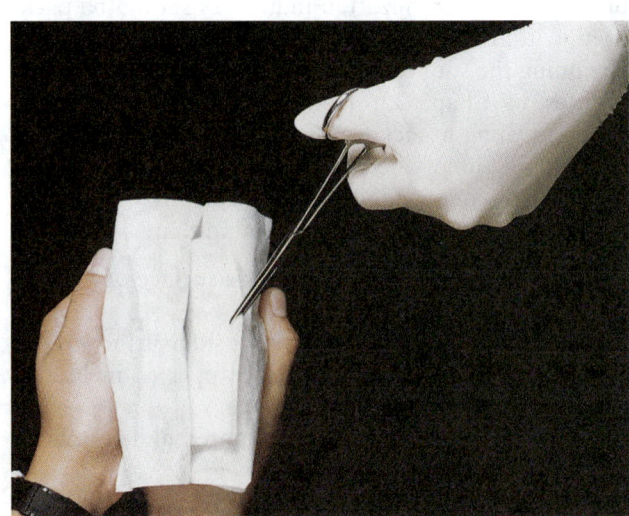

FIGURE 24-3
The physician may use forceps to remove small supplies.

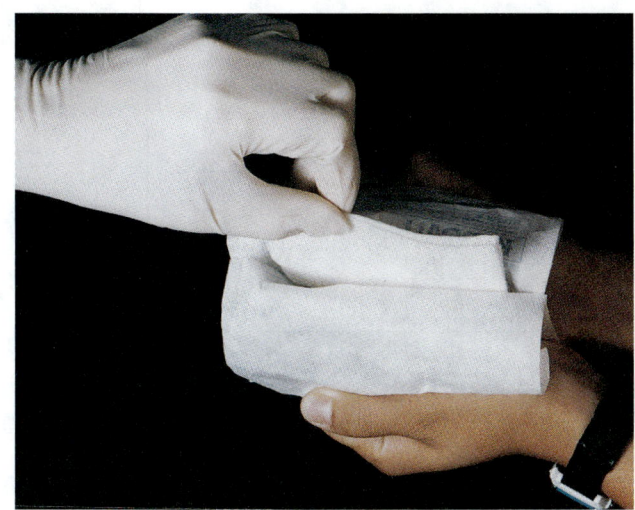

FIGURE 24-4
Sterile gloved hands may be used to remove small items.

In most cases, items in presterilized peel-back envelopes cannot be resterilized and must be discarded when opened even if not used. Because such items are relatively expensive to purchase, they should not be opened unnecessarily. A supply of items that might be needed during the procedure should be conveniently close to the area and added only if needed.

Checkpoint Question

2. What are three ways that contents of peel-back packages can be added to the sterile field?

➤ PREPARING THE PATIENT FOR MINOR OFFICE SURGERY

Patient Instructions and Consent

Many of the minor surgical procedures (eg, suture insertion or removal, incision and drainage, sebaceous cystectomy) that are performed in the medical office require only a full explanation of the procedure and informed consent. The patient either agrees and the procedure is performed, or the patient refuses and the procedure is not done.

In today's litigious society, physicians routinely obtain signed informed consent documents even for minor office procedures. Preprinted forms can be obtained or especially designed to contain all the information needed for informed consent and may be used for procedures requiring legal, witnessed signatures and for those requiring only that the patient review the procedure. Other forms can be rather general with blank spaces to add information relevant to the procedure to be performed. Both should provide spaces for the date and signatures of patient, physician, and witness(es) (Fig. 24-5).

Other data usually found in informed consent documents include procedure and purposes, expected results, possible side effects, risks, and complications. As noted in Chapter 3, Medicine and the Law, the medical assistant is not responsible for obtaining informed consent from the patient but will probably be required to witness the signing of the document by the patient. It is the physician's legal responsibility to obtain informed consent from the patient. If a procedure is performed on a date after the consent is signed, you may be asked to verify the consent at that time, but should not obtain the initial informed consent from the patient.

The patient may ask how long the procedure will last, what preparations are needed, if fasting is necessary, and other questions. You may answer queries of this nature for the patient after verifying the information with the physician. It is always a good practice to give specific written instructions to the patient for any necessary fasting or bowel preparation so that a procedure can be done on schedule and with no preventable risk to the patient. The physician may prescribe medication or may dispense medications to be taken by the patient at home before the surgery.

As with any patient instructions, you should notify the physician if the patient expresses confusion or misunderstanding. The patient should be encouraged to call the office should questions arise later.

Positioning and Draping

Before positioning the patient for a minor surgical procedure, have the patient void; this helps avoid discomfort during the procedure. Offer to help the patient remove whatever clothing is necessary to expose the operative site. Expose only the area necessary for the procedure to ensure the patient's privacy. Be aware that the air-conditioned office may become uncomfortably cool for patients. Additional sheets or a blanket may be added for comfort.

Assist the patient to assume a comfortable position on the examining table that offers exposure of and access to the operative site. Pillows may be used for comfort and support. Patients should not be expected to maintain uncomfortable positions, such as lithotomy or knee-chest, while waiting for the physician. They should be positioned only when the physician is ready to begin the procedure. (See Chap. 22, Physical Examination, for more information about positioning.) At the end of the procedure, assist the patient from the table, allowing as much time as needed. Often patients who did not need help removing clothing will require assistance dressing following minor surgery. Be aware of this and assist as necessary.

The type of procedure and the position in which the patient is placed for minor surgery will determine

---

SPECIAL CONSENT TO OPERATION OR OTHER PROCEDURE

PATIENT _____ PATIENT NUMBER _____

DATE _____ TIME _____

1. I HEREBY AUTHORIZE DOCTOR _____ AND/OR SUCH ASSIS-
   TANTS AS MAY BE SELECTED BY HIM, TO PERFORM THE FOLLOWING PROCEDURES(S):
   _____

   ON _____
       (NAME OF PATIENT) or (MYSELF)

2. THE PROCEDURE(S) LISTED ABOVE HAVE BEEN EXPLAINED TO ME BY DR. _____
   AND I UNDERSTAND THE NATURE AND THE CONSEQUENCES OF THE PROCEDURE(S).

3. I RECOGNIZE THAT, DURING THE COURSE OF THE OPERATION, UNFORESEEN CONDI-
   TIONS MAY NECESSITATE ADDITIONAL OR DIFFERENT PROCEDURES THAN THOSE SET
   FORTH. I FURTHER AUTHORIZE AND REQUEST THAT THE ABOVE NAMED SURGEON, HIS
   ASSISTANTS, OR HIS DESIGNEES PERFORM SUCH PROCEDURES AS ARE IN HIS PROFES-
   SIONAL JUDGMENT NECESSARY AND DESIRABLE, INCLUDING, BUT NOT LIMITED TO,
   PROCEDURES INVOLVING PATHOLOGY AND RADIOLOGY. THE AUTHORITY GRANTED UN-
   DER THIS PARAGRAPH SHALL EXTEND TO REMEDYING CONDITIONS NOT KNOWN TO
   DR. _____ AT THE TIME THE OPERATION IS COMMENCED.

4. I AM AWARE THAT THE PRACTICE OF MEDICINE AND SURGERY IS NOT AN EXACT SCI-
   ENCE AND I ACKNOWLEDGE THAT NO GUARANTEES HAVE BEEN MADE TO ME AS TO THE
   RESULTS OF THE OPERATION OR PROCEDURE.

5. TISSUE REMOVED DURING SURGERY SHALL BE SENT TO PATHOLOGY TO BE EXAMINED
   AND DISPOSED OF IN ACCORDANCE WITH THE RULES AND REGULATONS OF THE MED-
   ICAL STAFF OF CARTERET SURGERY CENTER.

_____   _____
Procedure has been discussed with patient. (Surgeon's Signature)   SIGNATURE OF PATIENT

PATIENT IS UNABLE TO SIGN BECAUSE   ❏ HE (SHE) IS A MINOR _____ YEARS OF AGE

            ❏ OTHER (SPECIFY) _____

_____   _____
WITNESS   PERSON AUTHORIZED TO SIGN FOR PATIENT

_____   _____
    RELATIONSHIP OF ABOVE TO PATIENT

FIGURE 24-5
Sample consent form.

---

the type of drapes used to expose the operative site and cover the patient. Disposable paper drapes are most commonly used in the medical office. They come in many different sizes and shapes, each suited for specific uses. Paper drapes can be used alone, in combination, or with separate drape sheets and towels. Fenestrated (window) drapes have an opening to expose the operative site while covering adjacent areas. Fenestrated drapes may be small, such as those used for suture insertion or removal, or rather large, as in lithotomy drapes used to cover the legs and lower abdomen but expose the perineal area. Some sterile drapes are combined with adhesive-backed clear plastic, which adheres to the patient's skin and eliminates the need for towel clamps, such as Backhaus clamps or nonperforating towel clamps (see Chap. 23, Instruments and Equipment, for illustrations of these clamps).

When removing contaminated drapes from the patient following a procedure, put on protective gloves and carefully roll the items in a direction away from the body, keeping the contaminated areas innermost.

This helps to surround the dirtier areas of the sheet with the cleaner area and helps prevent contaminated clothing. Because the sheets and towels will likely be contaminated with blood and/or bodily fluids, Standard Precautions must be followed (see Chap. 19, Asepsis and Infection Control.)

> **?** **Checkpoint Question**
> *3. What is a fenestrated drape?*

Preparing the Patient's Skin

The goal of preoperative skin preparation is to remove as many microorganisms from the skin as possible to decrease the chance of wound contamination. Skin preparation may range from simply applying an antiseptic solution to the skin to removing gross contamination and hair from the operative area. Hair can be removed with depilatory creams but often requires shaving the skin (Procedure 24-4).

➤ LOCAL ANESTHETICS

When office surgery of any kind is performed, the site is first anesthetized (numbed) with a local anesthetic to minimize the pain and discomfort felt by the patient.

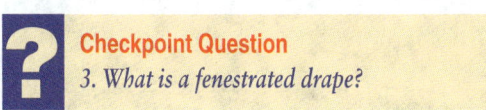

Charting Example

01/16/98	1400 Patient arrived for mole removal on left thumb. Patient was escorted to examining room. Patient instructed to wash hands with soap and water. Hands were dried. Antiseptic solution applied to thumb using a circular motion. Area was dried with sterile gauze. A sterile drape was applied. Patient was instructed not to touch sterile field —George Scott, CMA

Occasionally, when a wound contains imbedded debris that must be removed prior to repair, the local anesthetic will be injected before preparing the wound site to facilitate wound cleaning.

Lidocaine (Xylocaine), or xylocaine with epinephrine (0.5%–2%), are two of the many local anesthetics commonly used in the medical office. Others include lidocaine (Baylocaine), mepivacaine (Carbocaine), and bupivacaine (Marcaine). Epinephrine is added to local anesthetics to slow absorption by the body and lengthen its effectiveness; it is used when the physician anticipates a longer procedure.

There are two procedures used for the administration of local anesthesia. In one procedure, the assistant may draw the anesthetic for the physician, retaining the vial beside the syringe for the physician's approval. In this case, the anesthetic usually is given before the physician gloves for the procedure.

The second option is used if the physician gloves before the anesthetic is given. In this procedure, a sterile syringe will be included in the sterile field setup. When the physician is ready to administer the anesthetic, show the label, clean the stopper, and hold the vial while the physician draws the required amount into the syringe. There are many methods of holding the vial securely for the physician during this procedure. A team that works well together will develop a method that ensures that surgical asepsis is maintained.

➤ SCALPELS AND BLADES

Disposable scalpel blades with permanently attached handles are frequently used in the medical office. Less commonly seen in offices today are reusable scalpel handles with disposable blades attached. Figure 23-3 shows various types of scalpel handles and blades. Because of the possibility of serious injury to the assistant, the process of attaching or removing the blade should be performed very carefully and according to procedure. The blade should never be attached or removed by hand.

Attaching a Scalpel Blade

Scalpel blades, which are small and extremely sharp, are difficult to grasp with the fingers. To attach a blade to a scalpel handle, follow these steps:

1. Grasp the *blunt* side of the blade (*not* the sharp side) in the jaws of a hemostat held in the dominant hand (Fig. 24-6).
2. With the hemostat and blade in the dominant hand and the scalpel handle in the nondominant hand, slide the opening in the blade into the

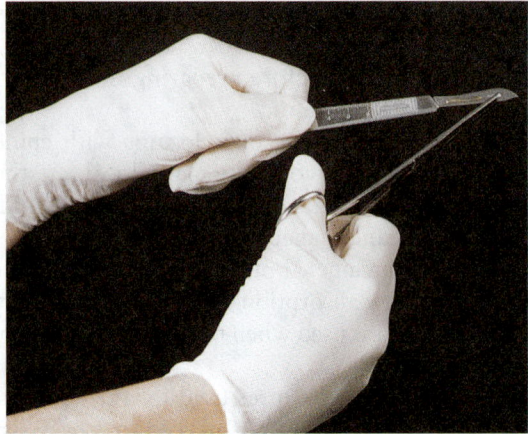

FIGURE 24-6
Place or remove a scalpel blade by grasping the blunt side with a hemostat.

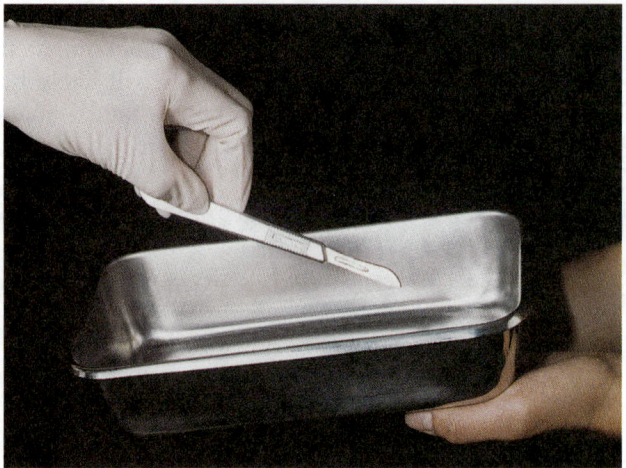

FIGURE 24-7
Instruments should be placed in a basin after use. They should never be tossed into a wash basin or returned to the field.

grooves in the handle tip in one smooth, continuous motion.

3. Note a click sound, which can be heard when the blade is correctly seated.
4. If the blade does not click, or if it does not lie flat against the handle tip, remove the blade with the hemostat and repeat the procedure. (To remove the blade, reverse the procedure.) Never place or remove blades without a hemostat. Instruments are available to remove blades in the safest manner possible.

Blades range in size for various procedures; the physician determines the size needed for any incision. Most medical office surgical procedures require the use of small-sized blades.

Discarding Sharps

When "sharps" are discarded from the surgical field, they should be placed in a basin rather than tossed into a sink or waste receptacle (Fig. 24-7). Contaminated instruments are not returned to the field, but must be cared for with safety in mind. For instance, when the physician has made the incision and no longer needs the scalpel, hold a basin to receive the soiled instrument. At the completion of the procedure, the instrument and other sharps from the field can be cared for or safely discarded into an appropriate sharps container.

➤ WOUND CLOSURE

Many types of wounds require closure to ensure rapid healing with minimal scarring. This is accomplished by bringing the edges of the wounds as closely together as possible in their original position (approximation). Skin closure procedures are performed after cyst or tis-

sue sample removal, in response to lacerating injuries, or anytime that skin surfaces require assistance in the healing process. Skin closures performed in the office include the insertion of sutures or the use of Steristrips. Supplies used to suture skin closure will include needles and sutures.

What If?
What if while you are separating a contaminated blade from a scalpel handle you accidentally cut your finger?

Remove your gloves and immediately wash your hands with an antiseptic solution. Then have the physician evaluate the wound. He or she may suggest that you perform a surgical scrub or irrigate the wound, or antibiotics may be ordered. The patient should be asked permission to obtain a blood sample to test for hepatitis and HIV. (State laws vary regarding the legality of health care workers demanding a blood sample for testing.) You should consider having the vaccine for hepatitis now to protect yourself from that disease. Many states require that health care workers be immunized at their employer's expense. Finally, be sure to notify your supervisor of any work-related injury so that it may be appropriately documented.

Needles

Needles used in minor office surgery are chosen for the type of surgery to be performed. Needles are classified by:

- Shape—curved or straight
- Point—tapered or cutting
- Eye—*atraumatic* (*swaged*) or **traumatic** (with an eye)

Round straight needles are called "domestic" needles; straight cutting needles are called "Keith" needles. Curved needles used in surgical procedures are almost always clamped in a needle holder before being handed to the physician. Straight needles (domestic or Keith) are not clamped in a needle holder, but are handed by the assistant to the physician with the point up. Straight needles are rarely used in the medical office.

Cutting needles are used on tough tissue such as skin. Round or tapered (noncutting) needles are used on tissues such as subcutaneous, peritoneum, or muscle.

Atraumatic, or **swaged needles** have suture material that has been mechanically attached to the needle by the manufacturer and do not require threading; they are called atraumatic because they cause less trauma as they pass through the tissues. Unlike atraumatic or swaged needles, threaded needles have an eye with a double thickness of suture that must be pulled through tissues. The double thickness of suture makes a larger, therefore more traumatic, opening in the tissues than a swaged suture. Swaged needles have the appropriate size suture material attached by the manufacturer.

Swaged needles are used far more often than any other type of needle in the medical office. It is considered rare to use any needle other than a curved, swaged needle in minor office surgery. Swaged needles are selected for a procedure according to the size and length of the suture material. The attached needle gauge is a corresponding size. When suture must be threaded through an eyed needle, both needle size and suture must be selected. Suture and needle selection is usually done by the physician; you should know your physician's preferences and anticipate needs whenever possible.

Sutures, needles, and suture/needle combinations are contained in peel-apart packages that are sterile on the inside so that they can be added to the sterile field (Fig. 24-8). This may be done by sterile transfer forceps, a sterile gloved hand, or by carefully flipping them onto the sterile field.

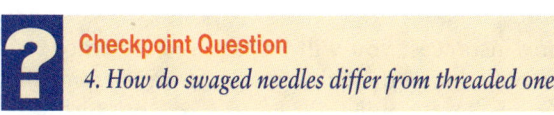

Checkpoint Question
4. How do swaged needles differ from threaded ones?

Sutures

Sutures are used to close wounds and incisions and to bring tissue layers into close approximation. Sutures come in various gauges (diameters) and lengths. Very

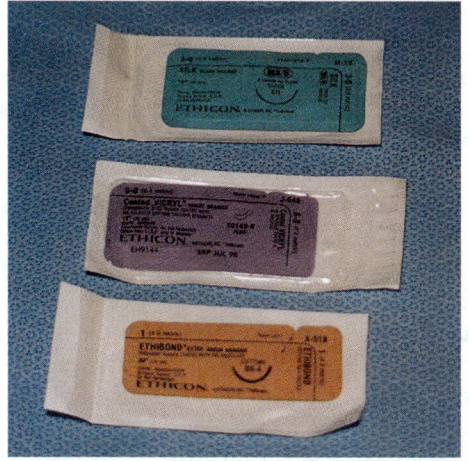

FIGURE 24-8
Suture material and suture needles are supplied in see-through packs, with the size of suture material and the type of needle listed on the packet. The inside of the packet is sterile.

large gauge (diameter) suture is given a number from 1 to 5; 5 is the largest. Sutures smaller than size 1 are expressed in zeros. Suture sizes, which become progressively smaller, range from 0 to 10, or smaller (ie, 1-0, 2-0, 3-0, and so forth). A very fine 10-0 suture, which is about the diameter of a human hair, is generally used for microsurgical procedures. When fine suture is needed, such as on the face and neck, 5-0 and 6-0 suture are commonly used. Very fine suture decreases obvious scarring and gives a better cosmetic result.

Sutures also come in absorbable and nonabsorbable forms. Absorbable suture, or catgut (made from the intestines of sheep or cattle), is readily broken down by body processes and usually does not require a removal procedure. There are two forms of absorbable gut suture: chromic, which is chemically treated to delay absorption for several days; and plain, which is not treated, and is the most quickly absorbed of the two. Absorbable sutures are used most frequently in the hospital setting during surgery on deep tissues.

Nonabsorbable sutures come in the greatest variety of brands, sizes, lengths, and swaged needles; they are the most versatile. Nonabsorbable sutures either remain in the body permanently or are removed after healing has occurred. Nonabsorbable sutures are used on the skin, intestines, or bone; to ligate larger vessels; to attach heart valves and various artificial and natural grafts. Nonabsorbable sutures are made from fibers (eg, silk, nylon, Dacron, cotton) and from stainless-steel wire.

Another form of nonabsorbable suture is the metal skin clip or staple; these may be made of stainless steel. There are very specialized types of metal clips made of sterling silver for use in neurosurgery and other procedures. When nonabsorbable sutures are used to close skin wounds, they must be removed when the wound has healed.

Depending on the location of the skin wound, sutures will remain in place for varying lengths of time: the head and neck may require 3 to 5 days, whereas the arms and legs may require 7 to 10 days.

Sutures are packaged individually, as are needles, in see-through peel-apart packages. These packages are labeled according to the type, size, and length of the enclosed suture material; whether it is absorbable or nonabsorbable; and the type of needle if this material is swaged. The insides of these packages are sterile until opened. Some are supplied in dual peel-apart packages so that the inside package can be reused if it has not been damaged or opened.

Assisting with Wound Closure

When a wound is sutured in the office, you will be required to set up a sterile field. The physician will inspect the wound and decide what type and size suture material to use. You may be required to assist the physician during the procedure.

Added to the sterile field may be items such as: surgical drapes, hemostats, needle holders, tissue (thumb) forceps, scissors (dissecting or operating), suture material (probably swaged suture/needle combinations), gauze sponges, sterile gloves, equipment to inject local anesthetic (syringe, needle, wipe, and anesthetic). If the physician requires assistance during the insertion of sutures, you will be required to scrub, glove, and pass instruments as needed during the procedure (see Chap. 19, Asepsis and Infection Control).

In almost all instances in the medical office, swaged needles will be used. If you are assisting, hand the needle to the physician in the functional position. The needle will be clasped in a needle holder for suturing. Click the **ratchets** (parts that lock together) twice for a secure hold. If the physician is right-handed, the suture material will extend to the right and the needle will point to the left. If the physician is left-handed, the reverse will be true.

Suture material must be cut during the procedure. This is usually be done by the physician. If you are scrubbed to assist, the scissors will be passed in a functional position, which means that you will grasp the closed blades with the handles downward. The physician will indicate when scissors are needed and expects the handles to be placed firmly in the palm with the blades pointing upward (Fig. 24-9). Thumb and tissue forceps will be passed in the opposite manner, tips downward when gripped by the physician. In all instances, the physician's personal preference will guide the assistant.

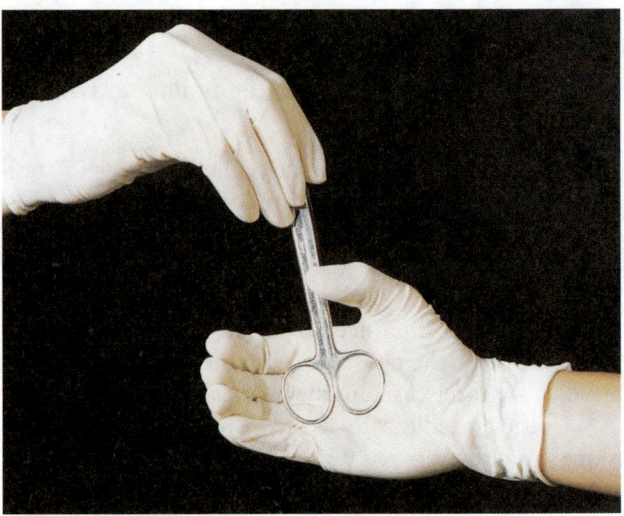

FIGURE 24-9
Instruments are passed in the functional position. Grasp the blades or tips and pass the instrument to the physician, with the handle to the palm.

Steri-strips

Steri-strips are adhesive skin closures used to **approximate** the edges of a small wound if sutures are not needed. Steri-strips are appropriate where there is little tension on the skin edges. The strips are placed transversely across the line of the wound to bring the wound edges in close approximation (Fig. 24-10). When removing Steri-strips, carefully lift the edges distal to the wound and pull gently toward the wound. Never pull the strips away from the wound as tension on the wound site may disrupt the healing process.

Checkpoint Question
5. *How do you hand a right-handed physician a needle for suturing?*

➤ ASSISTING WITH SUTURE REMOVAL

In many instances, you will be required to remove sutures from a wound. Patients should understand that there might be a "pulling" sensation during suture removal but there should not be pain. The area must first be cleaned with an antiseptic solution. Either gloved with sterile gloves or using a sterile transfer forceps, clean the area in a circular motion away from the wound or in straight wipes away from the suture line (Fig. 24-11). The wipe is discarded after each sweep

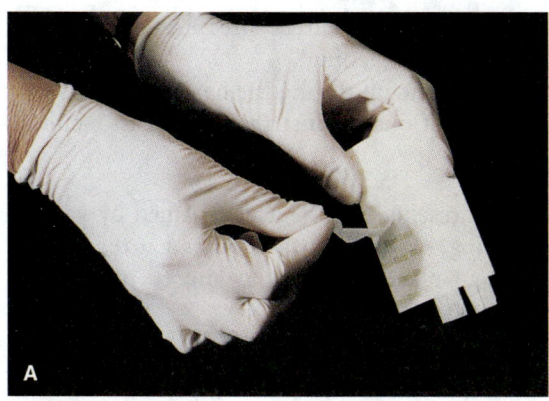

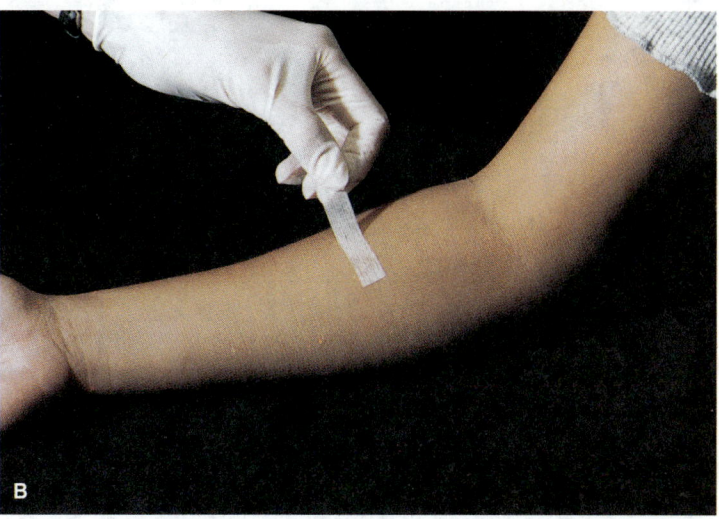

FIGURE 24-10
Steri-strips. (*A*) These light-weight lengths of porous tape are used for small sounds. (*B*) Steri-strips are placed transversely across a wound.

and a new one used for the next sweep across the area. Either sterile disposable suture removal kits, which contain all of the equipment needed for suture removal (Fig. 24-12), or sterile reusable equipment may be used (Procedure 24-5).

➤ ASSISTING WITH STAPLE REMOVAL

Following hospital surgery, many incisions will be closed with metal staples rather than fiber sutures. Patients frequently leave the hospital before the staples can

Charting Example

09/15/98	0945	Patient arrived for suture removal. Six sutures were removed from the left elbow. Wound appears to be healing; no drainage noted. Wound cleaned with antiseptic solution. ——John Robertson, RMA

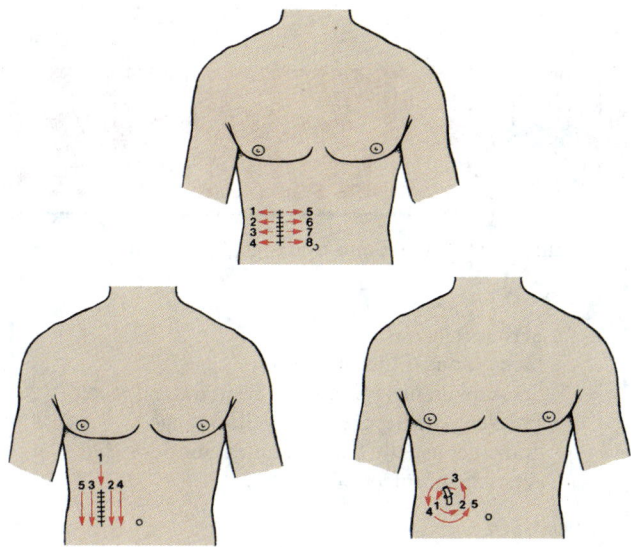

FIGURE 24-11
Clean the wound outward from the site following any of the numbered patterns shown here.

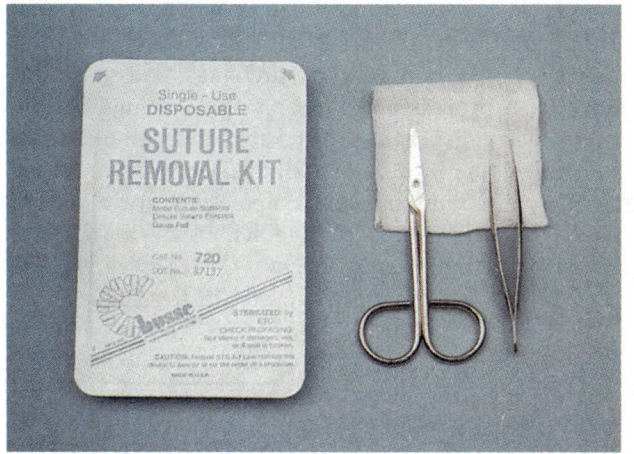

FIGURE 24-12
Suture removal kit.

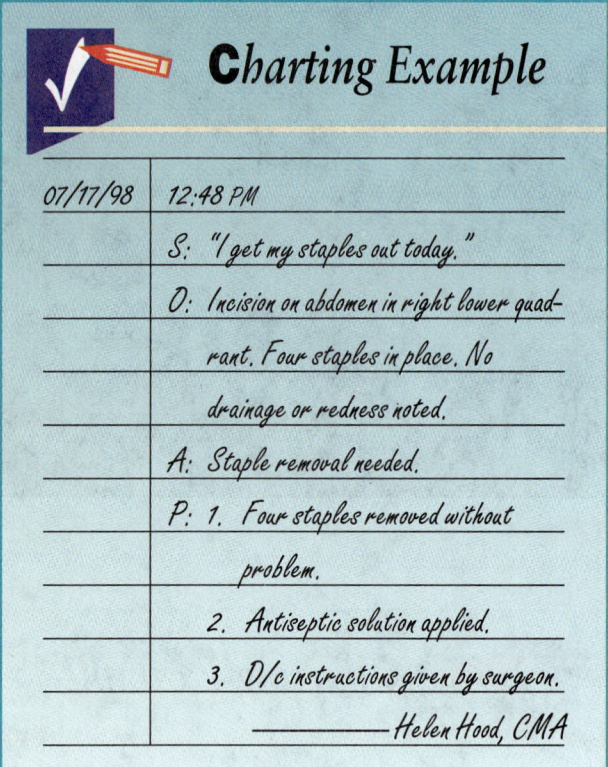

Charting Example

07/17/98	12:48 PM
	S: "I get my staples out today."
	O: Incision on abdomen in right lower quadrant. Four staples in place. No drainage or redness noted.
	A: Staple removal needed.
	P: 1. Four staples removed without problem.
	2. Antiseptic solution applied.
	3. D/c instructions given by surgeon.
	———— Helen Hood, CMA

be removed safely and need to return to the physician's office for their removal. Frequently it will be your responsibility to remove the staples. Most offices use staple removal kits similar to the kits supplied for suture removal. These include a special instrument for removing the staples rather than thumb forceps and suture scissors included in the suture removal kits. Some offices will assemble equipment on site (Procedure 24-6).

➤ STERILE DRESSINGS

Sterile dressings are items such as 4 × 4 absorbent gauze sponges, non-adhering dressings, and so on that have been processed for use on open wounds. Sterile dressings are generally prepackaged in small quantities but may come in bulk containers. They are manufactured in different sizes and shapes, each for a specific use. Dressings should be handled using sterile technique to maintain their sterility. Procedure 24-7 describes the steps for applying a sterile dressing.

A sterile dressing is considered contaminated, or unsterile, when it is damp or wet, its wrapper is damaged, it is outdated, or it is removed improperly from its wrapper or container. Sterile dressings are used directly over a wound to:

1. Cover and protect from contamination
2. Absorb drainage such as blood, serum, pus

3. Exert pressure (eg, direct pressure on an open wound to slow bleeding)
4. Hide disfigurement during the healing process
5. Hold medications against the wound to facilitate healing

A sterile dressing may be accompanied by various bandages (sling, cravat, roller, tubular gauze) to hold the dressing in place, protect the injured part, or restrict movement.
When you remove a sterile dressing or change an existing one (Procedure 24-8), carefully observe for any drainage or exudate and note this in the patient's chart (Box 24-1). Notify the physician when the wound is uncovered so that it can be examined and a decision made regarding appropriate healing. Box 24-2 discusses the types and phases of wound healing.

Checkpoint Question
6. When are sterile dressings used?

➤ BANDAGING

Bandages are strips of woven materials. Typically absorbent, they are used for many purposes, including:

1. Applying pressure to control bleeding
2. Holding a dressing in place
3. Protecting dressings and wounds from contamination
4. Immobilizing an injured part of the body
5. Supporting an injured part of the body

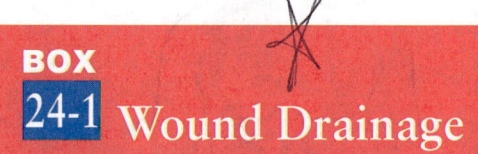

BOX 24-1 Wound Drainage

When observing wound drainage, be sure to note:

Color
- Serous (clear)
- Sanguinous (blood-tinged)
- Serosanguinous (pinkish or clear and red mixed)
- Purulent (white, green, or yellow-tinged drainage; usually has an unpleasant odor characteristic of infection)

Amount
- Copious (large amount)
- Medium (moderate amount)
- Scant (small amount)

BOX

24-2 **The Healing Process**

Types of Wound Healing

• *Healing by Primary Intention:* This simplest form of healing results from wounds that are closely approximated, allowing the entrance of little or no bacteria to complicate the process. The edges of the wound lie closely together, new cells form quickly to bind the site, and capillaries expand themselves across the tissue break to restore circulation to the tissues. There is usually little scarring.

• *Healing by Secondary Intention:* Granulation of tissue is present and the edges of the wound join indirectly. Because the area is not closely approximated, additional new cells are required to fill spaces in the lesion. Capillaries may not be able to reach across the gap to restore full circulation. Nerves may not rejoin, which results in diminished nerve stimulus through the area. A large scab forms to protect the area while healing goes on below it. Scarring is more severe than with Primary Intention Healing.

• *Healing by Tertiary Intention:* The wound initially is left open to fill in with granular tissue, then sutured at a later time. There is considerable scar formation.

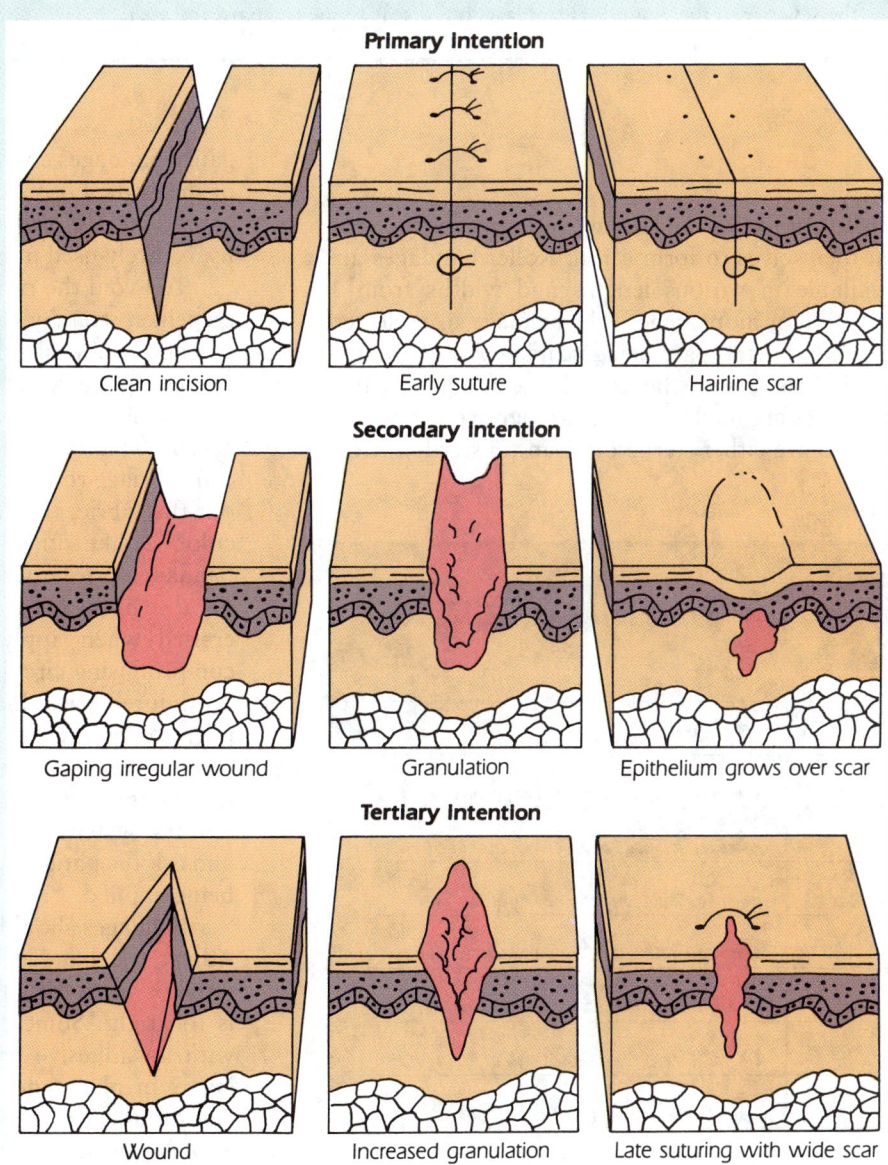

Primary Intention

Clean incision   Early suture   Hairline scar

Secondary Intention

Gaping irregular wound   Granulation   Epithelium grows over scar

Tertiary Intention

Wound   Increased granulation   Late suturing with wide scar

Types of wound healing.

continued

BOX 24-2 The Healing Process *(Continued)*

Phases of Wound Healing

- *Phase I (inflammatory, lag, or exudative phase)*: This phase usually lasts from 1 to 4 days. The body attempts to heal itself by increasing the circulation to the part and by beginning to reroute or repair the supplying vessels. The increased circulation brings with it more white blood cells to mount a defense against pathogens. Serum and red blood cells brought by the additional blood form a gluelike fibrin to plug the wound. As the fibrin dries, it pulls the edges of the wound closer together and forms a scab. Signs that this phase is working are edema from the tissue fluid, warmth from the extra blood, redness from the vasodilation, and pain from the pressure on the nerve endings caused by the edema.
- *Phase II (proliferative, healing, or granulation phase)*: This phase may last from several days to several weeks. The vessels continue to repair themselves and may reroute if damage is severe. The scab from phase I continues to dry and to pull the edges as closely together as possible.
- *Phase III (remodeling, maturation, or scarring phase)*: This phase may take from weeks to years, depending on the severity of the wound. Fibroblasts build scar tissue to guard the area.

Types of Bandages

- *Roller bandages* are soft woven materials wound on themselves to form a roll. Roller bandages are available in various lengths and widths from 1 inch to 6 or more inches. The bandage size selected depends on the part being bandaged and the desired thickness of the completed bandage. Most bandages are made of a porous, lightweight material and are either sterile or clean (unsterile). Most gauze bandages conform easily to angular surfaces of the body. Loosely woven standard cotton roller gauze, which is not stretchy and the edges fray easily, is rarely used in offices today.

   To avoid the problems of plain roller gauze, a crepelike, stretchy gauze is made to adjust to various body contours and resists unrolling much better than plain roller gauze. Kling or Conform are two brand names that are frequently used.
- *Elastic bandages*, such as the Ace brand, are special bandage rolls that have elastic woven throughout the fabric; they are generally brownish-tan in color. Unlike other types of roller gauze, elastic bandages can be washed and reused many times. Because of the elastic fibers, great care must be exercised when applying the bandage to prevent compromising circulation and still give support to the injured part. Elastic bandages should be applied so that there is no wrinkling of the concentric layers. Never stretch or pull on the elastic bandage during application to avoid applying it too tightly. Always watch for signs of impaired circulation and ask the patient for comments as the bandage is being applied.

   Bandages should fit snugly but not too tightly. Adjust the bandage accordingly if it seems too loose or when the patient expresses discomfort if it is too tight. Some elastic bandages are available with an adhesive backing, which helps keep the layers in place and provides a secure, snug, and comfortable fit.
- *Tubular gauze bandages* are used to enclose rounded body parts. The bandage resembles a hollow tube and is woven to give it an extremely

Charting Example

08/31/98	1:30 PM	Patient arrived in the office for sterile dressing change. Dressing was removed without problem. Ulcerated wound noted on right heel. Yellow drainage noted. Culture taken and physician notified. Wound cleansed with antiseptic solution. Sterile dressing applied. Patient to return in AM for dressing change.
		— Fran Williams, CMA

stretchy quality. It is used to enclose fingers, toes, arms, and legs and even the head and trunk. Tubular gauze bandages are available in various widths from 5/8 inch to 7 inches to fit any part of the body.

Tubular gauze is applied using a metal or plastic tubular framelike applicator. The applicator is available in various sizes and should be slightly larger than the body part to be covered. This enables the gauze to slide easily over the body part. Applicators are marked according to a size number that corresponds to the boxes of different size tubular gauze. Procedure 24-9 discusses the specific steps for applying a tubular gauze bandage.

Bandage Application Guidelines

When properly applied, bandages should feel comfortably snug and should be fastened securely enough to remain in place until removed. Bandages can be fastened with safety pins, adhesive tape, or clips, such as those supplied with elastic bandages. A patient's confidence in your professional ability is greatly enhanced when a bandage is applied that is comfortable, neat looking, and stays in place. Patients become understandably upset when bandages fall off through normal use. Below are general guidelines for applying bandages.

1. Observe the principles of medical asepsis to prevent the transfer of pathogens. Surgical asepsis is not necessary; the bandage may be used on the outside to cover a sterile dressing or may be used alone in cases where there is no open wound.
2. Keep the area to be bandaged and the bandage itself dry and clean because moisture may wick bacteria onto the area of concern. A moist bandage, which also encourages the growth of pathogens, will be uncomfortable for the patient.
3. Never place bandages directly over a wound. Sterile dressings are applied first and then are covered with a bandage for protection. The bandage should extend approximately 1–2 inches beyond the edge of the dressing.
4. Never allow skin surfaces of two body parts to touch each other because wound healing may cause opposing surfaces to adhere and result in scar tissue formation. For example, burned fingers are each dressed separately, but may be bandaged together.
5. Pad joints and any bony prominence to help prevent skin irritation caused by the bandage rubbing against the skin over a bony area.
6. Bandage the affected part in the normal position: joints should be slightly flexed to avoid muscle strain, discomfort, or pain. Otherwise, muscle

spasms may occur if the limb is made to assume an unnatural position.
7. Apply bandages beginning at the distal part and extending to the proximal part of the body. Bandage turns that extend distal to proximal aid in the return of venous blood to the heart and help make the bandage more secure.
8. Always communicate with the patient. If the patient complains that the bandage is too tight or too loose, adjust the bandage. The bandage should fit snugly, but if it is too tight it may impair circulation. If it is too loose, it may fall off.
9. When bandaging hands and feet, leave the fingers and toes exposed whenever possible to make it easier to check for circulatory impairment. If there is coldness, pallor, or cyanosis of the nail beds; or pain, swelling, numbness, or tingling of the toes or fingers, the bandage should be removed immediately and reapplied correctly.

Figure 24-13 illustrates various techniques for wrapping bandages.

Montgomery Straps

Surgical patients who are discharged from the hospital with draining wounds that will require frequent dressing changes will probably be dressed with Montgomery straps. This type of bandage consists of opposing pairs of straps, or tapes, with gauze ties that cross over thick layers of absorbent dressings (Fig. 24-14). When the dressings are soiled, the ties are loosened, the soiled dressings removed, and new dressings applied. The adhesive tapes, or straps, are not removed unless grossly soiled. Montgomery straps have many advantages over conventional dressings and bandages for the heavily draining wound, including ease of dressing change and maintenance of skin integrity at the operative site.

Checkpoint Question
7. When applying a bandage, at which end of the extremity must you begin? Why?

➤ COMMONLY PERFORMED OFFICE SURGICAL PROCEDURES

Two of the most frequently performed minor surgeries in the general medical office are the excision of skin lesions (moles, lentigines, keratoses, and skin tags) and the incision and drainage of abscesses. Incisions may be closed with sutures or may be left to heal without

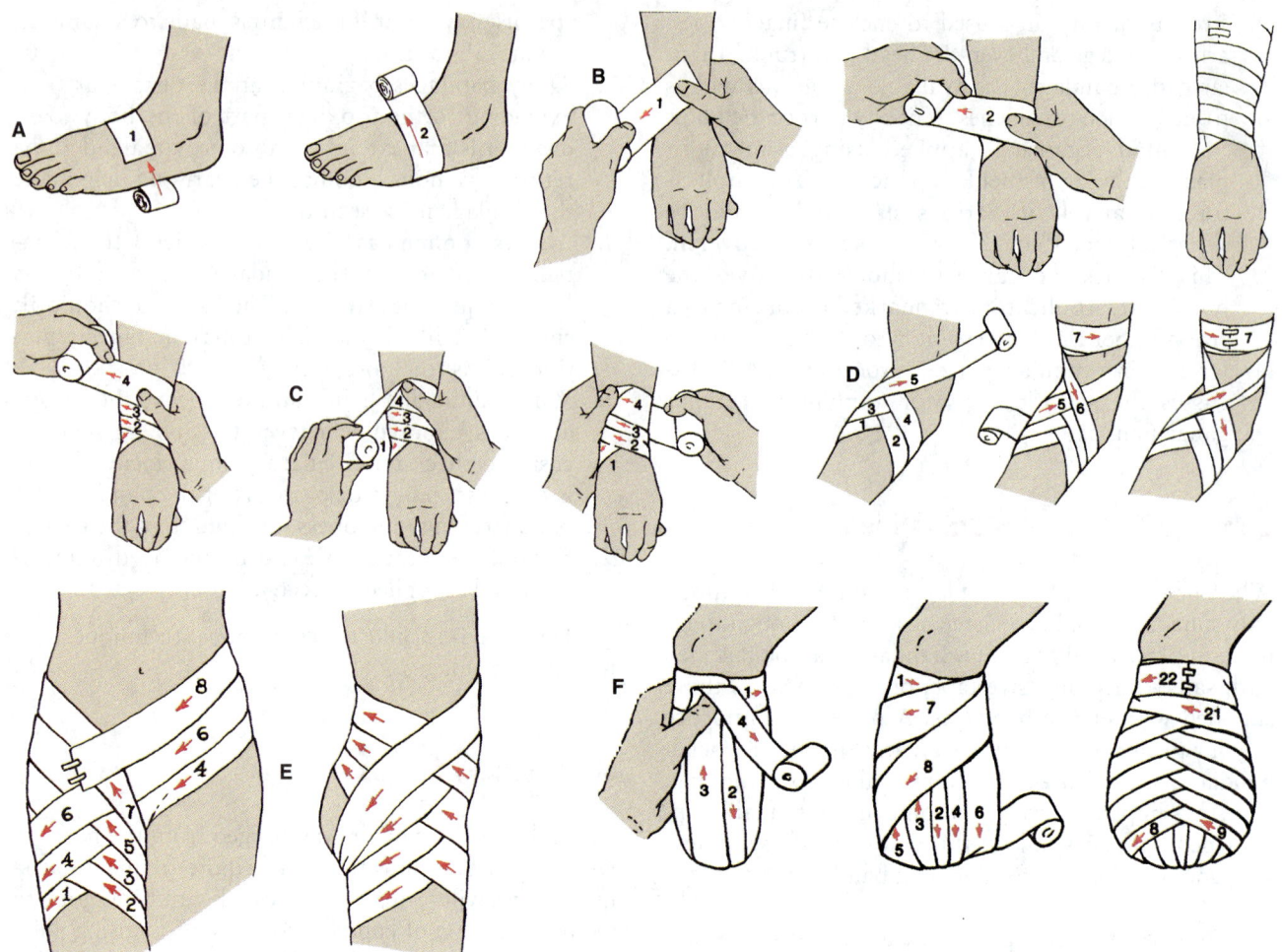

FIGURE 24-13
There are six basic techniques for wrapping a roller bandage. (A) A *circular turn* is used to anchor and secure a bandage when it is started and ended. It simply involves holding the free end
of the rolled material in one hand and wrapping it about the area, bringing it back to the starting point. (B) A *spiral turn* partly overlaps a previous turn. The overlapping varies from one-
half to three-fourths of the width of the bandage. Spiral turns are used when wrapping a cylindrical part of the body like the arms and legs. (C) A *spiral-reverse turn* is a modification of a
spiral turn. The roll is reversed halfway through the turn. This works well on tapered body
parts. (D) A *figure-of-eight turn* is best used when an area spanning a joint, like the elbow or
knee, requires bandaging. It is made by making oblique turns that alternately ascend and descend, simulating the number "8". (E) A *spica turn* is a variation of the figure-of-eight turn. It
differs in that the wrap includes a portion of the trunk or chest. (F) The *recurrent turn* is made
by passing the roll back and forth over the tip of a body part. Once several recurrent turns
have been made, the bandage is anchored by completing the application with another basic
turn like the figure-of-eight. A recurrent turn is especially beneficial when wrapping the stump
of an amputated limb.

interference depending on the size and position of the
wound. Surgical setups may be purchased prepackaged
with many of the supplies needed for minor excisional
procedures. Supplies listed with the procedures are
site-prepared and include sutures. Standard Precautions must be followed when assisting with these procedures.

Excision of a Lesion

Physicians may excise lesions with electrocautery (see
below) or with standard surgical equipment (Procedure
24-10). If the lesion does not require analysis, it can be
desiccated or fulgurated (see below). Many lesions are
referred to pathology for diagnosis after excision.

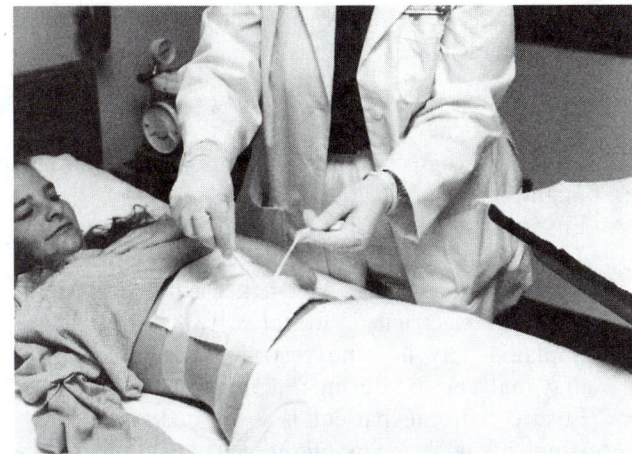

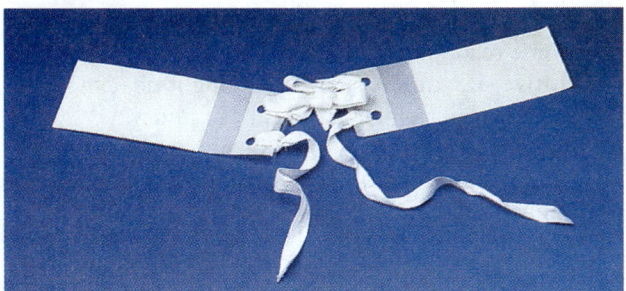

FIGURE 24-14
Montgomery straps or ties are used to prevent skin breakdown from frequent tape removal when dressings need to be changed often.

Incision and Drainage (I&D)

An abscess is a localized collection of pus in a cavity surrounded by inflamed tissue. It is the body's response to an infectious process when pathogens have entered through a break in the skin. Abscesses may be referred to as boils, furuncles (one lesion), or carbuncles (several lesions grouped closely together) and are very painful. The site must be incised and the infected material drained before healing can take place (Procedure 24-11).

➤ ELECTROSURGERY

Electrosurgery uses high-frequency, alternating electric current to destroy or cut and remove tissue. It is also used to **coagulate** small bleeding vessels. Electrosurgery is considered an alternative to traditional office surgery and is rapidly gaining favor for many procedures. An advantage of electrical surgery is the cautery effect produced by the electricity that seals small bleeding vessels and coagulates nearby cells to reduce bleeding and loss of cell fluid. Electrosurgical units use disposable **electrodes** (medium for conducting electrical current) tips of different sizes and shapes to deliver the desired amount of electric current to the tissues (Fig. 24-15).

The following procedures are considered to be electrosurgery:

- *Fulguration* destroys tissue using controlled electric sparks. As the physician holds the electrode tip 1–2 mm away from the site, a series of sparks destroys the superficial cells at the site.
- *Electrodesiccation* dries and separates tissue using an electric current. In this procedure, the electrode is placed directly on the site.
- *Electrocautery* causes quick coagulation of small blood vessels with the heat created by the electric

---

Charting Example

03/15/98	11:00 AM Patient arrived in the office with an abscess on left hand, third digit. Finger was prepped by the physician. Abscess was I & D. Patient tolerated procedure well. Tubular gauze dressing applied. Patient instructed to return for wound check in 3 days. Written instructions given to patient. Patient verbalized understanding of all instructions. ——Paula Abbe, RMA

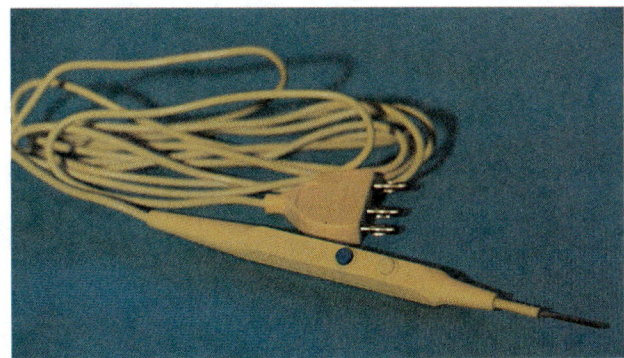

FIGURE 24-15
A disposable electrosurgical unit. The blade is designed to either cut or cauterize.

Patient Education: Instructions Following Minor Surgery

After minor surgery, instruct patients to report the following conditions:

- Excessive bleeding (additional teaching should include how to stop bleeding, eg, direct pressure, elevation)
- Redness, red streaks, or excessive swelling in the area
- Temperature elevation

Also explain that dressings must be kept clean and dry. If the dressing is to be changed, include instructions for dressing changes. Finally, make sure the patient understands the date, time, and place of suture or staple removal.

current. Electrocautery is commonly referred to as electrocoagulation.

- *Electrosection* is used for incision or excision of tissue. There is minimal bleeding with this type of procedure, but more damage can occur to surrounding tissues.

Medical offices frequently use electrosurgery to remove moles, cysts, warts, and certain types of skin and cervical cancers. Electrosurgical equipment includes various electrode tips, such as blades, needles, loops, and balls, each having specific uses.

During electrosurgery, your responsibilities are to ensure the safety and comfort of the patient and to pass the electrode to the physician as needed. As with all instruments, the electrode must be passed in its functional position. The electrode is handed with the tip in a downward position.

Safety Measures

Because electric current is delivered to the tip by the electrosurgical machine, great care should be exercised to prevent injuries. Although the device is always activated by the physician, it is possible to cause injury to the patient, physician, or medical assistant if the device is handled carelessly. Care must be taken to ground the patient before electrosurgery. Metal conducts electricity and can cause serious

burns. When assisting with electrosurgery, follow these safety measures:

- Ensure that all working parts are in good repair. The electrical current is carefully regulated; if the machine is defective, serious injury to the patient might occur.
- Ensure that all metal is removed from the patient. The patient must be asked if metal implants are present or if a cardiac pacemaker is in place. Metal conducts electricity and can cause burns. Metal implants may become very hot and pacemakers may malfunction during the procedure.
- Ensure that the patient is grounded with a pad supplied by the manufacturer. This should be attached at a site recommended by the manufacturer (some recommend placing the pad far from the operative site; others suggest placing it near the site). Improper placement can result in injury.
- Place the grounding pad firmly and completely against the patient's skin. A conducting gel must be applied to the pad and to the patient's skin or an adhesive-backed pad can be used to facilitate conduction through the grounding pad. Areas of skin against the pad that are not well connected will result in "hot spots" and may burn the patient.

Care of Equipment

Although tips in use today are usually disposable, reusable tips are still used in some offices. Reusable tips are processed in the autoclave. Reusable tips may be polished with steel wool if they become dull. Disposable tips should be discarded after use. Electrosurgical machines should be inspected periodically to ensure they are in good working order. The operating manual will suggest periods of maintenance to be performed by office staff and routine inspections by technicians trained to avoid potential malfunctions. Surfaces should be kept clean and dry; machines should be kept covered when not in use.

Checkpoint Question

8. Which type of electrosurgery is used for incision or excision of tissue?

➤ LASER SURGERY

Lasers are devices that focus high intensity light in a narrow beam to create extreme heat and energy. In medicine, lasers can be used to cut tissue and coagulate small bleeding vessels. There are many types of lasers, each with fairly specific applications in medicine. The more common types of lasers encountered in the medical office include:

- Argon laser—used for coagulation
- Carbon dioxide (CO_2) laser—used for cutting tissue
- Nd:YAG—used for coagulation and to separate warts and moles from surrounding tissues

Light from the laser is not usually visible. Colored filters are used to illuminate the laser's target, enabling the physician to direct the light to the affected area.

As with other electronic devices used in the medical offices, attention to care and handling of the laser will ensure that it is in good working order when it is needed. It is important to read and follow the manufacturer's recommended maintenance procedures described in the instruction manual that accompanies the equipment.

Everyone who is in the room while the procedure is in progress is required to wear goggles for eye protection. It is generally recommended that health care workers complete a training program before assisting with laser procedures to ensure that safety precautions are followed.

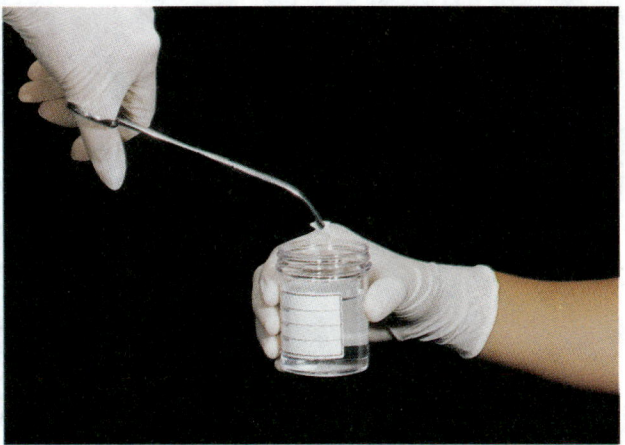

FIGURE 24-16
Tissue samples are placed in preservative by the physician.

➤ SPECIMEN COLLECTION DURING OFFICE SURGERY

Many minor office surgical procedures yield specimens that must be referred to a laboratory to be examined by a pathologist. Specimens include samples of tissue, wound exudate, foreign bodies, and so on.

The medical assistant usually chooses the proper container with the appropriate **preservative** (substance that delays decomposition) for the type of procedure being performed. The open container must be held steady to avoid touching the sides of the container as the physician drops the specimen into the preservative (Fig. 24-16).

The medical assistant is usually responsible for labeling the pathology request form with the correct patient and specimen data. Laboratory request forms usually require information such as patient name, age, sex, identification number or Social Security number, date, type of specimen to be examined, type of laboratory examination requested, and the physician's name or laboratory contract number. Specimens must be transported to the pathology laboratory as quickly as possible.

➤ POSTSURGICAL PROCEDURES

In preparation for the next patient, all used equipment must be discarded properly or transported to the equipment room for the sanitizing process before sterilization. The room must be cleaned as part of the procedure. Always put on gloves for environmental cleaning.

"Low-level disinfection" procedures should be followed as part of routine housekeeping between each patient use of the examining rooms to reduce the opportunity for cross-contamination between patients using the examination room. (See Chap. 19, Asepsis and Infection Control, for more information about levels of infection control.) Examining rooms should always be inspected prior to each use to ensure that the area has been properly cleaned after the previous patient.

Cleaning the Examination Table

Papers and sheets should be removed in a rolling movement so outside surfaces cover the interior of the bundle. Table covers and sheets should not come into contact with your clothing. Discard the sheets and covers appropriately. The surfaces of the table should be wiped down with an approved disinfectant solution and allowed to dry. Replace the covers and sheets for the next patient.

Cleaning the Operative Area

The surgical stand, sink, counter, examining table, and other surfaces used during the procedure should be wiped down with an approved disinfectant solution and allowed to dry before re-use. When environmental disinfection procedures are completed, examine the room with a critical eye to be sure that it is neat, clean, and ready for the next patient. Box 24-3 discusses proper waste disposal.

text continues on page 412

BOX 24-3 Proper Waste Disposal

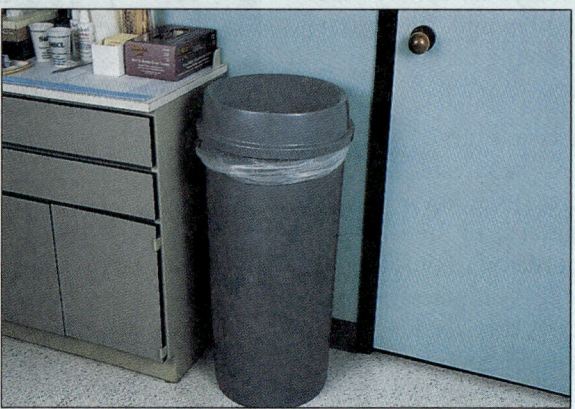

Regular waste container.

A regular waste container should only be used for disposal of "clean" waste material, such as paper, plastic, disposable tray wrapper, suture, unused gauze, or examining table paper liner. Small amounts of fluids, such as that poured off prior to adding a sterile solution to a sterile set-up, may also be disposed of here. To prevent leakage, large amounts of uncontaminated fluid should be discarded in the wash basin, not in plastic bags. NEVER discard sharps of any kind in plastic bags; these are not puncture resistant and injury may result even from careful handling. Bags should not be filled to capacity. When the plastic bag is about two thirds full it should be removed from its holder, the top edges brought together and secured with a twist tie. Remove the bag from the examining room and follow office procedure for disposal.

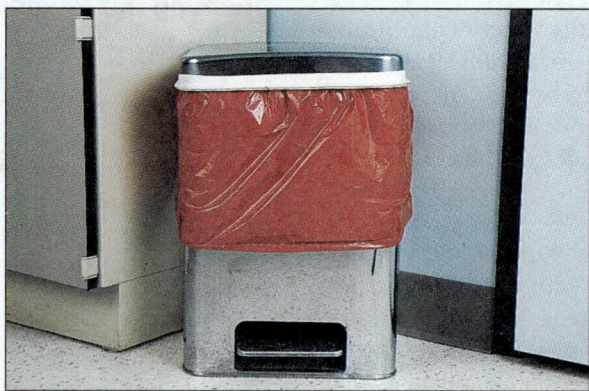

Biohazard waste container.

A biohazard waste container is reserved for the disposal of contaminated waste only. Such waste includes soiled dressings and bandages, soiled examining table paper, cotton balls, swabs, applicators, alcohol swabs, and gloves that have become soiled with, or exposed to, blood or body fluids. Other items that should be discarded in this type of container are used catheters or drains, wound packing, sutures, staples, orthopedic type pins, soiled tampons and sanitary napkins, ostomy bags, and any other object contaminated with blood or body fluids of any sort.

Procedure 24-1

Opening Sterile Surgical Packs

Equipment/Supplies

- surgical pack
- surgical stand

Steps	**Purpose**
1. Check the surgical procedure to be performed. Remove the appropriate tray or item from the storage area. Check the label for contents and expiration date. Check for tears or areas of moisture.	1. Packages that have passed the expiration date should not be used. Areas that have tears or are moist will contaminate the contents of the package.
2. Place the package, with the label facing up, on a clean, dry, flat surface, such as a Mayo or surgical stand.	2. Even though the field will be protected by a barrier undersurface, microorganisms must be kept at a minimum by using an area as free of pathogens as possible. The surgical stand makes it easy to move the field for the physician's convenience.
3. Without tearing the wrapper, carefully remove the sealing tape. If the package is commercially prepared, carefully remove the outer protective wrapper.	3. Many disposable packages are wrapped in a barrier wrap that will become the sterile field when properly opened. They are then sealed in see-through plastic film. Packages prepared in the medical office will be sealed using tape designed to indicate that the package has been through the autoclave procedure.
4. Loosen the first flap of the folded wrapper. Open the first flap by pulling it up, out and away; let it fall over the far side of the table.	4. By doing this, you avoid having to reach across the field again.

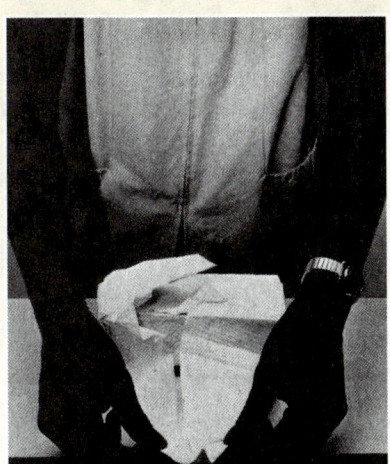

Step 4: Open the first flap.

5. Open the side flaps in a similar manner using the left hand for the left flap; right hand for right flap. Touch only the unsterile outer surface; do not touch the sterile inner surface.	5. This decreases movement over the sterile areas of the package.

Note: If it is necessary to leave the area after opening the field, cover the tray and its contents with a sterile drape. Also, discard any commercially wrapped items that are not used for the sterile procedure for which they were opened.

(continued)

Procedure 24-1   Opening Sterile Surgical Packs (continued)

Steps   **Purpose**

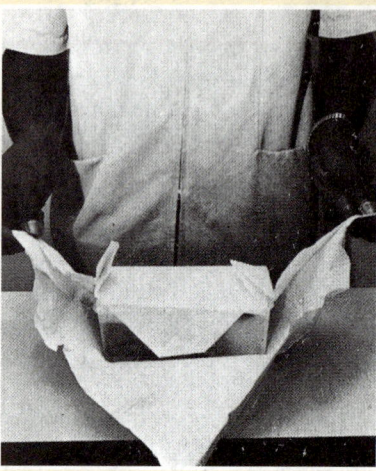

Step 5: Open the side flaps.

6. Pull the remaining flap down and toward you by grasping the unsterile outside surface only. By carefully following steps 3 through 5, the unsterile surface of the wrapper is now against the surgical stand; the sterile inside surface of the wrapper forms the sterile field.

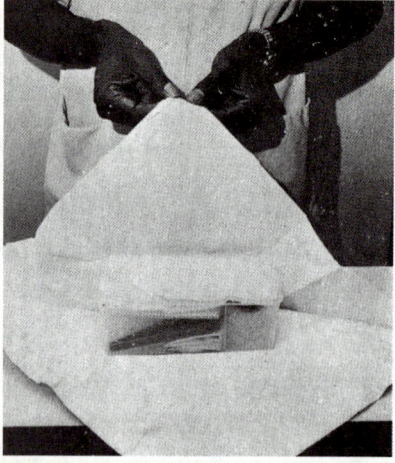

Step 6: Pull the remaining flap down and toward you.

7. Repeat steps 4 through 6 for packages with a second or inside wrapper. This sterile inside wrapper also provides a sterile field upon which to work. The field is now ready for additional supplies as needed or is ready for the procedure to begin.

Procedure 24-2 — Using Sterile Transfer Forceps

Equipment/Supplies
- forceps and container
- item(s) to be transferred

Steps	Purpose
1. Slowly lift the forceps straight up out of the container without touching the inside above the level of the solution or the outside of the container.	1. The area above the soaking solution and the rim are considered unsterile.
2. Hold the forceps with the tips down.	2. This avoids having the solution run toward the unsterile handles and then back to the grasping blades and tips, thus contaminating them.
3. Keep the forceps above waist level.	3. This prevents accidental and unnoticed contamination.
4. Pick up the article to be transferred and drop it onto the sterile field so that the forceps does not come in contact with the sterile field.	4. The forceps may still be moist from the soaking solution, which may cause microorganisms to wick from the surface below the sterile field.

Note: *Sterile transfer forceps that have been wrapped and autoclaved may be placed with tips on the sterile field with handles extending beyond the 1-inch contaminated perimeter. Doing this allows you to move objects around the field for the physician's convenience.*

Procedure 24-3 — Adding Sterile Solution to the Field

Equipment/Supplies
- container of sterile solution
- sterile set up

Steps	Purpose
1. As with any drug or medication, identify the correct solution by carefully READING THE LABEL.	1. The label should be checked three times to avoid errors: when taking the container from the shelf, before pouring the solution, and when returning the container to the shelf.
2. Check for an expiration date on the label; do not use the solution if it is out of date, if the label cannot be read, or if the solution appears abnormal. *Note:* Sterile water and saline bottles must be dated when opened and must be discarded if not used within 48 hours.	2. Out-of-date solutions may have changed chemically and deteriorated, and are no longer considered sterile.
3. If you are adding medications into the solution (eg, Xylocaine, a local anesthetic), show the medication label to the physician now.	3. This allows for verification of the contents.
4. Remove the cap or stopper. Hold the cap with the fingertips, with the cap opening facing downward,	4. If the cap becomes contaminated and is returned to the bottle, the contents are considered contami-

(continued)

Procedure 24-3   Adding Sterile Solution to the Field (continued)

Steps

to prevent accidental contamination of the inside. If it is necessary to put the cap down, place it with the opened end facing up. If you are pouring the entire contents of the container onto the sterile field, the cap may be discarded. Retain the bottle to keep track of amount added to the field and for charting purposes later. It can then be discarded.

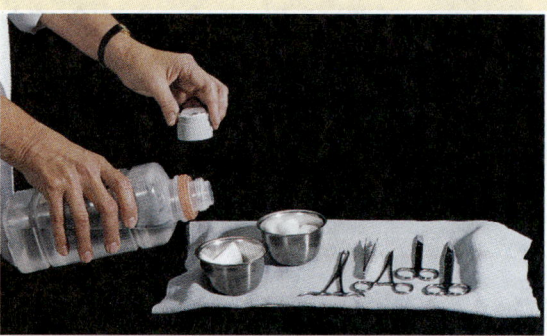

Step 4: Hold the cap facing downward to prevent contamination of the inside.

5. Grasp the container so that the label is facing the palm of the hand ("palm the label").

6. Pour a small amount of the solution into a separate container or waste receptacle.

7. Carefully and slowly pour the desired amount of solution into the sterile container from not less than 4 inches and not more than 6 inches above the container. The bottle of solution should never touch the sterile container or tray as this will cause contamination.

8. After pouring the desired amount of solution into the sterile container, recheck the label for contents and expiration date and replace the cap carefully to avoid touching the bottle rim with any unsterile surface of the cap.

9. Return the solution to its proper storage area and recheck the label again.

Purpose

nated. Placing the cap on a surface with the opening facing upward prevents contamination of the interior of the cap.

5. If solution runs down the side of the bottle in this position, it will not obscure the label.

6. The lip of the bottle is considered contaminated; pouring off this small amount cleanses the bottle lip.

7. Pouring the solution slowly reduces the chance of splashing and over-filling. Solution poured too quickly or from an improper height may splash. Touching the container to objects on the sterile field contaminates the field. If the solution splashes onto the field, a wicking action will cause contamination from the surface below.

8. This ensures accuracy. Careful replacement of the cap ensures that the contents remain sterile.

9. This ensures accuracy.

Procedure 24-4

Performing Hair Removal and Skin Preparation

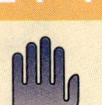

Equipment/Supplies

- nonsterile gloves
- shave cream or lotion
- new razor
- gauze or cotton balls and warm rinse water
- antiseptic
- sponge forceps

Note: Commercially packaged skin preparation kits are available with most of the listed items provided. Gloves must be worn for shaving to prevent contact with blood or body fluids if nicks or cuts occur. If the skin is not to be shaved, you will need only antiseptic solution, gauze or cotton balls, or antiseptic wipes.

Steps	Purpose
1. Wash your hands.	1. Handwashing aids infection control.
2. Assemble the equipment.	2. This ensures that all supplies are available. A new razor must be used for each patient to avoid the transmission of pathogens and to ensure the closest possible shave.
3. Greet and identify the patient. Explain the procedure and answer any questions.	3. This avoids errors in treatment, helps gain patient compliance, and eases anxiety.
4. Put on gloves.	4. Standard Precautions must be observed when contact with blood or body fluids is possible.
5. Prepare the patient's skin.	5.
a. If the patient's skin is to be shaved, apply shaving cream or soapy lather to the area to be shaved. Pull the skin taut and shave by pulling the razor across the skin in the direction of hair growth. Repeat this procedure until all hair is removed from the operative area. Rinse and pat the shaved area thoroughly dry using a gauze square.	a. Shaving cream or soapy lather on the skin reduces friction and helps prevent scratching the skin. Shaving in the direction in which the hair grows gives the closest shave while reducing the chance of nicking the skin. Rinsing removes soap residue and hair from the shaved area. Pat dry rather than rub to prevent abrasions. Using gauze squares for drying picks up stray hairs that might have been left behind during rinsing.
b. If the patient's skin is not to be shaved, rinse away any soapy solution used for general cleaning and dry the skin before applying antiseptic solution to avoid diluting the antiseptic.	
6. Apply antiseptic solution of the physician's choice to the skin surrounding the operative area using sterile gauze sponges, sterile cotton balls, or antiseptic wipes. With the gauze or cotton ball grasped in the sterile sponge forceps, wipe the skin in circular motions starting at the operative site and working outward. Discard each sponge after a complete sweep has been made. If the area is large or circles are not appropriate, the sponge may be wiped straight outward from the operative site, then discarded and the procedure repeated until the entire area has been thoroughly cleaned. At no time should a wipe that has passed over the skin be returned to the already cleaned area or to the antiseptic solution.	6. Discarding sponges after each stroke prevents contamination of the wound by microorganisms brought back to the area from the surrounding skin.

(continued)

Procedure 24-4 | Performing Hair Removal and Skin Preparation *(continued)*

Steps	Purpose
7. With dry sterile gauze sponges grasped in the sponge forceps, pat the area thoroughly dry. In some instances, the area may be allowed to air dry.	7. If the area is moist, the sterile drapes may become wet also, causing wicking to contaminate the operative site.
8. Instruct the patient not to touch or cover the prepared area.	8. This avoids contaminating the operative site, which would require repeating the procedure.
9. Drape the prepared area for the procedure or cover it with sterile drapes if the procedure will be delayed for a short time. Longer delays may require reapplication of the antiseptic solution.	

Procedure 24-5 | Removing Sutures

Equipment/Supplies

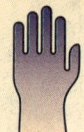

- thumb forceps
- antiseptic
- suture scissors
- sterile gloves
- gauze

Note: Sterile, disposable suture removal kits contain all of the needed equipment.

Steps	Purpose
1. Wash your hands.	1. Handwashing aids infection control.
2. Assemble the equipment.	2. This ensures that all supplies are available.
3. Greet and identify the patient. Explain the procedure and answer any questions.	3. This avoids errors in treatment, helps gain patient compliance, and eases anxiety.
4. If dressings have not been removed previously, do so (see Procedure 24-8). Properly dispose of dressings. Then clean the wound area as directed.	4. The skin must be as free of pathogens as possible before the removal of the sutures to prevent contamination of the wound.
5. Open the suture removal packet using surgical asepsis or set up a field for on-site sterile equipment. Put on sterile gloves.	5. Suture removal is a sterile procedure.
6. Note that the knots will be tied in such a way that one tail of the knot will be very close to the surface of the skin while the other will be closer to the area of suture that is looped over the incision.	
a. Grasp the end of the knot that is closest to the skin surface and lift, slightly and gently, up from the skin.	
b. Cut the suture below the knot as close to the skin as possible.	b. Cutting below the knot and close to the skin frees the knot at an area that has not been exposed to the outside surface of the body. The only part of the suture that will pull

(continued)

Removing Sutures (continued)

Steps	Purpose

through the tissues will be the suture that was under the skin surface.

c. Use the thumb forceps to pull the suture out of the skin with a smooth, continuous motion at a slight angle in the direction of the wound.

c. This avoids tension on the healing tissue.

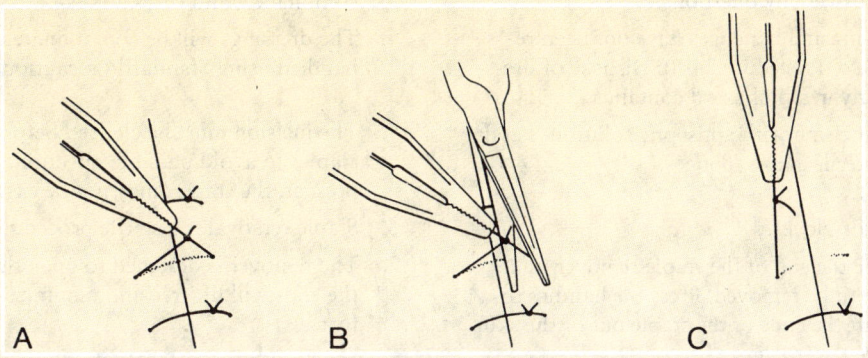

Step 6: (A) With the hemostat or forceps, lift the stitch upward and away from the skin surface. This permits the blades of the scissors to slide under the stitch (B) Cut the stitch near the skin. (C) Using the forceps, pull the freed stitch up and out.

7. Place the suture on a gauze sponge. Repeat the procedure for each suture.

7. This helps in counting the number removed; if six sutures previously inserted are now to be removed, there should be six sutures on the gauze sponge at the end of the procedure.

8. Clean the site with an antiseptic solution and, if the physician has indicated, cover with a sterile dressing.

8. Some wounds need to be protected for a while longer; some wounds will have healed well enough to be left uncovered.

9. Thank the patient and give appropriate instructions.

9. Courtesy encourages the patient to have a positive attitude about the physician's office.

10. Properly care for or dispose of equipment and supplies. Clean the work area. Remove gloves and wash your hands.

10. Standard Precautions must be followed.

11. Record the procedure, including the time, location of sutures, the number removed, and the condition of the wound.

11. Procedures are considered not to have been done if they are not recorded.

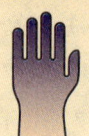

Procedure 24-6   Removing Staples

Equipment/Supplies

- antiseptic solution or wipes
- gauze squares
- sponge forceps
- instrument for removing staples
- sterile gloves

Steps	Purpose
1. Wash your hands.	1. Handwashing aids infection control.
2. Assemble the equipment.	2. This ensures that all supplies are available.
3. Greet and identify the patient. Explain the procedure and answer any questions.	3. This avoids errors in treatment, helps gain patient compliance, and eases anxiety.
4. If the dressing and bandages have not been removed, do so (Procedure 24-8). Dispose of dressings properly in a biohazard container.	4. The dressings will be contaminated and must be handled using Standard Precautions.
5. Clean the incision with antiseptic solution. Pat dry using dry sterile gauze sponges.	5. The incision must be cleaned before removing the staples to avoid possible infection. If exudate was present, the staples may not be easily visualized.
6. Put on sterile gloves.	6. Staple removal is a sterile procedure.
7. Gently slide the end of the staple remover under each staple to be removed. Press the handles together to lift the ends of the staple out of the skin and remove the staple.	7. The remover is designed to open the staple so that the ends will lift free and minimize patient discomfort.

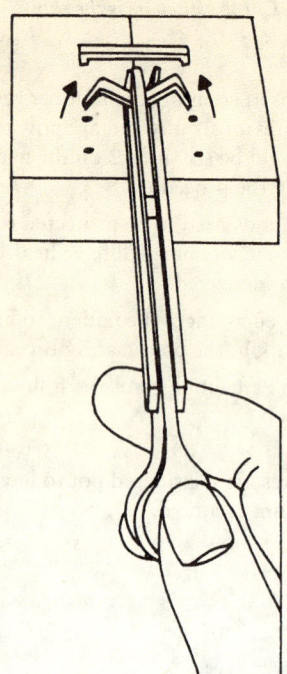

Step 7: Slide the end of the staple remover under each staple. Press the handles together to lift the ends of the staple out of the skin.

(continued)

Procedure 24-6   Removing Staples *(continued)*

Steps	Purpose
8. Place each staple on a gauze square as it is removed.	8. This helps in counting the staples. If three staples were inserted, then three staples should now be removed.
9. When all of the staples are removed, gently clean the incision as instructed for all procedures. Pat dry. Dress the site if required by the physician.	9. The area should be cleaned and dried before applying new dressings to avoid wicking microorganisms. The healing process may be far enough along to allow the wound to remain uncovered.
10. Thank the patient and give appropriate instructions.	10. Courtesy encourages the patient to have a positive attitude about the physician's office.
11. Properly care for or dispose of all equipment and supplies. Clean the work area. Remove gloves and wash your hands.	11. Standard Precautions must be followed.
12. Record the procedure.	12. Procedures are considered not to have been done if they are not recorded.

Procedure 24-7   Applying a Sterile Dressing

Equipment/Supplies

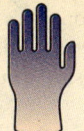

- sterile gloves
- dressings
- scissors
- appropriate bandages and tapes
- any medication to be applied to the dressing

Steps	Purpose
1. Wash your hands.	1. Handwashing aids infection control.
2. Assemble equipment.	2. This ensures that all supplies are available.
3. Greet and identify the patient. Ask about any tape allergies before deciding on the type of tape to use. With the size of the dressing and bandage in mind, cut or tear lengths of tape to secure the bandage. Set the tape aside in a convenient location.	3. Patients must be identified to avoid errors in treatment. Some patients are sensitive to the adhesive on tapes and may develop skin irritation. Many types of hypo-allergenic tapes are available to avoid this problem. Having tape prepared saves time and may prevent the dressing from slipping if tape must be torn after the dressing is applied.
4. Explain the procedure and instruct the patient to remain still during the procedure and to avoid coughing, sneezing, or talking until the procedure is complete.	4. Unexpected movements by the patient may result in contamination of the sterile supplies and the wound. Talking, coughing, and sneezing release droplets of moisture containing microorganisms from the respiratory tract which may contaminate the sterile field and the wound.

(continued)

Procedure 24-7 Applying a Sterile Dressing (continued)

Steps | **Purpose**

5. Open the dressing pack to create a sterile field. Observe the principles of surgical asepsis. Many packets are designed to be opened by the peel-apart method.

5. Observing sterile technique is necessary to ensure the sterility of the dressing after it has been opened. Packages of dressings are sterile on the inside surfaces; if opened in a manner that allows the inside of the package to remain sterile, the inner surface may be used as a sterile field on which the dressing may remain until it is needed.

6. a. If sterile gloves are to be used for the procedure, open the appropriate size package of sterile gloves. Using sterile technique, put on the gloves (see procedure for applying sterile gloves in Chapter 19, Asepsis and Infection Control).
   b. If using a sterile transfer forceps to apply the dressing (the "no-touch" method), use sterile technique to arrange the dressing on the wound site and do not touch the dressing or the site with the hands.

6. a. It is necessary to wear sterile gloves during a sterile procedure to prevent contamination of the dressings or wound site.
   b. Using proper technique avoids contamination of the dressings or the wound.

7. Using the already opened sterile dressings and principles of sterile technique, apply to the wound the number of dressings needed to properly cover and protect the wound. Sterile dressings must be carefully placed on the wound and not dragged over the skin into position.

7. If the dressing is dragged over the skin and into position, the dressing will be contaminated by microorganisms from the surrounding skin and may cause infection.

8. Apply the bandage so that it completely covers the sterile dressing and conforms to the patient's contours. The bandage should extend at least 1 inch beyond the border of the dressing.

8. The opportunity for wound contamination is greatly reduced when the dressing is placed so that it completely covers the wound from outside contaminants.

9. Apply the previously cut lengths of tape over the bandage in a manner that secures both bandage and dressing. Apply tape sufficiently to secure the bandage, but avoid overuse of tape. When the wound is completely covered, you may remove your gloves, or you may prefer to keep them on during the taping. Discard them in the proper receptacle.

9. Tape is used only to keep the dressings and bandages in place. Tape should not completely obscure the bandage, but should allow for the observation of any bleeding or drainage. Too much tape can cause perspiration to dampen the dressing and compromise sterility. Tape should not obstruct blood circulation. More tape used to secure dressings and bandages means more must be removed, which may cause discomfort to the patient.

10. When the patient is required to change dressings at home, provide appropriate instructions. Dressings and bandages should be kept clean and dry and changed when wet or soiled. Otherwise, dressings should be changed as frequently as instructed by the physician. *Note:* The physician will describe to the patient the signs of infection, such as redness, swelling, pain, or undue warmth at the site; what to do regarding excess bleeding or drainage; and how to manage any drains that might be present.

10. Microorganisms may be transported to the wound by capillary action when the dressing becomes wet or soiled. To decrease the chance of contamination and infection, dressings should be changed as they become wet or soiled in addition to the prescribed schedule.

(continued)

Procedure 24-7

Applying a Sterile Dressing (continued)

Steps	Purpose
11. Assist the patient from the examination table.	11. Patients may become dizzy or unsteady upon sitting up. To prevent falls, it is important to stay with the patient in case this occurs.
12. Properly care for or dispose of equipment and supplies. Disposable articles contaminated with blood or wound drainage require special disposal protocol. Clean the work area. (See Chapter 19, Asepsis and Infection Control.)	12. Standard Precautions must be followed.
13. Return reusable supplies (unopened sterile gloves or dressings, bandages, tape) to their appropriate storage areas; all others should be discarded correctly.	13. Unopened, reusable supplies should be returned to the appropriate storage areas for reuse. Discarding uncontaminated reusables is wasteful.
14. Record the procedure.	14. Procedures are considered not to have been done if they are not recorded.

Note: For the purposes of this procedure, it will be presumed that the skin and the lesion have been cleaned in the manner preferred by the physician. If medication is to be applied to the wound, it should be applied first to the dressing and then the dressing applied to the wound. This avoids touching the wound, which might cause discomfort to the patient.

Procedure 24-8

Changing an Existing Sterile Dressing

Equipment/Supplies

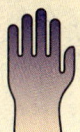

- sterile dressings and sterile gloves (for applying the new dressing)
- unsterile gloves (for removing the old dressing and bandage)
- skin antiseptic solution with sterile gauze squares or sterile cotton balls or premedicated antiseptic wipes of the physician's choice
- sterile basin (to receive the solution and gauze or cotton)
- tape, torn to appropriate lengths and set aside as in Procedure 24-7
- approved biohazard containers for contaminated waste

Steps	Purpose
1. Wash your hands.	1. Handwashing aids infection control.
2. Assemble the equipment.	2. This ensures that all supplies are available.
3. Greet and identify the patient. Explain the procedure and answer any questions.	3. This avoids errors in treatment, helps gain patient compliance, and eases anxiety.
4. Prepare a sterile field. If using a sterile container and solution, open the package containing the	4. This avoids wound contamination.

(continued)

Procedure 24-8   Changing an Existing Sterile Dressing (continued)

Steps	Purpose
basin using sterile technique and use the inside of the wrapper as the sterile field for the basin. Peel apart the wrappers for the gauze or cotton balls and flip them into the basin or use sterile transfer forceps to place them in the basin.	
5. Prepare antiseptic solution by first pouring off a small amount of the solution into a waste receptacle; then pour the solution from the stock bottle into the sterile container on the sterile field.	5. The first bit of solution to cross the mouth of the container should be poured away to remove any pathogens that may be in that area.
6. Instruct the patient not to talk, cough, sneeze, laugh, or move during the procedure.	6. Respiratory droplets may contaminate the sterile field. Movement may cause the field to be accidentally contaminated.
7. Wearing clean gloves, carefully remove the tape from the bandage. Tape must be removed by pulling it toward the direction of the wound. Large bandages that encircle a limb may first be cut with bandage scissors on the side of the limb away from the wound. Remove the old bandage and dressing. *Note:* If the dressing is difficult to remove because of dried wound exudate or blood, it may be soaked with sterile water or saline for a few minutes to loosen it for removing. Gently pull the edges of the dressing toward the center. Never pull on a dressing, that does not come off easily, the healing process will be disrupted. If this procedure does not loosen the dressing or causes undue discomfort to the patient, notify the physician immediately.	7. Gloves must be worn during any procedure involving contact with blood or body fluid. Tape pulled away from the direction of the wound may pull the healing edges of the wound apart.
8. Discard the soiled dressing in a biohazard container. Do not pass it over the sterile field.	8. The dressing will be soiled with blood and body fluid and must be considered potentially hazardous. Dressings passed over the sterile field will shed microorganisms and contaminate the area.
9. Inspect and observe the wound for degree of healing, amount and type of drainage, appearance of wound edges, and so on.	9. Inspections and observations are made now because following proper wound cleaning, most wound exudate will be removed. Make a mental note for charting when the procedure is complete.
10. Observing medical asepsis, remove and discard gloves. *Note:* At this point, the physician should inspect the wound before exudate or drainage is removed. Decisions must be made regarding the healing process. If a culture is ordered, it must be taken before the wound is cleaned to ensure the most reliable test results.	10. Proper removal of gloves helps prevent contamination.
11. Put on sterile gloves. Clean the area with the antiseptic solution of the physician's choice. Clean in a circular motion from the wound site outward. If a circular motion is not appropriate for this wound, use sweeps of the antiseptic-soaked gauze from the	11. The area must be cleaned before fresh dressings are applied. Returning the wipe to the wound area or the solution brings microorganisms from the surrounding skin to the open lesion.

(continued)

Procedure 24-8	**Changing an Existing Sterile Dressing** *(continued)*

Steps	**Purpose**
wound outward. Discard the wipe after each stroke. Never return the wipe to the antiseptic solution or to the skin after one sweep across the area.	
12. Replace the dressing using the procedure for sterile dressing application (Procedure 24-7).	
13. Record the procedure.	13. Procedures are considered not to have been done if they are not recorded.

Procedure 24-9	**Applying a Tubular Gauze Bandage**

Equipment/Supplies

- tubular gauze
- applicator
- tape
- scissors

Steps	**Purpose**
1. Wash your hands.	1. Handwashing aids infection control.
2. Assemble the equipment.	2. This ensures that all supplies are available.
3. Greet and identify the patient. Explain the procedure and answer any questions.	3. This avoids errors in treatment, helps gain patient compliance, and eases anxiety.
4. Choose the appropriate size tubular gauze applicator and gauze width. Manufacturers of tubular gauze supply charts with suggestions for the most appropriate size to use for various body parts.	4. The applicator and gauze should slip easily over the body part. Choose an applicator slightly larger than the part to be covered. The gauze designed to fit the chosen applicator will provide a secure fit.
5. Select and cut or tear adhesive tape in lengths to secure the gauze ends.	5. Tape ensures that the gauze will not slip off. Having it at hand before beginning the procedure saves time and effort.

6. Place the gauze bandage on the applicator in the following manner:
  a. Be sure the applicator is upright (open end up) and placed on a flat surface.
  b. Pull a sufficient length of gauze from the stock box; do not cut it at this time.
  c. Open the end of the length of gauze and slide it over the upper end of the applicator; continue pushing until all of the gauze needed for this procedure is on the applicator.	

(continued)

Steps

Purpose

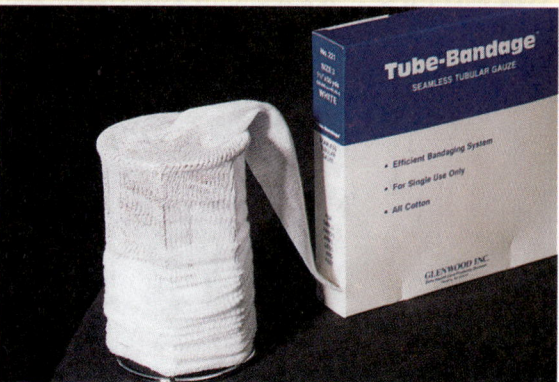

Step 6C: Place the applicator upright. Slide the end of the gauze over the applicator.

    d.   Cut the gauze when the required amount of gauze has been transferred to the applicator.

7.   Place the applicator over the distal end of the affected part (finger, toe, leg) and begin to apply the gauze. Hold it in place as you move to step 8.

8.   Slide the applicator containing the gauze up to the proximal end of the affected part. Holding the gauze at the proximal end of the affected part, pull the applicator and gauze toward the distal end.

7.   The application should begin distally and work proximally.

8.   This keeps the bandage from slipping. If the bandage is not held in place at the early stages of application, it may not completely cover the part.

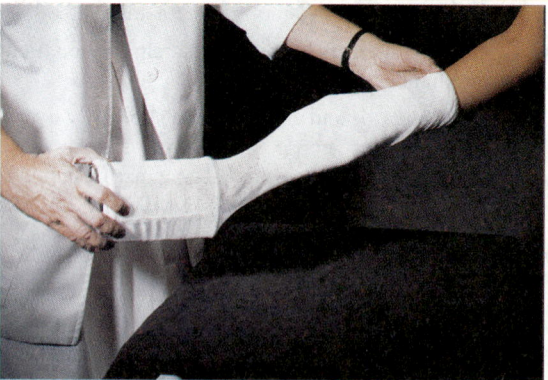

Step 8: Hold the gauze at the proximal end of the affected part and pull the applicator toward the distal end.

9.   Continue to hold the gauze in place. Pull the applicator 1–2 inches past the end of the affected part if the part is to be completely covered. In many instances, the gauze will not be required to extend beyond a limb and may cover only the area around the wound.

9.   The bandage will be secured at the distal end if the part is to be completely covered. If the distal portion of the limb is not to be covered, the bandage must extend at least 1 inch beyond the wound site to ensure adequate coverage.

(continued)

Steps	**Purpose**

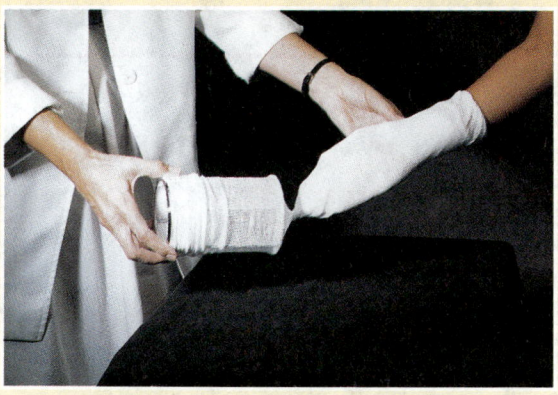

Step 9: Pull the applicator 1–2 inches past the affected part.

10. Turn the applicator one full turn to anchor the bandage.	10. The bandage will be securely held in place by the twist.
11. Move the applicator toward the proximal part as before.	11. This allows for a double layer of bandage for protection.

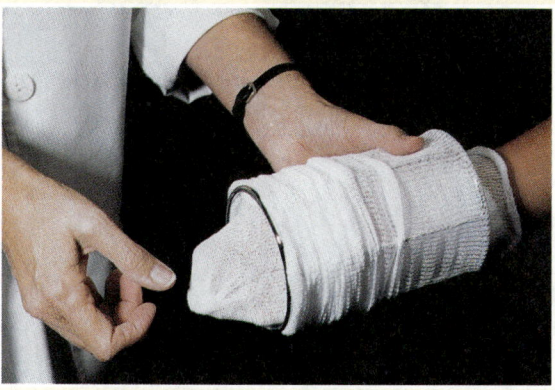

Step 11: Move the applicator toward the proximal part.

12. Move the applicator forward about 1 inch beyond the original starting point. Anchor the bandage again by turning it as before.	12. Anchoring provides a secure fit.

(continued)

Procedure 24-9 Applying a Tubular Gauze Bandage *(continued)*

Steps	Purpose

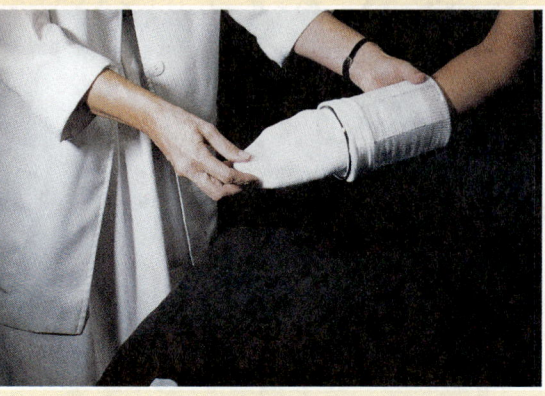

Step 12: Move the applicator forward about 1 inch beyond the original starting point.

13. Repeat the procedure until the desired coverage is obtained. The final layer should end at the proximal part of the affected area. Any extra length of gauze not needed can be cut from the applicator. Remove the applicator.

14. Secure the bandage in place with adhesive tape or cut the gauze into two tails and tie them at the base of the tear. Tie the two tails around the closest proximal joint. Use adhesive tape sparingly to secure the end if not using a tie.

13. The part should be adequately covered to protect the wound.

14. The bandage must be securely fastened to keep it in place until it must be changed.

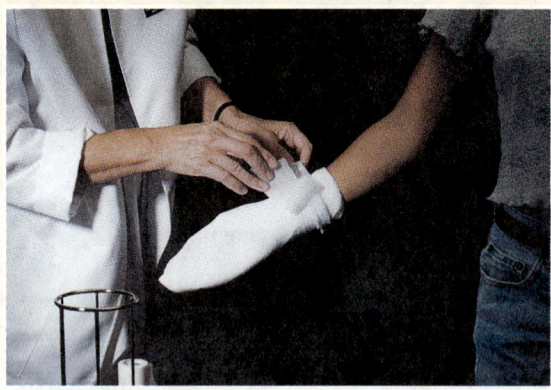

Step 14: Secure the bandage with adhesive tape.

15. Thank the patient and give appropriate instructions.

16. Properly care for or dispose of equipment and supplies. Clean the work area. Wash your hands.

17. Record the procedure.

15. Courtesy encourages the patient to have a positive attitude about the physician's office.

17. To ensure accurate documentation. Procedures are considered not to have been done if they are not recorded.

Assisting with Excisional Surgery

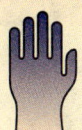

Equipment/Supplies

At the side
- sterile gloves
- local anesthetic
- antiseptic wipes

- adhesive tape
- bandages
- specimen container with completed laboratory request

On the field
- basin for solutions
- gauze sponges and cotton balls
- antiseptic solution
- sterile drape
- dissecting scissors or iris scissors

- scalpel blade and handle of physician's choice
- mosquito forceps
- tissue forceps
- needle holder
- suture and needle of physician's choice

Steps	Purpose
1. Wash your hands.	1. Handwashing aids infection control.
2. Assemble the equipment.	2. This ensures that all supplies are available.
3. Greet and identify the patient. Explain the procedure and answer any questions.	3. This avoids errors in treatment, helps gain patient compliance, and eases anxiety.
4. Set up a sterile field on a surgical stand with the at-the-side equipment close at hand. Cover the field with a sterile drape if necessary until the physician arrives.	
5. Position the patient appropriately.	5. The position required depends on the location of the lesion.
6. Put on sterile gloves or use transfer forceps for the aseptic process.	6. Sterile gloves or the "no touch" technique protects both the patient and you from contamination.
7. Cleanse the site with sterile antiseptic solution in the manner described for skin preparation (Procedure 24-4). *Note:* The physician may do this before gloving. Some physicians prefer that the site be cleaned and made ready by an assistant; others prefer doing it themselves after gloving and using the supplies on the field. In all instances, the physician's preference takes precedence over any outlined procedure.	7. The antiseptic discourages the entrance of micro-organisms into the wound.
8. The physician will perform the procedure; you may be asked to assist during the procedure. This usually involves adding supplies as needed, watching closely for opportunities to assist the physician and comforting the patient, or putting on sterile gloves and passing instruments to the physician from the field. *Note:* If the lesion is to be referred to pathology for analysis, you will be required to assist with the specimen container during the procedure.	
9. At the end of the procedure, dress the wound using the procedure for applying a sterile dressing (see Procedure 24-7).	9. The wound must be covered to protect the incision from contamination during the healing process.
10. Thank the patient and give appropriate instructions.	10. Courtesy encourages the patient to have a positive attitude about the physician's office.
11. Clean the examining room in preparation for the next patient. Discard all disposables in appropriate biohazard containers. Return unused reusable items to their proper places. Wash your hands.	11. Standard Precautions must be followed.
12. Record the procedure.	12. Procedures are considered not to have been done if they are not recorded.

Procedure 24-11 Assisting with Incision and Drainage (I & D)

Equipment/Supplies

At the side
- sterile gloves
- local anesthetic
- antiseptic wipes
- adhesive tape

On the field
- basin
- sterile cotton balls or gauze
- antiseptic solution
- sterile drape

- sterile dressings
- packing gauze
- bandages

(If the wound is to be cultured, a culture tube will also be included at the side.)

- syringes and needles for local anesthetic (unless the physician prefers that the site be numbed before gloving)
- commercial I & D set **or** scalpel, dissecting scissors or operating scissors, hemostats, tissue forceps, 4 × 4 gauze sponges, probe (optional)

Steps	Purpose
1–4. Follow steps 1–4 of Procedure 24-10: Assisting with Excisional Surgery.	
5. Position the patient appropriately.	5. The position required depends on the location of the abscess.
6–8. Follow steps 6–8 of Procedure 24-10: Assisting with Excisional Surgery.	
9. At the end of the procedure, dress the wound using the procedure for applying a sterile dressing (see Procedure 24-7).	9. The wound must be covered to avoid further contamination and to absorb drainage. The exudate is a hazardous body fluid requiring Standard Precautions.
10. Follow steps 10–12 of Procedure 24-10: Assisting with Excisional Surgery.	

SUMMARY

With the spiraling costs of health care, many procedures that once were performed in hospital settings are now being performed in the medical office. As a medical assistant, you will be required to become more proficient in minor surgical procedures as offices change to meet the needs of the patients. Continuing education, intensive and extensive research and reading in specialty health care, and on-the-job training will keep you current on the changes in the surgical field.

CRITICAL THINKING CHALLENGES

1. Dr. Brown has just informed Mrs. Levine that she should return tomorrow for office surgery. While you are alone with the patient, Mrs. Levine begins to cry and expresses great concern about the procedure. What should you do in this situation?

2. Review the anatomy of a hair follicle. Why are skin nicks more likely if the hair is shaved in the opposite direction as its natural growth?

3. Why would wounds in the head and face heal faster than those in the arms and legs?

4. Review the properties of epinephrine. Which of its actions would slow the absorption of medications in the tissues?

5. Why is it preferable for infected wounds to heal with delayed surface closure?

ANSWERS TO CHECKPOINT QUESTIONS

1. To maintain a sterile field, you must keep sterile packages dry, face the sterile field, keep sterile items above waist level, keep items in the middle of the field, avoid spills, do not cough or sneeze near the field, never reach

over the field, do not pass contaminated items over the field, and alert the physician if the field becomes contaminated.

2. Contents from a peel-back package can be added to a sterile field by sterile forceps, by a sterile gloved hand, and by flipping.

3. A fenestrated drape has an opening to expose the treatment site while covering adjacent areas.

4. Swaged (atraumatic) needles have the appropriate size suture material attached by the manufacturer. Threaded needles have an eye with a double thickness of suture that must be pulled through tissues.

5. To hand a right-handed physician a needle for suturing, place the needle in the needle holder, click the ratchets twice, and hand the needle holder with the suture material to the right and the needle to the left.

6. Sterile dressings are used to cover and protect a wound, absorb drainage, exert pressure, hide disfigurement, and hold medications against the skin.

7. Apply bandages beginning at the distal part and extending to the proximal part of the body. Bandage turns that extend distal to proximal aid in the return of venous blood to the heart and help make the bandage more secure.

8. Electrosection is the type of electrosurgery used for incision or excision of tissue.

SUGGESTIONS FOR FURTHER READING

Kozier, Barbara, and Erb, Glenora. (1993). *Techniques in Clinical Nursing*, 4th ed. Addison Wesley.

Scherer, J. C., Timby B. K. (1995). *Introductory Medical-Surgical Nursing*, 6th ed. Philadelphia: J.B. Lippincott.

Smeltzer, S., and Bare, B. (1996). *Brunner and Suddarth's Textbook of Medical-Surgical Nursing*, 8th ed. Philadelphia: Lippincott-Raven Publishers.

Smith-Temple, Jean, and Johnson, Joyce Y. (1994). *Nurse's Guide to Clinical Procedures*, 2nd ed. Philadelphia: J. B. Lippincott.

Timby, Barbara K. (1996). *Fundamental Skills and Concepts in Patient Care*, 6th ed. Philadelphia: Lippincott-Raven Publishers.

Pharmacology

Chapter Outline

Medication Names
Legal Regulations
    Food and Drug Administration
    Drug Enforcement Agency
Prescriptions
Sources of Drugs
Pharmacodynamics
Pharmacokinetics
    Absorption
    Distribution

    Metabolism
    Excretion
Drug Interactions
Medication Allergies
Sources of Information in Pharmacology
Summary
Critical Thinking Challenges
Answers to Checkpoint Questions
Suggestions for Further Reading

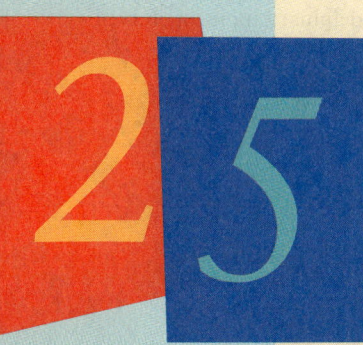

DACUM Components

1.2   Perform within ethical boundaries
1.3   Practice within the scope of education, training, and personal capabilities
2.1   Listen and observe
2.2   Treat all patients with empathy and impartiality
3.6   Locate resources and information for patients and employers
5.1   Document accurately
5.2   Determine needs for documentation and reporting
5.5   Dispose of controlled substances in compliance with government regulations
6.3   Inventory equipment and supplies

Chapter Competencies

Learning Objectives

Upon successfully completing this chapter, you will be able to:

1. Spell and define the Key Terms.
2. Identify chemical, trade, and generic drug names.
3. Name the regulations that historically have affected the manufacture, sale, and prescribing of medications.
4. List and explain the branches of the government that regulate both standard and controlled drugs.
5. List and identify the categories of controlled substances and give an example of each.
6. Describe the sources of drugs and give examples.
7. Explain how drugs are categorized by action and effect.
8. List factors that affect drug action.
9. Explain pharmacokinesis and describe the steps.
10. Describe how drugs may interact for an increased or decreased effect.
11. Explain and define terms related to drug effects.
12. List sources for information on pharmacology.

Key Terms

(See Glossary for definitions.)

antagonism
chemical name
drug
generic name
pharmacodynamics
pharmacokinesis
pharmacology
potentiation
synergism
trade name

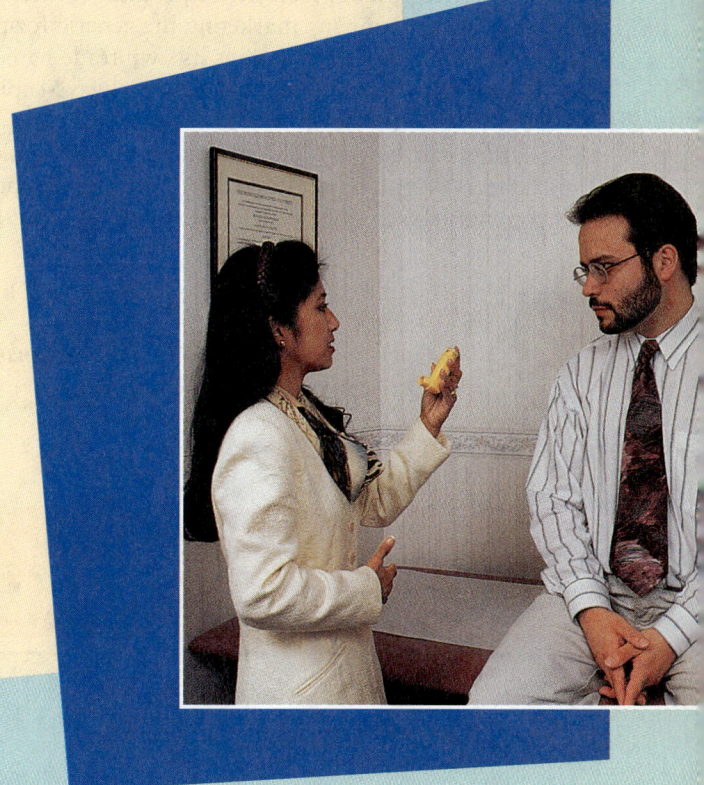

Pharmacology is the term given the study of drugs, their actions, dosages, and side effects. A **drug** is a chemical substance that, when administered, affects body function(s). Pharmaceutical companies are required to list the chemical compound, actions, dosages, adverse effects, indications, and contraindications of the medications they manufacture. Medications are available in many forms and are administered in various ways to produce therapeutic effects.

➤ MEDICATION NAMES

Most medications have a **chemical name** or an organic name, a **generic name**, and a **trade name** (Box 25-1). The chemical name, the first name given to any medication, identifies the chemical components of the drug. If the medication is primarily organic, such as digitalis, this name may be listed in addition to or in place of a chemical name. The generic name is assigned to the medication when it is manufactured during research and development. When the drug is available for commercial distribution by the original manufacturer, a brand name or trade name is given. The trade name is registered by the U.S. Patent Office and has the official mark of this office after its name. For 17 years, the manufacturer has the exclusive rights to produce the drug. After that time, other companies may combine the same chemicals and produce their own equivalent (generic) of the drug. Each company marketing the generic form of the trade name drug then assigns its own trade name to its generic equivalent. Trade names are always capitalized; generic names begin with lower case letters.

Drugs can be classified according to their actions and effects on the body. Table 25-1 provides examples of commonly prescribed drugs and their classifications.

Checkpoint Question

1. *What is the difference between a drug's chemical name and trade name?*

BOX 25-1 Drug Names

Chemical Name	7-chloro-1, 3-dihydro-1-methyl-5-phenyl-2H-1, 4-benzodiaxepin-2-one
Trade Name	Valium
Generic Name	Diazepam

➤ LEGAL REGULATIONS

Consumers in the United States are protected by federal regulations regarding drugs. The Pure Food and Drug Act was passed in 1906 and amended in 1938. The amended law, called the Federal Food, Drug, and Cosmetic Act, required that the safety of a drug must be proven before it is distributed to the public. An amendment, called the Durham-Humphrey Amendment, was passed in 1952. This addition banned many drugs from being dispensed without a prescription. The Kefauver-Harris Amendment of 1962 required testing of prescription and nonprescription medications for effectiveness before their release for sale.

Food and Drug Administration

The Food and Drug Administration (FDA) was established to review drug applications and petitions for food additives; to inspect facilities where drugs, cosmetics, and foods are made; and to remove unsafe drugs from the market. The FDA also ensures that the ingredients listed on food, drugs, and cosmetics are correct as labeled.

Drug Enforcement Agency

In 1970, the Controlled Substances Act was passed to regulate the manufacture and distribution of drugs whose use may result in dependency or abuse. This act also requires that anyone who manufactures, prescribes, administers, or dispenses such controlled substances must register annually with the United States Attorney General under the Bureau of Narcotics and Dangerous Drugs (BNDD).

The Drug Enforcement Agency (DEA) is a branch of the Justice Department designated to exercise strong regulatory control over all drugs listed by the BNDD. This authority extends to prescribing, refilling, and storing controlled substances in the medical office. The DEA is concerned with controlled substances only; medications not subject to abuse are not regulated by this agency. The DEA is also responsible for revising the list of drugs included in the Schedule of Controlled Substances (Table 25-2). Officials at regional DEA offices are available to answer any questions regarding the drugs under its control. As a medical assistant, you should make sure that the physician's office is on the DEA's periodic mailing list to keep abreast of changes.

text continues on page 419

Table 25-1

Classifications of Drugs

Therapeutic Classification	Effect or Action/Uses	Common Examples
Adrenergic blocking agents/antiadrenergics	Affect the alpha receptors of adrenergic nerves that control the vascular system; used to treat hypertension, cardiac arrhythmias, glaucoma	Metoprolol tartrate (Lopressor), propranolol hydrochloride (Inderal), timolol (Timoptic)
Adrenergics	Mimic the activity of the sympathetic nervous system; used to treat hypotensive episodes, bronchial asthma, cardiac arrest, heart block, ventricular arrhythmias, and allergic reactions	Epinephrine (Adrenaline), phenylephrine hydrochloride (Neo-Synephrine), ephedrine sulfate
Analgesics	Used to relieve pain; available in nonnarcotic and narcotic varieties (see also antipyretic and antiinflammatory agents)	Aspirin, acetaminophen (Tylenol), codeine
Anesthetics	Various actions and effects according to type of anesthesia indicated. Local anesthesia provides a pain-free state in a specific area or region; general anesthesia is administered to the patient with the aim of loss of consciousness	Procaine hydrochloride (Novocain), thiopental sodium (Pentothal), halothane (Fluothane)
Antacids	Neutralize or reduce the acidity of the stomach by combining with hydrochloric acid and producing salt and water	Magnesia (Milk of Magnesia), calcium carbonate (Tums)
Anthelmintics	Actions vary; prime purpose of anthelmintic drugs is to kill parasitic worms	Piperazine citrate, mebendazole (Vermox)
Antianginal agents	Promote vasodilation which relieves the symptoms of angina	Nitroglycerin, diltiazem hydrochloride (Cardizem)
Antianxiety agents	Act on subcortical areas of the brain; exact mechanism of action not fully understood; used in the short-term treatment of symptoms of anxiety	Alprazolam (Xanax), chlordiazepoxide (Librium), diazepam (Valium)
Antiarrhythmics	Various actions and effects; used to treat disturbances or irregularities of the heart rate, rhythm or both	Disopyramide (Norpace), procainamide hydrochloride (Pronestyl), esmolol (Brevibloc), bretylium tosylate (Bretylol), verapamil hydrochloride (Calan)
Antibiotics	Destroy, interrupt or interfere with the growth of microorganisms; used to treat bacterial infections	Penicillin, ampicillin, cefaclor, tetracycline, sulfadiazine
Anticoagulants and thrombolytics	Anticoagulants are used to prevent the formation of blood clots. Thrombolytics are used to dissolve blood clots	Heparin sodium, streptokinase (Streptase)
Anticonvulsants	Reduce the excitability of the nerve cells of the brain; used to treat convulsive disorders, epilepsy	Phenobarbital, clorazepate dipotassium (Tranxene), phenytoin (Dilantin), carbamazepine (Tegretol)
Antidepressants	Generally work to increase stimulation of the central nervous system; used in the management of various types of depression	Amitriptyline hydrochloride (Elavil), fluoxetine hydrochloride (Prozac), phenelzine (Nardil)
Antidiarrheals	Decrease intestinal peristalsis	Loperamide hydrochloride (Imodium A-D)
Antiemetic agents	Used to treat or prevent nausea or vomiting; some are also useful as antivertigo agents (used to treat or prevent motion sickness)	Dimenhydrinate (Dramamine), promethazine hydrochloride (Phenergan)
Antifungals	Destroy, slow or retard the growth of fungi; used to treat fungal infections	Ketoconazole (Nizoral), miconazole nitrate (Monistat 3 or 7)
Antihistamines	Used to counteract the effects of histamine on body organs and structures; used to treat allergies and allergic reactions. Some provide relief from nausea and vomiting; some have sedative effects	Chlorpheniramine maleate (Chlor-Trimeton), diphenhydramine hydrochloride (Benadryl), terfenadine (Seldane)
Antihypertensives	Act to lower blood pressure by increasing the size of arterial blood vessels; used in the treatment of high blood pressure	Methyldopate hydrochloride (Aldomet), prazosin (Minipress), propanolol hydrochloride (Inderal)
Antiinflammatory agents	Reduce irritation and swelling of tissues	Aspirin, acetaminophen (Tylenol), ibuprofen (Advil), naproxen (Naprosyn)
Antineoplastic agents	Slow the rate of tumor growth and delay metastasis; used to treat malignant diseases (cancer)	Cyclophosphamide (Cytoxan), mitoxantrone hydrochloride (Novantrone)
Antiparkinsonism agents	Used to treat the symptoms associated with parkinsonism	Benztropine mesylate (Cogentin), levodopa (Larodopa)

(continued)

Table 25-1

Classifications of Drugs (Continued)

Therapeutic Classification	Effect or Action/Uses	Common Examples
Antipsychotics (neuroleptics)	Exact mechanism not understood; used to treat various acute and chronic psychoses	Chlorpromazine hydrochloride (Thorazine), haloperidol (Haldol)
Antipyretics	Drugs that decrease body temperature	Aspirin, acetaminophen (Tylenol)
Antitussives, mucolytics, and expectorants	Antitussives relieve coughing, mucolytics loosen respiratory secretions, and expectorants aid in removing thick mucus from the respiratory passages; medications may have one or more combinations of the three; used to relieve the discomfort of upper respiratory infections	Codeine sulfate, diphenhydramine hydrochloride (Benylin Cough), guaifenesin (Entex)
Antivirals	Appear to inhibit viral replication. Antivirals are only effective against a small number of specific viral infections	Acyclovir (Zovirax), zidovudine (AZT)
Bronchodilators	Act to dilate the bronchi and allow more air to enter the lungs; used in the treatment of acute and chronic asthma, chronic bronchitis, and emphysema	Albuterol sulfate (Ventolin), metaproterenol sulfate (Alupent), theophylline
Cardiotonics	Increase the force of contraction of the myocardium of the heart; used in the treatment of congestive heart failure, atrial fibrillation, atrial flutter, and paroxysmal atrial tachycardia	Digoxin (Lanoxin), milrinone lactate (Primacor)
Cholinergic blocking agents/anticholinergics	Affect the autonomic nervous system; used to treat peptic ulcers, ureteral and biliary colic, and preoperatively to reduce secretions of the upper respiratory tract	Atropine sulfate, scopolamine hydrobromide, propantheline bromide (Pro-Banthine)
Cholinergics	Mimic the activity of the parasympathetic nervous system; used to treat glaucoma and myasthenia gravis	Neostigmine (Prostigmin), pilocarpine hydrochloride
Decongestants	Reduce swelling of the nasal passages to enhance drainage of the sinuses; used to treat nasal congestion	Oxymetazoline hydrochloride (Dristan), pseudoephedrine hydrochloride (Sudafed)
Diuretics	Increase the secretion of urine by the kidneys; used to release excess fluid in body tissues	Furosemide (Lasix), chlorothiazide (Diuril), methazolamide (Neptazane)
Emetics	Promote vomiting by acting on the chemoreceptor trigger zone of the medulla	Ipecac syrup
Histamine H_2 antagonists	Inhibit the action of histamine at the histamine H_2 receptor cells of the stomach, thereby reducing the secretion of gastric acid	Cimetidine (Tagamet), ranitidine (Zantac)
Hormones (female)	Used to prevent symptoms of menopause, female castration, ovarian failure, and amenorrhea; combinations of estradiol, norethindrone, and other hormones are used for contraception	Estradiol (Estraderm), medroxyprogesterone acetate (Provera)
Hormones (male)	Androgen therapy treats testosterone deficiency. Anabolic steroids are chemically related to androgens and promote the tissue-building process	Fluoxymesterone (Halotestin), nandrolone decanoate (Deca-Durabolin)
Immunologic agents (vaccines)	Stimulate the immune response to create protection against a specific disease or to supply ready-made antibodies which provide passive immunity	Pneumococcal vaccine, Influenza virus vaccine, Diphtheria and tetanus toxoids
Insulin and oral hypoglycemics	Injectable insulin is used to control type I diabetes mellitus. Type II diabetes mellitus can be controlled with oral hypoglycemics	Intermediate-acting insulin (NPH Insulin), long-acting insulin (Ultralente U), mixed insulin (Novolin 70/30), glipizide (Glucotrol), tolbutamide (Orinase)
Sedatives and hypnotics	Sedatives relax and calm, hypnotics induce sleep; available in barbiturate and nonbarbiturate varieties	Butabarbital; sodium, Phenobarbital, Chloral hydrate, Temazepam (Restoril)
Stimulants	Increase the activity of the central nervous system; used to increase respiration and to treat narcolepsy, attention deficit disorder, and exogenous obesity	Doxapram hydrochloride (Dopram), amphetamine sulfate, methamphetamine hydrochloride (Desoxyn)
Thyroid and antithyroid agents	Used to increase or decrease the amount of thyroid hormones manufactured and secreted into the body; used to treat hypothyroidism or hyperthyroidism	Levothyroxine sodium (T_4), (Levothroid), propylthiouracil (PTU)

Summarized from Scherer, J.C. and Roach, S.S., Introductory Clinical Pharmacology, 5th Edition. Philadelphia: Lippincott-Raven Publishers, 1996.

Table 25-2
Controlled Substances

Schedule	Description	Examples
I	These drugs have the highest potential for abuse and have no currently accepted medical use in the United States. There are no accepted safety standards for use of these drugs or substances even under medical supervision although some are used experimentally in carefully controlled research projects.	Opium, marijuana, lysergic acid diethylamide (LSD), peyote, mescaline
II	These drugs have a high potential for abuse. They have a current accepted medicinal use in the United States, but with severe restrictions. Abuse of these drugs can lead to dependence, either psychological or physiologic. Schedule II drugs require a written prescription and cannot be refilled or called into the pharmacy by the medical office. Only in extreme emergencies may the physician call in the prescription. A handwritten prescription must be presented to the pharmacist within 72 h.	Morphine, codeine, Seconal, cocaine, amphetamines, Dilaudid, Ritalin
III	These drugs have a limited potential for psychological or physiologic dependence. The prescription may be called in to the pharmacist by the physician and refilled up to five times in a 6-month period.	Paregoric, Tylenol with codeine, Fiorinal
IV	These drugs have a lower potential for abuse than those in Schedules II and III. They can be called into the pharmacist by a medical office employee and may be filled up to five times in a 6-month period.	Librium, Valium, Darvon, phenobarbital
V	These drugs have a lower potential for abuse than those in Schedules I, II, III, and IV.	Lomotil, Dimetane Expectorant DC, Robitussin-DAC

Five schedules, or categories, of controlled substances were established by the Bureau of Narcotics and Dangerous Drugs. Medications in the five schedules may be revised periodically after review.

Registration

When the physician registers with the U.S. Attorney General under the BNDD, a registration number (DEA number) is issued. Physicians are registered for a period of 3 years after application and acceptance. Near the end of the 3 years, the DEA will mail a renewal registration form to the physician. As a medical assistant, you will be responsible for maintaining professional records and licensure including this form. If the form does not arrive before the physician's registration expires, you must notify the DEA. The DEA does not take responsibility if the physician's registration expires. Instructions for completing the initial registration or a renewal are printed on the form. If medications are administered and dispensed by the same physician at different offices, a separate form must be completed for each site. The registration retires with the physician; it does not stay with the medical office.

Inventory

Controlled substances in Schedule II are received from suppliers using a Federal Triplicate Order Form DEA 222. Schedules III through V do not require triplicate forms, but invoices for receipt of these substances must be maintained for 2 years.

As controlled substances are received, they are listed on a special inventory form in the office. Their receipt should be signed by two employees. Every time a controlled substance leaves the medical office inventory, it must be recorded; include the drug name, patient, dose, date, ordering physician, and the employee who handled the procedure. At regular intervals decided at the site, two employees should reconcile the inventory list with the medications on hand and sign that both are correct. These inventory forms must be kept for 2 years.

If controlled substances are administered and dispensed, records must be maintained separate from the patients' charts and must be readily available for inspection by the authorities of the DEA. If only an occasional controlled substance is administered and none are dispensed, the procedure must be recorded on the patient's chart and be available for DEA review. If controlled substances are prescribed and not administered or dispensed, some states require only that the information be recorded on the patient's chart; others require that a separate file be kept of prescription copies of controlled substances.

The DEA number should not be preprinted on the prescription. Cautious physicians write it in rather than risk patients having easy access to it.

Most physicians avoid keeping controlled substances in their offices because of the risk of theft.

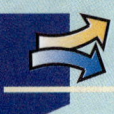

Ethical Tips

If you suspect that a physician or health care professional is illegally diverting controlled substances, you have an ethical and, in some states, a legal responsibility to report this suspicion. Gather and document evidence and reasons to suspect diversion of substances. You should have a clear and compelling case to present to the proper authorities. If a physician is involved, report this evidence to the Drug Enforcement Agency (DEA) and the American Medical Association (AMA). The state medical society should also be notified. If the suspected health care worker is not a physician, report it to the appropriate supervisor or superior. Most states have programs to assist the health care professional in obtaining appropriate help. In most instances, you may remain anonymous.

Controlled substances kept in the medical office must be locked in a safe or in a secure, locked box bolted to a shelf in a locked cabinet. The number of persons with access to the keys or to the cabinet should be limited. Many offices keep the DEA prescription pad, the state triplicate forms, and the inventory forms in the cabinet also.

If drugs are lost or stolen, the local law enforcement agency must be notified immediately. If drugs are expired and must be destroyed, two employees must witness the destruction of the medication and sign and date the form for destroyed substances. An option for the disposal of controlled substances requires that the regional DEA office send a representative to your office to retrieve and dispose of the drugs.

Checkpoint Question

2. What information needs to be documented when a controlled substance is administered?

➤ PRESCRIPTIONS

Medications may be administered (given in the office), dispensed (a supply given for later use), or prescribed (a written order to be filled by a pharmacist). An established protocol and traditional form must be followed when filling out the prescription:

Line 1. *Date.* Prescriptions must be filled within 6 months of the date listed.
Line 2. *Patient's name and address*
Line 3. *Superscription.* Includes the name of the medication, the desired form (eg, liquid, tablet) and the strength (eg, 250 mg, 500 mg).
Line 4. *Subscription.* Notes amount to dispense (eg, 60 tabs, 120 mL).
Line 5. *Signature.* Notes instructions for taking (eg, with meals, tid, qid).
Line 6. *Refills.* Notes number of times prescription can be refilled, generally no more than five times within 6 months, but this will vary.
Line 7. *Physician's signature.* Physicians are responsible for prescriptions written in their offices and should check and sign any that will be given to patients. The medical assistant may prepare the prescription for the physician, but it is in the best interest of all concerned for the physician to sign it.
Line 8. *Generic.* Some physicians will allow generic substitutes for certain medications but not for others.

All medications prescribed in the medical office must be documented in full on the patient's chart. Prescriptions that are called or faxed to the pharmacist must also be documented. The chart is a legal document and may be called into court in the event of legal action. If the medication order is not recorded, it will be presumed that the medication was never ordered. Figure 25-1 shows a sample prescription form.

Checkpoint Question

3. What does the superscription on the prescription indicate and how does this differ from the subscription?

➤ SOURCES OF DRUGS

Drugs are available from numerous natural sources such as plants, minerals, and animals. They may also be synthetic (prepared in the laboratory by artificial means). Table 25-3 lists a number of commonly prescribed drugs and their sources.

➤ PHARMACODYNAMICS

Drugs are commonly categorized by their action and effect on body function. **Pharmacodynamics** is the term used to describe the study of how drugs act within the body. All drugs cause cellular change (drug action) and a degree of physiologic change (drug effect).

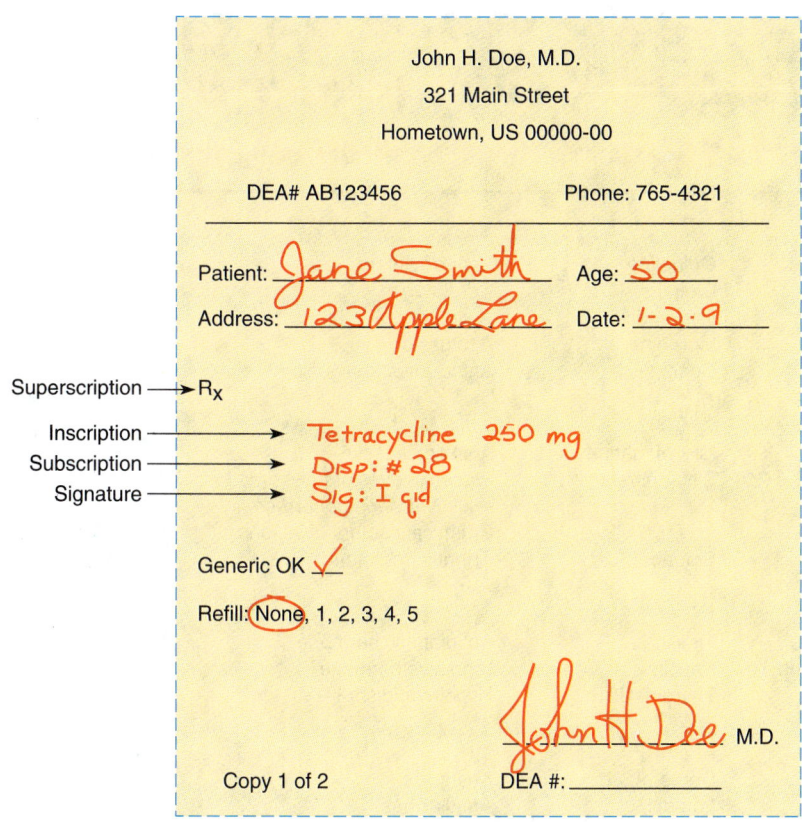

John H. Doe, M.D.
321 Main Street
Hometown, US 00000-00

DEA# AB123456   Phone: 765-4321

Patient: *Jane Smith*   Age: *50*
Address: *123 Apple Lane*   Date: *1-2-9*

Superscription → R_x

Inscription → *Tetracycline 250 mg*
Subscription → *Disp: # 28*
Signature → *Sig: I qid*

Generic OK ✓

Refill: (None), 1, 2, 3, 4, 5

John H. Doe M.D.

Copy 1 of 2   DEA #: _____

FIGURE 25-1
Sample prescription form.

An action of a drug administered for a local effect is limited to the area where it is administered. Drugs that exert local effects are ointments such as zinc oxide. A drug administered for a systemic effect is absorbed into the blood and then carried to the organ or tissue on which it will act. A systemic effect can be produced by administering drugs orally, sublingually, rectally, parenterally, transdermally, or by inhalation. (See Chap. 26, Preparing and Administering Medications, for more information.)

In addition, certain topical drugs will produce a systemic effect; these include drugs applied to the mucous membranes in the vagina, rectum, eyes, or nose. Because mucous membranes are bathed in watery solutions and are very vascular, they are more permeable than skin.

A number of factors can influence a drug's action in the body. These are described in Box 25-2.

➤ PHARMACOKINETICS

Drugs undergo numerous changes within the body from the time of transport from the site of administration until they are inactivated and excreted. **Pharmacokinesis** is the term given the study of the action of drugs within the body, from administration to excretion. Pharmacokinetic processes are described below.

Absorption

Absorption gets the drug into the bloodstream. Absorption usually occurs in the mucosa of the stomach, small intestine, mouth, rectum, the dermal layers of the skin, the subcutaneous tissue, or blood vessels in the muscles. If a drug is not administered correctly, it might be destroyed before it reaches its site of action. An example would be administering with a meal a medication that should only be given on an empty stomach.

Distribution

Distribution moves the drug from the bloodstream into the tissues and fluids of the body.

Metabolism

Metabolism is the physical and chemical alterations that the drug undergoes within the body. During the process of metabolism, the liver breaks down the drug

Table 25-3
Common Drugs and Their Sources

Source	Drug	Use
Plants		
Cinchona bark	Quinidine	Antiarrhythmic
Purple foxglove	Digitalis	Cardiotonic
Opium poppy	Paregoric	Antidiarrheal
	Morphine	Analgesic
	Codeine	Antitussive, analgesic
Minerals		
Magnesium	Milk of magnesia	Antacid, laxative
Silver	Silver nitrate	Placed in eyes of newborns to kill *Neisseria gonorrhoeae*
		Chemical cautery of lesions
Gold	Solganal	Arthritis treatment
Animal proteins		
Porcine or bovine pancreas	Insulin	Antidiabetic hormone
Porcine or bovine stomach acids	Pepsin	Digestive hormone
Animal thyroid glands	Thyroid, USP	Hypothyroidism
Synthetics		
	Demerol	Analgesic
	Lomotil	Antidiarrheal
	Gantrisin	Sulfonamide
Semisynthetic		
Escherichia coli bacteria and altered DNA molecules	Humulin	Antidiabetic hormone

BOX 25-2   Factors Influencing Drug Action

Age Elderly people have slower metabolic processes. Age-related kidney and liver dysfunctions also extend the break down and excretion times in these patients, so it is necessary to monitor the cumulative effects of drugs in the elderly. Children may have a more immediate response to drugs and therefore must be assessed frequently.

Weight Many drug dosages are calculated and administered according to the patient's weight. As a general rule, the larger the patient, the greater the dose; however, individual sensitivity to the effects of drugs will be taken into consideration.

Sex Women may react differently to certain drugs than men because of the ratio of fat/body mass or fluctuating hormone levels.

Existing Pathology If the body is compromised by a disease process, absorption, distribution, metabolism, and excretion may be altered.

Tolerance Some medications given over a long period of time may cause the body to become resistant to their effects, requiring larger doses to achieve the desired response.

NOTE: Medical assistants should *always* administer medications under the direct order of the physician. Under *no* circumstances should a medical assistant adjust a dosage unless specifically instructed to do so by the physician.

and alters it to more water-soluble by-products so it can be excreted by the kidneys. In the presence of hepatic disease, the liver may not be able to break down the drug properly for excretion by the kidneys. In this case, the patient may experience toxic effects caused by an accumulation of the drug in the liver or bloodstream. In some instances, drugs may bypass the metabolic processes. Some drugs reach the kidneys relatively unchanged; these drugs can be detected in the urine.

Excretion

Excretion eliminates the waste products of drug metabolism from the body. Most drugs are excreted by the kidneys. Unless the drug is excreted before a repeat dose is given, a cumulative effect can occur, possibly resulting in toxic levels of medications in the body.

Digoxin, a cardiotonic, has the potential for causing a toxic cumulative effect. If digoxin accumulates, the patient's heart rate may slow to a dangerously low level. For this reason, patients taking digoxin must be monitored. Digoxin levels in the blood are checked periodically to avoid toxicity. In some instances, the accumulation of the drug in the body may be the desired effect, to build a therapeutic blood level not possible without the cumulative effect.

If the kidneys are compromised by disease, medication may not be properly eliminated, adding to the danger of a cumulative effect and possible toxicity.

What If?

Mrs. Jones calls your office and asks that her prescription for digoxin be refilled. As you are talking with her, you pull her chart to record the call. What if, while reviewing her chart, you notice that she has not had digoxin levels determined as scheduled? How would you handle this situation?

Because digoxin may cause a toxic cumulative effect, it is important that patients taking this drug have their digoxin levels monitored regularly. Explain to Mrs. Jones that you will check with the physician regarding her request and that you will call her back. You should note your conversation in Mrs. Jones' chart, then place the chart on the physician's desk or discuss it personally at a convenient time. When the physician has made a decision, call Mrs. Jones with instructions for the drug's renewal and her course of action.

Checkpoint Question

4. What are the four pharmacokinetic processes? Explain each.

▶ DRUG INTERACTIONS

When two or more drugs are taken simultaneously, one drug may increase, decrease, or cancel the effects of the other. The following discussion explains common drug interactions and the terms used to describe these interactions. Table 25-4 lists other important drug-related terms you should know.

Synergism refers to two drugs working together. One drug helps the action of the other for an effect that neither produces alone. For example, small doses of Phenergan (a nonnarcotic sedative) and Demerol (a synthetic narcotic analgesic) are more effective for pain relief than the same dose or an increased dose of Demerol alone.

Table 25-4
Drug-Related Terms to Know

Term	Meaning
Therapeutic classification	States the purpose for the drug's use (eg, cardiotonic, anti-infective, antiarrhythmic)
Teratogenic category	Relates the level of risk to fetal or maternal health. These rank from Category A through D, with increasing danger at each level. Category X indicates that the particular drug should never be given during pregnancy.
Indications	Gives diseases for which the particular drug would be prescribed.
Contraindications	Indicates conditions or instances for which the particular drug should not be used.
Adverse reactions	Refers to undesirable side effects of the particular drug.
Hypersensitivity	Refers to an excessive reaction to a particular drug; also known as a drug allergy. The body must build this response; the first exposures may or may not indicate that a problem is developing.
Idiosyncratic reaction	Refers to an abnormal or unexpected reaction to a drug peculiar to the individual patient; not technically an allergy.

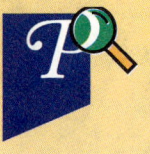

Focus on the Patient: Understanding Drug Dependence

Drug dependence, sometimes referred to as addiction, can be either physical or psychological. After the medication is stopped, a patient who is physically dependent will experience mild to severe physiologic symptoms that gradually decrease in intensity.

Patients who are psychologically dependent have acquired a need for the feeling brought on by the drug. After the drug is stopped, there will be no physiologic withdrawal; however, patients may experience depression for a time.

To prevent psychological dependence, physicians will sometimes substitute a placebo for the drug. Placebos are inactive substances that resemble the actual medication but contain no drugs. Sugar tablets or saline solution (for injections) are commonly used as placebos.

Potentiation describes the effect in which one drug prolongs or multiplies the effect of another drug. For example, Benemid (an antigout medication) is given with penicillin (an antibiotic) to delay its excretion and to build up a high level of penicillin in the blood.

Antagonism refers to an effect in which one drug decreases the effect of another. For example, Narcan (a narcotic antagonist) is used to treat some narcotic overdosages.

All of these examples of drug interactions are considered to be desirable interactions. However, on some occasions drug interactions produce undesirable effects. For example, sedatives and barbiturates given together can cause central nervous system depression (synergism). Tagamet, a gastric antisecretory drug, given with the antidepressant Tofranil will increase the levels of Tofranil in the blood (potentiation). Antacids taken with the antibiotic tetracycline prevent the absorption of tetracycline (antagonism).

? Checkpoint Question
5. How does synergism differ from antagonism?

➤ MEDICATION ALLERGIES

When gathering a patient's medical history (see Chap. 20, Medical History and Patient Assessment), you must always ask about allergies of any sort, particularly allergies to medications. Existing drug allergies must be noted prominently on the front of the patient's chart. Stickers are available with spaces to write the name(s) of the medication(s). These may also be posted on each page of the patient's order sheets.

If the patient is receiving allergy medications, or any medication that has a high incidence of allergic reactions (eg, penicillin), the patient must wait for 20 to 30 minutes and be rechecked before leaving the office. Leave the medication and the chart in the medication station until the patient has been checked and cleared to leave. The reaction, positive or negative, must be fully documented on the chart, including the lot number of the medication from the container. If a positive reaction is noted, it should be checked by the physician before the patient is allowed to leave the office.

Allergic reactions commonly noted include:

- redness and swelling at the injection site
- itching, either at the site or generalized
- dyspnea
- nausea
- dizziness

➤ SOURCES OF INFORMATION IN PHARMACOLOGY

The *Physician's Desk Reference* (PDR) is widely used as a reference for drugs in current use. The book is written to be used by physicians, but it is readily available in offices, libraries, and bookstores. It is clearly written to identify the drug's chemical name, brand name, and generic name. It also lists the properties, indications, contraindications, dosages, and so on.

The *United States Pharmacopeia Dispensing Information* (USPDI) consists of two paperback volumes providing drug information for the health care provider. It defines drugs in respect to sources, chemistry, physical properties, tests for identity, method of assay, storage, and dosage. It also provides directions for compounding and general use. The USPDI, however, does not contain photographs of the medications, and, unlike the PDR, which is sometimes distributed to physicians at no charge, must be purchased.

The *American Hospital Formulary Service* (AHFS) is distributed to practicing physicians and contains concise information arranged according to drug classifications.

Compendium of Drug Therapy is published annually and is distributed to practicing physicians. It includes photographs of the drugs and phone numbers of major pharmaceutical companies and poison control centers. It also includes copies of some package inserts.

SUMMARY

Medications are frequently given to patients to produce therapeutic effects. They are available in many forms and can be administered in various ways. Some medications, called controlled substances, may result in dependency and abuse. These drugs are strictly regulated by the federal government. As a medical assistant, you will need to keep abreast of the legal regulations concerning the manufacture, sale, and prescribing of medications. You also must understand the actions, effects, and interactions of drugs to effectively carry out a physician's medication orders.

CRITICAL THINKING CHALLENGES

1. How would you educate patients regarding prescribed medications? What type of information do they need to know? Is there anything that they do not need to know?
2. Using PDR, look up a medication that you have taken. (Your school's library will have a PDR.) What is the medication's chemical name? Explain what you learned about this medication that you did not already know. Is it a good idea for PDRs to be sold in bookstores for patients to buy? Justify your response.

ANSWERS TO CHECKPOINT QUESTIONS

1. A drug's chemical name identifies the chemical components of the drug; the trade name is the name under which the manufacturer distributes the drug commercially.

2. When a controlled substance is administered, you must document the drug name, patient, dose, date, ordering physician, and the employee who performed the procedure.
3. The superscription indicates the medication name, desired form, and strength. The subscription indicates the amount of medication to dispense.
4. The four pharmacokinetic processes are absorption, distribution, metabolism, and excretion. Absorption is the process by which the drug gets into the bloodstream. Distribution moves the drug from the bloodstream into body tissues and fluids. During metabolism, the drug undergoes chemical and physical changes within the body. The waste products of drug metabolism are eliminated during excretion.
5. Synergism refers to a drug interaction in which one drug helps another drug's action. Antagonism is a drug interaction in which one drug decreases another drug's effects.

SUGGESTIONS FOR FURTHER READING

Craven, R. F., & Hirnle, C. J. (1996). *Fundamentals of Nursing: Health and Human Function*, 2nd ed. Philadelphia: Lippincott-Raven Publishers.

Dawe, R. (1993). *Math and Dosage Calculations for Health Occupations*. New York: Glencoe.

Kozier, B., & Erb, G. (1993). *Techniques of Clinical Nursing*, 4th ed. Redwood City, CA: Addison-Wesley.

Lane, K. (1992). *Medications: A Guide for the Health Professions*. Philadelphia: F. A. Davis.

Scherer, J. C. & Roach, S. S. (1995). *Introductory Clinical Pharmacology*, 5th ed. Philadelphia: J. B. Lippincott.

Smeltzer, S. C., & Bare, B. G. (1996). *Brunner and Suddarth's Textbook of Medical-Surgical Nursing*, 8th ed. Philadelphia: Lippincott-Raven Publishers.

Taylor, C., Lillis, C., & LeMone, P. (1993). *Fundamentals of Nursing: The Art and Science of Nursing Care*, 2nd ed. Philadelphia: J. B. Lippincott.

Timby, B. (1996). *Fundamental Skills and Concepts in Patient Care*, 6th ed. Philadelphia: Lippincott-Raven.

Preparing and Administering Medications

Chapter Outline

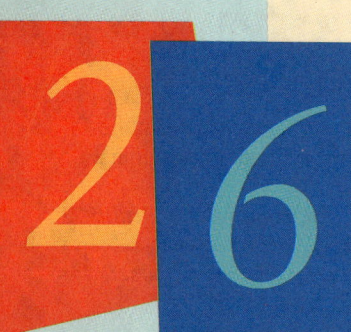

Common Abbreviations
Safety Guidelines
Seven Rights for Correct Medication Administration
Systems of Measurement for Medication Administration
    The Metric System
    The Apothecary System
Converting Measurements
    Metric to Metric
    Apothecary to Metric
Calculating Adult Dosages
    Ratio and Proportion
    The Formula Method
Calculating Pediatric Dosages
    The Nomogram
    Young's Rule
    Clark's Rule
    Fried's Rule
Medication Routes
Oral Administration
Procedure: Administering Oral Medications
    Sublingual Route
    Buccal Route
Procedure: Administering Sublingual or Buccal Medications
Mucosal Administration
    Rectal Route
    Vaginal Route
Dermal Administration
    Transdermal Medications
Procedure: Applying Transdermal Medications
Procedure: Applying Topical Medications
Parenteral Administration

Equipment Needed for Giving Injections
    Ampules
    Vials
    Cartridges
    Needles and Syringes
Procedure: Preparing an Injection
Types of Injections and Injection Sites
    Intradermal Injections
Procedure: Administering an Intradermal Injection
Procedure: Administering a Tine or Mantoux Test
    Subcutaneous Injections
Procedure: Administering a Subcutaneous Injection
    Intramuscular Injections
Procedure: Administering an Intramuscular Injection
    Z-Track Method of Intramuscular Injection
Procedure: Administering an Intramuscular Injection Using the Z-Track Method
Other Medication Routes
    Inhalation
    Intravenous (IV)
    Intra-arterial (IA)
    Intrathecal
    Intra-articular
Summary
Critical Thinking Challenges
Answers to Checkpoint Questions
Suggestions for Further Reading

DACUM Components

1.3   Practice within the scope of education, training, and personal capabilities
2.2   Treat all patients with empathy and impartiality
4.1   Apply principles of aseptic technique and infection control
4.13 Prepare and administer medications as directed by physician
4.14 Maintain medication records
5.1   Document accurately
7.2   Instruct patients with special needs

Chapter Competencies

Learning Objectives

Upon successfully completing this chapter, you will be able to:

1. Spell and define the Key Terms.
2. List safety guidelines for medication administration.
3. List and explain the "seven rights" of medication administration.
4. Explain the procedure for a charting error or a medication error.
5. Explain the differences between the oral and parenteral routes of medication administration and note why one method may be preferable to another in a specific situation.
6. Give examples of solid and liquid oral forms of medication.
7. List the parts of a syringe and name those parts that are to be kept sterile.
8. List the types of injections, their angles, and locate their sites.
9. Describe the needle lengths, gauges, and preferred site for each type of injection.
10. Describe how to calculate dosages using the metric and apothecary systems of measurement and how to convert measurements within and between systems.
11. Describe the various methods for calculating pediatric dosages.

Performance Objectives

Upon successfully completing this chapter, you will be able to:

1. Administer oral medications (Procedure 26-1).
2. Administer sublingual or buccal medications (Procedure 26-2).
3. Administer rectal medications.
4. Administer vaginal medications.
5. Apply transdermal medications (Procedure 26-3).
6. Apply topical medications (Procedure 26-4).
7. Prepare an injection (Procedure 26-5).
8. Administer an intradermal injection (Procedure 26-6).
9. Administer and read a tine or Mantoux test (Procedure 26-7).
10. Administer a subcutaneous injection (Procedure 26-8).
11. Administer an intramuscular injection (Procedure 26-9).
12. Administer an intramuscular injection using the Z-track method (Procedure 26-10).

Key Terms

(See Glossary for definitions.)

ampule	meniscus
diluent	nebulizer
gauge	vial
Mantoux	

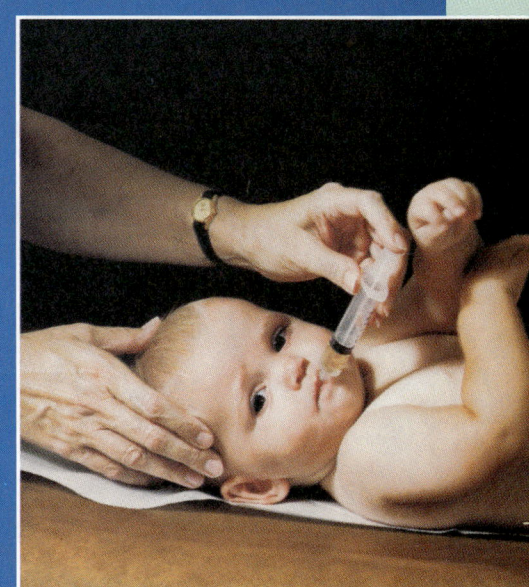

As a medical assistant, you may be responsible for administering medications under the supervision of the physician. It is important that you acquire a knowledge of medications, their uses and abuses, range of dosages, methods of administration, symptoms of overdosage, adverse effects, and untoward effects that may occur. Because medication administration is an exacting science and can be harmful to the patient when errors are made, you must perform this procedure with strict attention to safety.

➤ COMMON ABBREVIATIONS

You must be thoroughly familiar with the terminology, abbreviations, symbols, and signs used in prescribing and administering medications and in documenting such procedures. The abbreviations listed in Table 26-1 are among those most commonly used and should be memorized.

➤ SAFETY GUIDELINES

To ensure safety when administering medications, follow these guidelines:

1. Know the policies of your office regarding the administration of medications.
2. Give only the medication(s) that the physician has ordered in writing. Do not accept verbal orders.
3. Check with the physician if you have any doubt about a medication or an order.
4. Avoid conversations or other distractions while drawing up and administering medication. It is important to remain attentive during this task.
5. Work in a quiet, well lighted area.
6. Check the label when taking the medication from the shelf, when pouring it, and when replacing it on the shelf. This is known as the "three checks" for safe medication administration.
7. Place the order and the medication side by side to compare for accuracy.

Table 26-1
Abbreviations

Abbreviation	Meaning	Abbreviation	Meaning	Abbreviation	Meaning
aa	of each	IV	intravenous	qh	every hour
ac	before meals	kg	kilogram	q2h	every 2 hours
ad lib	as desired	L, l	liter	q3h	every 3 hours
AM, am	morning	lb	pound	qid	four times a day
amp	ampule	m, min	minim	qod	every other day
amt	amount	mcg, µg	microgram	qs	quantity sufficient
aq	aqueous	mEq	milliequivalent	qt	quart
bid	twice a day	ml, mL	milliliter	R	right, rectal
/c	with	n	normal	Rx	take, prescribe
cap	capsule	NaCl	sodium chloride	/s	without
cc	cubic centimeter	NKA	no known allergies	SC, subcu, subq, S/Q	subcutaneously
DC, disc, d/c	discontinue	noc	night	sig	label
disp	dispense	NPO	nothing by mouth	SL	sublingual
dl, dL	deciliter	NS	normal saline	sol	solution
dr	dram	OD	right eye	SOS	once if necessary
DW	distilled water	OS	left eye	sp	spirits
elix	elixir	OU	both eyes	ss	one-half
et	and	os	mouth	stat, STAT	immediately
ext	extract	oz	ounce	supp	suppository
fl, fld	fluid	p	after	syr	syrup
g, GM	gram	pc	after meals	tab	tablet
gr	grain	PM, pm	afternoon or evening	T, tbsp	tablespoon
gt(t)	drop(s)	po, PO	by mouth	t, tsp	teaspoon
h, hr	hour	prn, PRN	whenever necessary	tid	three times a day
hs, HS	hours of sleep	pt	pint	tinc	tincture
Id	intradermal	q	every	ung	ointment
IM	intramuscular	qd	every day		

8. Check strengths of the medication (eg, 250 mg versus 500 mg) and the routes (eg, ophthalmic, otic, topical).
9. Read labels carefully. Do not scan labels or orders.
10. Check the patient's chart for allergies to components of the medication.
11. Check the medication's expiration date.
12. Be alert for color changes, precipitation, odor, or any indication that the medication's properties have changed.
13. Measure exactly; there should be no bubbles.
14. Have sharps containers as close to the area of use as possible.
15. Put on gloves for all procedures that might result in contact with blood or body fluids.
16. Stay with the patient while oral medication is being taken. Watch for any reaction and record the patient's response.
17. Never return a medication to the container.
18. Never recap, bend, or break a used needle.
19. Never give a medication poured or drawn up by someone else.
20. Never leave the medication cabinet unlocked when not in use.
21. Never give the keys for the medication cabinet to an unauthorized person. Limit access to the medication cabinet by limiting access to the cabinet keys.

Checkpoint Question
1. When are the "three checks" for safe medication administration performed?

➤ SEVEN RIGHTS FOR CORRECT MEDICATION ADMINISTRATION

Medication errors should not occur during careful preparation or administration. By adhering to the policy of observing the "seven rights" during medication administration, you will eliminate the potential for many errors (Box 26-1). The "seven rights" include the following:

1. **Right patient.** Ask the patient to state his or her name. Some patients will answer to any name.
2. **Right time and frequency of administration.** Most medications are given immediately (stat) in the medical office.
3. **Right dose.** Check dosages. Many medications come in various strengths. Should it be 250 mg or 500 mg?
4. **Right route of administration.** Some medications may be formulated for various routes. Check the medication. Is it otic, ophthalmic, topical?

BOX 26-1 Medication Errors

Even if you are extremely careful, you may make an error when administering a medication. It is imperative that you report the error to the physician and that intervention measures start immediately. The error and all corrective actions must be documented thoroughly on the patient's chart. An incident report must be completed for the error and filed in the patient's chart as verification that all possible precautions were taken for the patient.

Errors made in charting medications must be corrected using a standard procedure. If you discover a charting error, mark it through with one line. Then mark the correction above the error and sign it.

P.O.   J. Smith, M.A.

Tetracycline 250 mg ~~I.M.~~ given stat as ordered. –
—— J. Smith, M.A.

---

5. **Right drug.** Many medication names are very much alike; for instance, Orinase and Ornade may be confused if care is not taken.
6. **Right technique.** Check how the medication is to be given. With food? With juice? Intramuscularly? Subcutaneously?
7. **Right documentation.** The medical record is a legal document. If the procedure is not documented, it is presumed that it was not performed.

All medications given in the office must be documented immediately with the medication name, dosage, route, site (if injected), and signed by the medical assistant. The patient's response may be charted as well when appropriate.

➤ SYSTEMS OF MEASUREMENT FOR MEDICATION ADMINISTRATION

The two systems most frequently used to measure medications for drug dosage are the metric and apothecary systems. Although often used by patients, household measurements are not accurate and should be avoided in the administration of medication (Box 26-2).

You may frequently find it necessary to convert from the apothecary to the metric system or to convert measurements within one of the systems. Although many medications are supplied in various dosages and in unit packs of the dosages most often ordered, occasionally you may be required to calculate a dosage by using mathematical equations. It will be necessary to

BOX 26-2 Household Measurements

Household measurements include cups, medicine droppers, teaspoons, and tablespoons. Some of the approximate equivalents to household measurements are:

1 teaspoon = 1 fluid dram = 5 mL
1 tablespoon = 1/2 fluid ounce = 4 fluid drams = 15 mL
2 tablespoons = 1 fluid ounce = 30 mL

Caution patients who will be using household measurements to avoid using table flatware and regular cups. Standard measuring spoons and cups are more accurate.

master the elements of the systems of measurement before calculations can be attempted.

The Metric System

The metric system is used throughout the world. Because the system is based on multiples of 10, decimals are often used but never fractions. In the metric system, the base unit of LENGTH is the METER (m). The base unit of WEIGHT is the GRAM (g or gm, either capitalized or lower case). LITER (L or l) is used to measure volume. Prefixes show a fraction of the base. Prefixes often used are:

- micro (0.000001)
- milli (0.001)
- centi (0.01)
- deci (0.1)
- kilo (1000)

For example, using the base unit of a GRAM, fractional measurements would be:

- microgram (mcg, μg)—one millionth of a gram
- milligram (mg)—one thousandth of a gram
- kilogram (kg)—1000 grams

(Decagram and centigram are not used in medication administration.)

Using the base unit of a METER (m = 39.37 inches), fractional measurements would be:

- millimeter (mm)—one thousandth of a meter (about 0.04 inches)
- centimeter (cm)—one hundredth of a meter (about 0.4 inches)

(Other measures are not used in medical practice.) Using the base unit of a LITER (l or L = approximately 1.06 quarts), fractional measurements would be:

- milliliter (ml, mL)—one thousandth of a liter (about 0.03 ounces)

(Other liquid measures are rarely used in medical practice.)

Note: One cubic centimeter takes up the same space as one milliliter. The measures are used interchangeably at times. An order may read 5 mL or 5 cc and the measure would be the same.

The Apothecary System

The apothecary system is used less frequently now than in the past and is gradually being replaced by the metric system. In the apothecary system, liquid measurements include DROP(S) (gt[t]), MINIM (min, m), FLUID DRAM (fl dr), FLUID OUNCE (fl oz), PINT (pt), QUART (qt), and GALLON (gal) (Fig. 26-1). Measurements for solid weights include GRAIN (gr), DRAM (dr), OUNCE (oz), and POUND (lb). Roman numerals may be used for smaller numbers, such as gr v or gtt ii. Fractions may be used when necessary, but never decimals.

Table 26-2 lists commonly used equivalents in the metric, apothecary, and household systems of measurement.

Checkpoint Question
2. What are three systems of measurement for medication administration? Which one should be avoided and why?

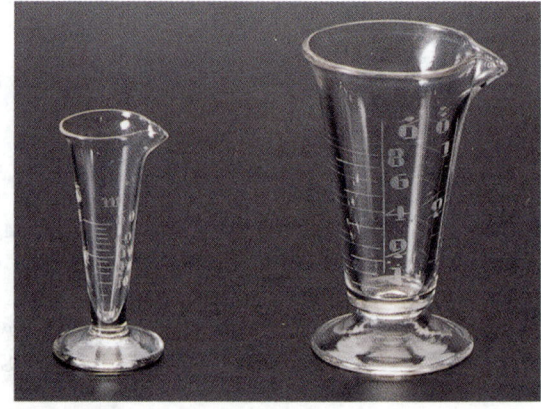

FIGURE 26-1
Apothecary measures. Minim glass (*left*) and dram/ounce glass.

Table 26-2
Most Commonly Used Approximate Equivalents*

Metric	Apothecary	Household
0.06 g	gr i	
0.06 mL	min i	1 drop
1.0 g	gr xv	
1.0 mL	min xv	⅛ tsp
5 mL	(1 dr) ℥ i	1 tsp
15 mL	(½ oz) ℥ ss	1 Tbs
30 mL	(1 oz) ℥ i	2 Tbs
500 mL	(16 oz) ℥ 16	1 pt
1000 mL	(32 oz) ℥ 32	1 qt

*There are many discrepancies among these approximate equivalents. For example, 30 mL is the accepted equivalent for 1 oz (29.57 mL is the exact equivalent); however, multiplying 5 mL per dram by 8 (℥ viii per ounce) results in an equivalent of 40 mL for 1 oz rather than the accepted equivalent of 30 mL = 1 oz.

Such discrepancies are inevitable when two systems are used whose equivalents are not exact. The discrepancies are within a 10% margin of error, which usually is acceptable in pharmacology.

From Taylor, C., Lillis, C., & Le Mone, P. (1993). Fundamentals of Nursing: The Art and Science of Nursing Care, 2nd ed., p. 1347. Philadelphia: J. B. Lippincott.

➤ CONVERTING MEASUREMENTS

Metric to Metric

In the metric system it is sometimes necessary to convert measurements to the same unit of measure. For example, the physician may order 0.5 g of medication, and the medication label reads 500 mg. To convert within the metric system, use the following rules:

- To change grams to milligrams, multiply grams by 1000 or move the decimal three places to the right.

  (Example: 0.5 g × 1000 = 500 mg)

- To change milligrams to grams, divide the milligrams by 1000 or move the decimal three places to the left.

  (Example: 500 mg ÷ 1000 = 0.5 gm)

- To change milligrams to micrograms, multiply the milligrams by 1000 or move the decimal three places to the right.

  (Example: 5 mg × 1000 = 5000 mcg)

- To change micrograms to milligrams, divide the micrograms by 1000 or move the decimal three places to the left.

  (Example: 500 mcg ÷ 1000 = 0.5 mg)

- To change liters to milliliters, multiply the liters by 1000 or move the decimal three places to the right.

  (Example: 0.01 L × 1000 = 10 mL)

- To change milliliters to liters, divide the milliliters by 1000 or move the decimal three places to the left.

  (Example: 100 mL ÷ 1000 = 0.1 L)

There is no conversion necessary when changing milliliters to cubic centimeters; they are approximately the same.

Apothecary to Metric

To convert from one system to another system, such as from the apothecary to the metric system, use the following rules:

- To change grains to grams, divide the grains by 15.

  (Example: gr 30 ÷ 15 = 2 gm)

- To change grains to milligrams, multiply the grains by 60. Use this rule when there is less than one grain.

  (Example: gr 1/4 × 60 = 15 mg)

- To change ounces to cubic centimeters (or mL), multiply the ounces by 30.

  (Example: 4 oz × 30 = 120 cc)

- To change cubic centimeters (or mL) to fluid ounces, divide the cc (or mL) by 30.

  (Example: 150 cc ÷ 30 = 50)

- To change kilograms to pounds, multiply the kilograms by 2.2.

  (Example: 50 kg × 2.2 = 110.0 lb)

- To change pounds to kilograms, divide the pounds by 2.2.

(Example: 44 lbs ÷ 2.2 = 20 kg)

- To change drams to milliliters (or cc), multiply the drams by 4.

    (Example: 3 drams × 4 = 12 mL)

- To change drams to cubic centimeters (or mL), multiply drams by 4.

    (Example: 2 drams × 4 = 8 cc)

- To change cubic centimeters to minims, multiply the cc by 15 or 16.

    (Example: 0.5 cc × 16 = 8 m)

- To change minims to cubic centimeters, divide the minims by 15 or 16.

    (Example: 30 m ÷ 15 = 2 cc)

Table 26-3 lists approximate equivalents in the metric and apothecary systems.

Table 26-3
Commonly Used Metric Units and Their Approximate Apothecary Equivalents

Metric	Metric	Apothecary
1 g	1000 mg	gr xv
0.6 g	600 mg	gr x
0.5 g	500 mg	gr viiss
0.3 g	300 mg	gr v
0.2 g	200 mg	gr iii
0.1 g	100 mg	gr iss
0.06 g	60 mg	gr i
0.05 g	50 mg	gr ¾
0.03 g	30 mg	gr ½ or gr ss
0.02 g	20 mg	gr ⅓
0.015 g	15 mg	gr ¼
0.016 g	16 mg	gr ¼
0.010 g	10 mg	gr ⅙
0.008 g	8 mg	gr ⅛
0.006 g	6 mg	gr ⅒
0.005 g	5 mg	gr 1/12
0.003 g	3 mg	gr 1/20
0.002 g	2 mg	gr 1/30
0.001 g	1 mg	gr 1/60
	0.6 mg	gr 1/100
	0.5 mg	gr 1/120
	0.4 mg	gr 1/150
	0.3 mg	gr 1/200

From Taylor, C., Lillis, C., & Le Mone, P. (1993). Fundamentals of Nursing: The Art and Science of Nursing Care, 2nd ed., p. 1347. Philadelphia: J. B. Lippincott.

➤ CALCULATING ADULT DOSAGES

Administration of medication is an exacting science; errors in calculation could prove fatal to the patient. There are two methods by which dosages are most frequently calculated: the ratio method and the formula method. It is important to note that measurements must be in the same system, either apothecary or metric, and in the same unit of measurement before a calculation can be made. When using the metric system, be careful to keep the decimal point in the correct position for calculation and be sure to convert fractions to decimals (eg, ½ should be converted to 0.5).

Ratio and Proportion

Proportion shows the relationship between two equal ratios. The first and fourth terms of a proportion are called the extremes. The second and third terms are called the means. In a proportion, the product of the means equals the product of the extremes. Ratio and proportion are sometimes used in dosage calculations. When the ratio and proportion method is used to calculate dosages the problem is set up as:

Dose on Hand : Known Quantity =
Dose Desired : Unknown Quantity

Example 1. The physician orders 250 mg erythromycin. On hand is 100 mg/mL. State the equation:

100 mg : 1 cc = 250 mg : X

Multiply the extremes = 100X.

Multiply the means = 250 mg.

250 = 100X

To arrive at X, divide 250 by 100.

250 ÷ 100 = 2.5.

In this example, you would administer 2.5 mL of erythromycin at 100 mg/mL.

Example 2. The physician orders phenobarbital 25 mg. On hand are 12.5-mg tablets. State the equation:

12.5 mg : 1 TAB = 25 mg : X

Multiply the extremes = 12.5X.

Multiply the means = 25 mg.

25 = 12.5

To arrive at X, divide 25 by 12.5.

25 ÷ 12.5 = 2

In this example, you would administer 2 tablets of phenobarbital.

The Formula Method

The formula method is written as:

$$\frac{\text{Desired}}{\text{On Hand}} \times \text{Quantity}$$

Example 1. The physician orders ampicillin 0.5 g. On hand is ampicillin 250 mg/capsule. How much ampicillin should be administered? Remember, both dosages must be in the same unit of measure. Change grams to milligrams following the rules for conversion within the metric system (eg, multiply the grams by 1000 or move the decimal three places to the right). To change 0.5 g to milligrams, multiply 0.5 by 1000. The answer is 500 mg.

$$\frac{500 \text{ mg (Desired)}}{250 \text{ mg (On Hand)}} \times 1 \text{ (Quantity)} = 2 \times 1 = 2$$

In this example, you would administer 2 capsules.

Example 2.

Desired: 0.35 g
On Hand: 700 mg/cc
How many cc?

Remember, measurements must be in equivalent units, so 0.35 g must be changed to milligrams (eg, multiply the grams by 1000 or move the decimal three places to the right. In this case, 0.35 g become 350 mg.)

$$\frac{350 \text{ mg}}{700 \text{ mg}} \times 1\text{cc} = \frac{1}{2} \text{ cc} = 0.5\text{CC}$$

Checkpoint Question

3. Before calculating dosages, what must be done with the measurements?

➤ CALCULATING PEDIATRIC DOSAGES

Several formulas are used for pediatric dosage calculation. The method considered to be the most accurate involves calculating dosage by body surface area (BSA) and requires a scale known as a nomogram. The following formulas are used in calculating dosage for infants and children.

The Nomogram

Pediatric dosages using the BSA are easily and accurately calculated on a nomogram such as the one illustrated in Figure 26-2. This method is considered to be one of the most accurate and can be used for children up to 12 years of age and for adults who are below normal percentiles for body weight. The nomogram chart estimates the BSA according to height and weight. BSA is expressed in square meters.

The chart has three columns. A straight line is drawn from the patient's height in inches or centimeters (column one) to the patient's weight in kilograms or pounds (column three). The straight line will then intersect on the BSA column (column two). This column gives the estimated BSA of the child. After obtaining the BSA average, the following formula is used:

$$\frac{\text{BSA in m}^2 \times \text{Adult Dose}}{1.7} = \text{Child's Dose}$$

Height		Surface Area	Weight	
feet	centimeters	in square meters	pounds	kilograms

FIGURE 26-2

Nomogram for estimating surface area of infants and young children. To determine the surface area of the patient, draw a straight line between the point representing the height on the left vertical scale and the point representing the weight on the right vertical scale. The point at which this line intersects the middle vertical scale represents the patient's surface area in square meters. (Courtesy of Abbott Laboratories.)

Example 1. The child weighs 65 lb, or 30 kg, and his height is 50 inches, or 128 cm. Therefore, his BSA is 1.02. If the adult dose is 250 mg, then:

$$\frac{1.02 \times 250}{1.7} \times 150 \text{ mg}$$

After obtaining the child's dose, use ratio and proportion or the short formula and compute the amount of medication to be administered from the amount on hand.

Young's Rule

Using Young's rule, the age of the child, divided by the age of the child plus 12, multiplied by the average adult dose equals the child's dose.

$$\text{Pediatric Dose} = \frac{\text{Child's age in years}}{\text{Child's age in years} + 12} \times \text{Adult Dose}$$

Young's rule is not used when the child is over the age of 12 years or under 12 months. If a child over 12 years is small enough to need a smaller dose, Clark's rule may be used.

Clark's Rule

This calculation is more accurate than Young's rule and allows for variations in body size and weight for different ages. Using Clark's rule, the weight of the child divided by 150 (presumed weight of average adult) multiplied by the average adult dose equals the child's dose.

$$\text{Pediatric Dose} = \frac{\text{Child's weight in pounds} \times \text{Adult Dose}}{150 \text{ pounds}}$$

For calculating dosages for infants less than 2 years of age, Fried's rule may be used.

Fried's Rule

This calculation is used only occasionally for children under 2 years of age and bases the dosage on age in months. In this case, the 150 used in calculations is the age in months of a 12½-year-old child and presumes that a child of that age would be eligible for an adult dose. Using Fried's rule, the child's age in months divided by 150 multiplied by the average adult dose equals the child's dose.

$$\text{Pediatric Dose} = \frac{\text{Child's age in months}}{150 \text{ months}} \times \text{Adult Dose}$$

Note: Young's, Clark's and Fried's rules are used less frequently than the BSA method of calculation.

Many medications that require careful calibration and that are based on weight are prepared with directions for administering a dosage per kilogram of body weight. Instructions for calculation will be included in the package insert. For instance, the insert may state: *Adults and children over 25 kg (55 lb), give 300 mg q 12 h per day in divided doses. Children less than 25 kg, give 25 mg/kg q 12 h per day in divided doses.*

Example 1. The child to whom this medication is to be given weighs 20 lb. This weight must be converted into kilograms. Remember that 1 kg is 2.2 lb; therefore, the child weighs 9 kg.

State the equation as follows: 25 mg/9 kg/day divided by 2 (medication is given twice in 24 hours).

$$25 \text{ mg} \times 9 = 225 \text{ mg/day} \div 2 = 112.5 \text{ q 12 h}$$

(In many cases it will be necessary to "round off" the dosage.)

Remember that some recommended doses are calculated for a day's total dose, then must be divided into recommended dose divisions, such as qid or bid. For example, the recommended dose for a 24-hour period may be 300 mg, but should be given in q 8 h increments of 100 mg each. A serious overdose might result if this final calculation step is not taken.

What If?
What if a child arrives at the medical office in cardiac arrest? How does the physician have time to calculate the child's body weight?

In such a situation, the physician does not have the time to perform the calculations and instead may rely on printed graphs that list precalculated emergency drug doses. Also, some hospital emergency departments use computer software that will automatically calculate and print a list of all pediatric emergency medications and their doses.

➤ MEDICATION ROUTES

Medication can be administered in many ways. The route of administration is chosen after considering many factors. Sometimes the route is chosen because of cost, safety, or degree of speed by which the drug will be absorbed into the system. Certain drugs may be administered by only one route. Some drugs may be toxic if given by a certain route, some may be effective only if given by a specific route, and sometimes absorption will only occur through one particular route.

➤ ORAL ADMINISTRATION

Of all of the medication routes, the oral route is the easiest and most preferred by patients; however, oral medication is usually slow to take effect and cannot be used for unconscious patients, those with nausea and vomiting, or those who are NPO (nothing by mouth).

Drugs given orally may be administered as tablets, capsules, pills, or liquids (Procedure 26-1). They are usually absorbed through the walls in the gastrointestinal tract.

Many drugs are available in unit-dose packages that contain the amount of the drug for a single dose and in the proper form for administration (Fig. 26-3). Unit-dose packages are labeled with the trade name, generic name, precautions, instructions for storage, and an expiration date. Liquid medications may be measured in a graduate, minim glass, medicine glass, or plastic cup.

Table 26-4 lists common solid and liquid forms of oral medications.

Sublingual Route

Medication given sublingually is placed under the patient's tongue; it must not be swallowed. The medication is dissolved by the saliva in the mouth and is absorbed directly into the bloodstream through the mucosa covering the sublingual vessels. The number of medications administered sublingually is limited. Cau-

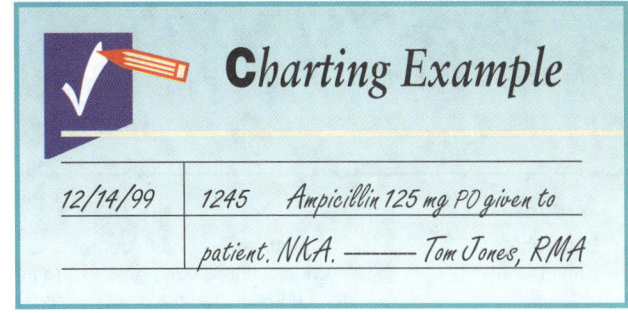

Charting Example

| 12/14/99 | 1245 | Ampicillin 125 mg PO given to |
| | | patient. NKA. ——— Tom Jones, RMA |

tion the patient not to eat or drink until the medication has totally dissolved.

Buccal Route

Medication given by the buccal route is placed in the pouch between the cheek and gum at the side of the mouth for absorption through the vascular oral mucosa. Few medications are manufactured for this route. The patient must not drink fluids until the medication is completely absorbed.

Procedure 26-2 describes the steps to follow for administration of sublingual or buccal medications.

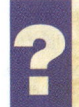

Checkpoint Question
4. What are the disadvantages of the oral route for medication administration?

MUCOSAL ADMINISTRATION

Many medications administered to the mucous membranes are designed for a local effect. Examples include local fungicides in vaginal suppositories or local irri-

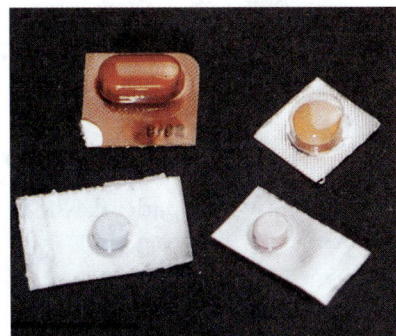

FIGURE 26-3
Unit dose packages.

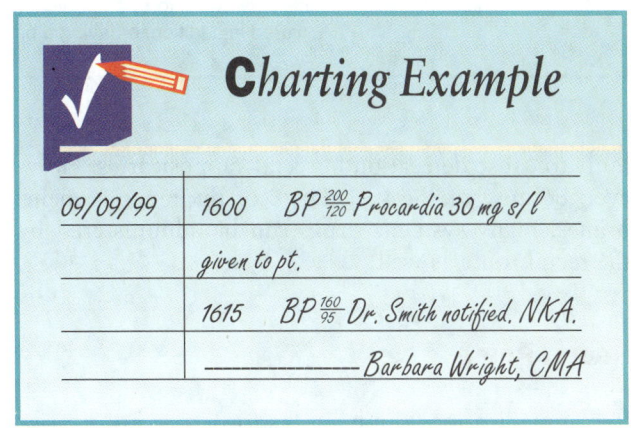

Charting Example

09/09/99	1600	BP $\frac{200}{120}$ Procardia 30 mg s/l
		given to pt.
	1615	BP $\frac{160}{95}$ Dr. Smith notified. NKA.
		——— Barbara Wright, CMA

Table 26-4
Forms of Oral Medications

Form	Description
Solids	
Buffered	Agents are added to decrease or counteract the medication's acidity to prevent gastric irritation.
Caplet	Medication is compressed into the shape of a capsule. It may be coated for ease in swallowing, but it does not have a gelatin covering.
Capsule	Powdered or granulated medication is enclosed in a gelatin capsule designed to dissolve in gastric enzymes or high in the small intestines.

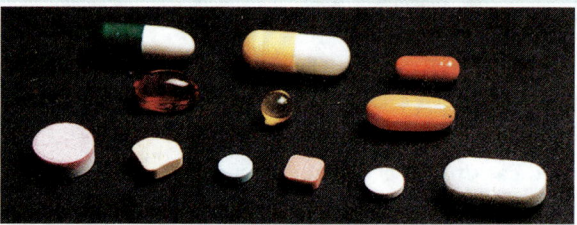

Oral medications. Tablets (*front*), gelcaps (*middle*), and capsules.

Enteric-coated tablet	A compressed dry form of a medication coated to withstand the gastric acidity and dissolve in the intestines. These may be medications that would be destroyed by the gastric enzymes or might be damaging to the gastric mucosa. Never crush or break enteric-coated tablets.
Gelcap	An oil-based medication is enclosed in a soft gelatin capsule.
Lozenge	A firm, compressed form of medication, usually for a local effect in the mouth or throat. Caution patients to let lozenges dissolve slowly and avoid drinking any fluids for a period of time after using the lozenge.
Powder	A finely ground form of medication; may be difficult for many patients to swallow.
Spansule or time-release capsule	Gelatin capsules are filled with forms of the medication that will dissolve over a period of time rather than all at once. Never open spansules unless this is recommended or allowed by the manufacturer.
Tablet	Medication is formed into many shapes and colors for easy identification. Tablets usually dissolve high in the gastrointestinal tract. These may be broken into halves only if they have been scored for that purpose (see photo).
Liquids	
Elixir	Medication is dissolved in alcohol and flavoring is added. These are less sweet than syrups and are usually preferred by adults. They should not be used for alcoholics or diabetics.
Emulsion	Medication is combined with water and oil. Emulsions must be thoroughly shaken to disperse the medication evenly.
Extract	This is a very concentrated form of medication made by evaporating volatile plant oils. Extracts may be administered as drops and are usually given in a liquid to disguise their strong taste.
Gel	Medication is suspended in a thin gelatin or paste base.
Suspension	Particles are dissolved in a liquid that must be shaken well before administering.
Syrup	This very sweet form of medication is used frequently for children's medications and is usually flavored in addition to having a high sugar content.

tants to cause defecation in rectal suppositories. However, because of the vascularity of the mucous membranes, many systemic drugs can be administered by the rectal route as well.

Rectal Route

Rectal medications can be in the form of suppositories or liquids (administered as a retention enema). They can provide a local effect or they may be absorbed through the rectal mucosa for a systemic effect. Rectal medications may be used for patients who are NPO or who have nausea and vomiting, but they are never used for patients who have diarrhea.

Most rectal suppositories use a cocoa butter or glycerin base that melts at body temperature (Fig. 26-4A). These should be inserted about 2 inches into the rectum, above the internal rectal sphincter to avoid the urge to evacuate (see Fig. 26-4B). If insertion is diffi-

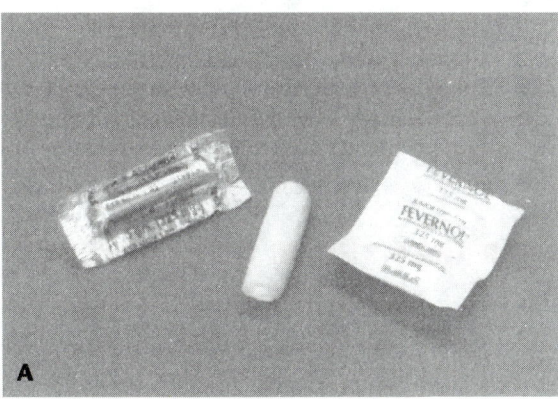

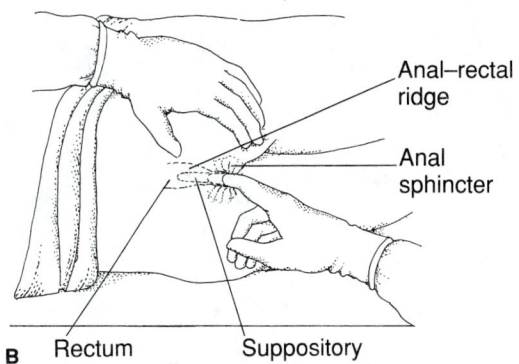

FIGURE 26-4
(*A*) These are examples of suppositories. They are made in a variety of sizes and shapes. (*B*) Rectal suppositories should be introduced into the anus well beyond the internal sphincter.

cult, lubricating gel may be applied, but never petrolatum (petrolatum interferes with absorption and is damaging to the mucosa). Never force the insertion of a suppository because this could be dangerous to the patient. At the very least, it would cause unnecessary discomfort.

Both enemas and suppositories should be retained by the patient for about 20 to 30 minutes before elimination.

Vaginal Route

Vaginal medications may be creams, tablets, cocoa butter-based suppositories, or solutions for douches. Examples include hormonal creams and antibiotic or antifungal preparations. Very few medications other than those for local effects are prescribed for the vaginal route. All are more effective if inserted the full length of the vagina, preferably into the posterior fornix (Fig. 26-5).

The patient should remain lying for a period of time after insertion; therefore, instructions may suggest that the medication be inserted at bedtime. For the patient's comfort, she may need a light pad to absorb drainage.

➤ DERMAL ADMINISTRATION

Dermal medications are applied to the skin. They include topical creams, lotions, and ointments and transdermal medications. Topical medications produce local-

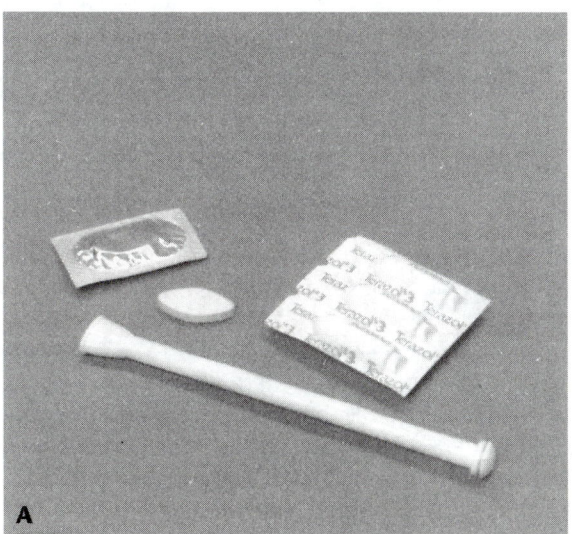

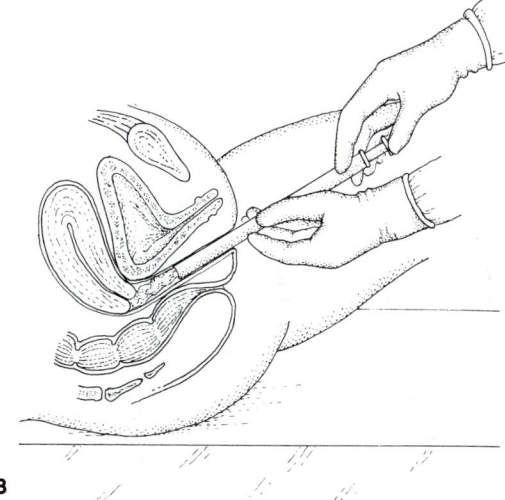

FIGURE 26-5
Insertion of vaginal medication. (*A*) Vaginal suppository and applicator. (*B*) Insertion of vaginal cream using an applicator.

Patient Education: Insertion of Suppositories

Some patients are not proficient with the insertion of suppositories and may require specific instructions or simple drawings. Medication errors have occurred because patients did not know the differences between their various orifices. Take a few moments to ensure that the patient understands the route of application, methods to make application easier (lubricating gel or warm water to moisten), and that the foil wrapper is to be removed and is not part of the treatment.

Remember: If you are helping the patient to insert either rectal or vaginal suppositories, or if you are administering solutions by either route, you must follow Standard Precautions and wear gloves.

ized effects, such as coating or soothing. Transdermal medications produce systemic effects.

Transdermal Medications

Medication administered transdermally is delivered to the body by absorption through the skin. Delivery is slow and maintains a steady, stable level of medication. Dermal patches are placed on the skin, usually on the chest or back, upper arm, or behind the ear (for prevention of motion sickness). Antiangina medications placed anywhere on the chest wall are effective by this route.

Procedure 26-3 describes the steps to follow in applying transdermal medication. Procedure 26-4 describes the steps to follow in applying topical medication.

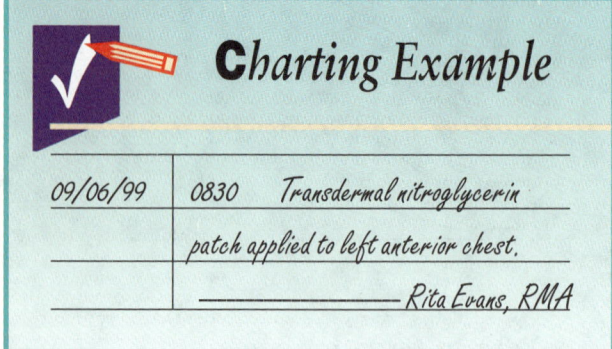

Charting Example

09/06/99	0830	Transdermal nitroglycerin
		patch applied to left anterior chest.
		— Rita Evans, RMA

Checkpoint Question
5. How do the effects of topical and transdermal medications differ?

➤ PARENTERAL ADMINISTRATION

If a patient is NPO, or if the drug cannot be absorbed through the gastrointestinal system, the parenteral route is used. Parenteral administration refers not only to injections, but to all the ways in which drugs are administered other than by swallowing for absorption in the gastrointestinal tract.

The intramuscular route is often used for this type of administration because the muscles are highly vascular and absorption is fairly rapid (see "Types of Injections and Injection Sites," p. 441). Administration by injection is the most efficient method of drug administration, but it can also be the most hazardous. The effects may be quite rapid, the medication cannot be retrieved, and, because the skin is broken, it is possible for infections to develop. You must use aseptic technique whenever administering medications by the injection route (Box 26-3).

If an injection is placed incorrectly, nerve damage could occur, or the penetration of blood vessels could cause formation of a hematoma. Incorrect placement of the needle during an intramuscular injection could cause the medication to be delivered intravenously.

➤ EQUIPMENT NEEDED FOR GIVING INJECTIONS

Medications used for injections are supplied in **ampules**, **vials**, and cartridges (Fig. 26-6).

BOX 26-3   Injections: Maintaining Sterility

The following parts of the hypodermic setup must be kept sterile:

- syringe tip
- inside of barrel
- shaft of plunger
- needle

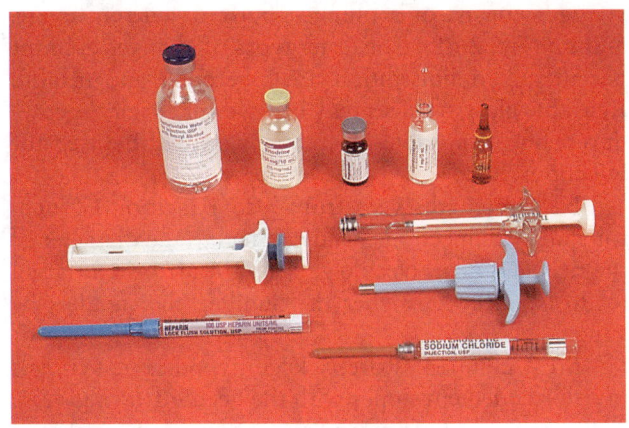

FIGURE 26-6
Ampules, vials, prefilled cartridges, and holders.

Ampules

Ampules are small, glass containers that must be broken at the neck to aspirate the solution into the syringe. When the ampule is opened, all medication from it must be either used or discarded. It must not be saved for later use because once the ampule is broken, sterility cannot be maintained.

Vials

Vials are glass or plastic containers sealed at the top by a rubber stopper. They may be single-dose or multiple-dose containers. The contents of vials may be in solution or in powder or crystal form, which requires reconstitution with a specific amount and type of **diluent** (diluting agent), usually sterile water or saline. Certain drugs such as Dilantin require a special diluent supplied by the manufacturer.

When a powdered drug is reconstituted, the following must be written on the label:

1. Date of the reconstitution
2. Initials of the person who reconstituted the drug
3. Diluent used

To reconstitute a dry form of medication, withdraw from the vial the amount of air that will be replaced by the diluent. Inject the required amount of diluent into the air space in the vial and not into the medication to avoid bubbles or foam. Withdraw the needle and gently roll the bottle between the palms to dissolve the medication. Shaking the bottle may cause bubbles.

Vials may be intended for multiple doses or for a unit dose. Vials intended for multiple dose use may be up to 50 mL and may be used repeatedly by entering through the rubber stopper to remove a portion of the solution. Unit-dose vials usually contain 1 to 2 mL and

all of the solution is removed for a single injection. Some single-dose vials are designed to include the dry form of the medication and the solution required for its reconstitution in separate compartments. Instructions for combining the two in these specially designed vials will be included by the manufacturer. These are usually to be reconstituted just before being administered.

Cartridges

Prefilled syringes contain a premeasured amount of a medication in a disposable cartridge with a needle attached. The prefilled cartridge and needle are placed in

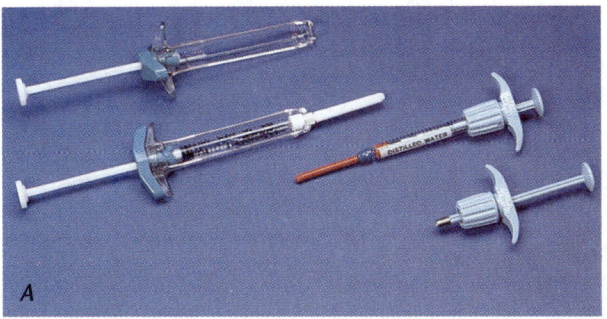

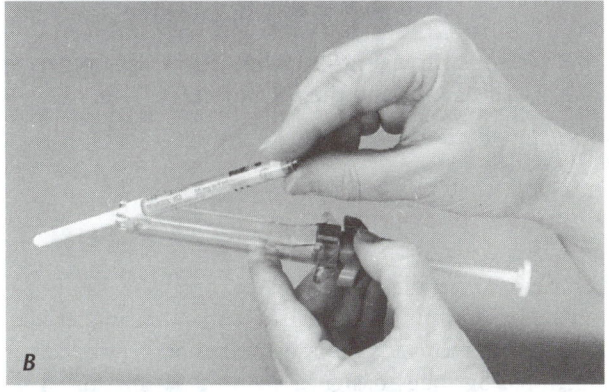

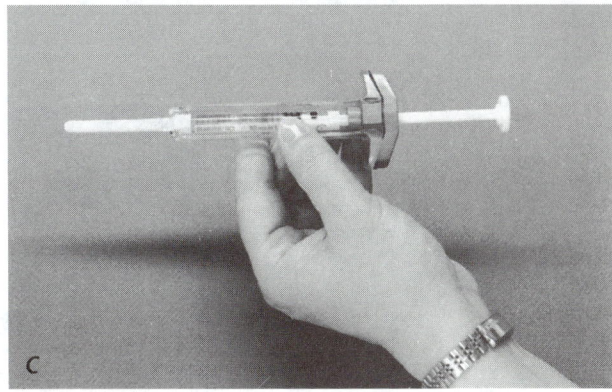

FIGURE 26-7
Prefilled syringes. (A) Prefilled medication cartridges and injector devices. (B) Inserting the cartridge into the injector device. (C) Ready for injection.

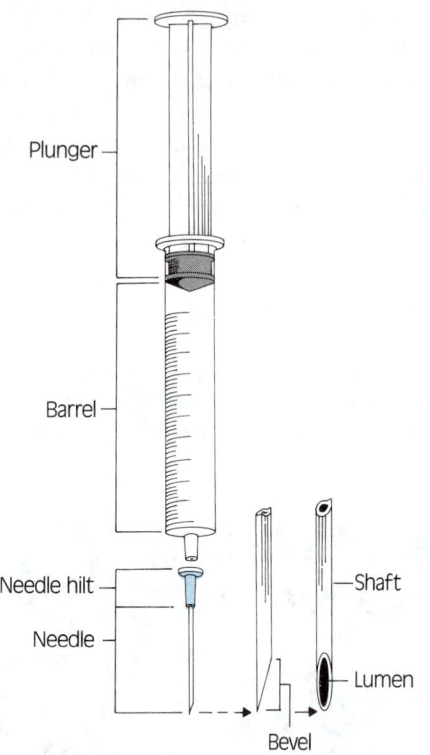

FIGURE 26-8
Parts of a syringe and needle.

a holder for administration (Fig. 26-7). Examples of units are the Tubex and the Carpuject.

Needles and Syringes

A variety of needles and syringes are used for injections. The 3- milliliter (mL) or cubic centimeter (cc) hypodermic syringe is the most common type used for injections. Syringes designed to hold 10 mL or more are usually used in the medical office for irrigation. All syringes consist of a plunger, body or barrel, flange, and tip (Fig. 26-8). The other types of syringes used for parenteral administration are tuberculin and insulin. Reusable glass syringes may be used for surgical procedures, but disposable plastic syringes will be used for injections.

Needle lengths vary from ⅜ to 1 inch or 1½ inch, for standard injections. **Gauge** refers to the diameter of the needle lumen. Needle gauge varies from 18 (large) to 30 (small); the higher the number, the smaller the gauge.

Most companies prepackage hypodermic syringes in color-coded envelopes with the needle attached (Fig. 26-9). Separate needles and syringes may be purchased as needed. This type of syringe may be used for either subcutaneous or intramuscular injections.

It is necessary to choose the package with a needle length and gauge appropriate for the route of the injection to be given. For example, an intramuscular injection requires a needle length of at least 1 inch, depending on the size of the patient and the fat/muscle ratio. The needle will vary from 20 to 25 gauge, depending on the medication to be administered. Thick medications, such as penicillin, are difficult to draw into a syringe using a small-gauge needle and will be supplied in a prefilled cartridge with the appropriate-sized needle. Subcutaneous injections are generally given using a short, small-gauge needle: 25 gauge ⅝ inch or 23 gauge ½ inch.

All hypodermic syringes are marked with 10 calibrations per milliliter or cubic centimeter on one side of the syringe. Each small line represents 0.1 (one-tenth) mL or cc. The other side of the syringe is marked in minims (Fig. 26-10).

The tuberculin (TB) syringe is narrow and has a total capacity of 1 mL or cc. There are 100 calibration lines marking the capacity. Each line represents 0.01 mL. Every tenth line is longer than the others to indicate 0.1 mL. TB syringes are used for newborn and pediatric doses, for intradermal skin tests, and

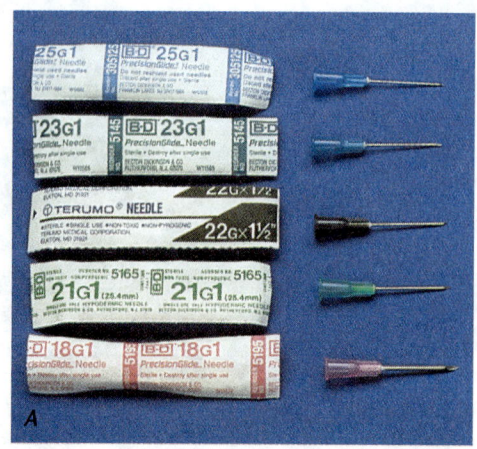

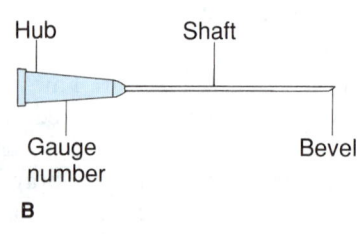

FIGURE 26-9
Needles. (*A*) Different gauges and lengths. (*B*) Parts of a needle.

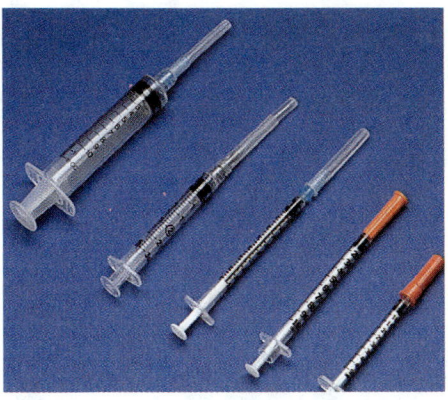

FIGURE 26-10
Syringes (*from top to bottom*): 10 mL, 3 mL, tuberculin, insulin, and low-dose insulin.

any time that minute amounts of medication are to be given.

The insulin syringe is used strictly for administering insulin to diabetic patients. It has a total capacity of 1 mL. The 1-mL volume is marked as 100 units (U) to represent the strength of 100 U insulin/mL when full. Each group of 10 U is divided by five small lines. Each line represents 2 U. A smaller insulin syringe with a capacity of 0.5 mL can be used when less than 50 U insulin is ordered. The smaller insulin syringe has 50 small calibration lines each representing 1 U insulin (Fig. 26-11).

Most of the insulin used today is U-100, which means that there are 100 U insulin in each mL (cc). It is important to remember that the insulin syringe must be marked U-100 to match the insulin used.

Procedure 26-5 describes the steps required for preparing an injection.

Checkpoint Question
6. *What are ampules and vials and how do they differ?*

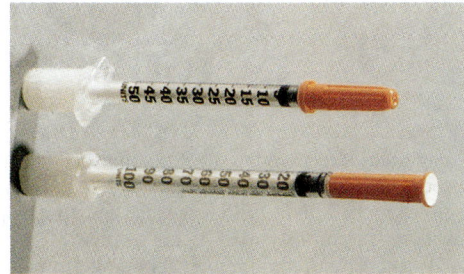

FIGURE 26-11
Insulin syringes. 50 units (*top*) and 100 units.

➤ TYPES OF INJECTIONS AND INJECTION SITES

Intradermal Injections

Intradermal injections are inserted at a 10°–15° angle, almost parallel to the skin surface (Fig. 26-12). When administered correctly, the needle will be slightly visible under the skin, and a small bubble (wheal or bleb) will be raised in the skin surface when the solution is injected. Recommended sites include the anterior forearm and across the back. Intradermal injections are used exclusively to administer skin tests, such as the tine or Mantoux tuberculin skin test or allergy tests.

The tine test is used for routine screening and is not considered as diagnostic as the Mantoux test. Both use purified protein derivative (PPD) from a live tuberculin bacillus culture to test for the presence of tuber-

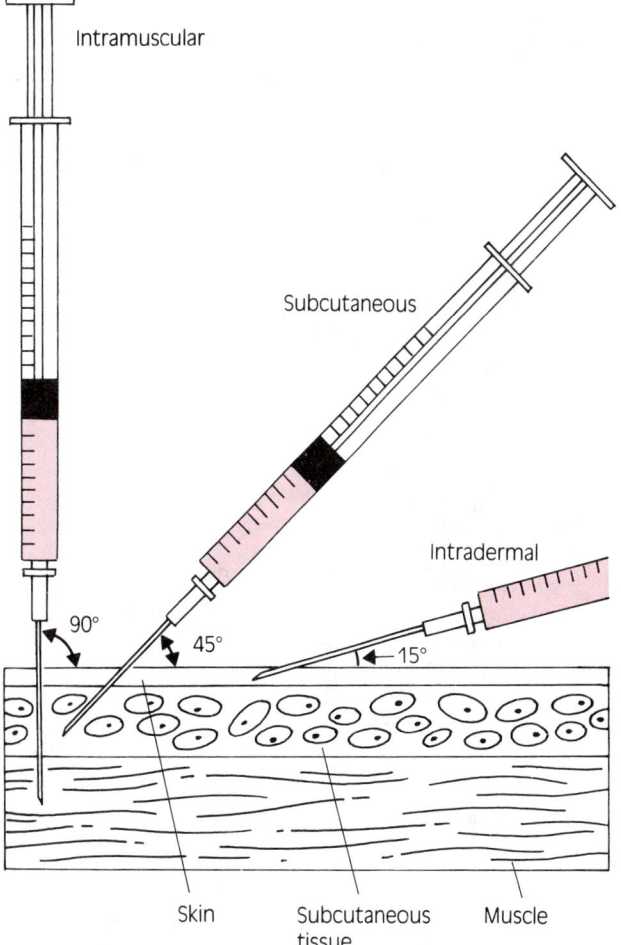

FIGURE 26-12
Comparison of the angles of insertion for intramuscular, subcutaneous, and intradermal injections.

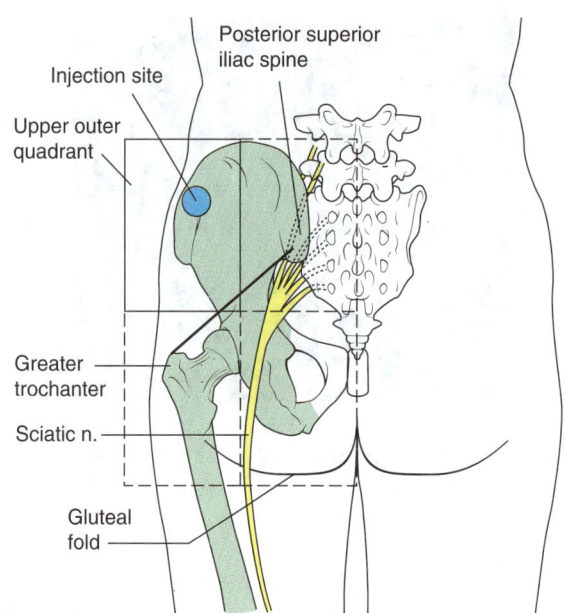

FIGURE 26-14
The dorsogluteal site for administering an intramuscular injection is lateral and slightly superior to the midpoint of a line drawn from the trochanter to the posterior superior iliac spine. Correct identification of this site minimizes the possibility of accidentally damaging the sciatic nerve.

Charting Example

| 05/04/99 | 1035 | Tine test administered intradermal to left forearm. Wheal noted. Pt. instructed regarding reading the results and will call the office on 05/07/99 with the results. ———— Paula King, CMA |

---

culin antibodies. A positive tine test is usually followed by a Mantoux test. A positive Mantoux reaction with induration greater than 10 mm will indicate the possibility of active or dormant tuberculosis or exposure to the disease. Further testing by sputum culture and x-rays are required for a definitive diagnosis.

Procedure 26-6 describes the steps for giving an intradermal injection. Procedure 26-7 describes how to administer the tine or Mantoux test.

Subcutaneous Injections

Subcutaneous injections are given into the fatty layer of tissue below the skin by positioning the needle and syringe at a 45° angle to the skin (see Fig. 26-12). The subcutaneous route is chosen for drugs that should not

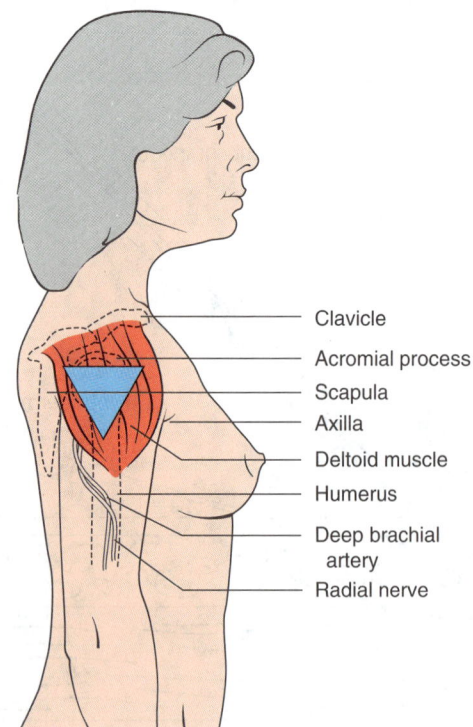

FIGURE 26-13
The deltoid muscle site for intramuscular injections is located by palpating the lower edge of the acromial process. At the midpoint, in line with the axilla on the lateral aspect of the upper arm, a triangle is formed.

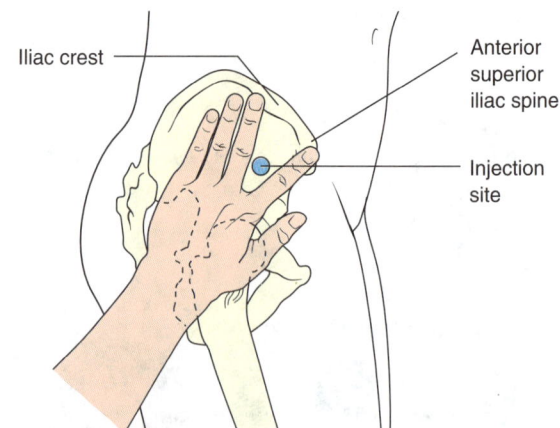

FIGURE 26-15
The ventrogluteal site is located by placing the palm on the greater trochanter and the index finger toward the anterior superior iliac spine. The middle finger is then spread posteriorly away from the index finger as far as possible. A "V" or triangle is formed by this maneuver. The injection is made in the middle of the triangle.

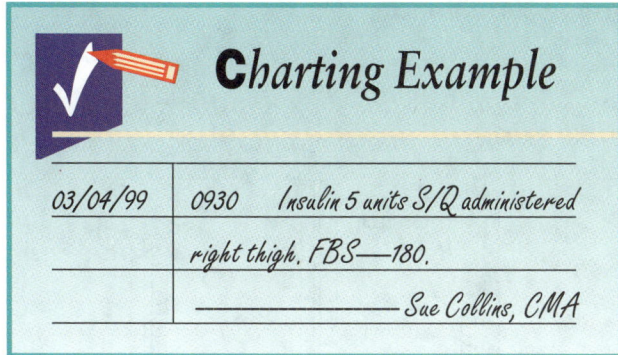

Charting Example

03/04/99	0930	Insulin 5 units S/Q administered
		right thigh, FBS—180.
		——— Sue Collins, CMA

be absorbed as rapidly as through the intramuscular or intravenous routes.

Common sites include the upper arm, thigh, back, and abdomen. Procedure 26-8 describes the steps for administering a subcutaneous injection.

Intramuscular Injections

Intramuscular (IM) injections are given into a muscle by positioning the needle and syringe at a 90° angle to the skin (see Fig. 26-12). Absorption of IM medications is fairly rapid because of the vascularity of

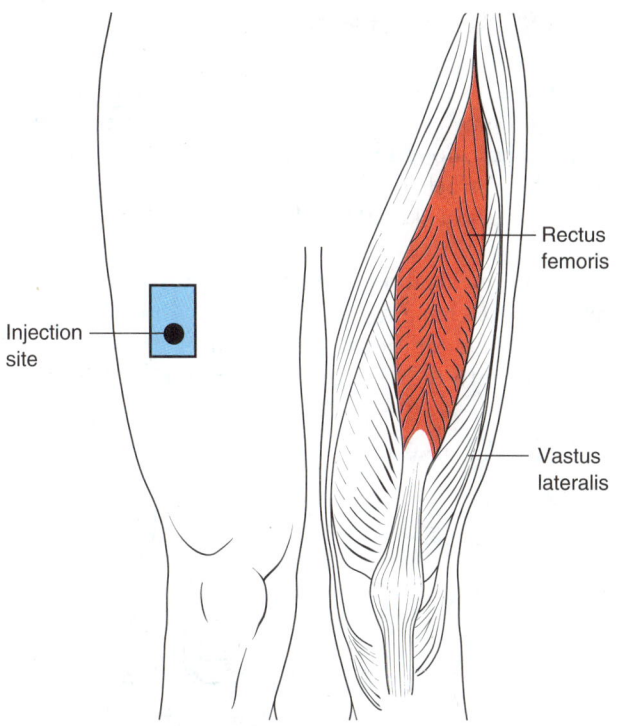

FIGURE 26-17
The rectus femoris site for intramuscular injections is used only when other sites are contraindicated.

muscle tissues. If absorption needs to be slower, the medication will be supplied mixed with an oil base rather than saline or water to prolong the absorption time.

Recommended sites include the deltoid (Fig. 26-13), dorsogluteal (Fig. 26-14), ventrogluteal (Fig. 26-15), and vastus lateralis (Fig. 26-16). The rectus femoris (Fig. 26-17) can also be used for giving intramuscular injections, but only when using the other sites is contraindicated. (It is recommended that no more than 1 mL be administered in the deltoid site.)

Procedure 26-9 describes the steps for administering an intramuscular injection.

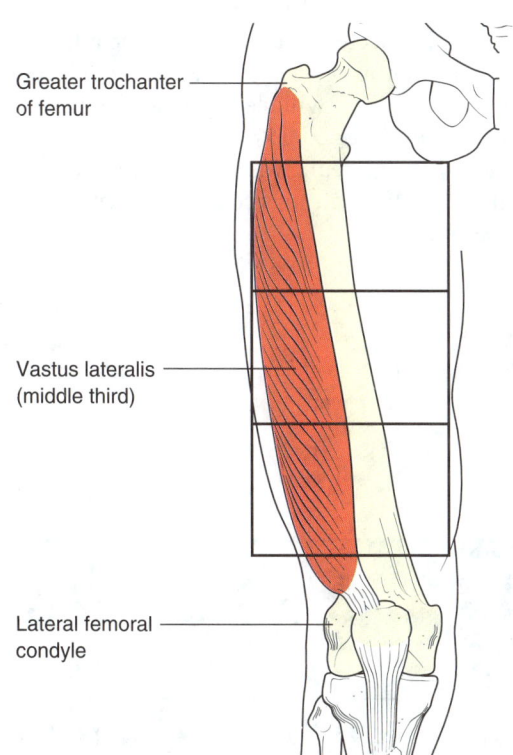

FIGURE 26-16
The vastus lateralis site for intramuscular injections is identified by dividing the thigh into thirds horizontally and vertically. The injection is given in the outer middle third.

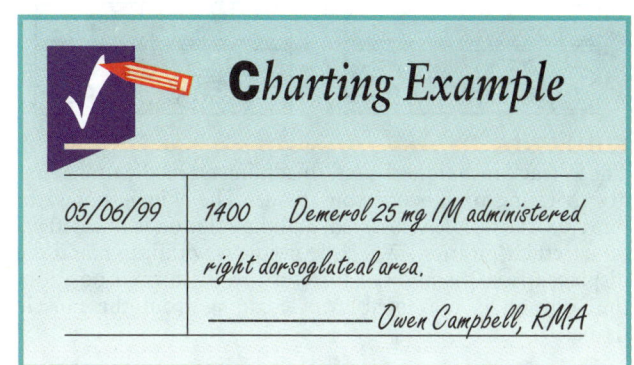

Charting Example

05/06/99	1400	Demerol 25 mg IM administered
		right dorsogluteal area.
		——— Owen Campbell, RMA

Z-Track Method of Intramuscular Injection

This method is used for IM administration of medications that may irritate or damage the tissues if allowed to leak back along the line of injection (Procedure 26-10). The Z-track method prevents leakage by sealing off the layers of skin along the route of the needle (Fig. 26-18).

If the medication is extremely caustic, directions may include changing the needle after drawing up the solution. The additional precaution of drawing up to 0.5 cc air into the syringe may be required. When the

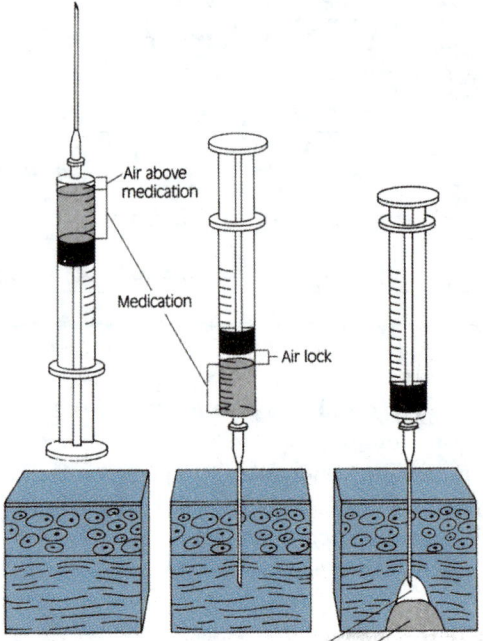

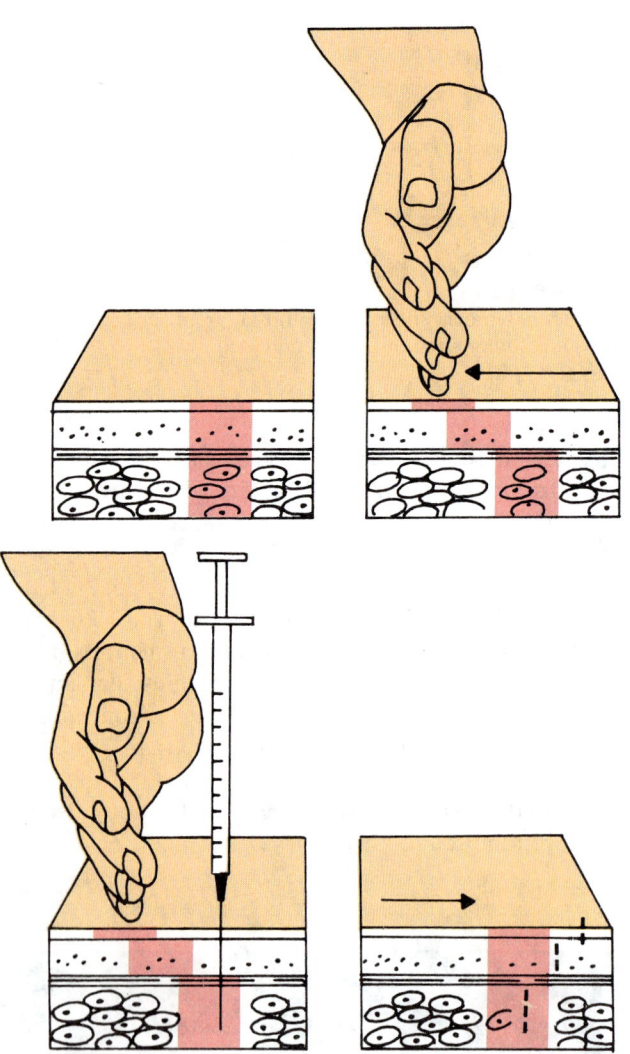

FIGURE 26-18
The Z-track technique is used to administer medications that are irritating to subcutaneous tissue. The skin is pulled to one side, the needle is inserted, and the solution is injected after careful aspiration. When the needle is withdrawn and the displaced tissue is allowed to return to its normal position, the solution is prevented from escaping from the muscle tissue.

FIGURE 26-19
An air bubble added to the syringe after the medication has been accurately measured helps to expel solution that is trapped in the shaft of the needle when the injection is given. It also helps to trap the injected solution in the intramuscular tissue.

medication is injected at a 90° angle, the additional air will rise to the top of the syringe and be injected after the medication. This will clear the needle and the path of the injection (Fig. 26-19).

The ventrogluteal, vastus lateralis, and dorsogluteal sites work well for the Z-track method; the deltoid does not.

Checkpoint Question
7. Name the types of injections. List possible sites for each type of injection.

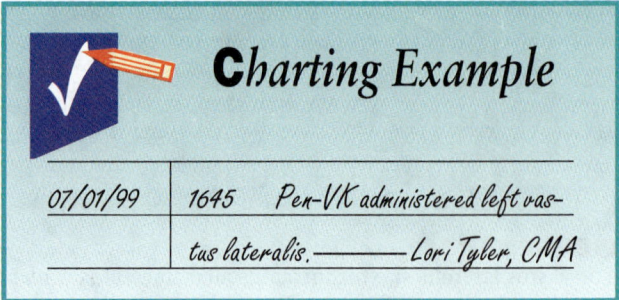

Charting Example

| 07/01/99 | 1645 | Pen-VK administered left vastus lateralis.———— Lori Tyler, CMA |

➤ OTHER MEDICATION ROUTES

Inhalation

Inhalation involves administration of medications, water vapors, or gases by inspiration of the substance(s) into the lungs. Medication is absorbed quickly through the alveolar walls into the capillaries. Existing pathology may make absorption difficult to predict. Patients with chronic pulmonary conditions may self-administer the medication with a hand-held **nebulizer**, which is an apparatus for producing a fine spray of medicated mist (Fig. 26-20).

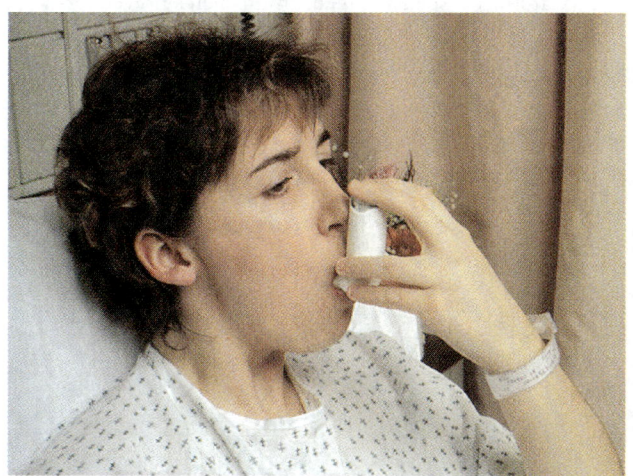

FIGURE 26-20
Nebulizer. A bottle of medication is attached to a mouthpiece. After the client exhales, the mouthpiece is gripped with the lips, and while the client takes a deep inhalation slowly, the bottle is firmly pushed down on the mouthpiece to release one dose of medication. (Photo © Ken Kasper.)

Intravenous (IV)

With this route, a sterile solution of a drug is injected into the body by venipuncture; larger amounts of medication in solution may be administered intravenously than by most other methods. Intravenous medication has the quickest action because it enters the bloodstream immediately. Only drugs intended for intravenous administration should be given by this route.

Intravenous medications are NEVER administered by medical assistants; physicians, nurses, or paramedics may administer intravenous medications.

Intra-arterial (IA)

Medications given using this route are administered into an artery and will have immediate effects. This method will never be used by medical assistants.

Intrathecal

Medication administered intrathecally is injected into the space within the spinal meninges. This route is usually confined to methods of anesthesia or analgesia.

Intra-articular

Medication given by this route is administered into a joint space. This route is used exclusively for treatment of joint pain.

text continues on page 467

Procedure
26-1

Administering Oral Medications

Equipment/Supplies

- medication
- medication tray
- disposable calibrated cup
- physician's instructions
- glass of water

Steps	Purpose
1. Wash your hands.	1. Handwashing aids infection control.
2. Assemble the equipment and supplies.	2. Doing this ensures that all of the materials are available.
3. Select the medication. Compare the label to the physician's instructions. Check the expiration date. Check the label three times: when taking it from the shelf, while pouring, and when returning to the shelf.	3. Carefully dispensing medications helps prevent errors. Outdated medication should not be administered to a patient.
4. Calculate the correct dosage to be given, if necessary.	
5. Remove the cap from the container, touching only the outside of the lid.	5. The inside of the lid will become contaminated if touched.
6. Remove the correct dose of medication from the container.	
a. *For solid medications*:	
(1) Pour the capsule or tablet into the bottle cap to prevent contamination of the cap and the medication. *CAUTION*: If the dosage requires that a scored tablet be broken, use a gauze square for breaking. Never break the tablet by using bare hands. Never crush enteric-coated tablets, and never open time-release capsules.	

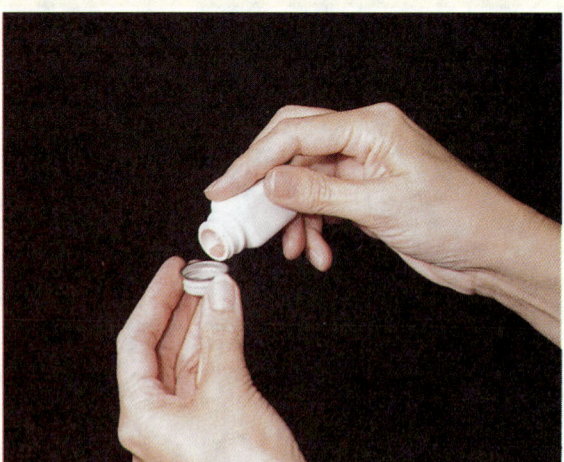

Step 6.a.(1): Pour the tablet into the bottle cap.

(continued)

Administering Oral Medications *(continued)*

Steps	Purpose

(2)   Transfer the medication to a disposable cup without touching the inside of the cup or the medication.

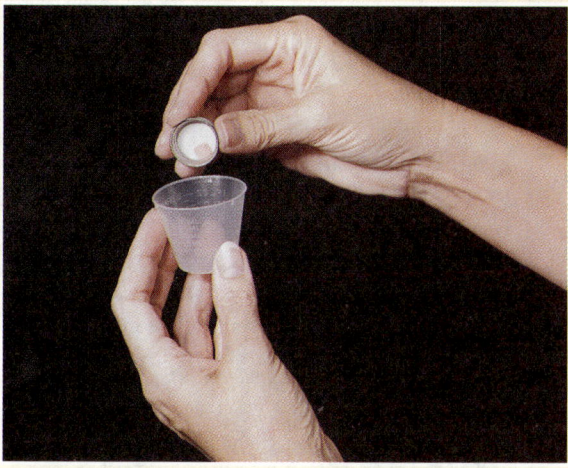

Step 6.a.(2): Transfer the medication to a disposable cup.

b.   *For liquid medications*:
(1)   Open the bottle lid and place it on a flat surface with the open end facing up to prevent contamination of the inside of the cap.
(2)   Palm the label to prevent liquids from dripping onto the label and obscuring the writing.

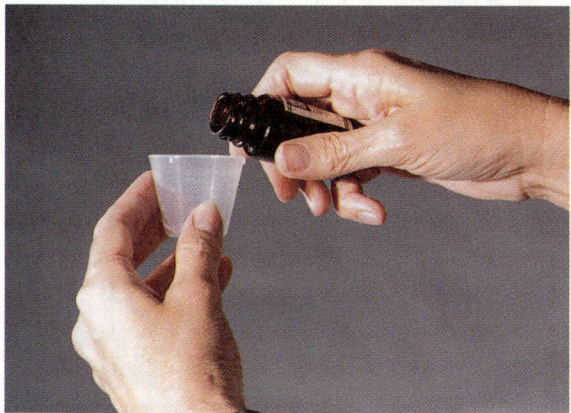

Step 6.b.(2): Palm the label.

(continued)

Procedure 26-1   Administering Oral Medications (continued)

Steps	Purpose
(3) With the opposite hand, place the thumbnail at the correct calibration on the cup. Holding the cup at eye level, pour the medication.	
(4) Read the level at the lowest level of the **meniscus,** the curved upper surface of the medication in the container. The lowest level of the meniscus gives the proper amount of medication.	
7. Greet and identify the patient. Explain the procedure. Ask the patient about medication allergies that might not be noted on the chart.	7. Identifying the patient prevents errors. Explaining the procedure helps ease anxiety and ensure compliance. Allergies may exist that have not been noted.
8. Give the medication to the patient.	
9. Give the patient a glass of water for swallowing the medication unless contraindicated.	9. Water helps the patient swallow the medication. However, water is contraindicated when giving medications intended for local effect (such as cough syrup or lozenges) or when giving buccal or sublingual medications, which are absorbed locally for a systemic effect and must not be swallowed (See Procedure 26-2).
10. Remain with the patient to be sure that all of the medication is swallowed. Observe any unusual reactions and report them to the physician. Record any unusual reactions on the patient's chart.	10. You cannot assume that the patient swallowed the medication unless you observe it. Unusual reactions may signal a developing hypersensitivity to the medication.
11. Thank the patient and give appropriate instructions.	11. Courtesy encourages the patient to have a positive attitude about the physician's office.
12. Wash your hands.	
13. Document the procedure.	13. Procedures are considered not to have been done if they are not recorded.

Procedure 26-2

Administering Sublingual or Buccal Medications

Equipment/Supplies

- medication
- medication tray
- disposable cup
- physician's instructions

Steps	Purpose
1–7. Follow steps 1–7 as described in Procedure 26-1, Administering Oral Medications.	
8. Administer the medication.	
a. *For sublingual medications*: Have the patient place the medication under the tongue.	
b. *For buccal medications*: Have the patient place the medication between the cheek and gum.	
9. Remain with the patient to be sure that the medication is *not* swallowed and is allowed to dissolve completely. Do not allow the patient to ingest any food or water until the medication is completely absorbed. Observe any unusual reactions and report them to the physician. Record any unusual reactions on the patient's chart.	9. You cannot assume that the medication was taken properly unless you observe it. Unusual reactions may signal a developing hypersensitivity to the medication.
10. Thank the patient and give appropriate instructions.	10. Courtesy encourages the patient to have a positive attitude about the physician's office.
11. Wash your hands.	
12. Document the procedure.	12. Procedures are considered not to have been done if they are not recorded.

Procedure 26-3   Applying Transdermal Medications

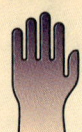

Equipment/Supplies

- medication
- medication tray
- physician's order

Steps	Purpose
1. Wash your hands.	1. Handwashing aids infection control.
2. Assemble the equipment and supplies.	2. Doing this ensures that all of the materials are available.
3. Greet and identify the patient. Explain the procedure. Ask the patient about medication allergies that might not be noted on the chart.	3. Identifying the patient prevents errors. Explaining the procedure helps ease anxiety and ensure compliance. Allergies may exist that have not been noted.
4. Select the site for administration and perform any necessary skin preparation. The sites are usually the upper arm, the chest or back surface, or behind the ear; these should be rotated. Ensure that the skin is dry, clean, and free of any irritation. Do not shave areas with excessive hair; trim the hair closely with scissors.	4. Shaving may abrade the skin and cause the medication to be absorbed too rapidly.
5. If there is a patch already in place, remove it carefully. Do not touch the inside of the patch to avoid absorbing any remaining medication. Discard the used patch in the trash container. Inspect the site for irritation. If there is a chance of contacting the medication with bare hands, wear gloves.	5. Touching the medication may cause it to be absorbed into your skin, causing undesirable reactions.
6. Open the medication package by pulling the two sides apart. Do not touch the area of medication.	
7. Apply the medicated patch to the patient's skin following the manufacturer's directions. Press the adhesive edges down firmly all around, starting at the center and pressing outward. If the edges do not stick, fasten with paper tape.	7. Starting at the center eliminates air spaces that may prevent contact with the skin.
8. Thank the patient and give appropriate instructions.	8. Courtesy encourages the patient to have a positive attitude about the physician's office.
9. Wash your hands.	
10. Document the procedure and the site of the new patch.	10. Procedures are considered not to have been done if they are not recorded.

Procedure 26-4   Applying Topical Medications

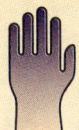

Equipment/Supplies

- medication
- medication tray
- physician's order
- washing solution (optional)
- tongue blade
- large cotton-tipped swab
- gloves
- dressing, bandage, tape (optional)

Steps	Purpose
1. Wash your hands.	1. Handwashing aids infection control.
2. Assemble the equipment and supplies. Check the medication label three times.	2. This ensures that all materials are available and prevents medication errors.
3. Greet and identify the patient. Explain the procedure. Ask the patient about medication allergies that might not be noted on the chart.	3. Identifying the patient prevents errors. Explaining the procedure helps ease anxiety and ensure compliance. Allergies may exist that have not been noted.
4. Assess the area to record observations regarding the condition of the skin.	4. Observations must be made before applying medication.
5. Put on gloves, in most instances.	5. Wearing gloves prevents contact with lesions or absorption of the medication through your skin.
6. If the area is soiled, clean the skin according to the steps for skin preparation outlined in Procedure 24-4: Performing Skin Preparation and Hair Removal in Chapter 24, Assisting with Minor Office Surgery.	6. Medication must be applied to clean skin.
7. If old medication remains in the area from a previous treatment, remove it by the same procedure.	7. New medication should not be applied over old medication.
8. If the lesion requires a dressing and bandage, apply the medication to the dressing using a tongue blade.	8. Medication is applied to the dressing, not to the wound, to avoid patient discomfort.
9. If the medication is to be applied directly to the area, lightly spread it with a tongue blade or a large cotton-tipped swab working from the center of the area outward.	9. Work from the cleanest area outward.
10. Use clean technique or medical asepsis if there are no open lesions. Use no touch technique or surgical asepsis if the skin is broken.	10. This avoids the spread of pathogens.
11. Bandage if necessary.	11. This protects the area.
12. Thank the patient and give appropriate instructions. Assist as needed.	12. Courtesy encourages the patient to have a positive attitude about the physician's office.
13. Clean the treatment room and dispose of equipment and supplies appropriately. Wash your hands.	13. This prevents the spread of pathogens.
14. Document the procedure.	14. Procedures are considered not to have been done if they are not recorded.

Procedure 26-5   Preparing an Injection

Equipment/Supplies

- medication
- medication tray
- antiseptic wipes
- appropriate-sized needle and syringe
- physician's instructions

Steps	Purpose
1. Wash your hands.	1. Handwashing aids infection control.
2. Assemble the equipment and supplies. Be careful to choose the needle and syringe according to the route of administration, type of medication, and patient's size.	2. Doing this ensures that all of the materials are available.
3. Select the proper medication. Check the expiration date and check the medication three times: when taking it from the shelf, while drawing it up, and when returning it to the shelf.	3. Never administer a medication that is out of date. Checking the medication ensures accuracy.
4. If necessary, calculate the correct dosage to be given.	
5. Open the sterile syringe/needle package. Assemble if necessary.	5. Needles and syringes often come preassembled in a package, or they may be purchased separately and assembled as needed.
6. Check to make sure the needle is firmly attached to the syringe by grasping the needle at the hub and turning it clockwise onto the syringe held in the other hand. Remove the needle guard.	6. A needle not firmly attached may become detached during the procedure.

Step 6: Grasp the needle at the hub and turn it clockwise.

7. Withdraw the correct amount of medication from the ampule or vial.
   a. *From an ampule*:
      (1) With the fingertips of one hand, tap the stem of the ampule lightly to remove any medication in or above the narrow neck.

(continued)

Procedure 26-5

Preparing an Injection (continued)

Steps	Purpose

(2) Place a piece of gauze around the ampule neck to protect your fingers from broken glass. Grasp the gauze and am-

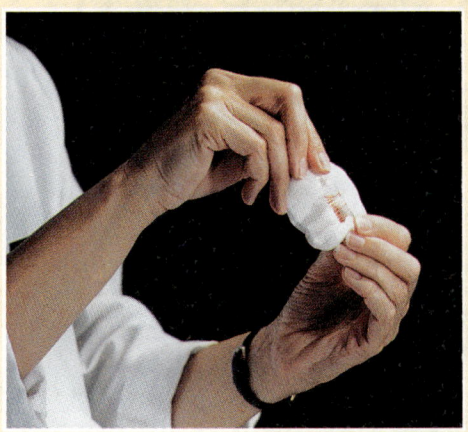

Step 7.a.(2): Grasp the gauze and ampule firmly.

pule firmly with the fingers. Snap the stem off the ampule with a quick downward movement of the gauze. Be sure to aim the break away from your face. Set the ampule top aside.

(3) Insert the needle lumen below the level of the medication. Withdraw the medication by pulling back on the plunger of the syringe without letting the needle touch the unsterile broken edge of the ampule to avoid contaminating the needle. Withdraw the desired amount of medication; set the ampule aside to dispose of properly.

(4) If there are air bubbles in the syringe, hold it vertically with the needle uppermost and tap the barrel gently with the fingertips until the air bubbles rise to the top. Draw back on the plunger to admit a small amount of air, then gently push the plunger forward to eject all of the air in the syringe. Do not eject any of the medication if only the required dosage has been drawn up. *Note*: Special needle adapters are available with filters to guard against the possibility of aspirating minute glass particles into the medication to be ad-

(continued)

Procedure 26-5   Preparing an Injection (continued)

Steps	Purpose

ministered. The adapter needle is discarded after drawing up the medication and the appropriate sized needle for the situation is then attached to the syringe for the administration of the medication.

b. *From a vial:*
(1) Cleanse the rubber stopper of the vial with the antiseptic wipe to avoid introducing bacteria into the medication.

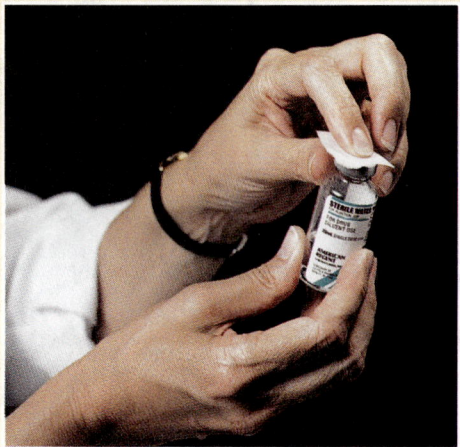

Step 7.b.(1): Clean the rubber stopper with an antiseptic wipe.

(2) Pull back on the plunger to aspirate an amount of air equal to the amount of medication to be removed from the vial.

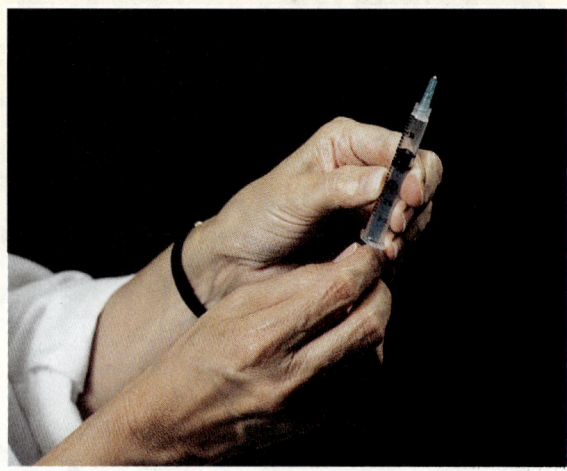

Step 7.b.(2): Pull back on the plunger.

(continued)

**Procedure
26-5**

Preparing an Injection *(continued)*

Steps	**Purpose**

(3) Insert the needle through the cleansed center of the stopper and above the level of the medication to prevent foam or bubbles from forming in the

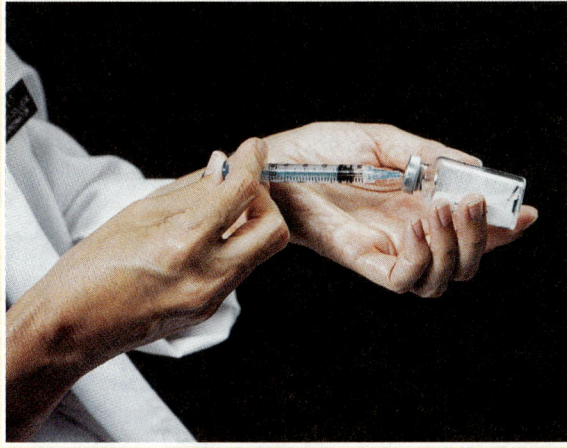

Step 7.b.(3): Insert the needle through the stopper.

medication. Inject the air from the syringe into the vial to avoid forming a vacuum in the vial, which would make withdrawal of the medication difficult.

(4) Invert the vial, holding the syringe at eye level. Aspirate the desired amount of medication into the syringe.

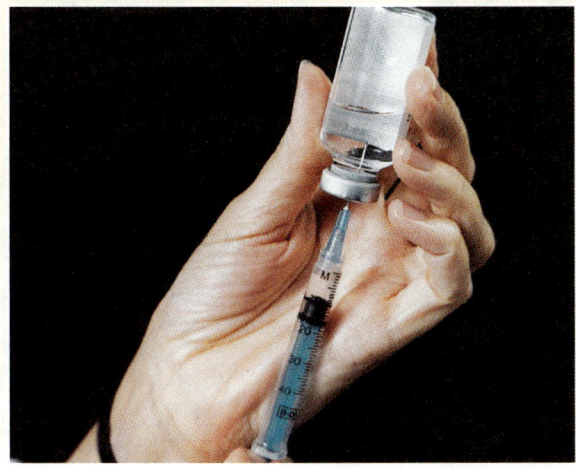

Step 7.b.(4): Invert the vial.

(continued)

Procedure 26-5   Preparing an Injection (continued)

Steps	Purpose
(5) Remove any air bubbles in the medication within the syringe by gently tapping with the finger tips on the barrel of the syringe held vertically. Remove any air remaining in the syringe by slowly pushing the plunger. Doing this allows the air to flow back into the vial to maintain the equalized pressure.	

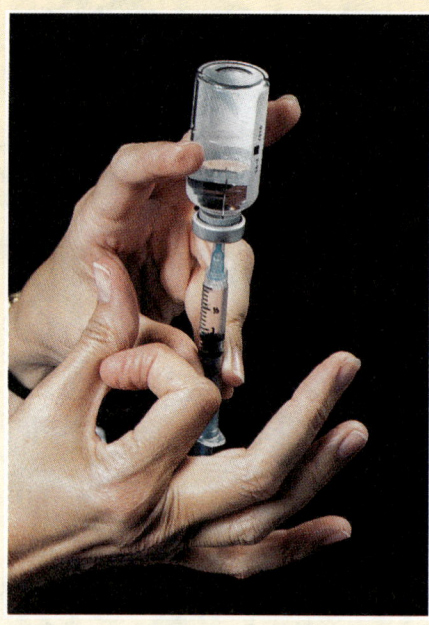

Step 7.b.(5): Tap on the barrel to remove air bubbles from the medication.

(continued)

Preparing an Injection (continued)

Steps	Purpose
8. Carefully recap the needle.	8. Needles are never recapped after administering the medication. The purpose of recapping a newly filled unused syringe is to protect the sterility of the needle.

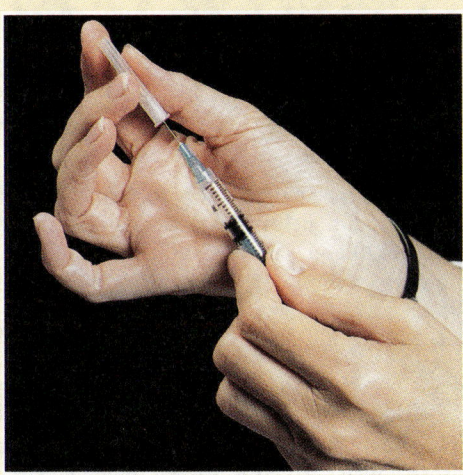

Step 8: Recap the needle.

9. Place the syringe with the medication on the medication tray with the physician's instructions. Place an antiseptic wipe on the tray for administering the medication. You are now ready to proceed with administering the specific type of injection ordered by the physician (see Procedures 26-6 to 26-10).

Procedure 26-6 Administering an Intradermal Injection

Equipment/Supplies

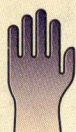

- medication
- medication tray
- antiseptic wipe
- appropriate-sized needle and syringe (generally a ⅜-inch 26–28-gauge needle
- on a tuberculin syringe to administer 0.1–0.2 mL)
- physician's instructions
- gloves

Steps	Purpose
1. Prepare the injection according to the steps in Procedure 26-5.	
2. Greet and identify the patient. Explain the procedure. Ask the patient about medication allergies that might not be noted on the chart.	2. Identifying the patient prevents errors. Explaining the procedure helps ease anxiety and ensure compliance. Allergies may exist the have not been noted.
3. Select the appropriate site for the injection. Recommended sites are the anterior forearm and the middle of the back. Make sure the entire site is exposed for safety and accuracy.	
4. Prepare the site by cleansing with an antiseptic wipe. Use a circular motion starting at the injection site and working toward to the outside. Do not touch the site after cleaning. If the site is grossly contaminated, wash it first with soap and water, then clean with an antiseptic wipe.	4. The site must be prepared by first removing microorganisms from the area. Wiping in a circular motion will carry the microorganisms away from the site. Touching the site after cleaning it will cause contamination.
5. Put on gloves.	5. Standard Precautions must be followed for protection against potential exposure to blood.
6. Remove the needle guard. Using your nondominant hand, pull the patient's skin taut.	6. Stretching the skin allows the needle to enter the skin with less resistance and secures the patient against movement.

Step 7: Insert the needle at a 10–15 degree angle.

(continued)

Procedure 26-6

Administering an Intradermal Injection (continued)

Steps	Purpose
7. With the bevel of the needle facing up, insert the needle at a 10–15 degree angle into the upper layer of the skin. When correctly placed for an intradermal injection, the needle will be slightly visible below the surface of the skin. It is not necessary to aspirate when performing an intradermal injection.	7. The needle should be inserted almost parallel to the skin to ensure that penetration occurs within the dermal layer. The bevel of the needle facing up will allow the wheal to be formed. If the bevel faces downward, no wheal will be formed and the medication may be absorbed into the tissues.
8. Inject the medication slowly by depressing the plunger. A wheal will form as the medication enters the dermal layer of the skin. Hold the syringe steady for proper administration.	8. Moving the needle once it has penetrated the skin will cause the patient to experience discomfort.
9. Remove the needle from the skin at the same angle at which it was inserted. Gently hold an antiseptic wipe over the site as the needle is withdrawn. Do not press or massage the site.	9. Withdrawing the needle quickly and gently at the angle of insertion reduces the chance of discomfort. Pressure on the wheal may cause the medication to be pressed into the tissues or out of the line of injection.
10. Dispose of the syringe and the needle in the approved container. Do not recap the needle. The sharps container should be placed where you have easy access to it after administration of an injection.	10. Discarding without recapping helps reduce the risk of an accidental needle stick.
11. Caution the patient not to massage the site.	11. Medication is not to be distributed into the tissues.
12. Remove gloves and wash your hands.	
13. Remain with the patient following the administration of an intradermal injection to observe for any unusual reactions. *Note*: If the patient experiences any unusual reactions, notify the physician immediately.	

14. Depending on the type of skin test administered, the length of time required for the body tissues to react, and the policies of the medical office, perform one of the following:
  a. Read the test results. Inspect and palpate the site for the presence and amount of induration.
  b. Tell the patient when to return (date and time) to the office to have the results read.
  c. Instruct the patient to read the results at home. Make sure the patient understands the instructions. Have the patient repeat the instructions if necessary.	

15. Document the procedure, the site, and the results. If instructions were given to the patient, document these also.	15. Procedures are considered not to have been done if they are not recorded.

Procedure 26-7

Administering a Tine or Mantoux Test

Equipment/Supplies

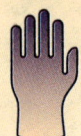

- tine applicator or tuberculin syringe with ⅜–½-inch, 26–27-gauge needle with 0.1 mL purified protein derivative
- millimeter ruler
- acetone wipe or alcohol wipe
- gloves

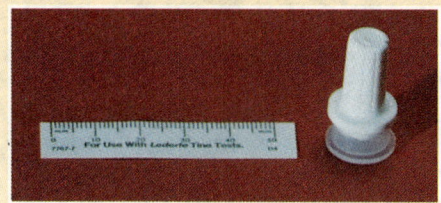

Tine applicator and millimeter ruler.

Steps	Purpose
1. Wash your hands.	1. Handwashing aids infection control.
2. For the tine test, obtain the tine applicator. For the Mantoux test, prepare the injection according to the steps in Procedure 26-5.	
3. Greet and identify the patient. Explain the procedure.	3. Identifying the patient prevents errors. Explaining the procedure helps ease anxiety and ensure compliance.
4. Assess the area of the forearm about 4 inches below the antecubital area.	4. Do this to ensure that the traditional site is appropriate and free of lesions.
5. Clean the area with outward, circular strokes with the acetone wipe. Allow to dry.	5. Cleaning from the area of injection outward carries the microorganisms away from the site. Allowing the area to dry prevents inoculation with the antiseptic. Acetone dries quickly, but alcohol may be used if allowed to dry completely.
6. Put on gloves.	6. Standard Precautions must be observed when there is any break in the integument.
7. Grasp the forearm with the nondominant hand to stretch the skin, to secure the site and to make it easier to pierce the skin.	7.
a. *For the Mantoux test*: Follow steps 7–9 of Procedure 26-6, Administering an Intradermal Injection.	a. The PPD must be inserted into the intradermal layer of the skin.
b. *For the Tine test*: Uncap the tester and press it into the skin.	b. The sharp tines of the tester must pierce the surface of the skin to introduce the PPD into the intradermal layer.

(continued)

Administering a Tine or Mantoux Test (continued)

Steps	**Purpose**

Step 7.b.: Press the tester into the skin.

Hold for 1–2 seconds, release the tension on the skin, and remove the tester.

8. Do not massage the site in either method. Cover the site gently and briefly with an alcohol wipe but do not press or wipe.

9. Properly care for or dispose of equipment and supplies. Remove gloves and wash your hands.

10. Advise the patient regarding returning for evaluation of the test or give instructions regarding the evaluation card to be completed in 48–72 hours and returned by mail. *Note*: If the patient is to return for evaluation of the test, read the results in a good light with the arm slightly flexed. Palpate from the outside area to the center of induration and measure using a millimeter ruler. Disregard erythema and measure only the area of induration. Record the results.

11. Record the procedure and site.

8. The testing material may be pressed into the lower layers or along the lines of injection.

9. This prevents the spread of pathogens.

10. Results must be documented.

11. Procedures are considered not to have been done if they are not recorded.

Procedure 26-8 — Administering a Subcutaneous Injection

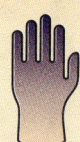

Equipment/Supplies

- medication
- medication tray
- antiseptic wipe
- appropriate-sized needle and syringe (generally a ½–⅝-inch, 24–28-gauge needle on a
- regular 2–3-mL syringe or tuberculin syringe)
- physician's instructions
- gloves

Steps	Purpose
1. Prepare the injection according to the steps in Procedure 26-5.	
2. Greet and identify the patient. Explain the procedure. Ask the patient about medication allergies that might not be noted on the chart.	2. Identifying the patient prevents errors. Explaining the procedure helps ease anxiety and ensure compliance. Allergies may exist that have not been noted.
3. Select the appropriate site for the injection. The upper arm, thigh, back, and abdomen are common sites for subcutaneous injections. Make sure the entire site is exposed for accuracy and safety.	3. Constricting clothing may cause an error in site identification.
4. Prepare the site by cleansing with an antiseptic wipe. Use a circular motion starting at the injection site and working toward the outside. Do not touch the site after cleaning. If the site is grossly contaminated, wash it first with soap and water, then clean with an antiseptic wipe.	4. The site must be prepared by first removing microorganisms from the area. Wiping in a circular motion will carry the microorganisms away from the site. Touching the site after cleaning it will cause contamination.
5. Put on gloves.	5. Standard Precautions must be followed for protection against potential exposure to blood.
6. Remove the needle guard. Using the nondominant hand, hold the skin surrounding the injection site in a cushion fashion.	6. Holding the skin up and away from the underlying muscle will ensure entrance into the subcutaneous tissues. Proper technique will help ensure that the subcutaneous tissue, not the muscle, is entered.
7. With a firm motion, insert the needle into the tissue at a 45-degree angle to the skin. Hold the barrel between the thumb and index finger of the dominant hand and insert the needle up to the hub into the tissue.	7. A quick, firm motion is less painful to the patient. Full insertion ensures that the medication is inserted into the proper tissue.
8. Remove your hand from the skin.	8. Removing your hand will prevent medication from being injected into compressed tissue, which causes pressure against nerve fibers and increases discomfort to the patient.
9. Holding the syringe steady, pull back on the syringe slightly. If blood appears in the syringe, a vessel has been entered. If this occurs, prepare a new injection and repeat steps 4–9.	9. Moving the syringe will cause discomfort to the patient. If medication intended for subcutaneous administration is administered into a vessel, the medication can be absorbed too quickly, producing undesirable results.
10. Inject the medication slowly and steadily by depressing the plunger.	10. If the medication is injected rapidly, pressure is created which will cause patient discomfort and may cause tissue damage.
11. Place an antiseptic wipe over the injection site and remove the needle at the same angle at which it was injected.	11. Withdrawing the needle quickly and at the same angle reduces patient discomfort. The antiseptic wipe helps prevent tissue movement when the needle is withdrawn.

(continued)

Steps	Purpose
12. Properly dispose of the syringe and needle into an approved sharps container. Do not recap the needle. The sharps container should be placed where you have easy access to it after giving the injection.	12. Discarding without recapping helps reduce the risk of an accidental needle stick.
13. Gently massage the injection site with the antiseptic wipe. Apply pressure to the site and cover with an adhesive bandage if needed. Heparin, sometimes given subcutaneously, is not massaged because it may cause excessive bleeding into the site.	13. Massaging helps distribute the medication into the tissues so that it can be more completely absorbed.
14. Remove your gloves and wash your hands.	
15. Remain with the patient to observe for any unusual reactions. An injection given for allergy desensitization requires that the patient remain in the office for at least 30 minutes to be observed for a reaction. Assist the patient from the examination table if necessary. *Note*: If the patient experiences any unusual reactions, notify the physician immediately.	15. Patient may become faint after an injection or may have an adverse reaction to the medication. Reactions to allergy injections may build over time and may cause anaphylaxis.
16. Thank the patient and give appropriate instructions.	16. Courtesy encourages the patient to have a positive attitude about the physician's office.
17. Document the procedure.	17. Procedures are considered not to have been done if they are not recorded.

Procedure 26-9 Administering an Intramuscular Injection

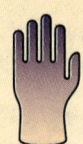

Equipment/Supplies

- medication
- medication tray
- antiseptic wipe
- appropriate-sized needle and syringe (generally a 1–2-inch, 20–23-gauge regular

- 2–5-mL syringes for the injection of up to 3 mL per site)
- physician's instructions
- gloves

Steps	Purpose
1. Prepare the injection according to the steps in Procedure 26-5.	
2. Greet and identify the patient. Explain the procedure. Ask the patient about medication allergies that might not be noted on the chart.	2. Identifying the patient prevents errors. Explaining the procedure helps ease anxiety and ensure compliance. Allergies may exist that have not been noted.
3. Select the appropriate site for the injection (see Figs. 26-14 through 26-18) and the appropriate syringe.	3. Major nerves and blood vessels may lie near the sites for intramuscular injections. Skill and accuracy are crucial.
4. Prepare the site by cleansing with an antiseptic wipe. Use a circular motion starting at the injection site and working toward the outside. Do not touch the site after cleaning. If the site is grossly contaminated, wash it first with soap and water, then clean with an antiseptic wipe.	4. The site must be prepared by first removing microorganisms from the area. Wiping in a circular motion will carry the microorganisms away from the site. Touching the site after cleaning it will cause contamination.
5. Put on gloves.	5. Standard Precautions must be followed for protection against potential exposure to blood.
6. Remove the needle guard. Pull the skin taut over the injection site using the thumb and index fingers of the nondominant hand. *Note*: Patients with meager muscle mass may require that you grasp the muscle and "bunch" it to ensure that the medication is inserted as deeply into the area as possible.	6. Pulling the skin taut allows for easier insertion of the needle and helps ensure that the needle enters muscle tissue. "Bunching" the muscle affords a deeper mass in a very thin patient.
7. Hold the syringe like a dart. Using a quick, firm motion, insert the needle at a 90-degree angle to the skin.	7. A quick, firm motion causes the patient less discomfort. A 90-degree angle ensures that the medication is injected into muscle tissue.

(continued)

Procedure 26-9

Administering an Intramuscular Injection *(continued)*

Steps	Purpose
8. Holding the syringe steady, pull back slightly on the plunger. If blood appears in the syringe, you must prepare a new injection and repeat steps 4–8.	8. Moving the syringe will cause discomfort to the patient. If the medication intended for an intramuscular injection is injected into a vessel, it will be absorbed too quickly, producing undesirable results.
9. Slowly inject the medication by steadily depressing the plunger of the syringe.	9. If the medication is injected too rapidly, it will cause discomfort and may cause tissue damage.
10. Place an antiseptic wipe over the injection site. Remove the needle quickly and at the same angle at which it was inserted.	10. Withdrawing the needle quickly and at the same angle reduces patient discomfort. The antiseptic wipe helps prevent tissue movement when the needle is withdrawn.
11. Properly dispose of the needle and syringe in an approved sharps container. Do not recap the needle. The sharps container should be placed where you have easy access to it after the injection has been administered.	11. Discarding the needle without recapping helps reduce the risk of an accidental needle stick.
12. Gently massage the injection site with an antiseptic wipe. Apply pressure to the site and cover with an adhesive bandage if needed.	12. Massaging helps distribute the medication into the tissues for better absorption.
13. Remove gloves and wash your hands.	
14. Remain with the patient to observe for any unusual reactions. Assist the patient off the examination table if necessary. *Note*: If the patient experiences any unusual reaction, notify the physician immediately.	14. Medications given intramuscularly may react quickly. The patient must be observed for reaction to the drug effects. Some patients become faint after injections.
15. Thank the patient and give appropriate instructions.	15. Courtesy encourages the patient to have a positive attitude about the physician's office.
16. Document the procedure, including the site of injection and any unusual patient reactions.	16. Procedures are considered not to have been done if they are not recorded.

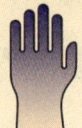

Procedure 26-10 Administering an Intramuscular Injection Using the Z-Track Method

Equipment/Supplies

- medication
- medication tray
- antiseptic wipe
- appropriate-sized needle and syringe
- physician's instructions
- gloves

Steps	Purpose
1–5. Follow steps 1–5 as described in Procedure 26-9; Administering an Intramuscular Injection. *Note*: The ventrogluteal, vastus lateralis, and dorso-gluteal sites work well for the Z-track method; the deltoid does not.	
6. Remove the needle guard. Rather than pulling the skin taut or grasping the tissue as you would for an intramuscular injection, pull the top layer of skin to the side and hold it with the nondominant hand.	6. By displacing the top layer of skin, the puncture route will be sealed when the layers of tissue slide back to their proper places.
7. Insert the needle to the hub at a 90-degree angle in a quick, dartlike motion.	
8. Aspirate by withdrawing the plunger slightly. If no blood appears, push the plunger in slowly and steadily. Count to 10 before withdrawing the needle.	8. This allows time for the tissues to begin absorption of the medication.
9. Cover the area with an antiseptic wipe. Withdraw the needle and release the skin. Most Z-track medications must not be massaged to avoid forcing the medication into upper tissues. Check the manufacturer's suggestions.	
10. Properly dispose of the needle and syringe in an approved sharps container. Do not recap the needle. The sharps container should be placed where you have easy access to it after the injection has been administered.	10. Discarding without recapping helps reduce the risk of an accidental needle stick.
11. Remove gloves and wash your hands.	
12. Remain with the patient to observe for any unusual reactions. Assist the patient off of the examination table if necessary. *Note*: If the patient experiences any unusual reaction, notify the physician immediately.	12. Medications given intramuscularly may react quickly. The patient must be observed for reaction to the drug effects. Some patients become faint after injections.
13. Thank the patient and give appropriate instructions.	13. Courtesy encourages the patient to have a positive attitude about the physician's office.
14. Document the procedure, including the site of injection and any unusual patient reactions.	14. Procedures are considered not to have been done if they are not recorded.

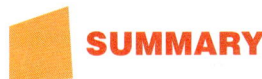

SUMMARY

The administration of medication will be one of the most challenging and exacting procedures performed in the medical office. Few other procedures require such intense concentration and attention to detail or include such potential for danger to the patient. You will be asked to practice interpersonal skills such as tact and diplomacy to make these procedures acceptable to the patient and to allay the anxiety felt by almost all patients during the administration of medications.

CRITICAL THINKING CHALLENGES

1. Create a conversion chart that you can carry with you to help with converting between the metric and apothecary systems.
2. Design a patient education brochure that will teach patients about taking oral medications.
3. You are giving an intramuscular injection. After inserting the needle, you aspirate by pulling back slightly on the plunger. As you do this, blood appears in the syringe. What has happened? What you should do?

ANSWERS TO CHECKPOINT QUESTIONS

1. The three checks are performed when the medication is taken from the shelf, when it is poured, and when it is put back on the shelf.
2. The three systems used to measure medications are the metric, apothecary, and household systems. Household measurements, which are often used by patients, should be avoided because they are inaccurate.
3. To accurately calculate dosages, you must ensure that the measurements are in the same system (either metric or apothecary) and in the same unit of measurement.
4. Oral medication typically takes effect slowly. Also, the oral route cannot be used for patients who are unconscious, for those with nausea and vomiting, and for those who are NPO.

5. Topical medications produce local effects; transdermal medications have systemic effects.
6. Ampules and vials are medication containers. An ampule is a glass container with a narrow neck; it must be broken to obtain the medication, which is in solution form. A vial is a glass or plastic container sealed with a rubber stopper; it contains medication in either solution or in dry form (eg, powder or crystals).
7. Types of injections include intradermal, subcutaneous, and intramuscular. Sites for intradermal injections include the anterior forearm and the back. Sites for subcutaneous injections include the upper arm, thigh, back, and abdomen. Sites for intramuscular injections include the deltoid, ventrogluteal, and vastus lateralis; the rectus femoris is used only when the other sites are contraindicated.

SUGGESTIONS FOR FURTHER READING

Boyer, M. J. (1994). *Math for Nurses: A Pocket Guide to Dosage Calculation and Drug Administration*, 3rd ed. Philadelphia: J. B. Lippincott.

Craven, R. F., & Hirnle, C. J. (1996). *Fundamentals of Nursing: Health and Human Function*, 2nd ed. Philadelphia: Lippincott-Raven Publishers.

Dawe, R. (1993). *Math and Dosage Calculations for Health Occupations*. New York: Glencoe.

Henke, G. (1995). *Med-Math: Dosage Calculation, Preparation and Administration*. 2nd ed. Philadelphia: J. B. Lippincott.

Kozier, B., & Erb, G. (1993). *Techniques of Clinical Nursing*, 3rd ed. Redwood City, CA: Addison-Wesley.

Lane, K. *Medications: A Guide for the Health Professions* Philadelphia: F. A. Davis, 1992.

Scherer, J. C., & Roach, S. S. (1995). *Introductory Clinical Pharmacology*. 5th ed. Philadelphia: J. B. Lippincott.

Smeltzer, S. C., & Bare, B. G. (1996). *Brunner and Suddarth's Textbook of Medical-Surgical Nursing*, 8th ed. Philadelphia: Lippincott-Raven Publishers.

Taylor, C., Lillis, C., & LeMone, P. (1993). *Fundamentals of Nursing: The Art and Science of Nursing Care*, 2nd ed. Philadelphia: J. B. Lippincott.

Timby, B. (1996). *Fundamental Skills and Concepts in Patient Care*, 6th ed. Philadelphia: Lippincott-Raven Publishers.

Diagnostic Imaging

Chapter Outline

X-rays and X-ray Machines
    Outpatient X-rays
Principles of Radiography
Patient Positioning
Examination Sequencing
Radiation Safety
Diagnostic Procedures
    Contrast Media Examinations
    Fluoroscopy
    Computed Tomography (CT, CAT
      Scan)
    Sonography (Ultrasound)
    Magnetic Resonance Imaging
      (MR, MRI)
    Nuclear Medicine

    Mammography
Teleradiology
Interventional Radiologic Techniques
Radiation Therapy
The Medical Assistant's Role in Radio-
    logic Procedures
    Patient Education
    Assisting With Examinations
    Handling and Storing of Radi-
      ographic Films
Transfer of Radiographic Information
Summary
Critical Thinking Challenges
Answers to Checkpoint Questions
Suggestions for Further Reading

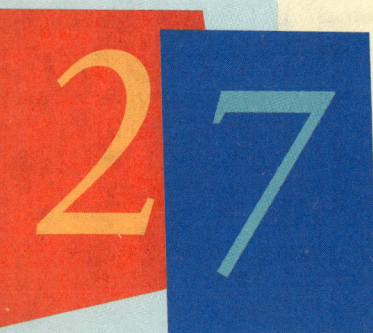

DACUM Components

1.3   Practice within the scope of education, training, and personal capabilities
1.5   Work as a team member
1.6   Conduct oneself in a courteous and diplomatic manner
2.2   Treat all patients with empathy and impartiality
2.5   Serve as liaison between physician and others
4.7   Prepare patients for procedures
4.8   Assist with examinations and treatments
7.2   Instruct patients with special needs

Chapter Competencies

Learning Objectives

Upon successfully completing this chapter, you will be able to:

1. Spell and define the Key Terms.
2. Explain the theory and function of x-rays and x-ray machines.
3. State the basic principles of radiography.
4. Describe routine and contrast media, computed tomography, sonography, magnetic resonance imaging, nuclear medicine, and mammographic examinations.
5. Explain the basic concepts of therapeutic techniques.
6. Describe the basic concepts of radiation therapy.
7. Explain the principles of radiology in a manner that can be used in patient education.
8. State the legal and ethical considerations involved in radiology.
9. Explain the role of the medical assistant in radiologic procedures.

Key Terms

(See Glossary for definitions.)

cassette
film
radiograph
radiographer
radiography
radiologist
radiology
radiolucent
radionuclide
radiopaque
tomography
x-ray

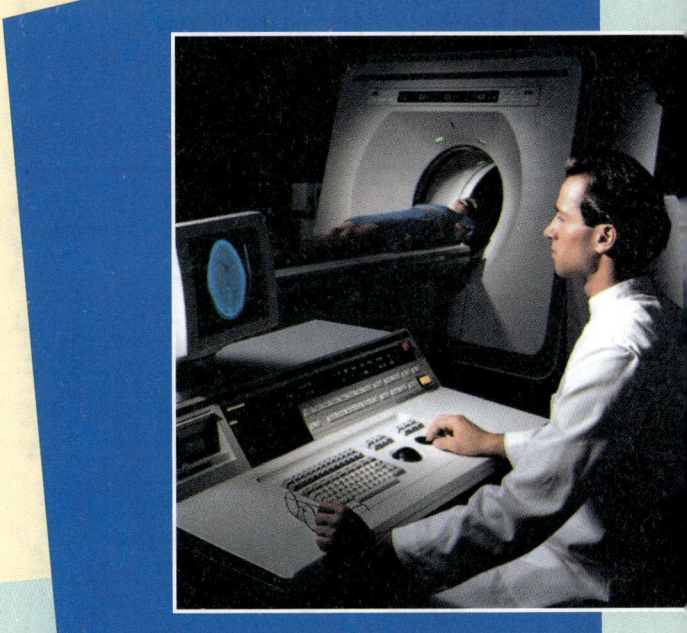

The discovery of x-rays in the late 19th century forever changed the practice of medicine. Today, **radiology** with its use of x-rays, radioactive isotopes and radiation, encompasses some of the most rapidly expanding diagnostic and therapeutic technologies. Routine x-ray imaging, computed tomography (CT) scans, sonography, magnetic resonance imaging (MRI), and nuclear medicine are commonly used diagnostic procedures in the fight against disease. Advances in radiation therapy continue to be at the forefront of the treatment for cancer.

Radiology continues to evolve through technologic changes that provide ever-increasing diagnostic information to physicians. As the technology advances, the need to adequately educate patients becomes even more important. As part of interacting with patients, medical assistants are often in the ideal position to assist in the educational process.

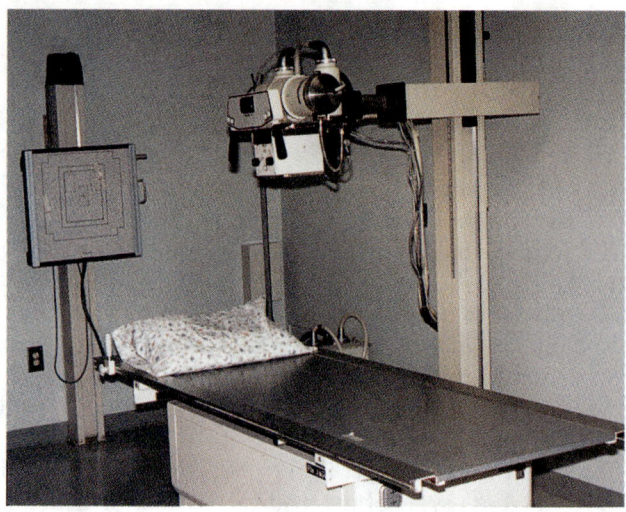

FIGURE 27-2
Permanently installed radiographic unit.

➤ X-RAYS AND X-RAY MACHINES

X-rays are high-energy electromagnetic radiation with several unique characteristics. They cannot be seen, heard, felt, tasted, or smelled. The rays travel at the speed of light and have the ability to penetrate fairly dense objects, such as the human body. This penetrating ability is what allows x-rays to be the diagnostic tools they are, creating two-dimensional shadow-like images on **film** that is similar to photographic film. The processed film containing a visible image is called a **radiograph** (Fig. 27-1). The process by which these films are produced is called **radiography**.

The production of x-rays occurs within the part of the machine called the x-ray tube. Electricity of extremely high voltage is applied to the tube, ultimately resulting in the production of x-rays. The x-rays exit the tube in one primary direction as a beam, through a collimator, the device used to control the size of the beam. The light seen by the patient is not part of the beam but is a positioning aid that demonstrates the area covered by the beam. A patient may hear noises coming from the tube area during an exposure, but these are made by the equipment, not the x-rays.

Today, x-ray machines are sophisticated and technologically advanced. Many are designed to work with computers to produce "digital" images of the body. Fluoroscopic units are capable of visualizing motion within the body. Most of the permanently installed radiographic units include a special table, some of which may be electronically rotated from the horizontal to the vertical position (Fig. 27-2).

Mobile radiographic units are designed to be moved to different areas of a hospital or clinic, to go to the patients' bedside or examination room when it is not advisable to transport the patient to the radiology area. This allows patients to have their studies done wherever they are being treated at that time: the emergency room, surgery, recovery room, in their bed in a hospital unit, or in an examining room. Mobile radiography is an essential part of critical care (Fig. 27-3).

Outpatient X-rays

Currently, the medical community is making a conscious effort to have as much patient treatment as possible done on an outpatient basis. In radiology, this has resulted in some medical offices (particularly special-

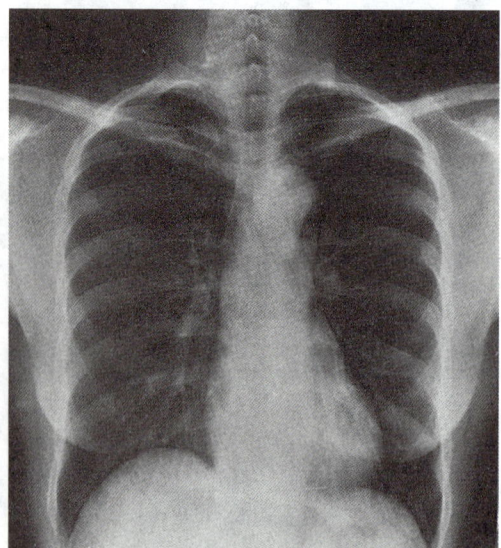

FIGURE 27-1
A radiograph of the chest.

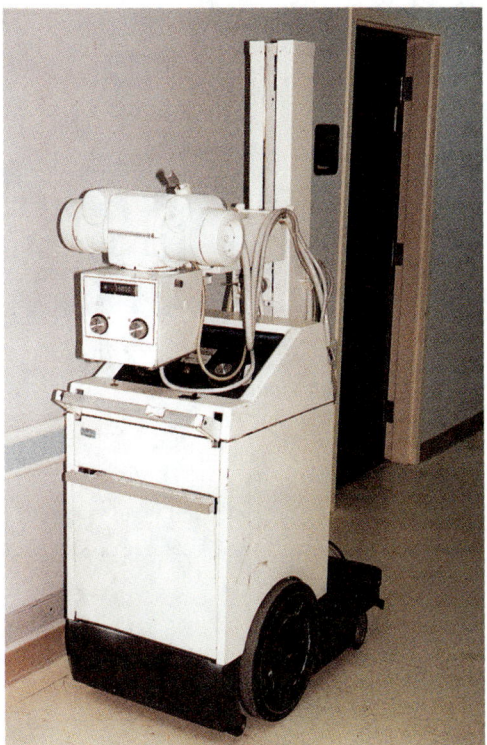

FIGURE 27-3
A mobile radiographic unit.

ties) having on-site x-ray equipment. Outpatient diagnostic imaging centers, separate from or a part of hospitals, have been created to offer these services. Many patients may have their radiographic examinations or procedures done in one of these settings.

Inpatients have their examinations done in the hospital or other resident care facility. Some companies specialize in providing minimal x-ray services to patients in nursing homes and other long-term care facilities, so that these patients do not have to be transported to hospitals.

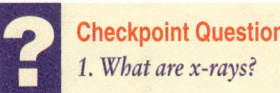

Checkpoint Question
1. What are x-rays?

► PRINCIPLES OF RADIOGRAPHY

The routine procedure for any radiographic examination generally includes:

1. Verifying the patient's identity and the examination to be performed.
2. Preparing the patient; may involve undressing as necessary to remove objects (snaps, buttons, hooks) that could show up on the radiograph, obscuring vital parts of the image.
3. Preparing the room by setting up the equipment and readying supplies.
4. Performing the procedure, including positioning the patient and making exposures.
5. Processing the images.
6. Interpreting the images (performed by a physician).
7. Filing the images.

Paperwork is a critical part of this procedure. Before an examination can be performed, a requisition must be completed by a physician or his or her authorized agent. Radiographic procedures should only be performed by or on the order of a licensed physician. After the images have been interpreted, a written report becomes part of the patient's medical record.

► PATIENT POSITIONING

The x-ray exposure on film is only a two-dimensional image. Because the human body is a three-dimensional structure, x-ray examinations usually require a minimum of two exposures taken at 90° to each other. For instance, a chest x-ray will require one exposure from the back and another from the side. Other examinations primarily interested in demonstrating joints will frequently involve the use of three or more exposures at different angles. These different angles of exposure are the basis for standard positioning for x-ray examinations (Box 27-1, Fig. 27-4).

► EXAMINATION SEQUENCING

Most radiographic procedures can be performed in any order of convenience. However, certain sequences are followed in specific situations. For example, patients who present with gallbladder symptoms may go through a series of procedures, progressing from the simple, noninvasive oral cholecystogram to the more complex operative cholangiogram.

Another example involves "barium studies," the name given to examinations that involve the administration of barium sulfate as a part of the procedure. A patient with gastrointestinal (GI) symptoms may undergo a series of barium-based studies to assist in a diagnosis. Because of the nature of the barium studies and the length of time required to eliminate the barium from the digestive tract, barium enemas are usually scheduled before upper GI examinations. If fiberoptic studies are ordered, it is imperative that these be scheduled before any procedure involving barium.

Because barium enemas involve filling only the large intestine with barium and because the large in-

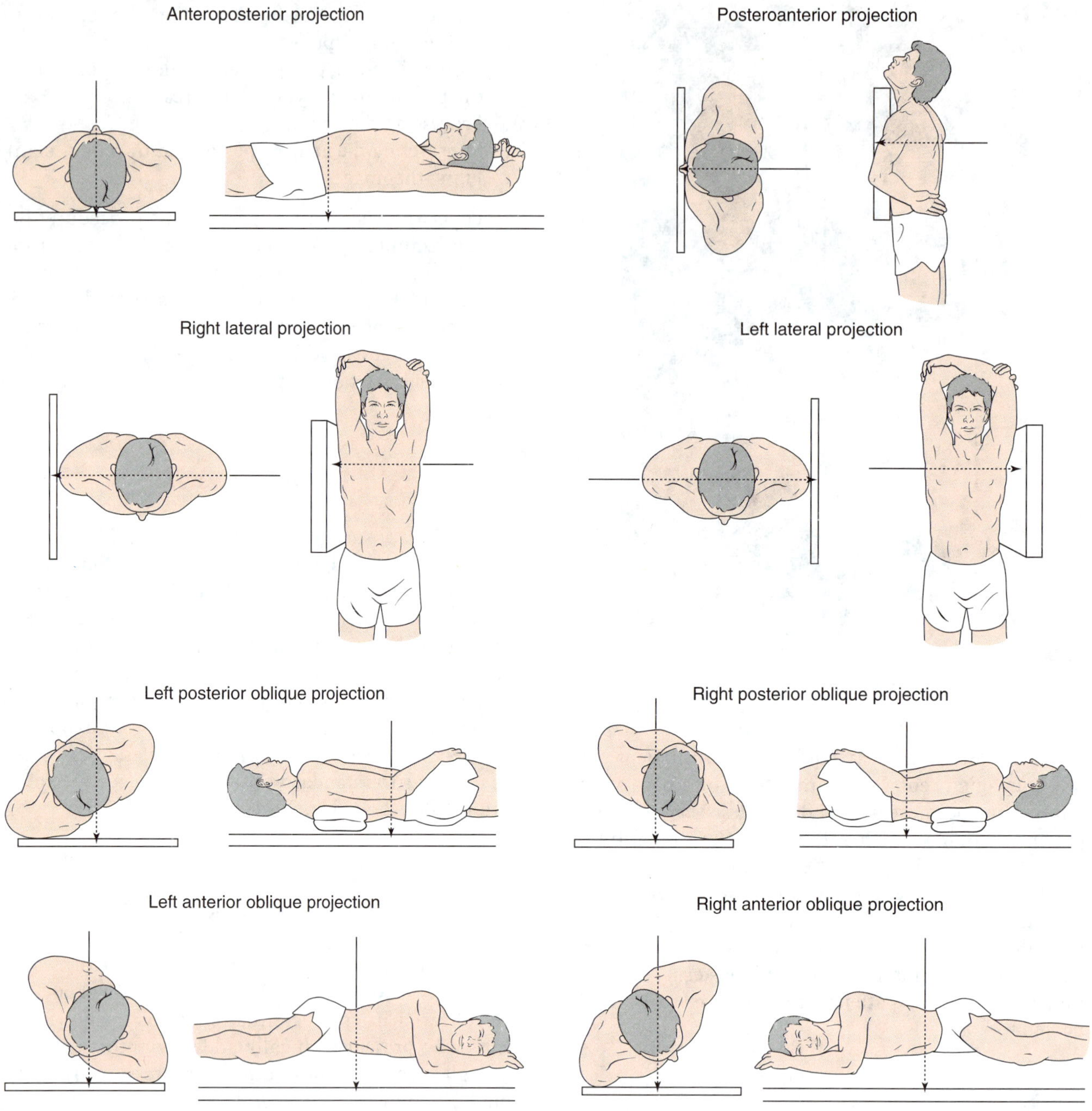

Anteroposterior projection

Posteroanterior projection

Right lateral projection

Left lateral projection

Left posterior oblique projection

Right posterior oblique projection

Left anterior oblique projection

Right anterior oblique projection

FIGURE 27-4
Standard positions for x-ray examinations.

testine is the last part of the GI tract, this barium can be eliminated more quickly so that other examinations can be attempted. If an upper GI examination is performed first, it may be days later before all the barium is out of the system, allowing other examinations to be performed. Any residual barium could obscure vital structures, preventing other examinations from contributing diagnostic information. The proper sequencing of barium enema first and upper GI last will usually provide diagnostic information in a shorter period of time.

Checkpoint Question
2. Why is a barium enema performed before upper GI studies?

➤ RADIATION SAFETY

Of primary concern to all radiation workers is the proper and safe use of radiant energy. The potential hazards of radiation have been known for many

BOX 27-1   Standard Terminology and Illustrations for Positioning and Projection

Radiographic View

Describes the body part as seen by an x-ray film or other recording media, such as a fluoroscopic screen. Restricted to the discussion of a *radiograph* or *image*.

Radiographic Position

Refers to a specific body position, such as supine, prone, recumbent, erect, or Trendelenberg. Restricted to the discussion of the patient's *physical position*.

Radiographic Projection

Restricted to the discussion of the *path of the central ray*.

Positioning Terminology

A. Lying down
   1. *Supine* — lying on the back
   2. *Prone* — lying face downward
   3. *Decubitus* — lying down with a horizontal x-ray beam
   4. *Recumbent* — lying down in any position
B. Erect or upright
   1. *Anterior position* — facing the film
   2. *Posterior position* — facing the radiographic tube
   3. *Oblique positions* — (erect or lying down)
      a. Anterior — facing the film
         i. *Left anterior oblique* — body rotated with the left anterior portion closest to the film
         ii. *Right anterior oblique* — body rotated with the right anterior portion closest to the film
      b. Posterior — facing the radiographic tube
         i. *Left posterior oblique* — body rotated with the left posterior portion closest to the film
         ii. *Right posterior oblique* — body rotated with the right posterior portion closest to the film

(© 1978, The American Registry of Radiologic Technologists, used with permission.)

---

years and warnings about x-ray radiation are usually posted in appropriate areas (Fig. 27-5). X-rays have the potential to cause cellular damage to the body, which may not manifest itself for years. The potential adverse effects are most critical for rapidly reproducing cells. Pregnant women, children, and adults of reproductive age are at the highest risk because of the rapid reproduction of the cells in these populations.

Radiation safety procedures generally directed toward patients include:

1. Reducing exposure amounts as much as possible.
2. Avoiding unnecessary examinations.
3. Limiting the area of the body exposed.
4. Shielding sensitive body parts from the radiation.
5. Evaluating the potential pregnancy status of female patients before performing examinations.

Safety procedures for radiation workers include:

1. Limiting the amount of time exposed to x-rays.
2. Staying as far away from the x-rays as possible, preferably behind a barrier.
3. Using all available shielding for protection, such as lead aprons, gloves, and barrier walls.

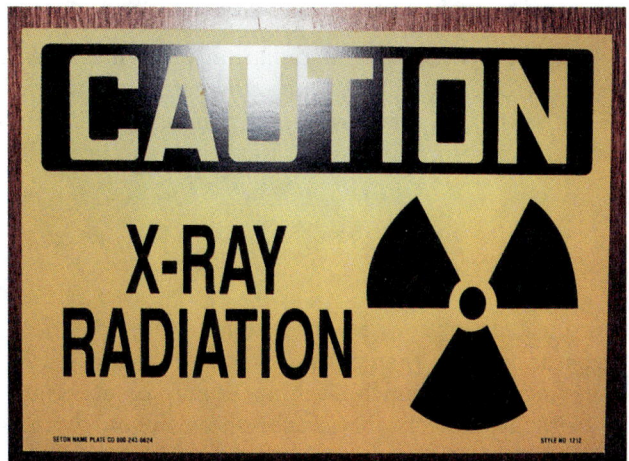

FIGURE 27-5
A posted x-ray warning sign.

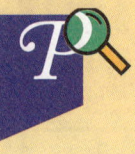

Focus on the Patient: Invading Personal Privacy?

When a radiographer (the technician who produces routine x-ray images) asks a female patient if she may be pregnant, or when signs in x-ray facilities instruct patients to inform someone if they may be pregnant, is personal privacy being invaded? No; these measures are not intended to invade privacy but to ensure the safety of the unborn. The embryo is most sensitive to radiation damage during the first 3 months of formation. This is also a time when a woman may be pregnant and not be aware of it. (The patient is not asked if she knows she is pregnant, only if there is a possibility that she might be.) To save the patient any embarrassment, proper precautions are usually taken, regardless of the answer. If the examination includes the abdominopelvic area, the precaution may be to delay the procedure until pregnancy status is determined medically.

If You Suspect You Are Pregnant, Please Notify the Technician

This is not an invasion of privacy, but an effort to provide protection for patients.

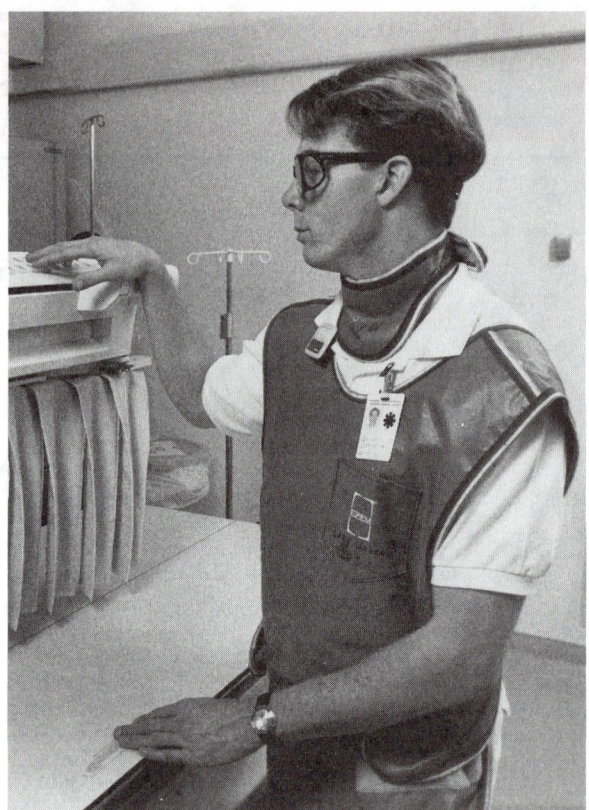

FIGURE 27-7
A radiographer wearing a dosimeter on the right collar, as well as protective glasses, an apron, and a thyroid shield.

4. Not holding patients during exposures. Sometimes small children need to be held to keep them still during an examination. A parent wearing a lead apron may be recruited for this procedure.
5. Wearing individual dosimeters, devices that record the amount of radiation to which the worker has been exposed (Fig. 27-6), and protective equipment (Fig. 27-7).
6. Ensuring proper working condition of the equipment to avoid having to repeat examinations.

For both patients and radiation personnel, these concerns can be summed up in what is called the ALARA concept: doing whatever is necessary to keep radiation exposure As Low As Reasonably Achievable.

➤ DIAGNOSTIC PROCEDURES

Routine examinations are those that require no patient preparation other than putting on a patient gown after removing only as much clothing as may be necessary to eliminate objects that might show up on the radiographs (eg, buttons, snaps, hooks). These are the most commonly performed examinations and are the most readily accepted by the patient. Routine radi-

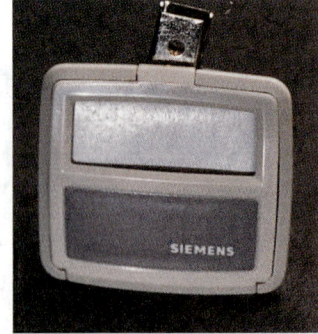

FIGURE 27-6
The dosimeter records the amount of radiation to which a worker has been exposed.

Table 27-1
Routine Radiographic Examinations by Body Region

Region	Patient Preparation
Trunk	Patient preparation includes disrobing of the appropriate area: chest, ribs, sternum, shoulder, scapula, clavicle, abdomen, hip, pelvis, sternoclavicular, acromioclavicular, sacroiliac joints
Extremities	Patient preparation includes removing jewelry or clothing that might obscure parts of interest: finger(s), thumb, hand, wrist, forearm, elbow, humerus, toe(s), foot, os calcis, ankle, lower leg, knee, patella, femur
Spine	Patient preparation includes disrobing of the appropriate area: cervical, thoracic, or lumbar spine; sacrum; coccyx
Head	Patient preparation includes removing eyewear, false eyes, false teeth, earrings, hairpins, hairpieces from appropriate area: skull, sinuses, nasal bones, facial bones/orbits, optic foramen, mandible, temporomandibular joints, mastoid/petrous portion, zygomatic arch

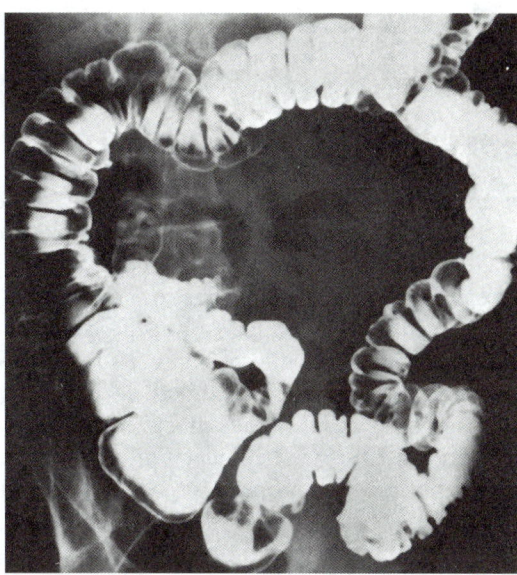

FIGURE 27-8
An x-ray of the large intestine with barium. The barium makes the large intestine show up as white on the radiograph.

ographic examinations are named for the part of the body involved (Table 27-1).

Contrast Media Examinations

Images are formed on the x-ray film as the rays either pass through or are absorbed by the tissues of the body. **Radiolucent** tissues permit the passage of x-rays; **radiopaque** tissues do not. Bone is dense, absorbs much of the radiation beam, and shows white on a radiograph. Air is not dense, does not absorb much radiation, and therefore shows dark on a radiograph. Other body tissues (such as muscle, fat, and fluid) show as varying shades of gray because of the way each tissue absorbs x-rays.

Within the abdomen, many structures having similar radiation absorption rates are superimposed on each other. This makes differentiating between structures, such as the components of the intestinal system, difficult. The use of radiopaque contrast media helps differentiate between body structures by artificially changing the absorption rate of a particular structure so that it may be distinctly visualized instead of blending in with adjacent structures. For example, barium sulfate absorbs radiation and shows white on a radiograph (Fig. 27-8).

There are different contrast medias for different applications. Iodinated compounds are used for many areas of the body, including the kidneys and blood vessels and for some computed tomography (CT) scans.

Patients who may have an intestinal perforation may be given an iodinated contrast media instead of barium because that material spilling into the peritoneum is much less troublesome to the patient than barium would be.

Contrast media may be introduced in several ways, such as by swallowing, by the intravenous route, or through a catheter. A barium sulfate mixture is swallowed for an upper GI series. Other contrast media are introduced intravenously or by means of a catheter for studies of the vascular system. Examinations using contrast media often are used not only to evaluate a structure but also to evaluate its function. The excretory urogram evaluates kidney structures as well as the organ's excretory functions.

Checkpoint Question
3. How do contrast media help in differentiating between body structures?

Of particular concern to patients is the preparation they must undergo before some contrast media examinations, especially barium studies. For contrast media to properly fill the intestinal tract, the intestine must be completely empty. For example, patient preparation for a barium study might include:

- Liquid diet only for the evening meal on the day before the examination
- Laxatives to help clean the intestinal tract
- Nothing by mouth (NPO) after midnight. This usually includes no gum chewing or cigarette smoking

because both activities increase gastric secretions that may interfere with the contrast media's ability to coat the wall of the intestine.

This general preparation could apply to any contrast media examination involving abdominal structures. Each facility may vary this to some extent. You should learn the specific preparations required for each procedure by each facility. It is to the advantage of the facility to provide its employees with this information to facilitate efficient and effective performance of x-ray procedures.

Examinations requiring that patients remain NPO past midnight should be scheduled as early in the morning as possible. If patients must remain NPO until late morning, they will be understandably upset.

If patients are not properly prepared for contrast studies, they may have to be rescheduled for another day and time and must go through the whole process again, sometimes adding cleansing enemas to the preparation. Explaining the importance of the preparation can be one of the most vital contributions a medical assistant can make to the patient's care in contrast examinations.

What If?
A patient who is scheduled to have a barium study has been kept waiting for over an hour. What if she asks you for a sip of water?

As a medical assistant, you must understand the reason for fasting and not give the patient anything by mouth just because it seems a benign request. Doing so could compromise the results and cause the patient to have to go through the whole process again. Give this explanation if you need to deny a patient's request for something to drink.

Table 27-2 lists common radiographic procedures that use contrast media. Some examinations included here are being replaced by other techniques such as CT, magnetic resonance imaging (MRI), and ultrasound in many institutions. Because they may still be performed, or may be referred to in a patient's medical record, they are included in this table.

Table 27-2
Common Radiographic Procedures

Examination	Contrast Media	Provides a Demonstration of:
Angiogram	Iodinated	Blood vessels; named for those studied (eg, femoral, carotid, aorta)
Arthrogram	Iodinated	Joint capsule and related structures, often with stress applied to joint
Barium enema	Barium/air	Large intestine, sometimes using air for additional contrast
Barium swallow	Barium	Esophagus as patient swallows barium
Bronchogram	Iodinated	Bronchial tree by instilling contrast medium through a tube
Cardiac	Iodinated	Heart; may include angiography
Cystogram	Iodinated	Urinary bladder after contrast medium introduced through catheter
Endoscopic retrograde cholangiopancreatogram (ERCP)	Iodinated	Biliary and pancreatic duct structures after introducing contrast medium through endoscopy
Excretory urogram	Iodinated	Kidney structures, ureters, and urinary bladder after intravenous (IV) injection of contrast medium
Hysterosalpingogram	Iodinated	Patency of oviducts by filling uterus and ducts with contrast medium
IV cholangiogram	Iodinated	Gallbladder and biliary ducts after administration of IV drip of contrast medium
Lymphogram	Iodinated	Lymphatic structures after contrast medium injection into vessels in feet
Myelogram	Iodinated	Subarachnoid space around spinal cord after injection of contrast medium via lumbar puncture
Operative cholangiogram	Iodinated	Gallbladder and biliary ducts with direct injection of contrast medium during surgery
Oral cholecystogram	Iodinated	Gallbladder and biliary ducts after patient ingests contrast pills
Percutaneous transhepatic cholangiogram	Iodinated	Biliary system after percutaneous introduction of needle through the liver to the bile duct
Retrograde pyelogram	Iodinated	Kidney structures by filling with contrast medium from catheter in distal ureter
Sialogram	Iodinated	Salivary glands after injection into ducts
Small bowel series	Barium	Small bowel by following contrast medium through from stomach to beginning of large intestine
T-tube cholangiogram	Iodinated	Biliary ducts through tube left in place after cholecystectomy
Upper GI series	Barium	Upper GI tract through the duodenum
Voiding cystourethrogram	Iodinated	Urinary bladder and urethra and voiding function

Fluoroscopy

Fluoroscopy, or fluoro studies, use x-rays to observe movement within the body. The movement may be of barium sulfate through the digestive tract, the beating of the heart, or the movement of contrast media through blood vessels or even through the heart itself. Fluoroscopy is also used as an aid to other types of patient treatments, such as reducing fractures or implanting pacemakers.

Computed Tomography (CT, CAT Scan)

Tomography is a procedure in which the x-ray tube and film move in relation to one another during the exposure, blurring out all structures except those in the focal plane. CT uses a combination of x-rays and computers to create cross-sectional images of the body. Some examinations are performed with contrast media, some without. Some units have the ability to create three-dimensional images (Fig. 27-9).

Sonography (Ultrasound)

Sonography uses high-frequency sound waves to create cross-sectional still or real-time (motion) images of the body, usually with the help of computers. This application is commonly used to demonstrate heart function or abdominal or pelvic structures. It is commonly used in prenatal testing to visualize the developing fetus. Many obstetricians routinely schedule at least one sonogram before the fourth month of pregnancy (Fig. 27-10).

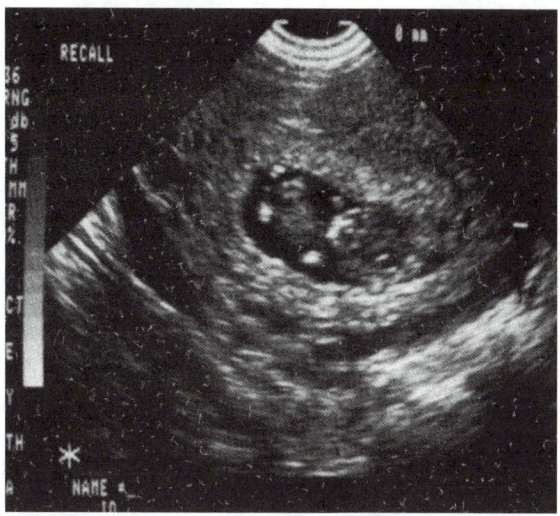

FIGURE 27-10
A sonogram showing an embryo 9 weeks after patient's last monthly period.

Magnetic Resonance Imaging (MR, MRI)

Magnetic resonance imaging uses a combination of high-intensity magnetic fields, radio waves, and computers to create cross-sectional images of the body. Some studies are performed with contrast media. Because MRI does not produce images using x-ray principles, but instead creates images based on the chemical makeup of the body, MR studies provide information unavailable by other means. MRI is commonly used for a variety of studies, including the central nervous system and joint structure. The patient must be prepared for lengthy procedures while in a closely enclosed machine making knocking and whirring noises. It is not unusual for patients with a fear of enclosed places to require a mild sedative before this procedure.

 **Checkpoint Question**
4. How does fluoroscopy differ from computed tomography and sonography?

Nuclear Medicine

Small amounts of **radionuclides** are injected into the body and are designed to concentrate in specific areas. Radionuclides are radioactive materials with a short life span. Sophisticated computerized "cameras" detect the radiation and create an image. This technique is commonly used to study the thyroid, brain, lungs, liver, spleen, kidney, bone, and breast. These examinations are called scans.

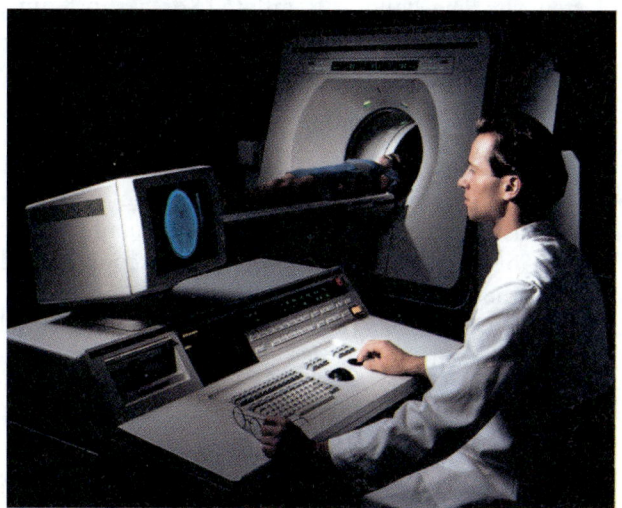

FIGURE 27-9
Computed tomography (CT) scanner. (Photograph courtesy of Philips Medical Systems)

Positron emission tomography (PET) is a sophisticated nuclear medicine study using specialized equipment to produce detailed sectional images of the body's physiological processes.

Single photon emission computed tomography (SPECT) is a nuclear medicine technology that produces sectional images of the body as detectors move around the patient.

Mammography

Mammography involves specialized x-rays of the breast and is used as a screening tool for breast cancer (Box 27-2). Compression of the breast is used to even the thickness, allowing a better diagnostic image. Needle localization studies using the information gained from the mammogram allow the physician to withdraw minute amounts of cells from suspicious areas in a minimally invasive procedure. Mammography has become a vital adjunct to biopsy procedures (Fig. 27-11).

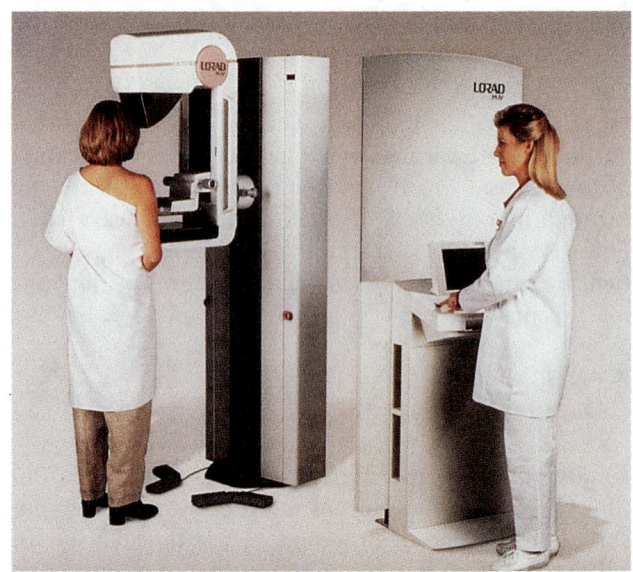

FIGURE 27-11
A patient being positioned for mammography. (LORAD M-IV mammography machine.)

➤ TELERADIOLOGY

The use of computed imaging and information systems can be mutually beneficial in medicine. Many institutions today have a picture archiving and communication system (PACS) that uses computers to store and transmit images. Digital images from a CT scan, for instance, can be transmitted via telephone lines to distant locations. This allows consultation with experts on a difficult case within a matter of minutes. Previously unavailable expertise can be brought to rural areas for greatly improved patient care. The result is improved patient care over large geographic areas, not just in specific locations. The name teleradiology has been coined to describe this "radiology over a great distance."

➤ INTERVENTIONAL RADIOLOGIC TECHNIQUES

Interventional radiologic techniques are designed to intervene in the normal process of specific disease conditions. For some patients, these therapeutic techniques can be so effective that the need for surgery will be eliminated. These interventional procedures, described below, may even be lifesaving.

Percutaneous transluminal coronary angioplasty (PTCA), also known as balloon angioplasty, is used to increase the size of the lumen of a coronary artery through the use of a balloon-tipped catheter. Under fluoroscopic guidance, the catheter is placed at a point of stenosis. The balloon is inflated for a short time, usually resulting in an increase in the lumen of the vessel. After deflation, the catheter is removed. Balloon angioplasties may be performed in almost any vessel.

Laser angioplasties use laser beams to remove deposits in vessels.

A *vascular stent* (a plastic tube or wire) placed in the stenosed area of the vessel is used to maintain the patency of the lumen of a vessel. Fluoroscopy is used to guide the stent.

Embolizations artificially embolize a blood vessel to stop active bleeding or to reduce or stop blood flow to diseased areas.

BOX 27-2 American Cancer Society Guidelines for Mammography Screening

- Mammography for women who do not have symptoms, such as palpable breast masses or masses found on prior radiological examination.
  If you are 40–49—every 1–2 years.
  If you are 50 or over, every year
- Screening mammogram by age 40

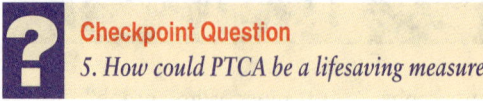

? Checkpoint Question
5. How could PTCA be a lifesaving measure?

➤ RADIATION THERAPY

A major force in the fight against cancer for many years has been radiation therapy. The use of high-energy radiation to destroy cancer cells can not only prolong the lives of many patients, it may even save lives. Used in conjunction with surgery, chemotherapy, or both, radiation is possibly the best known treatment for cancer. With an intensity sufficient to destroy cancer cells, the potential to damage some adjacent normal cells does exist. Therefore, treatments must be planned carefully and precisely.

Treatment planning involves the establishment of a precise regimen of therapy, dictating the frequency and amount of radiation to be used as well as the number of exposures during a given period. The exact area of the body to be exposed must be defined precisely so that each treatment is identical.

The therapy consists of placing the patient in the exact position described by the treatment plan and administering the exact amount of radiation. The patient usually has little to do but lie still.

Each patient's prognosis varies according to the specific situation. Most patients have some side effects, which may include hair loss, weight loss, loss of appetite, skin changes, and digestive system disturbances. Once the treatment plan is completed, most of the side effects disappear.

➤ THE MEDICAL ASSISTANT'S ROLE IN RADIOLOGIC PROCEDURES

Because medical assistants hold such a varied range of jobs related to patient care, they often are in ideal positions to help alleviate the anxiety patients feel. This may be done by giving patients information about examinations they do not understand, by making the patients feel comfortable enough to ask questions, and by providing answers to those questions in terms the patients can understand.

Patient Education

Patients who have had prior experience with the medical system have sometimes learned to overcome their anxieties and learned to find answers to their questions. No matter how much they have been through before, there is always something new, something they do not understand that can make them feel they have lost control of their situation. Being sensitive to the feelings of patients is one of the greatest talents anyone in medicine can possess and is a prime component of the medical assistant's training and personality.

Unfortunately, many patients are confronted with procedures they do not understand and do not know enough about to ask questions. Many undergo procedures as a spectator rather than a participant in their own health care. As a medical assistant, you can have an impact on a patient's emotional response to radiologic procedures by explaining what to expect, not in technical terms, but in simple, everyday language (Fig. 27-12). The technical aspects of radiology make it one of medicine's most difficult areas for patients to understand. The key to success in explaining these procedures to patients is simplicity, leaving the details to the experts.

Explaining the preparations for examinations and their importance is vital to the success of many procedures. Equally important may be an explanation of what to do after the procedure. The barium enema, for instance, can lead to constipation if the patient does not increase fluid intake after the examination. This simple direction can save the patient much postexamination distress.

Assisting With Examinations

As a medical assistant, you may assist with examinations by:

- Giving the patient instructions for appropriate undressing and assisting with clothing as needed.
- Assisting in positioning of the patient for the procedure, emphasizing to the patient the importance of remaining still and following breathing directions.

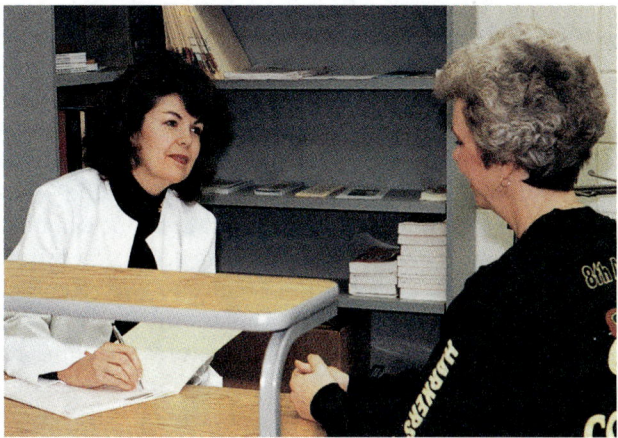

FIGURE 27-12
The medical assistant provides explanations of radiologic procedures that are easy to understand.

- Processing film in a darkroom, removing film from **cassettes** (lightproof film holders), placing film into an automatic processor, reloading new film into the cassette.
- Distributing or filing radiographs and reports.

Handling and Storing of Radiographic Films

Advancing technology and the need for quality control has led to automated processing and developing of film to eliminate the human error factor. Automated processing machines produce a film usually in less than 2 minutes. Processors vary by manufacturer, requiring that the medical assistant be proficient in the operation of the particular facility's equipment.

Unexposed film must be protected from moisture, heat, and light by storage in a cool, dry place, preferably in a lead-lined box. Film packets, exposed or unexposed, must be opened in a darkroom with only the darkroom light for illumination. The film is placed in a cassette for use in any area outside the darkroom. Intensifying screens in the cassette are used to reduce the amount of exposure required.

Special sleeves or envelopes of varying sizes are available for storing the properly labeled film. Film must be protected in a cool, dry area.

Checkpoint Question

6. How can medical assistants help with radiologic examinations?

➤ TRANSFER OF RADIOGRAPHIC INFORMATION

Radiography performed on site for use by the resident physician will remain as part of the patient's permanent record. In many cases, however, radiographic studies are performed at one site for consultation or referral to another site. X-ray films belong to the site where the study was performed, but the radiologist (physician who interprets the radiographs) or examining physician is generally required to return a written summary of the examination results to the referring physician. If the patient is a short-term referral, the examining physician will usually return the films to the referring physician. Patients with ongoing concerns who move from the area or who change physicians may request the information contained on their records and may obtain copies of the original radiographs.

Legal Tips

Follow these tips to help safeguard your patient and yourself:

- Be sure radiographic images are properly identified.
- Keep in mind that interventional procedures require a consent form, similar to those used for surgical procedures, to be signed by the patient.
- Remember that only physicians are legally permitted to make a diagnosis or interpret the radiographic images. If a patient asks you for the results of a radiographic study, you should not give any information unless directed to do so by a physician. The patient should be told in a calm, compassionate manner that only the physician is qualified to interpret the radiographs and that the physician will explain the results.
- Know your state laws regarding licensing for x-ray procedures. Many states now require the licensing of all personnel who perform x-ray procedures, which may exclude medical assistants from taking x-rays.

SUMMARY

Radiology is continually evolving as a tool to prevent, diagnose, and treat disease. As a medical assistant, you must understand the various diagnostic and therapeutic radiologic procedures described here. You also may be responsible for educating the patient about these procedures in general and about any particular preparations required. When assisting the physician, radiation safety precautions must be followed carefully for the protection of yourself and your patient.

CRITICAL THINKING CHALLENGES

1. A mother of a 6-year-old child voices concerns to you about the dangers of x-rays. How would you address her fears?
2. Summarize the key points of radiation safety, then write a policy booklet for new employees. Create a poster highlighting the most important points of radiation safety to hang in the staff lounge.
3. Constipation is a common problem among patients who have barium enemas. How could patient education diminish this problem? Develop a brief instruction sheet to give to these patients.

ANSWERS TO CHECKPOINT QUESTIONS

1. X-rays are high-energy electromagnetic radiation that travels at the speed of light. X-rays can penetrate fairly dense objects, such as the human body. They cannot be seen, heard, felt, tasted, or smelled.
2. Barium enemas involve filling only the large intestine with barium. Because the large intestine is the last part of the GI tract, this barium can be eliminated more quickly. If an upper GI examination is performed first, it may be days later before barium can be eliminated—thus delaying other examinations.
3. Contrast media helps differentiate between body structures by artificially changing the absorption rate of a particular structure so that it can be seen clearly instead of blending in with adjacent structures. For example, barium sulfate absorbs radiation and shows white on a radiograph.
4. Fluoroscopy uses x-rays to observe movement within the body. CT uses a combination of x-rays and computers to create cross-sectional images of the body. Sonography uses high-frequency sound waves to create cross-sectional still or real-time (motion) images of the body.
5. PTCA could save a patient's life by reopening the lumen of a coronary artery to allow sufficient blood flow to keep the heart muscle alive.
6. Medical assistants can help with radiologic examinations by providing instructing to patients, positioning patients, handling x-ray film, and distributing or filing radiographs and reports.

SUGGESTIONS FOR FURTHER READING

Andolina, V. F.; Lille, S. L.; Willison, K. M. (1992). *Mammographic Imaging: A Practical Guide*. Philadelphia: Lippincott-Raven.

Bontrager, K. (1993). *Textbook of Radiographic Positioning and Related Anatomy*, 3rd ed. Mosby-Year Book.

Carlton, R., & Adler, A. (1992). *Principles of Radiographic Imaging—An Art and a Science*. Albany, NY: Delmar.

Cullinan, A. M. (1994). *Producing Quality Radiographs*, 2nd ed. Philadelphia: J. B. Lippincott.

Cullinan, A. M. (1992). *Optimizing Radiographic Positioning*. Philadelphia: J. B. Lippincott.

Torres, L. S. (1993). *Basic Medical Techniques and Patient Care for Radiologic Technologists*, 4th ed. Philadelphia: J. B. Lippincott.

Medical Office Emergencies

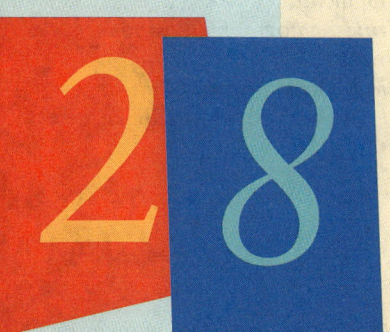

Chapter Outline

Emergency Medical Services System
Medical Office Emergency Procedures
  Emergency Action Plan
  Emergency Medical Kit
  Who Do I Call for Emergency
    Help?
  What Should Be Done Before the
    Ambulance Arrives?
  What Should Be Done When the
    Ambulance Arrives?
Patient Assessment
  Scene Survey
  Personal Protective Equipment
  Initial Approach to the Patient
  Primary Survey
Procedure: Managing an Adult Patient
    With a Foreign Body Airway
    Obstruction
Procedure: Performing Cardiopulmonary
    Resuscitation (One Rescuer)

  Secondary Survey
Types of Emergencies
  Shock
  Bleeding and Soft-Tissue Injuries
  Burn Injuries
  Musculoskeletal Injuries
  Cardiovascular Emergencies
  Neurologic Emergencies
  Allergic and Anaphylactic
    Reactions
  Poisoning
  Heat- and Cold-Related
    Emergencies
  Behavioral and Psychiatric
    Emergencies
Summary
Critical Thinking Challenges
Answers to Checkpoint Questions
Suggestions for Further Reading

DACUM Components

1.3 Perform within the scope of education, training, and personal capabilities
1.5 Work as a team member
1.8 Show initiative and responsibility
2.2 Treat all patients with empathy and impartiality
4.2 Take vital signs
4.3 Recognize emergencies
4.4 Perform first aid and CPR

Chapter Competencies

Learning Objectives

Upon successfully completing this chapter, you will be able to:

1. Spell and define the Key Terms.
2. Describe the role of the medical assistant in an emergency before the ambulance arrives.
3. Explain the purpose of the primary survey.
4. Identify the five types of shock and the management of each.
5. Describe how burns are classified.
6. Discuss the management of allergic reactions.
7. Discuss the role of the poison control center.
8. List the three types of hyperthermic emergencies and the treatment for each type.
9. Discuss the treatment of hypothermia.
10. Discuss the role of the medical assistant in managing psychiatric emergencies.
11. Explain the technique for managing an adult patient with a foreign body airway obstruction.
12. Explain the technique for performing cardiopulmonary resuscitation on an adult.

Performance Objectives

Upon successfully completing this chapter, you will be able to:

1. Manage an adult with a foreign body airway obstruction (Procedure 28-1).
2. Perform one-rescuer adult cardiopulmonary resuscitation (Procedure 28-2).

Key Terms

(See Glossary for definitions.)

anaphylactic shock	hyperthermia
anaphylaxis	hypothermia
cardiogenic shock	hypovolemic shock
contusion	neurogenic shock
ecchymosis	partial-thickness burn
frostbite	primary survey
full-thickness burn	seizure
heat cramps	shock
heat exhaustion	secondary survey
heat stroke	septic shock
hematoma	superficial burn

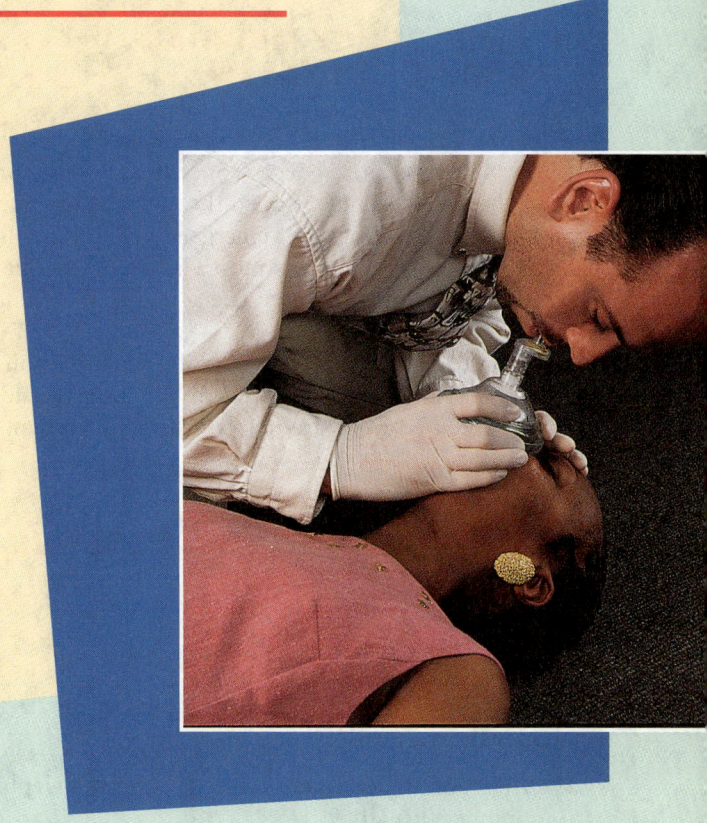

Emergency medical care is the immediate care given to the sick or injured person. When properly applied, it can mean the difference between life and death, rapid recovery and long hospitalization, or temporary disability and permanent injury. Emergency medical care in the medical office consists of furnishing temporary assistance until a basic or advanced life support ambulance or rescue squad, if needed, is obtained.

An emergency situation can occur anywhere and to anyone. For example, a patient who is being seen for a routine examination may collapse from a heart attack and require immediate cardiopulmonary resuscitation (CPR), or a coworker may forget to take her insulin and lapse into a diabetic coma, or an elderly person may fall down a flight of stairs. If first on the scene, the well prepared medical assistant can obtain important information and perform immediate lifesaving procedures before the ambulance or rescue squad arrives.

This chapter is not meant to provide a comprehensive study on all aspects of emergency care. Other chapters in this text should be read for details of various medical conditions. In addition, contact your local American Heart Association or American Red Cross chapter to obtain information about courses in first aid and CPR training.

➤ EMERGENCY MEDICAL SERVICES SYSTEM

The initial element of any emergency medical services (EMS) system is citizen access. Speedy access for emergency help has been developed through the use of 911 as a nationally recognized emergency telephone number. The EMS system at its most visible level is the arrival of the ambulance or rescue squad at the scene of the call.

The need for rapid, systematic intervention by medically trained personnel to care for the sick and injured patient is an integral part of the EMS system.

➤ MEDICAL OFFICE EMERGENCY PROCEDURES

Emergency Action Plan

Every medical office should have an emergency action plan. It should include:

- Appropriate emergency rescue service telephone number (usually 911)

- Location of the nearest hospital emergency department that provides 24-hour emergency care
- Telephone number of the local or regional poison control center in your area
- List of procedures of what to do in an emergency situation
- List of all personnel who are trained in CPR (this should include all office and medical staff)
- Location and list of contents of the emergency medical kit

Emergency Medical Kit

Along with the emergency action plan, proper equipment and supplies should be available to use in a medical emergency. General equipment and supplies used for routine procedures may vary depending on the medical office specialty. Equipment used for emergency situations, however, is fairly standard. This equipment should be made available for use and placed in a designated location that is accessible to all office staff. Standard supplies in an emergency medical kit are listed in Box 28-1.

Who Do I Call for Emergency Help?

Most communities have a 911 system for telephone access to report emergencies. The communications operator at a local emergency medical services (EMS) provider will answer the call, take the information, and alert the EMS, fire, or police departments as needed. In localities without the 911 system, emergency calls are usually made directly to the local ambulance, fire, or police department. The information is then routed to the appropriate agency. You should know which emergency system your community uses. The telephone numbers should be prominently displayed by all telephones in the medical office.

Some communities have what is called an enhanced 911 system. This system automatically identifies the caller's telephone number and location. If the telephone is disconnected or the patient loses consciousness, the communications operator will still be able to send emergency personnel to the scene.

Be sure to describe the emergency situation to the communications operator when you make the initial call. The operator will then know what level of emergency personnel and rescue equipment to send. Most of your emergency calls will probably be medical in nature. Ambulances are staffed by trained personnel who have met specific training and certification standards required by individual states.

BOX 28-1 Emergency Medical Kit and Equipment

These are standard supplies that can be used to make up a emergency medical kit:

Activated charcoal
Adhesive strip bandages, assorted sizes
Adhesive tape, 1- and 2-inch rolls
Alcohol (70%)
Alcohol wipes
Antimicrobial skin ointment
Chemical ice pack
Cotton balls
Cotton swabs
Disposable gloves, latex
Elastic bandages, 2- and 3-inch widths
Gauze pads, 2 × 2 and 4 × 4 inches
Roller, self-adhering gauze, 2- to 4-inch widths
Safety pins, various sizes
Scissors
Syrup of ipecac
Thermometer—1 oral, 1 rectal
Triangular bandages, 2 or 3
Tweezers

In addition to the kit contents listed above, the following equipment should be available:

Blood pressure cuff (pediatric and adult)
Stethoscope
Bag-valve-mask device with assorted size masks
Penlight
Portable oxygen tank with regulator
Oxygen masks
Suction unit

Additional equipment, if available:

Defibrillator
Intravenous equipment
Emergency drugs

What Should Be Done Before the Ambulance Arrives?

Whether confronted with a cardiac emergency or psychiatric crisis, the medical assistant must be able to coordinate a multitude of ongoing events while rendering patient care. Contributing to the complexity of decisions are such distractions as hysterical family members, arrival of emergency personnel, police directives, and language barriers.

Documentation is an important responsibility in patient care. The information given to emergency medical personnel should be as complete as possible. Information should include but not be limited to:

1. Basic identification information of the patient (eg, name, age, address, or location of patient contact)
2. Patient's chief complaint
3. Times of events (eg, responses, management technique, changes in patient condition)
4. Vital signs (blood pressure, pulse, and respiration)
5. Specific emergency management techniques rendered by the medical assistant (eg, cardiopulmonary resuscitation, bandaging, splinting, etc)

6. Observations (not subjective conclusions) of the patient's condition (eg, patient's speech was slurred, rather than drunk; patient unresponsive to loud verbal stimuli, rather than lethargic)

7. Any past medical history, medication, or allergies.

What Should Be Done When the Ambulance Arrives?

When emergency medical personnel arrive, escort the ambulance technician to the patient care area. Assist the technician as directed. Remove any obstacles, such as chairs or surgery stands, to allow room for stretchers and emergency personnel. Keep family members in the reception area or physician's private office. Calm other patients as needed.

Checkpoint Question

1. What six items should you attempt to document before the ambulance arrives?

➤ PATIENT ASSESSMENT

The two primary objectives in patient assessment are to identify and correct any life-threatening problems and to identify any associated problems, providing necessary care. As a result of information gained from the patient assessment, each step must be managed effectively before proceeding to the next. For example, the scene must be free from life-threatening hazards before proceeding to the primary survey. Airway, breathing, and circulation must be intact before taking a patient history, and the patient's history guides the secondary survey. This section provides a general review of the facets of patient assessment.

Scene Survey

The scene survey is the quick, yet observant, evaluation of potential hazards, mechanism of injury, and clues to medical illness that are provided by the patient's environment. For example, in an elderly person found at the bottom of a flight of stairs outside your office suite, a head or neck injury may be probable. Coffee ground-like emesis found near a person may be a clue to the presence of peptic ulcer disease and gastrointestinal hemorrhage.

Personal Protective Equipment

For each situation you encounter, it is important to use the appropriate precautions. Because it is impossible to identify patients who carry infectious diseases just by looking at them, all body fluids must be considered infectious and appropriate precautions taken at all times (see Chap. 19, Asepsis and Infection Control). Protective equipment should be accessible and available for easy access. Procedures should already be in place in your office protocol.

What If?
What if you encounter a person bleeding on the street and you do not have any protective equipment with you?

If the person is conscious, instruct him or her to cover the wound with a hand or piece of cloth and to apply pressure. You can also make a large bulky dressing with a piece of clothing and hold it on the area that is bleeding; of course, try to keep your hands from contacting blood. In many cases, it is up to you to decide whether or not to participate in a street emergency. However, some states have specific laws that require health care professionals to render emergency care. You should be aware of your state's law regarding emergency care and acting as a Good Samaritan.

Initial Approach to the Patient

In providing emergency care, do not assume that the obvious injuries are the only ones present because less noticeable injuries may also have occurred. Look for the causes of the injury, which may provide a clue as to the extent of physical damage. The medical assistant should be especially careful not to move the victim any more than necessary during the primary and secondary survey. Any unnecessary movement or rough handling should be avoided because it might aggravate undetected fractures or spinal injuries.

Primary Survey

The **primary survey** is always the first step once the medical assistant is at the patient's side. The primary survey is a rapid evaluation, less than 45 seconds, to determine the patient's status in the following areas:

- Responsiveness
- Airway
- Breathing
- Circulation

The purpose of the primary survey is to identify and correct any life-threatening problems. Although several procedures are shown in this chapter, it is not the purpose of this text to teach cardiopulmonary resuscitation (CPR). Such instruction can be acquired by taking a CPR course from a certified provider such as the American Red Cross or American Heart Association.

Responsiveness

The performance of the primary survey begins with attempts to awaken the patient by verbal and physical stimulation. Checking the patient's responsiveness should not be confused with the more specific level of consciousness, which is part of the more thorough secondary survey. State of responsiveness is quickly noting whether the patient is conscious or unconscious.

Airway

Depending on the circumstances, the airway should be opened by using the head-tilt/chin-lift or jaw-thrust method as described below and shown in Figs. 28-1 and 28-2. The jaw-thrust method is recommended if cervical injury is a possibility. Excessive movement, such as the head-tilt/chin-lift maneuver, could cause neurologic damage to an already injured spine.

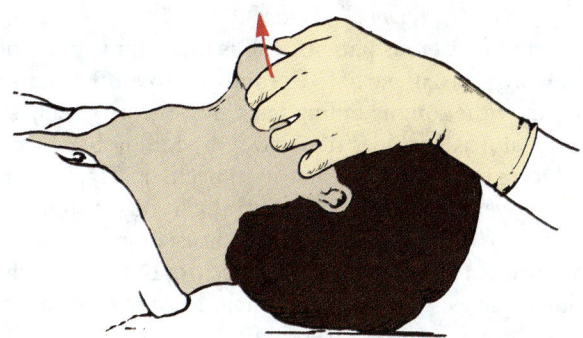

FIGURE 28-2
The jaw-thrust technique. The hands are placed on either side of the head. The fingers of both hands grasp behind the angle of the jaw, bringing it upward, as shown by the arrow.

The mouth should be quickly inspected for any obvious obstruction; prompt removal is essential before continuing the patient survey. The tongue falling back into the oropharynx is the most common cause of airway obstruction.

HEAD TILT/CHIN LIFT
The head-tilt/chin-lift method of opening the airway should be used on a patient who is not suspected of having a cervical spine injury. The patient's head should first be tilted back by placing one hand on the forehead and applying firm backward pressure. The other hand should be placed with the fingers under the bony part of the patient's lower jaw, near the chin, thus lifting the mandible and helping to tilt the head back (see Fig. 28-1).

JAW THRUST
The jaw-thrust method requires forward displacement of the jaw without any tilting of the head. This is the safest method of opening the airway and should always be used on a patient suspected of having cervical spine injury. The angles of the patient's jaw should be grasped with both hands, one on each side, displacing the mandible forward (see Fig. 28-2). The head should be supported without tilting it backward or turning it from side to side.

UPPER AIRWAY OBSTRUCTIONS
Damage, injury, or bypass of the upper airway may have significant consequences. For example, the patient who has a tracheostomy cannot filter air adequately, nor can inhaled air be humidified and warmed. Because the larynx has been bypassed, the cough reflex is also diminished, making the lower airway more vulnerable to foreign matter and mucous buildup. A number of other conditions can interfere with the function of the upper airway.

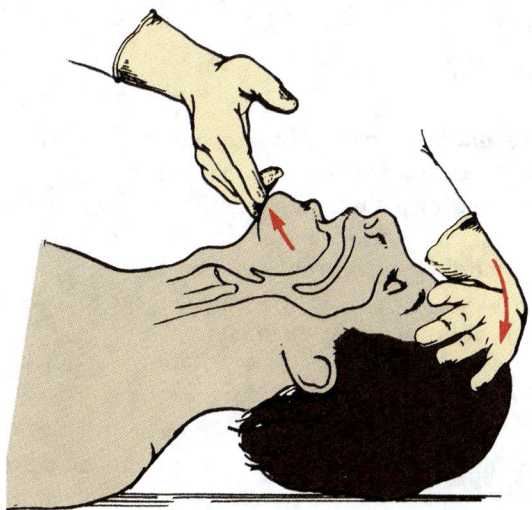

FIGURE 28-1
The head-tilt/chin-lift technique. The head is tilted backward with one hand (*down arrow*), while the fingers of the other hand lift the chin forward (*up arrow*).

OBSTRUCTION BY THE TONGUE

An unconscious patient who is in a supine position frequently has a partial or total airway obstruction caused by the tongue falling back into the oropharynx. The epiglottis occludes the airway by falling back over the laryngeal opening when its muscular attachments become weak. Patients with central nervous system depression from drugs, alcohol, or disease processes are more prone to this disorder because of poor tone in the facial muscles. Clinical signs include snoring respiration or total airway obstruction.

FOREIGN BODY ASPIRATION

Aspiration of foreign bodies has two effects on the airways. First, aspiration of any foreign material, including fluid, initiates a protective response that consists of sudden coughing and spasm of the airways. This spasm frequently causes labored or difficult breathing as well as wheezing in severe cases. It can produce partial or total airway obstruction. In addition, if the aspirated material is large enough it will cause a foreign body obstruction. Frequently, the object lodges in the larynx at the vocal cords because the adult airway is narrowest at this point.

As with obstruction by the tongue, foreign body aspiration in adults is associated most frequently with drug and alcohol ingestion or altered mental states, such as retardation or Alzheimer's disease. Often these patients have a decreased ability to feed themselves and a diminished gag reflex.

Management of Airway Disorders

After rapid assessment of the patient with airway compromise, immediate management must be started to establish and maintain an open airway. Various devices are available to assist in airway maintenance. Oropharyngeal and nasopharyngeal airways are used to open the upper airway and prevent the tongue from being an obstruction. Suction may be required to remove blood, mucus, or vomitus from the oropharynx.

Management techniques for airway obstruction are shown in Procedure 28-1.

Breathing

Once the airway is clear and secure, the patient's breathing is evaluated. You should watch the patient's chest while listening and feeling over the mouth and nose for adequate ventilation. If the patient is not breathing, artificial ventilatory support is given immediately. Any labored breathing is evaluated for the degree of distress involved.

Ventilation that is too slow, irregular, or too fast requires immediate intervention. The quality and pattern of breathing is simultaneously evaluated. Any obvious noises, such as stridor or wheezes, should be noted.

Circulation

Circulation is evaluated in either the adult or child by a check of the carotid pulse. The brachial pulse is used to evaluate circulation in the infant. If the patient has no pulse, external chest compressions should be performed. Any hemorrhage (profuse bleeding) should be observed and controlled.

If the pulse is present, the rate and quality are quickly noted. Perfusion (flow of blood through the tissues) is evaluated by skin temperature and moisture. Findings that indicate the presence of shock affect the steps of the secondary survey and ultimate patient management.

Management of Cardiopulmonary Resuscitation (CPR)

Although it is not the purpose of this text to teach CPR, it is important to describe some management techniques. The medical assistant is advised to use a face mask with a one-way valve or preferably a bag-valve-mask device when performing any rescue breathing. These devices should be in the emergency medical kit. The technique for performing CPR on an adult patient is described in Procedure 28-2.

Checkpoint Question
2. What is the purpose of the primary survey?

Secondary Survey

The **secondary survey** is an assessment tool for making correct decisions regarding patient care. The secondary survey includes a patient interview and a more thorough physical evaluation. Its aim is to find less obvious and less acute problems than those evaluated in the primary survey. Ideally, management follows as a logical extension of the examination.

Diagnostic Signs

Five diagnostic signs are necessary to gain an accurate impression during the secondary survey. They are:

1. General appearance. The patient's skin color and moisture, facial expression, posture, motor activity, speech, and state of awareness provide important clues about the patient's condition. Medic Alert bracelets or medicine bottles in pockets can

Procedure 28-1   Managing an Adult Patient With a Foreign Body Airway Obstruction

Steps	Purpose
1. Ask the patient, "Are you choking?"	1. If the patient is able to speak or cough, air is getting past the obstruction and the obstruction is not complete.
2. Give abdominal thrusts. Use chest thrusts for pregnant or obese victims.	2. Such thrusts can force air upward from the lungs into the airway with enough pressure to expel the foreign body.

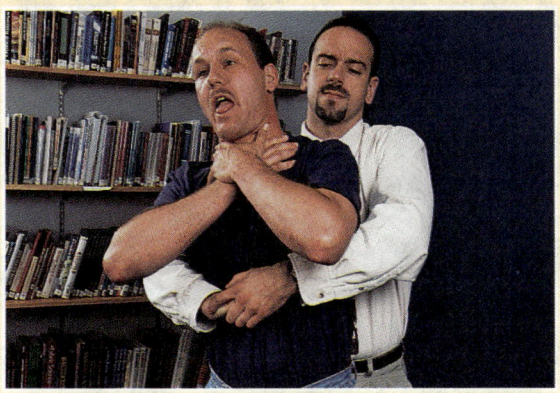

Step 2. Give abdominal thrusts.

3. Repeat thrusts until effective or the victim becomes unconscious.	3. Several thrusts may be necessary to expel the object.
4. If the victim is unconscious, activate the EMS system.	4. This will summon emergency personnel while you continue to provide assistance to the patient.
5. Perform a tongue-jaw lift followed by a finger sweep to remove the object.	5. With loss of consciousness, the object may become visible and may be removed.

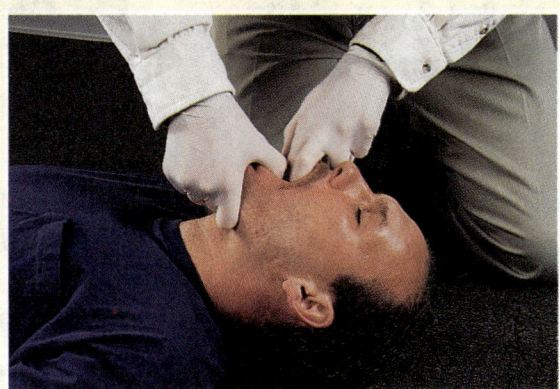

Step 5: Finger sweep.

6. Open the airway and try to ventilate. If the airway is still obstructed, reposition the patient's head and try to ventilate again.	6. Airway obstruction may be caused, in part, by improper head position.
7. Give up to five abdominal thrusts.	7. Such thrusts may expel the object.
8. Repeat steps 5 through 7 until effective.	

Procedure 28-2   Performing Cardiopulmonary Resuscitation (One rescuer)

Steps	Purpose
1. Establish patient unresponsiveness. Activate the EMS system.	1. You do not want to begin CPR unnecessarily if the patient does not require it. A call for help will summon emergency personnel.
2. Open the airway.	2. The airway must be opened to determine whether the patient is breathing.

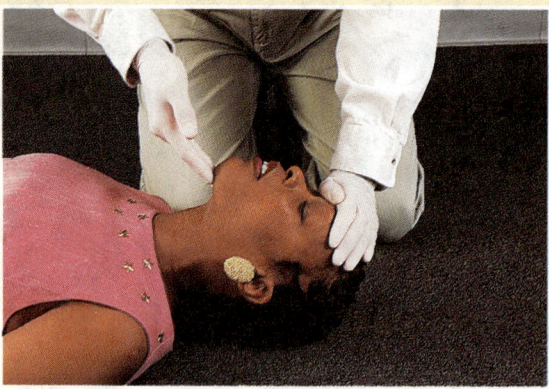

Step 2. Open the airway.

3. Give 2 slow breaths.	3. It is important to get as much oxygen as possible into the patient.

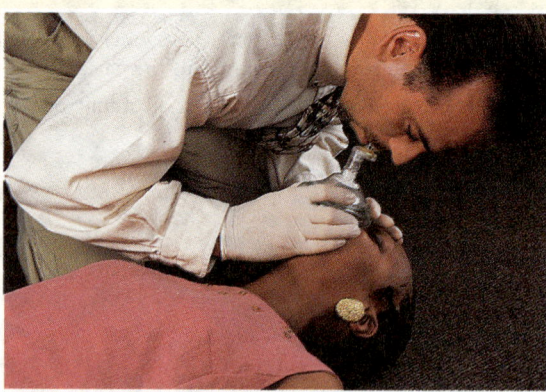

Step 3. Give two slow breaths.

(continued)

be helpful. The continuation of the secondary survey may confirm or deny initial suspicions seen by the patient's general appearance.

2. Level of consciousness. By the time you have completed the primary survey and noted the patient's general appearance, the level of consciousness may be apparent. The AVPU system is one example that uses a common language to describe the patient's level of consciousness. AVPU is an acronym that represents:

A = Awake and alert
V = Responds to voice
P = Responds only to pain
U = Unresponsive or unconscious

Procedure 28-2

Performing Cardiopulmonary Resuscitation (One rescuer) *(continued)*

Steps

Purpose

4. Check the carotid pulse. If no pulse is present, give cycles of 15 chest compressions and two breaths.

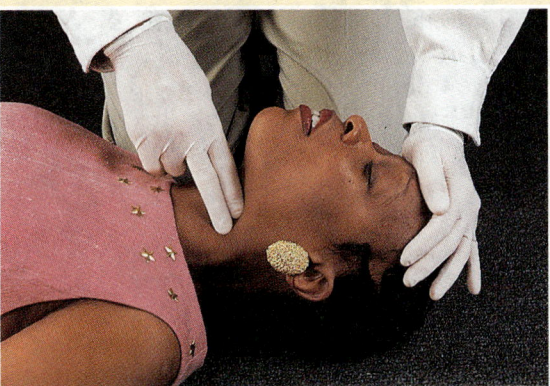

Step 4A: Check for pulse.

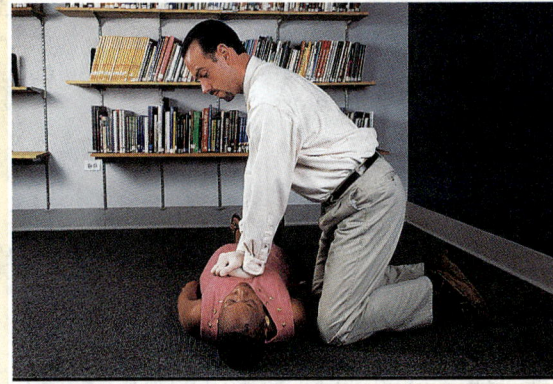

Step 4B: Begin CPR with chest compressions.

5. After giving four cycles of 15 chest compressions and 2 breaths (about 1 minute), check the patient's pulse. If no pulse is present, continue the 15:2 cycle, beginning with chest compressions.

3. Vital signs. The next step in the secondary survey is assessment of vital signs. Vital signs should be determined before further assessment in most patients. Each vital sign should include a proper measurement technique as well as appropriate interpretation of the readings. This interpretation should be based on both the initial reading and on serial measurements of each vital sign. The proper techniques and interpretation of the respiration, pulse, and blood pressure are described in Chap. 21, Anthropometric Measurements and Vital Signs.

4. Temperature. Temperature determination is important for patients with altered skin temperature or patients who have been exposed to environmen-

tal temperature extremes. Patients with a history of infection, chills, or fever and children with seizures should have their temperatures taken. Taking a temperature is discussed in Chap. 21, Anthropometric Measurements and Vital Signs.

5. Skin. An initial evaluation of the skin that included both temperature and moisture should have been noted during the primary survey. A more thorough look should now be taken. Skin is normally dry and somewhat warm. Moist, cool skin may indicate poor blood flow to the tissues and possible shock. The color of the skin should also be noted as an indication of the circulation near the surface of the body and oxygenation. Table 28-1 summarizes abnormal skin colors.

Physical Examination

The head-to-toe survey is organized as follows: head and neck, chest and back, abdomen, and extremities.

HEAD AND NECK

The head should be inspected and palpated. If a cervical spine injury is suspected, the spine should be immobilized immediately and the neck should not be manipulated while the head is being evaluated. The face should be examined for edema, bruising, bleeding, or fluid from the nose or ears. The mouth should be examined for loose teeth or dentures. In infants, the condition of the anterior fontanel should be noted.

The pupils can provide important clues in certain patients. All trauma patients and every patient with an altered level of consciousness or a neurogenic complaint or finding should have the pupils checked. The pupils should be examined for several items:

- Equal size
- Dilation in both eyes caused by darkness
- Constriction in both eyes caused by light
- Constriction that occurs rapidly
- Reaction to light that is equal

To evaluate these items, both eyes should be shaded from the light. Quickly shine a flashlight at each eye from an angle about 6 to 8 inches from the eye. The patient should not look directly into the light. Both pupils should quickly constrict.

CHEST AND BACK

The chest is evaluated to some degree when the patient's respirations are evaluated. A further inspection of the chest is necessary, especially in the trauma patient or in any patient with abnormal vital signs. The patient with a cardiac or respiratory complaint, finding, or history is also a candidate for a more thorough chest evaluation. Palpation of the chest and back may reveal tender areas that possibly indicate rib fractures.

ABDOMEN

The abdomen should be evaluated on all patients but particularly those with gastrointestinal symp-

Table 28-1
Abnormal Skin Colors and Causes

Color	Possible Cause	Possible Conditions
Pink	Vasodilation	Heat illness
		Hot environment
	Increased blood flow	Exertion
		Fever
		Alcohol consumption
White, pale	Decreased blood flow	Shock
		Fainting
	Decreased red blood cells	Anemia
	Vasoconstriction	Cold exposure
Blue	Inadequate oxygenation	Airway obstruction
		Congestive heart failure
		Chronic bronchitis
Yellow	Increased bilirubin	Liver disease
	Retention of urinary elements	Renal disease

From Jones S. A., Weigel, A., White, R. D., McSwain, N. E., Breiter, M. (1992). Advanced Emergency Care for Paramedic Practice. Philadelphia: J. B. Lippincott; p. 116.

toms or suspicion of blood or fluid loss as seen in vaginal bleeding, vomiting, or melena (blood in the stool). Inspection of the abdomen should be performed to observe for scars, bruises, or masses. A distended abdomen may indicate hemorrhage within the abdomen.

ARMS AND LEGS

The examination of the arms and legs is the last step of the head-to-toe survey. The arms and legs are inspected and palpated for swelling, deformity, or tenderness. Tremors in the hands should be noted. Comparing one side to another is necessary.

The neurologic status of the arms and legs is determined and tested for strength, movement, range of motion, and sensation. Muscle strength is checked by having the patient squeeze both of your hands. Leg strength may be determined by having the patient push the feet against your hand. The ability to move each arm or leg is simultaneously evaluated. Sensation is assessed by using a safety pin or other tool to determine the patient's response to pain. Throughout the examination, a comparison of both sides is essential.

Checkpoint Question

3. What are the five diagnostic signs that are evaluated in the secondary survey?

➤ TYPES OF EMERGENCIES

Shock

Shock is a lack of oxygen to the individual cells of the body. All of the body's tissues require oxygen for proper functioning—not just organs such as the heart and brain, which have an immediate response to lack of oxygenation.

The body initially adjusts for shock by increasing the strength of contractions of the heart, increasing the heart rate, and constricting the blood vessels. These acts all help to pump blood throughout the body in the best way possible. As shock progresses, the body has difficulty trying to adjust and eventually tissues and body organs will have such severe damage that the shock becomes irreversible. Box 28-2 lists the signs and symptoms of shock.

Types of Shock

Hypovolemic shock is caused by the loss of blood or other body fluids. If hypovolemic shock occurs due to blood loss it can also be called hemorrhagic shock.

BOX 28-2   Signs and Symptoms of Shock

- Restlessness or signs of fear
- Thirst
- Nausea
- Cool clammy skin
- Pale skin with cyanosis (bluish color) at the lips and earlobes
- Rapid and weak pulse
- Low blood pressure

Dehydration caused by diarrhea, vomiting, or heavy sweating can also lead to hypovolemic shock.

Cardiogenic shock is the most extreme form of heart failure, occurring when the function of the left ventricle is so compromised that the heart can no longer adequately pump blood to body tissues.

Neurogenic shock is caused by a dysfunction of the nervous system (as seen in spinal cord injury). The diameter of the blood vessels in the body can no longer be controlled. This leads to a dilation of the blood vessels. Once the blood vessels are dilated, there is not enough blood in the circulation to fill this need, thus causing shock.

Anaphylactic shock is an acute generalized allergic reaction that occurs within minutes to hours after the body has been exposed to a foreign substance to which it is oversensitive.

Septic shock is caused by a generalized infection of the bloodstream in which the patient appears seriously ill. It may be associated with an infection such as pneumonia or meningitis, or it may occur without an apparent source of infection especially in infants and children. History reveals that the patient may have become ill suddenly, or the illness may have developed over several days. Fever is present initially; however, hypothermia develops and is a clinical sign suggestive of sepsis.

Management of the Patient in Shock

Remember: Shock can be the result of many types of medical and trauma emergencies. The following should serve as a general guideline for managing a patient in shock.

1. Ensure an open airway and breathing.
2. Control bleeding.
3. Administer oxygen.
4. Immobilize for possible spinal injuries.
5. Splint fractures.

6. Prevent loss of body heat (use a blanket).
7. Transport to the closest hospital as soon as possible.

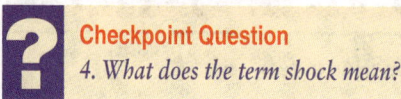

Checkpoint Question

4. What does the term shock mean?

Bleeding and Soft-Tissue Injuries

Soft-tissue injuries involve the skin and underlying musculature. An injury to these tissues is commonly referred to as a wound. Box 28-3 describes common soft-tissue injuries.

When a blunt object strikes the body, it may crush the tissue beneath the skin. Although the skin does not break, severe damage to tissue and blood vessels may cause bleeding within a confined area. This is called a closed wound.

Types of closed wounds include contusions, hematomas, and crush injuries. A **contusion** is a bruise. Blood collects under the skin or in damaged tissue. Swelling at the site may occur immediately or 24 to 48 hours later. As blood accumulates in the area, a characteristic black and blue mark, called **ecchymosis**, is seen. A blood clot that forms at the injury site is called a **hematoma**. Hematomas are generally caused when large areas of tissue are damaged. When a large bone such as the femur or pelvis is fractured, as much as a liter of blood can be lost in a confined space within the soft tissue. Crush injuries are usually caused by extreme external forces that crush both tissue and bone. Even though the skin remains intact, severe damage may occur to underlying organs.

In an open wound, the skin is broken and the patient is susceptible to external hemorrhage and wound contamination. An open wound may be the only surface evidence of a more serious injury, such as a fracture. Open wounds include abrasions, lacerations, major arterial lacerations, puncture wounds, avulsions, amputations, and impaled objects. When managing any patient with open wounds, follow Standard Precautions to protect yourself against disease transmission and to protect the patient from further contamination.

Management of Bleeding and Soft-Tissue Injuries

Management of open soft-tissue injuries includes controlling bleeding by direct pressure and elevation. Sterile gauze should be used to cover the wound. Elevation

---

BOX 28-3   Types of Soft-Tissue Injuries

- **Abrasion** is the least serious type of open wound. It is little more than a scratching of the surface of the skin. All abrasions, regardless of size, are extremely painful because of the nerve endings involved.
- **Laceration** results from the snagging or tearing of tissues that leaves a jagged wound that bleeds freely. Skin tissues may be partly or completely torn away, and the laceration may contain foreign matter that can lead to infection. An example of a laceration would be a wound caused by a broken bottle or a jagged piece of metal.
- **Major arterial laceration** can cause significant bleeding if the sharp or jagged instrument also cuts the wall of a blood vessel, especially an artery. If uncontrolled, major arterial bleeding can result in shock and death.
- **Puncture wound** can result from a number of causes, such as from sharp, narrow objects like knives, nails, and ice picks. Punctures also can be caused by high-velocity penetrating objects, such as bullets. A special care of the puncture wound is the *impaled object wound*, in which the instrument that causes the injury remains impacted in the wound. The object could be anything—a stick, piece of glass, a knife, a steel rod—that penetrates any part of the body.
- **Avulsion** is the tearing loose of a flap of skin, which may either remain hanging or tear off altogether. Avulsions usually bleed profusely. Most often, the patient who presents with an avulsion works with machinery. Home accidents that involve lawn mowers and power tools are common.
- **Amputation** is caused by the ripping, tearing force of industrial and automobile accidents, which is often great enough to tear away or crush limbs from the body.

of the affected part above the level of the heart is effective in the control of both pain and bleeding.

Management of amputations includes controlling bleeding but also preserving the severed part. The severed part should be put in a plastic bag. Place the first bag in a second plastic bag and seal it shut. The second bag provides added protection against moisture loss. Place the sealed bags in a container of ice or ice water; never use dry ice.

An impaled object requires careful immobilization of the patient and the injured part. Any motion of the impaled object can cause additional damage to the surface wound and, particularly, the underlying tissues.

Burn Injuries

The four major sources of burn injury are thermal, electrical, chemical, and radiation. *Thermal burns*, also called heat burns, are a result of heat conducted by hot liquids, solids, and superheated gases, as well as flame burns from fire. *Electrical burns* are caused from contact with low- or high-voltage electricity. Lightning injuries are also considered electrical burns. *Chemical burns* result when wet or dry corrosive substances come in contact with the skin. The amount of injury with a chemical burn depends on the concentration and quantity of the chemical agent. *Radiation burns* are similar to thermal burns and can occur from overexposure to ultraviolet light (sunburn) or from the heat of an atomic explosion.

Classification of Burn Injuries

Classification of burn injuries depends on the depth or tissue layers of the skin involved. Factors that determine the depth of the burn include the agent of burn, temperature, and length of time exposed. Burns are classified as superficial (first-degree), partial-thickness (second-degree), and full-thickness (third-degree). Table 28-2 describes the characteristics of burns according to depth.

Table 28-2
Characteristics of Burns According to Depth

Depth of Burn and Causes	Skin Involvement	Symptoms	Wound Appearance	Recuperative Course
Superficial (First-Degree)				
Sunburn Low-intensity flash	Epidermis	Tingling Hyperesthesia (super sensitivity) Pain that is soothed by cooling	Reddened; blanches with pressure Minimal or no edema	Complete recovery within a week Peeling
Partial-Thickness (Second-Degree)				
Scalds Flash flame	Epidermis and part of dermis	Pain Hyperesthesia Sensitive to cold air	Blistered, mottled red base; broken epidermis; weeping surface Edema	Recovery in 2–3 weeks Some scarring and depigmentation Infection may convert it to third-degree
Full-Thickness (Third-Degree)				
Flame Prolonged exposure to hot liquids Electric current	Epidermis, entire dermis, and sometimes subcutaneous tissue	Pain free Shock Hematuria (blood in the urine) and possibly, hemolysis (blood cell destruction) Possible entrance and exit wounds (electrical burn)	Dry; pale white, leathery, or charred Broken skin with fat exposed Edema	Eschar sloughs Grafting necessary Scarring and loss of contour and function Loss of digits or extremity possible

From Smeltzer, S. C., Bare, B. G. (1996). *Brunner and Suddarth's Textbook of Medical-Surgical Nursing, 8th Ed.* Philadelphia: Lippincott-Raven; p. 1550.

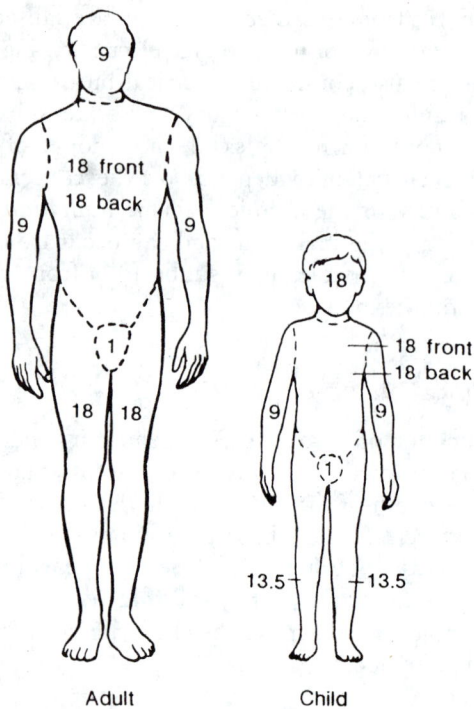

FIGURE 28-3
The rule of nines.

Calculation of Body Surface Area

The extent of body surface area (BSA) burned is most commonly estimated by a method called the rule of nines. This method calculates the percentage of body surface occupied by individual sections of the body. To fully determine the extent of BSA burned, the percentage of superficial, partial-thickness, and full-thickness burns should be recorded. This process, however, is not practical in the out-of-hospital setting.

RULE OF NINES

The **rule of nines** is the most common method of determining the extent of burn injury (Fig. 28-3). With this technique, in the adult, 9% of the skin is estimated to cover the head and each upper extremity, including front and back surfaces. Twice as much, or 18%, of the total skin area covers the front and back of the trunk and each lower extremity, including front and back surfaces. The area around the genitals, called the perineum, represents the additional 1% of BSA. In the infant or child, the percentages remain the same with the exception of the head, which is 18%, and each lower extremity, which is 13.5% of total BSA. The rule of nines works well in adults but does not reflect the various anatomic differences seen in children.

Management of the Burn Victim

The following should be used as management guidelines for burn victims:

1. Eliminate the source of the burn.
2. Assess the patient's airway, breathing, and circulation.
3. Remove all jewelry and clothing necessary to evaluate the burn.
4. Wrap the patient in a clean, dry sheet.
5. Administer oxygen.
6. Keep the patient warm.
7. Treat the patient for shock.
8. Transport the patient to the hospital.

> **? Checkpoint Question**
> *5. What are the four major sources of burn injuries?*

Musculoskeletal Injuries

Injuries to muscles, bones, and joints are some of the most common problems encountered in providing emergency care. The seriousness of these injuries varies widely from simple injuries, such as a fractured finger, to major life-threatening conditions, such as an open femur fracture or compromising spinal injuries. Injuries to muscle, tendons, and ligaments occur when a joint or muscle is either torn or stretched beyond its normal limits. Fractures and dislocations are usually associated with external forces, although some may occur through disease, such as bone degeneration.

Caring for patients with strains, sprains, fractures, and dislocations is described in Chap. 31, Caring for Patients With Musculoskeletal Disorders.

Management of Musculoskeletal Injuries

It is often difficult to distinguish between strains, sprains, fractures, and dislocations in an emergency situation. Therefore, in most cases, assume that the area is fractured and immobilize it accordingly. Proper splinting technique involves immobilizing above and below the fracture site. Splinting helps prevent further injury to soft tissues, blood vessels, or nerves from sharp bone fragments and relieves pain by stopping motion at the fracture site.

Never attempt to reduce (put back in place) a dislocated area. You may, however, in a severely deformed limb, gently realign it before splinting. This may be required when an angulated injury to the arm or leg cannot be fit into a rigid splint or if a pulse is absent distal to (below) the fracture site. Realignment is nothing more than pulling gently in line with the normal bone position. If there is pain or resistance to this procedure, splint the fracture as it is.

TYPES OF SPLINTS

Any device used to immobilize a fracture or dislocation is a splint. A splint may be soft or rigid. It can be improvised from almost any object that can provide stability. There are several kinds of commercially available splints, such as a traction splint, air splint, wire ladder splint, and padded board splint.

Cardiovascular Emergencies

Cardiovascular disease accounts for nearly one million deaths each year in the United States. The most common problem is coronary artery disease, which usually leads to chest pain and eventually to heart attack (myocardial infarction) if left untreated. Approximately two-thirds of sudden deaths due to coronary artery disease occur out of the hospital, and most occur within 2 hours of the onset of cardiovascular symptoms. Many of these deaths can be prevented by prompt basic or advanced life support, including rapid access to the emergency medical services system, bystander cardiopulmonary resuscitation (CPR), and early defibrillation.

If CPR is initiated promptly and the patient is successfully and rapidly defibrillated, survival chances are good. Defibrillation can be performed with manual, automatic, or semiautomatic external defibrillators. Manual defibrillation requires interpretation of a monitor or rhythm strip. Defibrillation using automatic or semiautomatic devices will analyze the rhythm and either automatically defibrillate or advise the operator to defibrillate.

Neurologic Emergencies

A seizure is caused by an abnormal discharge of electrical activity in the brain. During a seizure attack, bizarre muscle movements, strange sensations, and a complete loss of consciousness can occur. A seizure is not a disease but a manifestation or symptom of an underlying disorder.

In assessing the patient having a seizure, priority must be given to responsiveness, airway, breathing, and circulation. In certain types of seizure, the patient experiences a period of unconsciousness and, therefore, is unable to protect the airway. Frequently, these patients vomit during the seizure. Also, they have a tendency to bite their tongue. Thus, particular attention and care should be given to clearing and maintaining the airway. Patient history is an important factor in the assessment of these patients. It should include information about past seizure disorders, frequency of the attacks, prescribed medications, and regularity in taking medications. Further, history of head trauma is a significant finding. Other important aspects to explore include alcohol and drug abuse, recent fever, stiff neck (as seen in meningitis), and a history of heart disease, diabetes, or stroke.

Care of the patient should always begin with opening and securing an airway. In maintaining the airway of the patient having a seizure, objects should never be forced between the patient's teeth. Padded tongue blades or bite sticks may cause further complications, such as broken teeth, vomiting, aspiration, and laryngeal spasm.

After gaining control of the airway, perhaps the most important thing you can do for a patient who is having a seizure is to protect the patient from injury. The patient will rarely need to be restrained. Placing the patient on the side will help secretions drain from the mouth and is an easier position to suction the patient, if necessary.

Allergic and Anaphylactic Reactions

This section addresses allergic reactions, including the severe form, anaphylaxis. Anaphylaxis (or anaphylactic reaction) causes the most emergency department visits related to allergies. It is an acute generalized allergic reaction that occurs within minutes to hours after the body has been exposed to a foreign substance to which it is oversensitive. This anaphylactic reaction has systemic signs and symptoms that are exaggerated from a simple allergic reaction.

The exact incidence of anaphylactic reactions is difficult to pinpoint. Estimates in a study in the United States determined that 1% to 2% of all patients who receive penicillin have some form of allergy to the drug and that 1 in 50,000 injections of penicillin results in death. Estimates of anaphylactic death from insect stings number at least 50 per year.

As explained in Chap. 36, Caring for Patients With Immune Disorders, the immune response is a positive adaptive response. It is designed to guard the body against dangerous foreign substances, such as infections and antigens. In this normal immune response, the protective cells of the body recognize dangerous intruders, fight them, and destroy them. The allergic reaction, on the other hand, is an oversensitive and harmful response against foreign substances that may actually be harmless. The protective cells overestimate the danger of the harmless intruder and may produce needless damage to body tissue.

Common Allergens

An allergen is a substance that gives rise to hypersensitivity or allergy. Allergen groups include drugs, insect venom, food, and pollen. The causative agent may be injected, ingested, absorbed through the skin or mucous membranes, or even inhaled. A patient may experience symptoms within seconds after exposure to an allergen, or the reaction may be delayed for several hours.

Signs and Symptoms

The initial signs and symptoms typically occur with severe itching, a feeling of warmth, tightness in the throat or chest, or a rash. Cardiovascular collapse and shock can occur if the situation becomes worse. The primary rule for any exposure is that the earlier the onset of symptoms after exposure, the more severe the reaction is likely to be.

Management of Allergic and Anaphylactic Reactions

Because the primary cause of death in anaphylaxis is airway obstruction, the medical assistant must observe closely for signs of airway involvement. Choking or tightness in the neck and throat may signal this danger. In addition to the upper airway, the entire respiratory system frequently is involved. The patient may exhibit wheezing, shortness of breath, coughing, spitting up blood (hemoptysis), or pulmonary edema. A fast heart rate (tachycardia), low blood pressure (hypotension), pale skin, dryness of the mouth, sweating, and other classic signs of shock may be seen. The patient is likely to be anxious, and reassurance is an important part of the immediate intervention.

Medic Alert tags can be lifesaving, particularly for patients who have severe anaphylactic reactions. The tags are available as a bracelet or necklace and have engraved medical information.

Some allergic reactions are mild, without respiratory problems or signs of shock. These simple reactions can be managed with giving the patient oxygen (2–4 L/min) by nasal cannula or simple face mask. If respiratory involvement occurs without shock, the physician may order that epinephrine (1:1000) be given subcutaneously. In the patient with a severe anaphylactic reaction who is in shock, more aggressive therapy is indicated. Along with administering oxygen, the physician may order intravenous epinephrine (1:10,000). Monitoring the cardiac rhythm and additional drug therapy may be required. The primary goal of therapy in the patient with a severe anaphylactic reaction is to restore respiratory and circulatory function.

> **? Checkpoint Question**
> 6. What is the primary cause of death in anaphylaxis?

Poisoning

The likelihood that one will be exposed to toxins in the home or workplace is increasing. Over-the-counter and prescription medications are common in the home. About-two thirds of physician visits result in a prescription. Household chemicals are a hazard, many times designed to have a pleasant odor and color. Industrial chemicals offer another dimension of potential toxic exposures. These chemicals may involve a single victim or may create a triage problem in a hazardous materials incident.

Overall, most toxic exposures occur in the home. Almost 50% of exposures reported occur in children between the ages of 1 and 3 years. About 90% of all reported poisonings are accidental. In adolescents and adults, intentional toxic exposures can occur. Although deaths from poisoning and drug overdose are not frequent, intentional toxic exposures tend to have a higher death rate and result in more serious symptoms than accidental exposures or adverse drug actions.

Poison Control Center

When information about a poisoning or drug overdose is not readily available, the poison control center is a valuable resource. Poison control centers are designed to answer questions from health care professionals and the public. Many times, they can evaluate a nontoxic or mildly toxic exposure by telephone, instruct the caller in the use of syrup of ipecac to induce vomiting, and check on the progress by follow-up telephone calls. In questionable or more potentially serious toxic exposures, the poison control center can be consulted from the emergency scene (ie, physician's office).

The American Association of Poison Control Centers has established standards and recognizes regional poison control centers throughout the country. These centers are staffed by physicians, nurses, and pharmacists who are specifically trained or experienced in collecting information from a caller and retrieving information from many sources. Exactly how and when a poison control center is consulted should be part of the medical office's protocol.

Management of Poisoning Emergencies

Few toxic substances have specific antidotes. As a result, management of the poisoning emergency is aimed at the signs and symptoms present and organ systems involved. Decontamination and prevention of further absorption is done once the patient is relatively stable and initial priorities have been addressed.

Heat- and Cold-Related Emergencies

Temperature is one of the many variables to which the body adjusts in the process of maintaining equilibrium. As warm-blooded animals, human beings depend on the ability to limit core body temperature within a range of several degrees. This range centers around a normal core temperature, measured rectally, or 37.6°C (99.6°F). Peripheral temperature is usually lower, as seen by a normal value of 37°C (98.6°F) for oral readings. The definition of normal thus varies with location. Temperature also fluctuates over a range of several degrees under entirely healthy circumstances. To take advantage of the body's temperature as an assessment tool, both rectal and oral thermometers should be available.

Several conditions disrupt the normal heat-regulating mechanisms of the body. They are divided into two main categories, hyperthermia and hypothermia.

Hyperthermia

Hyperthermia refers to the general condition of excess body heat. Correct management depends on assessment of underlying causes.

Heat cramps result from profuse sweating. Most often, the cramping follows a period of physical exertion in a hot environment. Heavy sweating leads to high sodium losses, and at some point, the sodium deficit compromises muscle function. The cramps are a consequence of sweating, a healthy compensatory mechanism, and usually present without evidence of more severe problems.

The patient complains of cramps most commonly in the calves of the legs and in the abdomen. Cramps may occur in the hands, arms, and feet. The patient's skin is cool and usually wet. Mental status and blood pressure should be normal although an increased pulse rate is common.

Heat cramps signal the need for cooling and rest. In uncomplicated cases, the patient is often able to take fluid by mouth, but nausea may make intravenous infusion of 0.9% sodium chloride the desired management. If the patient is able to take fluid by mouth, add ½ to 1 teaspoon of salt per pint of water or fruit juice or give one of the commercial electrolyte solutions, such as Gatorade. Cramps can sometimes be prevented entirely with similar oral intake before physical exertion. Salt tablets are not recommended because they may cause nausea.

Heat exhaustion results most often from physical exertion in the heat without adequate fluid replacement. Body temperature usually remains normal or only slightly above normal. Patients often present with central nervous system symptoms, such as headache, fatigue, dizziness, or syncope. Skin is typically moist, and the pulse rate is high. Skin color, blood pressure, and respiratory rate are all variable depending on the degree to which the body is able to hold off the distress. Patients with later stages of heat exhaustion have pale skin, low blood pressure, and increased respiratory rate.

Management used for heat cramps may suffice in the early stages of heat exhaustion, but any hint of decreased mental status or unstable vital signs demands closer attention. Aggressive cooling measures must be used, as described for heat stroke, if rectal temperature is above 39°C (102°F).

Heat stroke is a true emergency. The body is no longer able to compensate for the rise in body temperature. Core body temperature threatens brain damage as it rises rapidly past 41°C (105°F). Heat stroke victims can deteriorate quickly to coma. They often have seizures, and the skin is classically hot, flushed, and dry, although gradual onset, age, and other factors can alter this sign. Vital signs rise initially, then drop later, resulting in cardiopulmonary arrest.

Heat stroke demands rapid cooling. The patient should be moved quickly to a cool area, clothing removed, and cold water, ice, or wet sheets placed on the patient's body. Concentrate on the core surface areas where the ability to cool central blood is greatest: the scalp, neck, axillae, and groin. The patient should be given oxygen and placed on a cardiac monitor. Transport to the hospital with continued cooling en route is required.

Hypothermia

The body's core temperature can drop several degrees in the normal course of body function. Even when the heat loss is not routine, the body usually tolerates a 3° to 4° drop without symptoms. Hypothermia is an abnormally low body temperature, with rectal readings below 35°C (95°F). Internal metabolic factors and heat loss to the external environment can lead to hypothermia. The rate of onset of hypothermia is variable. Very cold air and immersion in cold water can cause rapid drops in core temperature.

Basic management of hypothermia includes handling the patent gently, removing wet clothing, and covering the patient to prevent further cooling. Give warm oral fluids only if evidence of active rewarming is seen. The patient should be alert and able to swallow easily before taking fluids. The patient must be able to control shivering to achieve active rewarming. Avoid drinks that contain caffeine (coffee and tea), which constricts peripheral blood vessels, and alcohol, which dilates them. Warm beverages with sugar, such as hot chocolate, can be given to begin replacement of the

Focus on the Patient: Recognizing Groups at High Risk for Hypothermia

Heat loss can be more serious in groups at high risk for hypothermia.

Children, particularly newborns and infants, have heat-regulating systems that are not completely developed, and their ratio of skin surface/body mass is higher than that of adults. Both of these factors predispose them to rapid heat loss.

The elderly tend to lose heat gradually. Their heat-balancing mechanisms and other defense systems that would otherwise protect them from excessive heat loss lose sensitivity with age. Additional risks for the elderly may include poor circulation, physical immobility, the tendency of friends and family to dismiss early mental changes as senility, and other factors such as malnutrition and poorly heated homes. Hypothermia in the elderly can develop over a period of days in indoor surroundings that feel comfortable to the young healthy adult.

fuel the body needs to restore normal heat production. No oral fluids should be given to patients with changing levels of consciousness.

Frostbite

Windy, subfreezing weather creates the greatest risk for frostbite. Frostbite occurs when small body parts with a high ratio of surface area/tissue mass (fingers, toes, ears, and the nose) are exposed to extreme cold. Larger areas of the extremities are vulnerable in more profound cooling. This cold exposure causes tissues to freeze and for cells to eventually die.

The type and duration of contact are the two most important factors in determining the extent of frostbite injury. Touching cold fabric is not nearly as dangerous as coming into direct contact with cold metal, particularly if the hands are wet or even damp. In the latter case, the skin usually is cemented instantly to the cold metal and is torn off when the hand is removed. The combination of wind and cold is a dangerous freezing factor.

Superficial frostbite appears as firm and waxy gray or yellow skin in an area that loses sensation after

hurting or tingling. Prolonged exposure can lead to blistering and eventually *deep frostbite*, which most often afflicts hands and feet. No warning symptoms appear after the initial loss of feeling. Freezing progresses painlessly once the nerve endings are numb. Skin becomes inelastic and the entire area feels hard to the touch.

Superficial frostbite can be managed by warming the affected part with another body surface, for example, placing an ungloved hand over a cold spot on the cheek. Management for more than superficial frostbite is rapid rewarming after any system-wide hypothermia has been corrected. Deep frostbite should only be managed in the hospital to prevent further damage. Immerse the frozen tissue in lukewarm water (41°C [105°F]) until the tissue becomes pliable, and color and sensation return. Because this effect may take at least 20 minutes in most cases, transport to the hospital should not be delayed. Dry heat, cold therapy, massaging, and any handling that breaks blisters are harmful actions.

Apply dry sterile dressings and handle gently after thawing. If rewarming is not attempted, the frostbitten part should be bandaged with dry sterile dressings and the patient transported to the hospital. Frostbitten flesh also shares burned tissue's vulnerability to infection, so care should be taken to keep the affected part as clean as possible.

All frostbite victims should be assessed for signs of hypothermia as well. Clothing offers good protection against weather only if it is loose enough to avoid restricting circulation. Tight gloves, cuffs, boots, and straps add to the danger.

Behavioral and Psychiatric Emergencies

It is important to remember that psychological distress may be mild, moderate, or severe in nature. The degree of intensity determines the type and amount of intervention necessary. When working with a behavioral problem in a patient, the medical assistant should know what constitutes a psychiatric emergency and what is better classified as an emotional crisis. A psychiatric emergency is any situation in which patients' moods, thoughts, or actions are so disordered or disturbed that they have the potential to produce danger, harm, or death to themselves or to others if the situation is not quickly controlled.

An emotional crisis, on the other hand, is a situation with much less intensity. It is distressing but in most cases is not likely to end in danger, harm, or death if not responded to immediately. However, if neglected entirely, an emotional crisis may escalate to a full psychiatric emergency.

A true behavioral emergency, like a medical emergency, has an element of serious threat to it. Without immediate intervention, true behavioral emergencies can end in injury or death to the patient or to someone else near the patient. Urgent behavioral situations usually require some form of professional intervention; the patient should be transported to a hospital for evaluation. The nonemergency cases have a far less degree of urgency attached to them. Nonemergency situations are less likely to result in potentially dangerous behaviors. Kindness, reassurance, and general support are usually sufficient until specialized services are available.

SUMMARY

The role of the medical assistant has evolved into a complex occupation that combines elements of medicine with interpersonal and communicative skills. As a professional, the medical assistant interacts in many situations with a vast number of people. As with many areas of emergency care, it is often less important to accurately diagnose the specific problem than to recognize the need for expedient transport for definitive care. Chances are you will probably not encounter a life-threatening emergency in the medical office. If you do, the proper knowledge and training in handling an emergency could mean the difference between life and death.

CRITICAL THINKING CHALLENGES

1. When an emergency occurs, the patient's family members may become anxious and, in some cases, emotionally distraught. How would you help to calm an anxious family member?

2. Reread the "What If?" question in this chapter. Analyze how you would respond to such a situation.

ANSWERS TO CHECKPOINT QUESTIONS

1. Before the ambulance arrives you should document basic identification information, chief complaint, times of events, vital signs, techniques used to treat the patient, and any observations.
2. The purpose of the primary survey is to identify and correct any life-threatening problems.
3. The five diagnostic signs of the secondary survey are general appearance, level of consciousness, vital signs, temperature, and skin appearance.
4. Shock is defined as the lack of oxygen to the individual cells.
5. The four major sources of burn injuries are thermal, electrical, chemical, and radiation.
6. The primary cause of death from anaphylaxis is airway obstruction.

SUGGESTIONS FOR FURTHER READING

Grant, H. D., Murray, R. H., & Bergeron, D. J. (1990). *Brady Emergency Care,* 5th ed. Englewood Cliffs, NJ: Brady Division of Prentice Hall.

Harwood-Nuss, A. L. & Luten, R. C. (1995). *Handbook of Emergency Medicine.* Philadelphia: J. B. Lippincott.

Jones, S. A., et al. (1992). *Advanced Emergency Care for Paramedic Practice.* Philadelphia: J. B. Lippincott.

Assisting With Diagnostic Tests and Therapeutic Procedures for Common Disorders

Introduction to Anatomy and Physiology

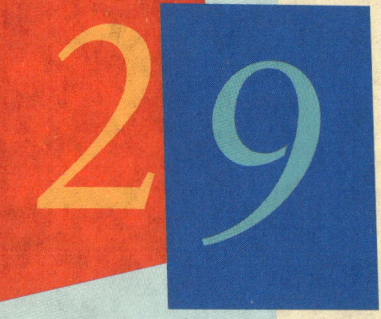

Chapter Outline

Organization of the Body
    Chemicals
    Cells
    Tissues
    Organs
    Body Systems
General Plan of the Body
    Anatomic Position
    Body Planes

    Locations and Positions
    Body Cavities
    Areas and Regions
Homeostasis
Summary
Critical Thinking Challenges
Answers to Checkpoint Questions
Suggestions for Further Reading

Chapter Competencies

Learning Objectives

Upon successfully completing this chapter, you will be able to:

1. Spell and define the Key Terms.
2. Describe in ascending order the organization of the body, beginning at the atomic level and advancing to the systemic level.
3. Describe a cell and its components.
4. List the nine abdominal regions and name the organs included in each.
5. List the body cavities and their contents.
6. Describe the systems, the organs involved in each system, and the function of each system.
7. Define the anatomic position.
8. Explain the meaning of the terms homeostasis and positive and negative feedback.

Key Terms

(See Glossary for definitions.)

abdominal regions
anatomic position
anatomy
cell
element
homeostasis
negative feedback
organ
physiology
planes
positive feedback
quadrants
system
tissues

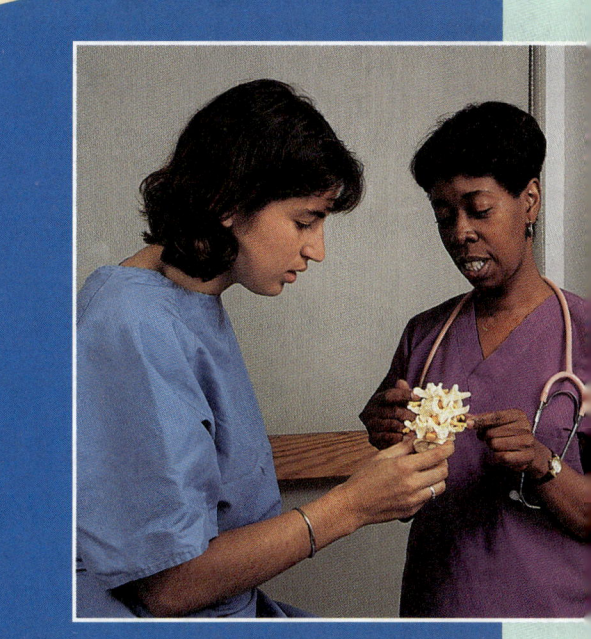

To function effectively in the medical field, you will need an understanding of the human body and how it works. To achieve this goal, you must study the body's normal structures and functions. Anatomy refers to the study of the body's structure; physiology is the study of the body's functions. Knowledge of the body in its normal state will enable you to evaluate and understand abnormal conditions observed and described in the medical practice.

➤ ORGANIZATION OF THE BODY

Beginning at the most basic atomic structure, the body progresses through levels of organization that interact to maintain the functions necessary for life (Fig. 29-1).

Chemicals

The atom is the smallest component of an element that contains the physical properties of that element. An element is a substance made up of only one type of atom.

For example, iron is an element. It may be broken down into individual iron atoms, but no other type of atom will be contained in the element. Everything in the world is made up of atoms in a multitude of arrangements.

An atom consists of a *nucleus* with positively charged *protons* and usually an equal number of neutral particles called *neutrons*. These are orbited by negatively charged *electrons* (Fig. 29-2). Positives and negatives attract each other, each possessing a property that the other needs. This attraction keeps the protons and electrons in constant motion and holds them close in an arrangement that resembles a galaxy with a sun (the nucleus) and orbiting planets (the electrons).

Each of the more than 100 elements currently identified (eg, iron, calcium, phosphorus, and so on) has a specific number of protons, neutrons, and electrons. The numbers are always consistent for each atom to be identified as a particular element. Each atom is given a number based on the number of protons in the nucleus. No other atom will have this number of protons. For instance, all hydrogen atoms have one proton and one electron, all carbon atoms have six of each, and all oxygen atoms have eight of each.

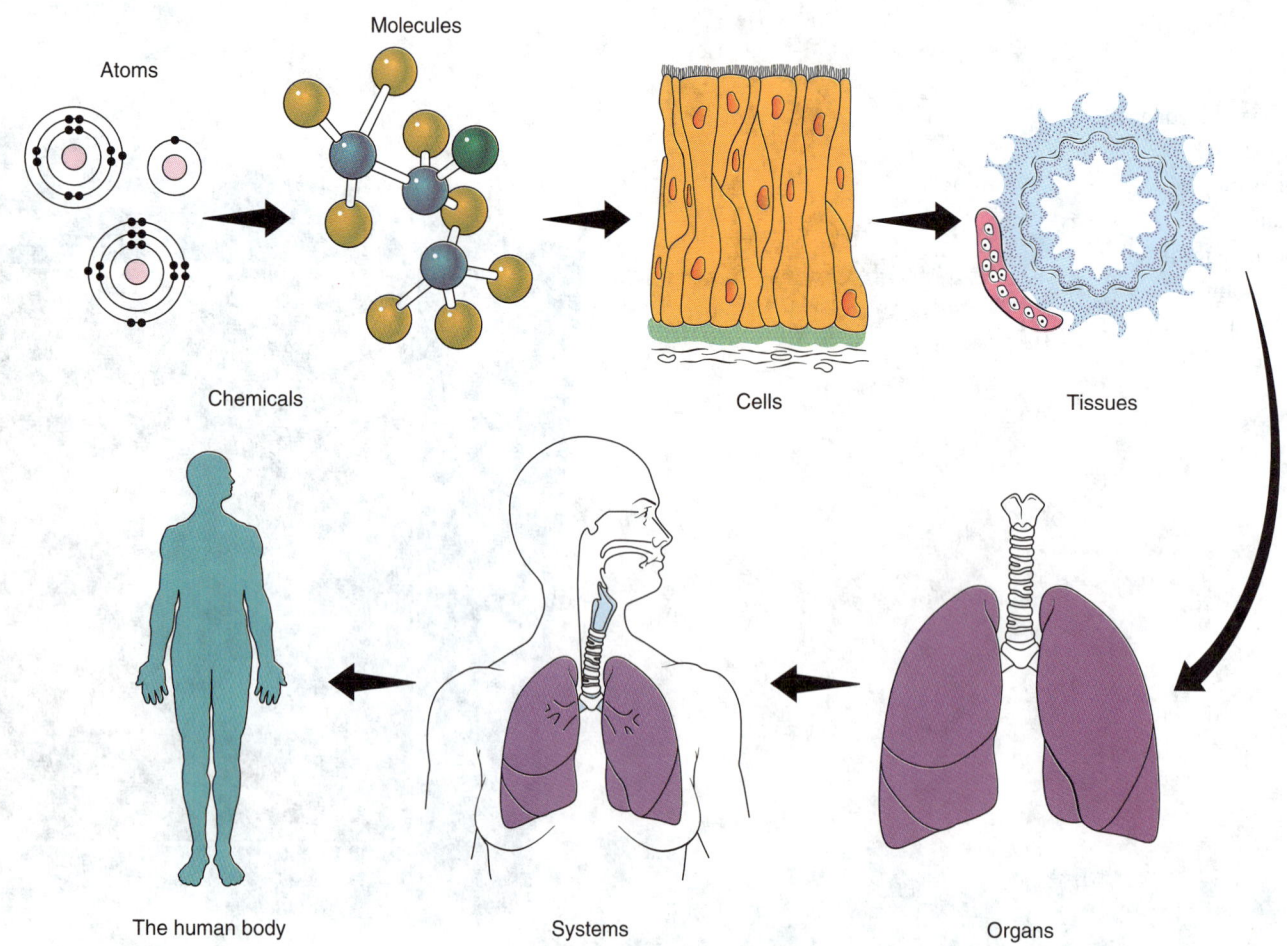

FIGURE 29-1
The body's level of structural organization.

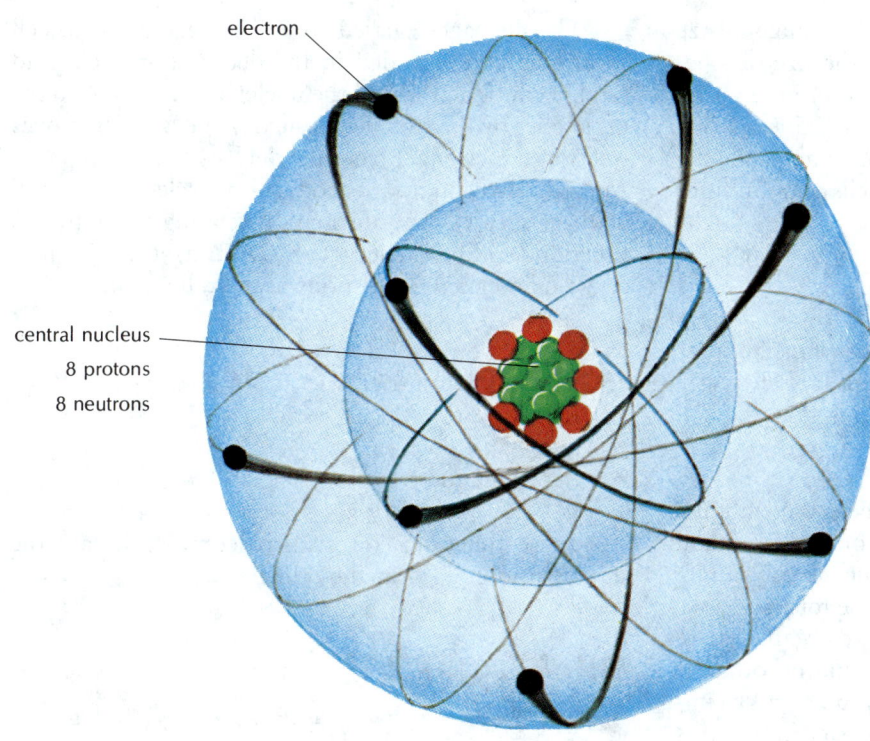

electron

central nucleus
8 protons
8 neutrons

FIGURE 29-2
Representation of the oxygen atom. Eight protons and eight neutrons are tightly bound in the central nucleus, around which the eight electrons revolve.

Each atomic element is also designated by a symbol (Table 29-1). The symbol may be an abbreviation of the element's name, such as O for oxygen or H for hydrogen. Or it may be an abbreviation of the element's Latin name, such as Fe for iron (from the Latin ferrum) or K for potassium (from the Latin kalium).

The arrangement of the atoms within their structure is consistent, with electrons always orbiting the nucleus in a certain pattern. The first orbit around the nucleus will hold only two electrons and the concentric orbits beyond will hold up to eight. If the outer orbit has fewer than eight electrons, the atom will look for another with fewer than eight to complete the outer orbit. If the atoms attracted to each other completely share the outer eight, they will form a very stable union. For example, sodium has an arrangement of 2-8-1 and chloride has 2-8-7, which means that chloride needs one electron to complete its outer orbit and sodium needs seven. When these two elements meet, they bond and become the very stable molecule known as sodium chloride or salt. A molecule is the combination of two or more atoms usually into something other than the original element.

To maintain life functions, atoms and molecules arrange and rearrange themselves constantly within the cells and the body fluids. The exchange of oxygen for carbon dioxide would not be possible nor would the transmission of nerve impulses or the release of body wastes without this effort to balance the normal composition of the internal environment. These minute elements are the basis of all physiologic functions within the body.

Cells

After the simplest structural level of the atom, combining then to the molecule, the body is organized in an orderly manner of ever-increasing complexity.

The cell—the fundamental unit of all living tissue—is a complex arrangement of chemicals designed

Table 29-1		
Common Chemical Elements		

Name	*Symbol*	*Atomic Number*
Hydrogen	H	1
Carbon	C	6
Nitrogen	N	7
Oxygen	O	8
Sodium	Na	11
Phosphorus	P	15
Sulfur	S	16
Chlorine	Cl	17
Potassium	K	19
Iron	Fe	26

These elements are essential to life. Our body functions depend on the interaction of their properties.

to carry out specific activities. Body cells range in size from the relatively large ovum, about the size of a period on this page (or 1000 μm), to the infinitely tiny red blood cells, which are only about 7.5 μm. Cell shapes range from the basic round shape normally associated with cells to the long nerve cells and multinucleated muscle cells.

No matter the shape, size, or function, each cell has three main parts: the cell membrane, the cytoplasm, and the nucleus.

Cell membranes are composed of phospholipids (phosphorus and fatty substances) and are selectively permeable. Selective permeability means that the cell membranes allow necessary substances to move in and wastes to move out, but the cytoplasm and the cell components are kept inside. Within the cell membrane is the cytoplasm, which contains the organelles (small organs) that move about and carry out the cell's functions (Fig. 29-3). If the cell is responsible for the manufacture of an enzyme or a hormone, the organelles are designed to create just that substance and no other. If the cell is responsible for the transmission of nerve impulses, its cellular components are designed for this purpose (Table 29-2).

The messages carried from one generation of cell to another are encoded in the deoxyribonucleic acid (DNA) contained within the nucleus and relayed to the organelles by the ribonucleic acid (RNA), which moves freely as a messenger from the nucleus to the cell parts. At each division, or reproduction cycle, of the cell (called *mitosis*), the information relating to that cell's functions will be carried by the DNA as it divides into two daughter cells. Functions of the cell include:

*   Respiration
*   Digestion of nutrients
*   Elimination
*   Energy production
*   Reproduction

These functions, on a microscopic scale, are the same as those performed by the body.

Checkpoint Question

1. *What are the three main parts of the cell and their functions?*

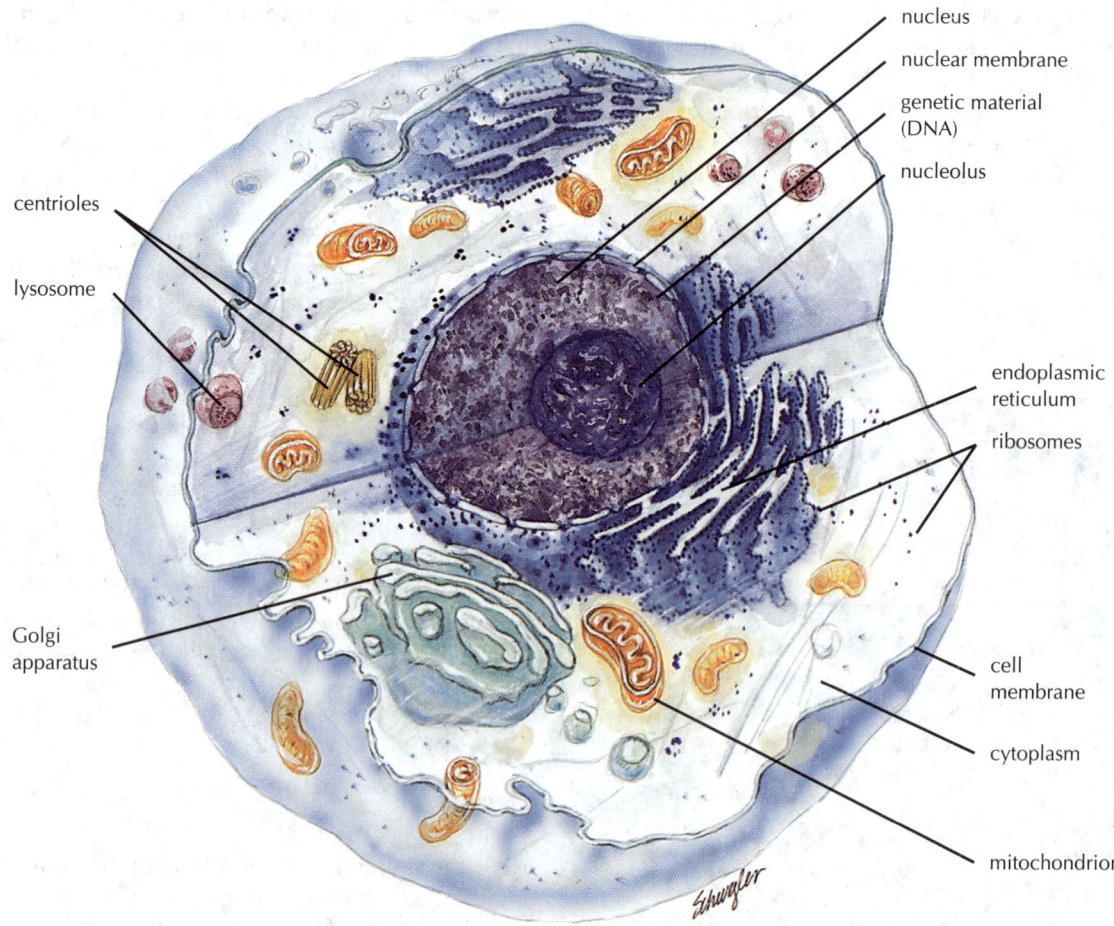

FIGURE 29-3
Diagram of a typical animal cell showing the main organelles.

Table 29-2
Cell Structures

Name	Description	Function
Cell membrane	Outer layer of the cell; composed mainly of lipids and proteins	Limits the cell; regulates what enters and leaves the cell
Cytoplasm	Colloidal suspension that fills cell	Holds cell contents
Nucleus	Large, dark-staining body near the center of the cell; composed of DNA and proteins	Contains the chromosomes with the genes (the hereditary material that directs all cell activities)
Nucleolus	Small body in the nucleus; composed of RNA, DNA, and protein	Needed for protein manufacture
Endoplasmic reticulum (ER)	Network of membranes in the cytoplasm	Used for storage and transport; holds ribosomes
Ribosomes	Small bodies in the cytoplasm or attached to the ER; composed of RNA and protein	Manufacture proteins
Mitochondria	Large organelles with folded membranes inside	Convert energy from nutrients into adenosine triphosphate
Golgi apparatus	Layers of membranes	Put together special substances such as mucus
Lysosomes	Small sacs of digestive enzymes	Digest substances within the cell
Centrioles	Rod-shaped bodies (usually 2) near the nucleus	Help separate the chromosomes in cell division
Cilia	Short, hairlike projections from the cell	Create movement around the cell
Flagellum	Long, whiplike extension from the cell	Moves the cell

Tissues

Body **tissues** are made up of a collection of similar cells and their supporting structures acting together to perform a particular function (Table 29-3). Tissues differ from each other by their cell shape and size, by the type and amount of supporting material between the cells, and by their specific functions. The four basic types of tissue are: epithelial, connective, muscular, and nervous (Fig. 29-4).

Organs

An **organ** is more complex than a tissue and is formed by various tissues and cells working together to perform a specific function. For example, the heart is an organ made of special cardiac conduction cells formed into muscular tissue that work in a coordinated effort to pump blood throughout the body. Another example is the ovary, which is a collection of specialized cells capable of reproducing the species and contained

Table 29-3
Tissue Types and Functions

Type	Functions	Examples
Epithelial	Covers body surfaces Lines cavities Forms glands	Skin surfaces, respiratory and gastrointestinal tracts, genitourinary system
Connective	Holds other tissues together Forms and supports all parts of the body Protects body parts	Fibrous, reticular, fatty (or adipose), bone, cartilage, blood
Muscular	Maintains posture Generates bone movement Helps produce heat to regulate body temperature	Skeletal, cardiac, smooth, involuntary muscles
Nervous	Conducts nerve impulses and messages to and from the brain Regulates body functions	Central and peripheral nervous systems

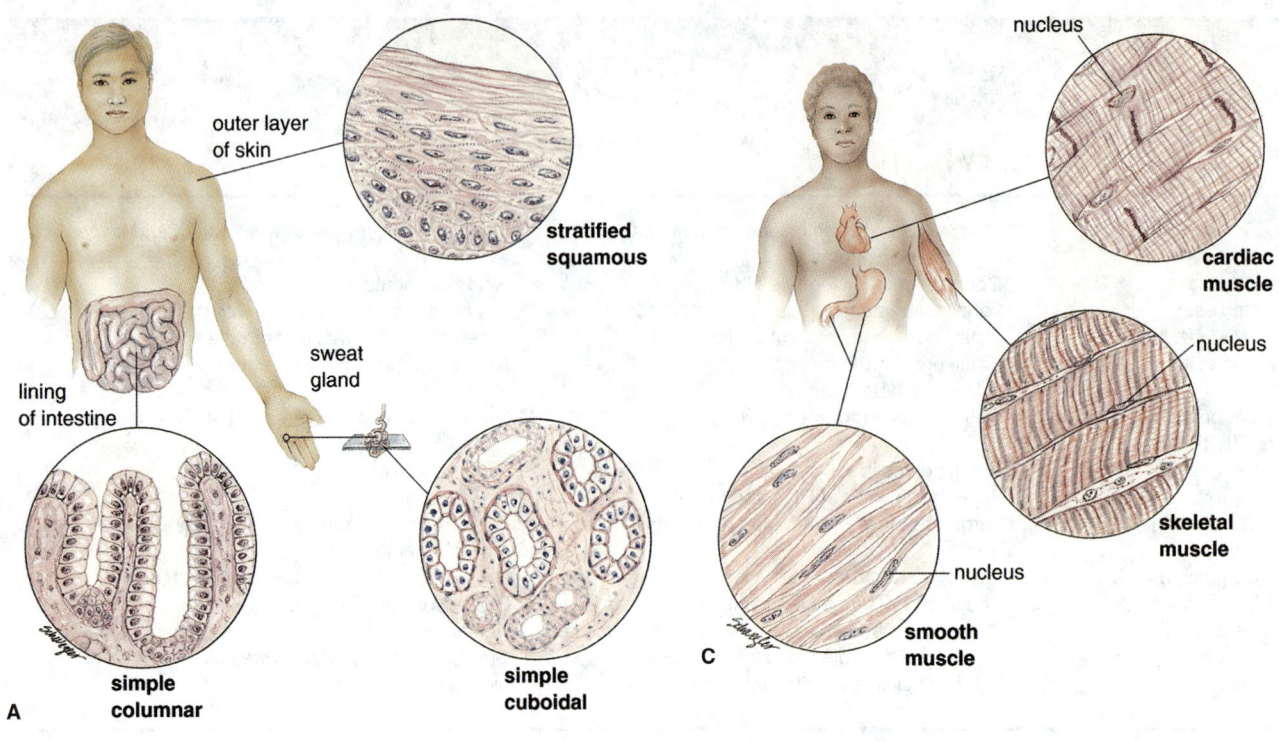

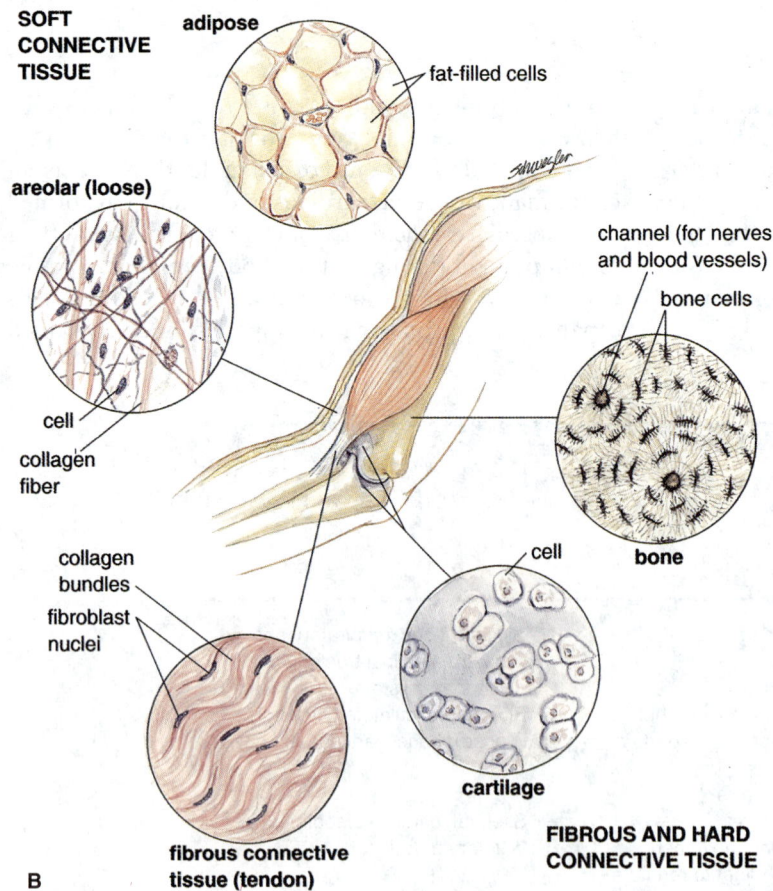

FIGURE 29-4

Illustration showing four types of tissue. (**A**) Three types of epithelium. (**B**) Connective tissue. (**C**) Muscle tissue.

within tissue designed to nurture and mature the cells as needed for ovulation.

Some organs are found in pairs, such as the kidneys and the lungs. Each one of the paired organs can function independently, if necessary, after injury to or surgical removal of the organ. The liver, pancreas, spleen, and brain are so specialized that they can maintain near-normal functioning with over 30% of the organ damaged or excised.

Body Systems

A body system is composed of a group of organs that work together to perform a specific function for the body. For example, the nervous system includes the brain, the spinal cord, and the nerves. These organs function as a system to coordinate body activity through nerve stimulation. The circulatory system includes the heart, blood vessels, and blood, all working together to transport nutrients and wastes (Table 29-4).

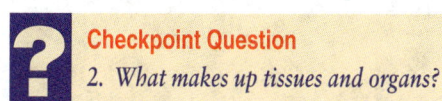

Checkpoint Question

2. What makes up tissues and organs?

➤ GENERAL PLAN OF THE BODY

As a medical assistant, you must be able to accurately locate the various organs and structures to specifically describe the details of your observations and assessments. References must be consistent across the profession to avoid confusion in describing location, direction, position, and so on. The following discussion outlines the acceptable standards of references set by the allied health professions.

Anatomic Position

Anatomic position refers to a standing position with the body erect, facing forward, feet pointed forward and slightly apart, arms down at the sides with the palms facing forward and the thumbs outward. Anatomic position will always be the reference for direction, distance, or movement. Remember also that the patient will be facing you, so that the patient's right will be on your left.

Body Planes

Planes are imaginary lines drawn through the body and used to facilitate the study of individual organs or

Table 29-4
Body Systems and Functions

System	Organs	Functions
Circulatory	Heart, blood, and blood vessels	Carries oxygen and nutrients to the cells and removes waste
Endocrine	Pituitary, pineal body, thyroid, parathyroid, thymus, adrenal, ovaries, testes, islets of Langerhans (in pancreas)	Produces hormones that regulate body processes
Gastrointestinal	Salivary glands, teeth, tongue, pharynx, esophagus, stomach, intestines, liver, gallbladder, pancreas	Digests, transports, and absorbs nutrients Eliminates solid wastes
Integumentary	Skin, hair, nails, sweat and oil glands	Protects against infection Helps regulate body temperature Eliminates some waste
Musculoskeletal	Muscles, bones, joints, ligaments, tendons	Protects and supports the body Makes movement possible Produces some blood cells
Nervous	Brain, spinal cord, nerves	Coordinates body activity through nerve stimulation
Respiratory	Nose, pharynx, larynx, trachea, bronchi, lungs	Brings oxygen into the body and eliminates carbon dioxide
Reproductive	Male: testes, urethra, prostate gland, penis, and related structures Female: breasts, ovaries, uterus, vagina, and related structures	Regulates reproduction, sexual activity, and sexual identity
Urinary	Kidneys, ureters, urinary bladder, urethra	Eliminates liquid wastes

of the body as a whole. There are three planes at right angles to each other. These are:

1. *Transverse.* A line drawn from side to side horizontal to the floor divides the body into inferior and superior portions.
2. *Sagittal.* A line drawn through the body from the head to the feet divides the body into right and left. A mid-sagittal line divides the body exactly into halves.
3. *Frontal.* A line drawn from the head to the feet divides the body into front and back, or anterior and posterior (also referred to as ventral and dorsal).

Body planes locate areas on the body from left to right, from back to front, and from top to bottom (Fig. 29-5).

Locations and Positions

References to locations and positions on the body are made from the anatomic position (see above). With a transverse plane, the body is divided into superior and inferior sections. The heart is superior to the stomach, for example. The frontal plane divides the body into anterior (front) and posterior (back), or ventral (front) and dorsal (back). The chest is anterior, for example, and the spine is posterior. Positions and locations may also be described using the following terms:

- *Medial* (close to the midline of the body). The heart is medial to the lungs.
- *Lateral* (away from the midline, to the side of the body). The arms are lateral to the chest.
- *Superficial* (close to the surface). The epidermis is the most superficial layer of skin.
- *Deep* (far from the surface). The abdominal lymph nodes are deep within the peritoneum.
- *Proximal* (close to the point of origin). The elbow is proximal to the wrist.
- *Distal* (further from the point of origin). The ankle is distal to the knee.

Checkpoint Question

3. *How many body planes are there? Name and describe each one.*

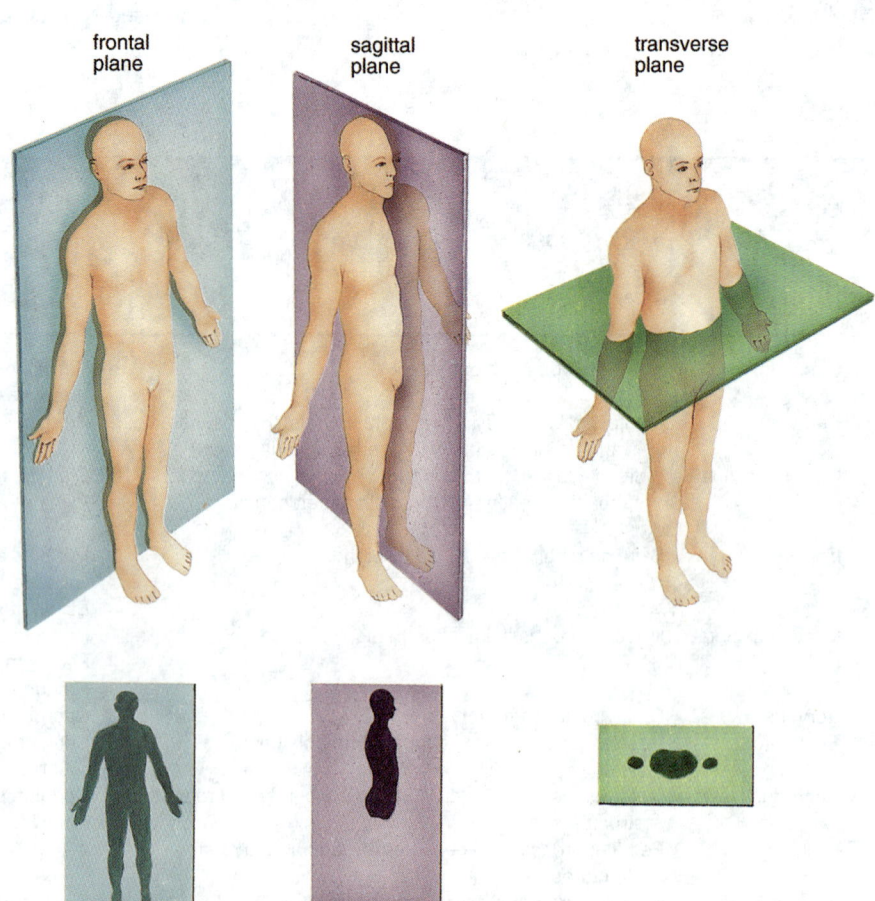

FIGURE 29-5
Planes of division.

Body Cavities

The body has two major cavities, the ventral cavity and the dorsal cavity, that contain a compact arrangement of internal organs (Fig. 29-6). The dorsal cavity is further divided into the cranial cavity, which contains the brain, and the vertebral cavity, containing the spinal cord. The ventral cavity is the larger of the two and is further divided into more specific areas:

- The *thoracic cavity* contains the heart, lungs, esophagus, trachea, and large blood vessels.
- The *abdominal cavity* contains the stomach, most of the intestines, the liver, the gallbladder, the pancreas, and the spleen. The abdominal cavity is further divided into a retroperitoneal (behind the peritoneum) cavity, which contains the kidneys and ureters.
- The *pelvic cavity* lies below the abdominal cavity and contains the bladder, the rectum, and the internal reproductive system.

The thoracic and the abdominal cavities are divided by the diaphragm—a thin, very muscular layer that assists with respiratory movements. All of the abdominal organs are maintained in place by the omenta, layers of peritoneum that stretch from the upper posterior wall of the abdominal cavity and loop around the organs to keep them in place.

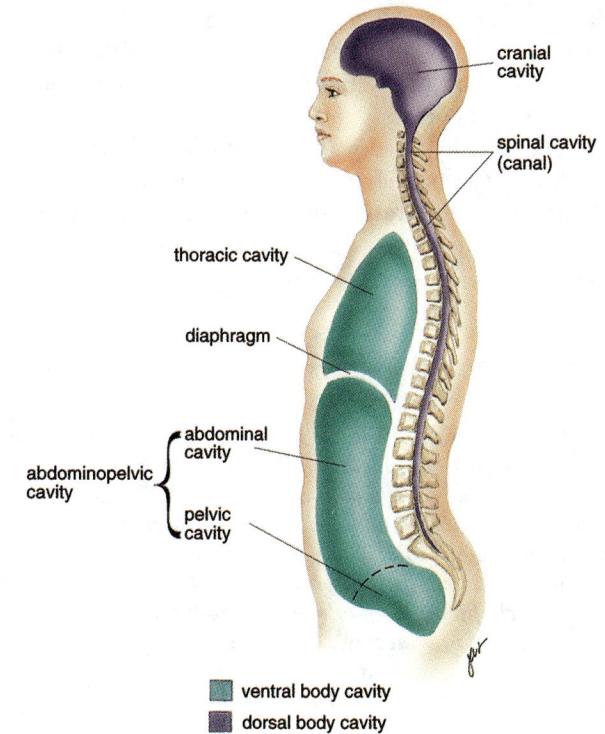

FIGURE 29-6
Side view of the body cavities.

Labels: cranial cavity; spinal cavity (canal); thoracic cavity; diaphragm; abdominal cavity; abdominopelvic cavity; pelvic cavity; ventral body cavity; dorsal body cavity

Areas and Regions

Locations and positions may be described by the region involved. For instance, a patient complaining of neck pain has pain in the cervical region. Pain in the groin may be described as inguinal pain. Some of the more common areas and regions are listed in Box 29-1.

Because the abdominal cavity is so large an area, it is divided into nine areas—called the **abdominal regions**—to provide more accurate means of identifying underlying organ and structure locations. The three central regions include the:

- Epigastric region, located just below the breastbone
- Umbilical region, the area around the umbilicus (naval)
- Hypogastric region, the lowest of the midline regions

At each side are the right and left hypochondriac regions, just below the ribs; the right and left lumbar regions; and the iliac, or inguinal regions. With this information, it is possible to be precise in identifying the exact location of a patient's abdominal complaints (Fig. 29-7).

BOX 29-1   Body Areas and Regions

Axillary	armpit
Brachial	upper arm
Buccal	between the cheek and gum
Cardiac	in the region of the heart
Cervical	neck
Cranial	head
Femoral	thigh
Gastric	stomach (not abdomen)
Hepatic	liver
Iliac	hip
Inguinal	groin
Lumbar	small of back
Mammary	breast
Occipital	back of the head
Pectoral	chest
Perineal	floor of the pelvis
Plantar	sole of the foot
Popliteal	behind the knee
Pulmonary	lungs
Sacral	base of the spine
Temporal	side of the head

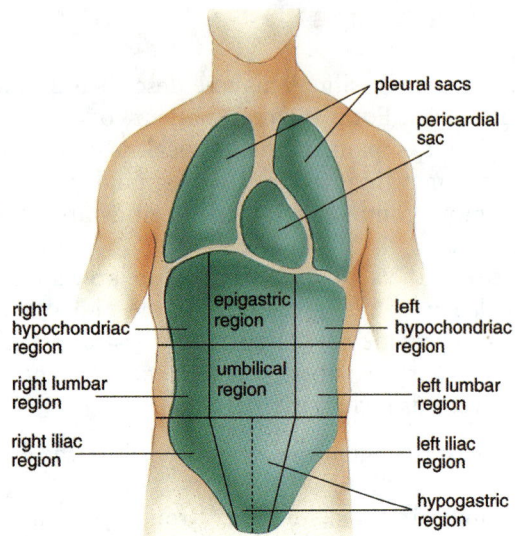

FIGURE 29-7
Nine abdominal regions.

What If?

A patient presents complaining of a "stomach-ache." What if, when asked to point where it hurts, the patient says "right down here" and points to the mid-abdominal area?

Be aware that many people confuse the term "stomach" with the term "abdomen" when describing the location of a complaint. Using the anatomic position and the regions, you can correctly interpret the position of incorrectly described symptoms.

The abdomen also may be divided into **quadrants**, or four parts. These are the right and the left upper quadrants and the right and left lower quadrants. These areas are also important in reporting findings and preparing documentation.

 Checkpoint Question
4. *Why is the abdominal cavity divided into nine regions?*

➤ HOMEOSTASIS

Homeostasis is the means by which the body maintains a relative constancy of its internal environment to survive. Some of the functions maintained by homeostasis can tolerate a fairly wide range. For example, the body will do fairly well with a blood glucose level between 60 and 100 mg/dL, but it cannot tolerate a blood pH (acid–base balance) lower than 7.35 or higher than 7.45. If either of those values ventures away from a normal range, the body mechanisms will begin to work to bring them back into acceptable ranges. Homeostasis manages the constant fluctuations of the body functions by keeping the internal environment within relatively narrow boundaries.

Feedback refers to the information that comes to the body's sensors from the internal or external environment. Feedback either stimulates or depresses the mechanisms that maintain homeostasis.

Positive feedback is an increase in a body function in response to a stimulus. Positive feedback reinforces, rather than opposes, the change that is occurring. Clot formation in response to an injury is an example of positive feedback.

Negative feedback works against a change and is a stabilizing mechanism. An example of negative feedback shows how the system is used to maintain homeostasis of blood carbon dioxide (CO_2) concentration. As CO_2 levels increase, the respiratory rate increases to permit CO_2 to exit the body in increased amounts through expired air. Without this homeostatic mechanism, the body's CO_2 content rapidly rises to toxic levels and may result in death. Consider also a change in body temperature. If the temperature sensors perceive the environment as too cool, shivering will generate warmth; if it is perceived as too warm, vasodilation will rush blood to the periphery for cooling to reduce the core temperature.

The healthy person's homeostasis can maintain a balance between the negative and the positive feedback. This homeostatic balance is necessary for continued health and an ongoing steady internal environment.

 ### SUMMARY

The body is organized in an orderly manner of increasing complexity from chemicals to cells to tissues to organs to systems to make up the whole living body. The description of the body and its components has been standardized to be instantly recognizable by any health care professional in reporting assessment and observation.

This chapter will enable you to continue with the more detailed study of anatomy and physiology. The descriptions presented will lead to a better understanding of the body parts and their locations. This information will be invaluable in developing observation skills and in interpreting and recording medical material.

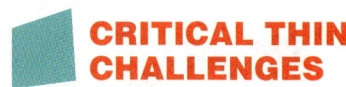

CRITICAL THINKING CHALLENGES

1. You have been asked to give a brief presentation to a group of students on the organization of the body. Develop a presentation that describes the body's organization in an ascending order. At what level would you start? At what level would you end?
2. While transcribing dictation from the physician, you note the following statements:
   - A bullet was surgically removed from the thoracic cavity. It was lodged in the superior aspect of the esophagus.
   - An incision was made medially in the right hypochondriac region.
   - The 3-cm laceration was sutured. It was located medial and proximal to the left knee.
   - Draw a stick figure to illustrate the correct location of each ailment described.
3. Compare and contrast the forms of regulatory feedback. Include several examples of each.

ANSWERS TO CHECKPOINT QUESTIONS

1. The three main parts of the cell are the cell membrane, cytoplasm, and nucleus. The cell membrane regulates what enters and leaves the cell through selective permeability. The cytoplasm holds the organelles that are responsible for the cell's function. The nucleus contains the chromosomes.
2. Tissues are made up of a group of similar cells working together. Organs are formed by different tissues working together to perform a specific function.
3. There are three body planes. The transverse plane is a line drawn from side to side horizontal to the floor that divides the body into inferior and superior positions. The sagittal plane is a line drawn through the body from the head to the feet to divide the body into right and left. The frontal plane is a line drawn from the head to the feet to divide the body into front and back, or anterior (ventral) and posterior (dorsal).
4. The abdominal cavity is divided into nine regions because it is so large and to provide a more accurate means of identifying and locating organs and structures.
5. Feedback refers to the information that comes to the body's sensors from the internal or external environment. It either stimulates or depresses homeostatic mechanisms.
6. Positive feedback is an increase in body function in response to a stimulus. Negative feedback works against a change and is a stabilizing mechanism.

SUGGESTIONS FOR FURTHER READING

Carpenito, L. (1993). *Nursing Diagnosis.* Philadelphia: J. B. Lippincott.

Memmler, R. L., Cohen, B. J., & Wood, D. L. (1996). *The Human Body in Health and Disease,* 8th ed. Philadelphia: Lippincott-Raven.

Memmler, R. L., Cohen, B. J., & Wood, D. L. (1992) *Structure and Function of the Human Body,* 5th ed. Philadelphia: J. B. Lippincott.

Smeltzer, S., & Bare, B. (1996). *Brunner and Suddarth's Textbook of Medical-Surgical Nursing,* 8th ed. Philadelphia: Lippincott-Raven.

Caring for Patients With Integumentary Disorders

Chapter Outline

Function of the Integumentary System
Structure of the Integumentary System
    Epidermis
    Dermis
    Subcutaneous Tissue
Common Integumentary Disorders
    Bacterial Skin Infections
    Viral Skin Infections
    Fungal Skin Infections
    Parasitic Skin Infestations
    Inflammatory Reactions
    Disorders of Wound Healing
    Disorders Caused by Pressure
    Alopecia
    Disorders of Pigmentation
    Skin Cancers
Common Diagnostic Procedures and the
    Medical Assistant's Role
    Wound Cultures
    Skin Biopsy

Urine Melanin
Wood's Light Analysis
Allergy Skin Testing
Tuberculin Skin Testing
Schick Test
Warm and Cold Applications
    Precautions
Procedure: Applying Cold
Procedure: Applying a Warm or Cold
    Compress
Procedure: Using a Hot Water Bottle or
    Commercial Hot Pack
    Soaks and Sitz Baths
Procedure: Assisting With Therapeutic
    Soaks
Summary
Critical Thinking Challenges
Answers to Checkpoint Questions
Suggestions for Further Reading

DACUM Components

1.3   Practice within the scope of education, training, and personal capabilities
1.6   Conduct oneself in a courteous and diplomatic manner
2.2   Treat all patients with empathy and impartiality
4.1   Apply principles of aseptic technique and infection control
4.5   Prepare and maintain examination and treatment area
4.7   Prepare patients for procedures
4.8   Assist physician with examinations and treatment
7.3   Teach patients methods of health promotion and disease prevention

Chapter Competencies

Learning Objectives

Upon successfully completing this chapter, you will be able to:

1. Spell and define the Key Terms.
2. List the major components of the integumentary system.
3. Describe the functions of the integument.
4. Recognize common skin disorders.
5. Describe common diagnostic procedures.
6. List precautions to observe during the application of warm or cold treatment.
7. Prepare the patient for examination of the integument.
8. Assist the physician with examination of the integument.
9. Understand how to instruct the patient on proper procedures for self-administering warm or cold applications at home.

Performance Objectives

Upon successfully completing this chapter, you will be able to:

1. Apply cold packs (Procedure 30-1).
2. Apply warm or cold compresses (Procedure 30-2).
3. Use a hot water bottle or commercial hot pack (Procedure 30-3).
4. Assist with therapeutic soaks (Procedure 30-4).
5. Obtain a wound culture.

Key Terms

(See Glossary for definitions.)

alopecia	erythema	scale
abscess	exudate	sebaceous gland
adipose	fascia	seborrhea
allergen	fissure	sebum
arrector pili	keratin	*Staphylococcus*
benign	macule	stratum corneum
blister	malignant	stratum germinativum
boil	melanin	*Streptococcus*
bulla	melanocyte	subcutaneous
collagen	neoplasm	sudoriferous gland
comedo	nodule	urticaria
cyst	papilloma	verruca
dermatitis	papilloma virus	vesicle
dermatophytosis	papule	wheal
dermis	pediculosis	Wood's light
elastin	pruritus	
epidermis	pustules	

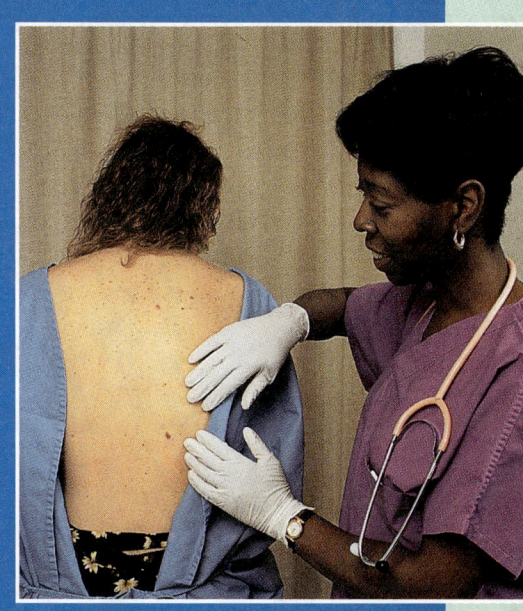

The skin, or integument, is the largest organ of the body. It has many functions and plays a vital role in maintaining homeostasis. This chapter covers the structure and function of the integument and its accessories, common skin disorders, and the role of the medical assistant in the examination and treatment of diseases of the integumentary system.

FUNCTION OF THE INTEGUMENTARY SYSTEM

One of the most important functions of the integumentary system is to protect the underlying tissues and organs of the body from the external environment. Unbroken skin provides a protective barrier that prevents the entrance of microorganisms and is the body's first line of defense against infection. In addition, the skin protects the body from mechanical injury, damaging substances, and the ultraviolet rays of the sun.

The integument assists in the regulation of body temperature. Increased sweat production in a warm environment lowers body temperature as sweat evaporates. Blood vessels in the skin dilate (vasodilation), bringing interior heat close to the body's surface to cool the body. In a cold environment, the blood vessels constrict (vasoconstriction) to conserve heat and shunt blood to the internal organs. In this way, the body's temperature tends to be maintained within a normal range.

The skin contains separate receptors for each of the cutaneous sensations such as heat, cold, pain, touch, and pressure. It contains glands that secrete substances to prevent drying of the skin, hair, and ear canal. It is a storage site for fat, glucose, water, and certain salts. It excretes water, some salts, and waste products through the sweat glands. It converts cholesterol to vitamin D when exposed to ultraviolet rays. It cushions the body and its waterproof surface prevents or regulates the loss or entry of fluids.

The integumentary system consists of the skin and its accessory organs, which include the hair, nails, sweat and oil glands, and the cutaneous nerve supply. The entire system defends against disease and helps to control temperature and regulate homeostasis.

Checkpoint Question
1. How does the integument help to control body temperature?

STRUCTURE OF THE INTEGUMENTARY SYSTEM

The skin is arranged in three basic layers: the **epidermis** (outer layer), the **dermis** (middle layer), and the **subcutaneous** tissue, which is beneath the skin. Each layer contains structures that perform specific functions for defense or homeostasis (Fig. 30-1).

Epidermis

The epidermis is the outer covering of the skin. It is comprised of epithelial tissue and contains no blood vessels. The epidermis is relatively thin except in areas

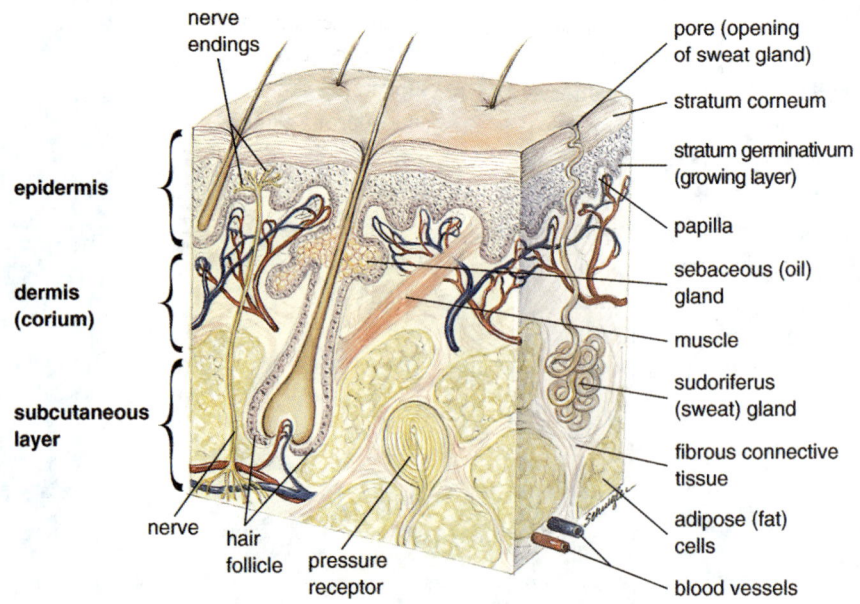

FIGURE 30-1
Cross section of the skin.

subjected to pressure, such as the palms of the hands and soles of the feet. Because of friction here, the rate of new cell production is greater than in other surfaces and thick ridges called a callus may be formed.

The epidermis has two important layers. The outermost layer is called the **stratum corneum**, sometimes called the horny layer. Below this is the **stratum germinativum**.

Stratum Corneum

The cells of the stratum corneum are composed of **keratin**, a nonliving waterproof substance that prevents loss of body fluid. These cells are constantly lost or worn off by friction or exposure to the environment, such as by bathing or from clothing.

Stratum Germinativum

The stratum germinativum is the layer which, when intact and unbroken, provides protection against invading microorganisms. The acidity of the cells in this layer assists in destroying many of the microorganisms that come into contact with it, thus providing another avenue of protection. The cells of the stratum germinativum are constantly producing new skin cells by mitosis to replace those lost from the body surface.

Melanocytes are located in this layer. These cells produce **melanin**, a skin pigment. The activity of melanocytes is one of the inherited genetic characteristics. The amount of melanin produced determines the darkness of our skin. Light-skinned people produce less melanin; dark-skinned people produce more. Exposure to the ultraviolet rays of the sun increases melanin production and temporarily results in darker skin. Dark skin provides good protection for the stratum germinativum from damage by ultraviolet rays.

Dermis

The dermis is the middle layer of the skin. It is fibrous connective tissue made up of protein substances called **collagen** and **elastin**. Collagen provides strength and elastin provides elasticity.

Papillary Layer

The papillary layer, which separates the epidermis and dermis, is richly supplied with capillaries. This blood supplies oxygen and nutrients to the stratum germinativum in the epidermis as well as to the structures in the dermis.

Arterioles located in the dermis, assisted by the nervous system, aid in maintaining body temperature with their ability to constrict or dilate in response to the environment.

Sensory Receptors

Receptors for touch, pressure, heat, cold, and pain are located in the dermis. Each sensation has a specific receptor to detect information about the external environment. The number of receptors present in an area determines how sensitive that area is.

Hair Follicles

Hair is found everywhere on the body except the soles, the palms, the lips, and the nipples. The base of each hair follicle is called the hair root and is located in the dermis. Capillaries provide oxygen and nutrients for new cell production. The hair shaft projects from the skin surface at an angle. It is made up of hard, nonliving, keratinized cells.

Attached to each follicle is the **arrector pili** or pilomotor muscle that contracts when the environment is cool, causing "goose bumps" as the skin tightens around the hair and the hair shaft is pulled erect. Oil glands open into hair follicles, helping to maintain moisture in the hair.

Hairs in the eyelashes and eyebrows help keep perspiration and dust out of the eyes. Nasal hair filters dust from the air that we breathe in. Hair on the scalp provides insulation against heat lost through the vascular surfaces of the head.

Nail Follicles

Specialized follicles at the ends of the fingers and toes produce nails. New cells are formed in the matrix, called the nail bed, which is composed of living tissue. The nail beds produce keratinizing cells that push to the surface and adhere to one another. As they are pushed to the surface, the cells die so that the nails are composed of hard, keratinized dead cells.

Nails protect the ends of our fingers and toes from injury. When the nails are injured or lost, new nails will continue to be formed as long as the nail bed remains intact.

Sebaceous Glands

The **sebaceous glands**, or oil glands, open directly on the skin surface or into a hair follicle. Sebaceous glands secrete **sebum**, a thick, oily substance that acts as "waterproofing" for the skin. It lubricates the skin, keeping it soft to prevent drying and cracking. Muscle movement and the movement of the skin across underlying tissues pushes sebum up from the glands to the skin surface.

Focus on the Patient: Dealing with Adolescents

Adolescents are acutely aware of their body appearance and any imperfections that they may have. The presence of acne can be a major concern for a teenager. Here are some tips for dealing with adolescents:

Be understanding of their need for acceptance from their peers.
Avoid condescending language. For example, never say, "It is *only* a pimple." To the teenager, this is a significant problem.
Help the adolescent feel involved in making health care decisions. It will help to discuss health care issues in terms appropriate to their level of understanding.
Give discharge instructions to both the adolescent and the caregiver, but focus the conversation to the young patient to ensure a feeling of participation.

Adolescents often have hyperactive sebaceous glands, which contribute to acne. Older adults have dry and fragile skin resulting from hypoactivity of these glands.

Sudoriferous Glands

The **sudoriferous glands** are also known as sweat glands. They have a coiled base in the dermis, which extends as a tiny tube to form a pore in the skin through which sweat is excreted from the body. In the axillae and the groin, sudoriferous glands open into a hair follicle, rather than into a pore. Sweat, or perspiration, is made up mostly of water, some salts, and waste products. Through the sweat glands, the integumentary system helps the urinary system to maintain water balance and eliminate wastes.

Sudoriferous glands are located all over the body but are especially numerous in the axillae, on the palms and soles, and on the forehead. They are controlled by the nervous system. They may be activated by heat, pain, fear, and fever. Evaporation of perspiration from the body surface is an effective means of cooling the body.

One other function of the dermis is the conversion of a type of cholesterol to vitamin D when the body is exposed to ultraviolet rays. Vitamin D is necessary for the absorption of calcium and phosphorus from the small intestine.

Subcutaneous Tissue

The subcutaneous tissue, also called the superficial fascia (fibrous membrane tissue), connects the dermis to the underlying muscles.

The subcutaneous tissue contains collagen, elastin, blood vessels, and white blood cells that migrate throughout the tissues to search for and destroy pathogens. **Adipose** tissue is also located here. Adipose tissue stores fat as a potential energy source, cushions bony prominences, and helps to conserve body heat. The amount of adipose tissue varies from person to person and in thickness from one area of the body to another.

Checkpoint Question

2. What are the three layers of the skin? Briefly describe each.

➤ COMMON INTEGUMENTARY DISORDERS

A number of integumentary disorders are manifested by lesions, or abnormalities in skin tissue (Fig. 30-2). These lesions may be primary or secondary (resulting from primary lesions).

Bacterial Skin Infections

Impetigo

Impetigo is a contagious bacterial infection of the skin that is usually seen in young children. It may be caused by *Staphylococcus* or *Streptococcus* organisms, types of bacteria commonly implicated in skin diseases. The lesions produced are usually seen on the face, neck, and exposed areas of the body. They appear on the superficial layers of the skin as:

- **macules**—small, flat skin discolorations (see Fig. 30-2*A*)
- **vesicles**—small fluid-filled sacs (see Fig. 30-2*D*)
- **bullae**—large fluid-filled sacs (see Fig. 30-2*E*)
- **pustules**—pus-filled sacs (see Fig. 30-2*F*).

There are patches of exudative vesicles that produce honey-colored crusts (see Fig. 30-2*K*). These vesicles leave red areas when the crusts are removed.

Treatment involves washing the area two to three times a day and applying a topical antibiotic. Oral an-

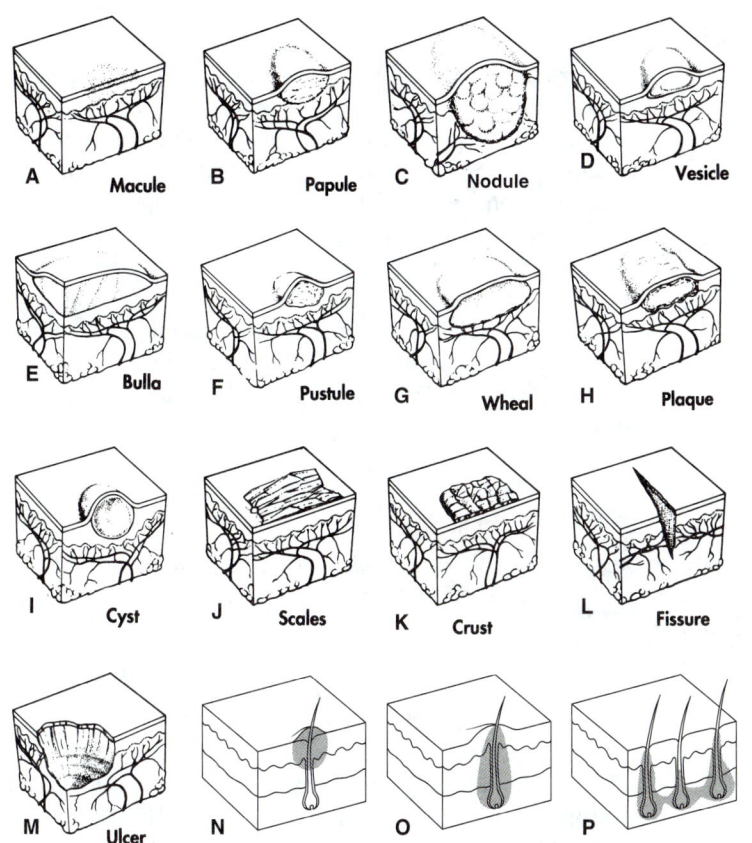

FIGURE 30-2

Skin lesions. *Primary lesions:* (*A*) Macule. Flat, circumscribed discoloration. (*B*) Papule. Solid, elevated palpable lesion smaller than 1 cm; colors vary. (*C*) Nodule. Raised, solid lesion larger than 1 cm. (*D*) Vesicle. Small elevation filled with clear fluid. (*E*) Bulla. Large vesicle or blister; larger than 1 cm. (*F*) Pustule. Lesion containing pus. (*G*) Wheal. Transient elevation of the skin caused by edema of the dermis and surrounding capillary dilatation. (*H*) Plaque. Solid, elevated lesion on skin or mucosa; larger than 1 cm. (*I*) Cyst. Tumor that contains semisolid or liquid material. *Secondary lesions:* (*J*) Scales. Heaped up, horny layer of dead epidermis. (*K*) Crust. Covering formed from serum, blood, or pus drying on the skin. (*L*) Fissures. Cracks in the skin. (*M*) Ulcer. Lesion formed by local destruction of the epidermis and part of the underlying dermis. *Other lesions:* (*N*) Superficial folliculitis. Localized infection of hair follicle. (*O*) Furuncle. Acute inflammation deep within hair follicle. (*P*) Carbuncle. Infection involving subcutaneous tissues around several hair follicles.

tibiotics may be prescribed for severe cases. Scratching must be discouraged. Towels, washcloths, and bed linens should be kept separate and must be washed daily to prevent spread of the disease. Individuals at risk for developing impetigo are those in poor health, those with conditions such as anemia or malnutrition, and those with poor hygiene.

Folliculitis

Folliculitis is a superficial infection of a hair follicle (see Fig. 30-2*N*). It is characterized by itching, burning, and pustule formation. Treatment is aimed at promoting drainage and healing. Saline soaks or compresses are ordered for 15 minutes twice a day. A topical anti-infective followed by application of a dressing is also recommended three times a day.

If folliculitis is left untreated, it may lead to **abscess** formation. An abscess is formed when a small sac of pus accumulates at the site of inflammation. The causative agent of these infections is often *Staphylococcus aureus.*

Furuncle

A furuncle, or **boil,** is a deep-seated infection of a hair follicle (see Fig. 30-2*O*). Friction and pressure at the site may contribute to its formation. A hard, painful **nodule** (mass) forms (see Fig. 30-2*C*), enlarges for several days, then erupts with pus oozing from one site. Treatment of a furuncle includes application of moist heat to assist in "ripening" it or bringing it to a head. Often an incision and drainage (I & D) procedure is performed.

Carbuncle

A carbuncle consists of an interconnected group of hair follicles or several furuncles joined together in a mass (see Fig. 30-2*P*). The subcutaneous tissue in the surrounding area is also involved. These are hard, round, extremely painful swellings that take from several days to a week to enlarge. They eventually soften and erupt, discharging pus from several sites. When the skin sloughs away, a scarred cavity remains. The patient usually has an accompanying fever.

Treatment involves use of a systemic antibiotic, applications of moist heat, and incision and drainage once the lesion has matured. A topical anti-infective and loose bandages are applied. The site may require a wick to remain in the cavity for several days to facilitate healing by secondary intention.

Cellulitis

Cellulitis is a spreading infection of the connective tissue. It is caused by an infection of an already existing wound. The skin becomes hot, red, and edematous. A systemic anti-infective usually provides rapid and successful treatment.

Viral Skin Infections

Herpes Simplex

Herpes simplex infections are also called cold sores or fever blisters. (A blister is a collection of fluid in or beneath the epidermis.) The lesions, which appear on the lips, mouth, face, and nose, are small vesicles grouped together on a red base. They eventually erupt, leaving a painful ulcer, then a crust. They cause burning and stinging and may be precipitated by other infections, menstruation, fatigue, trauma, stress, or exposure to the sun.

Fever blisters are caused by herpes simplex virus I. They are recurrent and no effective treatment eliminates or controls the disease. Acyclovir has shown promise in reducing the severity of the disease, but it does not offer a cure. Treatment is aimed at relieving discomfort with topical ointments.

Herpes Zoster

It is commonly believed that herpes zoster, or shingles, is caused by the same virus that causes chickenpox. After exposure to chickenpox, the virus may lie dormant in the body for years until reactivated. It spreads down the length of a nerve to the skin, causing redness, swelling, and pain. After about 48 hours, a band of lesions develops, which begin as **papules**, small, red, solid elevations on the skin (see Fig. 30-2*B*). These progress to vesicles and pustules, then dry crusts. The lesions last for several weeks. Scarring and alterations in pigmentation are common. Pain often remains after the lesions have disappeared, in some cases as long as several months.

Shingles commonly appear on the face, back, and chest. Lesions are frequently unilateral. The disorder usually occurs in adults. The virus remains dormant in the nervous system of anyone who has had the disease and may recur in times of physical or emotional stress.

Treatment includes narcotic analgesics for the discomfort, or nerve blocks for severe pain. Locally, calamine lotion may be used. The area must be protected from air and the irritation of clothing. Acyclovir is sometimes used to alleviate the severity of the disease.

Verruca

A **verruca** is a wart. Warts are squamous cell **papillomas** (benign skin tumors) that appear as rough, raised lesions with a pitted surface. Warts occur singly or in groups and may be found anywhere on the skin or mucous membranes. They commonly appear on the fingers or hands. Warts vary in size, shape, and appearance, and are thought to be caused by papillomaviruses.

Treatment of warts includes removal with keratolytic agents, liquid nitrogen, podophyllum resin, laser therapy, or surgery. They also may disappear spontaneously.

Fungal Skin Infections

The most common fungal infections of the skin (**dermatophytosis**) are caused by a group of fungi molds called dermatophytes. There are several and treatment is similar. The group of fungal diseases called tinea is collectively known to the lay public as ringworm.

Tinea Capitas

Tinea capitas affects the scalp. It is contagious and appears most frequently in children. It is characterized by round, gray, **scale** patches (dried skin flakes) and areas of **alopecia** (baldness). There are usually no symptoms, with the exception of light itching.

Tinea Corporis

Tinea corporis, or tinea circinata, is exhibited on non-hairy portions of the body. It is characterized by itchy, red rings that are clear in the center with a scalelike border (see Fig. 30-2*J*). It is frequently found on the face and arms.

Tinea Cruris

Tinea cruris is known in lay terms as "jock itch." The lesions, which cause marked itching, are red macules with clear centers and scalelike borders. They are found on the skin in the groin area and the gluteal folds.

Tinea Pedis

Tinea pedis, or athlete's foot, is characterized by itching, burning, and stinging between the toes and on the soles. The lesions may appear as red, weepy vesicles, as chronic dry scales, or as **fissures** (cracklike lesions) between the toes (see Fig. 30-2L).

Tinea Unguium

Tinea unguium, also known as onychomycosis, causes thickening, discoloration, and crumbling of the nails, most often the toenails. It is difficult to cure and will take months of local antifungal preparations and oral griseofulvin for severe cases.

Tinea Versicolor

Tinea versicolor, also known as pityriasis versicolor, is not caused by dermatophytes. It is not known exactly what sort of fungus is the causative agent. The disease exhibits as a multicolor rash generally over the upper trunk. It is more common in young people in warm weather and is chronic. It varies from macular to raised, round or oval, from darkly pigmented to depigmented, and is slightly scalelike. There are usually no symptoms. Diagnosis of tinea versicolor is by **Wood's light**, an ultraviolet light that, when used in a darkened room, shows abnormalities in the skin as fluorescent colors. Treatment is with selenium sulfide daily for 7 days, antifungal creams or lotions, and griseofulvin for severe cases.

All of the tineas are treated with topical antifungal powders, creams, or shampoos and oral griseofulvin. Inflamed lesions may be treated with wet compresses or soaks. General measures for treating fungal infections and preventing transfer is to keep the area clean and dry because fungi thrive in moist conditions. Clothing should be loose fitting and laundered daily. Socks and underclothing should be changed frequently. Clothing should not be shared with others. Shower shoes should be worn in public showers and pools.

Checkpoint Question
5. What is the difference between tinea capitas and tinea pedis?

Parasitic Skin Infestations

Scabies

Scabies is a contagious skin disorder caused by the itch mite, *Sarcoptes scabiei*. It is spread by direct contact.

The itching caused by the mite is worse at night when the female burrows under the epidermis to lay her eggs. The lesions are small red vesicles or pustules that occur between the fingers, at the inner wrist, elbows, axillae, waist, and groin.

Treatment for scabies is aimed at disinfestation. For adults, 1% lindane cream or lotion is applied from the neck down at bedtime. One application of Elimite cream is effective and is the drug of choice for children. All bedding and clothing for the whole family should be laundered daily until the infestation is clear.

Pediculosis

Pediculosis is an infestation of the skin with lice. Lice may be found in three body areas: the scalp (head lice), the body (body lice), or the pubic hairs ("crabs"). Wherever they are found, itching is intense and the skin often becomes secondarily infected from scratching. Lice feed on human blood and lay eggs (nits) on body hairs or in clothing fibers. Nits may be seen on hair shafts close to the skin or in seams of clothing.

Pediculosis is commonly seen among populations with overcrowding and poor hygiene. The disorder is transmitted through physical contact with an infested person, by sitting on an infested toilet seat, or by sharing a comb, brush, clothing, or bedding that is infested. γ-Benzene hexachloride creams, lotions, or shampoos are used for all types of pediculosis. All clothing and linen must be dry cleaned or washed in hot water and ironed. Sealing items in plastic bags for 30 days or heating to 140°F will eliminate lice on items that cannot be laundered.

Inflammatory Reactions

Eczema

Eczema is an inflammatory skin disorder generally involving only the epidermal layer. It is more common in children than adults. It is characterized by itching, which may be prolonged. The lesions vary at different stages but generally begin as red patches, proceed to weepy vesicles, and end up as dry scale crusts. They appear on the face, neck, bends of knees and elbows, and the upper trunk. They usually run a chronic course of exacerbations.

The causes of eczema are many and varied, depending on the individual. Causes include:

- Food allergies to fish, eggs, and milk products
- Medication or chemical allergies
- Sensitivity to irritating soaps, household cleaning products, deodorants, and perfumes
- Inhalants such as pollen, dust, or animal dander

- Poor circulation to a part
- Ultraviolet rays

Treatment involves removing the cause and promoting healing of the lesions. The causative agent should be avoided if it is known. The patient should maintain good hydration and keep the skin well moistened with emollients. A humid environment is recommended. Only one warm, not hot, bath should be taken daily with a nondrying soap. The skin should be patted dry and a topical emollient should be applied immediately. Scratchy clothing should be avoided.

Exudative lesions are treated with soaks, baths, or wet dressings for 10 to 30 minutes three or four times daily. Domeboro, Aveeno, or bicarbonate are good for these purposes. Topical corticosteroid lotions, creams, or ointments are usually applied twice a day. Bandages should be used at night to protect against scratching. Antihistamines may be necessary for severe **pruritus** (itching). For scales, a steroid ointment is recommended. Systemic corticosteroids, such as prednisone, are recommended only in severe cases.

Seborrheic Dermatitis

Seborrheic **dermatitis** (skin inflammation) is also known as **seborrhea**, which is an overproduction of sebum. It is a chronic dermatitis resulting in greasy yellow scales primarily on the scalp, where it is referred to as seborrheic dandruff. Underlying redness and pruritus may be present. The eyelids, face, chest, back, umbilicus, and body folds may also be affected. It is felt that seborrhea is caused by a genetic predisposition and a combination of hormones, nutrition, infection, or stress. It is treated with shampoos and topical corticosteroid lotions.

Urticaria

Urticaria, or hives, is characterized by acute inflammatory reaction of the dermis. It begins with itching, followed by **erythema** (redness) and swelling. The **wheals** (see Fig. 30-2G) that develop have a pale center with a red edge. They resemble a mosquito bite and each lasts only a few hours. They appear in clusters anywhere on the body. Hives are self-limiting, lasting from a few days to a few weeks.

The most common causes are:

- Foods such as shellfish, strawberries, tomatoes, citrus fruits, eggs, and chocolate
- Inhalants such as feathers or animal dander
- Chemicals, cosmetics, and medications
- Sunlight
- Insect bites or stings
- Heat, cold, or pressure on the skin
- Infection
- Stress

Treatment involves reducing the inflammation. The cause should be avoided if known. Antihistamines are usually given to reduce itching and swelling. A short course of prednisone is sometimes ordered. Starch or Aveeno baths twice a day may make the patient more comfortable. Epinephrine is given if symptoms of urticaria develop rapidly and are associated with dyspnea.

Acne Vulgaris

Acne vulgaris is an inflammatory disease of the sebaceous glands. Its cause is not known. It commonly occurs during adolescence and is characterized by pimples, **comedos** (blackheads), **cysts** (fluid sacs beneath the skin) (see Fig. 30-2I), and scarring. The lesions usually occur on the face, neck, upper chest, back, and shoulders. Overactive sebaceous glands cause excessive sebum to become trapped in the follicle, producing a dark substance that results in a blackhead. Leukocytes accumulate and pus production results.

Treatment for acne includes a regimen of Retin-A, benzoyl peroxide, and tetracycline. Sunlamp treatments are sometimes used to dry the lesions. Accutane may be prescribed for severe acne that does not respond to ordinary treatments.

Psoriasis

Psoriasis is a chronic inflammatory skin disorder characterized by bright red plaques (see Fig. 30-2H) covered with dry, silvery scales. The cause is unknown. Psoriasis is usually found on the scalp, elbows, knees, base of the spine, palms, soles, and around the nails. There are usually no vesicles and itching varies from mild to severe. It cannot be completely cured and recurrences are likely. Exacerbations are common during cold weather, stress, or pregnancy. It is usually a chronic disorder and is difficult to treat.

Treatment includes tar preparations and topical steroid creams or ointments. Exposure to ultraviolet B light three times a week is also used.

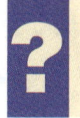
Checkpoint Question
6. What is urticaria and which layer of the skin does it affect?

Disorders of Wound Healing

Cicatrix

A cicatrix is scar tissue that forms erratically and causes distortion of the wound. It usually occurs late in wound healing. It is an especially frequent occurrence after extensive burns. It may cause deformity and immobility of joints because it is less elastic than normal tissue.

Keloids

Keloids, an overproduction of scar tissue, occur as a complication of wound healing. The scar tissue forms as a result of excessive collagen accumulation. A raised nodule is formed that does not resolve with time. The cause is unknown. It occurs most frequently in young women, especially during pregnancy, and in African Americans. The most common sites are the neck and shoulders. Injections of cortisone are sometimes effective in treating keloids.

Disorders Caused by Pressure

Callus and Corn

A callus, sometimes called a callosity, is a raised painless thickening of the epidermis. It is caused by pressure or friction on the hands and feet. A corn is a hard, raised thickening of the stratum corneum on the toes. It results from chronic friction and pressure, especially from poorly fitting shoes. The pressure compresses the dermis, making it thin and tender and causing pain and inflammation. Soft corns can form between the toes.

The treatment for calluses and corns should begin with relieving pressure. Shoes should be made of soft leather and fit properly. Liners may be inserted in shoes to relieve pressure. Bandages and corn pads are also available to correct the problem. Sometimes surgical intervention or chemical peeling with a keratolytic agent are recommended.

Decubitus Ulcers

Decubitus ulcers are also called bedsores or pressure sores. Decubiti are ulcers of the skin caused by prolonged pressure to an area of the body, usually over a bony prominence (see Fig. 30-2M). The pressure impairs blood supply and nutrition to the area. The most common sites are over the sacrum and hips, but they may also be seen on the back of the head, ears, elbows, heels, and ankles. They are most often seen in aged, debilitated, and immobilized patients. Bedridden patients are at risk for developing decubiti unless they are turned frequently to relieve pressure and the bed linen is kept clean and dry. Special mattresses, pads, and pillows are useful in prevention.

Decubitus ulcers are graded, or staged, according to the degree of involvement (Table 30-1). Treatment consists of topical antibiotic powders and adhesive ab-

Table 30-1
Staging or Grading Scale for Decubitus Ulcers

Stage	Description
I	Red skin that does not return to normal when massaged or when pressure is relieved. 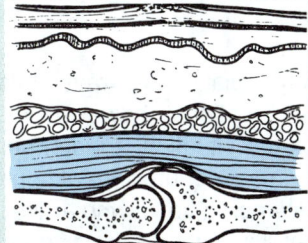
II	Skin is blistered, peeling, or cracked superficially. 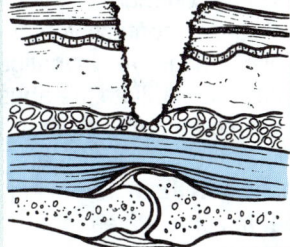
III	Skin is broken with loss of full thickness; subcutaneous tissue may be damaged; serous or bloody drainage may be present. 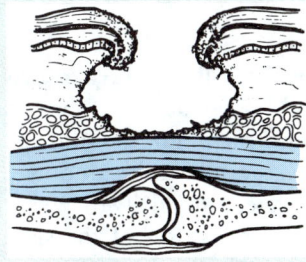
IV	Deep, crater-like ulcer with destruction of subcutaneous tissue; fascia, connective tissue, bone, or muscle are exposed and may be damaged. 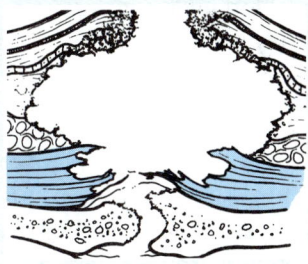

sorbent bandages and dressings. Deep infections may require systemic antibiotics and possible surgical debridement.

What If?

What if your elderly patient comes into the office with multiple decubitus ulcers? What should you do?

The geriatric population is always at risk for developing skin ulcerations; however, the physician must assess the situation to determine if the patient is receiving adequate care at home to prevent such breakdowns. Patients who arrive in a medical office with multiple ulcers in different stages of healing may be in situations of abuse or neglect. Elder abuse is less often identified, but some experts believe it is as common as child abuse. If you suspect elder abuse, contact your local Department of Social Services. An investigation will be initiated that may substantiate the abuse (requiring referral to law enforcement) or that may identify ways to alleviate the situation (caregiver education, respite care) without removing the patient from the home. In some states, not reporting elder abuse is against the law. The physician can be fined or other penalties can be imposed.

Intertrigo

Intertrigo is a disorder of skin breakdown that occurs in the body folds of obese persons. The combination of heat, moisture, and friction of the skin against itself in these areas causes the skin to break down. Humid climates and poor hygiene are likely to aggravate the condition. Erythema and fissures of the skin result. The patient experiences itching, stinging, and burning.

Treatment for intertrigo involves proper hygiene and an attempt to keep the area clean and dry. Talcum powder or cornstarch is often recommended. Antibacterial or antifungal lotion or powder is necessary if secondary infection is present.

Alopecia

Alopecia refers to baldness. It may occur from physical trauma, systemic diseases (eg, lupus erythematosus, lymphomas, or hypothyroidism), bacteria or fungal infections, chemotherapy, excessive radiation, or genetic predisposition, as in male pattern baldness.

Baldness caused by scarring and male pattern baldness are permanent and cannot be reversed. For other causes of baldness, treatment of the underlying disorder often results in new hair growth.

Disorders of Pigmentation

Albinism

Albinism is a genetically determined condition in which there is a partial or total absence of the pigment, or melanin, in the skin, hair, and eyes. The skin is pale, the hair is white, and irises appear pink. The skin will not tan and is prone to sunburn. Eye problems are frequent because no pigment is present to protect the underlying structures from the ultraviolet rays of the sun. Albinism has no treatment.

Vitiligo

Vitiligo is a progressive, chronic destruction of melanocytes. It is thought to be an autoimmune disorder in patients with an inherited predisposition. The depigmented areas occur as white patches that sometimes have a hyperpigmented border. It usually occurs in exposed areas of the skin.

There is currently no effective method for treating vitiligo. Patients are advised to protect the areas from the sun because they are prone to sunburn in the absence of melanin. Waterproof cosmetics may be used to cover the areas.

Leukoderma

Leukoderma is the localized loss of skin pigment that results from damage caused by skin trauma. It is more common in African Americans. Frequent causes of leukoderma include contact with caustic chemicals or the healing of burns or infection.

Nevus

A nevus, also known as a birthmark or mole, is a congenital pigmented skin blemish. It is usually circumscribed and may involve the epidermis, connective tissue, nerves, or blood vessels. Nevi are usually benign (not cancerous) but may become malignant (cancerous); patients should be cautioned to watch for changes in the color, size, and texture of any nevus. Bleeding and itching should also be reported (Box 30-1).

? Checkpoint Question

7. What are four disorders of pigmentation? Briefly describe

BOX 30-1 American Cancer Society

On the lookout for malignant melanoma

Its incidence has doubled since 1980, and currently, melanoma accounts for over 6000 deaths a year. Melanomas are usually pigmented, elevated skin lesions and frequently develop in a new or existing mole. The key to treatment of this potentially deadly cancer is early detection of changes in size, color, shape, elevation, texture, or consistency of any pigmented area—old or new—in any spot or bump (see illustrations below). By becoming familiar with what is normal for you, you'll be more apt to notice what is abnormal.

The eventual outcome of melanoma is governed by how deeply it has invaded the skin, which also determines how aggressively the cancer will be treated. That early detection can work to cut the mortality rate is clearly evident in the 90%-plus cure rate of malignant melanoma in Queensland, Australia, where an enormous incidence of the cancer led to excellent public education and screening campaigns. The cure rate in the United States is about 20%.

Mole patrol

Mole inspection becomes simpler if you keep in mind the American Cancer Society's ABCD rule for distinguishing a normal mole or other skin blemish from an abnormal one.

Normal   *Abnormal*

Asymmetry. One-half of the mole does not match the other.

     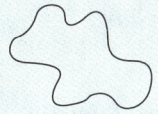

Border. The edges are irregular—ragged, notched, or blurred.

Color. The color is not uniform, but may be differing shades of tan, brown, or black, sometimes with patches of red, white, or blue.

     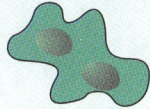

Diameter. The mole is larger than the size of a pencil eraser—about 6 mm or a quarter of an inch—or is increasing in size.

From *Harvard Medical Letter,* June 1991, p. 4, American Cancer Society

Skin Cancers

Basal Cell Carcinoma

Basal cell carcinoma is a slow-growing cancer that appears most frequently on exposed areas of the body, usually the face, but may also be found on the shoulders and chest, where sebaceous follicles are abundant. The lesions have a waxy appearance with a depressed center and a rolled edge where blood vessels may be apparent. Metastasis almost never occurs, but if left untreated, the lesions will grow locally and may ulcerate and damage surrounding tissues (Fig. 30-3).

Basal cell carcinoma is the most common malignant tumor of the skin of whites. It commonly occurs in blond, fair-skinned men over age 40. Prolonged exposure to ultraviolet light or x-rays are thought to be predisposing factors for the development of basal cell carcinoma.

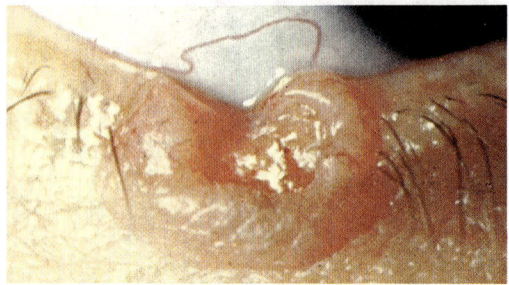

FIGURE 30-3
Basal cell carcinoma.

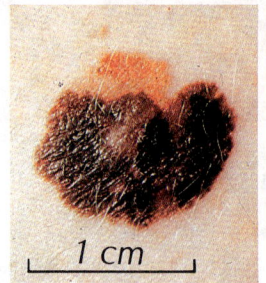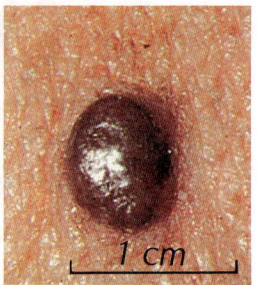

FIGURE 30-5
Malignant melanoma. (*Left*) Superficial melanoma. (*Right*) Nodular melanoma.

The most common treatment for basal cell carcinoma is surgical removal. Radiation therapy and cryosurgery are alternative treatments.

Squamous Cell Carcinoma

Squamous cell carcinoma is slightly less common than basal cell carcinoma. It may occur in any squamous epithelial area of the body, such as the lungs, cervix, or anus, but is more frequently found on the skin (Fig. 30-4). Squamous cell carcinoma is a slow-growing, malignant **neoplasm** (tumor). The lesions are firm, red, horny or prickly, and painless and range widely in size. Those on exposed areas are thought to result from exposure to the sun. Those on areas not normally exposed, such as mucous membranes, are thought to be the result of frequent irritation. Treatment is the same as that used for basal cell carcinoma. Although basal cell carcinoma is not generally metastatic, squamous cell carcinoma, in contrast, will spread readily through underlying and surrounding tissues.

Malignant Melanoma

Malignant melanoma is a cancer of the skin that forms from melanocytes. Lesions vary from macules to nodules and often have an irregular border and a variety of colors (Fig. 30-5). Mixtures of white, blue, purple, and red are the most common. The tumor grows both in

radius and in depth into the dermis. In about 30% to 35% of cases, it grows in a preexisting nevus.

Malignant melanoma, which is thought to be caused by excessive exposure to sunlight, is the leading cause of death due to skin disease. It is the ninth most common cancer. The incidence is 1 in 105 individuals in the United States. The peak age for malignant melanoma is between 50 and 70. Those at highest risk for developing the disease have blond or red hair, fair skin, blue eyes, and a tendency to sunburn and spend a lot of time out of doors (Box 30-2).

Treatment for malignant melanoma is surgical removal after a biopsy, possibly including lymph re-

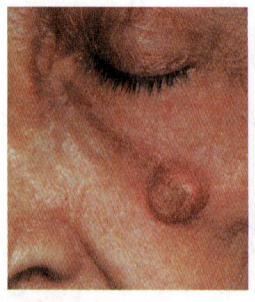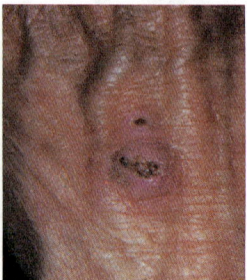

FIGURE 30-4
Squamous cell carcinoma.

BOX 30-2 Effects of Sunlight on the Skin

Exposure to the sun's ultraviolet rays is the major cause of skin cancers. In addition, ultraviolet rays cause sunburn and premature aging of the skin.

The incidence of skin cancers has risen dramatically in the last 20 years. This is thought to be due to the lack of sunscreen use and the increased tendency of people to spend more leisure time in the sun and sunbathing.

Primary prevention consists of limiting exposure to ultraviolet light by wearing proper clothing and using sunscreens. Exposure to the sun is not recommended during the five peak hours of the day, from 10:00 AM to 3:00 PM. A sunscreen with at least a 15 SPF (sun protective factor) is considered good protection in blocking ultraviolet rays. Most sunscreens contain PABA (*p*-aminobenzoic acid), which causes allergy in many people. However, a number of PABA-free sunscreens are available.

The use of sunlamps and tanning beds should be avoided.

moval. Prognosis depends on the depth of the tumor. Tumors over 1.5 mm often metastasize to the lymph nodes, liver, lungs, and brain (see Box 30-1).

> **Checkpoint Question**
> *8. Which is more likely to metastasize—basal cell or squamous cell carcinoma?*

COMMON DIAGNOSTIC PROCEDURES AND THE MEDICAL ASSISTANT'S ROLE

Examination of the skin is performed mostly by inspection. This may be aided by palpation and the use of a diascope, a clear glass plate that allows the examiner to observe skin changes when pressure is applied.

Many skin lesions can be diagnosed by the characteristic size, shape, and distribution on the skin. However, laboratory studies may be necessary to confirm a diagnosis. The medical assistant will be required to assemble equipment as directed by the physician, obtain informed consent, and properly direct the specimens to appropriate laboratories. Standard Precautions must be observed when handling such specimens.

As the medical assistant, you will be responsible for preparing the room and the patient for the examination. Gowning and draping should be appropriate to the patient's symptoms and body part to be examined.

During the examination, you will aid the physician by ensuring that the lighting is directed properly, handing necessary instruments and equipment, assisting in obtaining wound cultures, maintaining asepsis, and applying topical medications and dressings. Skin lesions must be protected from further infection by using medical asepsis or surgical asepsis as indicated. Again, Standard Precautions must be observed.

You will aid the patient in position changes and try to make the patient as comfortable as possible. To protect the patient's privacy, only those body parts being examined are to be exposed.

After the examination, instruct the patient about home care, remove all soiled and contaminated supplies, and clean the room in the usual manner.

Wound Cultures

A wound culture consists of obtaining a specimen of wound **exudate** (drainage), which is then examined under a microscope to diagnose bacterial or fungal

infection. To obtain a wound culture, follow these steps:

1. Wash your hands and put on gloves.
2. If a dressing is present, remove it and dispose of it appropriately. Assess the wound for signs of infection by observing the color, odor, and amount of exudate.
3. Obtain a sample by either swabbing or aspirating the exudate. *For swabbing*: Obtain a sterile culture tube and remove the swab. Insert the swab into the exudate, being sure to saturate the swab (Fig. 30-6). Place the swab in the culture tube and crush the ampule of transport medium (Fig. 30-7). Label the culture tube appropriately and send it to the laboratory. *For aspirating*: Use a 1- to 5-mL syringe with needle removed to aspirate a sample of exudate, which is then placed in the culture tube for transport to the laboratory.
4. Clean the wound and apply a sterile dressing according to the steps in Procedure 24-7: Applying a Sterile Dressing, in Chapter 24, Minor Office Surgery.
5. Remove the gloves and wash your hands.

Skin Biopsy

The purpose of a skin biopsy is to remove a small piece of tissue from a lesion so that it may be examined under a microscope to differentiate between benign and malignant growths. A local anesthetic and sterile asepsis are used.

There are three types of skin biopsies: excision, punch, or shave biopsy. In an excision biopsy, the entire lesion is removed for study. When a punch biopsy is done, a small section is removed from the center of the lesion. A shave biopsy cuts the lesion off just above the skin line.

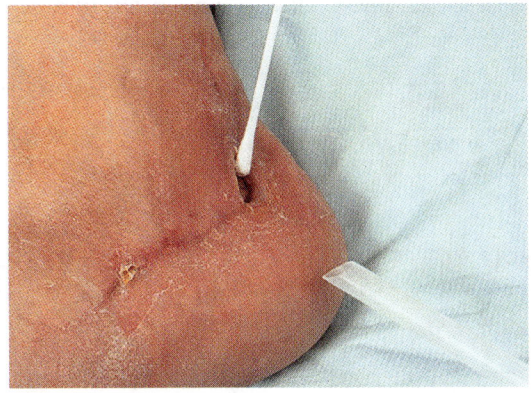

FIGURE 30-6
Insert culture swab into wound to obtain sample.

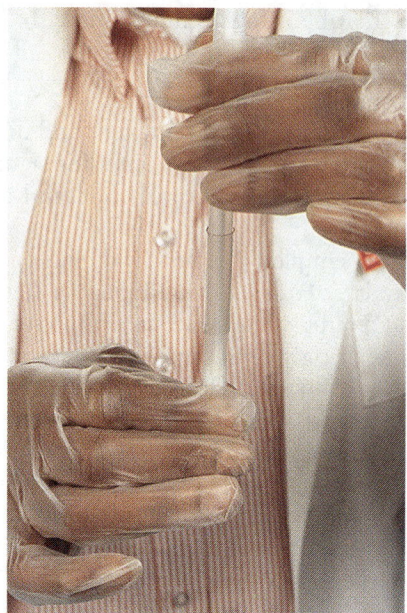

FIGURE 30-7
Crush ampule of medium.

Urine Melanin

A urine test to detect the presence of melanin is done with a random sample of urine from the patient. The specimen is allowed to sit for 24 hours and then examined under a microscope. Melanin is not normally present in the urine unless the patient has a malignant melanoma.

Wood's Light Analysis

Wood's light is a black (ultraviolet) light. When it is directed 4 to 5 inches from the patient's skin in a darkened room, abnormalities in the skin and hair appear as fluorescent colors. It is used to detect fungal and bacterial infections, scabies, or alterations in pigment.

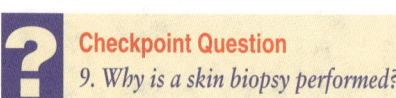

Checkpoint Question
9. Why is a skin biopsy performed?

Allergy Skin Testing

Scratch test

Scratch or puncture tests are usually done on the outer surface of the upper arm or back to detect allergies. The skin surface is labeled or numbered in rows

1½ to 2 inches apart. A short scratch is then made with a needle or lancet and a drop of various **allergens** (substances that produce allergic reactions) is placed on each scratch or puncture. Fifty or more tests may be done at a time and a certain pattern is followed so that the site of each allergen is identified. The test sites are examined after 15 to 20 minutes. A positive test for allergy to a substance is indicated by the development of a wheal at a site. Patients should not leave the office for at least 30 minutes after allergy testing so they can be observed for delayed allergic reactions (Box 30-3).

Intradermal Tests

Intradermal tests are done by injecting 0.01 to 0.02 mL of specific allergen extract intradermally on the anterior forearm. (See Chap. 26, Preparing and Administering Medications, for the procedure for intradermal injections.) Ten to 15 tests may be done on each arm. These are thought to be a more accurate method of testing for allergies than the scratch or puncture method.

Patch Tests

Patch tests, skin tests to identify allergens, are often done to determine the cause of contact dermatitis. A small amount of suspected allergen is placed on the anterior forearm, covered with cellophane, and taped down. Twenty to 30 tests may be done at a time. Results are read after 24 to 48 hours.

BOX 30-3   **Allergy Testing Safety Precautions**

Allergy testing is usually performed by a trained technician in a controlled setting. The possibility of anaphylaxis is remote but must be considered. A well equipped and current emergency cart or tray must be on site and as close to the testing sites as possible. A basic setup includes:

- injectable epinephrine with syringes and needles
- various sizes of airways and intubation devices
- oxygen and masks or ambubags
- tourniquet

Additionally, some sites may require tracheotomy equipment, defibrillators, electrocardiography machines, and intravenous equipment.

Tuberculin Skin Testing

Tuberculin skin tests (Mantoux and tine tests) are used to screen for previous infection by the tuberculin bacillus, *Mycobacterium tuberculosis.*

- The Mantoux test consists of an injection of a minute amount of purified protein derivative (PPD) of the tuberculin bacillus given intradermally in the anterior forearm.
- The tine test is performed with a device that holds four tines, or prongs, impregnated with old tuberculin (OT) or PPD. This is pressed briefly into the anterior forearm. (Refer to Chap. 26, Preparing and Administering Medications, for the procedure for administering the Mantoux and tine tests.)

Tuberculin skin tests are read between 48 and 72 hours. A test is considered positive if redness and induration are present. The diameter of the area should be measured in millimeters, usually with a guide provided by the manufacturer of the testing material. A positive test is usually indication for a follow-up chest x-ray and sputum studies.

Schick Test

The Schick test is an intradermal skin test for diphtheria sensitivity or immunity. A small amount of diphtheria toxin is injected in the anterior forearm. The test is read at 24 hours, 48 hours, and 4 to 7 days. Inflammation and induration at the site indicates a positive reaction. This test is not used routinely in the United States.

➤ WARM AND COLD APPLICATIONS

Because of the time involved in properly performing warm or cold soaks or compresses, these procedures are not often performed in the office setting. It will frequently be the medical assistant's responsibility to instruct patients who will be administering the treatments at home. Patients should understand the purpose for the procedure, the full performance of the procedure, the expected results, and precautions or danger signs.

Treatments may be warm or cold, moist or dry. Table 30-2 discusses types of heat and cold treatments and the purposes for each.

Precautions

The body quickly adapts to temperatures; for example, water in a pool feels cool at first, but the body soon becomes accustomed to the temperature. The water is no warmer, the body has simply adapted. By this reasoning, patients can be made to understand that it is not necessary to increase the temperature of treatments when they can no longer feel the initial benefits.

The body responds to extremes of temperature for extended periods of time by exerting an opposite effect, called the rebound phenomenon. For example, beyond 30 minutes, heat applied to an area will cause vasoconstriction rather than vasodilation. Therefore, applications left on for longer periods of time than recommended will have an opposite effect than the one intended by the physician.

Heat applied to a large part of the body will decrease blood pressure due to peripheral vasodilation. Conversely, cold applied to large areas may cause the blood pressure to increase due to the shunting effect of vasoconstriction.

Some areas are more sensitive to heat than others. For example, areas of thin skin with few nerve receptors will not feel heat as quickly as the palms but because of the fragile skin in this area will be more likely to burn. The very young with immature nervous systems and the elderly with impaired nervous systems are more likely to suffer burns. Individuals with impaired mental states, such as the confusional states, are more prone to burns. Preexisting pathology with compromised skin may also present a risk of burns.

Table 30-3 provides additional guidelines for proper use of heat and cold.

Temperature levels will vary by the length of application, method of application, the patient's general condition, and the condition of the skin. Temperature should be kept generally within the following guidelines:

- Warm—from tepid, 95/98°, to a very warm 115°
- Cold—from neutral, 93/95°, to a very cold 50°

text continues on page 540

✓ 📝 *Charting Example*

07/16/98	1400	Cold pack applied to left lower leg. Pack removed at 1430. No mottling, pallor, or redness noted. Pt. states pain is less. Pt d/c to home by physician. ——*Maria Sefferin, RMA*

Table 30-2

Heat and Cold Treatments: Types and Purposes

Dry Heat	Moist Heat	Purposes	Dry Cold	Moist Cold	Purposes
Heat Treatments			**Cold Treatments**		
Hot water bottle, heating pad, thermal pad, disposable heat pack, heat lamp	Compresses, warm packs, soaks, sitz bath	Relieve muscle spasm or tension Relieve pain Hasten healing by increasing blood flow to a part Provide local or systemic warming	Ice bag, ice collar, disposable cold pack	Compresses, cold soaks	Limit initial edema by decreasing capillary permeability (*Caution*: Cold retards relief of existing edema by decreasing blood flow to the part.) Decrease bleeding or hemorrhage Decrease inflammation formation Relieve pain by numbing the nerve pathways Provide local or systemic cooling

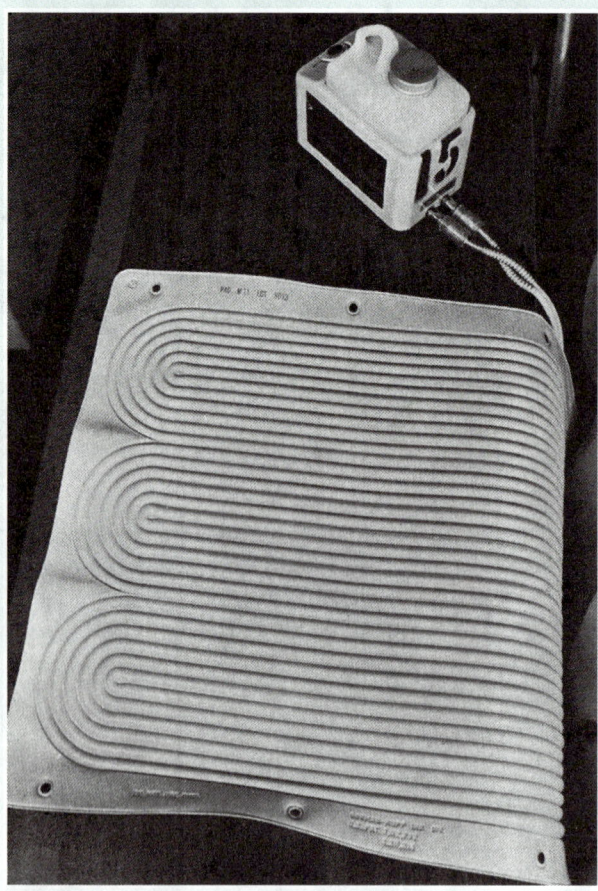

The Aquathermia (Aqua-K) pad is an electrical device that can be set to maintain water at a constant temperature and circulate it through the coils of the plastic pad. The pad can be used to provide dry heat, or it can be placed over moist dressing to provide moist heat.

Table 30-3
Proper Use of Heat and Cold: When *not* to Use Heat or Cold—and Why

Do not *use heat*:
- Within 24 h after an injury because it may increase bleeding
- For noninflammatory edema because increased capillary permeability will allow additional tissue fluid to build up
- In cases of acute inflammation because increased blood supply will increase the inflammatory process
- In the presence of malignancies because cell metabolism will be enhanced
- Over the pregnant uterus because incidences of genetic mutation have been linked to heat applied to the gravid uterus
- On areas of erythema or vesicles because it will compound the existing problem
- Over metallic implants because it will cause discomfort

Do not *use cold*:
- On open wounds because decreased blood supply will delay healing
- In the presence of already impaired circulation because it will further impair circulation

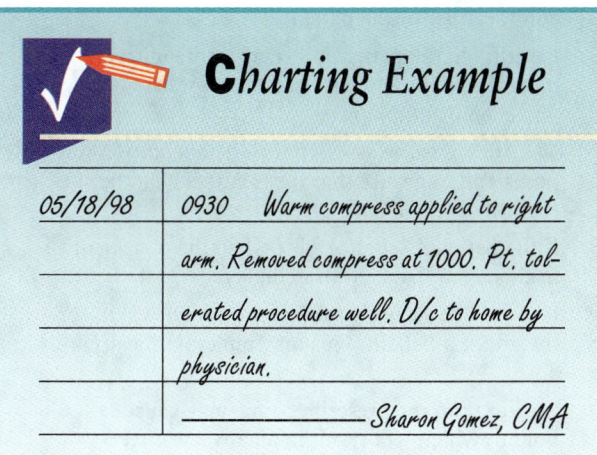

Charting Example

| 05/18/98 | 0930 | Warm compress applied to right arm. Removed compress at 1000. Pt. tolerated procedure well. D/c to home by physician. |
| | | —————— Sharon Gomez, CMA |

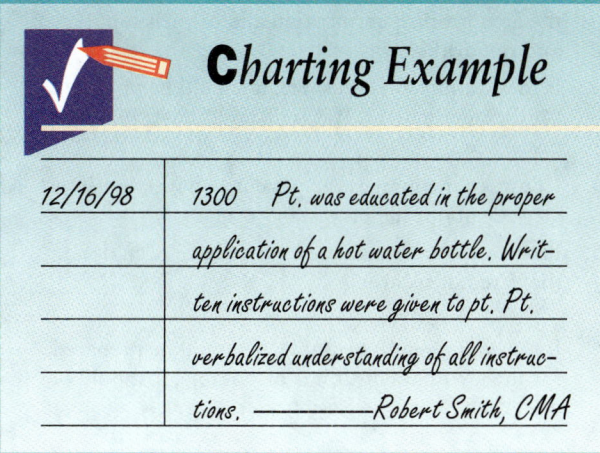

Charting Example

| 12/16/98 | 1300 | Pt. was educated in the proper application of a hot water bottle. Written instructions were given to pt. Pt. verbalized understanding of all instructions. ——————Robert Smith, CMA |

Patient Education: Heating Pads

Heating pads are not used in the office setting but may be recommended for home use. The patient must be aware of the potential for injury if strict guidelines are not followed. Share the safety tips below with your patient.

1. Be aware that most heating pads are equipped with a cover to ensure comfort and safety. If one is not provided, wrap the pad in a soft cover.
2. Do not fold or bend the pad; wires may break or short if not kept in alignment.
3. Do not pin the pad; pins may cause malfunction if they come in contact with wiring.
4. Never place pads under the body; heat may build up as it is reflected from the surface below and cause burns.
5. Set the temperature to be comfortably warm at first touch; do not turn the temperature up again as the body adjusts. (Explain to the patient in terms that can be understood the concept of adaptation to heat or cold and the dangers in ignoring warnings and guidelines.)
6. Alert the patient to the recommended time frame for heat treatments and the need for circulation to return to normal at intervals.

Procedure 30-1

Applying Cold

Equipment/Supplies

- ice bag or ice collar or disposable cold pack
- cover
- ice chips or small cubes
- gauze or tape

Steps	Purpose
1. Wash your hands.	1. Handwashing aids infection control.
2. Assemble the equipment and supplies, checking the bag or collar for leaks. If using a commercial cold pack, read the manufacturer's directions.	2. Check for leaks to avoid wetting and chilling the patient. Small bits of ice help the container conform to the patient's contours better than large pieces. The cover will add to the patient's comfort.
3. Fill the container about two-thirds full. Press it flat on a surface to express excess air from within. Seal the container.	3. If the container is too full of ice or air it will not conform to the patient's contours.
4. If using a commercial pack, activate it now.	
5. Cover the bag.	5. The cover will absorb condensation and be more comfortable for the patient.
6. Greet and identify the patient. Explain the procedure.	6. Identifying the patient prevents errors in treatment. Explaining the procedure helps ease anxiety and ensure compliance.
7. Assess the area.	7. The area must be assessed for documentation purposes and to ensure that the treatment can be successfully completed.
8. Ensure the patient's comfort.	8. If the patient is comfortable when the treatment begins, compliance is more likely.
9. Secure the appliance with gauze or tape.	9. It should be securely against the patient's skin for the greatest benefit. Pins may puncture the appliance.
10. Apply for no longer than 30 minutes.	10. Longer than the prescribed time may cause rebound, which will result in an adverse effect.
11. Assess the area for mottling, pallor, redness or pain.	11. Adverse effects should be reported to the physician immediately.
12. If the treatment is to be reapplied, wait 1 hour.	12. Circulation must be allowed to return to normal in the area for proper nutrition and oxygen supply and removal of wastes.
13. Properly care for or dispose of equipment and supplies. Wash your hands.	13. If the equipment is reusable, it should be prepared for the next patient. If it is disposable, it should be discarded.
14. Thank the patient and provide appropriate instructions.	14. Courtesy encourages the patient to have a positive attitude about the physician's office.
15. Document the procedure, the results, the patient's reactions, and any comments appropriate to the situation.	15. Procedures are considered not to have been done if they are not recorded.
16. Properly care for equipment as appropriate to the situation.	16. If the equipment is reusable, it should be prepared for the next patient. If it is disposable, it should be discarded.

Note: *Ice bags are used for larger areas; ice collars are used for smaller areas. Disposable cold packs are convenient and safe for most uses.*

Procedure 30-2

Applying a Warm or Cold Compress

Equipment/Supplies

- appropriate solution, warmed to recommended temperature
- absorbent material of the physician's choice
- waterproof barriers and insulators
- thermometer
- hot water bottle or cold pack
- clean or sterile basin
- sterile gloves or sterile transfer forceps, if appropriate

Steps	**Purpose**
1. Wash your hands.	1. Handwashing aids infection control.
2. Assemble the equipment and supplies. Pour the solution into the basin. Check the temperature of the solution.	2. This ensures that all of the materials are available. The solution must fall within the guidelines to avoid injury to the patient.
3. Greet and identify the patient. Explain the procedure.	3. Identifying the patient prevents errors in treatment. Explaining the procedure helps ease anxiety and ensure compliance.
4. Ensure patient comfort and privacy.	4. The patient is more likely to remain still for the procedure if comfort is ensured. Privacy must always be provided.
5. Protect the undersurface and clothing with waterproof barriers.	5. Wet bedding and clothing are uncomfortable for the patient and may cause chilling.
6. Press or wring out excess moisture from the absorbent material. If using sterile procedure, this may be done with sterile gloves or with two sterile transfer forceps.	6. Compresses should be moist but not dripping to avoid wetting the patient.
7. Touch the compress to the area lightly and observe the patient's reaction or ask for a response.	7. Applying too rapidly to a compromised skin surface may cause pain or discomfort.

Step 7. Gently touch the wet compress to the affected site.

8. Check the surface of the skin.	8. If response to the solution is immediate, the temperature may be inappropriate.
9. Gently arrange the compress over the area and conform the material to the patient's contours. Insulate the compress with waterproof barriers.	9. Unless the material is against the skin, temperature will not be transferred to the area of concern. Insulating the area will retard temperature loss and will avoid wetting the patient.

(continued)

Procedure 30-2   Applying a Warm or Cold Compress *(continued)*

Steps	Purpose
10. Check frequently for moisture and temperature. Hot water bottles or ice packs may be used to maintain the temperature.	10. The temperature needs to stay fairly constant. If the material dries out, benefits will be lost.
11. Discontinue after 30 minutes. Wait 1 hour before reapplying.	11. Treatment longer than 30 minutes may result in rebound. The circulation should be allowed to return to normal for periods of time to avoid tissue damage.
12. Discard disposable materials and appropriately disinfect reusable equipment. Wash your hands.	12. Equipment should be available for the next use. Cross contamination must be avoided.
13. Document skin color, patient reaction, assessment of the area, and performance of the procedure with time, temperature, and solution.	13. Procedures are considered not to have been done if they are not recorded.

Note: *Review Chapter 19, Asepsis and Infection Control, for gloving procedures or use of transfer forceps if an open lesion is present and if sterile technique is required for this procedure.*

Note: *Warm compresses will speed the suppuration process to increase healing. Cold compresses will slow bleeding and decrease inflammation.*

Procedure 30-3   Using a Hot Water Bottle or Commercial Hot Pack

Equipment/Supplies

* hot water bottle or commercial hot pack
* cover
* thermometer

Steps	Purpose
1. Wash your hands.	1. Handwashing aids infection control.
2. Assemble equipment, being sure to check the hot water bottle for leaks.	2. This ensures that all of the materials are available. Checking for leaks avoids wetting the patient.
3. Fill bottle about two-thirds full with water at appropriate temperature. Check temperature with thermometer.	3. If bottle is too full, it will not conform to the patient's contours. If water is too warm, it may cause tissue damage; if it is too cool, maximum benefits will not be achieved.
4. Place the bottle on a flat surface with the opening up and "burp" it by pressing out the excess air.	4. Excess air will prevent the bottle from conforming to the patient's contours.

(continued)

Procedure 30-3   Using a Hot Water Bottle or Commercial Hot Pack (continued)

Steps	Purpose

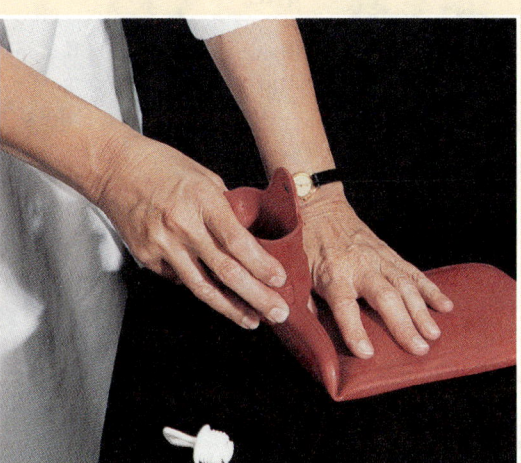

Step 4: Express air from the bottle before capping.

5. If using a commercial hot pack, follow the manufacturer's directions for activating it.

6. Wrap and secure the pack or bottle before placing on the patient's skin.

6. Covering the bag will increase the patient's comfort and help to prevent burns.

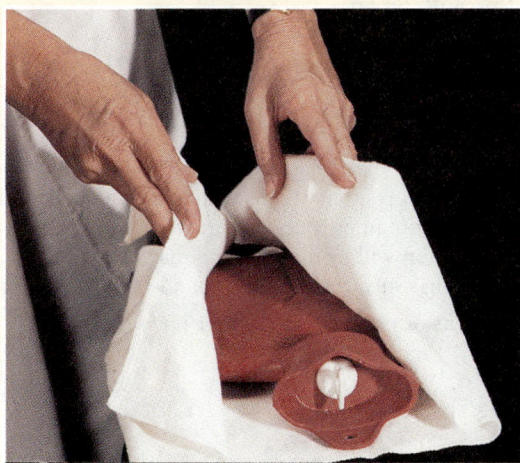

Step 6A: Wrap and secure the bag before placing on the patient's skin.

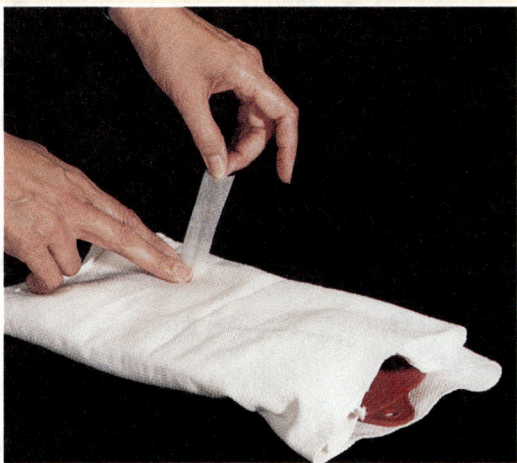

Step 6B: Continued

7. Greet and identify the patient. Explain the procedure.

7. Identifying the patient prevents errors in treatment. Explaining the procedure helps ease anxiety and ensure compliance.

(continued)

Procedure 30-3: Using a Hot Water Bottle or Commercial Hot Pack *(continued)*

Steps	Purpose
8. If continuous heat has been ordered, follow the physician's instructions; otherwise, remove after 30 minutes. Assess the area every 10 minutes.	8. General orders recommend removing sources of heat or cold after 30 minutes to avoid rebound and to allow circulation to return to normal.
9. Report pallor (an indication of rebound), excessive redness (indicates temperature may be too high for this lesion), swelling (indicates that capillary permeability may contribute to tissue damage).	9. Treatment may have to be reevaluated for this patient.
10. Caution the patient that the body will adapt to the temperature and that it is not necessary to continually increase the temperature to achieve maximum benefits.	10. This protects the patient from injury.
11. Document the time, temperature, patient comments, skin and lesion assessment and any observations.	11. Procedures are considered not to have been done if they are not recorded.

Procedure 30-4: Assisting With Therapeutic Soaks

Equipment/Supplies

- container large enough to comfortably contain the part to be soaked
- solution
- towels (for padding surfaces and drying the part)
- thermometer

Steps	Purpose
1. Wash your hands.	1. Handwashing aids infection control.
2. Assemble the equipment and supplies.	2. This ensures that all of the materials are available. If the container is uncomfortably small, proper application will be difficult and may cause muscle spasms. Surfaces should be padded for comfort.
3. Fill the container with the solution and check the temperature with thermometer. (The proper temperature is usually below 110° because of the large surface involved and the possibility of blood pressure changes with vasodilation and vasoconstriction.)	3. Burns or other tissue damage must be avoided.
4. Greet and identify the patient. Explain the procedure.	4. Identifying the patient prevents errors in treatment. Explaining the procedure helps ease anxiety and ensure compliance.
5. Slowly lower the part into the container and check for the patient's reaction. Arrange the part comfortably and in easy alignment. Check for pressure areas and pad the edges. The bottom may also be padded for comfort.	5. Immersing too quickly can be shocking to the patient. If the patient is not comfortable, muscle spasms or strain may result.

(continued)

Procedure 30-4	Assisting With Therapeutic Soaks *(continued)*

Steps   **Purpose**

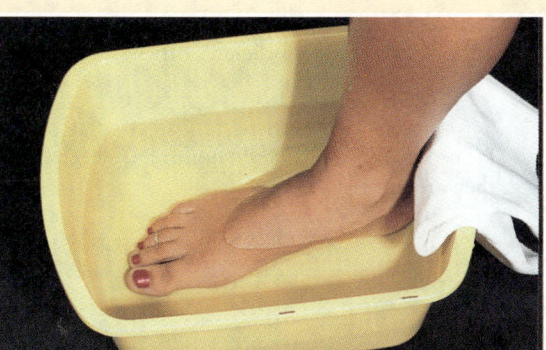

Step 5: The basin should be large enough to immerse the entire limb. Pad the edge for comfort.

6. Soak for the prescribed period of time.

7. Check every 5–10 minutes for the proper temperature. If additional water or solution must be added to maintain the temperature, remove a quantity of the solution. With your hand between the patient and the stream of solution, add the required amount and swirl it quickly through the container.

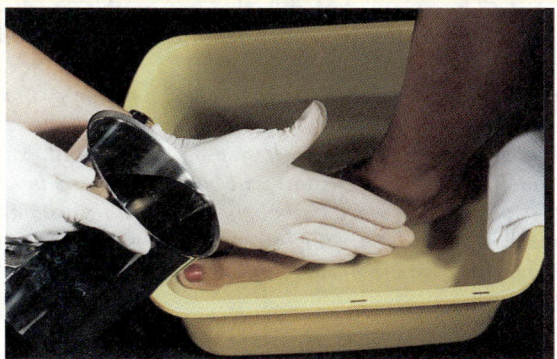

Step 7: Shield the patient's skin when adding warm water to the soak.

8. Soak for the prescribed time, usually 15–20 minutes.

9. Carefully dry the part.

10. Assess the area.

6. Soaking too long may result in tissue damage or the rebound effect.

7. The proper temperature must be maintained for maximum benefit. Avoid pouring the solution or water against the patient.

8. Soaking for longer may result in rebound or in tissue damage.

9. The area may be sensitive to brisk rubbing after the treatment but must be dried to prevent chilling the patient or causing discomfort by remaining wet.

(continued)

Procedure 30-4 — Assisting With Therapeutic Soaks *(continued)*

Steps	Purpose
11. Thank the patient and provide appropriate instructions.	11. Courtesy encourages the patient to have a positive attitude about the physician's office.
12. Properly care for or dispose of equipment supplies. Wash your hands.	
13. Document the time, the solution, the temperature, the state of the lesion or area, patient reactions and your observations.	13. Procedures are considered not to have been done if they are not recorded.

Procedures 30-1, 30-2, and 30-3 describe the steps for applying cold, applying warm or cold compresses, and using a hot water bottle or commercial hot pack. For all of the following procedures, observe Standard Precautions as necessary.

Soaks and Sitz Baths

Treatments may require that parts of the body be immersed in warm water or solutions for periods of time (Procedure 30-4). Disposable sitz bath containers are available at all medical supply stores for soaking the perineal area. They are equipped with detailed instructions from the manufacturer. If an extremity is to be soaked at home, the patient can use a Styrofoam chest to soak limbs. The chests are waterproof and are fairly large and deep and easy to clean. A towel draped over

the opening will help to maintain the temperature of the treatment.

 **Checkpoint Question**

10. How does the body respond to prolonged exposure to temperature extremes?

 SUMMARY

As the largest and certainly the most visible organ of the body, the skin and its accessories offer the first glimpse into the total state of health. Clear skin glowing with health indicates a good general state of wellness; pallor, cyanosis, or dry, scalelike skin indicates poor general health. Assessment of the integument is the first step of any physical examination. The medical assistant will be exposed to many examples of integumentary pathologies listed in this chapter and must learn to identify the forms of skin lesions significant in diagnosing the presenting illness.

 CRITICAL THINKING CHALLENGES

1. Sunlight or ultraviolet rays are needed to convert vitamin D necessary for calcium and phosphorus absorption. Why would it be important that children be exposed to sunlight regularly during their growing years?
2. Why would molds and fungi thrive in a public shower or pool? Consider the factors needed for microorganisms to thrive.
3. Why would hot water be contraindicated in cases of eczema?

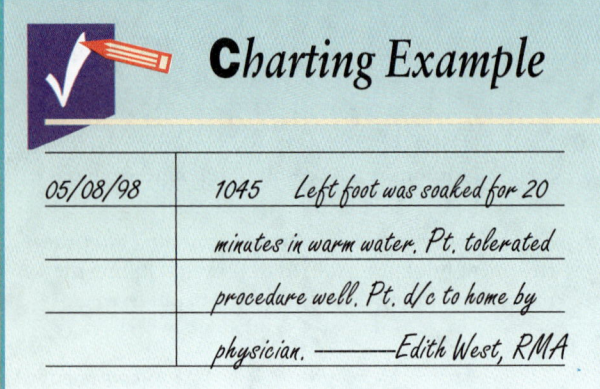

Charting Example

| 05/08/98 | 1045 | Left foot was soaked for 20 minutes in warm water. Pt. tolerated procedure well. Pt. d/c to home by physician. ———Edith West, RMA |

ANSWERS TO CHECKPOINT QUESTIONS

1. The integument helps control body temperature through vasodilation and vasoconstriction. When the body is hot, blood vessels in the skin dilate, bringing interior heat close to the body's surface. When the body is cold, the vessels constrict to conserve heat.

2. The three basic layers of the skin are the epidermis (outer layer), the dermis (middle layer), and the subcutaneous tissue (connects the dermis to underlying muscles).

3. Folliculitis, furuncle, and carbuncle are bacterial skin infections that develop in the hair follicles. Folliculitis is a localized infection of a hair follicle. A furuncle is an infection deep within the hair follicle. A carbuncle is an infection involving subcutaneous tissue around several hair follicles.

4. Herpes zoster, also known as shingles, is believed to be caused by the same virus that causes chickenpox. This virus can lie dormant for years after initial exposure. When reactivated, the virus spreads down a nerve to the skin, resulting in redness, swelling, pain, and eventual development of lesions.

5. Tinea capitas is a fungal skin infection that affects the scalp; tinea pedis is a fungal infection that affects the feet (it is also known as athlete's foot).

6. Urticaria (also known as hives) is an acute inflammatory reaction of the dermis; it is characterized by itching and the development of wheals.

7. Four pigmentation disorders are albinism (partial or total absence of pigment in the skin, hair, and eyes), vitiligo (chronic destruction of melanocytes), leuko-derma (localized loss of pigment), and nevus (pigmented skin blemish).

8. Squamous cell carcinoma will spread through underlying and surrounding tissues.

9. A skin biopsy is used to examine a lesion for benign and malignant cells.

10. After prolonged exposure to temperature extremes, the body exerts the opposite effect. For example, heat applications lasting longer than 30 minutes will cause vasoconstriction rather than vasodilation. This is called the rebound phenomenon.

SUGGESTIONS FOR FURTHER READING

Craven, R. F., & Hirnle, C. J. (1996). *Fundamentals of Nursing: Health and Human Function*, 2nd ed. Philadelphia: Lippincott-Raven Publishers.

Professional Guide to Diseases, 4th ed. (1992). Springhouse, PA: Springhouse Corporation.

Schroeder, S. A., et al. *Current Medical Diagnosis and Treatment*. (1992). East Norwalk, CT: Appleton & Lange, 1992.

Smeltzer, S. C., & Bare, B. G. (1996). Brunner and Suddarth's *Textbook of Medical-Surgical Nursing*, 8th ed. Philadelphia: Lippincott-Raven Publishers.

Taylor, C., Lillis, C., & LeMone, P. (1993). *Fundamentals of Nursing: The Art and Science of Nursing Care*, 2nd ed. Philadelphia: J. B. Lippincott.

Timby, B. (1996). *Fundamental Skills and Concepts in Patient Care*, 6th ed. Philadelphia: Lippincott-Raven.

Walter, J. B. (1992). *An Introduction to the Principles of Disease*, 3rd ed. Philadelphia: W. B. Saunders.

Caring for Patients With Musculoskeletal Disorders

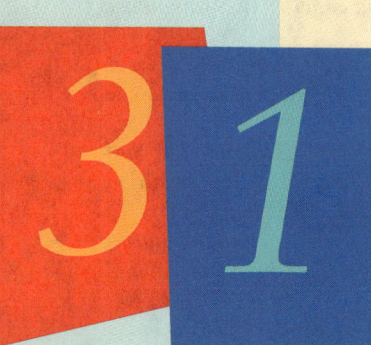

Chapter Outline

Structure and Function of the Musculoskeletal System
    The Skeletal System
    Joints
    Cranial Structures
    Major Skeletal Structures and Their Movements
    The Muscular System
Common Musculoskeletal Disorders
    Sprains
    Dislocations
    Fractures
    Abnormal Spinal Curvatures
    Herniated Intervertebral Disk
    Rotator Cuff Injury
    Adhesive Capsulitis (Frozen Shoulder)
    Bursitis
    Tendinitis
    Lateral Epicondylitis (Tennis Elbow)
    Carpal Tunnel Syndrome
    Dupuytren's Contracture
    Chondromalacia Patella

    Plantar Fasciitis
    Foot Deformities
    Gout
    Osteoarthritis
    Rheumatoid Arthritis
    Muscular Dystrophy
    Osteoporosis
    Bone Tumors
Common Diagnostic Procedures
    Physical Examination
    Diagnostic Studies
Ambulatory Aids and the Medical Assistant's Role
    Crutches
    Procedure: Measuring a Patient for Axillary Crutches
    Procedure: Teaching a Patient Crutch Gaits
    Canes
    Walkers
Summary
Critical Thinking Challenges
Answers to Checkpoint Questions
Suggestions for Further Reading

DACUM Components

1.3   Practice within the scope of education, training, and personal capabilities
1.6   Conduct oneself in a courteous and diplomatic manner
2.2   Treat all patients with empathy and impartiality
4.8   Assist physician with examinations and treatments
7.2   Instruct patients with special needs

Chapter Competencies

Learning Objectives

Upon successfully completing this chapter, you will be able to:

1. Spell and define the Key Terms.
2. Describe the structure and function of the skeletal and muscular systems.
3. Identify the axial and appendicular skeletons.
4. List and describe the five types of bones.
5. Describe the curves of the spinal column using the appropriate terminology.
6. Explain the role of the intervertebral disks.
7. Name the three types of joints and give examples of each.
8. Name and locate the major muscles of the body.
9. List and describe types of fractures.
10. List and describe disorders of the musculoskeletal system.
11. Identify and explain diagnostic procedures of the musculoskeletal system.
12. List and describe types of ambulatory aids.

Performance Objectives

Upon successfully completing this chapter, you will be able to:

1. Prepare a patient for casting.
2. Assist the physician with cast application.
3. Apply a triangular arm sling.
4. Measure a patient for axillary crutches (Procedure 31-1).
5. Instruct a patient in the use of various crutch gaits (Procedure 31-2).

Key Terms

(See Glossary for definitions.)

amphiarthroses
ankylosing
   spondylitis
antagonist
appendicular
   skeleton
arthrogram
arthroplasty
axial skeleton
bursae
callus
cancellous
contracture
contusion
diarthroses
electromyography

embolus
epiphyseal end
   plate
fixator
goniometer
insertion
interosseus
   membrane
intrinsic
iontophoresis
kyphosis
ligament
lordosis
meniscus
myofibrils
olecranon fossa

olecranon process
origin
Paget's disease
phonophoresis
prime mover
prosthesis
reduction
scoliosis
sesamoid
striated
synarthroses
synergist
tendons
tonus

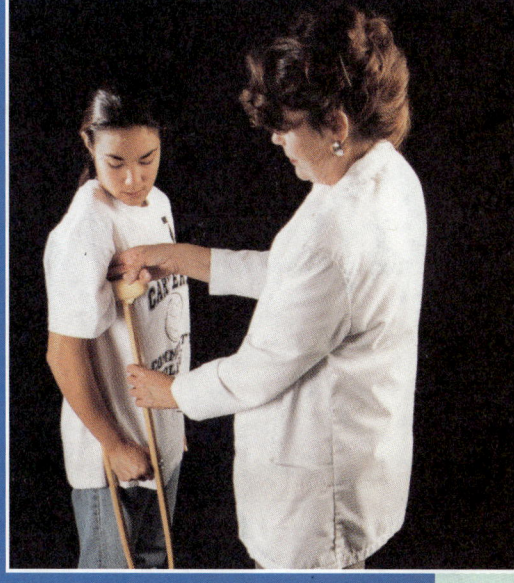

Muscles allow movement of the body parts through contraction and relaxation. Bones provide the framework on which muscles and their supporting structures are attached. Because both systems depend on each other to function, they are often referred to as a single system—the musculoskeletal system. The integrity of the entire system is required for normal body movement.

➤ STRUCTURE AND FUNCTION OF THE MUSCULOSKELETAL SYSTEM

The Skeletal System

The adult human has 206 named bones. These bones are grouped into two distinct structures known as the **axial skeleton** and the **appendicular skeleton** (Fig. 31-1). The axial skeleton—consisting of the 80 bones of the head,

thorax, and trunk—is a fairly rigid structure that supports and connects the two halves of the body. It includes the skull, the vertebral column, the thorax, and the hyoid bone. There are no long or short bones in the axial skeleton (see "Types of Bones," below).

The appendicular skeleton consists of the remaining 126 bones and provides a freely movable frame for the arms and legs. It includes the shoulder and pelvic girdles and all the bones of the arms, wrists, hands, thighs, legs, and feet. There are no irregular bones in the appendicular skeleton (see "Types of Bones," below). Fractures are more common in the appendicular skeleton; however, they are more serious in the axial skeleton (see "Common Musculoskeletal Disorders," below).

Types of Bones

The skeletal system consists of five types of bones: long, short, flat, **sesamoid**, and irregular.

Long bones are the largest bones in the body and make up most of the appendicular skeleton. Their length is greater than their width. These bones are tubular shaped with bulbous ends. The humerus and femur are long bones.

Short bones, unlike long bones, are generally more equal in height, length, and width. They usually articulate (join or attach) with more than one bone. The wrist and ankle bones are short bones.

Flat bones are thin bones with broad surfaces. Despite their name, these bones are more curved than flat. The scapula and ilium are flat bones.

Sesamoid bones are small bones that develop within **tendons** (tough, flexible fibers that bind muscle to bone), protecting them from undue wear and tear. They also change a tendon's angle of attachment to increase the leverage of the muscle force. The patella is a sesamoid bone.

Irregular bones are of mixed shapes and varieties that do not fit into the other categories. Vertebrae are classified as irregular bones.

Bone Structure

Bone is the hardest of all living tissue. Because bones are made up of different types of tissue, they are considered organs. Bone is composed of one-third organic (living) material, which provides elasticity and allows for partial deformation to help distribute forces, and two-thirds inorganic (nonliving) material, which provides strength and hardness.

Bone strength and integrity are maintained by a complex system that rebuilds osteocytes (bone cells) as they age and weaken. Osteoclasts are specialized cells that break down nonfunctional osteocytes and recycle

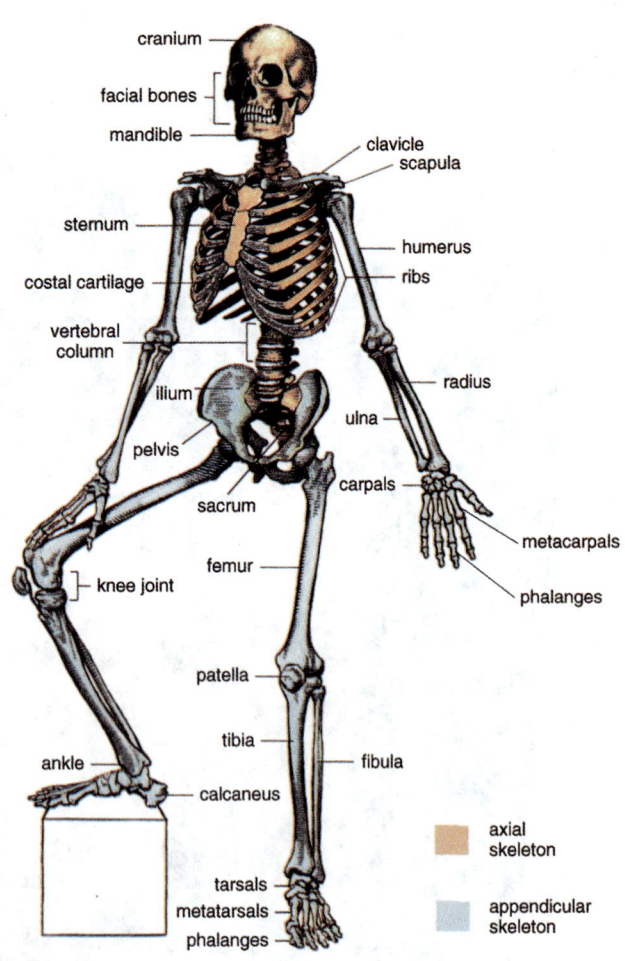

FIGURE 31-1
The skeleton.

cranium
facial bones
mandible
clavicle
scapula
sternum
humerus
costal cartilage
ribs
vertebral column
ilium
radius
pelvis
ulna
sacrum
carpals
femur
metacarpals
knee joint
phalanges
patella
tibia
ankle
fibula
calcaneus
axial skeleton
appendicular skeleton
tarsals
metatarsals
phalanges

the reusable components to rebuild new osteoblasts, the embryonic cells that will become mature osteocytes. Healthy bones are constantly removing old bone cells and building new ones.

Bone is either compact or **cancellous**. Compact bone is hard and dense and makes up the outer shell. Cancellous bone, which is porous and spongy, makes up the inside portion—a lattice-work space filled with marrow. Yellow marrow consists of fat cells and connective tissue. Red marrow fosters the production of blood cells.

Blood cell production occurs primarily in the epiphysis. The epiphysis is located at each end of a long bone; it is wider than the shaft (Fig. 31-2). Bones grow by producing new bone at the **epiphyseal end plate**. In children, this plate is easily seen on x-ray. It is not seen in adults, however, indicating that growth has stopped. If injury occurs at the epiphyseal end plate during the growth years, the bone may no longer grow causing one limb to be shorter than the other.

The diaphysis is the shaft of the long bone. It is composed mainly of compact bone, making it very hard and strong. Its hollow center, called the medullary canal, lightens the weight of the bone. It contains yellow marrow and the blood vessels that supply the bone with nutrients. The metaphysis is the flared end of the diaphysis. It is mostly cancellous bone and supports the epiphysis.

Bones are covered by a tough fibrous layer called the periosteum. It is the life support system for the bone, providing the cells that form new bone after a fracture. It is well supplied with sensory nerves, which is the reason damage to a bone is so painful. Bones have a great capacity for healing themselves, more so than most other body structures.

Bones have various projections and depressions that serve various purposes. Table 31-1 describes the main bony landmarks and features.

Bone Function

Bones support the body and act in response to the contraction of skeletal muscles, making movement possible.

Their overall functions include:

- Providing a supportive framework for the body
- Providing leverage for muscles
- Protecting vital organs
- Allowing for calcium metabolism and storage
- Facilitating blood cell production

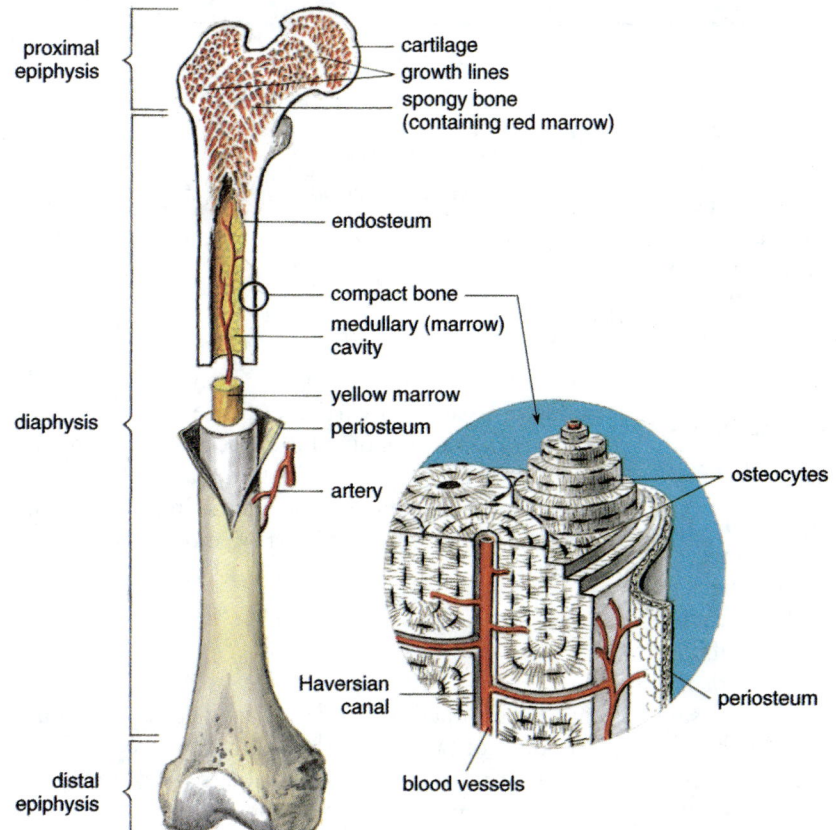

proximal
epiphysis

cartilage
growth lines
spongy bone
(containing red marrow)

endosteum

compact bone
medullary (marrow)
cavity

yellow marrow
periosteum

diaphysis

artery

osteocytes

Haversian
canal

periosteum

distal
epiphysis

blood vessels

FIGURE 31-2
The structure of a long bone; the composition of compact bone.

Table 31-1	
Bony Landmarks and Features	
Bones are marked with various projections and depressions that serve a multitude of purposes. The main landmarks and features are listed below.	
Landmark	*Features*
Condyle	A rounded projection on a bone that anchors ligaments and articulates with adjoining bones (eg, the olecranon condyle that fits into the olecranon fossa at the elbow to allow the forearm to straighten)
Crest	A ridge or long projection on a bone (eg, the iliac crest)
Epicondyle	A projection on a bone above the condyle (eg, the medial and lateral epicondyles at the elbow)
Facet	A smooth surface for articulation (eg, the facets of the vertebrae)
Foramen	An opening into a bone (or any body structure) as a passageway (eg, the foramen magnum at the base of the skull for the passage of the spinal cord)
Fossa	A hollow or depression in a bone, usually for the articulation of another bone (eg, the olecranon fossa that receives the olecranon process of the ulna to allow the forearm to straighten)
Head	The topmost part of a structure, the proximal end of a bone (eg, the head of the femur)
Neck	A constricted section, usually just below the head of a body part or a bone (eg, the neck of the femur)
Process	A projection or natural outgrowth of bone (eg, the acromion process)
Sinus	A hollow space within a bone; may serve to make the bone lighter (eg, the paranasal sinuses)
Spine	A sharp, bony process (eg, the sharp dorsal projection on a vertebra)
Suture	Union between nonmovable articulations (eg, the cranial sutures)
Tubercle	A small elevation on bone, usually for the attachment of muscles (eg, the greater tubercle of the humerus)
Tuberosity	Another name for a tubercle (eg, tibial tuberosity)

All bones have particular functions. For example, the skull protects the brain and is a framework for the face. The ribs and sternum support the chest wall and protect the contents of the thorax. The scapula (shoulder blade) is joined to the humerus, the longest bone in the arm, which is attached at the elbow to the radius and the ulna (bones of the forearm). The wrist has eight carpal bones that attach to the metacarpals (bones of the hand), which attach to phalanges (bones of the fingers). All of these bones are necessary for the many movements involving the hands and arms.

The ilium and the ischium are the major bones of the pelvis. The femur (thigh bone) is the longest, strongest, and heaviest bone in the body. It attaches to the tibia, the longer bone of the lower leg. The patella (kneecap) covers this joint and protects it. The fibula articulates with the tibia and, at its distal end, forms the lateral ankle bone. The foot has seven tarsal bones, five metatarsal bones, and the toes, which are called the phalanges (like the fingers). All of these bones work together to keep us upright and give us mobility.

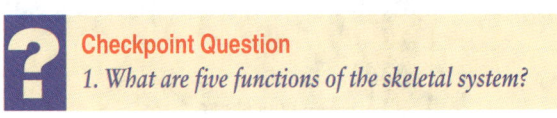

Checkpoint Question
1. What are five functions of the skeletal system?

Joints

Joints hold the bones together. They are formed by connective tissue and cartilage, dense fibrous connective tissue that is capable of great tension and pressure (Box 31-1). In some joints, the bones are held together so tightly that little movement occurs. In those joints in which the bones are held loosely, more movement is possible.

Types of Joints

Joints are grouped into three main types, according to the amount of movement they allow.

Synarthroses are immovable joints. They are formed by the direct union of bone to bone by dense fibrous tissue. Examples are the skull joints.

BOX 31-1   Types of Cartilage

- *Hyaline cartilage* is articular cartilage, covering the ends of opposing bones. It has no blood supply and gets its nutrients from the synovial fluid. It cannot heal itself when damaged.
- *Fibrocartilage* functions as a shock absorber and fills the gap between two bones. In the knee, it is called the meniscus; in the shoulder, the labrum.
- *Elastic cartilage* allows for specific movements. In the symphysis pubis it allows for birth, and in the larynx its motion is important for speech.

Amphiarthroses, slightly movable joints, are formed when two bones are joined directly by fibrocartilage or hyaline cartilage. Examples are the symphysis pubis and sacroiliac joint. Synarthrotic and amphiarthrotic joints function primarily to provide stability.

Diarthroses, or synovial joints, allow the bones to move freely in relation to one another because no structures directly connect the two bony surfaces (Table 31-2). The bones are connected indirectly to each other by **ligaments** that form a joint. Synovial joints make up the majority of the joints of the body. Examples include the shoulder, elbow, and knee.

The cavity of a synovial joint is filled with synovial fluid, which lubricates the joint, absorbs shock, reduces friction between the bones, and allows free, painless movement. It also nourishes the cartilage. The joint is surrounded by a capsule consisting of strong fibrous tissue that holds the joint together. The articular surface is smooth and covered with cartilage. The bones are held together and supported by ligaments; these are flexible but not elastic. The flexibility allows movement, and the absence of elasticity provides protection for the joint.

Bursae are small, padlike sacs that surround some joints. They are filled with a clear synovial fluid. Bursae are found in areas of excessive friction, such as under tendons and over bony prominences. Their primary purposes are to reduce friction between moving parts and to help to prevent damage.

Joint Movement

The body is constantly moving and changing position. Movement in a joint occurs in a plane around an axis. The body has three planes—sagittal, frontal, and transverse—in which activity occurs. (See Chap. 29, Introduction to Anatomy and Physiology, for a discussion of body planes.) Various joint motions are described below and illustrated in Fig. 31-3.

In the sagittal plane:

- Flexion—bending one bone on another, causing a decrease in the angle of the joint (eg, bending the elbow or the knee)
- Extension—straightening the joint, causing an increase in the joint angle. Extension usually returns the part of the body to the anatomic position.
- Hyperextension—straightening the body part beyond the anatomic position (eg, bending backward or raising the leg behind oneself)

In the frontal plane:

- Abduction—movement away from the midline of the body
- Adduction—movement toward the midline of the body

In the transverse plane:

- Rotation—movement around a fixed point. Internal or medial rotation occurs when the ball in a ball-and-socket joint moves into the joint (eg, reaching into one's back pocket). External or lateral rotation occurs when the ball moves back and away from the joint (eg, patting the back of the head). Internal and external rotation occur only in the shoulder and hip joint.

Circumduction combines all the movements, causing the distal end of the extremity to make a wide circle while the proximal end makes a small circle (eg, arm movements in swimming).

Some movements are specific to certain joints. For example, supination of the forearm occurs when the palms are turned up toward the face. Conversely, pronation occurs when the palms are turned down and away. Inversion occurs, for instance, when the foot is turned inward at the ankle so that the bottom of the big toe can be seen. Eversion is movement in the opposite direction. Dorsiflexion usually involves the foot or hand and describes a movement that shortens the angle at the back of the hand or top of the foot so that they point upward. The opposite is plantar flexion, which shortens the angle between the palm and the wrist, or pulls the foot downward to point the toes.

Range of Motion

Normal range of motion is the amount of motion possible in a joint within the limits of its anatomic structure. Many conditions can affect joint range, such as degenerative changes, injury, inflammation, disease, fractures, tumors, dislocations, nerve damage, deformities, and congenital anomalies (birth defects). When joint motion is limited, the joint is hypomobile. If

Table 31-2
Types of Joints

Type	Description	Movement	Examples
Fibrous (immovable)	No synovial cavity Bones held together by fibrous tissue	No motion, or "give" only	Bones of skull fitted together with teethlike projections (sutures), roots of teeth in sockets of the maxillae and mandible
Cartilaginous (slightly movable)	No synovial cavity Bones held together by cartilage	Slight degree of flexibility	Intervertebral joints, costal cartilage, attachments of first 10 ribs to sternum, symphysis pubis
Synovial (freely movable) Gliding	Synovial cavity and articular cartilage present One bone slides over another Surrounding structures restrict the motion	Freely movable Gliding motion without any angular or circular movements	Types of synovial joints listed below Joints between carpal bones, tarsal bones, the sternum and clavicle, and the scapula and clavicle
Hinge	Spool-shaped process fits into concave socket	Motion like a door on a hinge; permits flexion and extension	Finger, elbow, and knee
Pivot	Arch-shaped process fits around peglike process	Motion like turning a doorknob; permits rotation	Joint between the first and second cervical vertebrae allows rotation of the head from side to side; joint between the head of the radius notch of the ulna allows for supination and pronation of the palms
Condyloid	Oval-shaped condyle of one bone fits into an elliptical cavity of another bone	Allows motion in two planes at right angles, permits flexion, extension in one plane, abduction, adduction in another plane	Radiocarpal joint of wrist
	Articular surface of one bone is saddle-shaped and the articular surface of the other bone is shaped like a rider sitting in the saddle	Movements are side to side and back and forth; permits flexion, extension, abduction, adduction	Carpometacarpal joint of thumb, ankle
Ball-and-socket Ball-and-socket	Ball-like surface of one bone fitted into a cuplike depression of another bone	Rotating motions; permits widest range of motion: flexion, extension, abduction, adduction, rotation, circumduction	Shoulder and hip joints

From Jones, S. A., Weigel, A., White, R. D., McSwain, N. E., Breiter, M. (1992). Advanced Emergency Care for Paramedic Practice. *Philadelphia: J.B. Lippincott; p. 364.*

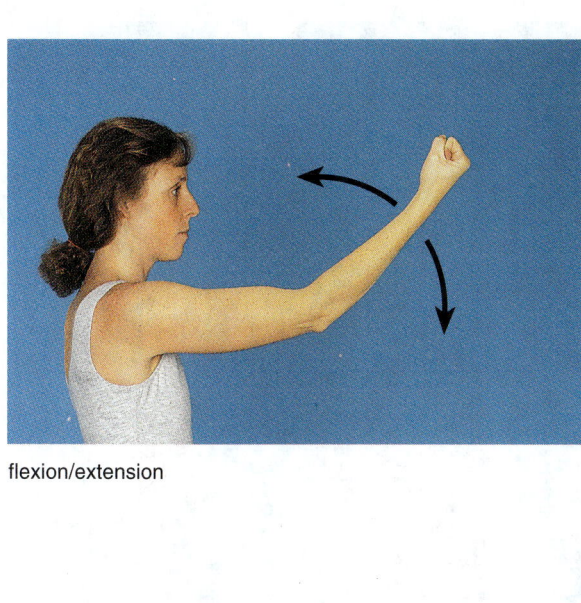

flexion/extension

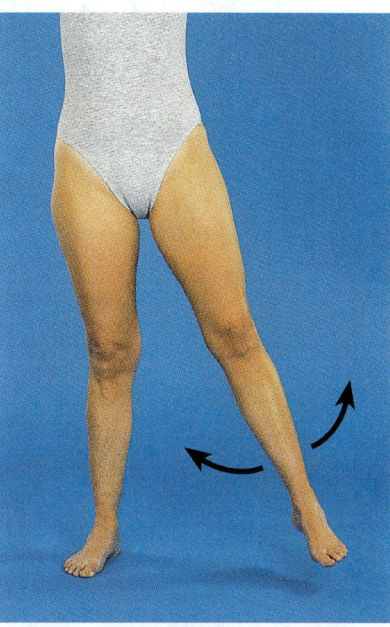

abduction/adduction

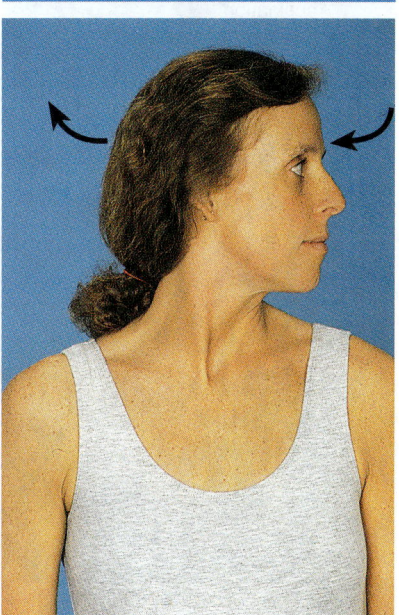

circumduction

rotation

FIGURE 31-3
Normal range of motion of selected joints.

movement is loose or greater than normal, the joint is hypermobile and is usually unstable.

The more complex the joint, the more likely it is to be affected by injury, degenerative processes, and disease. Anything that alters or disturbs the function of a specific part of a joint can eventually affect every part of the joint itself and its surrounding structures.

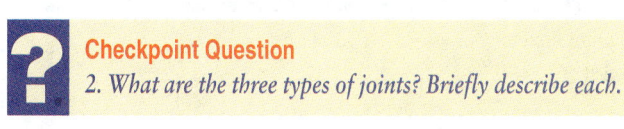

Checkpoint Question
2. What are the three types of joints? Briefly describe each.

Cranial Structures

The skull is considered to be two structures: the facial bones and the cranium.

The facial bones form the framework to give the face its shape. The *mandible*, the only movable bone in the skull, hinges at the temporomandibular joint (TMJ), forms the lower jaw, and holds our lower teeth (Fig. 31-4). The *maxillae* are two fused bones in the upper jaw that hold the upper teeth and form the anterior hard palate. The two *palatine* bones form the posterior hard palate. If the maxillae and palatine bones

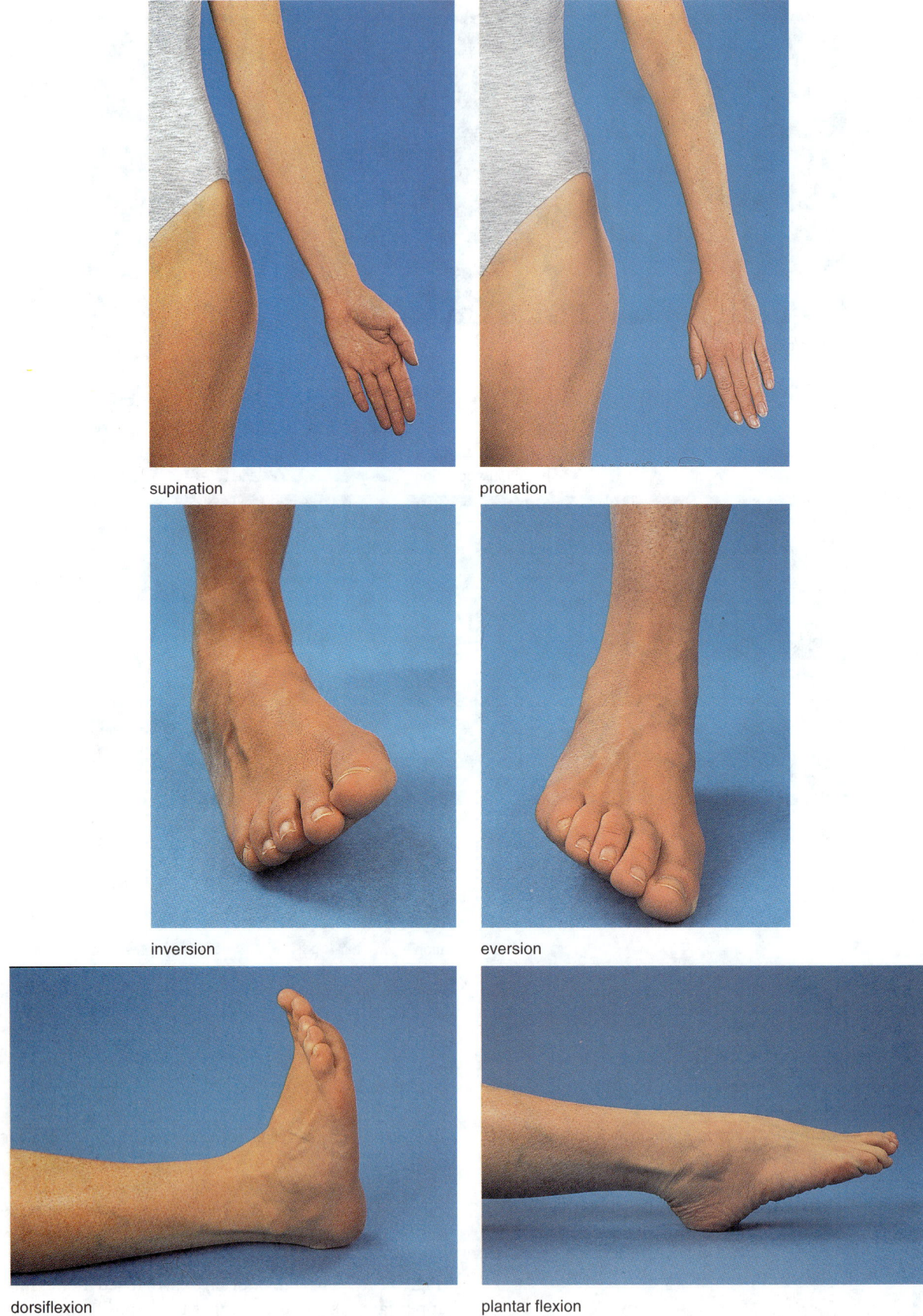

supination

pronation

inversion

eversion

dorsiflexion

plantar flexion

FIGURE 31-3 *(Continued)*

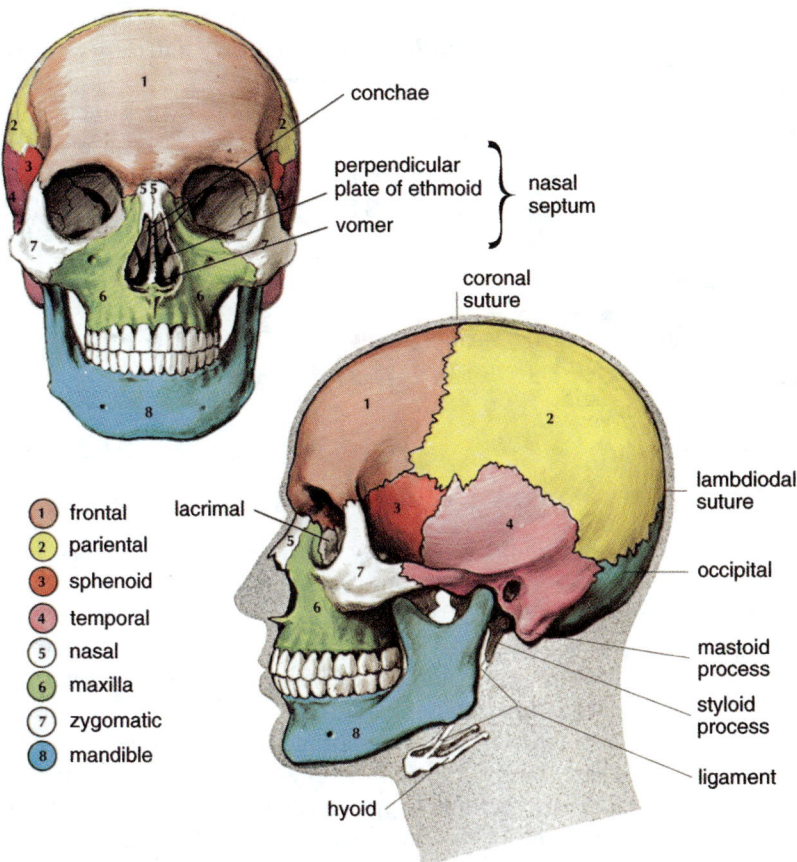

FIGURE 31-4
The skull, from the front and from the left.

fail to fuse in the fetus, a cleft palate or hare lip will result, depending on the severity of the defect. The maxillae contain the maxillary sinuses. The *nasal* bones form the bridge of the nose and the *vomer* supports the lower nasal septum. The *zygomatic* bones are referred to as the cheekbones. On the lateral walls of the nasal cavity are the *conchae* (also part of the ethmoid bone in the cranium). When covered with mucous membrane, these structures are called the turbinates and are part of the respiratory system. Part of the medial eye socket is formed by the *lacrimal* bone that contains a channel for the tear duct to drain into the nasal cavity. The *hyoid* bone is considered part of the skull but joins with no other bone and is supported by the posterior attachment of the tongue.

The bones of the cranium form the floor of the brain pan and the protective outer structure of the skull. The forehead is formed by the *frontal* bone and contains the frontal sinuses. The *parietal* bones extend across the top and down the sides of the cranium. The *temporal* bones meet the parietal bones at the sides of the cranium and continue to enclose part of the base of the brain. Each contains a mastoid sinus and the structures of the ear (see Chap. 33, Caring for Patients With Sensory Disorders). The *ethmoid* bone encloses the medial eye socket, part of the nasal cavity and, with the *sphenoid* bone, forms part of the base of cranium.

The *occipital* bone is at the back of the skull and extends anteriorly to include part of the base. It also contains the foramen magnum, the opening through which the spinal cord and its structures exit the skull.

Major Skeletal Structures and Their Movements

The following discussion provides a description of the various joint structures and the specific kinds of movements permitted by each.

Vertebral Column (Spine)

The vertebral column (Fig. 31-5) is made up of 33 vertebrae and numerous joints. The vertebrae house the spinal cord. They are separated from each other by 23 intervertebral disks, which make up 25% of the length of the spinal column. The vertebrae and their disks absorb and transmit the shock of running, walking, and jumping and keep the spine flexible for a high degree of mobility.

The four natural curves in the spine allow for great flexibility and significantly more strength (10 times) and resilience than that of a straight rod. These include:

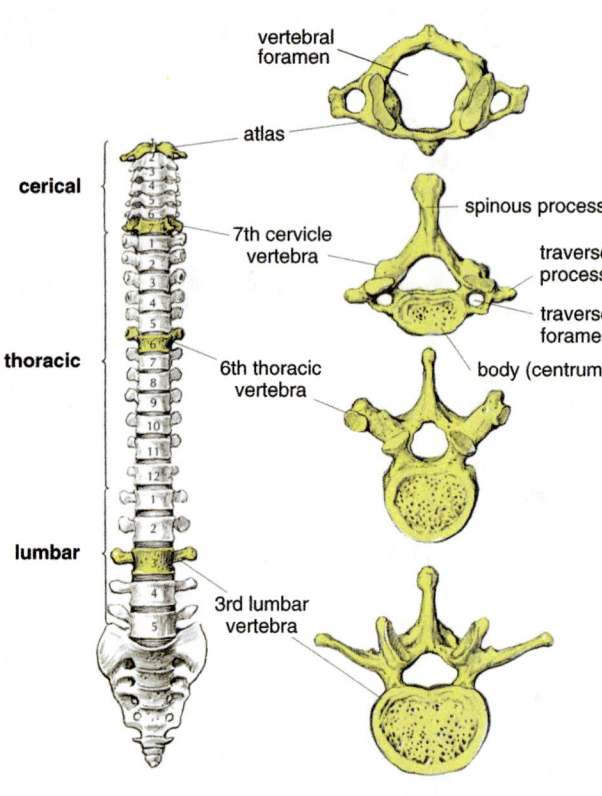

vertebral foramen

atlas

cerical

7th cervicle vertebra

spinous process

traverse process

traverse foramen

thoracic

6th thoracic vertebra

body (centrum)

lumbar

3rd lumbar vertebra

front view of vertebral column   **vertebrae from above**

FIGURE 31-5
Front view fo the vertebral column; vertebrae from above.

- Cervical curve (projects anteriorly)
- Thoracic curve (projects posteriorly)
- Lumbar curve (projects anteriorly)
- Sacral curve (projects posteriorly)

One of the most important spinal joints involved for mobility is the facet joint. It is the point of posterior articulation between the vertebrae above and below. Each vertebra moves through four facet joints. The alignment of the facet joint determines the amount of rotation and other movements possible in the spine. Because of the shape of the facet joints, most of the flexion and extension occurs in the lumbar spine; most of the rotation and lateral side bending occurs in the thoracic spine.

Two vertebrae in the cervical spine differ from the others in shape and function. They are the first cervical (atlas) and second cervical (axis) vertebrae. The head rests on the ring-shaped atlas, which has no body or spinous process. The axis forms the pivot on which the atlas rotates. Both support the weight of the head and allow for rotation.

Many strong ligaments and structures support and protect the spine. The most important are the anterior longitudinal ligament and the posterior longitudinal ligament, which help to prevent too much forward or backward bending of the spine.

Back strains are a leading cause of work-related injury among health care professionals because of the lifting, moving, and twisting often required while caring for patients. Box 31-2 offers some tips for avoiding back strain.

? Checkpoint Question
3. What are the four natural curves of the spine?

Shoulder

The shoulder, a ball-and-socket joint, is the most mobile joint in the body, allowing movement in three planes around three axes. It is made up of the head of the humerus articulating with the glenoid fossa (hollow or depression) of the scapula. Its articulating surface is surrounded by a joint capsule that is formed by an outer fibrous membrane and an inner synovial membrane. The joint capsule, the rotator cuff muscles, and surrounding support structures provide stability to the joint. (The rotator cuff is formed by the tendons of insertion of four muscles that hold the joint surfaces together during joint motion.)

The shoulder joint is capable of many movements, including horizontal abduction, horizontal adduction, and circumduction. Because it is so mobile, it is also one of the most unstable and easily injured joints in the body.

Elbow

The elbow, a hinge joint, is made up of the articulation of the humerus with the radius (lateral) and the ulna (medial). Flexion and extension are the only movements that occur in the elbow. The elbow is prevented from more than a few degrees of hyperextension by the fit of the **olecranon process** of the ulna into the **olecranon fossa** of the humerus. The radius and the ulna articulate at both the proximal and distal ends. These pivot joints allow pronation and supination of the forearm as the radius pivots around the ulna. Ligaments and **interosseous membranes** help to stabilize and reinforce these joints.

Wrist

The complex structure of the wrist allows for flexion, extension, ulnar deviation, radial deviation, and a combination of all these movements known as circum-

BOX 31-2   Avoiding Back Strain

You can prevent back strain by using good body mechanics.

- When lifting a heavy object, keep the object close to your body. Never lift an object with extended arms.
- Never lift and twist at the same time. Lift the object, then reposition your feet by pivoting or taking two steps to turn.
- Learn the proper methods for transferring patients in and out of wheelchairs, stretchers, and examining tables.
- Bend your knees, not your back, when lifting.
- Ask for assistance from coworkers when you must lift or move obese patients or heavy objects.
- Maintain proper posture at all times; slouching causes muscle strain.
- Learn to use mechanical lifting devices, such as the Hoyer lift.

If you do sustain an injury at work, inform your supervisor immediately and document what happened. Complete an incident report in accordance with the facility's policy.

duction. Rotation does not occur at the wrist. The midcarpal joints allow gliding motions and aid wrist movement. The wrist is supported by ligaments and a joint capsule. The structures of the palm are protected by the palmar fascia. The flexor muscles generally originate on the medial epicondyle and the extensors on the lateral epicondyle of the humerus. They insert on the metacarpals.

Hand

The hand performs the most intricate and specialized movements of the musculoskeletal system. Because the hand is the most significant point of function for the arm, all other joints of the upper extremity function mainly to place the hand in the many diverse positions necessary for it to accomplish its intended activities.

The thumb, the first digit, accounts for 50% of hand function. Its actions occur in different planes than do other joints. The thumb's carpal-metacarpal joint is a saddle-shaped joint that allows flexion, extension, abduction, adduction, opposition, and reposition. The fingers, the second through fifth digits, have four joints each. The carpal-metacarpal joints provide stability for the fingers. The metacarpal-phalangeal joints (knuckles) allow for flexion, extension, abduction, and adduction. The proximal interphalangeal joints and the distal interphalangeal joints can only flex and extend.

The thumb is shorter than the fingers because it has only three joints; however, this allows for greater function with opposition (touching the thumb to the little finger). It also allows the hand to grasp.

The muscles that control the precision movements and fine motor activities of the hand are known as **intrinsic** muscles because they have both of their attachments, origin and insertion, in the hand.

Hip

The hip, a ball-and-socket joint, is important for weight bearing and walking. Like the shoulder, it allows for flexion, extension, abduction, adduction, rotation, and circumduction. Unlike the shoulder, however, it is stable but not nearly as flexible.

The acetabulum is the socket of the hip joint. It receives the ball of the femur and is surrounded by a cylindrical joint capsule. The joint is strong and stable because the acetabulum is deep enough to hold most of the femoral head and is surrounded by three strong ligaments, the most important of which is the iliofemoral ligament. This ligament splits into two parts and is commonly known as the "Y" ligament. A person can maintain the upright position without using any muscles by thrusting the hips forward and resting on the Y ligaments. In this way, it is possible for an individual with paraplegia (paralysis of both lower extremities) to maintain the standing position using long leg braces.

The remaining structures of the pelvis include the *ilium*, the upper flared portion; the *ischium*, the posterior base of the pelvis; the *pubis*, the anterior portion fused with cartilage; and the *sacrum*, which is considered part of the vertebral column.

Knee

The largest joint in the body, the hinged knee joint allows for flexion and extension. It also has a rotational component that is caused by a small amount of rotation of the femur on the tibia and vice versa. "Locking" the knee into extension allows one to stand for long periods without using the muscles.

The patella is an integral part of the knee joint. It lies inside the quadriceps tendon and primarily protects the joint and increases the mechanism by which the quadriceps muscles facilitate lower leg movement.

Two important sets of ligaments stabilize the knee joint. These are the collateral and the cruciate ligaments. The medial and lateral collateral ligaments attach to both sides of the knee and support the sides of the joint. The long, cylindrical, lateral collateral ligament is strong and not easily injured; however, injuries to the broad, flat, medial collateral ligament are common. The cruciate ligaments are located inside the joint capsule and cross obliquely front to back (anterior cruciate) and back to front (posterior cruciate).

Because many tendons surround the knee, there are 13 bursae whose primary purpose is to reduce friction. The surface directly behind the knee is known as the popliteal space through which the arteries and nerves pass. The major muscles of support for the knee are the quadriceps (knee extension), hamstrings (knee flexion), and gastrocnemius muscles (calf muscle). The latter combines with the soleus muscle to form a common tendon known as the Achilles tendon, which attaches on the heel bone (calcaneus). These serve to point the toes downward and help to propel the body forward while walking.

The knee joint is often injured because it is supported entirely by muscles and ligaments and has no bony stability. It is also one of the most stressed joints because it lies between the two longest bones in the body.

Ankle and Foot

The only true weight-bearing bone of the ankle is the tibia. It is the larger of the two bones of the lower leg and is medial to the fibula. The ends of the bones are called the medial and lateral malleoli (ankle bones). The muscles in the foot and ankle allow for dorsiflexion and plantar flexion.

Weakness of these muscles, especially the tibialis anterior muscle, results in foot drop or a "flat, slap-footed" gait in which the person is unable to heel strike while walking and cannot clear the floor with the toes when swinging the leg forward while walking. The ankle is the most frequently injured joint in the body. The lateral ligaments are damaged more often than the medial ligaments.

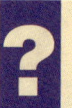

Checkpoint Question

4. What kind of joint is the knee? What are its two primary movements?

The Muscular System

Types of Muscle Tissue

Muscle tissue makes up 40% to 50% of body weight. Muscles attached to bone are usually under conscious control and are called voluntary muscles. These muscles are composed of **myofibrils**, tiny threadlike structures with dark and light bands called striations. There are three types of muscle tissue, each with its own purpose and characteristics.

STRIATED OR SKELETAL MUSCLE

Most of the body's muscles are **striated** skeletal muscles (Fig. 31-6). The striations are the light and dark muscle fibers called myosin (thick fibers) and actin (thin fibers) that slide back and forth across each other with contraction and relaxation.

Skeletal muscles are under voluntary control, are attached to bones, and facilitate movement. The muscles of the arms and legs are examples of skeletal muscles. The fibers of skeletal muscles can be aligned parallel with the line of pull, thus producing greater mobility, or they may be aligned at oblique angles for greater strength.

Very rarely does a skeletal muscle act alone. It may act as a **prime mover** at a joint or it may work in cooperation with other muscles to perform a movement (**synergist**). It may fix or stabilize a joint (**fixator**) rather than cause it to move, or it may prevent movement by opposite muscles acting on a joint (**antagonist**).

SMOOTH MUSCLE

Smooth muscles are found in the wall of the hollow organs and viscera. They are present in the blood vessels and the large lymphatic vessels. Smooth muscle is controlled by the autonomic nervous system (see Chap. 32, Caring for Patients With Neurologic Disorders). Smooth muscles act in breathing, dilating pupils, contracting the uterus during childbirth, and moving food through the intestines. They are characterized by slow, rhythmic contractions.

CARDIAC MUSCLE

Cardiac muscle is also controlled by the autonomic nervous system. In the heart these nerves regulate the activity of the specialized heart muscle, ensuring that the normal cardiac pacemaker and conductor cells

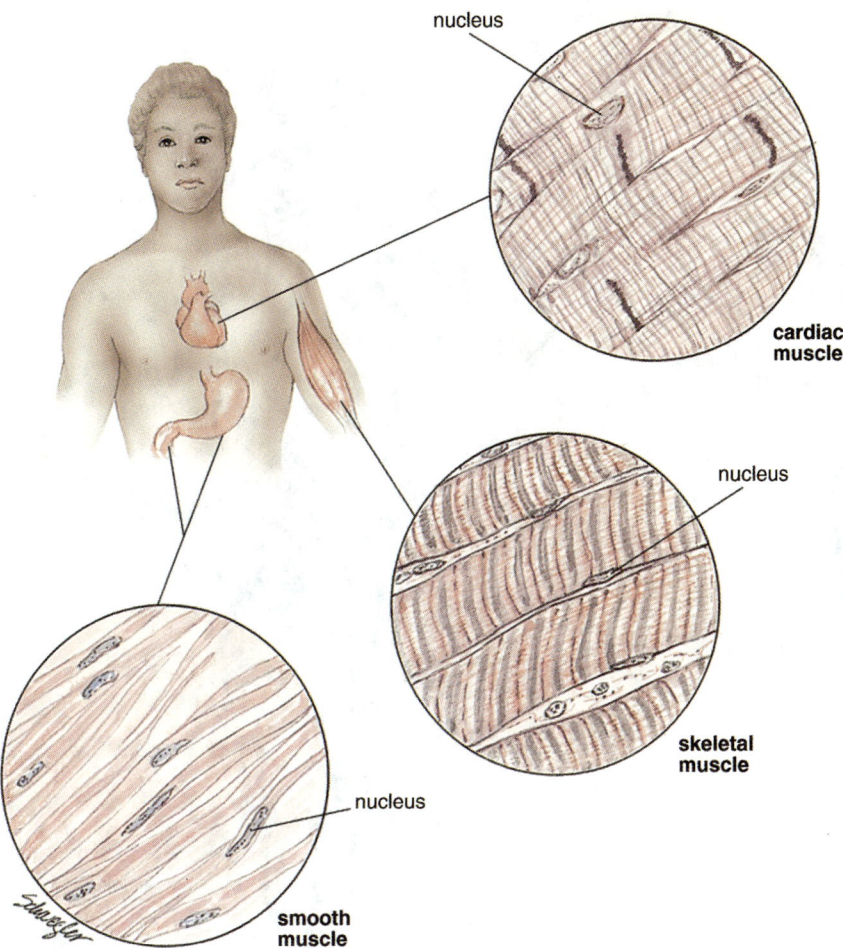

FIGURE 31-6
Muscle tissue.

keep the heart beating over 100,000 times daily. Cardiac muscle fibers make up the walls of the heart and usually do not regenerate.

Muscle Structure

Muscles are attached to bones by tendons, which aid the body's mobility and stability. If the body had no muscles, the skeleton would collapse when placed in the erect position. When muscles are unable to function due to injury or disease, a person is unable to stand or walk independently. Figure 31-7 provides an anterior and posterior view of the muscles of the body.

Tendons begin within the muscles as part of the connective tissue surrounding individual muscle fibers. They extend and join to become the tough, flexible fibers that bind the whole muscle mass to its accompanying bone. Tendons can be cylindrical or flattened. Some tendons are encased in heavy fibrous sheaths for protection if they are subject to friction or pressure, such as when they

pass between muscles, between bones, or through tunnels between bones. A broad tendinous sheet that attaches some muscles to bone is called an aponeurosis. The abdominal muscles, which arise from both sides of the body and attach to the midline where there are no bones, are attached to an aponeurosis called the linea alba (white line). The umbilicus lies within the linea alba.

Checkpoint Question

5. What connects muscle to bone? What connects bone to bone?

Muscle Function

Muscle tissue has four unique important properties:

- Irritability—the ability to respond to stimulus
- Contractibility—the ability to shorten

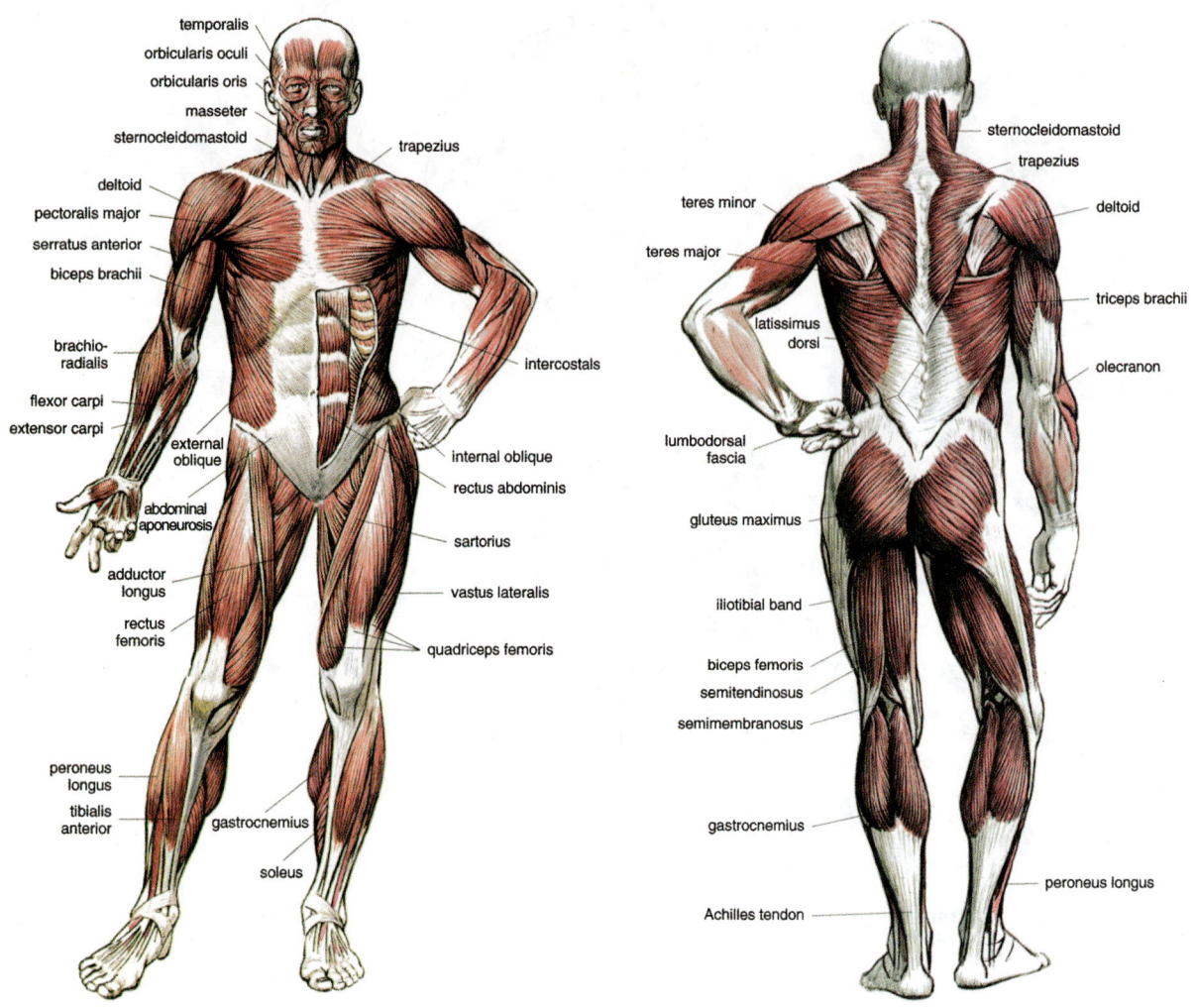

FIGURE 31-7

Muscles of the body. (*A*) Anterior (front) view. (*B*) Posterior (back) view.

- Extensibility—the ability to lengthen or stretch on the application of force
- Elasticity—the ability to return to its normal length when the shortening or stretching force is removed

Muscles function by contracting and relaxing. Their function depends on their bony attachments, arising from one bone and inserting on another, usually crossing one or more joints. The end of the muscle that stays relatively fixed is said to be the **origin** of the muscle. The more movable end is the **insertion** of the muscle.

Muscles are capable of shortening to flex their bony attachments or may be stretched to extend these attachments. The force built up within a muscle is referred to as tension, which is required for a muscle to contract. The general steady, partial contraction of skeletal muscles, called **tonus**, helps us to remain upright and is maintained by an intact neurologic system. If the stimulus is disrupted, as in paralysis, the tension in the unaffected muscles will pull the body toward the unaffected side.

Muscles are complex and more adaptable than joints. A joint can be replaced, but no replacement for muscles has been found. The characteristics of a muscle can change in response to the demands placed on it. For example, weight lifting results in increased muscle size, whereas endurance training increases the capacity of the muscles to perform for long periods of time.

Lack of use over a short period of time (as little as 3 weeks) can cause muscles to atrophy (waste away). Muscles are resilient in that they can be stretched, tightened, molded, strengthened, and enlarged.

Table 31-3 lists the muscles and their locations and functions.

➤ **COMMON MUSCULOSKELETAL DISORDERS**

Orthopedists and physical therapists specialize in treating musculoskeletal disorders and are often asked to provide appropriate treatment and rehabilitation proce-

Table 31-3
Review of Muscles

Name	Location	Function
Muscles of the Head and Neck		
Orbicularis oculi	Encircles eyelid	Closes eye
Levator palpebrae superioris	Back of orbit to upper eyelid	Opens eye
Orbicularis oris	Encircles mouth	Closes lips
Buccinator	Flesh part of cheek	Flattens cheek; helps in eating, whistling, and blowing wind instruments
Temporal	Above and near ear	Closes jaw
Masseter	At angle of jaw	Closes jaw
Sternocleidomastoid	Along side of neck, to mastoid process	Flexes head, rotates head toward opposite side from muscle
Muscles of the Upper Extremities		
Trapezius	Back of neck and upper back, to clavicle scapula	Raises shoulder and pulls it back, extends head
Latissimus dorsi	Middle and lower back, to humerus	Extends and adducts arm behind back
Pectoralis major	Upper, anterior chest, to humerus	Flexes and adducts arm across chest; pulls shoulder forward and downward
Serratus anterior	Below axilla on side of chest to scapula	Moves scapula forward; aids in raising arm
Deltoid	Covers shoulder joint, to lateral humerus	Abducts arm
Biceps brachii	Anterior arm, to radius	Flexes forearm and supinates hand
Triceps brachii	Posterior arm, to ulna	Extends forearm
Flexor and extensor carpi groups	Anterior and posterior forearm, to hand	Flex and extend hand
Flexor and extensor digitorum groups	Anterior and posterior forearm, to fingers	Flex and extend fingers
Muscles of the Trunk		
Diaphragm	Dome-shaped partition between thoracic and abdominal cavities	Dome descends to enlarge thoracic cavity from top to bottom
Intercostals	Between ribs	Elevate ribs and enlarge thoracic cavity
External and internal oblique; transversus and rectus abdominis	Anterolateral abdominal wall	Compress abdominal cavity and expel sustances from body; flex spinal column
Levator ani	Pelvic floor	Aids defecation
Sacrospinalis	Deep in back, vertical mass	Extends vertebral column to produce erect posture
Muscles of the Lower Extremities		
Gluteus maximus	Superficial buttock, to femur	Extends thigh
Gluteus medius	Deep buttock, to femur	Abducts thigh
Iliopsoas	Crosses front of hip joint, to femur	Flexes thigh
Adductor group	Medial thigh, to femur	Adducts thigh
Sartorius	Winds down thigh, ilium to tibia	Flexes thigh and leg (to sit cross-legged)
Quadriceps femoris	Anterior thigh, to tibia	Extends leg
Hamstring group	Posterior thigh, to tibia and fibula	Flexes leg
Gastrocnemius	Calf of leg, to calcaneus	Extends foot (as in tiptoeing)
Tibialis anterior	Anterior and lateral shin, to foot	Dorsiflexes foot (as in walking on heels); inverts foot (sole inward)
Peroneus longus	Lateral leg, to foot	Everts foot (sole outward)
Flexor and extensor digitorum groups	Posterior and anterior leg, to toes	Flex and extend toes

From Memmler, R. L., Cohen, B. J., Wood, D. L. (1996). The Human Body in Health and Disease, 8th ed. Philadelphia: Lippincott-Raven; p. 125.

dures when a condition warrants specialized care. The most common disorders of the musculoskeletal system are sprains, dislocations, fractures, joint disruption, and degeneration. The musculoskeletal system reacts to injury or disease with pain (Box 31-3), swelling, inflammation, deformity, or limitation of range and function.

Sprains

Injury to a joint capsule and its supporting ligaments is called a sprain. (In contrast, injury to a muscle and its supporting tendons is called a strain.) Damage to muscle, ligament, or tendon fibers may result in joint instability. If the ligament is completely torn, it is unable to efficiently stabilize the joint. Common symptoms are inflammation and pain.

Applying ice at the time of injury helps reduce swelling and pain. For mild sprains, treatment includes exercise to prevent joint stiffness and muscle atrophy. Therapeutic devices and compression wraps reduce swelling. Moderate sprains must be treated with care to prevent further injury because the ligaments have been weakened. Healing takes 6 to 8 weeks. Severe sprains often require surgery and take much longer to recover.

In the spine, facet joint sprain can cause pain not only at the point of difficulty, but also radiating into an extremity (radicular pain) due to impingement on the nerve root that passes close to the joint.

In the knee, injury to the anterior cruciate ligament greatly compromises the joint's stability. The knee becomes swollen and painful, unstable, and has limited motion. Complete tears require surgery and extensive rehabilitation. This kind of injury most commonly is caused by strong, forced hyperextension of the knee. The menisci, crescent-shaped fibrocartilage located on the proximal tibia, serve primarily as shock absorbers for the knee joint. Because they have no blood supply, they cannot repair themselves and usually require arthroscopic surgery (surgery through punctures into the joint to insert a scope rather than through an incision) to remove the torn parts. The medial **meniscus** is more often injured than the lateral meniscus.

Injury to the Achilles tendon is extremely painful and limits the ability to walk. A complete tear usually requires surgery followed by immobilization.

BOX 31-3   Relieving Musculoskeletal Pain

To relieve pain in acute, soft-tissue strains, sprains, and inflammations, rest or immobilization or both may be needed. Because painful movement may cause further damage to the injured tissue, restriction of movement may also be required. This can be accomplished by bed rest and by the use of casts, braces, slings, splints, collars, Ace wraps, or corsets. If weight bearing is painful or inadvisable due to fractures or musculoskeletal pathology, ambulatory aids (eg, canes, walkers, or crutches) may be used. (See "Ambulatory Aids and the Medical Assistant's Role" for more information.)

The use of hot moist packs, heating pads, or warm baths can help increase circulation, relax spasms, or ease sore muscles. Ice packs help prevent swelling, decrease inflammation, and reduce **contusions,** which may occur when there is a direct blow on a muscle.

With contusions, the capillaries (small blood vessels) rupture and bleed into the tissue. Swelling and inflammation may result. Reduction of the bleeding is crucial and is accomplished by applying cold packs and a pressure bandage. Immobilization to prevent further injury is also important. Within a few days, pain-free exercises and heat applications should be introduced to begin the healing process.

Generally, movement should begin as soon as possible after a soft-tissue injury to maintain a healthy joint and resilient muscles. Gentle active or passive movement in the pain-free range, mild joint mobilization, traction, or exercise are effective in maintaining normal range, function, and strength.

Dislocations

Dislocation of a joint, called a luxation, occurs when the end of the bone is displaced from its articular surface. It can be caused by trauma or disease, or it may be congenital (eg, congenital hip dislocation in infants). Common sites for dislocations include the shoulders, elbows, fingers, hips, or ankles.

A subluxation is a partial dislocation in which the bone is pulled out of the socket, but all joint structures maintain their proper relationships. It can be the result of weakness, decreased muscle tone, gravity, or neurologic deficit. The muscles bear most of the responsibility for preventing subluxation. Subluxations are often seen in the weakened shoulder joints of stroke patients. In children, a common subluxation site is the elbow. The injury, termed "nursemaid's elbow," results from a sudden and forceful longitudinal pull on an extended arm. It is often caused by a parent or caregiver pulling on the child's outstretched arm. The injury is usually painless and is identified by lack of arm movement. Reductions of the elbow are usually not difficult and do not require pain medications or surgery. Parental teaching should be done in a nonjudgmental manner. Parents often feel guilty for this injury and should be consoled accordingly.

Common symptoms of dislocations include pain, pressure, limited movement, and deformity. Numbness and loss of pulse to the part can also occur. Treatment may include reduction and immobilization of the joint. The patient may be taught exercises to strengthen supporting muscles to avoid recurrences.

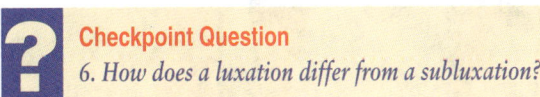

? Checkpoint Question
6. How does a luxation differ from a subluxation?

Fractures

A fracture is a break or a disruption in a bone. Causes include falls or other trauma, disease, tumors, and unusual stress. There are many types of fractures, each presenting with its own set of problems (Table 31-4). However, all fractures have one symptom in common: pain. Other manifestations include swelling, hemorrhage, lack of movement or unusual movement, contusions, and deformity of the body part involved.

Treatment involves **reduction** (correction) by placing the broken ends into proper alignment. Casting, splinting, wrapping, and taping are means of obtaining a closed reduction. If it is not possible to obtain proper alignment by a closed reduction, surgery is required and

the procedure is called an open reduction. Fractures in the shoulder joint are serious injuries because the immobilization necessary for healing causes adhesions in the capsule, resulting in a severe loss of motion and function.

Casts

Fractures must be immobilized to facilitate healing in the proper alignment. In many instances, both proximal and distal joints are included in the cast to further ensure that movement is restricted. Box 31-4 describes various types of casts. The casting material used can be either plaster or fiberglass.

The traditional *plaster* bandages are impregnated with calcium sulfate crystals and are supplied as rolls of material in widths (eg, 2–6 inches) appropriate to a variety of sites. When water is added to the dry rolls of bandage, a chemical reaction generates heat that may be uncomfortable to the patient for a short time, usually less than 30 minutes, but is necessary to produce a rigid dressing when dry. The bandage will mold smoothly to the casting site as it is applied.

The cast will be rather soft until it is fully dry, which can take as long as 72 hours. Patients must be cautioned not to exert pressure on the drying cast to avoid pressure sores from indentations. The cast must be kept dry at all times.

Because of its lighter weight, water resistance, and durability, *fiberglass* is rapidly becoming the material of choice for casting. The polyurethane additives harden in minutes, eliminating the extended drying time. After the cast has set, the material will not soften when wet but must be dried to prevent skin lesions. The fabric has a more open weave than plaster, which helps maintain skin integrity.

ASSISTING WITH CAST APPLICATION.

Position the patient comfortably before the procedure begins. Drape to expose only the part to be casted to avoid unnecessary exposure and protect other skin areas from the casting material. The part should be clean and dry; lesions, if present, should be attended and dressed appropriately before casting (see Chap. 24, Assisting With Minor Office Surgery, for the procedure for dressing a wound).

Assemble the following items:

- Tubular-shaped soft fabric stocking material large enough to encircle the limb
- Roller padding, also called sheet wadding
- Casting material
- Bucket of cool or tepid water
- Plaster or cast knife (Fig. 31-8)
- Utility gloves

text continues on page 562

Table 31-4
Types of Fractures

Type	Description
Simple or closed	A break in the bone that does not protrude through the skin. It is usually treated with a closed reduction.
Compound or open	A break in the bone in which the broken end protrudes through the skin; infection is a major concern. Surgery is often required to reduce a compound fracture.
Spiral	A fracture that occurs with torsion or twisting type injuries. It appears to be "S" shaped on x-ray.
Impacted	A fracture in which one bone segment is driven into another.
Greenstick	A common injury in children involving a partial or incomplete break in which only one side of a bone is broken like a "green stick."
Transverse	A fracture that is at right angles to the axis of the bone. It is generally caused by an excessive bending force or a direct hit on the bone.
Oblique	A fracture that is slanted across the axis of the bone.
Comminuted	A fracture occurring when a bone is fragmented, usually by a great deal of direct force. A comminuted fracture is difficult to reduce because of the many pieces of bone that must be held in proper alignment. Because it is more complicated to treat a fracture if the articular surface is involved, surgical intervention is usually required. Severe soft-tissue damage frequently accompanies this type of fracture because the force necessary to cause the fracture is so great that it causes a small explosion within the soft tissue.
Compression	Results from damage to the bone by the application of a strong force against both ends, such as a fall. Vertebrae are susceptible to compression fractures, especially in the elderly.
Depressed	A fracture of flat bones (usually the skull), causing the fragment to be driven below the surface of the bone.
Avulsion	A fracture caused by a strong force applied to the bone by the sharp, twisting-pulling motion of the attached ligaments or tendons.
Pathologic	These types of fractures are usually the result of a disease process such as osteoporosis (brittle bone), **Paget's disease** (a chronic skeletal disease in the elderly with bowing of the long bones), bone cysts, tumors, or cancer.

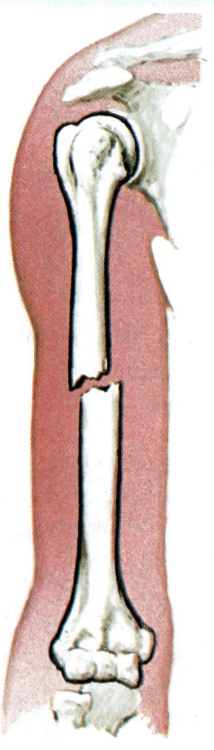

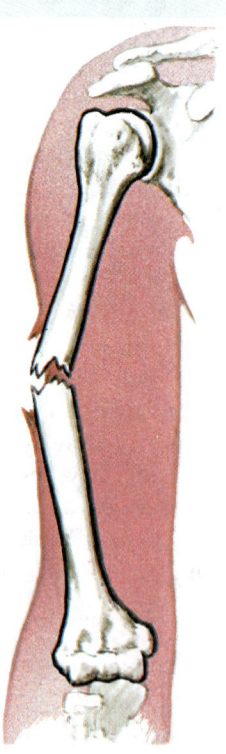
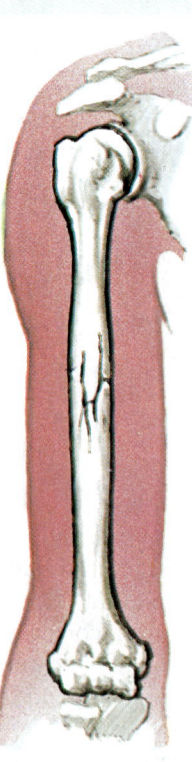
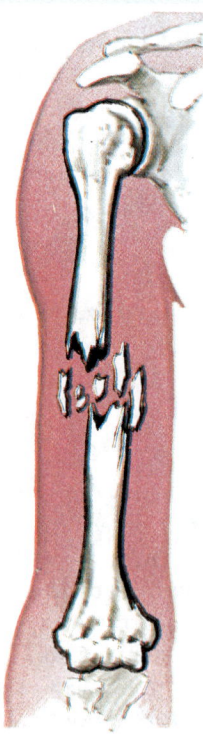

closed   open   greenstick   comminuted

Types of fractures.

(continued)

Table 31-4
Types of Fractures (Continued)

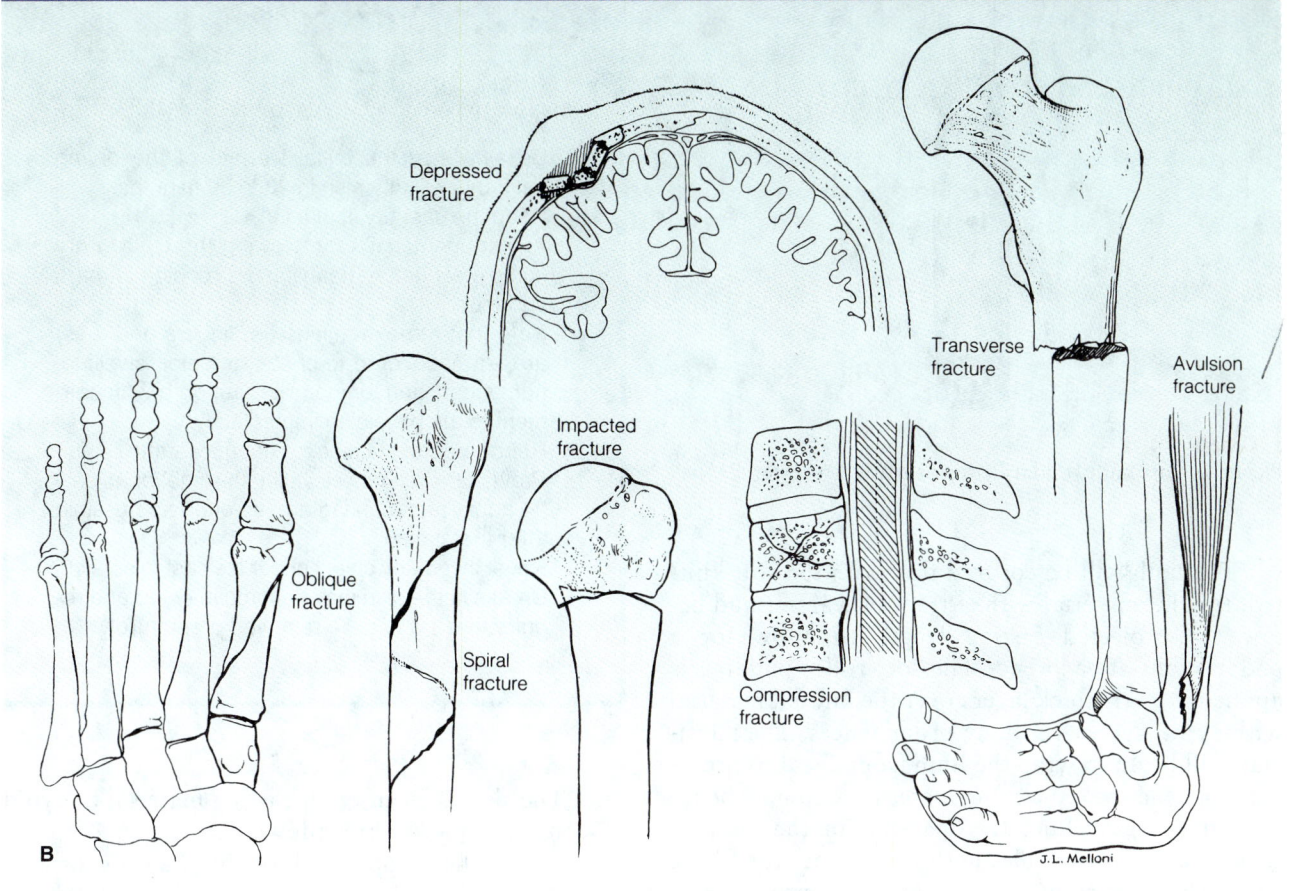

B

J. L. Melloni

**BOX
31-4   Types of Casts**

- *Short arm cast* extends from below the elbow to mid-palm.
- *Long arm cast* extends from the axilla to the mid-palm; the elbow is usually at a 90° angle.
- *Short leg cast* extends from below the knee to the toes; the foot is in a natural position.
- *Long leg cast* extends from the upper thigh to the toes; the knee is slightly flexed and the foot is in a natural position.
- *Walking cast* may be either a short leg cast or a long leg cast; the cast is extra strong to bear weight and may include a walking heel.
- *Body cast* encircles the trunk, usually from the axilla to the hip.
- *Spica cast* encircles part of the trunk and one or two extremities.

Note: Body and spica casts are not usually seen in the medical office because transporting these patients as outpatients is very difficult.

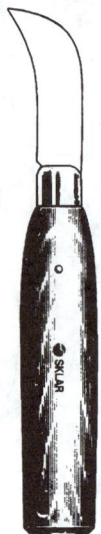

FIGURE 31-8
Plaster or cast knife. (Sklar Instruments, Westchester, PA)

The limb will be covered first with the soft knitted, tubular material with extra fabric above and below the projected casting length to allow for a padded fold at each end. The soft roller padding is applied in fairly thick layers over the knitted material with extra layers over bony prominences. The physician will begin to wrap the limb from distal to proximal with the soaked casting material. You may be responsible for soaking the material in the cool or tepid water until bubbles no longer form around the rolls. The rolls should be pressed, not wrung, until they are wet through but not dripping and should be handed to the physician as needed. Utility gloves should be worn to protect your hands from the material. When the site is adequately covered, rough edges are trimmed with the plaster knife and the knitted fabric is folded back to form cuffs at each

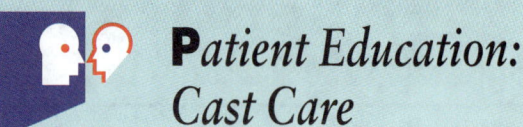

Patient Education: Cast Care

Instruct patients with casts to:

- Be aware of the initial warmth of the drying cast; this will diminish in 20 to 30 minutes.
- Keep the cast dry, if plaster.
- Avoid indentations by allowing the cast to dry completely before handling or propping on hard surfaces.
- Note that the extremities (ie, fingers and toes) are left uncovered to check for color, swelling, numbness, and temperature; report any impairment to the physician immediately.
- Report odors, staining, or undue warmth.
- Prevent swelling by elevating the limb for at least 24 hours after casting and as often as possible after that time.
- Never insert any object under the cast to scratch. Breaks in the skin may become infected and require that the cast be removed prematurely.

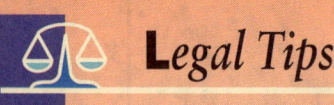

Legal Tips

Casts that are applied improperly can lead to nerve and vascular damage, resulting in permanent loss of function to the extremity. (In extreme situations, a surgical amputation may be required.) To ensure proper patient care and to avoid potential lawsuits, it is essential that distal extremity circulation be assessed and documented before and after reductions and casting.

end. The skin is cleansed of casting material to avoid discomfort and skin breakdown.

Because the unsupported weight of a short or long arm cast may put undue stress and strain on the shoulder muscles, slings are ordered to relieve and redistribute the weight. Slings are also used in situations that do not require a cast but do require that the arm be immobilized to facilitate healing. Box 31-5 describes the steps for applying a sling.

CAST REMOVAL

Cuts are made in the cast through its length on opposite sides, dividing it into halves. An electric oscillating circular saw known as a cast cutter is used. Assure the patient that this will not cut the skin. Protect your eyes from flying particles and caution the patient also. The cast will be split apart with a cast spreader. The padding will be cut with utility scissors. The patient should be warned that the skin will be pale and dry and the muscle will be wasted from disuse. The skin will be sensitive to touch and temperature. Creams and lotions will alleviate the dryness and physical therapy will restore muscle tone. (See Chap. 23, Instruments and Equipment, for illustrations of an oscillating saw, plaster shears, and a plaster spreader.)

BOX 31-5 Applying a Triangular Arm Sling

Follow these steps to apply a triangular arm sling.

1. Position the affected limb with the hand at slightly less than a 90° angle so that the fingers are a bit higher than the elbow. (This position helps reduce swelling.)
2. Place the triangle with the uppermost corner at the shoulder on the unaffected side (extend the corner across the nape), the middle angle at the elbow of the affected side, and the final lowermost corner pointing toward the foot of the unaffected side.
3. Bring up the lowermost corner to meet the upper corner at the side of the neck, *never* at the back of the neck (to avoid discomfort).
4. Tie or pin the sling. Secure the elbow by fitting any extra fabric neatly around the limb and pinning.
5. Check the patient's level of comfort and distal extremity circulation.
6. Document the appliance in the patient's chart.

Note: Fitted canvas slings with buckles or Velcro are also available.

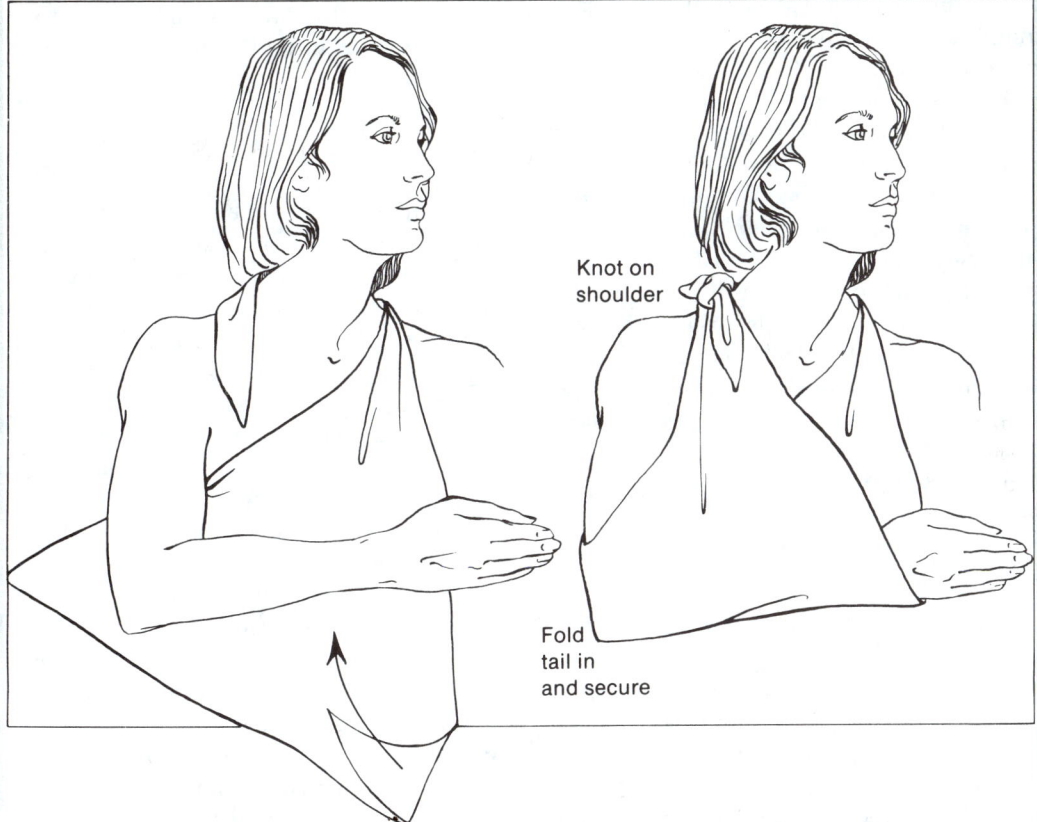

Knot on shoulder

Fold tail in and secure

Arm sling. Place one end of the triangle over the unaffected shoulder. Bring the other end of the triangle over the affected shoulder. Tie or pin the ends to one side of the neck. Fold the corner flat at the elbow and secure with safety pins.

Checkpoint Question
7. *What is the difference between an open and closed reduction?*

Healing of Fractures

The most important criterion for successful healing of a fracture is an adequate blood supply. The blood secretes an important gluelike substance known as **callus**, which is deposited around the break. Callus holds the ends of the bones together; with time the callus turns to bone. Cells mold the callus and smooth the fracture site to close to its original size. Immobilization of the fracture site allows the molding and reshaping process to occur successfully.

If the blood supply is inadequate, delayed union or nonunion may occur. If damage is sufficient (eg, soft tissue, vascular, or neurologic) or if severe trauma, disease, tumor, or complications are involved, amputation may be necessary. Amputation is a drastic measure that is performed only when all other avenues are exhausted. A **prosthesis** enables the amputee to resume functional activities such as walking, grasping, or holding.

A potentially life-threatening complication of a fracture of the long bones is a fat **embolus**, which results from the release of fat droplets from the yellow marrow of these bones. If the embolus becomes lodged in the coronary or pulmonary vessels, or in a large vessel in the brain, it can totally block the vessel causing an infarction and resulting in death. The elderly require longer periods for healing. Prosthetic joint replacements may be necessary if bone restructuring won't be adequate (Box 31-6).

What If?
What if your patient has a cervical fracture?

Fractures to the cervical spine can be life-threatening or seriously disabling. There are seven cervical vertebrae. Fractures to cervical one (C-1), the most superior vertebra, tend to be fatal unless immediately and aggressively treated by emergency services personnel before transport to a trauma center. Fractures to cervical two (C-2) and three (C-3) often result in permanent or long-term respiratory dependency. Vertebrae fractures of cervical four through seven will result in various levels of paralysis and motor impairment. If you suspect a patient has a cervical fracture or other vertebral fractures, immobilize the patient and call for emergency personnel. Never move the patient unless the patient is in immediate danger. The ambulance technicians will properly immobilize the patient for transport to a hospital where radiographic tests will diagnose the extent of the injury.

Abnormal Spinal Curvatures

Exaggerated or abnormal curvatures of the spine affect the posture and the alignment of the shoulders and hips (Box 31-7). An abnormally deep lumbar curvature is referred to as **lordosis** or swayback. Abnormal thoracic curvature, particularly the upper portion, is called **kyphosis** or hunchback. A side-to-side or lateral curve is called **scoliosis**; this is relatively common during adolescence (Fig. 31-9).

Treatment involves the use of devices (eg, braces) to assist with the straightening of the curve to a more normal position. Transcutaneous muscle stimulation devices cause the muscles on one side to contract and draw the spine into its proper position.

Herniated Intervertebral Disk

The lumbar spine is one of the most frequently injured parts of the body because it absorbs the body's full weight and the weight of anything that is carried. Because most of the movement in the lumbar spine occurs at the L-4 to L-5 and L-5 to S-1 segments, most herniated disks are seen at these levels, but injury can also occur anywhere in the spine.

A herniated disk occurs when the soft center of the disk (nucleus) ruptures through its tough outer layer to protrude into the spinal canal, sometimes pressing on the spinal cord. It is usually caused by severe trauma, degenerative changes, or strenuous strains. Common symptoms include severe back pain, numbness in the extremities, spasms, weakness, and limitation of movement. Flexion will cause pain to radiate into the extremities, and extension will be restricted and cause pain at the spinal segment. The straight leg raise test will be positive for pain at 45 degrees to 60 degrees. A flattened lumbar curve and a lateral shift are not uncommon. On x-ray, the disk space may be narrowed.

Bone strength throughout the body is diminished during periods of confinement or inactivity; therefore, total bed rest is no longer the treatment of choice for the majority of musculoskeletal disorders, including herniated disks. Activity will be limited by pain. Patients are instructed to perform simple ankle pumps and encouraged to take short walks from room to room. Therapy, traction, massage, and mild extension exercises will help

text continues on page 567

BOX
31-6 Bone Healing in the Elderly

A fracture of the femur in the elderly raises special concerns. Bone-repairing osteoblasts are less able to use calcium to restructure bone tissue at any site in the elderly, but the neck of the femur, the most common fracture site, is especially vulnerable to delayed or imperfect healing due to poor blood supply. Fractures through this area, involving the femoral head or neck or just inferior to the greater trochanter, may require hip **arthroplasty** or total hip replacement.

Hip joint replacement prostheses are usually metal or polyethylene molded to conform to the joints they are designed to replace. Total hip replacement, usually used for degenerative joint disease or rheumatoid arthritis, replaces the head and neck of the femur and the acetabular surface. Knee replacement replaces both the head of the tibia and the distal epiphysis of the femur.

Early repair and return to mobility prevents contractures and atrophy of the supporting muscles. Postoperative ambulation prevents many of the complications associated with prolonged confinement in the elderly, such as pathologic fractures, static pneumonia, and renal calculi.

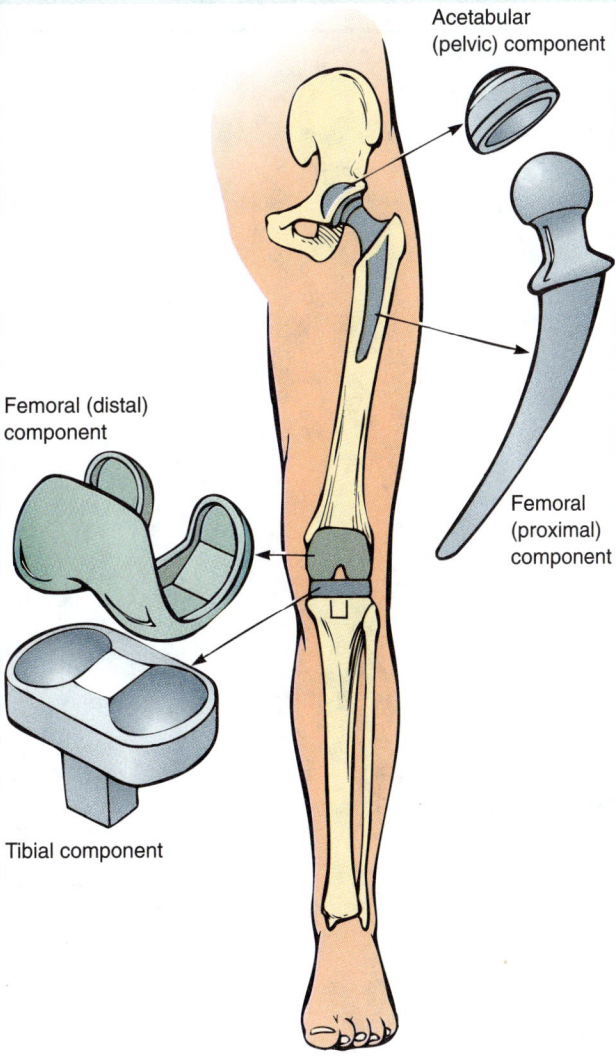

Acetabular (pelvic) component

Femoral (distal) component

Femoral (proximal) component

Tibial component

Hip and knee replacement.

BOX 31-7 Posture and Back Pain

Poor posture can lead to back pain, and pain and injury can lead to poor posture. Also, as people age, natural changes occur in the body that may affect posture. For example, the disks become less resilient and give in to forces such as gravity and body weight. Muscles are less flexible, and degenerative changes occur in the spine. In addition, more sedentary life-style causes weakness and shortening in some muscles, and overstretching in others. The most common posture faults are the forward head posture and rounded shoulders.

In patients with poor posture, the bones are not aligned properly, and the muscles, joints, and ligaments become strained and stressed. Weak, tight, and inflexible muscles cannot support the back's natural curves. Years of poor posture can affect the position and function of the vital organs.

Maintaining good posture—or correcting poor posture—can help reduce a bulging disk or relieve the biomechanical stress caused by poor skeletal alignment, thus greatly aiding musculoskeletal system functioning.

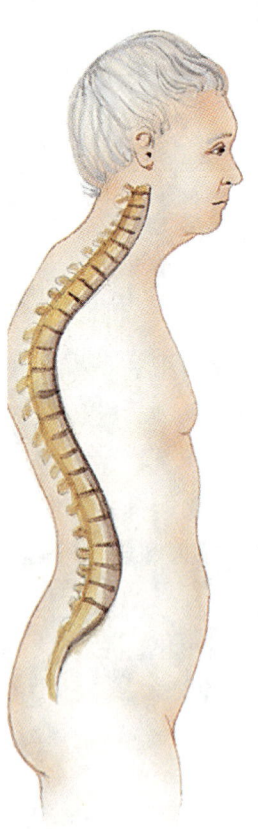

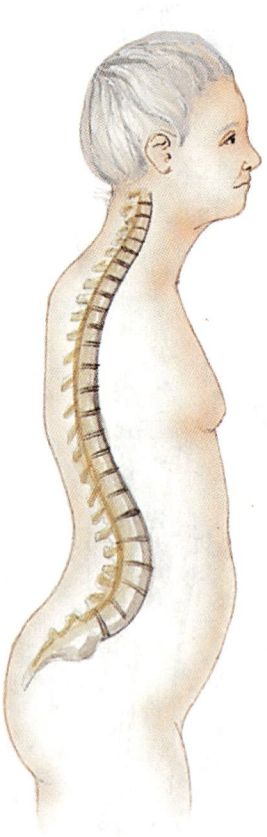

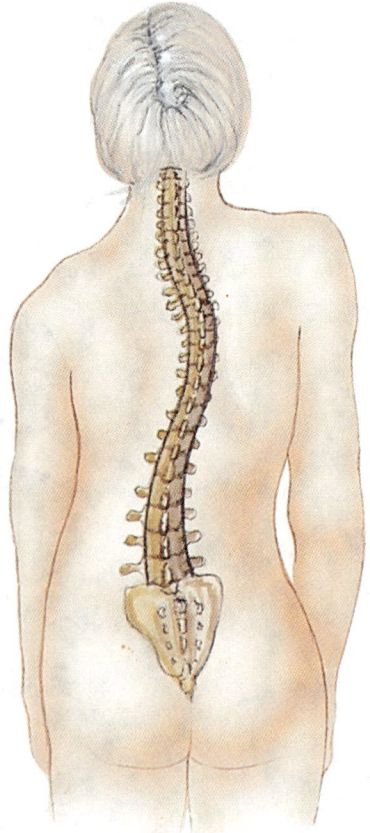

kyphosis   lordosis   scoliosis

FIGURE 31-9
Abnormalities of the spinal curves.

to relieve muscle guarding, which causes a compression force on the disk. Most disk herniations and bulges can be treated successfully without surgery. Severe, unremitting pain, numbness, and progressive weakness of an extremity are indications for surgery.

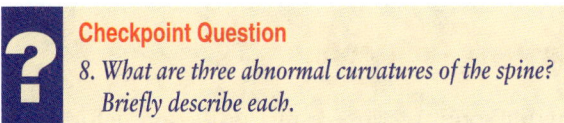

? Checkpoint Question
8. What are three abnormal curvatures of the spine? Briefly describe each.

Rotator Cuff Injury

Injury to the rotator cuff muscles in the shoulder can cause severe pain, weakness, and loss of function. Surgical intervention is often necessary because the tendons do not heal on their own. An extended period of postoperative rehabilitation is usually needed to increase range and strength and to regain the use of the shoulder. Professional athletes, particularly baseball pitchers, are prone to rotator cuff injuries.

Adhesive Capsulitis (Frozen Shoulder)

This condition affects the entire shoulder joint and its capsule. It involves a **contracture** (binding by shortening) of the joint structures, which usually results from a fracture or disease process that prevents movement. Anything that causes pain or restricts motion (eg, tendinitis, bursitis, nerve damage, strokes, sprains, or strains) can lead to a frozen shoulder.

Contractures develop when the joint is immobilized causing the collagen fibers to stick to each other, thereby limiting the movement in the joint. Adhesions and additional collagen are produced in response to injury, thus resulting in a painful, tight, and constricted capsule.

The shoulder movements most restricted are abduction and external rotation. Because full active range of motion is not possible, weakness and atrophy are often present. Prolonged immobility can lead to joint degeneration. Women commonly find it difficult to fix their hair; men complain of the inability to reach their wallets in their back pockets.

Treatment consists of administration of anti-inflammatory medications, heat or cold applications, ultrasound, mobilization (gentle gliding of the joint surfaces) or manipulation, and stretching exercises. The recovery process is slow and typically painful. Contractures in the joints are often preventable with proper management and by moving the joint through a full range of motion each day.

Bursitis

The subdeltoid bursa lies between the deltoid muscle (the muscle that covers the cap of the shoulder) and the joint capsule. The subdeltoid bursa is the most common site for bursitis, an inflammation of the bursa. Other frequent sites are the olecranon process, the trochanter, the heel, and the prepatellar bursae. The most common symptom is pain during range-of-motion movement. In subdeltoid bursitis, pain occurs in the mid-range of abduction but not at the beginning or end of the range. Pain occurs when the inflamed bursa is pinched between the head of the humerus and the clavicle during abduction.

Treatment for bursitis usually consists of administration of anti-inflammatory medication, rest, heat or cold applications, ultrasound to promote healing, range-of-motion exercises, and activities within the pain-free range.

Tendinitis

Tendinitis is inflammation of the tendons. This disorder and others involving inflammation of contractile tissue or their attachments (eg, myositis [muscles] and tenosynovitis [sheaths covering the tendon]) usually occur after strains, sprains, overuse, or overstretching of the tissue. Pain does not occur with passive movement. Active movement is painful, and resistance to movement is intensely painful because the tissue must contract during active and resisted movement. Localized tenderness is usually present. The most common site for tendinitis in the shoulder is at the supraspinatus tendon (one of the rotator cuff muscles). Palpation over the tendon will elicit exquisite pain. Sometimes tendons will contain calcium deposits (calcific tendinitis).

Treatment consists of rest, heat or cold applications, ultrasound, **iontophoresis** (electrical transfer of ions), massage, and transverse friction massage (deep massage across the fibers of the tendons). Achilles tendinitis can be treated with medication, immobilization, ice massage, ultrasound or iontophoresis, and gentle stretching exercises.

Lateral Epicondylitis (Tennis Elbow)

Lateral epicondylitis, often called tennis elbow, is a common elbow injury involving a sprain or strain of the tendons of origin of the wrist and finger extensor muscles. Symptoms include extreme pain with extension of the wrist (such as when trying to lift a cup or glass) and exquisite pain on palpation over the extensor tendons at the elbow joint. Resistance to wrist extension and supination are the diagnostic tests for tennis elbow because both movements greatly increase the pain.

Treatment consists of ice applications, **phonophoresis** (ultrasound with cortisone) or iontophoresis, avoiding movements that cause the pain, use of a forearm strap just distal to the elbow joint to take the pressure off the tendon, transverse friction massage, and gentle passive exercise to maintain mobility. In prolonged, extreme cases, surgery may be indicated.

Carpal Tunnel Syndrome

A repetitive motion injury, carpal tunnel syndrome occurs when the carpal bones and transverse carpal ligaments compress the median nerve at the wrist. Symptoms include numbness in the thumb and the index and middle fingers, pain, and weakness. Often, pain awakens the patient at night.

Diagnostic tests for carpal tunnel syndrome include Phalan's test, in which holding the wrist in flexion reproduces the symptoms; Tinel's test, in which the wrist is held in hyperextension and the transverse carpal ligament is thumped, thereby causing tingling into the hand and fingers; and nerve conduction velocity tests. Treatment can be conservative (eg, administration of anti-inflammatory medications and immobilization) or can require surgical release of the transverse carpal ligament.

Dupuytren's Contracture

Dupuytren's contracture results in flexion deformities of the fingers, most often the ring and little fingers, caused by contractures of the palmar fascia due to the proliferation (overgrowth) of fibrous tissue. Function is lost because the fingers cannot be straightened. Dupuytren's contracture is easily diagnosed by sight and palpation. Surgery is often required to release the contractures. Stretching of the tight structures in the early stages may help to slow the progression.

Chondromalacia Patella

Chondromalacia patella is a degenerative disorder affecting the cartilage underlying the kneecap. It usually occurs in young women or in athletes who perform running, jumping, and bicycling activities. A common complaint is pain when walking down stairs or getting out of a chair. Rest, therapy, bracing or taping, and exercises can help to relieve the symptoms.

Plantar Fasciitis

This disorder, the most frequent cause of pain in the bottom of the foot, is often associated with heel spurs on the calcaneus. Deep palpation over the plantar (sole) surface of the heel bone will elicit pain. Treatment of choice is a foot orthosis (splint or heel pad) to support the arch and distribute the weight evenly. Heat, massage, and ultrasound are often effective. Surgery is rarely done because of the high incidence of recurrence.

Foot Deformities

Bunions, corns, and calluses form on the toes at pressure points or over points of excessive, prolonged friction. They are usually caused by poorly fitting shoes. Treatments of choice include well fitting shoes, pads, and topical medications. Hallux valgus, a great toe deformity, results in lateral deviation of the toe, which is painful. It can be caused by excessive pressure on the foot, most often from shoes that are too narrow. In the

---

Focus on the Patient: Living With Carpal Tunnel Syndrome

Patients who are diagnosed with carpal tunnel syndrome should be questioned regarding their work environment. This syndrome is common among typists, computer operators, assembly line workers, or other professions that demand frequent grasping, twisting, and flexion of the wrist. Many job sites can be re-engineered to be worker friendly. For example, caution a patient who is a typist to maintain good body alignment at all times in a properly proportioned and well constructed chair. Palm supports for computer keyboards decrease the degree of wrist flexion. Advise the patient to take breaks and, if possible, to alternate computer work with other tasks. A physical therapist may offer range-of-motion exercises that the patent can do throughout the day to alleviate wrist tension and may also assist with suggestions for changes in the working environment. Always consult the physician before making patient referrals.

early stages, hallux valgus can be corrected with straightening devices and properly fitting shoes. Surgery may be required for severe bone deformities.

Gout

Gout, a metabolic disease involving an overproduction of uric acid, usually affects the joint of the great toe. Gout presents as a painful, hot, inflamed joint; symptoms progressively worsen unless treated. Periods of remission and exacerbation may occur. The condition may become chronic and can lead to multijoint involvement with chronic pain, degeneration, and deformity. Symptoms are relieved by avoidance of purine-rich foods and alcohol-related products. Medication to prevent uric acid formation or foster its excretion from the body also may be prescribed.

Osteoarthritis

Osteoarthritis, or degenerative joint disease (DJD), is caused by wear and tear on the weight-bearing joints in which the articular cartilage degenerates and the ends of the bones enlarge. This overgrowth of bone intrudes into the joint cavity, causing pain and restricted movement. If the articular cartilage is inflamed, it is called osteochondritis.

Treatment includes administration of anti-inflammatory medications, intra-articular corticosteroid injections, and use of ambulatory aids (eg, crutches, cane, walker) to decrease joint stress.

Rheumatoid Arthritis

Rheumatoid arthritis is a systemic autoimmune disease that attacks the synovium of the joint. Ultimately, it leads to inflammation, pain, stiffness, and crippling deformities. It usually begins in the non–weight-bearing joints but eventually affects most of the joints of the appendicular skeleton.

Rheumatoid arthritis of the spine is also called Marie-Strumpell disease, or **ankylosing spondylitis**, and is characterized by extreme forward flexion of the spine and tightness in the hip flexors. Rheumatoid arthritis in children is known as Still's disease.

Checkpoint Question

9. How does osteoarthritis differ from rheumatoid arthritis?

Treatment involves rest, hot and cold applications, physical therapy, and administration of anti-inflammatory medications.

Muscular Dystrophy

The congenital disorders collectively known as muscular dystrophy are characterized by varying degrees of progressive wasting of skeletal muscles. There is no neurologic involvement. The wasted, weakened muscles tend to be hypertrophic. The most common type, Duchenne's, is apparent in early childhood and is usually fatal by young adulthood. Mixed forms of muscular dystrophy occur in the middle adult years and are rapidly fatal. Several forms, such as facioscapulohumeral and limb girdle dystrophy, progress slowly from a childhood onset and result in varying degrees of disability. Duchenne's, facioscapulohumeral, and limb girdle dystrophies are genetically transmitted; the cause of the mixed form is not known.

Diagnosis is based on family and patient history. Electromyography and muscle biopsy are used to rule out neurologic involvement. The characteristic signs are frequently the most obvious diagnostic indicators of the disease. There is no known cure for any form of muscular dystrophy.

Osteoporosis

If the rate of bone resorption by osteoclastic activity is greater than bone formation by osteoblasts, bones become lacy and porous rather than dense and solid. Porous bones deficient in calcium and phosphorus are brittle and vulnerable to fractures. The cause may be dietary with general deficiencies in calcium, vitamin D, or phosphorus, or may be a primary progressive inability to metabolize calcium brought on by estrogen deficiency in elderly women, a sedentary life-style, alcoholism, liver disorders, or rheumatoid arthritis.

There are few signs other than a gradual loss of stature with progressive kyphosis; the most severe sign is spontaneous, nontraumatic fractures. Diagnosis includes bone scans, densitometry (measuring the density of the bones), thyroid and parathyroid studies, and serum calcium and phosphorus determinations.

Treatment involves preventing fractures by increasing appropriate levels of exercise. Estrogen is usually prescribed for postmenopausal women if therapy can begin within 3 to 5 years of menopause. Calcium and vitamin D supplements are beneficial to arrest the progression but will not cure the underlying degenerative factors.

Bone Tumors

Bone tissue is rarely the primary site for malignancies but is frequently a secondary site for metastasis. Primary osteosarcomata occur most often in young men although they may occur less frequently at any age in either sex. Osteogenic sarcomata originate in the bony tissue; nonosseous tumors seed to the bones from other primary sites. Ewing's sarcoma, originating in the marrow and invading the shaft of the long bones, is a common form of nonosteogenic sarcoma.

There is no known cause, but theories suggest that rapid development of bone tissue during growth spurts is a predisposing factor. Bone pain is the most common early sign. The pain is more intense at night, is usually dull and centered at the site, and is not relieved by resting the body part. Depending on the site, the mass may be palpable through the skin and muscles.

Biopsy is the definitive diagnostic route after bone scans suggest the need. Treatment is excision of the tumor including a large margin of surrounding bone structure and nearby lymph nodes. Chemotherapy and radiation are usually indicated also.

➤ COMMON DIAGNOSTIC PROCEDURES

Physical Examination

The physician's evaluation of the musculoskeletal system will usually include an assessment of the patient's structure and function, movement, and pain. An important part of the evaluation involves the patient history, which includes the patient's description of the events and circumstances that led to the decision to seek medical help.

The physician observes the patient's overall physical state by noting how the patient walks, sits, stands, and moves. Concentrating on the area of concern, the physician then evaluates the problem by visual inspection, palpation, and diagnostic tests or reports. Pain and limited or compromised functions are warning signals. Strength also affects function and is a part of any musculoskeletal evaluation. Other important considerations are skin color, temperature, tone, and tenderness; abnormal findings might indicate underlying pathology.

Diagnostic Studies

The most frequently used tools for detecting disorders of the musculoskeletal system are radiology and diagnostic imaging, which are used for diagnosing fractures, dislocations, and degeneration or diseases of the bones and joints. Other radiographic studies include **arthrograms**, which show joint pathology, and myelograms, which help detect intervertebral disk conditions. A bone scan analyzes bone growth, density, age, tumors, or other pathology.

Computed tomography (CT) scans and magnetic resonance imaging (MRI) reveal soft-tissue pathology, such as tumors, metastatic lesions, strokes, and ruptured or bulging disks.

Electromyography (EMG) and nerve conduction velocity (NCV) tests measure the health and fitness of the nerves as they relate to conduction of nerve impulses and muscle function.

Goniometry is the measurement of the amount of movement available in a joint by a protractor-like device called a **goniometer**.

A bone or muscle biopsy is also a valuable diagnostic tool. It allows intense examination of the tissue under a microscope to determine cell damage, neoplasms (tumor or growth), or other types of diseases.

Checkpoint Question

10. What are 10 procedures that can be used to diagnose musculoskeletal disorders?

➤ AMBULATORY AIDS AND THE MEDICAL ASSISTANT'S ROLE

Patients may lose their ability to move normally due to accidents and injuries, disease processes (eg, cerebrovascular accidents), neurologic or muscular defects, or degeneration. Patients who require assistance to maintain mobility may use crutches, canes, or walkers. Medical assistants often are responsible for teaching

BOX 31-8 Safety Tips for Using Ambulatory Aids

- Check the rubber tips frequently and replace worn tips immediately. (Most ambulatory aids require rubber tips although some walkers are equipped with rollers.)
- Check screws and bolts frequently; tighten as needed.
- Remove scatter rugs and small pieces of furniture that may cause falls.

patients how to use these kinds of ambulatory aids safely (Box 31-8).

Crutches

Crutches may be either wooden or tubular aluminum. The most common form is the axillary crutch, which extends from the patient's axillae to the floor, with hand rests to distribute the weight to the palms. The Lofstrand or Canadian crutch is usually aluminum and reaches just to the forearms, with a metal cuff to maintain its posi-

text continues on page 577

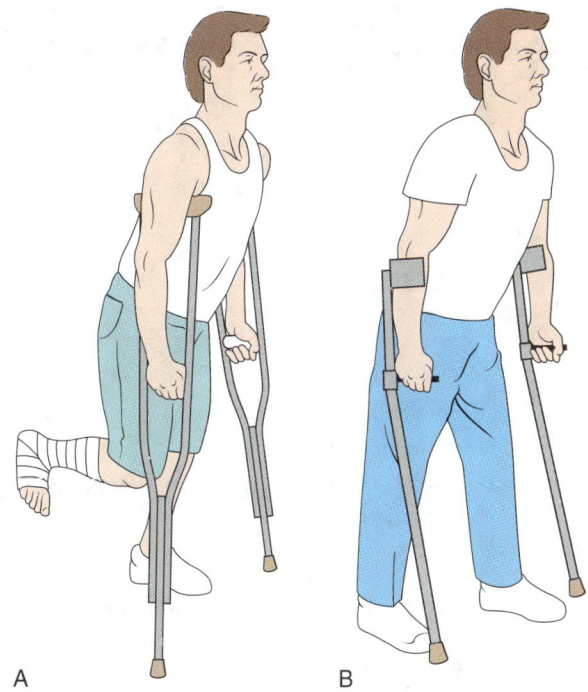

A   B

FIGURE 31-10
Types of crutches. (*A*) Axillary crutches. (*B*) Lofstrand, Canadian or forearm crutches.

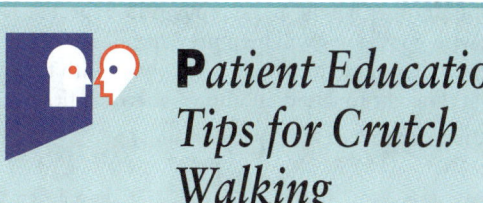

Patient Education: Tips for Crutch Walking

To go up stairs:

- Stand close to the bottom step.
- With weight on the hands, step up to the first step with the unaffected leg.
- Bring the affected side and the crutches up to the step at the same time.
- Resume balance before proceeding to the next step.
- *Remember:* The good side goes up first!

To descend stairs:

- Stand close to the edge of the top step.
- Bend from the hips and knees to adjust to the height of the lower step. *Do not* lean forward (leaning forward may cause a fall).
- Carefully lower the crutches and the affected limb to the next step.
- Next, lower the unaffected leg to the lower step and resume balance. If a handrail is available, hold both crutches in one hand and follow the steps above.
- *Remember:* The affected foot goes down first!

To sit:

- Back up to the chair until you feel the edge on the backs of the legs.
- Move both crutches to the hand on the affected side and reach back for the chair with the hand on the unaffected side.
- Lower yourself slowly into the chair.

Charting Example

| 09/15/99 | 4:30 PM. Patient fractured left distal tibia. Fracture reduced and casted by Dr. Miranda. Postreduction—left toes warm to touch and pink in color. Able to wiggle toes. Patient fitted for axillary crutches—2 finger breadths below the axillae. Handgrips adjusted keeping elbows flexed at 30-degree angle. Two-point gait demonstrated. Patient returned demonstration without problem. Written instructions given to patient on crutch walking. Verbalized understanding of all instructions. ——— Tamika Burton, RMA |

Measuring a Patient for Axillary Crutches

Equipment/Supplies

- crutches with tips
- pads for the axillae and hand rests, as needed
- tools to tighten bolts

Steps	Purpose
1. Wash your hands.	1. Handwashing aids infection control.
2. Assemble the equipment.	2. This ensures that all supplies are available.
3. Greet and identify the patient.	3. This helps avoid errors in treatment.
4. Ensure that the patient is wearing low-heeled shoes with safety soles.	4. To obtain proper height measurement. Low-heeled shoes with good soles will help prevent falls. While using crutches, patients should wear shoes with the same heel height to avoid an improper crutch fit.
5. Have the patient stand erect. Support the patient as needed.	5. Providing support ensures patient safety.
6. Have the patient hold the crutches naturally with the tips about 2 inches in front of and 4–6 inches to the side of the feet. This is called the tripod position, and all crutch gaits start from this position (see Procedure 31-2: Teaching a Patient Crutch Gaits).	
7. Using the tools as needed, adjust the central support in the base so that the axillary bar is about 2 finger-breadths below the patient's axillae. Tighten the bolts for safety when the proper height is reached.	7. If the axillary bar presses on the axillae, nerve damage may occur. If it is too low, the crutches will be difficult to manage.

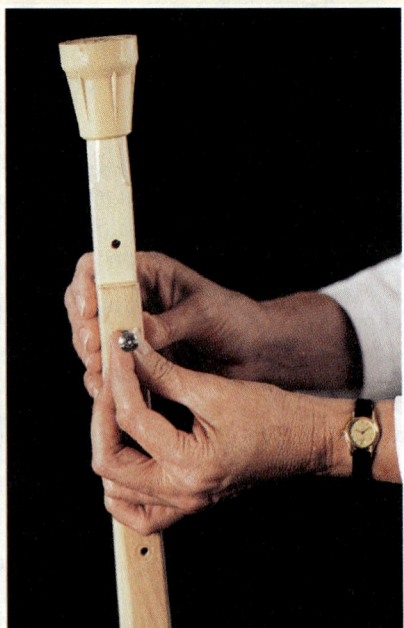

Step 7A: The crutches may be adjusted to the patient's height by removing the wing nut and bolt and moving the extension.

Step 7B: Tighten the bold securely.

(continued)

Procedure 31-1 Measuring a Patient for Axillary Crutches (continued)

Steps	Purpose
8. Adjust the handgrips by raising or lowering the bar so that the patient's elbow is at a 30-degree angle when the bar is gripped. Tighten bolts for safety.	8. Handgrips that are too high or low will compromise safety and may cause nerve pressure.

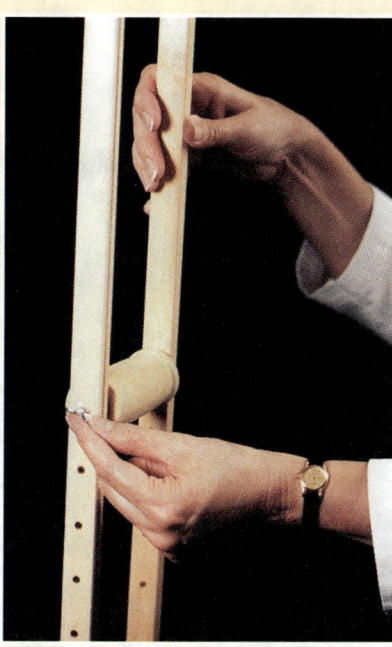

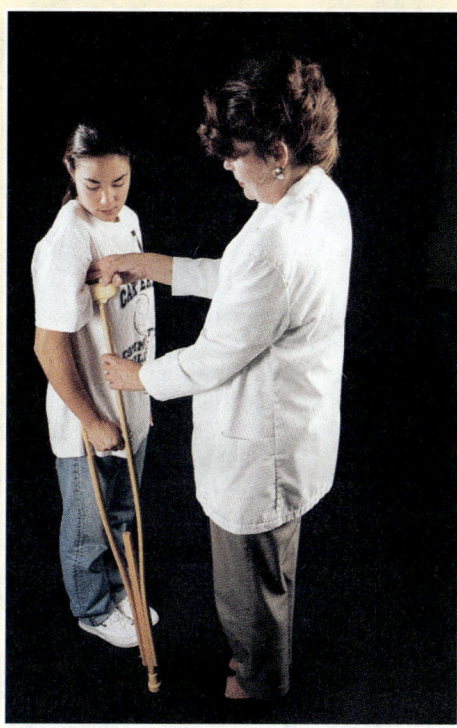

Step 8A: The hand rests are adjusted by raising or lowering along the shaft of the crutch.

Step 8B: Crutches are properly adjusted when the patient's elbow is at a 30-degree angle and two fingers can be inserted at the axillae.

Steps	Purpose
9. If needed, pad axillary bars and handgrips with soft material to prevent friction.	
10. Thank the patient and give appropriate instructions.	10. Courtesy encourages the patient to have a positive attitude about the physician's office.
11. Properly care for or dispose of equipment and supplies. Wash your hands.	
12. Record the procedure.	12. Procedures are considered not to have been done if they are not recorded.

Procedure 31-2   Teaching a Patient Crutch Gaits

The gait chosen will depend on the patient's weight-bearing ability, coordination, and general state of health. All gaits start with the tripod position (see Procedure 31-1: Measuring a Patient for Axillary Crutches).

Steps	Purpose
1. Wash your hands.	1. Handwashing aids infection control.
2. Have the patient stand up from a chair. To do this, the patient holds both crutches on the affected side, then slides to the edge of the chair. The patient pushes down on the chair arm on the unaffected side, then pushes to stand. Weight should be rested on the crutches until balance is restored.	
3. Ensure that the crutches are in the tripod position.	3. To ensure safety and proper balance, crutches should be in this position before proceeding with any gait.
4. Have the patient begin the appropriate gait. a. *Three-point gait:* This gait is the most commonly used gait for crutch training. This gait is used when only one leg can be used for weight bearing or when only partial weight bearing is allowed on the affected leg. Amputees, those with injury to one leg, or patients who have had limb surgery will use this gait. This gait requires coordination and upper body strength. (1) The affected leg can be held clear of the floor or used in concert with crutches. Both crutches are moved forward with the unaffected leg and the affected leg bearing the weight. (2) With the weight supported by the crutches, the unaffected leg is brought past the level of the crutches. (3) The steps are repeated. b. *Two-point gait:* This gait requires partial weight bearing and good coordination. Two points will be raised, and two points will be on the floor in this gait. (1) The right crutch and left foot are moved forward. (2) As these points rest, the right foot and left crutch are moved forward. (3) The steps are repeated. c. *Four-point gait:* This gait is the slowest and safest of the gaits. At least three points are on the ground at all times. The patient must be capable of partial weight bearing. Patients with degenerative diseases, spasticity, and poor coordination will use this gait.	

(continued)

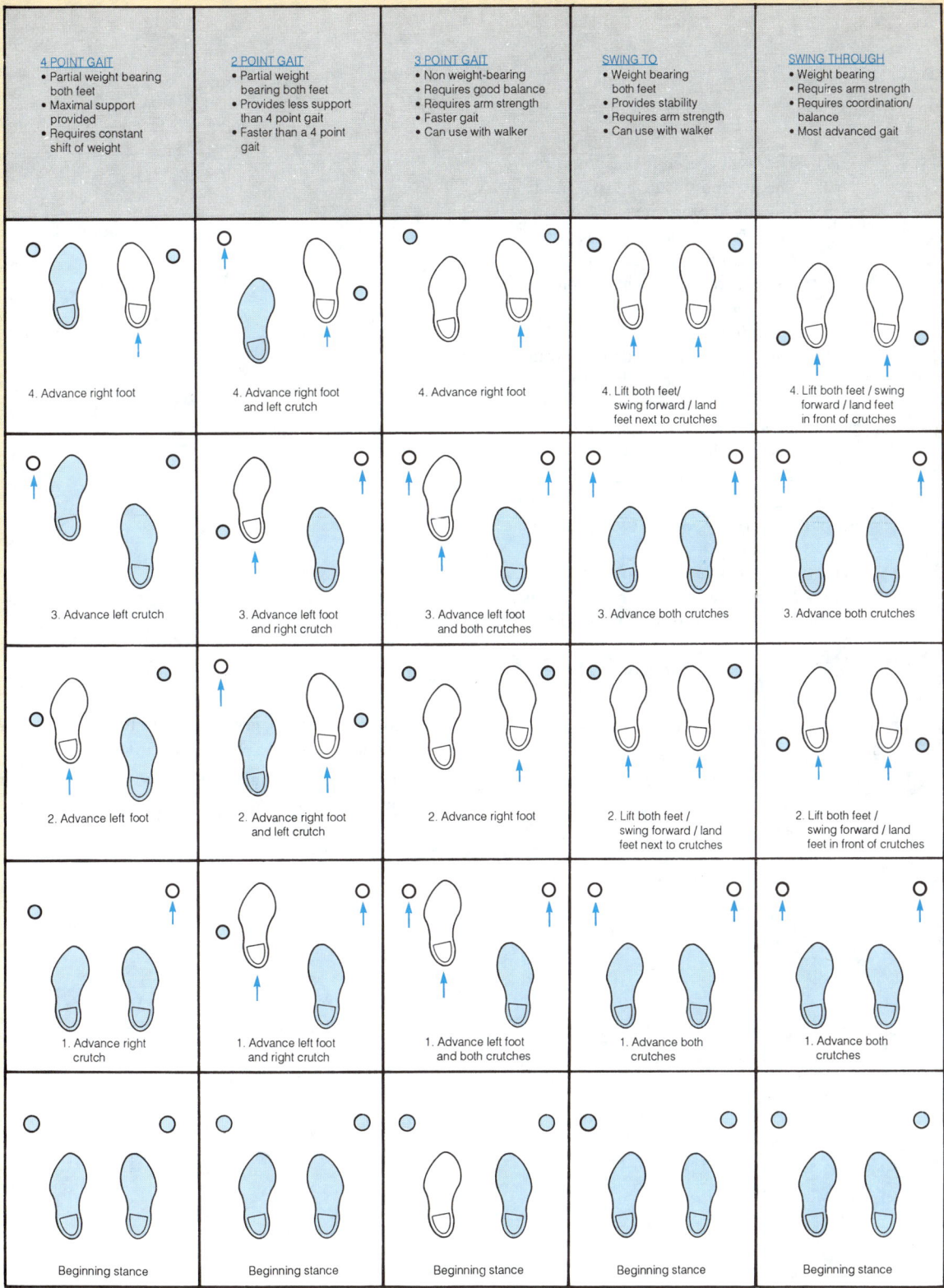

4 POINT GAIT	2 POINT GAIT	3 POINT GAIT	SWING TO	SWING THROUGH
• Partial weight bearing both feet • Maximal support provided • Requires constant shift of weight	• Partial weight bearing both feet • Provides less support than 4 point gait • Faster than a 4 point gait	• Non weight-bearing • Requires good balance • Requires arm strength • Faster gait • Can use with walker	• Weight bearing both feet • Provides stability • Requires arm strength • Can use with walker	• Weight bearing • Requires arm strength • Requires coordination/balance • Most advanced gait
4. Advance right foot	4. Advance right foot and left crutch	4. Advance right foot	4. Lift both feet / swing forward / land feet next to crutches	4. Lift both feet / swing forward / land feet in front of crutches
3. Advance left crutch	3. Advance left foot and right crutch	3. Advance left foot and both crutches	3. Advance both crutches	3. Advance both crutches
2. Advance left foot	2. Advance right foot and left crutch	2. Advance right foot	2. Lift both feet / swing forward / land feet next to crutches	2. Lift both feet / swing forward / land feet in front of crutches
1. Advance right crutch	1. Advance left foot and right crutch	1. Advance left foot and both crutches	1. Advance both crutches	1. Advance both crutches
Beginning stance	Beginning stance	Beginning stance	Beginning stance	Beginning stance

Crutch gaits.

(continued)

Procedure 31-2   Teaching a Patient Crutch Gaits (continued)

Steps	Purpose

(1) The right crutch moves forward.
    (2) The left foot is moved to a position just ahead of the left crutch.
    (3) The left crutch is moved forward.
    (4) The right foot moves to a position just ahead of the right crutch.
    (5) The steps are repeated.
  d. *Swing-through gait:*
    (1) Both crutches are moved forward.
    (2) With the weight on the hands, the body swings through to a position ahead of the crutches.
    (3) The crutches are moved ahead.
    (4) The steps are repeated.
  e. Swing-to gait: This gait may be used until the patient is ready for the swing-through gait.
    (1) Both crutches are moved forward.
    (2) With the weight on the hands, the body swings to the level of the crutches.
    (3) The crutches are moved ahead.
    (4) The steps are repeated.	

5. Thank the patient and give appropriate instructions.	5. Courtesy encourages the patient to have a positive attitude about the physician's office.
6. Wash your hands and record the procedure.	6. Procedures are considered not to have been done if they are not recorded.

on the arms and a covered hand grip to distribute the weight (Fig. 31-10). The Lofstrand allows the patient to release and use his hands without losing the crutches. These work well for patients who will require crutch use for a long period of time or who have poor coordination.

Procedures 31-1 and 31-2 describe how to measure a patient for axillary crutches and how to teach a patient various crutch gaits. The display offers patient education tips for ascending and descending stairs with crutches and for sitting down safely.

Canes

Canes are used when the patient needs extra support and stability, but requires only a small measure of assistance with weight bearing. The standard cane may be used when the patient needs very slight assistance. The tripod (three legs) or quad cane (four legs) is useful when the patient needs greater stability (Fig. 31-11). The tripod and quad canes can stand alone if the patient needs free hands and can find other support. They tend to be bulkier and heavier, but because they offer greater

stability and safety, they are good choices for patients who need greater support than the standard cane.

To measure for the proper cane length, have the patient stand erect. The cane should be level with the patient's greater trochanter, and the patient's elbow should be bent at a 30 degree angle.

To walk with a cane, the patient should:

1. Position the cane on the unaffected side, about 4 to 6 inches to the side and about 2 inches ahead of the foot.
2. Advance the cane and the affected leg together.
3. Bring the unaffected leg forward to a position just ahead of the cane.
4. Repeat the steps.

Walkers

Walkers are comfortable aids for the elderly or others with weakness or poor coordination. They consist of a lightweight aluminum frame in an open square. Because walkers are somewhat bulky, maneuvering in close quarters can be difficult. The walker frame should be level with the patient's hip, and the patient's elbow should be bent at about a 30 degree angle (Fig. 31-12).

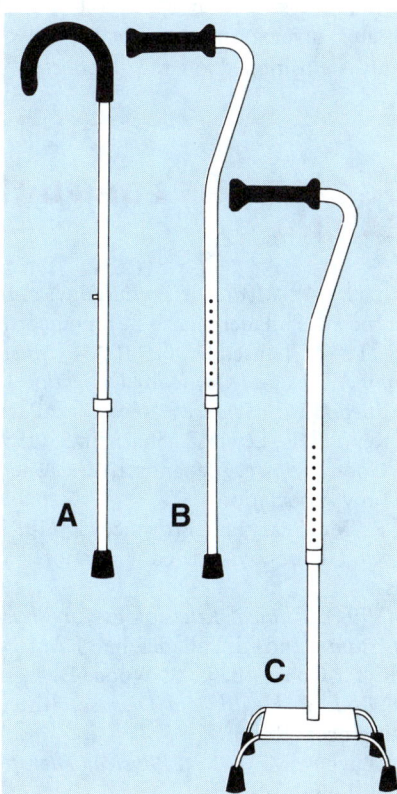

FIGURE 31-11
Three types of canes. (A) Single-ended canes with half-circle handles are recommended for patients requiring minimal support. (B) Single-ended canes with straight handles are recommended for patients with hand weakness. (C) Three- or four-prong canes are recommended for patients with poor balance.

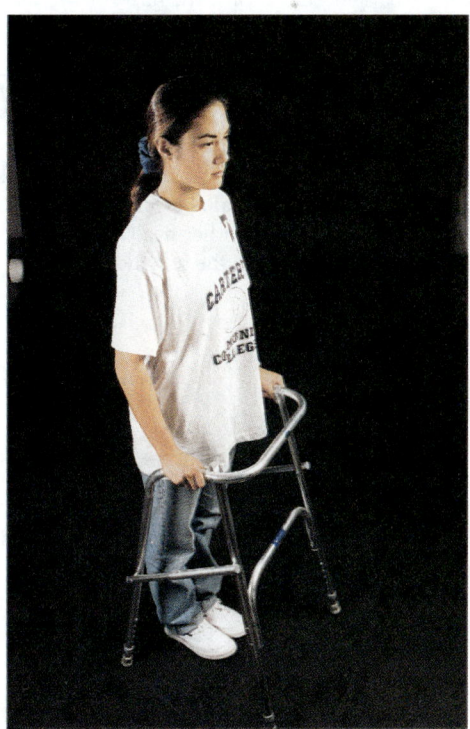

FIGURE 31-12
A properly adjusted walker.

To use a walker, the patient should:

1. Stand erect and move the walker ahead about 6 inches.
2. Using an easy walking gait with hands on the walker grips, step into the walker.
3. Move the walker ahead again.
4. Repeat the steps.

 Checkpoint Question
11. On which side of the body is the cane positioned?

 ## SUMMARY

The musculoskeletal system provides support and protection for vital organs and allows movement and mobility. The skeleton is the frame on which muscles are attached. Bones are held together by joints, which provide stability and flexibility. Muscles enable the body to stand upright, to move, and to perform specific and detailed functions requiring strength and dexterity. The integrity of the entire musculoskeletal system allows for safe, pain-free, and normal movement.

 ## CRITICAL THINKING CHALLENGES

1. Create a patient education brochure for the use of ambulatory aids. Be sure to include a brief description of the purpose of each aid along with the procedure steps.
2. The youth baseball league playoffs care coming to your town and you are asked to participate in the first aid station. What kinds of orthopedic injuries would you expect to see and why? Develop a list of the first aid supplies that you would want to have available and explain the reasons for your selections. What other health care professionals would you want to have at the first aid station with you?

 ## ANSWERS TO CHECKPOINT QUESTIONS

1. The skeletal system provides a supportive framework for the body, provides leverage for the muscles, protects vital organs, allows for calcium metabolism and storage, and facilitates blood cell production.
2. Types of joints are synarthroses (immovable), amphiarthroses (slightly movable), and diarthrosis (freely movable).

3. The four natural curves of the spine are the cervical, thoracic, lumbar, and sacral curves.
4. The knee is a hinge joint. Its two primary movements are flexion and extension.
5. Tendons connect muscle to bone. Ligaments connect bone to bone.
6. Luxation is a complete dislocation; subluxation is a partial dislocation.
7. An open reduction involves surgery; a closed reduction does not.
8. Abnormal spinal curvatures include scoliosis (lateral curve), kyphosis (hunchback), and lordosis (swayback).
9. Osteoarthritis is a degenerative joint disease caused by wear and tear on the weight-bearing joints in which the articular cartilage degenerates and the ends of the bones enlarge. Rheumatoid arthritis is a systemic autoimmune disease that attacks the synovium of the joint, ultimately leading to inflammation, pain, stiffness, and crippling deformities. It usually begins in the non–weight-bearing joints, but eventually affects most of the joints of the appendicular skeleton.
10. Ten procedures that can be used to diagnose musculoskeletal disorders are physical examination, computed tomography scans, magnetic resonance imaging, electromyography, nerve conduction velocity, goniometry, arthrograms, myelograms, bone scans, and x-rays.
11. The cane is positioned on the unaffected side of the body.

 ## SUGGESTIONS FOR FURTHER READING

Cohen, B. J. (1994). *Medical Terminology: An Illustrated Guide*, 2nd ed. Philadelphia: J. B. Lippincott.

Colburn, G. L., & Lause, D. B. (1993). *Musculoskeletal Anatomy: A Text and Guide for Dissection for Students in the Allied Health Sciences*. New York: Parthenon.

Iglarsh, A., Kendall, F., Lewis C., Sharman S. (1994). *The Secret of Good Posture*. Alexandria, VA: American Physical Therapy Association.

Kendall, F. P., McCreary, E., Provance, P. (1993). *Muscles Testing and Function*, 4th ed. Baltimore: Williams & Wilkins.

Lippert, L (1994). *Clinical Kinesiology for Physical Therapist Assistants*, 2nd ed. Philadelphia: F.A. Davis.

Memmler, R. L., Cohen, B. J., & Wood, D. L. (1996). *The Human Body in Health and Disease*, 8th ed. Philadelphia: Lippincott-Raven.

Scully, R. & Baynes, M. (1989). *Physical Therapy*. Philadelphia: J. B. Lippincott.

Wolf, R. (1991). *The Rehabilitation Specialists Handbook*. Philadelphia: F. A. Davis.

Caring for Patients With Neurologic Disorders

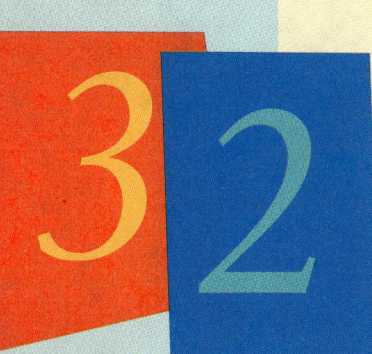

Chapter Outline

Structure and Function of the Nervous System
Structure of a Neuron
Nervous System Communication
Central Nervous System
The Brain
Spinal Cord
Peripheral Nervous System
Cranial Nerves
Spinal Nerves
Autonomic Nervous System
Sympathetic System
Parasympathetic System
Common Nervous System Disorders
Infectious Disorders
Degenerative Disorders
Seizure Disorders
Developmental Disorders

Trauma
Brain Tumors
Headaches
Common Diagnostic Tests for Nervous System Disorders
Physical Examination
Radiologic Tests
Electrical Tests
Lumbar Puncture
Procedure: Assisting With a Lumbar Puncture
Prenatal Screening
Pediatric Testing
Summary
Critical Thinking Challenges
Answers to Checkpoint Questions
Suggestions for Further Reading

DACUM Components

1.3   Practice within the scope of education, training, and personal capabilities
1.6   Conduct oneself in a courteous and diplomatic manner
2.2   Treat all patients with empathy and impartiality
4.1   Apply principles of aseptic technique and infection control
4.7   Prepare patients for procedures
4.8   Assist physician with examinations and treatments
4.10 Collect and process specimens
5.1   Document accurately
7.3   Teach patients methods of health promotion and disease prevention

Chapter Competencies

Learning Objectives

Upon successfully completing this chapter, you will be able to:

1. Spell and define the Key Terms.
2. Differentiate between the functions of the central, peripheral, and autonomic nervous systems.
3. Explain the reflex arc.
4. Identify the three main components of the brain and list their individual functions.
5. Compare the functions of the parasympathetic and sympathetic systems.
6. Identify infectious diseases that involve the nervous system.
7. Identify physical and emotional effects of degenerative nervous system disorders.
8. Describe the medical assistant's role in caring for a patient having a seizure.
9. List potential complications of a spinal cord injury.
10. Name common diagnostic procedures for nervous system disorders and briefly explain each.

Performance Objective

Upon successfully completing this chapter, you will be able to:

1. Assist with performance of a lumbar puncture (Procedure 32-1).

Key Terms

(See Glossary for definitions.)

afferent
alpha-fetoprotein
amniocentesis
arachnoid
autonomic
axon
basal ganglia
cerebellum
cerebrum
concussion
convulsion
cranium
dendrite
diencephalon
dura mater

dysphagia
dysphasia
efferent
electroencephalogram
 (EEG)
gyri
hypothalamus
insula
medulla oblongata
meninges
meningocele
midbrain
migraine
myelogram
myelomeningocele

neuron
neurotransmitter
parasympathetic
pia mater
pons
Queckenstedt test
Romberg test
seizure
spina bifida occulta
sulci
sympathetic
synapse
thalamus

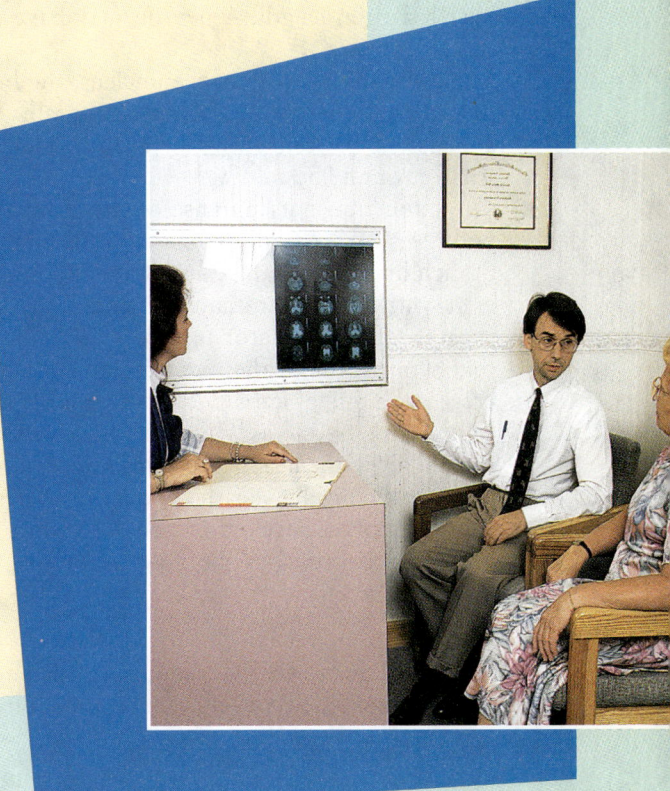

The nervous system is the chief communication and command center for all parts of the body. Its responsibilities range from controlling vital homeostatic functions to processing memory and logical thought.

The nervous system has two divisions: the central nervous system (CNS) and the peripheral nervous system (PNS). The CNS is composed of the brain and spinal cord and is the body's command center. Messages are relayed to and from the CNS by the cranial and spinal nerves that make up the PNS. A division of the PNS, the **autonomic** nervous system, functions automatically without conscious awareness. Respiratory and circulatory rates, blood pressure, and digestive processes are controlled by the autonomic nervous system (Fig. 32-1).

➤ STRUCTURE AND FUNCTION OF THE NERVOUS SYSTEM

Structure of a Neuron

The fundamental functioning units of the nervous system are special cells called neurons, designed to carry electrical nerve impulses. A neuron is composed of three main parts: **dendrite**, **axon**, and cell body (Fig. 32-2).

1. The dendrite conducts impulses *toward* the cell body. Dendrites range from less than an inch to over a foot in length. A neuron may have one or more dendrites.
2. The cell body consists of the nucleus, the brain of the cell, and the cytoplasm, which contains the organelles of the cell. (See Ch. 29, Introduction to Anatomy and Physiology)
3. The axon transmits impulses *away* from the cell body. A neuron has only one axon that may then branch into collateral axons. Some axons are covered with a cellular material called the myelin sheath, a fatty insulator formed by Schwann cells that wraps around the axon at intervals and increases the rate of impulse conduction. Myelinated cells are referred to as white cells because the fatty sheath gives them a white appearance. Neurons without the myelin sheath conduct impulses more slowly than the myelinated cells. They are called gray cells because, in the absence of the myelin sheath, they appear gray in color.

Neurons located outside of the CNS are combined in pathways to form what is commonly called a nerve. Nerves are classified according to their functions:

- Sensory (**afferent**) nerves conduct impulses to the brain.
- Motor (**efferent**) nerves conduct impulses away from the brain.

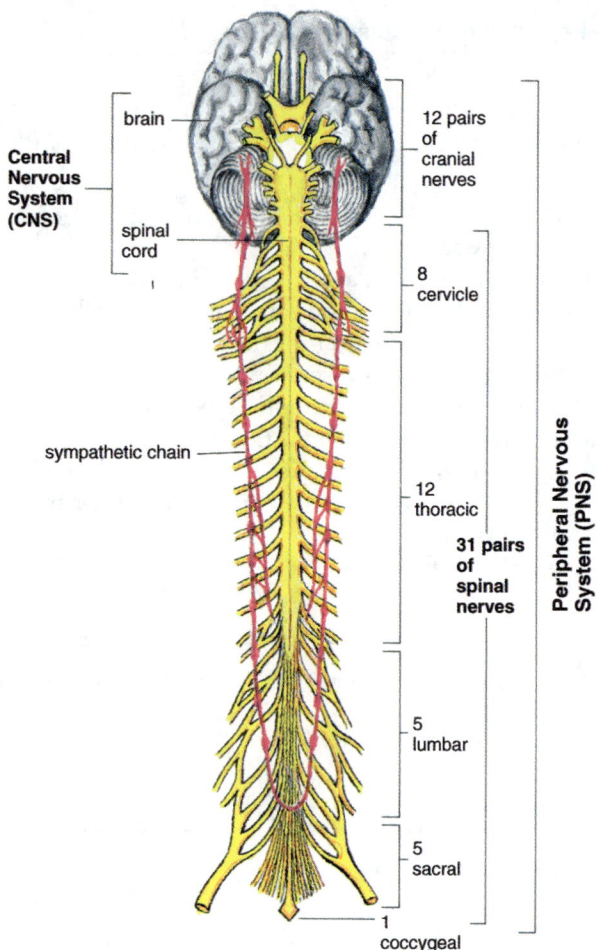

FIGURE 32-1
Anatomic division of the nervous system.

- Mixed nerves are capable of both motor and sensory functions.

Nervous System Communication

Because communication within the internal environment is essential for life, the nervous system must be able to communicate with itself and with the rest of the body systems. It does so in two ways—through **synapses** (the junction of two neurons) and reflexes.

Neurons transmitting impulses do not actually touch the receiving neuron. They are divided by a small space, called a synapse, between the axon of one neuron and the dendrites and cell body of the next neuron. Communication between neurons occurs when a message is released by the axon of one neuron and then "jumps" across the synapse to the dendrite of another. Chemicals called **neurotransmitters** transport messages across the synapse in the form of an electrical charge. Neurotransmitting substances include epinephrine (adrenaline), norepinephrine (noradrenaline), acetyl-

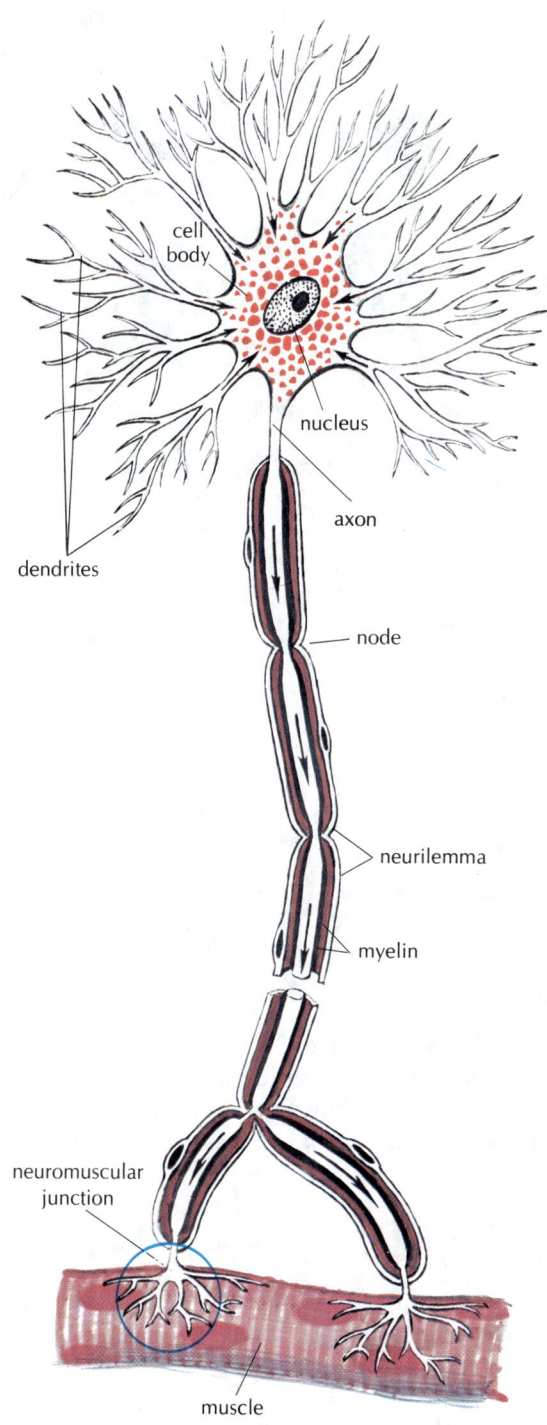

to a given stimulus. Reflex arcs are tested during routine office visits in what is commonly called reflex testing. The most common example is the tapping of the knee with a reflex hammer. Listed below is the sequence of events in this instance:

1. The skin of the knee is stimulated by a tap with a percussion hammer just below the patella. (The knee is usually flexed and dangling.)
2. The sensory neuron transmits the impulse along the dendrite to the cell body of the neuron.
3. The sensory axon carries the impulse to the spinal cord.
4. The message is interpreted within the spinal cord and communicated back by the motor neuron dendrite. A nerve pathway ascending the spinal column begins sending the information to the brain for grading and interpretation while the reflex impulses are flashing toward the peripheral motor neuron responsible for the muscles of the knee area.
5. The message is received and processed by the cell body of the motor neuron and passed on to the axon.
6. The motor neuron axon stimulates the muscles in the knee to contract, causing movement to occur before the brain has had time to interpret the message sent by the ascending spinal nerves that the blow or knee tap has occurred.

Although the reflex arc sounds highly technical, it occurs without our conscious awareness and the results are evident in milliseconds (Fig. 32-3).

 Checkpoint Question
1. How does communication between two neurons occur?

➤ CENTRAL NERVOUS SYSTEM

The central nervous system (CNS) consists of the brain and the spinal cord. The brain is situated in the skull and is protected by the strength of the **cranium**. The spinal cord begins at the base of the brain and travels through the vertebral column until about the second lumbar vertebra, referred to as L-2.

The Brain

Protective Coverings

The brain is covered by three layers of connective tissue called the **meninges**, which completely enclose the brain and spinal cord.

FIGURE 32-2
Diagram of a motor neuron. The break in the axon denotes length. The arrows show the direction of the nerve impulse.

choline, and dopamine. Neurotransmitters rely on the presence of electrolytes, specifically sodium, potassium, and chlorine, to conduct the electrical impulse through the cell body to the point of synapse.

Internal communication also occurs through the reflex arc. A reflex is the body's involuntary response

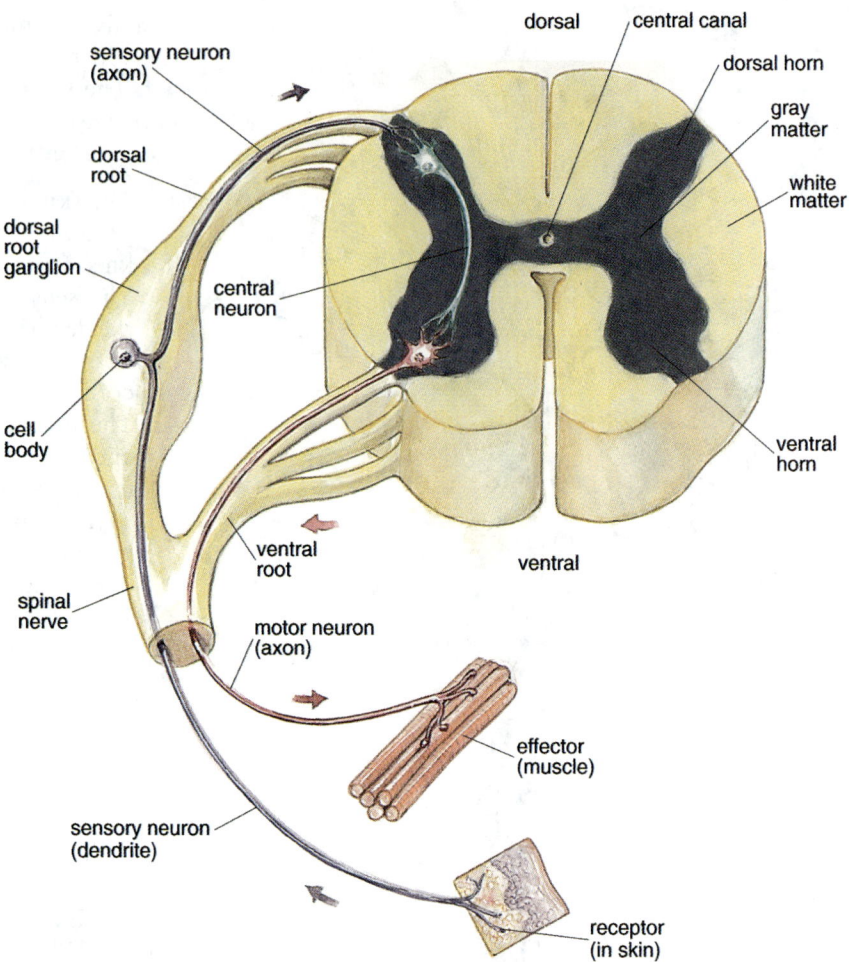

FIGURE 32-3
Reflex arc showing the pathway of impulses and a cross section of the spinal cord.

1. The outermost layer, the **dura mater**, is composed of fibrous tissue and is the thickest and toughest protective layer.
2. The middle layer, the **arachnoid**, is loosely attached to the dura mater by fine fibers that allow movement of cerebrospinal fluid (CSF) in the spaces between the membranes. This layer is responsible for cushioning and protecting the brain and spinal cord from external injury.
3. The innermost layer, the **pia mater**, is closest to the brain. It is a very thin membrane of connective tissue that weaves in and out of the grooves in the brain carrying most of the brain's blood supply.

Cerebrospinal Fluid

The brain is cushioned by CSF, which is formed in spaces deep within the brain called ventricles. CSF is filtered from the bloodstream and contains water and nutrients to nourish the tissues of the brain and spinal cord. It is clear and colorless, unless a disease process is present. CSF circulates from the ventricles out to the meninges, through the spinal cord, and

back to the brain spaces. It is then reabsorbed into the bloodstream to be replenished by newly filtered fluid. CSF levels remains fairly constant; an elevation indicates the presence of a disease process or trauma (Fig. 32-4).

Major Divisions of the Brain

The brain has three main divisions or components: the cerebrum, brain stem, and cerebellum.

CEREBRUM

The **cerebrum** is the largest part of the brain. It is composed of the right and left hemispheres, the corpus callosum, and the **diencephalon**, which lies beneath the hemispheres. It is important to note that the right hemisphere of the brain controls the left side of the body, and vice versa. The hemispheres are covered with an outer layer of nerve tissue called the cerebral cortex, also referred to as the gray matter. The cerebral cortex appears gray because the neurons in this area are not myelinated. This gray matter forms valleys that are called **sulci** and ridges that are called **gyri**. Under

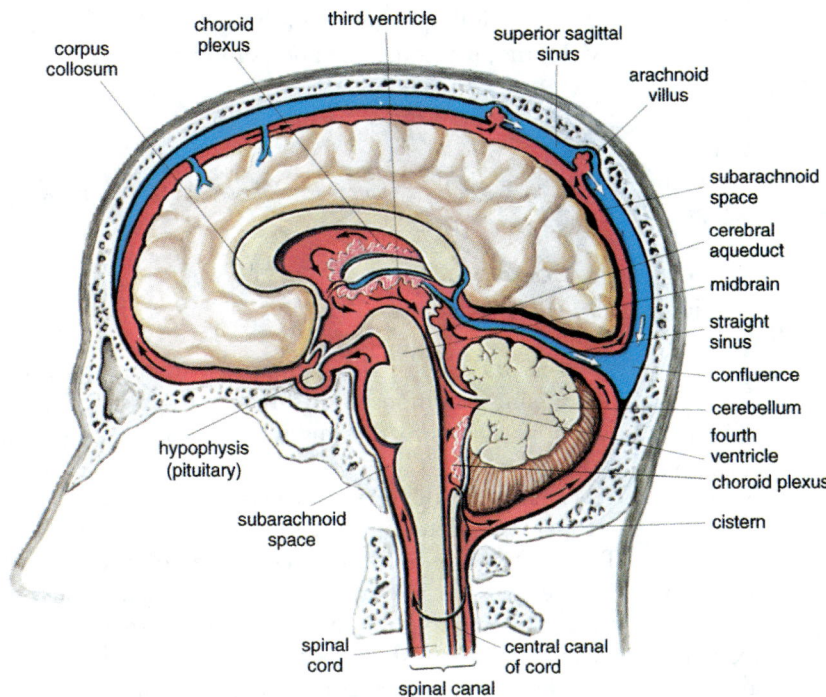

FIGURE 32-4
Flow of cerebrospinal fluid (CSF) from choroid plexuses back to the blood in dural sinuses is shown by the black arrows; flow of blood is shown by the white arrows.

the gray matter is white matter consisting of myelinated axons covered with fatty Schwann cells and dendrites that connect the areas of the cerebrum to one another and to other parts of the brain (Fig. 32-5).

Located deep in the white matter of each hemisphere is a band of gray matter called the **basal ganglia**. The basal ganglia neurons secrete a fluid called dopamine, one of the neurotransmitters essential for controlling body movement and facial expressions.

The cerebral cortex has many functions. As the brain's "memory bank," it sorts and stores knowledge for recall. It facilitates thought processes, judgment, word association, and the highest reasoning powers.

The cerebral cortex is divided into four areas or lobes. Each lobe is bilateral and is divided centrally by the longitudinal fissure. Each is associated with certain functions and is named according to the cranial bone under which it lies.

1.   The frontal lobe lies below the frontal bone in the cranium and is the largest lobe. One of its main functions is generating impulses for voluntary move-

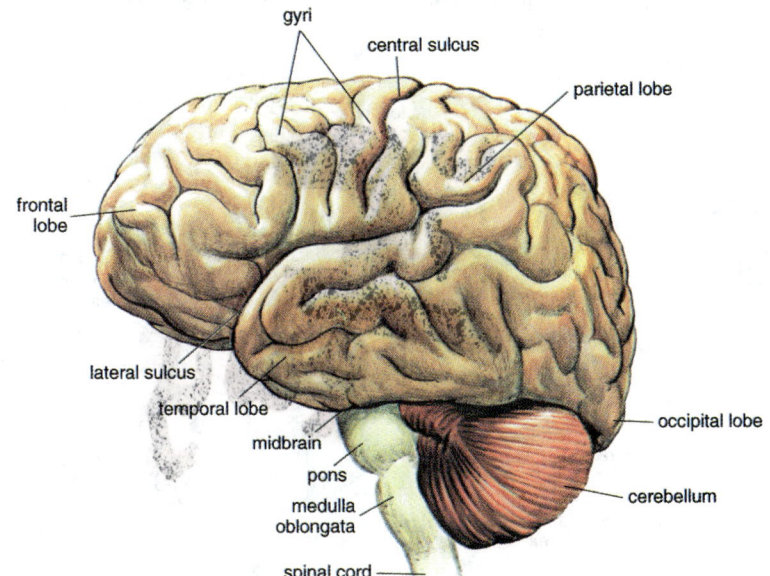

FIGURE 32-5
External surface of the brain showing the main parts and some of the lobes and sulci of the cerebrum.

ment. Other functions include intellectual reasoning, abstract thinking, and speech control.

2. The parietal lobe is found below the parietal skull bones. Its main function is sensory interpretation. It receives impulses from the nerves in the skin for touch, pain, and temperature and from the lingual papillae for taste. This lobe also interprets shapes, distances, and sizes.

3. The temporal lobe is located beneath the temporal bone. Its main function is sound interpretation within its auditory area. Also within this lobe is the olfactory area, which analyzes the stimuli perceived by the olfactory nerve bulbs in the nose.

4. The occipital lobe is located at the base of the cerebrum. Its main function is interpreting visual stimuli received from the optic nerve (Fig. 32-6).

Recent research has revealed the existence of an additional lobe, called the **insula**, which is thought to be responsible for visceral, or body organ, functions.

Under the gray matter of the cerebral cortex is the white matter. In it lies a band of nerve fibers called the corpus callosum responsible for connecting the two hemispheres and transmitting information back and forth between them.

Between the two hemispheres lies the diencephalon. It is made of two parts called the **thalamus** and the **hypothalamus**. Most sensory impulses arrive by way of the thalamus. The thalamus sorts the impulses and sends them to the correct areas of the cerebral cortex for interpretation. Located below the thalamus is the hypothalamus, which is responsible for regulating body temperature, appetite, sleep patterns, and assisting with autonomic responses. It also helps regulate various body functions, including heart rate and blood pressure. In addition, the hypothalamus (in close cooperation with the pituitary) helps regulate several hormones, including secretion of the antidiuretic hormone (ADH) that maintains the body's fluid balance.

Checkpoint Question

2. *What are the four lobes of the cerebral cortex and their functions?*

BRAIN STEM

The brain stem, although apparently one continuous organ, is composed of three overlapping areas of function. They are the **midbrain**, **pons**, and **medulla oblongata**.

The midbrain serves primarily as a relay center for messages that control certain eye and ear reflexes. This part of the midbrain is composed of gray matter. The rest of the midbrain, made up of white matter, transmits impulses from the cerebrum to the other parts of the brain stem, cerebellum, or spinal cord.

The pons is a key communication center, relaying messages between the cerebellum and the entire nervous system. The pons also helps control some of the involuntary muscles used for breathing. In addition, the pons has control over the reticular formation cycle (also referred to as the reticular activating network), which initiates and maintains alertness and awareness. This mechanism wakes us when a threatening sound is perceived, even in deep sleep.

The medulla oblongata—perhaps the most important part of the brain in terms of life maintenance—contains three vital centers that regulate breathing, heart rate, and blood pressure. The respiratory center regulates the muscles used for breathing. The cardiac center regulates heart rate and the force of contractions of the heart muscle. The vasomotor center regulates blood

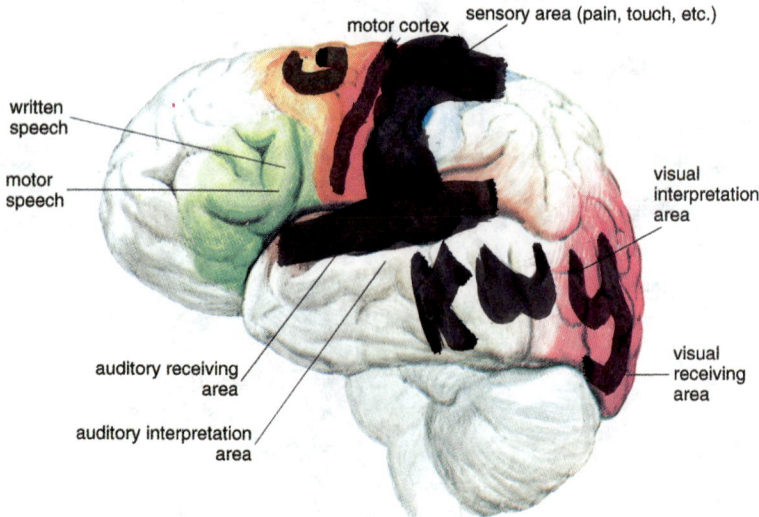

FIGURE 32-6
Functional areas of the cerebral cortex.

pressure by controlling the smooth muscles of the blood vessels, causing either vasoconstriction or vasodilation.

CEREBELLUM

The **cerebellum** is composed of both gray and white matter. It has three basic involuntary functions:

1. *Maintaining equilibrium.* Equilibrium is required for standing, sitting, walking, and all body position changes. The cerebellum coordinates equilibrium by receiving the impulses from the semicircular canals in the inner ear and from various proprioception receptors in the body.
2. *Regulating muscle tone.* The cerebellum ensures that all muscles are ready for impulse reaction. If muscle response is compromised, the state of *tonus* (the condition that maintains the upright position with a state of partial muscle contraction) will collapse, causing paralysis.
3. *Ensuring muscle coordination.* The cerebellum is responsible for the quality of movement of the voluntary muscles.

The cerebellum gives the body its grace and coordination, translating impulses from the cerebrum into muscle movement. Essentially, the cerebrum tells the muscles what to do, and the cerebellum tells them how to do it.

Spinal Cord

The spinal cord is located in the vertebral column. It consists of both gray and white matter for transmitting impulses to and from the brain. The gray matter forms two columns called the ventral and the dorsal horns (see Fig. 32-3). This formation gives the gray matter an "H" appearance. The nerve cell bodies are located here. The white matter fills the rest of the cord and houses the nerve tracts and fibers.

The spinal cord has three distinct functions: sensory, motor, and reflex control. The sensory function carries messages to the brain by way of ascending nerve pathways. The motor function carries messages away from the brain or spinal cord by way of descending nerve pathways. The reflex function requires a stimulus, transmission of the stimulus, and a response. This is possible through connections with a sensory neuron, a connecting or associative neuron, and a motor neuron.

➤ PERIPHERAL NERVOUS SYSTEM

Both the brain and the spinal cord have nerves that transmit impulses. These nerves, called the cranial and spinal nerves, make up the peripheral nervous system (PNS).

Cranial Nerves

The brain is connected to the body through a set of 12 cranial nerves (Fig. 32-7). Cranial nerves function as either sensory, motor, or mixed nerves. Sensory cranial nerves are responsible for functions such as smell, taste, hearing, touch, pain, and vision. The motor cranial nerves are related to both involuntary and voluntary muscle movements and to gland functions. The cranial nerves have specific names and are numbered using Roman numerals. Sensory cranial nerves are I, II, VIII; motor nerves are III, IV, VI, XI, XII; and the mixed are V, VII, IX and X (Table 32-1).

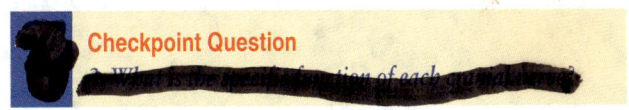

Checkpoint Question

Spinal Nerves

The spinal cord has 31 pairs of spinal nerves. Each nerve is attached to the spinal cord by a dorsal and a ventral root. The dorsal root carries the sensory impulses; the ventral root carries the motor impulses. Therefore, all spinal nerves are mixed nerves (Fig. 32-8). The nerves are numbered by their exit between the vertebrae. The area served by each spinal nerve is referred to as a dermatome.

➤ AUTONOMIC NERVOUS SYSTEM

The autonomic nervous system is a specialized part of the PNS and works without conscious control. It regulates the action of the heart, certain glands, and the smooth muscle hollow organs. It is divided into two systems: **sympathetic** and **parasympathetic**. These systems work to either stimulate certain body functions or to reduce activity (Fig. 32-9).

Sympathetic System

The sympathetic system dominates in times of intense physical or mental stress, automatically producing certain stimuli to the vital organs (ie, the "fright, flight, or fight response"). For example, the following responses help to ensure survival:

1. The adrenal glands are stimulated to produce epinephrine, or adrenaline, a hormone required for the response to stress.
2. Because the brain and muscles need more oxygen to respond to the emergency, the heart rate increases and the force of each contraction becomes

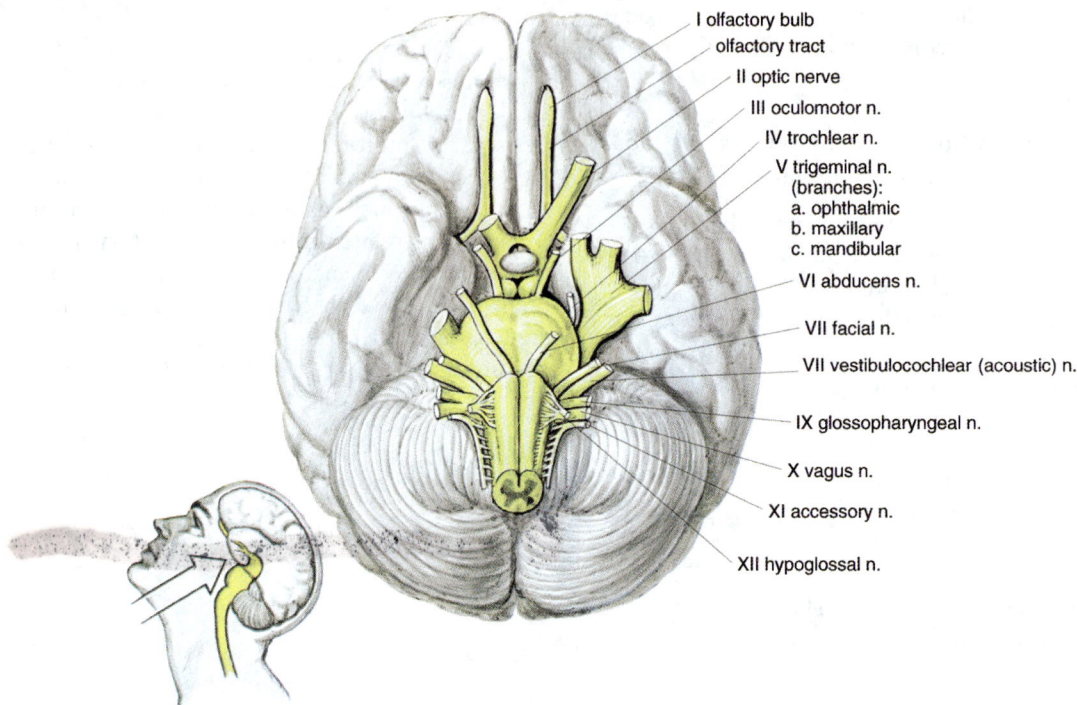

I olfactory bulb
olfactory tract
II optic nerve
III oculomotor n.
IV trochlear n.
V trigeminal n.
(branches):
a. ophthalmic
b. maxillary
c. mandibular
VI abducens n.
VII facial n.
VII vestibulocochlear (acoustic) n.
IX glossopharyngeal n.
X vagus n.
XI accessory n.
XII hypoglossal n.

FIGURE 32-7
Base of the brain showing cranial nerves.

Table 32-1
Cranial Nerves

Nerve (Number)	Type	Functions	Methods for Examining Nerve
Olfactory (I)	Sensory	Sense of smell	Test each nostril for smell reception and interpretation
Optic (II)	Sensory	Sense of vision	Test vision for acuity and visual fields
Oculomotor (III)	Motor	Pupil constriction Raise eyelids	Test pupillary reaction to light and ability to open and close eyelids
Trochlear (IV)	Motor	Downward inward eye movement	Test for downward and inward movement of the eye
Trigeminal (V)	Motor	Jaw movements—chewing and mastication	Ask client to open and clench jaws while palpating the jaw muscles
	Sensory	Sensation on the face and neck	Test face and neck for pain sensations, light touch, temperature
Abducens (VI)	Motor	Lateral movement of the eyes	Test ocular movement in all directions
Facial (VII)	Motor	Muscles of the face	Ask the client to raise eyebrows, smile, show teeth, puff out cheeks
	Sensory	Sense of taste on the anterior two-thirds of the tongue	Test for the taste sensation with various agents
Acoustic (VIII)	Sensory	Sense of hearing	Test hearing ability
Glossopharyngeal (IX)	Motor	Pharyngeal movement and swallowing	Ask the client to say "ah," and have client yawn to observe upward movement of the soft palate; elicit gag response; note ability to swallow
	Sensory	Sense of taste on the posterior one-third of the tongue	Test for taste with various agents
Vagus (X)	Motor	Swallowing and speaking	Ask the client to swallow and speak; note hoarseness
Accessory (XI)	Motor	Movement of shoulder muscles	Ask the client to shrug shoulders against your resistance
Hypoglossal (XII)	Motor	Movement of the tongue; strength of the tongue	Ask the client to protrude tongue; ask client to push tongue against cheek

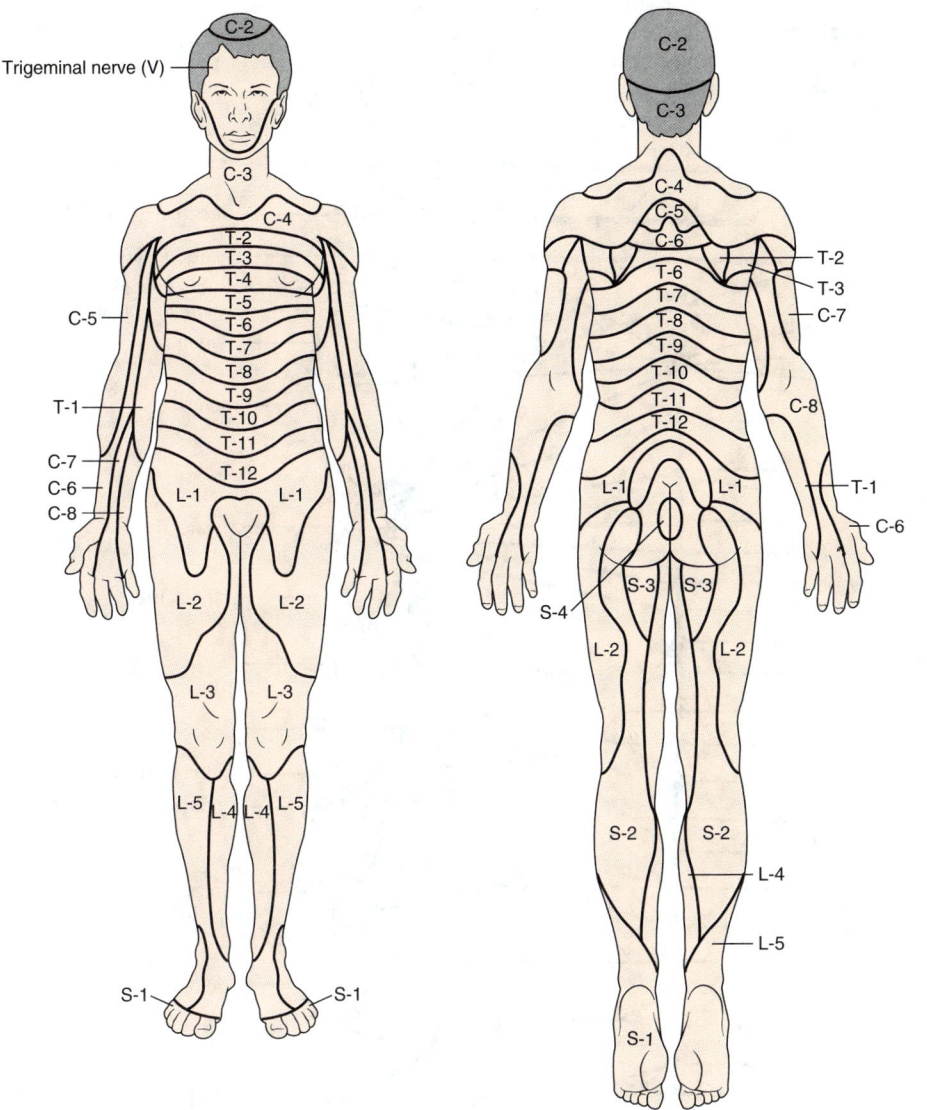

FIGURE 32-8
Spinal dermatomes.

stronger. (This is due to the effect of epinephrine on the cardiovascular system.)

3. The bronchioles dilate in response to the epinephrine, and the respiratory rate increases to allow more oxygen into the lungs.
4. Blood pressure increases to speed blood to areas that must respond to the stressor.
5. Metabolism increases for extra glucose to supply energy for the crisis.
6. The pupils dilate, allowing more visual information to be gathered.
7. The gastrointestinal muscles and kidneys slow to conserve energy and shunt blood where it is most needed.
8. Sweat glands are stimulated to produce perspiration.
9. The blood vessels in the skin constrict to shunt blood away from the skin and to the vital organs.

10. The arrector pili muscles contract, pulling hair follicles upright and causing "goose bumps."

Parasympathetic System

In contrast to the sympathetic system, the parasympathetic system is involved with nonemergency automatic functions. Under normal circumstances or after the stress of a crisis, the following mechanisms take over:

1. The heart slows and the bronchioles constrict with the decreased physiologic need.
2. Saliva production increases and becomes thinner, allowing easier food digestion and nutrient absorption.
3. Blood flow increases to the stomach to aid digestion and nutrient absorption.

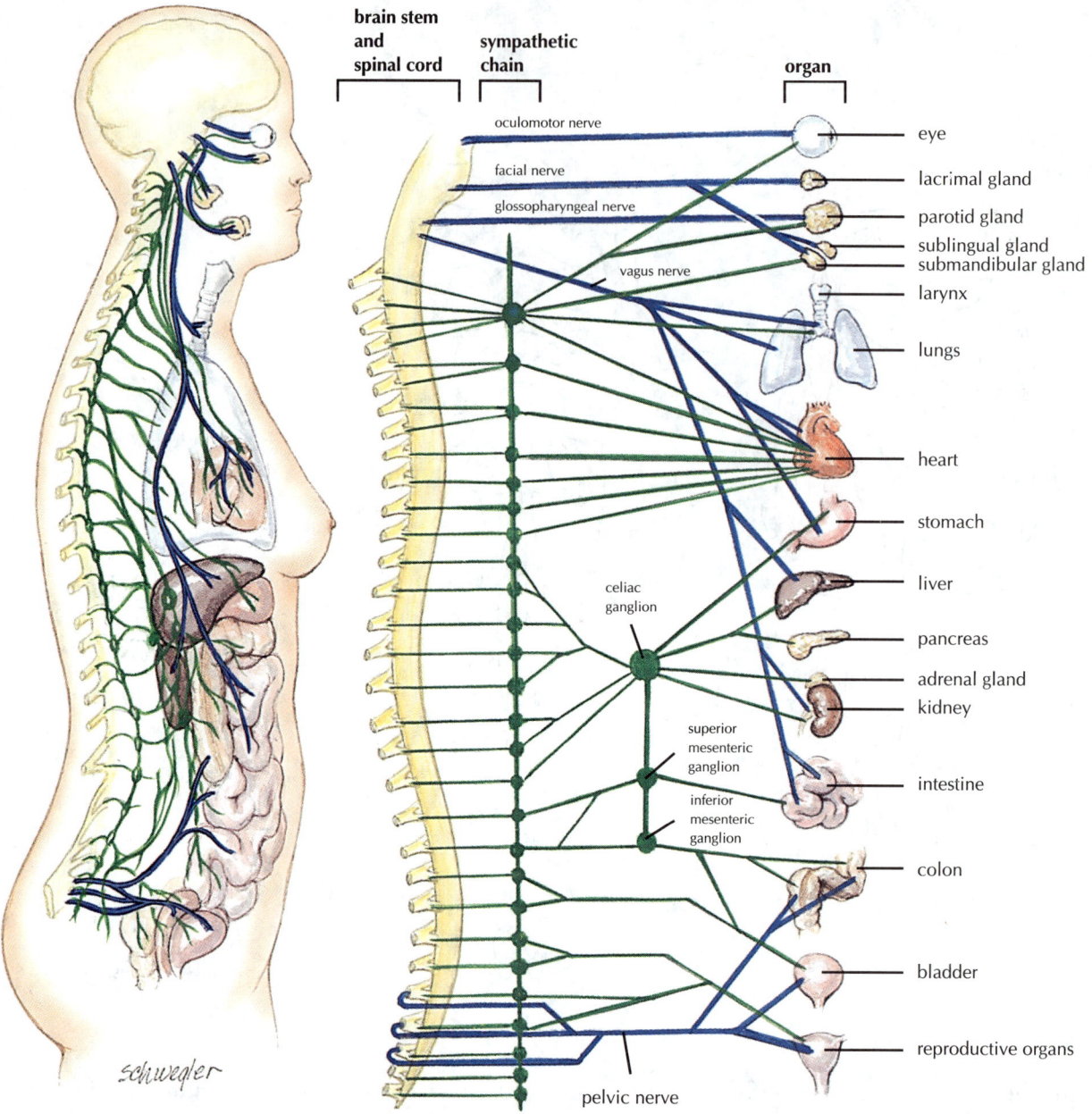

FIGURE 32-9

Autonomic nervous system (only one side is shown). The sympathetic system is shown in green; the parasympathetic system is shown in blue.

4. Kidneys resume urine production and excretion.

Table 32-2 compares body responses to a sympathetic and parasympathetic stimulus.

➤ COMMON NERVOUS SYSTEM DISORDERS

The complexity of the nervous system makes it subject to many disorders. These disorders, which range from minor inconveniences to lethal diseases, can be organized into the following groups: infectious, degenera-

tive, convulsive (seizures), developmental, traumatic, neoplastic, and headaches.

Infectious Disorders

Meningitis

This disorder is characterized by inflammation of the meninges covering the spinal cord and the brain. It can result from either a bacterial or a viral infection. Viral meningitis is usually not life-threatening and is short lived, but bacterial meningitis is often severe and may

Table 32-2

Autonomic Nervous System—Body Response to Sympathetic and Parasympathetic Stimulus

	Sympathetic Stimulus	Parasympathetic Stimulus
Blood Vessels to:	Response	Response
Skeletal muscles	Dilation	Constriction
Skin	Constriction	No effect
Respiratory	Dilation	Constriction
Digestive tract	Constriction	Dilation
Pupils	Dilation	Constriction
Heart	Increased rate	Decreased rate
Bronchi (lungs)	Dilation	Constriction
Sweat glands	Stimulation	No effect
Kidneys	Decreased output	No effect
Liver	Glucose release	No effect
Adrenal medulla	Stimulation	No effect

be fatal. The infectious process is usually precipitated by upper respiratory, sinus, or ear infections. Because these infections occur frequently in children, they are the most likely age group to develop meningitis. Meningitis also can result from head trauma in which an open area allows the organisms to enter the nervous system.

The patient with meningitis will present with a variety of symptoms, including nausea, vomiting, fever, headaches, and a stiff neck. The patient may complain of photophobia (intolerance to lights). A rash with small, reddish purple dots may appear. As patients become sicker, they may slip into a coma and **seizures** (involuntary contractions of voluntary muscles) may occur.

To diagnose meningitis, the physician will usually order a complete blood count (see Chap. 46, Hematology). If the white blood cell count is high, a lumbar puncture (see below) is performed and cerebrospinal fluid (CSF) is analyzed to determine the infectious organism. The treatment of meningitis is based on the organism. For viral meningitis, fluids and bed rest are encouraged. Bacterial meningitis is treated with antibiotics and generally requires hospitalization.

To identify other potential carriers, a thorough patient history is taken. The local health department must be notified of the diagnosis; some states require that an infectious disease form be completed. Depending on the type of meningitis, others who have had contact with the patient may be treated prophylactically.

Checkpoint Question

4. How does the treatment of viral meningitis differ from that of bacterial meningitis?

Encephalitis

Encephalitis is an inflammation of the brain. Frequently, it results from a viral infection that follows varicella (chickenpox), measles, or mumps. A strain of the virus is transmitted by mosquitoes. This type is primarily seen on the eastern and gulf coasts. Symptoms for all forms include drowsiness, headaches, and fever. Seizures and coma may occur in the later stages. Diagnosis is made through a lumbar puncture (see below) and analysis of CSF.

Treatment requires hospitalization for intravenous fluid therapy and supportive care. The prognosis is usually good if the diagnosis is made early and treatment begins quickly.

As with meningitis, the local health department should be notified to identify those who may have been exposed.

Poliomyelitis

Commonly called polio, this highly resistant virus affects the brain and spinal cord. It can live outside the body for several months, making it almost impossible to eliminate once it has appeared in a community. It is transmitted by direct contact and usually enters by the mouth. In the United States, its incidence has been greatly reduced as a result of aggressive immunization programs. However, because not all children have received the proper schedule of immunizations, and because some adults have not been immunized at all, concern about the disease still exists.

In the acute phase, the patient will complain of a stiff neck, fever, headaches, and a sore throat. Nausea, vomiting, and diarrhea may also be noted. As the disease progresses, paralysis may develop. Muscle atrophy occurs, leading to eventual deformities. If the respiratory muscles are affected, the patient will be unable to breathe without artificial assistance.

A new dimension to the disease, postpoliomyelitis muscular atrophy (PPMA) syndrome, has been documented in some individuals who had polio as children. These patients often present with symptoms similar to those that signaled the onset of the original disease. They usually complain of muscle weakness and a lack of coordination. Typically, patients with PPMA are treated on an outpatient basis with supportive care. No cure is known.

During the acute stage of polio, treatment is palliative and supportive. After the primary illness has resolved, treatment is based on rehabilitation with a strong emphasis on physical and occupational therapy. To increase mobility, patients are fitted for mechanical supports (eg, braces and splints). Some patients may need to wear these devices indefinitely. Emotional support is important for these patients, particularly those with PPMA. They often require counseling to reconcile themselves to body image changes caused by the deformities and to allay fear of dependency and loss of autonomy.

Activities aimed at preventing polio are essential. As a medical assistant, you may be responsible for patient education regarding immunizations and the importance of keeping these current. (Polio immunizations are currently given at 2, 4, 6, and 15 months and repeated at 4–6 years of age.) The polio immunization is usually an oral weakened or attenuated vaccine. Persons on chemotherapy or steroidal therapy, transplant recipients, and those who are immunocompromised have been known to contract polio through contact with stools and saliva of recently immunized children. Therefore, children living with immunosuppressed individuals should receive a killed injectable form of the vaccine to avoid shedding the live, weakened virus through their digestive system.

Tetanus

This disorder, commonly called lockjaw, is an infection of nervous tissue caused by the tetanus bacilli *Clostridium tetani*, which live in the intestinal tract of animals and are excreted in their feces. The organisms are found in almost all soil. The bacilli enter the body through puncture wounds or open areas in the skin. Wounds caused by farm equipment in which manure is present are at very high risk for developing tetanus. All deep, dirty wounds should be treated as high risk for tetanus.

Tetanus has a very slow incubation period; it may be present in the body for up to 14 weeks before signs and symptoms occur. Initial symptoms include spasms of the voluntary muscles, restlessness, and stiff neck. As the disease progresses, seizures and **dysphagia** (difficulty swallowing) occur. The facial and oral muscles contract, leaving the mouth sealed with the teeth clenched tightly. The respiratory muscles become paralyzed. The disease is typically fatal.

Prevention is the best defense against tetanus. Wounds should be properly cleaned immediately. Dead tissue around the wound must be removed, and antibiotics should be given if the wound is contaminated with bacteria. Immunizations against tetanus are given prophylactically in infancy at 2, 4, 6, and 15 months, and repeated at age 4 to 6 years and every 10 years for life. If the infection is caused by an animal bite, and the tetanus immunizations are not current, tetanus immune globulin (TIG) is given. Patients who develop tetanus require rapid hospitalization and aggressive antibiotic therapy with supportive care. The prognosis is guarded when tetanus has fully developed.

Rabies

Rabies is transmitted by animal saliva through a bite wound. Animals that most commonly transmit rabies are skunks, squirrels, raccoons, bats, dogs, cats, and foxes. Children are at higher risk for rabies because they are the most likely to be bitten by such animals.

The incubation period for rabies ranges from 10 days to many months. Initial symptoms include fever, general malaise, and body aches. As the disease progresses, mental derangement, paralysis, and photophobia develop. The patient's saliva becomes extremely profuse and sticky and the throat muscles begin to spasm, making swallowing difficult or impossible and causing profuse drooling. (The phrase "foaming at the mouth" has been used to describe this.) Muscle spasms of the throat occur at the sight of water, resulting in hydrophobia. If rabies reaches the brain, it is fatal.

Treatment for bite wounds must be aggressive. After the wound is cleaned, the patient should receive antibiotics and prophylactic vaccine therapy consisting of the human diploid cell vaccine and a rabies immune globulin vaccine.

All animal bites must be reported to the city or county animal control center. If possible, the animal should be quarantined and evaluated for behavioral changes. If the animal is domestic, a complete veterinary history must be obtained. A copy of the animal's rabies tag and certificate, if available, should be placed in the patient's chart.

Reye's Syndrome

This devastating nervous system illness is seen in children after a typical viral illness, commonly varicella (chickenpox). Studies have found that the use of aspirin in combination with a viral illness increases the risk of developing Reye's syndrome. No other antifebrile agents have been implicated in this disorder.

Typical symptoms are vomiting and lethargy. A small red macular rash may occur. Later symptoms include seizures and coma. Diagnosis is made through a variety of blood testing, such as ammonia levels, clotting times, aspartate aminotransferase and alanine aminotransferase, and liver functions.

Patients with Reye's syndrome require rapid hospitalization and aggressive antibiotic therapy and supportive care. The prognosis is good if the diagnosis is made early.

Degenerative Disorders

Multiple Sclerosis (MS)

In MS, the myelin sheaths degenerate and are replaced with plaques, which impair nerve impulse conduction. The cause of MS is unknown although possible origins include a viral infection, autoimmunity, immunologic responses, or genetic predisposition.

Multiple sclerosis is more commonly seen in women between the ages of 20 and 40 (Box 32-1). The disease is characterized by remissions and exacerbations. The rate of progression varies greatly among patients.

Typically, patients will present with complaints of progressive loss of muscle control. They may also complain of loss of balance, shaking tremors, and poor muscle coordination. Tingling and numbness can also be first signs. **Dysphasia** (difficulty speaking) may be another symptom. As the disease progresses, bladder dysfunction and complaints of visual disturbances are common. Patients may also develop nystagmus (involuntary rapid movement of the eyeball in all directions).

Treatment for MS is palliative. Physical therapy is critical to maintain mobility; its goal is to limit the extent of muscle deterioration and to promote existing muscle strength. As the disease progresses, the patient will be fitted for prosthetic appliances such as crutches to assist with ambulation. Drug therapy includes muscle relaxants and steroids.

BOX 32-1 Multiple Sclerosis: A Case Study

Barbara Smith, age 28, is happily married with two children, ages 6 months and 4 years. She has had no past medical pathology and has always considered herself healthy. However, for the past month she has had complaints of general weakness and lack of muscle control. She is finding it hard to do the routine household chores. At first she attributed her tiredness to her young children, but as symptoms grew worse she decided to seek medical attention.

Anticipating that her physician would prescribe "vitamins and rest," she was shocked when Dr. Fernandez diagnosed multiple sclerosis. He determined this through his physical examination and history taking. Filled with concern, Barbara questions Dr. Fernandez about the disease and her prognosis, and he provides her with explanations.

Dr. Fernandez also describes the symptoms that Barbara will eventually develop and further explains there is no definitive cure, only palliative treatments such as physical and occupational therapy, muscle relaxants, steroids, and the application of prosthetic appliances.

Dr. Fernandez arranges an appointment for Barbara and her husband to return to the office within the week for a further evaluation and discussion. At that visit, Dr. Fernandez explains the diagnosis of multiple sclerosis and answers the husband's questions. He also supplies Barbara with local support group telephone numbers.

Over the next 10 years, Barbara has many remissions and exacerbations. She is now confined to a wheelchair and has great difficulty in performing the activities of daily living. She is assisted at home by a nurse.

Dr. Fernandez, Barbara, and her husband begin to make plans for the future. Dr. Fernandez explains the term advance directive. "An advance directive is a statement in advance of what your health care wishes are. Part of it is the living will in which you can state whether you would like to be placed on a feeding tube, breathing machine, or whether you would want cardiopulmonary resuscitation performed." Dr. Fernandez further explains that another part of the advance directive is the assignment of a health care surrogate. "This is a person you assign to be your spokesperson for health care decisions," he says.

Barbara and her husband make their wishes known to Dr. Fernandez and have formal documents made through an attorney. At the end, Barbara and her husband feel great relief that they have had an opportunity to openly and honestly discuss their individual feelings and that personal arrangements have been made.

A large part of caring for patients with MS involves providing psychological support. This disease affects persons in the "prime of life." Patients may have young children at home and so must struggle with emotional concerns regarding long-term welfare for the family. Eventually, sexual dysfunction occurs, and spouses may have difficulty dealing with this symptom. Many support groups and counselors specialize in providing therapy for persons affected by debilitating diseases; share this information with patients as appropriate.

Amyotrophic Lateral Sclerosis (ALS)

Commonly known as Lou Gehrig's disease, ALS causes the progressive loss of motor neurons. It is a terminal disease with no known etiology. There is a strong familial connection. Typically, ALS is seen most often in middle-aged men. It begins with loss of muscle mobility in the forearms, hands, and legs, then progresses to the facial muscles, causing dysphasia and dysphagia that worsen over time. Death usually occurs in 3 to 5 years after the onset of symptoms.

Treatment of ALS involves instituting patient comfort measures and providing family education. As the disease progresses, it becomes increasingly difficult to maintain a patent airway. The family must be instructed in preventing and managing choking. Often, advance directives will be discussed with the family and patient.

Seizure Disorders

Seizures are involuntary contractions of voluntary muscles. (They are commonly called **convulsions** by the lay public.) Seizures have many causes, including chemical imbalances, trauma, pregnancy-induced hypertension, tumors, and withdrawal from drugs or alcohol. However, many seizures prove to be idiopathic (resulting from no known cause).

Epilepsy is the most common form of seizure disorder. The onset of epilepsy may appear in early childhood or at any life stage. Diagnosis is made through electroencephalographic (EEG) studies, blood tests, and radiologic tests.

Epileptic seizures are characterized as either petit mal or grand mal. Petit mal seizures, also called "absence seizures" or "partial seizures," are briefer in duration than grand mal seizures and usually occur only in childhood. The child may appear to "fall asleep" or drift away momentarily. Some muscle twitching may occur. The child awakes and continues the interrupted activities without delay. Petit mal seizures may go undetected for many years.

Grand mal seizures or tonic-clonic seizures, are more involved than petit mal seizures. Generally, the patient will go through three phases:

1. The first phase involves an aura or warning that a seizure is impending. The aura may include tingling in the extremities, visual signs (such as flashing lights), or perception of a particular taste or odor. Not all patients have auras, but those who do usually experience the same aural phenomena each time.
2. The second phase is the complete loss of consciousness with extensive muscle twitching or contractions, which may be violent. The patient falls to the ground and usually loses control of bladder and bowel functions.
3. The third phase is the postictal state. During this phase, the patient slowly regains consciousness but will remain drowsy for an extended time.

The primary treatment during the actual seizure involves preventing injury to the patient (Table 32-3). Epilepsy is treated with various pharmacologic agents. When providing patient teaching, instruct patients to take these medications every day as prescribed, never missing a dose. Many epileptic patients who become stabilized and seizure free on medication feel they no longer need the medication. Remind these patients that stopping the medication may lead to the recurrence of seizures.

A patient who has seizures is allowed to have a driver's license; however, each state has specific regulations requiring that patients be seizure free for a particular length of time (eg, 2 years) to qualify.

Checkpoint Questions

5. *How do petit mal seizures differ from grand mal seizures? Describe the typical progression of a grand mal seizure.*

Febrile Seizures

These kinds of seizures occur in a small number of children, most commonly between the ages of 6 months and 3 years. Children suffering febrile seizures must have a complete physical and neurologic examination to rule out the possibility of an organic origin for the seizures. Children generally outgrow febrile seizures by age 6 or 7, with no other seizure activity after this time.

Treatment involves gently returning the body temperature to a more manageable level. Cool compresses are preferable to ice baths or alcohol sponges, which

Table 32-3
Action STAT: How to Care for an Actively Seizing Patient

Action	Rationale
Place the patient on the floor and remove nearby objects (chairs, tables, electrical cords, and so on).	This will prevent additional injury from falling. Removing all obstacles in the way of the patient will also decrease injuries.
Protect the patient's head.	The convulsions will be very strong. It is possible for the patient to sustain brain injury or skull fractures from falling to the floor.
Put nothing in the patient's mouth while actively seizing.	It is a myth that the tongue will be swallowed. By forcing an object into the mouth, teeth may be broken, the airway may be obstructed, or oral damage may occur. After the seizure, an oral airway may be inserted by emergency personnel or the physician if necessary.
Provide privacy to the patient.	This can be very embarrassing for the patient. Usually incontinence occurs. Try to have other patients escorted to other waiting areas, or screen the seizing patient from view.
Get physician assistance.	Sometimes medications are needed to control the seizure. Some patients will be transferred to the hospital.
Place the patient in the recovery position after the seizure is over.	It is common for a postseizure patient to vomit. If the patient is in the side-lying position, vomitus will not be aspirated and the airway is kept open.

The first exposure to a seizing patient may be frightening for the entire health care team. Remember to maintain professionalism at all times.

Focus on the Patient: Coping With Febrile Seizures

Febrile seizures can be very scary for parents of small children. Here's how you can help parents cope:

- Reassure the parents that febrile seizures are common in young children and that they generally are not chronic in nature.
- Allow the parents to be involved in the care of the child. Once the child is stabilized, urge the parents to hold and comfort the child.
- Provide easy-to-understand explanations for all procedures.
- Encourage parents to verbalize their fears.

You, too, will probably be very anxious in this situation; however, you must remain calm and demonstrate confidence in handling the situation.

may cause hypothermia. To avoid Reye's syndrome, salicylates should not be given.

Focal (Jacksonian) Seizures

This type of seizure begins as a small localized seizure that spreads to adjacent areas. For instance, the small seizure may begin in the fingers and spread to the hand and arm. The cause of focal seizures must be researched to prevent the progression to generalized seizures.

Developmental Disorders

Neural Tube Defects

Many abnormalities may occur during the embryonic and fetal stages of development. As the neural tube develops in the embryo, it will grow and expand as the embryo matures. Tissue closes over the tube and evolves into the components of the CNS. If a developmental failure occurs on the proximal (upper) portion, anencephaly, or absence of a brain, will result.

An abnormality in development in the distal, or caudal, end of the neural tube will result in spina bifida. **Spina bifida occulta** is the most benign form. In this condition, the posterior laminae of the vertebrae fail to close, typically at L-5 or S-1. There are usually no external signs of a deformity; only a skin dimple or dark tufts of hair may be present. A **meningocele** occurs when the meninges protrude through the spina bifida. In spina bifida with **myelomeningocele**, the most severe form, the spinal cord and meninges protrude externally (Fig. 32-10). The main treatment is surgical intervention. Prognosis is based on the extent of spinal cord involvement.

Hydrocephalus

Hydrocephalus occurs when excessive CSF is present in the arachnoid and ventricular spaces of the brain. Although it occurs more commonly in children as the result of a defect in CSF production or absorption, hydrocephalus sometimes occurs in adults as a result of tumors or trauma. Treatment involves surgical insertion of a shunt, which reroutes the excessive CSF from the brain to the right atrium of the heart or the peritoneal cavity. The prognosis is usually good if treated aggressively in the early stages, before CNS damage has occurred.

Cerebral Palsy

Cerebral palsy is the term used to describe a group of neuromuscular disorders that result from CNS damage sustained during the prenatal, neonatal, or postnatal periods. Although cerebral palsy is not progressive, the damage may become more obvious as developmental delays are discovered. Impairment may range from slight motor dysfunction to catastrophic physical and mental disabilities. Prognosis varies with the site of the damage and its severity.

Treatment is supportive and rehabilitative. Currently, no cure exists.

Trauma

Traumatic injuries are the most common among the young to middle-age groups. Traumatic injuries are the number one killer for individuals between ages 1 and 24.

Traumatic Brain Injuries

The pediatric population is particularly at risk for head trauma. A child's head is large in proportion to the rest of the body. Therefore, as children fall (as they do frequently), gravity will pull the head to the ground first. Children are also more prone to traumatic injuries because their reflex systems are immature.

Traumatic injuries to the brain include concussions, contusions, or intracranial hemorrhages. A concussion is a nonlethal brain injury that results from blunt trauma. The patient may experience a momentary loss of consciousness but returns to an awake and alert status promptly. A contusion is more serious and involves a focal alteration of cerebral circulation. Hemorrhages and extravasation of blood and fluid can result. Loss of consciousness will result and brain damage may occur. Intracranial hemorrhages involve the bleeding of a vessel inside the skull due to trauma, congenital abnormalities, or aneurysms. (See Chap. 35, Caring for Patients With Cardiovascular Disorders, for more information about aneurysms.)

Traumatic brain injuries are diagnosed through radiographic studies. Treatment for contusions and hemorrhages can involve surgery, drug therapy, and supportive care. The prognosis for all brain injuries de-

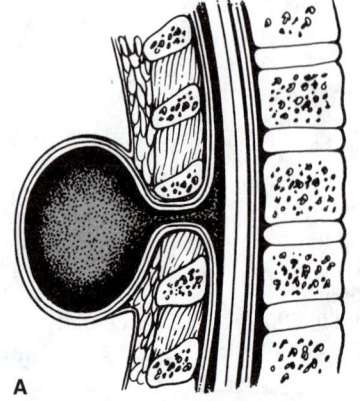
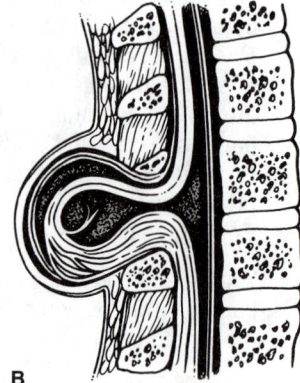

FIGURE 32-10
Types of spina bifida. (A) Meningocele. (B) Meningomyelocele.

A

B

Table 32-4
Spinal Cord Injuries

Level of Injury	Resulting Disabilities
Cervical 1–2	Unable to breathe on own
	No neck muscle control
Cervical 3–4	May be able to manipulate electric wheelchair with mouth piece
	Some neck control possible
Cervical 5	Uses wheelchair with hand controls
	Self-feeds with hand splints
	Good elbow flexion
Cervical 6	Transfers to wheelchair and bed with little or no assistance
	Good shoulder control
Cervical 7	Transfers independently to wheelchair and bed
	Self-feeds with no special devices
Thoracic 1–4	Able to move from wheelchair to floor with little or no assistance
	Normal upper extremity function
Thoracic 5–Lumbar 2	Total wheelchair independence
	Limited ambulation with bilateral leg braces and crutches
Lumbar 3–4	Ambulation with short leg braces with or without crutches
Lumbar 5–Sacral 3	Able to ambulate on own with no equipment, if good foot strength is present

pends on the extent of damage and the location of the injury.

Spinal Cord Injuries

Spinal cord injuries are most common among individuals 15 to 35 years of age. Most often, spinal cord in- juries are due to trauma from motor vehicle accidents, diving accidents, or falls. Spinal cord injuries may be either complete, in which the cord is transected and no neurologic abilities remain below the point of injury, or incomplete, in which the cord is spared with minor to severe neurologic disabilities below the point of in- jury (Table 32-4). The higher in the spinal cord the in- jury, the more serious the complications for the patient (Table 32-5). There is no cure at this time.

In caring for patients with spinal cord injuries, the initial consideration is to prevent further damage. Ac- cident victims with suspected spinal cord injuries must be kept immobile until proper emergency medical ser- vices personnel are present. Treatment in the emer- gency department is focused on stabilization.

In the physician's office, patients in the posttrauma period receive follow-up treatment and evaluation. These patients are continuously monitored for changes in their reflexes and evaluated for physical therapy. The goal of long-term care is to prevent complications, which can include skin ulcerations (pressure ulcers), hypostatic pneumonia, bladder infections, contrac- tures, and depression. Most of the physical complica- tions will be treated with physical therapy and good care; the mental and emotional complications will re- quire intensive therapy by counselors who specialize in treating patients with debilitating disorders.

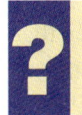

Checkpoint Question
6. How does a complete spinal cord injury differ from an incomplete one?

Brain Tumors

Brain tumors may be either malignant or benign; many are secondary or metastatic sites. If the brain tumor is the primary site, it is named for the site of origin (eg,

Table 32-5
Types of Paralysis

Type	Causes	Result
Hemiplegia	Cerebrovascular accident, trauma to one side of the brain, tumors	Paralysis on side of body opposite involvement
Paraplegia	Spinal cord trauma, spinal tumors	Paralysis of any part of the body below the point of involvement
Quadriplegia	Spinal cord trauma, spinal tumors	Paralysis of all limbs (usually cervical or high thoracic vertebra involvement)

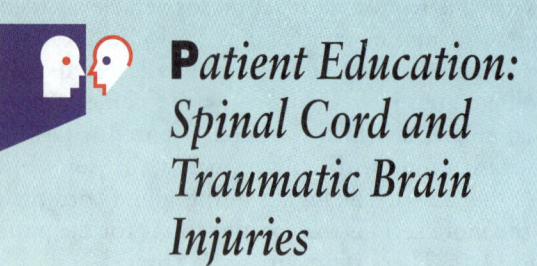

Patient Education: Spinal Cord and Traumatic Brain Injuries

Spinal cord and traumatic brain injuries are very common among young people. Both types of injuries can produce serious and even fatal results. As a medical assistant, you must take an active role in educating your community, patients, and friends about the prevention of these injuries. Education may include instructions such as:

- Use seat belts for all passengers.
- Secure infants and young children in approved car seats.
- Avoid alcohol when participating in sporting activities and driving.
- Obey traffic signs and speed limits.
- Avoid illicit drug use or any medication that impairs awareness.
- Wear helmets while bicycling and riding motorcycles.

glioma, meningioma, medulloblastoma). Both malignant and benign tumors can produce serious complications for the patient because of the limited space inside the cranium.

Generally, the patient will present with vague complaints of headaches, blurred vision, personality changes, or memory loss. In more advanced cases, seizures, blindness, and dysphagia may be evident. The type of tumor and its location will affect the presenting symptoms, their severity and onset, and the prognosis.

Diagnosis is made primarily through radiologic studies. The treatment can include surgery, radiation therapy, chemotherapy, or a combination of radiation and chemotherapy.

Headaches

It is estimated that 70% of the population experiences headaches. Headaches may have a variety of origins including stress, trauma, bone pathology, infections (eg, sinus), or vascular disturbances. In many instances, the etiology will never be known.

Migraine headaches are one of the most common types of headaches. These can be triggered by stress,

high altitudes, smoking, certain smells, or ingested chemicals (caffeine, alcohol, certain food additives), but in many situations the cause is unknown. Patients who have migraines may complain of an aura before the onset. Symptoms usually include a unilateral temporal headache, photophobia, diplopia, and nausea. Generally, headaches are treated with analgesics, and the patient may be instructed to rest in a dark, quiet room. Propanolol (Inderal) and ergotamine derivatives have shown promise in headache prevention for patients with frequent, debilitating migraines.

Other common types of headaches include:

- *Tension headaches.* These are associated with contraction of the muscles of the neck and scalp due to stress. The treatment involves muscle relaxants, analgesics, and reversing the precipitating factors.
- *Cluster headaches.* Theses are similar to migraine headaches but typically occur at night. They are usually of short duration but may recur as often as four or five times a night for several weeks and then not again for weeks or months. They are associated with stress and tension. Treatment requires muscle relaxants, analgesics, and relieving the stressful situation.

➤ COMMON DIAGNOSTIC TESTS FOR NERVOUS SYSTEM DISORDERS

The physician may perform a variety of tests to evaluate a patient's neurologic status. These tests may be invasive or noninvasive and may include radiologic and electrical tests as well as physical examinations.

Physical Examination

The physical examination is a key component in diagnosing nervous system disorders and includes the following evaluations:

- Mental status and orientation
- Cranial nerve assessment
- Sensory and motor functions
- Reflex assessment

The patient's mental status is evaluated by routine questioning to establish mental alertness and orientation. For example, the examiner may ask the patient to count to 10 and to state the president's name and the current year.

Cranial nerves are assessed according to the methods discussed in Table 32-1. For example, visual acuity may be tested on a chart such as the Snellen eye chart.

Sensory function is tested with the pin versus soft brush method for spinal nerves and cranial nerves. The instrument commonly used is the Buck neurologic hammer (see Fig. 22-1 in Chap. 22, Physical Examination). With the patient's eyes closed, the physician uses the pin or brush to determine the patient's ability to distinguish between sensations. The physician evaluates sensory reception and determines if there is a reception difference on either side of the body.

Motor functioning is tested by watching the patient walk. Many disorders can be detected by observing a patient's gait. Part of this assessment will include the **Romberg test**. The patient is asked to stand with feet together and with eyes closed. A positive Romberg sign is noted if the patient sways or is unsteady.

The last part of the examination includes reflex testing (Table 32-6). Figure 32-11 depicts the correct method for tendon reflex testing. Reflexes are scored using this scale:

0—No response
1+—Diminished response
2+—Normal
3+—Brisker than normal
4+—Hyperactive with clonus, which is the repetitive jerking of a muscle and indicates a neurologic disorder

Radiologic Tests

The most common examples of noninvasive radiologic tests include computed tomography (CT) scan and magnetic resonance imaging (MRI). These tests may also be done with a contrast medium or dye. The contrast medium helps differentiate between the soft tissue areas of the nervous system and the tumors, lesions, or hemorrhages that may blend in with their supporting tissues (see Chap. 27, Diagnostic Imaging).

A **myelogram** is an invasive form of radiologic test in which dye is injected into the CSF. The spinal cord is then filmed and various abnormalities can be detected. The blood vessels of the brain can be visualized on x-ray by injecting a dye through a femoral artery catheter threaded up to the carotid artery in a test called a cerebral angiogram.

Radiography of the skull may be used to rule out many possible disorders and is diagnostic for fractures and malformations.

Electrical Tests

An **electroencephalogram (EEG)** is a noninvasive test that records electrical impulses in the brain. A variety of electrodes are placed on the patient's scalp and tracings of brain wave activity are recorded. Typically, the patient is given a mild sedative to induce a quiet state.

Checkpoint Question
7. *What are the differences between a myelogram and an EEG?*

Lumbar Puncture

A lumbar puncture is used to diagnosis infectious, inflammatory, or bleeding disorders. A needle is inserted into the subarachnoid space at the level of L-4 to L-5, below the level of the spinal cord (Fig.

Table 32-6 Reflex Testing			
Reflex	*Method of Testing*	*Expected Response*	*Localization*
Brachioradialis	Tapping the styloid process of radius	Flexion of elbow	C-5 and C-6
Biceps	Tapping on biceps tendon	Flexion of elbow	C-5 and C-6
Triceps	Tapping on triceps	Extension of elbow	C-7
Patellar	Tapping on patellar tendon	Extension of leg	L-2 and L-4
Achilles	Tapping on Achilles tendon	Plantar flexion of foot	S-1
Corneal	Light touch on the corneoscleral corner	Closure of eyelid	Cranial nerves V and VII

C, cervical; L, lumbar; S, sacral

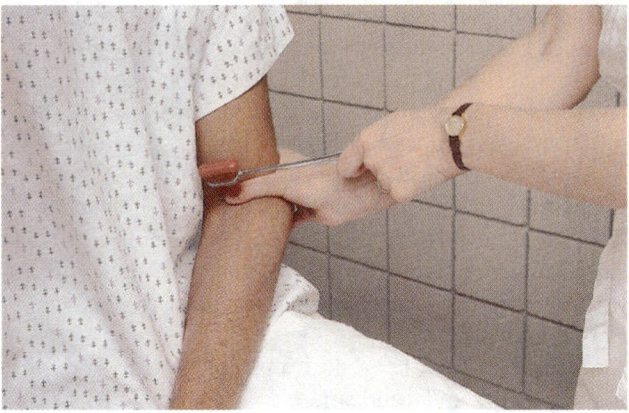

A Biceps reflex

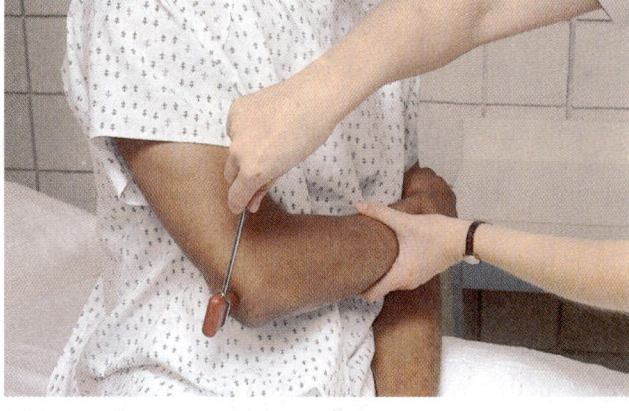

B Triceps reflex

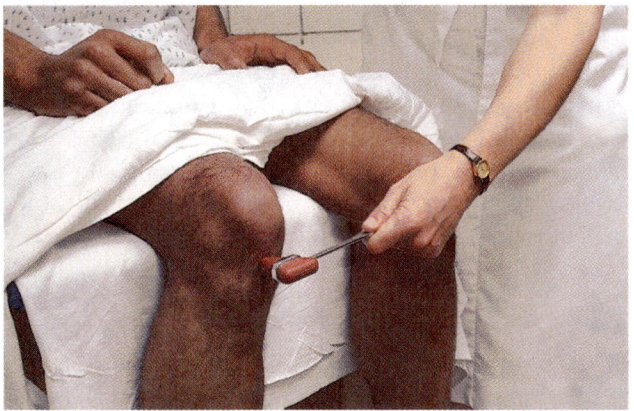

C Patellar reflex

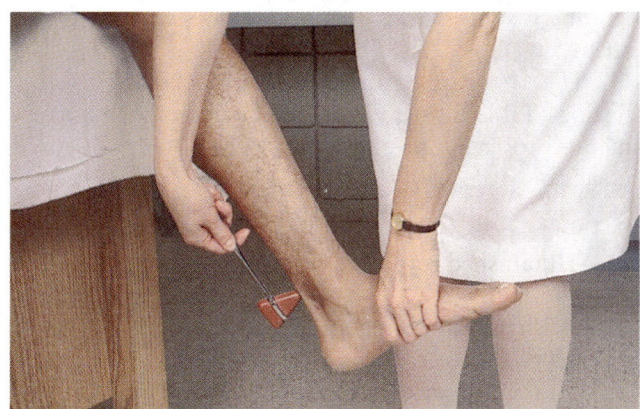

D Ankle or Achilles reflex

FIGURE 32-11
Techniques for eliciting major tendon reflexes.

32-12). CSF is removed and may be tested for glucose, protein, bacteria, cell counts, and the presence of red blood cells to indicate intracranial bleeding. It may also be evaluated to determine intracranial pressure. In addition, the presence of an obstruction in the CSF flow can be determined through the **Queckenstedt test**.

If a lumbar puncture is performed in the medical office, the medical assistant's responsibility includes assisting the patient into a side-lying, curled position or a supported, forward-bending sitting position. These are difficult and uncomfortable positions to maintain. You may help the patient to relax in these positions by encouraging slow, deep breathing. Procedure 32-1 describes the steps for assisting the physician with a lumbar puncture.

Patients must rest lying flat for 6 to 12 hours after a lumbar puncture and may require intravenous fluids and pain medications for the severe headaches that are often experienced. For these reasons, the lumbar puncture is more commonly performed in outpatient clinics than in the medical office.

Prenatal Screening

Great strides have been made in diagnosing fetal abnormalities early in gestation. During the first trimester, a procedure called chorionic villus sampling may be performed to detect chromosomal abnormalities. In this test, a small tissue sample is taken from the embryonic implantation site for analysis.

At 16 to 18 weeks of gestation, a routine blood test for **alpha-fetoprotein** (AFP) is done to assess development of the neural tube, which will evolve into the brain and spinal cord. AFP is a substance produced by the embryonic yolk sac and later by the fetal liver. Elevated AFP levels *may* indicate nervous system deformities. Falsely elevated samples can be caused by more than one fetus or incorrect gestational dates. A positive AFP result is often followed by an **amniocentesis**. In this invasive procedure, a needle is inserted through the abdomen into the gravid uterus to remove fluid from the amniotic sac. The fluid is analyzed for a variety of nervous system and sex-linked disorders.

An ultrasound allows the physician to see the brain and spinal cord of the developing fetus. Many CNS disorders can be detected by this method, including spina bifida and anencephaly.

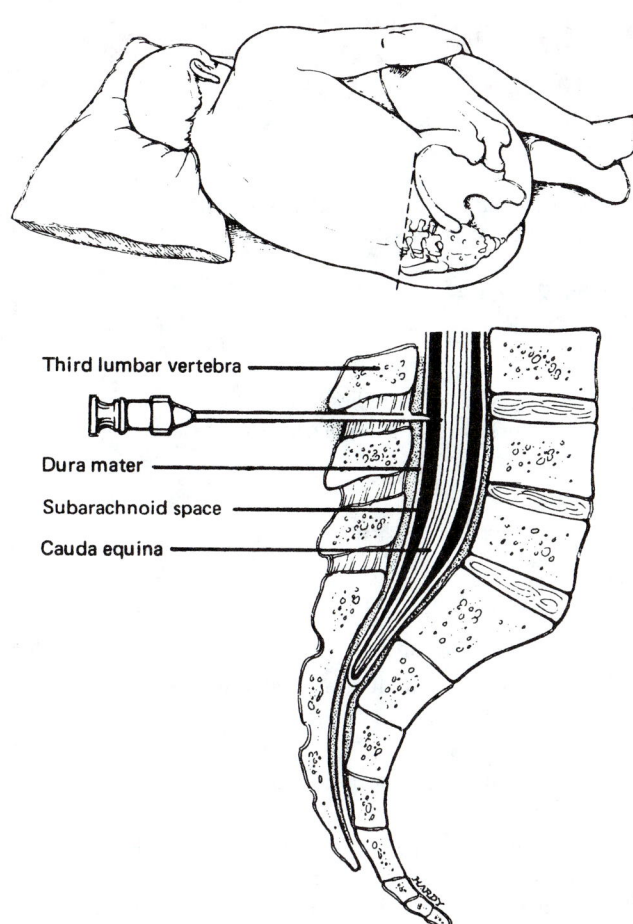

FIGURE 32-12
Technique for lumbar puncture. The interspaces between L-3 and L-5 are just below the line connecting the anterior-superior iliac spines.

Third lumbar vertebra

Dura mater

Subarachnoid space

Cauda equina

What If?

You are working in an obstetrician's office and have been asked to draw a blood sample from a pregnant patient to test for AFP. What if the patient seems anxious about the test?

Allow the patient to voice any concerns and encourage her to ask questions about the test. Explain that AFP is a test to determine abnormalities of the CNS in the developing fetus. If the test results are positive, an amniocentesis will likely be performed to obtain additional information.

Pediatric Tests

The nervous system is immature at birth. Cortical function develops slowly and cannot be completely tested until early childhood. During regular visits to the pediatrician, the infant is tested for infantile automatisms—reflexes found in the newborn that disappear later in childhood. Examples include the Moro (or startle) reflex and the rooting reflex (see Chap. 49, Pediatric Patients). The absence of infantile automatisms, or the

text continues on page 604

✓ Charting Example

02/12/99	0830 Patient positioned and draped for lumbar puncture, BP 120/80,
	P-86, R-18. Dr. Alexander performed LP.
	0900 LP completed. Pt tolerated procedure well. CSF sent to the lab.
	Post LP vitals: 114/74, P-76, R-16. Pt resting comfortably.
	0930 Pt denies discomfort. No n/v. No leakage at LP site.
	Pt and wife were given d/c instructions.
	Verbalized understanding. Pt d/c by Dr. Alexander.
	— Barbara Ryan, CMA

Procedure 32-1

Assisting With a Lumbar Puncture

Equipment/Supplies

On the sterile field
- 3–5-inch lumbar needle with a stylet (physician will specify gauge and length)
- gloves for the physician
- gauze sponges
- test tubes

- spinal fluid manometer with a 3-way stopcock adapted (if CSF pressure is to be measured)
- fenestrated drape
- sterile drape
- antiseptic

On the side
- local anesthetic and syringe
- adhesive bandages
- sterile gloves (if not included on the field)
- examination gloves for the assistant

- skin preparation supplies
- blood pressure cuff (if Queckenstedt test is to be performed)

Steps	Purpose
1. Wash your hands.	1. Handwashing aids infection control.
2. Assemble the equipment. (Most offices stock the equipment in a purchased disposable tray or a site-prepared setup.)	2. This ensures that all of the materials are available.
3. Gather personal protective equipment (eg, gloves, face shield, impervious gown) as needed.	3. Standard precautions must be followed.
4. Identify the patient and explain the procedure. Check that the consent form is signed and posted on the chart. Explain that the puncture will be made below the level of the spinal cord and should present no danger to the patient. Warn the patient not to move during the procedure. Tell the patient that the area will be numbed but that pressure may still be felt after the local anesthetic is administered.	4. Identifying the patient prevents errors in treatment. Explaining the procedure helps ease anxiety and ensures compliance. Although there is little chance of damage to the cord, movement may cause the patient injury and will probably contaminate the field.
5. Have the patient void.	5. This will decrease the level of discomfort during the procedure.
6. Direct the patient to disrobe and put on a gown with the opening in the back.	6. The back must be exposed for the procedure.
7. When the physician is ready, open the field (follow the steps described in Procedure 24-1, Opening Sterile Surgical Packs, in Chap. 24, Assisting With Minor Office Surgery) and assist with the initial preparations.	
8. Prepare the skin if this is not done as part of the sterile preparation. Many physicians prefer to prepare the skin using a sterile forceps after gloving. If this is the preferred procedure, you may be required to add sterile solutions to the field (follow the steps in Procedure 24-3, Adding Sterile Solution to a Sterile Field in Chap. 24, Assisting With Minor Office Surgery). Assist as needed with administration of the anesthetic.	

(continued)

Procedure 32-1   Assisting With a Lumbar Puncture (continued)

Steps	Purpose
9. Assist the patient into the appropriate position. *For the side-lying position:* • Stand in front and help by holding the knees and top shoulder. Have the patient move so the back is close to the edge of the table. *For the forward-leaning, supported position:* • Stand in front and rest your hands on the patient's shoulders as a reminder to remain still. Have the patient breathe slowly and deeply.	9. These positions widen the space between the vertebrae to allow entrance of the needle. Your presence will help ensure that there is no movement during the procedure.
10. Throughout the procedure, observe the patient closely for signs such as dyspnea or cyanosis. Monitor the pulse at intervals and record the vital signs after the procedure. Note mental alertness, any leakage at the site, nausea, and vomiting. Assess lower limb mobility.	
11. When the physician has the needle securely in place, help the patient to straighten slightly to ease tension and to allow a more normal CSF flow. The physician may now use the stopcock and spinal fluid manometer to determine the intracranial pressure.	
12. If specimens are to be taken, put on gloves to receive the potentially hazardous body fluid. Label the tubes in sequence as you receive them. Label them also with the patient's identification and place them in biohazard bags.	12. The first tube may be more likely to contain contaminants.
13. If the Queckenstedt test is to be performed, you may be required to press the veins of the neck with your hands, first the right, then the left, then both sides, each for ten seconds, while the physician measures the pressure with the stopcock and manometer. In an alternate method, the physician places a blood pressure cuff around the patient's neck before gloving for the procedure and instructs you to inflate the cuff to 22 mmHg for 10 seconds while he measures the pressure with the manometer.	13. The Queckenstedt test helps determine the presence of an obstruction in the CSF flow. Normally the pressure will rise and drop rapidly during the procedure. If an obstruction is present, the rise and return to normal may be very slow or there may be no response to the external application of pressure.
14. At the completion of the procedure, cover the site with an adhesive bandage and assist the patient to a flat position. The physician will determine when the patient is ready to leave the examining room and the office.	14. Many patients experience severe headaches after the procedure and must be monitored during the recovery period.
15. Route the specimens as required. Clean the room and care for or dispose of the equipment as needed. Wash your hands.	15. Standard Precautions must be followed throughout the procedure.
16. Chart all observations and record the procedure.	16. Procedures are considered not to have been done if they are not recorded.

Note: *Before beginning, assess the lumbar region. If the site is very hairy, it may be necessary to shave the skin before the procedure. (Follow the steps for skin preparation and hair removal in Procedure 24-4 in Chap. 24, Assisting With Minor Office Surgery.) Strict asepsis must be observed to reduce the risk of introducing microorganisms into the nervous system.*

continuation of these reflexes beyond infancy, suggests potential CNS dysfunction and requires further testing.

Specific gross and fine motor coordination can be tested from birth through childhood by the Denver Developmental Screening Tests (DDST), which evaluate motor, sensory, and language development and social skills. DDST are usually performed at routine intervals throughout early childhood at well-child visits. The DDST do not measure intelligence levels.

SUMMARY

The nervous system is complex and works with both conscious and unconscious functions. It allows us to perform the activities of daily living, records our memories, helps us think rationally, moves us through our external environment safely, and coordinates our internal environment. It has two major divisions: the CNS and the PNS. Nervous system disorders can be grouped into several types: infectious, degenerative, convulsive, developmental, traumatic, neoplastic, and headaches. Common diagnostic tests include radiologic studies (eg, CT scan and MRI), EEG, physical examinations, prenatal screening, lumbar puncture, and skull x-rays. Although many positive strides are being made in the diagnosis and care of neurologic disorders, medical assistants must be aware that neurologic disorders can be physically and psychologically devastating for patients and their families.

CRITICAL THINKING CHALLENGES

1. Your patient has a spinal cord injury below C-5. Describe the functions of the spinal nerves above and below that point of injury. Explain what symptoms this patient might experience.
2. A 3-year-old girl comes into the office with varicella zoster (chickenpox). She has a fever, and the physician orders acetaminophen. The child's mother asks, "Why can't she have aspirin instead?" How would you respond?

ANSWERS TO CHECKPOINT QUESTIONS

1. Communication between two neurons occurs when a message released by one axon jumps across the synapse to the next dendrite.
2. The frontal lobe is responsible for motor functions, reasoning, thinking, and speech. The parietal lobe is responsible for touch, pain, temperature, and interpretation of spatial concepts. The temporal lobe is responsible for interpreting sounds and smells. The occipital lobe is responsible for interpreting visual stimuli.
3. The specific function of each cranial nerve is as follows:
    - I. Olfactory—sensory—sense of smell
    - II. Optic—sensory—vision
    - III. Oculomotor—motor—eye muscles
    - IV. Trochlear—motor—eye muscles
    - V. Trigeminal—mixed—facial sensations, jaw muscles
    - VI. Abducens—motor—eye movements
    - VII. Facial—motor—expressions, sense of taste
    - VIII. Acoustic—sensory—hearing and balance
    - IX. Glossopharyngeal—mixed—taste, swallowing, salivation
    - X. Vagus—mixed—visceral functions and respirations
    - XI. Accessory—motor—neck and shoulder muscles
    - XII. Hypoglossal—motor—tongue movements
4. For viral meningitis, fluids and bed rest are encouraged. For bacterial meningitis, antibiotics are prescribed and hospitalization may be required.
5. Petit mal seizures are briefer in duration than grand mal seizures and usually occur only in childhood. Grand mal seizures are more involved than petit mal seizures and encompass three phases. The first phase involves an *aura*, or warning that a seizure is impending. The second phase is the complete loss of consciousness. During the third phase, the *postictal* state, the patient slowly regains consciousness.
6. A complete spinal cord injury involves total transection of the spinal cord; no neurologic abilities remain below the point of injury. An incomplete spinal cord injury is one in which the cord is spared, with minor to severe neurologic disabilities below the point of injury.
7. An EEG is a noninvasive, electrical test of brain waves. A myelogram is an invasive, radiologic test in which dye is injected into the CSF to help detect abnormalities.

SUGGESTIONS FOR FURTHER READING

Adams, R. D., Victor, M. (1993). *Principles of Neurology*, 5th ed. New York: McGraw-Hill.

Bullock, B. L., Rosendahl, P. P. (1992). *Pathophysiology*, 3rd ed. Philadelphia: J. B. Lippincott.

Craven, R. F., Hirnle, C. J. (1992). *Fundamentals of Nursing*. Philadelphia: J. B. Lippincott.

Greenberg, D. A., Aminoff, M. J., Simon, R. P. (1993). *Clinical Neurology*, 2nd ed. East Norwalk, CT: Appleton & Lange.

Memmler, R. L., Cohen, B. J., Wood, D. L. (1992). *Structure and Function of the Human Body*, 5th ed. Philadelphia: J. B. Lippincott.

Memmler, R., Cohen, B., & Wood, D. (1996). *The Human Body in Health and Disease*, 8th ed. Philadelphia: Lippincott-Raven.

Porth, C. M. (1994). *Pathophysiology: Concepts of Altered Health States*, 4th ed. Philadelphia: J. B. Lippincott.

Rosedahl, C. B. (1995). *Textbook of Basic Nursing*, 6th ed. Philadelphia: J. B. Lippincott.

(1992). *Professional Guide to Diseases*, 4th ed. Springhouse, PA: Springhouse.

Caring for Patients With Sensory Disorders

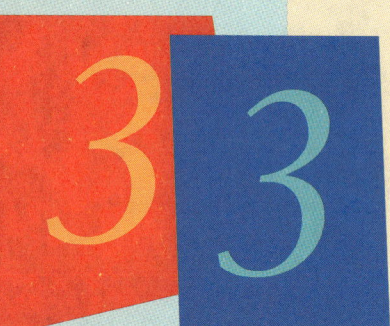

Chapter Outline

The Eye
    Basic Structure and Function
    Common Disorders
    Common Diagnostic Studies and
        Therapeutic Procedures and the
        Medical Assistant's Role
Procedure: Measuring Distance Visual
        Acuity
Procedure: Measuring Color Perception
Procedure: Instilling Eye Medication
Procedure: Irrigating the Eye
Procedure: Removing a Foreign Object
        From the Eye
The Ear
    Basic Structure and Function
    Common Disorders
    Common Diagnostic Studies and
        Therapeutic Procedures and the
        Medical Assistant's Role

Procedure: Irrigating the Ear
Procedure: Instilling Ear Medication
The Nose
    Basic Structure and Function
    Common Disorders
    Common Diagnostic Studies and
        Therapeutic Procedures and the
        Medical Assistant's Role
Procedure: Instilling Nasal Medication
Other Senses
    Taste
    Smell
    Touch
Summary
Critical Thinking Challenges
Answers to Checkpoint Questions
Suggestions for Further Reading

DACUM Components

1.3   Practice within the scope of education, training, and personal capabilities
1.6   Conduct oneself in a courteous and diplomatic manner
2.2   Treat all patients with empathy and impartiality
4.1   Apply principles of aseptic technique and infection control
4.5   Prepare and maintain examination and treatment area
4.7   Prepare patients for procedures
4.11 Perform selected tests that assist with diagnosis and treatment
5.1   Document accurately
7.3   Teach patients methods of health promotion and disease prevention

Chapter Competencies

Learning Objectives

Upon successfully completing this chapter, you will be able to:

1. Spell and define the Key Terms.
2. Locate and describe the anatomic structures of eye, ear, and nose.
3. Describe the function of the organs associated with each structure.
4. List and define several diseases associated with the eye, ear, and nose.
5. Identify common diagnostic procedures associated with the eye, ear, and nose.
6. Describe patient education procedures associated with the eye, ear, and nose.
7. Identify other senses and give their importance in assessing patient wellness.

Performance Objectives

Upon successfully completing this chapter, you will be able to:

1. Prepare a diagnostic set for use in the examination of the eye, ear, and nose.
2. Measure distance visual acuity with a Snellen chart (Procedure 33-1).
3. Measure close (or near) visual acuity with a Jaeger chart.
4. Measure color perception with an Ishihara color book (Procedure 33-2).
5. Perform tonometry.
6. Instill eye medication (Procedure 33-3).
7. Irrigate the eye (Procedure 33-4).
8. Remove a foreign object from the eye (Procedure 33-5).
9. Perform impedance audiometry.
10. Irrigate the ear (Procedure 33-6).
11. Instill ear medication (Procedure 33-7).
12. Instill nasal medication (Procedure 33-8).

Key Terms

(See Glossary for definitions.)

adnexa	optician
astigmatism	optometrist
cerumen	otoscope
decibel (db)	presbyopia
hyperopia	refract, refraction
intraocular pressure	retinal degeneration
myopia	tactile
ophthalmologist	tinnitus
ophthalmoscope	URI

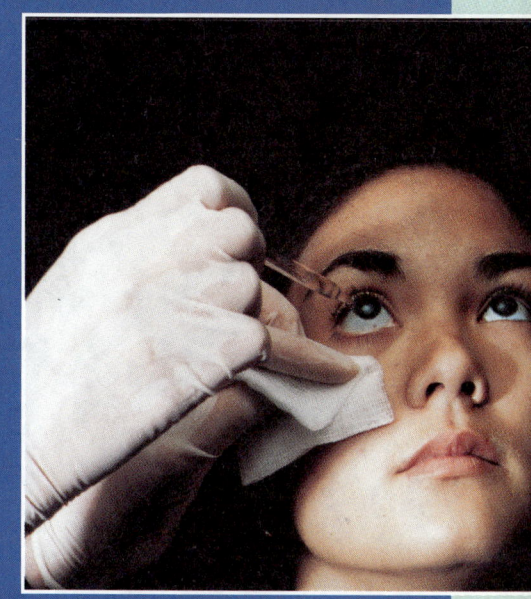

The sensory organs maintain our contact with the environment. They add richness and pleasure to our lives and warn us of danger. The main external senses include sight, hearing, taste, smell, and touch. The various stimuli are transmitted by the afferent nerves to their designated destinations in the brain for interpretation.

➤ THE EYE

Basic Structure and Function

The eye is the organ of sight. The right and left eyes individually imprint an image on the optic center of the brain located in the occipital area. These singular images are then combined into one overlapping image by the brain to provide three-dimensional sight.

Approximately five-sixths of the eyeball fits into a bony orbit, by which it is protected. The eyeball is hollow and consists of three layers: the scleral-corneal layer, the choroid layer, and the retina (Fig. 33-1).

The sclera, also known as the "white of the eye," makes up the majority of the outer cover of the eye and is connected to the cornea, the anterior one-sixth, to form the fibrous tunic of the eye. The cornea is transparent and covers the iris and pupil. It has a greater curvature than the sclera to **refract** (bend) the light as it enters. Both the sclera and cornea are very sensitive and vascular and are covered with a mucous membrane called the conjunctiva that continues to the edges of the lids.

Between the scleral-corneal layer and the retina lies the choroid layer. This middle layer is highly vascular and extends to the ciliary body, which controls the shape of the lens. The lens lies directly behind the iris and changes shape to assist in the focusing process. The iris is the pigmented section of the eyeball. It contains a black center known as the pupil, actually just an empty space, which regulates the amount of light

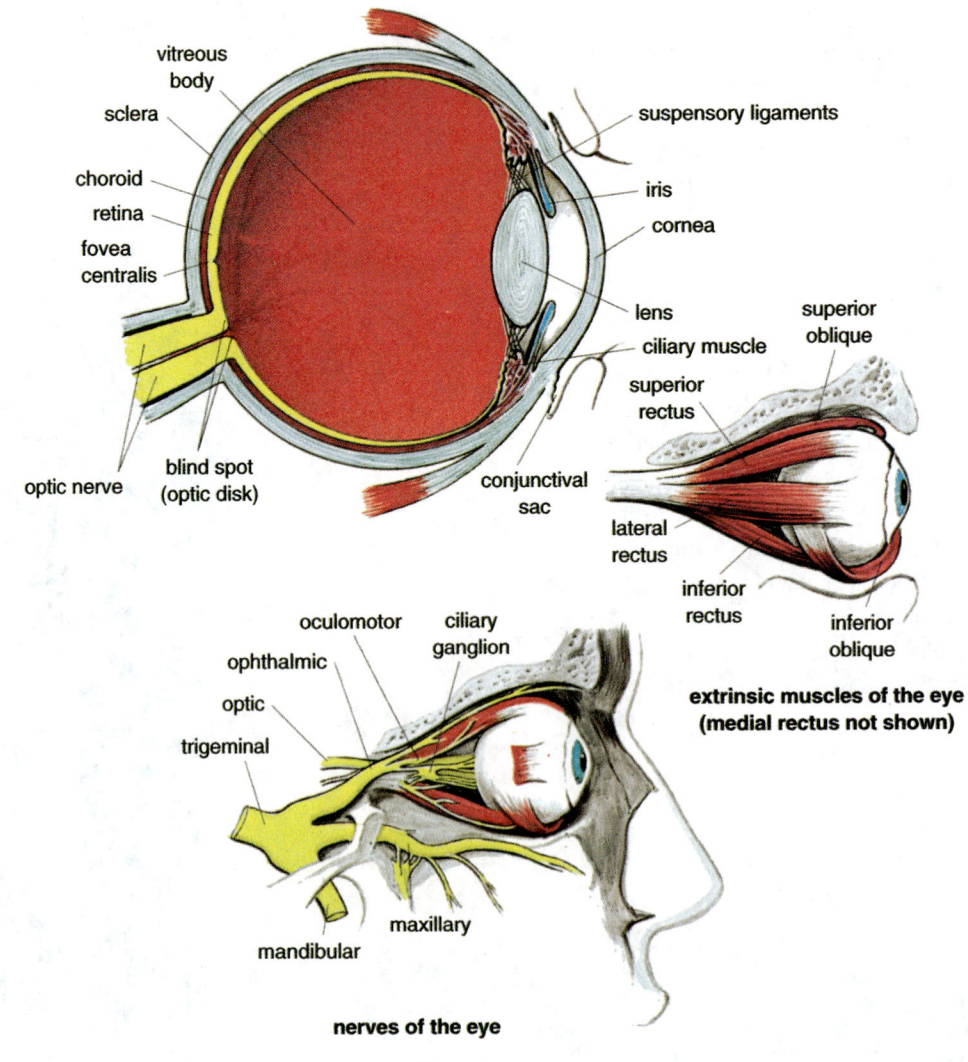

FIGURE 33-1
The eye.

nerves of the eye

allowed to enter the eye. The iris is a smooth muscle that adjusts automatically to control the amount of light reflected onto the retina. The vascularity of the choroid layer makes it dark like the lining of a camera to absorb rather than reflect the entering light.

The retina, the innermost layer of the eye, functions primarily to form images. The rods and cones are nerve cells contained in the retina. Rods are responsible for shadings of light and dark but form no clear images. Cones are for color reception and require bright light. Cones record the three primary colors of red, blue, and green. Variations of colors are registered when the cones perceive bits of color on more than one receptor. For instance, violet may be recorded in part on the red receptors and on the blue receptors and then is perceived by the brain as a combination of both colors.

The rods and cones are most concentrated in the fovea centralis, a small depression with great sensitivity exactly at the posterior of the eye opposite the lens. All receptive nerve fibers and vessels enter and exit just medial of the fovea at the optic disk, also known as the blind spot. The disk has no receptors of its own.

There are two chambers containing fluid within the eye. *Aqueous humor* is a liquid similar to cerebrospinal fluid and formed from the blood that circulates through the eye. This fluid passes forward between the iris and the lens into the anterior chamber. It drains from there back into the bloodstream through the canal of Schlemm. The **intraocular pressure** (pressure within the eyeball) is produced mainly by the aqueous humor.

Vitreous humor, a jelly-like substance, fills the posterior chamber behind the lens. Vitreous humor maintains the shape of the eye and helps with image refraction. This fluid is also produced by special cells within the eye from plasma fluid and is returned to general circulation as needed to maintain a homeostatic intraocular environment.

The optic nerve transmits impulses from the rods and cones to the brain's visual centers located in the cerebral cortex.

Checkpoint Question
1. Where are the rods and cones located and what are they responsible for?

The Adnexa

In addition to the eye itself, visual accessory structures (**adnexa**) include the lids, the lashes, and the lacrimal

apparatus. The lids blink reflexively and are a protective device. Normally the blink reflex is triggered about 25 times a minute. Blinking increases with the need for moisture from tears.

The lacrima helps keep the conjunctivae moist as tears wash across from the excretory gland at the upper, outer rim of the bony orbit. Tears flow across the eye as the lids blink and deliver them to the puncti in the inner cantha (corner) of the upper and lower lids. The puncti drain into the lacrimal canaliculi, then to the lacrimal sac, then into the nasolacrimal ducts, and empty into the nasal passages through the turbinates. If the lacrimal glands produce more tears than the apparatus can channel away, the tears are shed onto the cheeks. Tears are salty and are slightly bacteriocidal as a protection against microorganisms. Figure 33-2 shows the lacrimal apparatus.

Musculature

The eye requires the intrinsic (inside) muscles to change the shape of the lens for refraction and the pupil for the entrance of light. This is controlled by the autonomic nervous system.

The extrinsic (outside) muscles are responsible for eye movement and must coordinate movements in the field of vision. There are six per eye and each is responsible for moving the eye into position very quickly. The initial movement to fix on an object is voluntary, then the involuntary focusing takes over on command of the optic center to define the image.

Paralysis or dysfunction of any of the intrinsic or extrinsic muscles causes focus to be poor and may result in diplopia (double vision) with an eventual loss of vision.

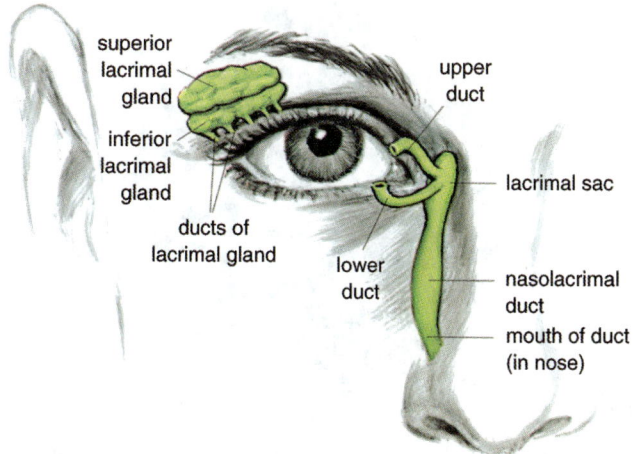

FIGURE 33-2
Lacrimal apparatus.

Process of Sight

Light waves are given off by all objects and are transmitted through the cornea, aqueous humor, lens, vitreous humor and to the retina, then through the optic nerve to the occipital lobe of the cerebral cortex. The rays are bent, or refracted, by the curvature of the cornea and lens to reduce the image to a fine point on the fovea centralis. If the object is out of focus to the occiput, efferent impulses change the shape of the lens or the position of the extrinsic muscles to sharpen the image.

Common Disorders

The eye is a complex, highly developed organ. Any of its many components may malfunction or be the object of infection or disease. A few of the many eye disorders that you may encounter in the medical office are described below.

Cataract

A cataract is an opacity of the lens that leads to a decrease in visual acuity (Fig. 33-3). Cataracts are usually bilateral and are more commonly seen in the elderly. Some infants are born with congenital cataracts, sometimes as a result of first trimester maternal rubella. Occasionally, trauma to the lens or chemical toxicity will cause clouding of the lens.

The symptoms are a gradual blurring and loss of vision. A sign for the observer is a milky opacity at the pupil rather than the normal black opening. Ophthalmoscopy will reveal the white area behind the pupil if

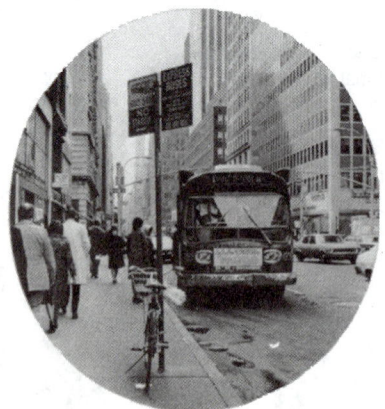

FIGURE 33-3
Cataract vision—diminished acuity from an opacity of the lens. The field of vision is unaffected but the individual has an overall haziness of the view.

it is not fully advanced enough to be seen by the observer without diagnostic aids.

Surgery is beneficial in 95% of the patients and is usually an outpatient procedure. The opaque lens is removed by any of several effective methods, such as emulsification or capsular extraction. In some cases, an intraocular lens is implanted where the lens has been removed; in other instances the vision is corrected by contact lenses or special glasses.

Sty or Hordeolum

A sty or hordeolum is a staphylococcal infection of any of the glands of the eyelids, causing redness, swelling, and pain. Warm compresses will hasten suppuration; topical drops or ointments attack the microorganism. You may be responsible for teaching the patient the procedure for applying warm compresses and instilling drops or ointment.

Conjunctivitis

Conjunctivitis is a common infectious disease of the conjunctiva caused by several forms of bacteria, chlamydia, or viruses. It may also be caused by allergens or irritants without an infectious process. Many of the pathogens will cause unilateral conjunctivitis; allergic conjunctivitis will almost always be bilateral.

Signs and symptoms include tearing and occasionally exudate and pain. Bacterial conjunctivitis, or "pink eye," is highly contagious and will spread through schools and day-care centers quickly. It is spread by contact as the host child rubs the itching eyes, handles toys and books, and passes them and the disease to the next child who comes in contact with the pathogen. Treatment must address the specific pathogen. The patient, parents, and day care providers must be taught good hygiene to prevent disease spread.

Checkpoint Question
2. What is the difference between a sty and conjunctivitis?

Corneal Ulcer

A corneal ulcer is the eroding away of the corneal surface, leaving scar tissue that may lead to visual disturbances or blindness. Corneal ulcers are caused by several types of bacteria, fungi, viruses, and protozoa, or by trauma, allergens, or toxins. Signs and symptoms include tearing, pain on blinking, and sensitivity to light. A visual examination with a penlight will show an irregular corneal surface. A fluorescein dye will stain the perimeter of the ulcer to confirm the diagnosis. Treatment includes rest to the eyeball and antibiotic therapy.

Retinopathy

Retinopathy refers to any disease or disorder affecting the retina. A decrease in the blood supply to the highly vascular retina will cause **retinal degeneration**, pathologic changes in the cell structure that impair or destroy the retina's function. The causes include atherosclerosis that impedes the blood flow to the retina, the microcirculatory changes associated with diabetes or sickling disease, or vascular changes from long-term hypertension. Depending on the cause, the loss of vision may be sudden or gradual. The loss of vision may be preceded by small intraocular hemorrhages, night blindness, or loss of central visual fields. If small vessels rupture and scar, they may pull against the retina and cause retinal detachment. Treatment depends on the cause. Some forms of retinopathy respond well to treatment; others will progress to full blindness.

Glaucoma

Glaucoma is actually a group of disorders that result in increased intraocular pressure. As aqueous humor is formed in the posterior chamber just in front of the lens, it flows through the pupil to the anterior chamber, just behind the cornea. It is eventually filtered into the canal of Schlemm and is returned to the general circulation. Any pathology that impedes the outflow of aqueous humor will cause the pressure to increase, either very gradually or quite suddenly. The gradual form may present with mild pain, halos around lights, and loss of peripheral vision (Fig. 33-4). The acute form presents with pain and inflammation, eye pressure, and even nausea and vomiting. Blindness may result within days of the onset of acute glaucoma.

Treatment for chronic glaucoma includes parasympathomimetics or diuretics. Acute glaucoma may require an iridectomy to remove part of the iris to increase the outflow of the humor.

Refractive Errors

These comprise the most common of all eye problems, resulting in either hyperopia, myopia, astigmatism, or presbyopia.

Hyperopia, also known as farsightedness, is the result of an eyeball that is too short from front to back to allow the lines of vision to reflect distinctly on the fovea centralis. Objects must be held far from the face to focus the image on the retina.

Myopia, also known as nearsightedness, results when the eyeball is too long. The lines of vision con-

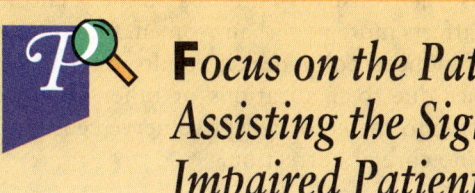

Focus on the Patient: Assisting the Sight-Impaired Patient

Follow these tips to assist a sight-impaired patient.

- Ask the patient how you can help and follow the patient's requests and suggestions. Many sight-impaired patients know best what they need.
- When escorting the patient, offer your arm. Tell the patient the approximate length of the hallway and advise the patient of any turns, eg, *"It should be about 20 steps and then we'll take a right."* Avoid steps if possible, but if you must assist a sight-impaired patient up or down stairs, advise the individual of the number of steps. Many patients prefer to hold the railings for balance.
- If the patient has a guide dog, do not approach the dog without first speaking to the patient and receiving approval.
- If the patient needs extensive teaching on a particular subject, suggest using a tape recorder to record the instructions.

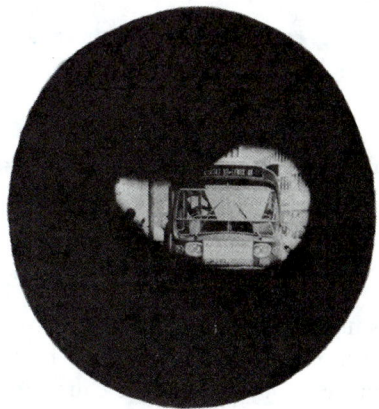

FIGURE 33-4
Glaucoma. Advanced glaucoma involves loss of peripheral vision but the individual still retains most of his central vision.

verge before they reach the fovea centralis and begin to diverge again at the fovea. Objects must be held close to the face to focus the image far back on to the retina.

Astigmatism is unfocused refraction of light rays on the retina. It results from lens or corneal irregularities. If the cornea is not smooth, images refracted through it will not project sharply onto the retina but will look much like peering through wavy glass.

Presbyopia refers to vision changes resulting from age. It does not involve the length of the eyeball but is the result of loss of lens elasticity. The lens must be made to adjust thicker or thinner to refract light from near or far on to the retina. As the eye grows older, the ciliary bodies that hold and adjust the lens and the lens themselves all lose youthful elasticity and will no longer accommodate near vision; far vision may be unaffected. Symptoms usually begin gradually around age 40. Most adults are affected to some degree by age 50.

All refractive errors are treated with corrective lenses (Fig. 33-5). An **optometrist** is a trained specialist who can measure for errors of refraction and prescribe lenses. An **optician** is a trained specialist who grinds lenses to fit refraction corrective lens prescriptions written by either an optometrist or an **ophthalmologist,** a medical doctor who treats eye disorders.

Checkpoint Question

3. What are four common refractive errors? Briefly explain each.

Strabismus

Strabismus is a misalignment of the eye movements, usually caused by muscle incoordination. Strabismus may be:

- Esotropic (also known as cross eye or convergent)
- Exotropic (also known as wall eye or divergent)
- Hypotropic (deviation downward)
- Hypertropic (deviation upward)

Strabismus may be concomitant if both eyes move together or nonconcomitant if they move independently. Treatment depends on the cause and may only require patching, or covering, the good eye to require the affected eye muscles to strengthen. In some cases, surgery may be required to correct the deviant muscle.

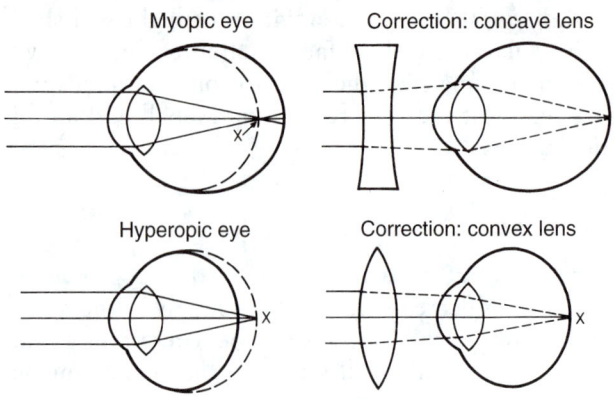

FIGURE 33-5
The myopic eye with concave corrective lens. The hyperopic eye with convex corrective lens.

Color Deficit

Color deficit is an absence of or defect in color perception. Red, green, or blue perception or any combination of colors may be impaired or absent. The term color deficient or color deficit is commonly used rather than referring to the disorder as a type of blindness.

The disorder is usually inherited on the X chromosome and affects more men than women. Occasionally, chemically induced color deficit results from damage to the cones due to medications or other substances that are toxic to the color receptive nerve cells. Color deficit has no cure or correction.

Dacryocystitis

Dacryocystitis refers to an infection of the tear sac. In adults, dacryocystitis usually results from an obstruction of the nasolacrimal duct. Infants may present with an atresia (closing off) or an infection. Because the duct is closed, the normal flow of tears cannot drain into the puncta and through to the nose, causing constant tearing. The area may be swollen and tender; a purulent discharge from the puncta may develop.

Cultures are ordered if infection is suspected. Treatment includes palliative soaks and local or systemic antibiotics. If atresia is the cause, dilation or probing may open the sac.

Common Diagnostic Studies and Therapeutic Procedures and the Medical Assistant's Role

Almost all offices use **ophthalmoscopes** and **otoscopes.** An ophthalmoscope is a lighted instrument used to visually examine the inner surfaces of the eye.

It is often referred to as the "eye to the heart" of the patient. In many instances its use can alert the physician to a number of vascular and prehypertensive conditions as well as to many intraocular conditions. It is an important part of the everyday "diagnostic set" used in the office. The otoscope, an instrument used to visually examine the ear, is another part of the diagnostic set. Otoscopes have probe covers, which may be reusable or disposable.

Commonly, the base of the diagnostic set is one instrument, which houses a rechargeable battery with interchangeable heads (Fig. 33-6). Some offices are equipped with electrical, wall-mounted instruments.

Preparing a Diagnostic Set

Follow the steps below to prepare a diagnostic set:

1. Assemble the equipment.
2. Check to determine that the lights in the instruments are functioning by illuminating them.
3. Place and remove the ophthalmoscope, otoscope, and illuminated tongue-blade holder, if used, to check the readiness of each. Press firmly and twist to place or remove the head. The small red button at the connection is held down as the rim is rotated to keep the light on. Reverse the procedure to turn it off.
4. Place tongue blades and disposable ear specula on a covered tray for the physician's use.

5. Have extra light bulbs available for replacement during the examination if needed.

Visual Acuity Testing

Far vision is tested using the Snellen chart or any other of the far vision testing devices available. These charts are hung 20 feet away from the patient at eye level in an area with good lighting and few distractions (Procedure 33-1). Normal vision (20/20) means that the patient can read at 20 feet what the normal eye should see from that distance.

The figures on the charts—letters, numbers, or a series of Es—are progressively smaller to test levels of perception. For patients who cannot read or who are not English-speaking, an "E" chart, also called the tumbling E chart, may be used. A picture chart is often used for children (Fig. 33-7).

If a child is to be tested, spend a few moments familiarizing the child with the objects on the chart. Some children may have no point of reference for some of the objects. For example, if the picture is of a Collie dog and the child has never seen one, the illustration may not be recognized as a dog. Children are frequently tested at 10 feet rather than at 20 feet because they do not focus well at distances and are easily distracted within the line of vision. Enlist a parent or coworker to help with the eye cover.

Near vision is tested by using the Jaeger system. The Jaeger is a series of ever smaller lines to test at what point the patient can no longer discern the letters. Rather than checking for the ability to distinguish

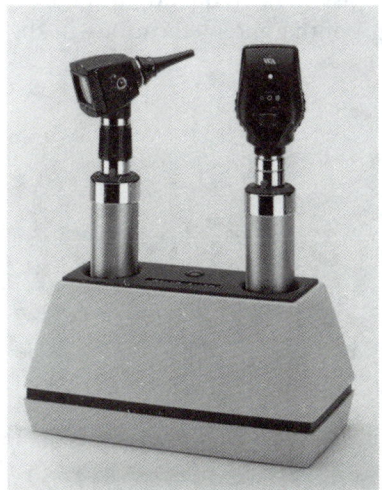

FIGURE 33-6
The diagnostic set includes an ophthalmoscope and an otoscope in a recharging base. The heads are interchangeable. Many physicians will use one base and change heads as needed. This otoscope has a reuseable speculum cover in place. (Courtesy of Welch-Allyn.)

Charting Example

05/14/99	9:30 AM Patient arrived in the office
	complaining of occasional blurred vision in
	the left eye. Patient does not wear eye-
	glasses. Last eye exam was 5 years ago.
	Visual acuity: OD 20/60-1, OS 20/40-2.
	Patient squinting throughout procedure.
	———— Karen Keeney, CMA

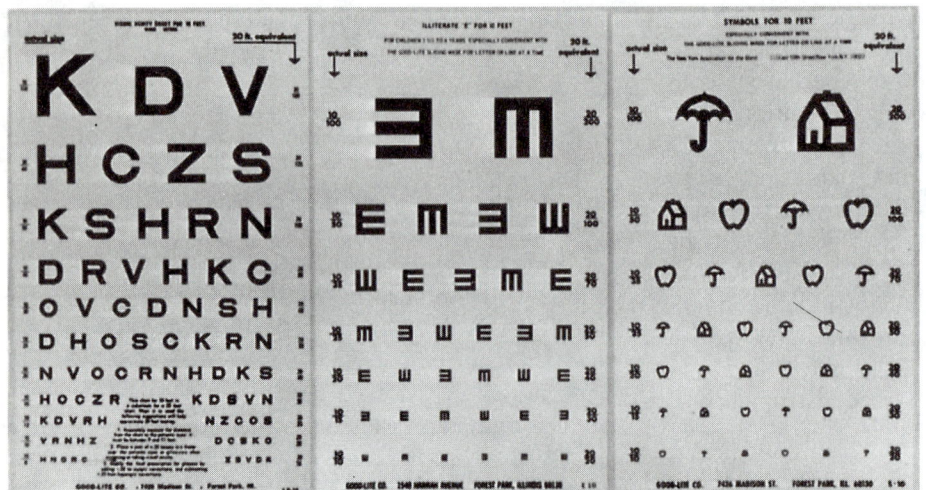

FIGURE 33-7
These are various Snellen charts used to test distant vision. The charts in the center and at far right are used for very young children and illiterate adults.

objects at a distance, the Jaeger tests for difficulties at a near reading level. *The Jaeger is usually used for patients over age 40 and suspected of presbyopia or for those with hyperopia.* The steps are:

1. Hold the card containing lines of text or pictures of Es to be evaluated about 14 to 16 inches from the patient's face at a comfortable reading level.
2. Start by covering the patient's left eye (for consistency of testing).
3. Record the last line read with no errors.
4. Repeat the procedure to test the left eye. If corrective lenses are worn, record this on the patient's record also.

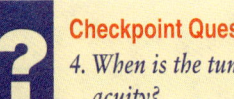

Checkpoint Question
4. When is the tumbling E chart used to test visual acuity?

Color Perception

The Ishihara method is used to test for color perception (Procedure 33-2). It consists of a series of color plates with many four-colored dots forming a number, a letter, or a pattern of contrasting color within the arrangement of dots (Fig. 33-8). Patients with deficient color perception will be unable to find the design within the plate.

Tonometry

Using a tonometer such as the Schiotz or the applanation, the physician measures tension or pressure within

a site—in this case, intraocular pressure. The anterior eye is anesthetized with drops and the instrument is moved against the cornea to measure how much pressure is required to produce an indentation (tonometer) or to flatten a small area of the cornea (applanation) (Fig. 33-9).

Gonioscopy

Using the gonioscope, the physician measures the angle formed by the anterior chamber of the eye between the iris and the cornea. This method is used to diagnose the cause of glaucoma.

Instilling Eye Medications

The medical assistant frequently has the responsibility of instilling ophthalmic medications in the office and

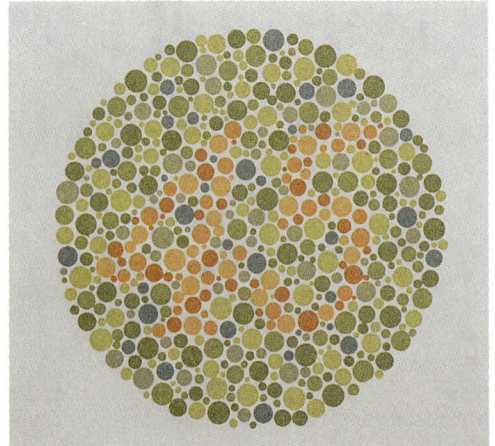

FIGURE 33-8
Ishihara color plate (© B. Proud).

Charting Example

05/14/99	11:20 AM Color perception measured
	by Ishihara method. Patient stated he
	understood the procedure and success-
	fully identified Plate #1. Patient iden-
	tified all plates except Plate #9=X.
	Dr. Barker notified.
	————————— Jack Crosby, CMA

of educating the patient about the procedure for home use. Instillations treat infection or irritation, dilate the pupil for retinal examination, and apply anesthetic for treatment or testing (Procedure 33-3).

Other Ophthalmic Procedures

To remove exudates and debris and relieve inflammation, eye irrigations are performed (Procedure 33-4). Sometimes, foreign objects lodge in the eye. The physician must remove objects that are embedded, but the

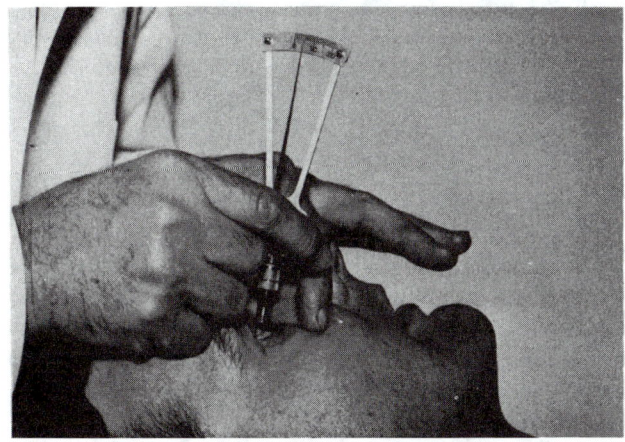

FIGURE 33-9
Tonometry. After a local anesthetic is instilled into the eye, the Schiotz tonometer is gently rested on the eyeball. The indicator measures the ocular tension in millimeters of mercury. (Courtesy of F. H. Rofy, M.D.)

medical assistant can remove loose debris (Procedure 33-5).

➤ THE EAR

Basic Structure and Function

The ear is the organ of hearing. It is divided into three sections: external ear, middle ear, and inner ear (Fig. 33-10). The inner ear also functions to maintain balance.

The pinna or auricle is also known as the external ear. It is made of cartilage and is shaped to collect and channel sound waves through the auditory canal to the eardrum, or tympanic membrane. The lining of the auditory canal is made of modified sweat glands that are referred to as ceruminous glands. Earwax, or **cerumen**, is a protective mechanism for the ear.

The tympanic membrane separates the external and middle ear sections. The middle ear contains three small bones known collectively as the ossicles. The first is the malleus or hammer. Sound waves from the eardrum initiate a reaction in the attached malleus and are then transmitted to the next tiny bone, the incus or anvil. Vibrations from the anvil move the third bone, the stapes or stirrup, so named for its recognizable shape.

Charting Example

03/02/99	1440 Dr. Howser ordered Cor-
	tisporin eye drops to OD. Patient has
	NKA. Cortisporin 2 gtt administered
	into OD. Patient instructed to close
	eyeball and roll eye to disperse medica-
	tion. Patient educated in proper proce-
	dure for instilling eye medications. Pa-
	tient verbalized understanding.
	————————— Charles White, CMA

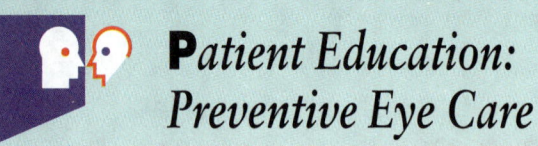

Patient Education: Preventive Eye Care

Preventive care of the eye is a vital component of patient education. Regular eye checkups, proper care of contact lenses, control of diabetes and hypertension, annual tonometer or "puff-of-air" checks for glaucoma each year after age 40, and proper attention to eye injuries are important aspects of eye health maintenance.

Patients should be advised to wear sunglasses with ultraviolet protection during any sun exposure to protect against ultraviolet ray damage to the eyes. Children should also be fitted for sunglasses to protect immature eyes from sun damage.

Rubbing the eyes should be avoided. This spreads infection from person to person and can damage the cornea if small foreign objects are introduced into the eye. Wearing eye goggles during procedures can prevent disease transmission and injury from foreign bodies.

The auditory or eustachian tube connects the middle ear with the nasopharynx. This tube opens during swallowing and equalizes pressure in the middle ear.

The third section is divided into two parts called the cochlea and the semicircular canals. The two send the impulses for hearing (cochlea) and motion (semicircular canals) to the brain. The cochlea is attached to the stapes at the oval window, a thin membrane that moves as the stapes vibrate with transmitted waves. These sound waves are translated into nerve impulses by tiny hairlike processes in the cochlea that act as receptors for the organ of Corti, which sends the impulses through the acoustic nerve to the brain.

The semicircular canals, also known as the vestibular apparatus, are three half-circles set at right angles to each other. They are filled with a fluid called endolymph and lined with microscopic hairs. As the body position changes, the endolymph moves back and forth in the canals. This movement bends the hairs, which send to the brain the message regarding its current position. This function works closely with the visual images projected by the eyes. If the eyes perceive the horizon to be slanted and the semicircular canals transmit the message that the body is upright, the disorientation may lead to nausea; this is the reason many people experience motion sickness. If the vestibular apparatus is impaired or if an inner ear disorder is present, the patient will experience vertigo (moving sensation).

Charting Example

10/31/99	1330
	S: "I got some laundry detergent in my eyes."
	O: 22-year-old woman. Both eyes appear red and teary. Dr. Burns in to see patient. Eye irrigation ordered.
	A: Chemical irritation both eyes.
	P: 1. Both eyes irrigated with 1000 mL normal saline. Tolerated procedure well.
	2. Preventive education instructions given to patient. Patient verbalized understanding of teachings ———————— Tamika Roberts, CMA

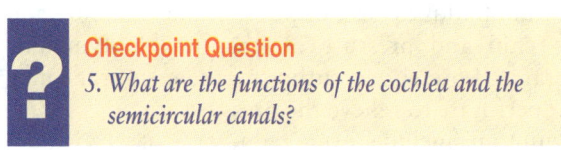

Charting Example

07/15/99	0935 Patient arrived in office complaining of a metal chip in his OD Occurred on the job at 0900. Dr. Spruce removed the foreign object. Neosporin ointment instilled in OD Eye patch applied. Patient instructed to wear goggles on job site as needed. Patient verbalized understanding of teaching.
	———————— John Smith, RMA

? Checkpoint Question
5. What are the functions of the cochlea and the semicircular canals?

Transmission of Sound

Sound waves are produced by vibrations, such as the movement of air across the larynx, plucking the strings of a guitar, or slamming a door. The waves are caught by the pinna and channeled through the auditory canal to the tympanic membrane, which vibrates as the waves strike against it. The vibrations move the malleus, then the incus, then the stapes. The stapes move with the waves and transmit the impulse to the oval window, which moves the endolymph within the cochlea. The movement of the fluid is picked up by the tiny hairs of the organ of Corti. The waves are transmitted as impulses through the auditory nerve to the temporal lobe of the brain for interpretation.

Common Disorders

Hearing loss is a frequent outcome of diseases and disorders of the ear and can occur at any age. Congenital disorders, trauma, disease, and environmental noise can all result in hearing loss.

Ceruminosis

Also known as impacted earwax, ceruminosis is a frequent reason for diminished hearing. Cerumen is usually soft and moist and leaks out in such small amounts that it is unnoticed. Occasionally the cerumen may be hard and dry, or excess hair within the ear canal may hold the wax in, causing it to build up against the eardrum.

The presenting symptoms may be a gradual hearing loss or **tinnitus**, an extraneous noise heard in one or both ears. Otoscopy shows the obvious reason. The wax may be softened by warm oil ear drops or hydrogen peroxide and may be removed by an ear curet (refer to Chap. 23, Instruments and Equipment, for an illustration of a Buck ear curet) or by gently washing with an irrigating device (Fig. 33-11).

Conductive and Perceptual Hearing Loss

These disorders are the two categories of hearing impairment. In conductive loss, sound waves are not appropriately transmitted to the oval window and to the cochlear level. Perceptual, or sensorineural, loss involves transmission from the oval window through to the receptors in the brain. Many patients present with a combination of both, called mixed deafness.

Causes of hearing loss may include heredity with predisposing factors to deafness; infections, particularly of the middle and inner ear; trauma; ototoxic drugs that affect the eighth cranial nerve; some neurologic diseases; exposure to loud noises; and presbycusis, also known as "old ear," which usually results from otosclerosis or a hardening of the joints between the ossicles.

Diagnosis involves the various audiometric tests as described. Treatment addresses the underlying cause. A stapedectomy may be performed for otosclerosis with a replacement for the impaired joint. Cochlear implants are gaining favor for those whose loss involves impairment in the cochlear receptors. Cochlear implants are relatively new; the next few years will probably see as much improvement in this resource for the hearing impaired as has been made in the quality of hearing aids since their invention.

Conductive hearing loss can be treated successfully in most instances with hearing aids; however, perceptual loss is far more difficult to correct. If perceptual loss is due to tumor on the eighth cranial nerve, surgical removal of the tumor may be required. These tumors, although usually benign, tend to recur and often occur bilaterally.

What If?

What if your patient asks you if a hearing aid could help her? What would you tell her?

Hearing aids improve hearing ability, but they do not restore the ability to hear by 100%. The purpose of the aid is to amplify sound waves. Not all patients are good candidates for hearing aids. For example, patients who have permanent nerve damage generally will not have significant improvement with standard hearing aids.

There are two basic types of aids: bone conduction receivers sit behind the ear and press against the skull; air conduction receivers fit into the auditory canal. The size and type of hearing aid is based on the patient's specific condition and need. Binaural (both ear) aids are available and often can be fitted into eyeglasses for a less conspicuous appearance.

Patients need to understand that a hearing aid will improve hearing, not correct it. Teach patients about maintenance requirements so they can keep the device in good working condition and explain how to adjust the volume control. Have the patient speak to the physician regarding any concerns about the purchase and use of a hearing aid.

Checkpoint Question

6. How would you differentiate between conductive and perceptual hearing loss?

Meniere's Disease

Meniere's disease, a degenerative condition, affects the inner ear and upsets the body's ability to maintain equilibrium in addition to a loss of hearing. The symptoms include vertigo, sensorineural hearing loss, and tinnitus. Severe symptoms may lead to nausea and vomiting. Caution the patient to avoid situations that could cause falls.

Periods of remission are followed by periods of exacerbation. Many of the symptoms can be treated with palliative medication. If the symptoms persist and increase or become incapacitating, it may be necessary to destroy the organs of the inner ear. A cure is usually immediate, but the patient will be irreversibly deaf.

Otitis Externa

Also known as swimmer's ear, otitis externa is an inflammation or infection of the external ear. It is common in the summer and is caused by any number of pathogens that grow in the warm, moist ear canal. It is best treated by antibiotics, either topical or systemic, warm compresses, and pain relief medication.

The presenting symptom is pain on movement of any of the adjoining structures around the ear, jaw, auricle, and so on. Otoscopy will reveal a red, swollen ear canal. Debris must be gently washed from the area using the procedure outlined. Preventive therapy of applying an alcohol solution after swimming can help avoid this problem. Encourage patients who are prone to otitis externa to wear earplugs while swimming and to avoid using any objects to clean the ears, such as swabs or hairpins.

Otitis Media

Otitis media, an inflammation or infection of the middle ear, frequently results from an upper respiratory infection (URI). Pathogens responsible for pharyngitis, nasopharyngitis and the common cold frequently travel through the warm, moist eustachian tube to the hospitable middle ear. As infection increases, the mucous membranes of the eustachian tubes swell, closing off the opening to the middle ear. With no way to drain, fluid builds up as a response to the infection and causes pain and pressure on the flexible tympanic membrane. If pressure is sufficient, the membrane may tear or perforate to relieve the pressure.

Symptoms include severe pain, fever of varying degrees, and mild hearing loss. Infants may be fussy and tug at their ears. Any elevation in a child's temperature should be a warning to check for otitis media. Diagnosis is usually made by otoscopy, which may reveal a reddened bulging tympanic membrane. Bubbles can sometimes be seen behind the thin membrane. Treatment requires antibiotics to subdue the infection and analgesics for the pain. Decongestants may reduce some of the swelling. In severe chronic cases, a myringotomy may be performed to relieve pressure. Tubes may be inserted through the tympanic membrane and remain several months to equalize pressure if the problem persists.

Children have very short, almost horizontal eustachian tubes. For some children, virtually every cold and cough forces microorganisms into the middle ear, causing seemingly endless infections. The problem is compounded for children who are put to bed with a bottle of milk or formula. The milk acts as a hospitable medium for bacteria to grow.

Otosclerosis

Otosclerosis affects all of the ossicles, but most particularly the stapes bone, and is thought to be hereditary.

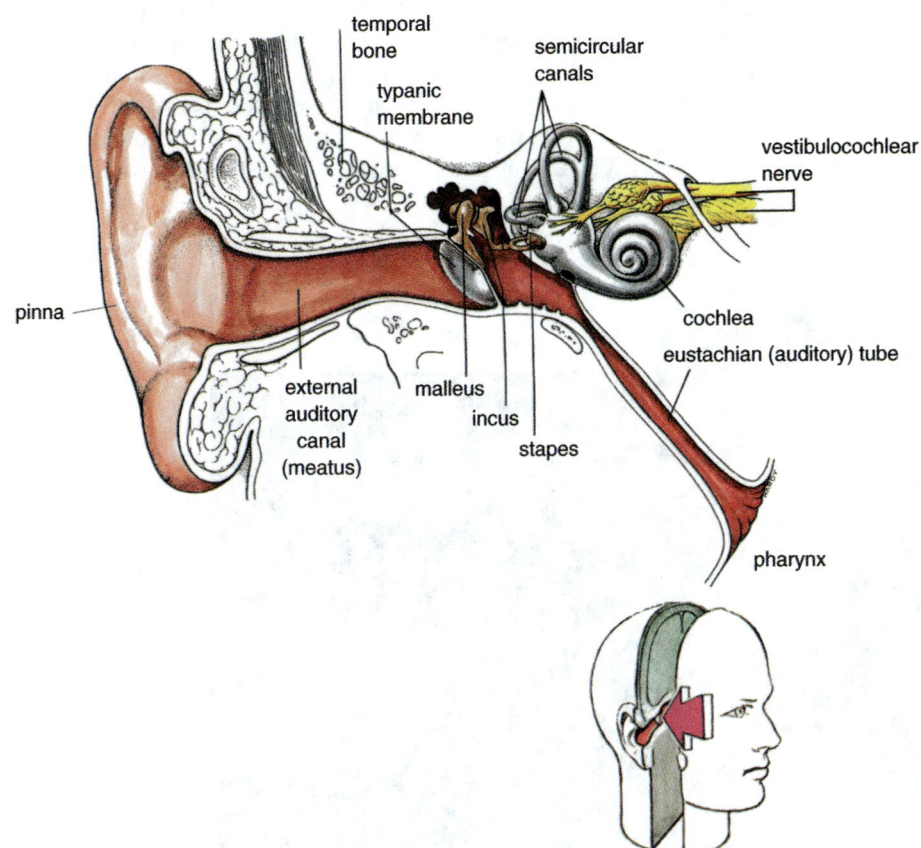

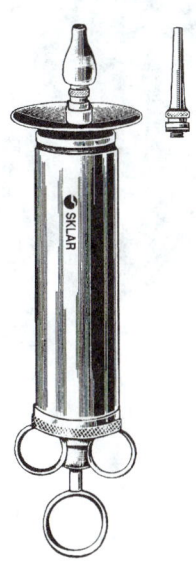

FIGURE 33-10
The ear, showing the external, middle, and internal subdivisions. (Chaffee EE, Lytle IM: *basic Physiology and Anatomy.* 4th ed, p 227. Philadelphia, JB Lippincott, 1980)

It causes loss of hearing in the low tones and is treatable with use of hearing aids. A stapedial prosthesis may also be implanted through microscopic surgery to replace the sclerotic joint and allow movement.

Common Diagnostic Studies and Therapeutic Procedures and the Medical Assistant's Role

Visual Examination

By using an otoscope, the physician can view the auditory canal and the eardrum. Disposable specula or specula covers are used most often. The otoscopic attachment is frequently used interchangeably with the base used for the ophthalmoscope.

Audiometry

An audiometer can be used to detect hearing loss by using earphones and producing pure tones of various decibel (db) levels and various frequencies. (Decibel is a unit for measuring the intensity of sound.) The results of the test are recorded by the audiometer on a

FIGURE 33-11
The ear syringe is used to gently irrigate the external auditory canal. Devices used to irrigate interdental spaces are also used to flush the canal. (Sklar Instruments, Westchester, PA)

special graph. Speech audiometry uses voice tones rather than pure tones to assess hearing. Impedance audiometry evaluates tympanic membrane and ossicle mobility. A probe is inserted into the auditory meatus and emits tones of various intensity that bounce back to the probe receiver. If the tympanic membrane and ossicles are normal, the movement is transmitted and rebound is picked up by the receiver to produce a curve on the graph. If the tympanic membrane and ossicles are less mobile than normal, much of the sound transmitted bounces back and is reflected back to the instrument to produce a distinct curve on the graph. Figure 33-12 illustrates the steps for performing impedance audiometry.

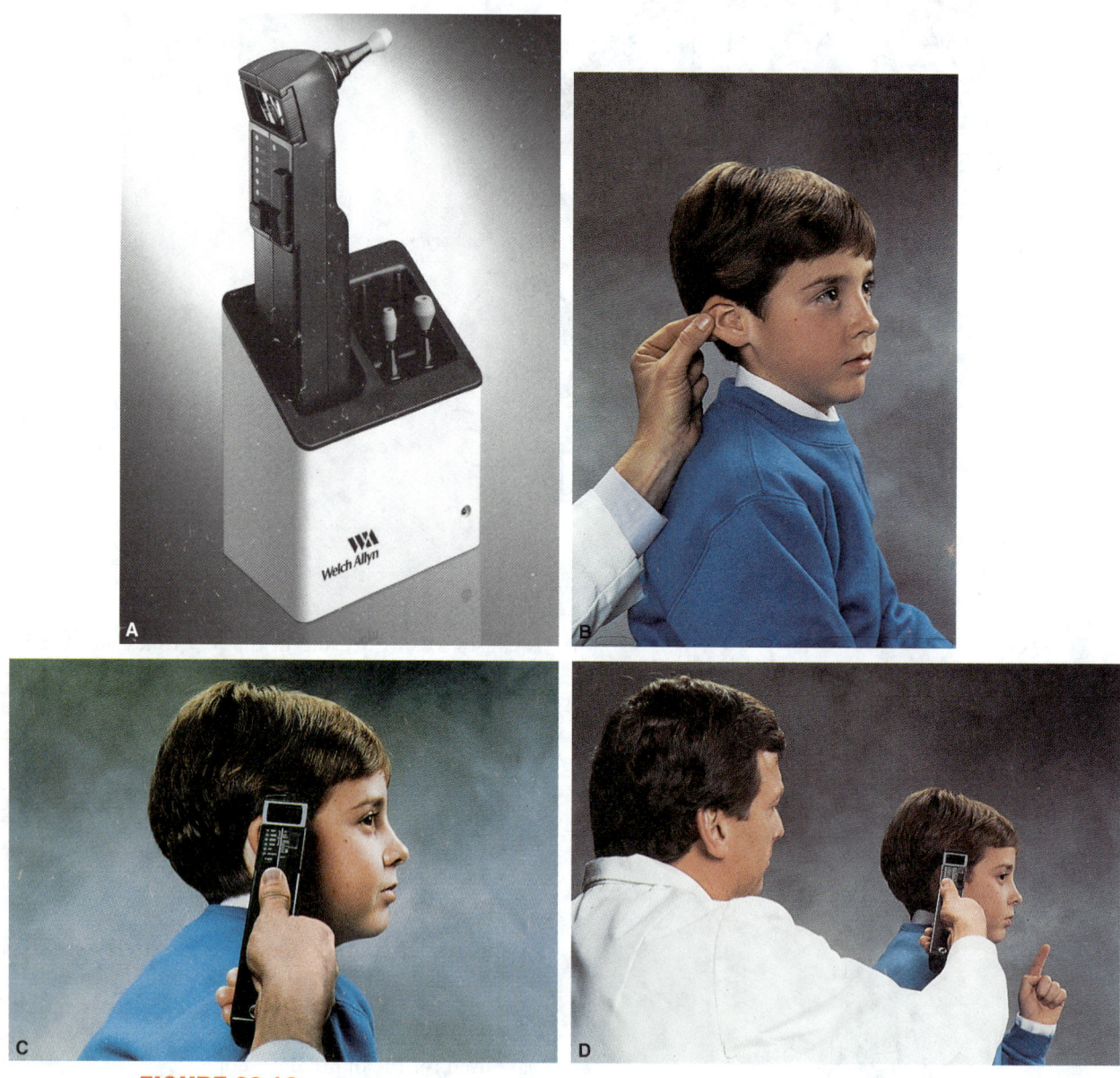

FIGURE 33-12

Audiometry. (A) Audioscopes with a light source allow a visual inspection of the ear canal and tympanic membrane before and during the examination. There is a pretone for patient practice and a random tone option for objectivity. The design of the tip eliminates the need for bulky ear phones. (B) Seat the patient in a quiet room. Attach a speculum to fit the patient's external auditory meatus. Instruct the patient in the procedure. Retract the pinna: up and back for adults; down and back for children. (C) Turn the instrument on and select the screening level. Insert the scope into the ear canal and visualize the canal and the tympanic membrane. (D) Depress the "start" button. Observe the tone indicators and the patient's responses. Screen the other ear. If the patient fails to respond at any frequency, rescreening is required. If the patient fails rescreening, referral may be indicated. (Courtesy of Welch-Allyn.)

Tympanometry

This works like the impedance audiometer but uses air pressure rather than tones to produce the graph. Figure 33-13 illustrates the steps for performing tympanometry.

Know hearing tests

Rinne Test

By using a tuning fork on the mastoid bone then moving it to the external auditory meatus, testing for a conductive hearing loss is performed.

Weber Test

This test uses a tuning fork on the midline of the forehead to differentiate between conductive and sensorineural loss.

Irrigations and Instillations

Ear irrigations (Procedure 33-6) are performed to relieve pain, to remove debris or foreign objects, or to apply topical solutions. Ear instillations (Procedure 33-7) are usually in the form of local anesthetics for the pain of otitis externa or otitis media, or topical antibiotics for otitis externa.

Patient Education: Otologic Disorders

Teach patients to recognize symptoms of otologic disorders and to report them promptly to the physician. Proper attention at the early stage of an infection or injury can often prevent serious or irreversible damage.

Instruct patients to avoid trying to clean the ears with cotton applicators or any other device. This drives cerumen deeper into the ear and creates more of an impaction than is already present.

Children should be instructed not to place small objects such as beans, peas, or small parts of toys into their ears because they may become lodged and require surgery to remove.

Caution parents to complete all antibiotic treatment for children's ear infections even though the symptoms may subside. The infection may be present for awhile after the patient is asymptomatic. Ear recheck appointments should be kept as scheduled to ensure that the child is free of infection.

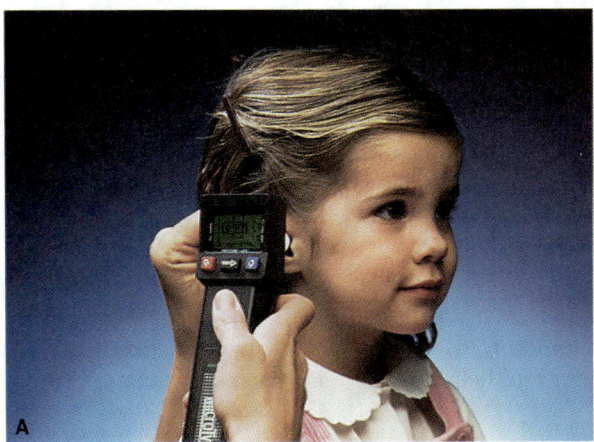
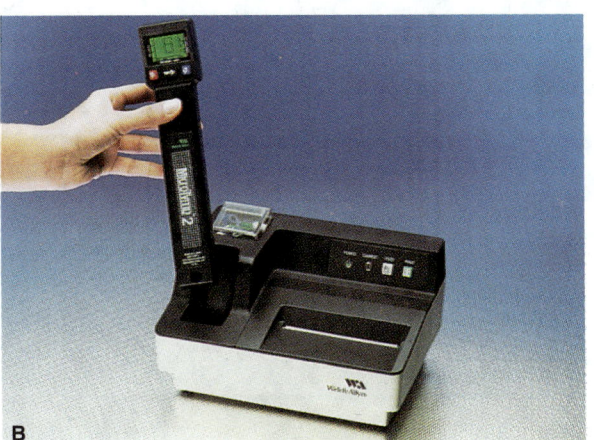

FIGURE 33-13
Microtymp 2 Tympanometric Instrument. This tympanometric instrument is light-weight and portable and provides a hard copy printout of many middle ear disorders. (*A*) Press the button, then insert the probe tip in the ear. Watch the LCD screen as it completes the tympanogram in about 1 second. (*B*) Return the handle to the printer/charger and a printout appears in 5 seconds. (Courtesy of Welch-Allyn.)

Charting Example

06/07/99	1230
	S: "I put a piece of corn in my ear."
	O: 30-month-old boy tugging on left ear. Mother states this occurred 20
	minutes ago. Kernel observed with otoscope. Tympanic membrane intact.
	A: Foreign object in left ear.
	P: 1. Left ear irrigated with 500 mL normal saline. One kernel of corn
	removed. Patient tolerated procedure well. Postirrigation ear
	canal clear. Tympanic membrane intact.
	2. Mother and child educated on prevention techniques.
	3. Dr. Rogers d/c patient to home. ———— Robin Low, RMA

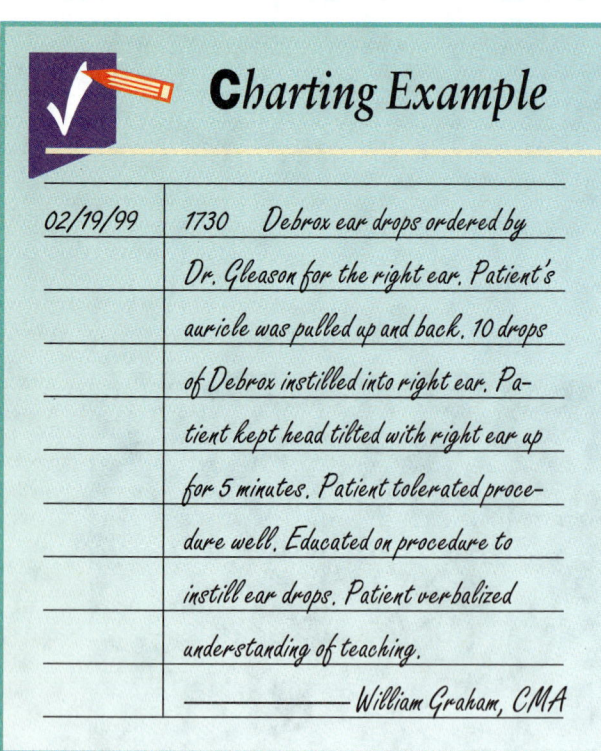

Charting Example

02/19/99	1730	Debrox ear drops ordered by
		Dr. Gleason for the right ear. Patient's
		auricle was pulled up and back. 10 drops
		of Debrox instilled into right ear. Pa-
		tient kept head tilted with right ear up
		for 5 minutes. Patient tolerated proce-
		dure well. Educated on procedure to
		instill ear drops. Patient verbalized
		understanding of teaching.
		———— William Graham, CMA

? Checkpoint Question
7. What is an audiometer used for and how does it work?

➤ THE NOSE

Basic Structure and Function

The nose is the primary organ of intake for oxygen and output for carbon dioxide. The external nares are the openings through which oxygen is inhaled and carbon dioxide is exhaled. Cartilage gives the nose its shape and makes the external structures flexible. The nasal cavity is separated by a nasal septum into right and left cavities.

Small hairlike projections covering virtually all surfaces of the nasal structures are called cilia and move secretions along to the throat for swallowing. The nasal surface area is increased by the presence of turbinates on the lateral surfaces of the nasal cavities. The mucous membranes of the turbinates cover the bones called conchae. This area moistens, warms, and filters the air that enters the nares.

The four sinuses—frontal, ethmoidal, sphenoidal, and maxillary sinuses—open into the nasal cavities within the folds of the turbinates. They make the skull lighter and help give the voice its resonance.

Process of Smell

The olfactory nerves are contained in the olfactory bulbs at the uppermost surface of the nasal cavity

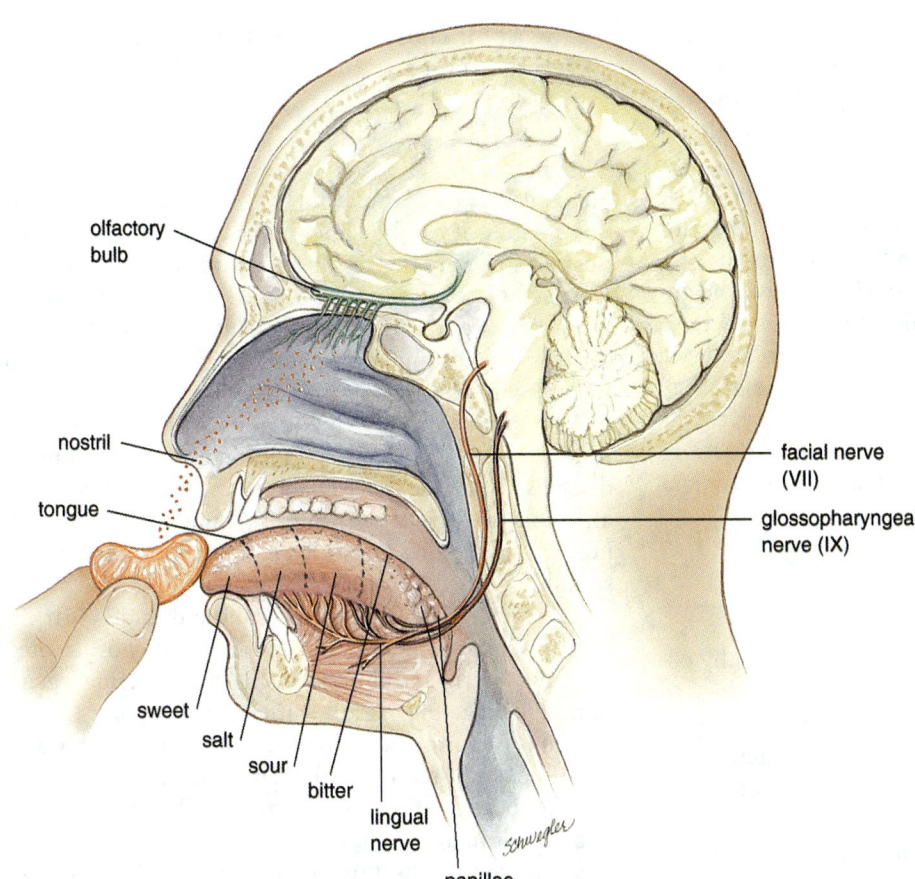

FIGURE 33-14
Organs of taste and smell.

(Fig. 33-14). Free olfactory nerve endings project into the mucous membranes and are specific for various types of smells. All scents or chemicals must be moistened by mucus to be perceived by the nerve endings. The impulses caused by the chemicals against the specific nerve endings travel by the olfactory tract to the thalamic and olfactory centers for interpretation. This area of the brain through which the nerve tract passes is so vital to associative memory and thought processes that smells can trigger an array of emotions from fear to joy and can stimulate appetite or cause nausea.

Loss of the sense of smell has an adverse effect on appetite and consequently on nutrition for patients with disease processes involving the nose or the transmission or perception of olfactory nerve impulses. The sense of smell tires easily; the initial perception of an odor diminishes as much as 50% within several minutes. The ability to discern odors is lost with age and plays an important part in the loss of appetite for the elderly.

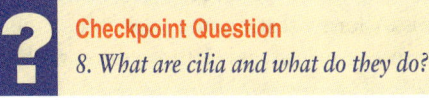

Checkpoint Question
8. What are cilia and what do they do?

Common Disorders

Allergic Rhinitis

Allergic rhinitis involves inflammation of the mucous membranes of the nasal passages and usually results from exposure to allergens. Symptomatic treatment is usually offered during peak pollen seasons. It is also known as hay fever or seasonal allergic rhinitis when it appears in response to seasonal plant pollens. If the symptoms are present year round, it is referred to as perennial allergic rhinitis and is usually a reaction to household irritants such as dust mites and pet dander. The signs are obvious with paroxysmal sneezing, intense rhinorrhea, congestion, and watery reddened eyes.

Diagnosis usually involves history and differential diagnosis. Mucous secretions may reveal an increase in immunoglobulin E in response to the allergens. An allergist may isolate the offending protein by skin testing. Allergy treatment involves exposure to the allergen in minute doses to desensitize the immune reaction.

Cleft Palate

Cleft palate is a separation of the palatine bones that divide the internal nose from the mouth. It is a congenital condition that requires surgery to correct. The abnormality occurs during the second embryonic month as the face is forming. Although a predisposition is present in some families, it is not strictly a familial pattern.

Cleft palate may or may not involve the entire palate area. If the defect involves only the posterior palate, surgery may be simple and will not require facial plastic surgery. The defect may also involve the anterior palate and may extend into the facial structure. If the lip is involved, the defect is referred to as "hare lip," and may be unilateral or bilateral. The defect may be complete and extend from the oral cavity to the nasal cavity all the way from the anterior surfaces to the posterior surfaces. Such defects will require extensive surgery over a period of years.

Epistaxis

Commonly known as nosebleed, epistaxis generally occurs as a result of trauma, but it may be secondary to other disorders. Hypertension, malignancies, polyps, and the fragile capillaries associated with pregnancy are other contributing factors. Bleeding beyond 10 minutes after treatment begins is considered severe. Diagnosis requires a history and inspection with a nasal speculum. History of severe epistaxis requires nasal packing or a balloon catheter that may remain from several hours to days. If the bleeding is secondary to anticoagulant therapy, adjustment of the medication may be required. Cautery to an exposed vessel helps if that is the only cause.

Immediate therapy involves having the patient sit upright with the head slightly forward to avoid postnasal drainage that may lead to nausea. Compress the nares against the septum for 5 to 10 minutes with either ice or a cold, wet compress. Advise the patient to remain still and not to blow the nose until the physician feels that all danger is past.

Nasal Polyps

Nasal polyps are small hanging pendulous tissues that obstruct breathing. They are easily treated by surgery, including laser treatments. Polyps are usually produced in the mucous membranes of the nasal passages as a response to long-term allergies. Symptoms include a feeling of fullness or congestion and occasionally a nasal discharge. Diagnosis will require direct examination with a nasal speculum or x-ray of the nasal structures. Treatment may involve corticosteroids by topical application or injection into the polyps. The underlying allergy must be treated as well to prevent

recurrence. If conservative treatment is not effective, surgery is required.

Sinusitis

Sinusitis is the inflammation of one or more of the sinus cavities. It can be either acute or chronic. Acute sinusitis is usually the result of an upper respiratory infection and is fairly easily resolved. Chronic sinusitis is more persistent and more difficult to control. Either form is more common when bacteria are forced into the warm moist sinus during nose blowing.

Symptoms include the obvious signs of upper respiratory infection with the addition of a purulent nasal discharge and face pain. Diagnosis requires direct visualization, x-rays of the sinuses, punctures of the sinuses to withdraw a specimen for culture, and ultrasound.

Serious complications of brain and middle ear infection may occur if the condition is not treated promptly with antibiotics to kill the infecting agent. Total blockage may result if the disorder is not treated and may require surgical procedures such as a Caldwell-Luc, or a nasal window procedure, to puncture the wall between the nose and the involved sinus cavity to allow drainage. Ephedrine nose drops are often used to shrink the mucosal tissue. (Procedure 33-8 describes the steps for instilling nasal medication.) A newer treatment is the use of steroidal nasal sprays. Acute sinusitis responds to antibiotic therapy within 7 to 10 days. For chronic sinusitis, therapy may have to be instituted for 4 to 6 weeks.

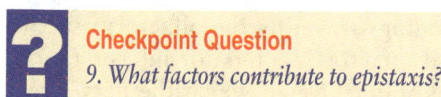

Checkpoint Question
9. What factors contribute to epistaxis?

Common Diagnostic Studies and Therapeutic Procedures and the Medical Assistant's Role

Many tests for the nose require direct visualization, including gross inspection and use of the illuminated otoscope (part of the diagnostic set). Diagnostic imaging (radiography and computed tomography scanning) may be used for the nasal sinuses, for traumatic injuries, and for congenital problems. Nose and throat cultures may also be ordered for differential diagnosis (see Chap. 37, Caring for Patients With Respiratory Disorders, for the procedure for obtaining a throat culture). Allergy testing may be performed for chronic rhinitis. A noninvasive procedure with a

---

Charting Example

02/02/99	1045 Patient complaining of dry, itchy nares. Patient uses hot air for home heating. Saline nasal spray ordered by Dr. Thomas. Both nostrils were sprayed while the patient took deep breaths. Patient was instructed in the need to keep nasal passages open and clear. Home humidification was suggested. Patient verbalized understanding of teachings. —— Carmen Simon, CMA

Patient Education: Nasal Disorders

Patients need to be aware of any changes in normal breathing patterns. It is imperative to have early symptoms of any nasal disorder treated as soon as possible to prevent complications. Children should be instructed to never place small pieces of toys or items such as dried beans or peas into the nares. These can be aspirated into the lungs and cause respiratory distress or aspiration pneumonia.

Instruct patients about the rebound phenomena of nasal sprays and drops. If used without the advice of a physician, these medications may become addictive. The nasal mucosa responds to the withdrawal by becoming congested if not routinely treated with the offending chemicals. Nasal preparations should never be used more than four times a day for 3 days unless specified by the physician.

---

fiberoptic sinus endoscope may be performed after numbing the patient's nose with a light anesthetic spray. Rhinoplasty is the surgical repair of the nose either to correct actual structural damage or for cosmetic purposes.

➤ OTHER SENSES

Taste

Taste receptors are located all across the tongue, through the mouth, and into the pharynx and larynx (see Fig. 33-14). The receptors require that food be moistened with saliva to be perceived. (Think of how tasteless food becomes when the mouth is dry.) The various chemical components of food are picked up by specific areas of the tongue:

- Sweet—tip of the tongue
- Sour—sides of the tongue
- Salt—edges of the tongue
- Bitter—back of the tongue

Some of the receptors pick up painful stimuli also, as in highly caustic foods such as certain peppers and ginger. The receptors tire quickly, which explains why we frequently move bits of hard candy from side to side to renew the taste. The gustatory center of the brain is in the center of the parietal lobe. Lesions in the brain can be traced by assessing a patient's taste perception.

Smell

Taste perception is closely associated with the sense of smell. Foods that have no odor have less taste than those that are also perceived by smell. The perception of both smell and taste diminishes with age and interferes with nutrition for the elderly.

Touch

Specialized receptors are scattered throughout the body to receive impulses for heat or cold, pressure, vibration, pain, touch, or position (Fig. 33-15). Each receptor is designed to register and transmit just that particular sensation. For instance, the pacinian corpuscles are **tactile** organs that are specific for deep pressure and vibrations but do not transmit heat or cold (Table 33-1). Nerves in the muscles, joints, and tendons transmit the position of our body parts: *Is my*

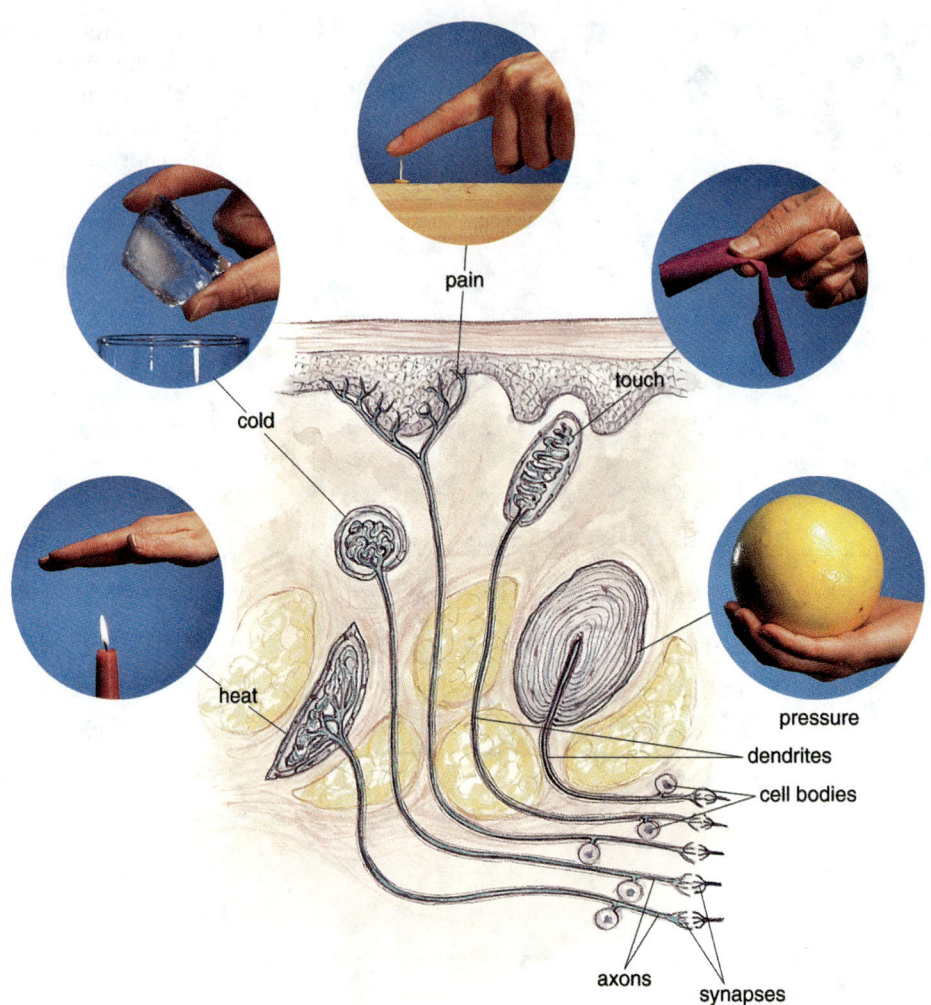

FIGURE 33-15
Diagram showing the superficial receptors (end-organs) and the deeper cell bodies and synapses, suggesting the continuity of sensory pathways into the central nervous system (CNS).

arm by my side or over my head? Am I standing or lying? These nerves are called proprioceptors and help coordinate our movements.

Pain Perception

Although we may learn to accept the perception of pain, we never adapt as we do to scents or tastes. The last painful stimulus is frequently as intolerable as the first, unlike some of our other perceptions. Pain is one of our most important protective devices. If we did not feel pain, we would be less aware of injury or disease. Pain receptors are found everywhere in our body but somewhat less viscerally.

Pain may be physiologic, implying that it is actually caused by an organic disorder, or it may be psychological, referring to pain that is perceived without the presence of an identifiable source. Whether or not

pain has an organic basis, it is no less real to the patient and must be treated with the same care and compassion.

Referred Pain

It is sometimes difficult for the physician to determine the source of pain by the symptoms reported by the patients. Many patients who are experiencing a myocardial infarction will complain of pain in the arms, shoulders, back, or jaw, rather than around the heart. Patients experiencing gallbladder attacks may complain of shoulder pain. These two examples are called referred pain. Theories suggest that the brain does not expect pain to be felt viscerally so it assigns the origin of the pain to a body part fairly close to the source. The medical assistant must record and report all symptoms of pain exactly as the patient describes them.

Table 33-1		
Tactile Organs		
Receptor	**Location**	**Sensation**
Pacinian corpuscles	Scattered throughout most of the surface of the body, including beneath the skin, mucous membranes, and serous tissues and around joints	Deep pressure and vibrations
Ruffini's corpuscles	Dermal layers of the skin and subcutaneously in the fingertips	Touch and pressure
Meissner's corpuscles	Upper layers of the skin, concentrated in the lips and fingertips	Fine touch
Krause's end bulbs	Dermal layer and subcutaneous tissues and lips	Touch and cold

Note: *Many free nerve endings present throughout the skin and mucosa register pain, gross touch, heat, or cold.*

Open-ended questions must be pursued, such as: *"How long have you felt this pain?" "Describe how it feels. What makes it better or worse?"* The physician will correlate the pain with the physical and laboratory findings to arrive at a diagnosis.

Pain Treatment

Pain may be treated by many means. Some of the accepted methods mask the perception of pain, others deaden the source area, and some are used to confuse the brain into feeling something other than pain.

Pain medications will mask the pain but will not usually relieve the source pathology. Surgery may help to remove the source of the pain. If removal is not possible, nerves to the area may be severed.

Transcutaneous electrical nerve stimulation (TENS), cold, and pressure are used to override the transmission of pain and confuse the pain receptors but will not treat the source of pain. Music, hypnosis or autohypnosis, imaging, and so on distract the patient from the pain but will not cure the source.

Checkpoint Question
10. *What is the difference between physiologic and psychological pain?*

text continues on page 638

Procedure 33-1

Measuring Distance Visual Acuity

Equipment/Supplies

- eye chart
- paper cup or eye paddle

Steps	Purpose
1. Wash your hands.	1. Handwashing aids infection control.
2. Prepare the examination room. Make sure the area is well lighted. A distance marker should be measured 20 feet from the chart; the chart must be at eye level.	2. The room must be well lighted to elicit the best response. All visual acuity tests require a distance of 20 feet for consistency of results.
3. Greet and identify the patient. Explain the procedure.	3. Identifying the patient prevents errors in the treatment. Patients who understand the procedure are more likely to be compliant, resulting in a more accurate test result.
4. Position the patient in a standing or sitting position at the 20 foot marker.	4. The patient may stand or sit, if necessary, as long as the chart is at eye level and the patient is 20 feet away from the chart.
5. Ask if the patient wears glasses or contact lenses. Mark the record accordingly.	5. Office policy will state whether examinations will include corrective lenses. The patient record should indicate if the patient wore corrective lenses for the test.
6. Have the patient cover the left eye with the eye paddle. Instruct the patient to keep both eyes open.	6. The testing routinely starts with the left eye covered for consistency in testing. The eyes must be covered alternately by an opaque object. The hand may not be used to avoid pressure against the eye or peeking through the fingers. Squinting to close one eye changes the vision.
7. Stand beside the chart and point to each row as the patient reads aloud the indicated lines, starting with the 20/200 line.	7. It is generally best to start at about the second or third row to judge the patient's response. If these lines are read easily, move down to smaller figures. If the patient has trouble reading the larger lines, the physician should be notified.
8. Record the smallest line the patient can read error free and note as OD (ocularis dexter). The numbers are listed on the side of the chart. For instance, if the patient reads line five with one error for the right eye, record as OD 20/40 -1. Your physician may prefer that only those lines read without error be counted as correct.	
9. Repeat the procedure with the right eye covered and record as in step 8, using OS (ocularis sinistra). If the patient squints or leans forward, record this observation on the patient record.	
10. Thank the patient and give appropriate instructions.	10. Courtesy encourages the patient to have a positive attitude about the physician's office.
11. Wash your hands.	
12. Document the procedure.	12. Procedures are considered not to have been done if they are not recorded.

Procedure 33-2   Measuring Color Perception

Equipment/Supplies

- Ishihara color plates
- gloves

Steps	Purpose
1. Wash your hands and put on gloves.	1. Gloves in this case are not for the protection of the patient or worker, but for the protection of the color plates. Oils from the hands can cause the colors to deteriorate and interfere with testing.
2. Identify the patient and explain the procedure by the first plate. Hold the plate about 30 inches from the patient.	2. The first plate should be obvious to all patients and serves as an example.
3. Ensure that the patient is in a comfortable sitting position in a quiet, well lighted room. Indirect sunlight gives the best illumination. (Sunlight should not shine against the plates; the colors fade with bright lights.)	
4. Be aware that patients who wear glasses or contact lenses may keep them on.	4. The Ishihara is testing color acuity, not visual acuity. Corrective lenses will not interfere with accurate test results.
5. Follow directions on the chart with the right eye, then the left eye.	
6. Thank the patient and give appropriate instructions.	6. Courtesy encourages the patient to have a positive attitude about the physician's office.
7. Record the results of the test by noting what the patient reports as being seen on each plate, using the plate number and the answer given by the patient. If the patient cannot distinguish the pattern, record as Plate #3 = X. Record any squinting or tearing or any hesitation or guesses indicating that the patient was not sure of what was being perceived.	7. Procedures are considered not to have been done if they are not recorded.
8. Store the book in a closed, protected area to protect the integrity of the colors.	

Procedure 33-3 Instilling Eye Medications

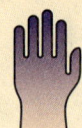

Equipment/Supplies

- physician's order
- medication
- sterile gauze
- tissues
- gloves

Steps	Purpose
1. Wash your hands and put on gloves.	1. Handwashing aids infection control. Gloves must be worn when there is potential exposure to body fluids.
2. Obtain the physician's order, the correct medication (check the label three times as directed in Chap. 26, Preparing and Administering Medications), sterile gauze, and tissues.	2. The medication must specify ophthalmic use. Medications formulated for other uses may be harmful if used in the eye.
3. Greet and identify the patient. Explain the procedure. Ask the patient about allergies not recorded in the chart.	3. Identifying the patient prevents errors in treatment. Patients who understand the procedure are more cooperative and compliant.
4. Position the patient comfortably.	4. The patient may be lying or sitting with the head tilted slightly back and positioned with the affected eye slightly downward to avoid the medication running into the unaffected eye.
5. Pull down the lower eyelid with sterile gauze and have the patient look upward.	5. Pulling down the lower lid exposes the conjunctival sac to receive the medication. If the patient is looking up and away from the medication, the blink reflex may not be triggered.
6. Instill the medication.	6.
a. *Ointment:* Discard the first bead of ointment. Place a thin line of ointment across the inside of the lower eyelid, moving from the inner canthus outward. Release the tube by twisting slightly. Do not touch the tube to the eye.	a. The first bead is considered contaminated. Placing the ointment into the sac avoids touching the eye with the tip of the ointment tube. Twisting the tube releases the ointment.
b. *Drops:* Hold the dropper close to the conjunctival sac (about ½ inch away) but do not touch the patient. Release the proper number of drops into the sac. Discard any medication left in the dropper.	b. Discarding the remaining medication avoids contaminating the remainder of a multiple dose container.

Step 6b.: Release the drops into the sac.

(continued)

Procedure 33-3   Instilling Eye Medications (continued)

Steps	Purpose
7. Have the patient gently close the eyelid and roll the eye to disperse the medication.	
8. Wipe up any excess medication with the tissue. Instruct the patient to apply light pressure on the puncta for several minutes.	8. Pressing the puncta prevents the medication from running to the nasolacrimal sac and duct.
9. Thank the patient and give appropriate instructions.	9. Courtesy encourages the patient to have a positive attitude about the physician's office.
10. Properly care for or dispose of equipment and supplies. Clean the work area. Wash your hands.	10. This prevents the spread of microorganisms.
11. Record the procedure.	11. Procedures are considered not have been done if they are not recorded.

Procedure 33-4   Irrigating the Eye

Equipment/Supplies

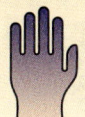

- small sterile basin
- towels
- emesis basin
- sterile irrigating solution at about 100°F
- sterile bulb syringe
- tissues
- sterile gloves

Steps	Purpose
1. Wash your hands and put on sterile gloves.	1. Handwashing aids infection control. Gloves must be worn when there is potential exposure to body fluids. The eyes may be easily damaged by infection.
2. Assemble the equipment and supplies. Check the solution label three times as recommended for medication administration. Make sure the preparation is for ophthalmic purposes. *Note:* If both eyes are to be treated, use separate equipment for each to avoid cross-contamination.	2. Solutions used for the eye must be sterile, must be formulated for ophthalmic use, and should be just above body temperature to avoid patient discomfort.
3. Greet and identify the patient. Explain the procedure.	3. Identifying the patient prevents errors in treatment. Patients who understand the procedure will be more cooperative and complaint.
4. Position the patient comfortably, either sitting with head tilted with the affected eye downward or lying with the affected eye downward.	4. With the affected eye downward, there is less chance of contamination running into the unaffected eye.
5. Drape the patient with a protective barrier to avoid wetting the clothing.	

(continued)

Procedure 33-4   Irrigating the Eye *(continued)*

Steps	Purpose
6. Place the emesis basin against the upper cheek near the eye with the towel under the basin. With clean gauze, wipe from the inner cantha outward to remove debris from the lashes.	6. Debris from the lashes might be washed into the eye.
7. Separate the lids with the thumb and forefinger of the nondominant hand. The dominant hand holding the syringe with solution may be lightly supported on the bridge of the patient's nose parallel to the eye to steady the hand.	
8. Gently irrigate from the inner to the outer canthus, holding the syringe 1 inch above the eye. Use gentle pressure and do not touch the eye. The physician will order the period of time required for the irrigation.	8. The solution must flow across from the inner to the outer cantha to avoid washing pathogens into the puncta. With the syringe 1 inch above the eye there is little chance of touching the eye and causing patient discomfort.

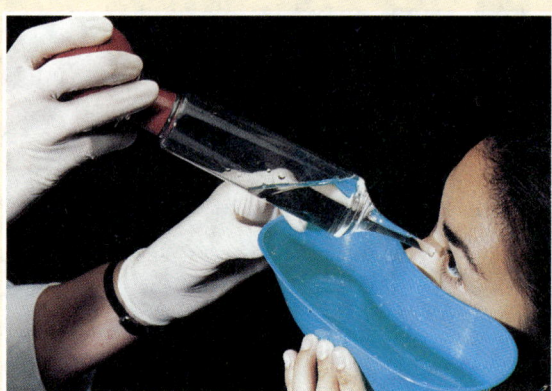

Step 8: Hold the syringe one inch above the eye.

Steps	Purpose
9. Use tissue to wipe up any excess solution from the patient's face.	
10. Properly dispose of equipment or sanitize as recommended and remove the gloves. Wash your hands.	10. This prevents the spread of microorganisms.
11. Thank the patient and give appropriate instructions.	11. Courtesy encourages the patient to have a positive attitude about the physician's office.
12. Record the procedure on the patient record, including the length of the procedure, type and strength of the solution, which eye, and any observations.	12. Procedures are considered not to have been done if they are not recorded.

Note: *Eye irrigations can be performed using a Morgan lens, which consists of a plastic applicator that is placed directly on the eyeball (similar to a contact lens). An attachment to the lens connects to an irrigating solution, which runs in and irrigates the eye. One advantage to the system is that it prevents blinking during irrigation. Before using a Morgan lens, carefully read the manufacturer's instructions.*

Procedure 33-5 — Removing a Foreign Object From the Eye

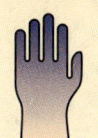

Equipment/Supplies

- sterile, cotton-tipped applicator
- sterile water or saline
- sterile medicine dropper or small bulb syringe
- tissues
- sterile gauze
- gloves

Steps	Purpose
1. Wash your hands and put on gloves.	1. Handwashing aids infection control. Gloves must be worn when there is potential exposure to body fluids.
2. Assemble the equipment and supplies.	2. This ensures that all supplies are available.
3. Greet and identify the patient. Explain the procedure.	3. Identifying the patient prevents errors in treatment. Patients who understand the procedure are more likely to be cooperative and compliant.
4. With the gauze against the cheek, pull down the lower eyelid and check for the object. If it is seen, moisten the applicator with the water or saline and gently try to remove the object.	
5. If the object is not found on the lower lid, grasp the lashes of the upper lid and pull gently upward, checking for the upper surfaces of the eye for the object.	
6. Perform an eye irrigation if necessary, following the steps in Procedure 33-4.	
7. Wipe up any excess liquid with the tissue.	
8. Thank the patient and give appropriate instructions.	8. Courtesy encourages the patient to have a positive attitude about the physician's office.
9. Properly care for or dispose of equipment and supplies. Clean the work area. Wash your hands.	9. This prevents the spread of microorganisms.
10. Record the procedure and any observations on the patient's chart.	10. Procedures are considered not to have been done if they are not recorded.

Note: *Imbedded objects must be removed by a physician but loose debris may be removed by the medical assistant.*

Procedure 33-6 — Irrigating the Ear

Equipment/Supplies

- ear irrigation syringe or irrigating device
- emesis basin or ear basin
- waterproof barrier
- otoscope
- irrigation solution at no more than 100°F
- bowl for solution
- unsterile gauze

Steps	Purpose
1. Wash your hands.	1. Handwashing aids infection control.
2. Assemble the equipment and supplies.	2. This ensures that all supplies are available. Ear irrigation is not a sterile procedure. A temperature of more than 100°F may be uncomfortable for the patient.
3. Greet and identify the patient. Explain the procedure.	3. Identifying the patient prevents errors in treatment. Explaining the procedure helps ease anxiety and ensure patient compliance. Ear irrigations are not usually painful but the flow of the solution may be uncomfortable. The patient will be more cooperative if this is understood.
4. Position the patient comfortably in an erect position.	
5. View the affected ear with an otoscope to locate the problem. *Adults:* Gently pull up and slightly back to straighten the auditory canal. *Children:* Gently pull slightly down and back to straighten the auditory canal. *Note:* Do not irrigate if the tympanic membrane appears to be perforated without checking with the physician; solution may be forced into the middle ear through the perforation. Remove any obvious debris at the entrance of the canal before beginning the irrigation.	5. The area of treatment must be visualized before irrigation begins. If debris from the external auricle is not removed, it may be washed into the canal.

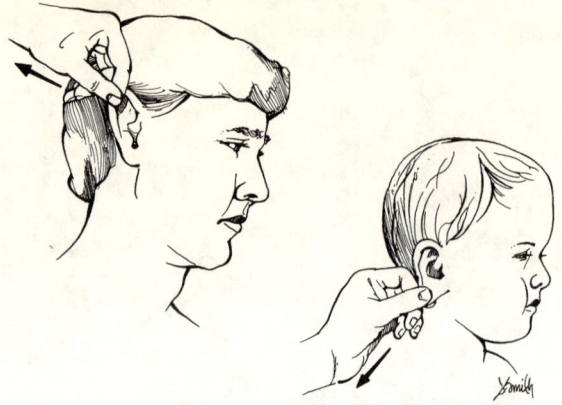

Step 5: The shape of the ear canal changes with growth. To allow better inspection, position the ear as illustrated.

(continued)

Procedure 33-6   Irrigating the Ear *(continued)*

Steps	Purpose
6. Drape the patient with a waterproof barrier.	6. Wet clothing would be uncomfortable for the patient.
7. Tilt the patient's head toward the affected side.	7. Tilting the head downward will facilitate the flow of solution.
8. Place the drainage basin next to the affected ear.	
9. Fill the syringe or turn on the irrigating device.	
10. Gently position the auricle as described above with the nondominant hand.	10. The canal must be straightened for either visualization or treatment.
11. With the dominant hand, place the tip of the syringe into the auditory meatus and direct the flow of solution gently upward toward the roof of the canal.	11. Directing the flow against the upper surface will avoid pressure against the tympanic membrane and will facilitate the outflow of solution.

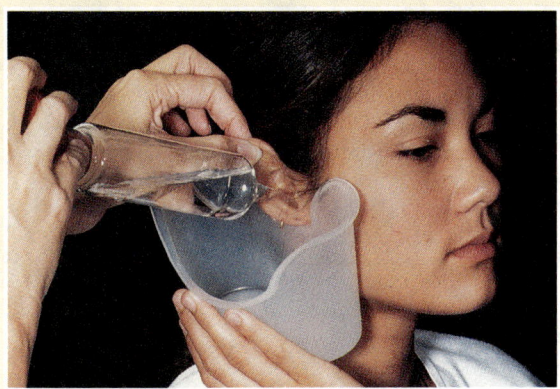

Step 11: Place the syringe tip into the auditory meatus.

Steps	Purpose
12. Continue irrigating for the prescribed period of time.	
13. Dry the patient's external ear with gauze. Have the patient sit for awhile with the affected ear downward to drain the solution.	13. Allowing the solution to remain in the ear will be uncomfortable.
14. Inspect the ear with the otoscope to determine the results.	14. It may be necessary to repeat the procedure, and it is always necessary to inspect the area to record the results.
15. Thank the patient and give appropriate instructions.	15. Courtesy encourages the patient to have a positive attitude about the physician's office.
16. Properly care for or dispose of equipment and supplies. Clean the work area. Wash your hands.	16. This prevents the spread of microorganisms.
17. Record the procedure on the patient's chart.	17. Procedures are considered not to have been done if they are not recorded.

Procedure 33-7 Instilling Ear Medication

Equipment/Supplies

- medication with dropper
- cotton balls

Steps	Purpose
1. Wash your hands.	1. Handwashing aids infection control.
2. Assemble the equipment.	2. This ensures that all supplies are available.
3. Check the medication three times as specified for medication administration. It must specify otic preparation.	3. Medication for otic instillation must be formulated for that purpose.
4. Greet and identify the patient. Explain the procedure.	4. Identifying the patient prevents errors in treatment. Explaining the procedure helps ease anxiety and ensure compliance.
5. Have the patient seated with the affected ear tilted upward.	5. The medication must be allowed to flow through the canal to the area of concern.
6. Draw up the ordered amount of medication.	
7. *Adults:* Pull the auricle slightly up and back to straighten the S-shaped canal. *Children:* Pull the auricle slightly down and back to straighten the S-shaped canal.	
8. Insert the tip of the dropper without touching the patient's skin and let the medication flow along the side of the canal.	8. Touching the patient will contaminate the dropper. The medication should flow gently to avoid patient discomfort.

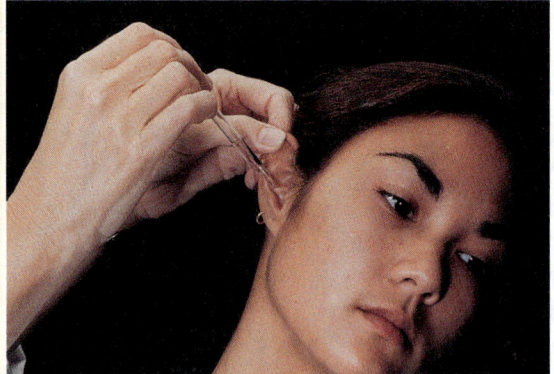

Step 8: Insert the tip of the dropper.

9. Have the patient sit or lie with the affected ear upward for a short while.	9. The medication should rest against the tympanic membrane for as long as possible.
10. If the medication is to be retained, insert the cotton ball slightly into the external auditory meatus without force.	10. A wick will help keep the medication in the canal. Force could be painful to the patient.
11. Thank the patient and give appropriate instructions.	11. Courtesy encourages the patient to have a positive attitude about the physician's office.

(continued)

Procedure 33-7

Instilling Ear Medication *(continued)*

Steps	Purpose
12. Properly care for or dispose of equipment and supplies. Clean the work area. Wash your hands.	12. This prevents the spread of microorganisms.
13. Record the procedure in the patient's chart.	13. Procedures are considered not to have been done if they are not recorded.

Procedure 33-8

Instilling Nasal Medication

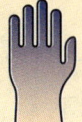

Equipment/Supplies

- medication order
- medication (drops or spray)
- nonsterile tissues
- gloves

Steps	Purpose
1. Wash your hands.	1. Handwashing aids infection control.
2. Assemble the equipment and supplies. Check the medication label three times.	2. This ensures that all supplies are available. Preparations for use in the nasal passages must be formulated for these surfaces.
3. Greet and identify the patient. Explain the procedure. Ask the patient about allergies not documented.	3. Identifying the patient prevents errors in treatment. Explaining the procedure helps ease anxiety and ensures compliance. Nasal instillations are uncomfortable but should not be painful; patients will be more cooperative if they understand the procedure.
4. Position the patient in a comfortable recumbent position. Extend the patient's head beyond the edge of the examination table or place a pillow under the patient's shoulders. Support the patient's neck to avoid strain as the head is tilted back.	4. The patient must be properly positioned to reach the upper nasal passages.
5. Administer the medication.	5.
a. Administer nose drops by holding the dropper upright just above each nostril and dropping the medication one drop at a time without touching the nares. Keep the patient in recumbent position for 5 minutes.	a. Touching the dropper to the nostril will contaminate the dropper. For effective treatment, the patient must allow the medication to reach the upper nasal passages.
b. Administer nasal spray by having the patient sit up. Place the tip of the bottle at the nare opening without touching the patient's skin or nasal tissues and spray as the patient takes a deep breath.	b. The medication must reach the upper passages; if the patient breathes out, much of the medication will be exhaled.

(continued)

Procedure 33-8   Instilling Nasal Medication *(continued)*

Steps	Purpose
6. Wipe any excess medication from the patient's skin with tissues.	6. Excess medication around the nares will be uncomfortable.
7. Thank the patient and give appropriate instructions.	7. Courtesy encourages the patient to have a positive attitude about the physician's office.
8. Properly care for or dispose of equipment and supplies. Clean the work area. Remove gloves. Wash your hands.	8. This prevents the spread of microorganisms.
9. Record the procedure on patient's chart.	9. Procedures are considered not to have been done if they are not recorded.

SUMMARY

Working with the nervous system is a fascinating medical specialty. With the invention of radiologic imaging and scanning devices, the development of microsurgery, and the seemingly infinite array of new technology, the medical profession is rapidly opening up the complexity of this system that oversees the maintenance of our life functions. The senses are our window into the world around us and a glimpse of the interconnection between what we perceive and how we respond.

CRITICAL THINKING CHALLENGES

Pamela Martin calls your general practice office on Monday regarding her son Brian, age 8. She states that on Saturday, he began having a runny nose and sore throat. His temperature was only 99.4°F so she has been giving him acetaminophen every 4 hours. This morning he awoke screaming and tugging at his right ear and has a temperature of 102.4°F.

As you decide how to handle this call, consider the following questions:

1. Would you see the child today or schedule him on Tuesday because Mondays are extremely busy?
2. On what facts would you base your decision?
3. Would you seat the child in the waiting room with other patients? What factors would influence this decision?
4. What pieces of equipment would you have prepared for the child's examination and why?

ANSWERS TO CHECKPOINT QUESTIONS

1. The rods and cones are nerve cells contained in the retina. Rods are responsible for light and dark shadings. Cones are responsible for color reception.
2. A sty is an infection of the glands of the eyelids; conjunctivitis is an infection of the conjunctiva, the mucous membrane that covers the sclera and cornea.
3. Four common refractive errors are hyperopia (farsightedness), myopia (nearsightedness), astigmatism (unfocused refraction of light rays on the retina), and presbyopia (age-related vision changes).
4. The tumbling E chart is used for patients who cannot read or who do not speak English.
5. The cochlea transmits sound waves into nerve impulses and the semicircular canals aid balance and coordination.
6. Conductive hearing loss stops the flow of sound wave vibrations in the area before the cochlea. Perceptual hearing loss stops the flow of nerve impulses from the cochlea to the brain.
7. An audiometer is used to detect hearing loss. The patient wears earphones and listens for pure tones of various decibel levels and various frequencies. The results of the test are recorded by the audiometer on a special graph.
8. Cilia are small, hairlike projections covering virtually all surfaces of the nasal structures. They move secretions along to the throat for swallowing.

9. Hypertension, malignancies, polyps, and the fragile capillaries associated with pregnancy are factors that contribute to epistaxis.

10. Physiologic pain is caused by an organic disorder; psychological pain is perceived by the patient without the presence of an identifiable source.

SUGGESTIONS FOR FURTHER READING

Memmler, R. L., Cohen, B. J., & Wood, D. L. (1996). *The Human Body in Health and Disease*, 8th ed. Philadelphia: Lippincott-Raven Publishers.

(1992). *Professional Guide to Diseases*, 4th ed. Springhouse, PA: Springhouse.

Rosdahl, C. B. (1995). *Textbook of Basic Nursing,* 6th ed. Philadelphia: J. B. Lippincott.

Scherer, J. C. & Timby, B. K. (1995). *Introductory Medical-Surgical Nursing,* 6th ed. Philadelphia: J. B. Lippincott.

Smeltzer, S., & Bare, B. (1996). *Brunner and Suddarth's Textbook of Medical-Surgical Nursing,* 8th ed. Philadelphia: Lippincott-Raven Publishers.

Timby, B. K. (1996). *Fundamental Skills and Concepts in Patient Care,* 6th ed. Philadelphia: Lippincott-Raven Publishers.

Caring for Patients With Endocrine Disorders

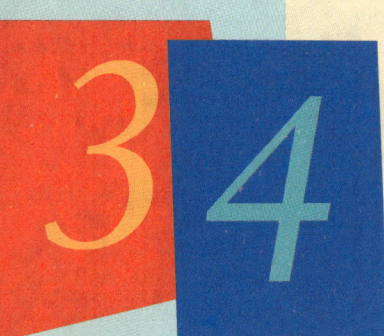

Chapter Outline

Structure and Function of the Endocrine System
   Pituitary
   Thyroid
   Parathyroids
   Thymus
   Adrenals
   Pancreas
   Pineal Body
   Gonads
Common Endocrine Disorders
   Hypopituitarism
   Hyperpituitarism
   Diabetes Insipidus
   Goiter
   Hypothyroidism
   Hyperthyroidism

   Hypoparathyroidism
   Hyperparathyroidism
   Thymic Abnormalities
   Hypoadrenocorticalism
   Hyperadrenocorticalism
   Diabetes Mellitus
   Diabetic Ketoacidosis
   Diabetic Coma and Insulin Shock
   Gonadal Abnormalities
Common Laboratory Tests and Diagnostic Procedures and the Medical Assistant's Role
Summary
Critical Thinking Challenges
Answers to Checkpoint Questions
Sugggestions for Further Reading

DACUM Components

1.3   Practice within the scope of education, training, and personal capabilities
1.6   Conduct oneself in a courteous and diplomatic manner
2.2   Treat all patients with empathy and impartiality
4.1   Apply principles of aseptic technique and infection control
4.10 Collect and process specimens
4.11 Perform selected tests that assist with diagnosis and treatment
7.3   Teach patients methods of health promotion and disease prevention

Chapter Competencies

Learning Objectives

Upon successfully completing this chapter, you will be able to:

1. Spell and define the Key Terms.
2. Locate and identify the glands of the endocrine system.
3. State the hormones secreted by each gland, their actions, and their the target tissues.
4. Identify abnormal conditions resulting from deficient and excessive hormone secretions.
5. Identify abbreviations, laboratory tests, and clinical procedures related to endocrinology.
6. State current treatments for common endocrine disorders.

Key Terms

(See Glossary for definitions.)

Addison's disease
corticoid
cretinism
diabetes insipidus
dwarfism
endemic
eunuchoidism
exophthalmic goiter
gigantism
goiter
glucocorticoid
glycosuria

Graves' disease
hormone
hypercalcemia
hyperglycemia
hyperplasia
hypoglycemia
insulin-dependent
    diabetes mellitus
    (IDDM)
ketoacidosis
ketones
myxedema

non–insulin-
    dependent diabetes
    mellitus (NIDDM)
polydipsia
polyphagia
polyuria
pruritus
radioimmunoassay
tetany
thyrotoxicosis
vasopressin

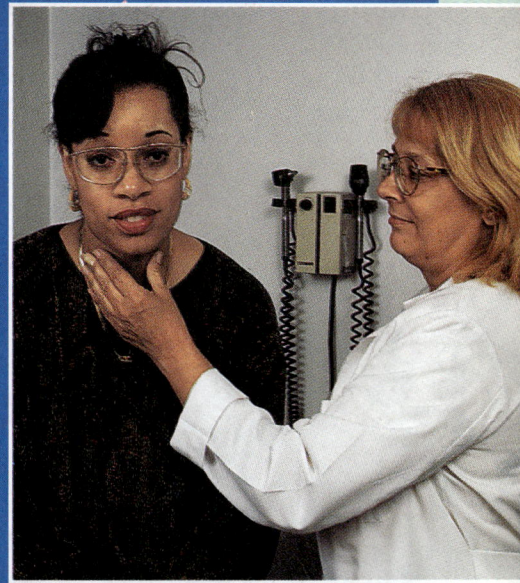

Together with the nervous system, the endocrine system regulates body functions. Although the control exerted by the nervous system is immediate and directed at a specific (usually short-term) response, the endocrine system regulates chemical metabolism for a longer-acting, more widespread response. **Hormones** are the chemical regulators, or messengers, of the endocrine glands. Some hormones stimulate system-wide metabolic processes; others are specific for a particular tissue.

The endocrine glands differ from the body's other glands (exocrine glands) because they are ductless, secreting hormones directly into the bloodstream for transmission rather than requiring direct access to the target tissue. Hormones circulate through the bloodstream to act on target tissues and exert specific regulatory effects.

Homeostatic regulation keeps hormone levels within specific ranges. Negative feedback alerts endocrine glands to the need for increased or decreased secretion. Some glands operate within a limited range to maintain almost constant hormonal levels; other glands function by cyclic or rhythmic fluctuations, as exemplified by estrogen and progesterone release during the menstrual cycle.

➤ STRUCTURE AND FUNCTION OF THE ENDOCRINE SYSTEM

The glands of the endocrine system include:

- Pituitary
- Thyroid
- Parathyroids
- Thymus
- Adrenals
- Pancreas
- Gonads

The pineal body is also included in the endocrine system although some sources do not consider it technically a gland (Fig. 34-1).

A description of each gland and its particular regulatory role follows. Table 34-1 lists the glands and provides a summary of their principal functions.

Pituitary

The pituitary gland (also known as the hypophysis) is the master gland and is responsible for controlling many components of the endocrine system. It is lo-

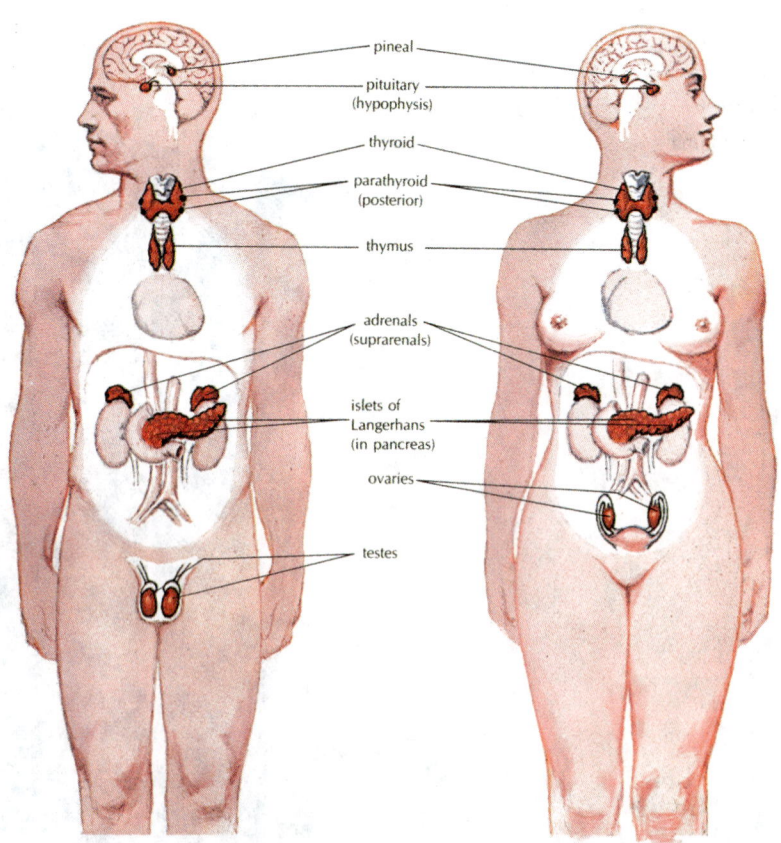

pineal
pituitary (hypophysis)
thyroid
parathyroid (posterior)
thymus
adrenals (suprarenals)
islets of Langerhans (in pancreas)
ovaries
testes

FIGURE 34-1
The main hormone-secreting organs.

Table 34-1
The Major Endocrine Glands and Their Hormones

Gland	Hormone	Principal Functions
Anterior pituitary	GH (growth hormone)	Promotes growth of all body tissues
	TSH (thyroid-stimulating hormone)	Stimulates thyroid gland to produce thyroid hormones
	ACTH (adrenocorticotropic hormone)	Stimulates adrenal cortex to produce cortical hormones; aids in protecting body in stress situations (injury, pain)
	PRL (prolactin)	Stimulates secretion of milk by mammary glands
	FSH (follicle-stimulating hormone)	Stimulates growth and hormone activity of ovarian follicles; stimulates growth of testes; promotes development of sperm cells
	LH (luteinizing hormone); ICSH (interstitial cell-stimulating hormone) in males	Causes development of corpus luteum at site of ruptured ovarian follicle in female; stimulates secretion of testosterone in male
Posterior pituitary	ADH (antidiuretic hormone; vasopressin)	Promotes reabsorption of water in kidney tubules; stimulates smooth muscle tissue of blood vessels to constrict
	Oxytocin	Causes contraction of muscle of uterus; causes ejection of milk from mammary glands
Thyroid	Thyroid hormone (thyroxine and triiodothyronine)	Increases metabolic rate, influencing both physical and mental activities; required for normal growth
	Calcitonin	Decreases calcium level in blood
Parathyroids	Parathyroid hormone	Regulates exchange of calcium between blood and bones; increases calcium level in blood
Adrenal medulla	Epinephrine and norepinephrine	Increases blood pressure and heart rate; activates cells influenced by sympathetic nervous system plus many not affected by sympathetic nerves
Adrenal cortex	Cortisol (95% of glucocorticoids)	Aids in metabolism of carbohydrates, proteins, and fats; active during stress
	Aldosterone (95% of mineralocorticoids)	Aids in regulating electrolytes and water balance
	Sex hormones	May influence secondary sexual characteristics in male
Pancreatic islets	Insulin	Aids transport of glucose into cells; required for cellular metabolism of foods, especially glucose; decreases blood sugar levels
	Glucagon	Stimulates liver to release glucose, thereby increasing blood sugar levels
Testes	Testosterone	Stimulates growth and development of male sexual organs (testes, penis, others) plus development of secondary sexual characteristics such as hair growth on body and face and deepening of voice; stimulates maturation of sperm cells
Ovaries	Estrogens (eg, estradiol)	Stimulate growth of primary female sexual organs (uterus, tubes, etc.) and development of secondary sexual organs such as breasts, plus changes in pelvis to ovoid, broader shape
	Progesterone	Stimulates development of secretory parts of mammary glands; prepares uterine lining for implantation of fertilized ovum; aids in maintaining pregnancy

cated at the base of the brain, protected in a saddle-like bone structure called the sella turcica, just beneath the hypothalamus. It is a small, bilobed gland, with the anterior lobe forming the largest portion of the gland.

The pituitary is controlled by the hypothalamus through a connection called the infundibulum. The anterior lobe of the pituitary is responsible for the majority of the body's hormonal control. The posterior lobe is a storage area for two hormones that are produced in the hypothalamus and retained within the lobe until needed. Several pituitary hormones act directly on tar-

get tissue or organs to produce the necessary reaction. Others, called tropic hormones, stimulate the target tissue or organs to secrete hormones from within the local tissues (Fig. 34-2).

Anterior Lobe

A number of hormones are secreted by the pituitary's anterior lobe. Human growth hormone (GH or HGH), also known as somatotropin hormone (STH), stimulates growth by promoting protein metabolism.

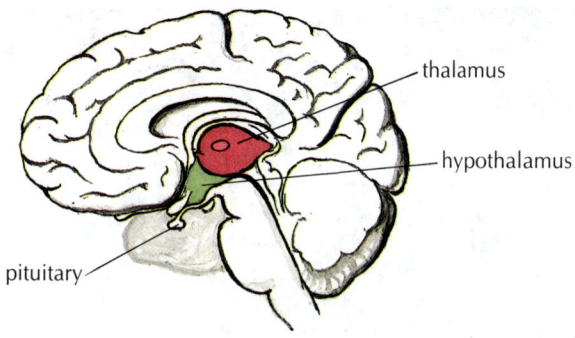

FIGURE 34-2
Diagram showing the relationship among the thalamus, hypothalamus, and pituitary (hypophysis).

Growth is stimulated until the epiphyseal ends of the long bones have sealed. (See Chap. 31, Caring for Patients With Musculoskeletal Disorders, for more information on long bones and bone growth.) The hormone then acts to ensure proper tissue replacement and repair.

Gonadotropic hormones include luteinizing hormone (LH), interstitial cell-stimulating hormone (ICSH), and follicle-stimulating hormone (FSH). LH acts on ovarian tissue to stimulate ovulation, to develop the corpus luteum, and to liberate progesterone in the female. ICSH stimulates the interstitial cells of the testes to produce testosterone. In females, FSH acts on the ovarian follicles to stimulate the production of estrogen and growth of the ova. In males, FSH acts on the tissue of the testes to initiate sperm production.

Thyroid-stimulating hormone (TSH) functions to maintain the thyroid gland and stimulates it to produce the thyroid hormones.

Adrenocorticotropic hormone (ACTH or corticotropin) stimulates the secretion of adrenal corticosteroids by the adrenal cortex.

Prolactin (PRL) controls proliferation of the mammary glands and stimulates milk production.

Melanocyte-stimulating hormone (MSH) controls the intensity of skin pigmentation.

Posterior Lobe

The two hormones stored in the pituitary's posterior lobe are oxytocin and antidiuretic hormone (ADH).

Oxytocin promotes contractions of the uterine muscle during labor and involution. In the postpartum period, oxytocin also affects the mammary glands and causes the "let down" reflex or ejection of milk.

Also known as **vasopressin**, ADH increases reabsorption of water by the kidneys (Fig. 34-3).

Checkpoint Question
1. *What are the anterior and posterior lobes of the pituitary gland responsible for?*

Thyroid

The thyroid is a yellowish or amber-red lobulated, shield-shaped organ located in the neck near the junction of the larynx and trachea. It consists of two lateral lobes that lie on either side of the trachea and are connected by an isthmus that crosses anterior to the second and third tracheal rings. The blood supply to the thyroid is extremely rich; more blood flows through this gland in proportion to its size than through any of the body's other organs.

Iodine is essential to the production of the three thyroid hormones:

- Thyroxine (T_4)
- Triiodothyronine (T_3)
- Calcitonin

The thyroid hormones T_4 and T_3 are iodine-containing amino acids that stimulate cellular metabolism and promote growth. Their primary action is regulating the metabolic rate. They directly increase the rate of oxidation of foodstuffs within the cells, accelerating the rate of sugar absorption and directing the liver to convert glycogen to glucose as needed for energy. They also regulate mineral and protein metabolism to supply energy needed for cell growth and maintenance of life functions.

Calcitonin inhibits the release of calcium and phosphates from the bones to the blood, thereby decreasing the circulating calcium. In balance with the parathyroid hormone (see below), calcitonin maintains blood and bone calcium composition. Calcitonin is essential to normal bone development, to maintaining the balance of calcium available for impulse transmission in the nervous and muscular systems, and to clot development in the circulatory system.

Checkpoint Question
2. *How does the thyroid affect blood calcium levels?*

Parathyroids

There are usually four parathyroids, two on each side, situated on and more or less intimately connected with the posterior thyroid. (The actual number of parathyroids can range from 2 to 10.) The parathyroids pro-

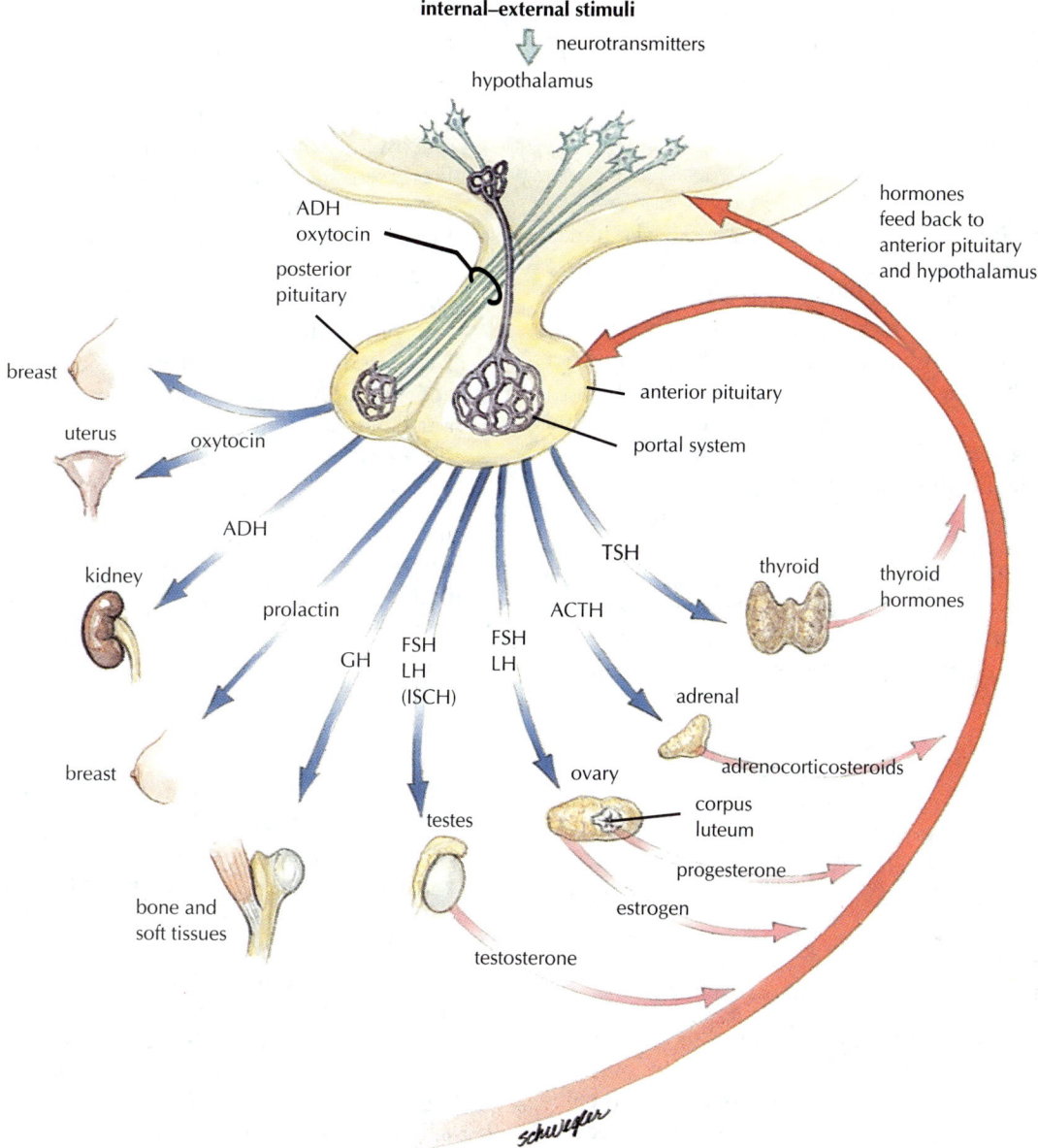

FIGURE 34-3
Pituitary gland and its relations with the brain and target tissues. Hypothalamic-releasing hormones influence the anterior pituitary through a portal system. Tropic hormones from the anterior pituitary affect the working of various other glands. The hypothalamus communicates with the posterior pituitary through tracts.

duce parathormone, also known as the parathyroid hormone (PTH).

Parathyroid hormone has a vital role in metabolizing calcium and phosphorus and regulating calcium in blood and tissues. It has two target sites:

1. Kidneys—PTH promotes the renal excretion of phosphate by decreasing reabsorption, thereby causing the serum phosphorous levels to decrease.

2. Bone tissue—PTH causes bone tissue to break down through increased osteoclastic activity. This breaking down of bone cells is necessary to return stored calcium to the general circulation when blood calcium levels are low.

It is vital that the parathyroids work together with the thyroid (calcitonin) to maintain bone strength. If either gland malfunctions, bone health and available calcium will be compromised.

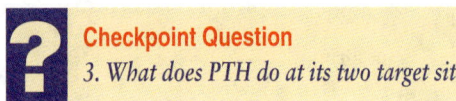

Checkpoint Question
3. What does PTH do at its two target sites?

Thymus

The thymus is composed of two elongated, flask-shaped lobes, which occupy a region just above the heart where the chest cavity narrows at the base of the neck. The two glands are joined to one another by connective tissue, which also covers each gland, forming a distinct capsule around the inner mass of lymphoid tissue.

The thymus is a prominent organ at birth and reaches its greatest size at puberty, after which it undergoes a gradual regression. During regression, the thymic tissue is usually replaced by fat, so that the adult thymus is composed largely of fat and connective tissue. The thymus is believed to be vital to the development of the immune response in children. It produces thymosin, which is most important in the production and maturation of lymphocytes and the development of immunity.

Adrenals

The adrenals, also referred to as the suprarenal glands, are two pyramid-shaped structures lying close to the upper pole of the kidneys. The two glands usually differ somewhat in size, and there is also a difference in size between the glands in men and women. Each gland consists of two functionally distinct parts:

- Medulla—the central portion of the gland, which is closely associated with the central nervous system
- Cortex—a surrounding zone of tissue, which comprises eight to nine times the volume of the medulla

The functions of the adrenal medulla and adrenal cortex are completely unrelated.

Adrenal Medulla

The only function of the adrenal medulla is the secretion of epinephrine (adrenaline) and norepinephrine (noradrenaline) in response to sympathetic nervous system stimulation. Epinephrine is secreted in response to need, as in the fright-flight-fight syndrome (see Chap. 32, Caring for Patients With Neurologic Disorders, for more information). It has cardiovascular effects, exerting a constricting action on arteries, veins, and capillaries. The vasomotor effect, however, is not the same in all areas. For example, the blood vessels of the brain and muscles react only slightly to epinephrine, whereas those of the adrenal glands, thyroid, and placenta do not react at all.

Epinephrine effects include:

- Contraction of arterioles, which increases blood pressure
- Conversion of glycogen stored in the liver to glucose, which is rushed to muscle tissue for energy
- Increased heart rate, which results in more blood for emergency response
- Increased cellular metabolism, which boosts energy output
- Dilation of the bronchi, which supplies more oxygen for metabolism
- Decreased intestinal movement and activity and contraction of the cardiac, pyloric, ileocecal, and anal sphincters
- Increased numbers of blood components and lymphocytes

Because epinephrine mimics the effect of the sympathetic nervous system, it is often referred to as a sympathomimetic substance. Norepinephrine is also a product of the adrenal medulla and is produced in response to stressors.

Adrenal Cortex

The adrenal cortex affects almost all body systems and is necessary to maintain life. Excision of the adrenal medulla is not fatal. However, complete removal of both adrenals, with loss of the cortical hormones, leads to death in a short period of time. Approximately 28 steroid hormones have been separated from cortical extracts, but only 6 or 7 have been identified by their physiologic activity. These are called **corticoids** and their effects are called "corticoid effects."

Glucocorticoids regulate conversion of amino acids to maintain a carbohydrate reserve for energy. These hormones use sugar in times of stress for immediate energy and rely on carbohydrates for longer-term energy needs. They help suppress inflammation and may be used to treat acute or chronic inflammatory processes. Hydrocortisone made from the glucocorticoid cortisol is widely used for this purpose.

Mineralocorticoids help regulate electrolyte balance. They target the kidneys to control the sodium reabsorption and potassium secretion. Aldosterone is this group's major hormone.

The sex hormones arise from the adrenal cortex and assist estrogen and testosterone in establishing secondary sexual characteristics.

Checkpoint Question
4. How do the functions of the adrenal medulla and adrenal cortex differ?

Pancreas

The pancreas is located in the upper left quadrant of the abdominal cavity, extending from the curve of the duodenum to the spleen. The pancreas functions in both the gastrointestinal and endocrine systems. The bulk of the pancreas produces an external secretion, or enzyme, concerned with digestion. Within the pancreas are groups of cells—called the islets of Langerhans—that produce two endocrine hormones. The islets of Langerhans contain alpha and beta cells. Alpha cells produce glucagon, and beta cells produce insulin.

Glucagon stimulates the liver to change glycogen to glucose and to increase fat conversion and amino acid production for use as energy. The process, called gluconeogenesis, is the conversion of excess amino acids into simple carbohydrates that may aid cell respiration. The overall effect of glucagon is to raise the blood glucose level and to make energy stores available for metabolic needs. Glucagon secretion is stimulated by hypoglycemia (low blood glucose level).

Insulin production is stimulated by hyperglycemia (high blood glucose level). Insulin secretion removes glucose from the circulation and facilitates its transfer through cell membranes. Insulin increases the liver's ability to convert excess sugar into fatty acids for storage as fat cells. The effect of insulin is to lower blood glucose levels.

Checkpoint Question

5. How is glucagon secretion stimulated, and what are its effects?

Pineal Body

Situated within the brain, this glandlike structure is fairly large in children but, like the thymus, diminishes with age. The main purpose of the pineal body seems to be the production of the hormone melatonin, which is thought to play a part in the onset of puberty. Melatonin levels decrease in the presence of daylight and increase at night. This fluctuation is thought to be responsible for our diurnal rhythms that urge us to sleep at night and awake with daylight.

Gonads

The gonads include the ovaries and the testes. The ovaries are located in the pelvic cavity on each side of the uterus. The testes are located in the scrotum, a sac of skin between the upper thighs. (See Chap. 40, Caring for Patients With Disorders of the Male Reproductive System, and Chap. 41, Caring for Patients With Obstetric and Gynecologic Disorders, for more information about these organs.)

In the ovaries, estrogen (estradiol) is produced by the follicle cells. Estrogen stimulates:

- Maturation of the ova
- Proliferation of blood vessels in the endometrium
- Development of secondary sexual characteristics
- Growth of the duct system of the mammary glands
- Growth of the uterus
- Disposition of fat subcutaneously in the hips and thighs

Estrogen also promotes the closure of the epiphyses of the long bones and is believed to lower blood levels of cholesterol and triglycerides. Estrogen gets its stimulus from the anterior pituitary's follicle-stimulating hormone (FSH). Progesterone prepares and maintains the uterus during pregnancy.

In the testes, testosterone is produced by the interstitial cells in response to the anterior pituitary's interstitial cell-stimulating hormone (ICSH). Testosterone promotes maturation of sperm in the testes. Testosterone stimulates:

- Development of secondary sexual characteristics
- Growth of the reproductive organs
- Growth of facial and body hair
- Growth of the larynx and the deepening of the voice
- Growth of the skeletal muscles

Testosterone also brings about closure of the epiphyses of the long bones.

Table 34-2 classifies the many hormones produced by the endocrine glands according to their various functions.

➤ COMMON ENDOCRINE DISORDERS

Because many normal body processes depend on appropriate hormone levels, either a deficiency (hyposecretion) or excess (hypersecretion) of hormones can result in altered functioning.

Hypopituitarism

Hypopituitarism is a deficiency of the anterior pituitary hormones. It may be caused by injury or atrophy of the gland, or it may result from certain types of tumors.

Table 34-2
Functional Classification of Hormones

Function	Hormone	Major Source
Control of water and electrolyte metabolism	Aldosterone	Adrenal cortex
	Antidiuretic hormone (ADH)	Posterior pituitary
	Calcitonin	C cells, thyroid
	Parathyroid hormone	Parathyroid
	Angiotensin	Kidney
Control of gastrointestinal function	Cholecystokinin	Gastrointestinal tract
	Gastrin	Gastrointestinal tract
	Secretin	Gastrointestinal tract
Regulation of energy, metabolism, and growth	Glucagon	Alpha cells, pancreatic islets
	Insulin	Beta cells, pancreatic islets
	Growth hormone	Anterior pituitary
	Thyroid hormones	Thyroid gland
Neurotransmitters	Dopamine	Central nervous system
	Epinephrine	Adrenal medulla
	Norepinephrine	Adrenal medulla and nervous system
Reproductive function	Chorionic gonadotropins	Placenta
	Estrogens	Ovary
	Oxytocin	Posterior pituitary
	Progesterone	Ovary
	Prolactin	Anterior pituitary
	Testosterone	Testes
Stress and control of inflammation	Glucocorticoids	Adrenal cortex
Tropic hormones (regulation of other hormone levels)	Adrenocorticotropic hormone (ACTH)	Anterior pituitary
	Follicle-stimulating hormone (FSH)	Anterior pituitary
	Luteinizing hormone (LH)	Anterior pituitary
	Thyroid-stimulating hormone (TSH)	Anterior pituitary

Hypopituitarism that occurs before puberty is manifested chiefly by a retarded growth rate. If it begins very early in life, **dwarfism** will result. A person with dwarfism is extremely short but has normal body proportions. Because growth hormone (GH) can be produced using genetic engineering, it can be used to stimulate growth in children with this disorder.

Adult hypopituitarism may be classified according to whether the various anterior pituitary hormones are selectively or completely deficient. If all the hormones are deficient, for example, the condition is called panhypopituitarism. If a selective deficiency exists, the condition is named for the specific deficiency. For instance, a deficiency in the gonadotropic hormones will lead to **eunuchoidism** (loss of secondary sexual characteristics) in the male.

Hyperpituitarism

Hyperpituitarism is marked by excess production of human growth hormone (HGH). If this occurs during childhood or adolescence, the result is a form of hyperpituitarism called **gigantism** (excessive size and stature). Normally, HGH is active only up to the time of maturity, when the epiphyseal lines on the long bones seal. Oversecretion of HGH increases bone length, and sometimes its width, in excess of normal growth before closure of the epiphyses. In some instances, a suppression of gonadotropic hormones occurs. If this happens, the testes and adrenals in the male or the adrenals in the female do not develop as in normal puberty. Consequently, epiphyseal closure, which is dependent on the male hormone, fails to occur. The result is that the individual reaches a height of 7 or 8 feet.

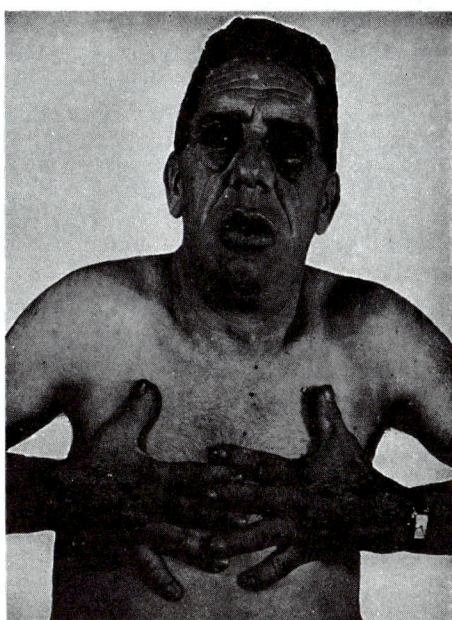

FIGURE 34-4
A patient with acromegaly.

Associated metabolic changes are attributed to a generalized pituitary hyperfunction. If the pituitary malfunctions in any of its responsibilities, it may malfunction in all areas, causing widespread pathology. If pituitary hyperfunction occurs near the end of puberty or in adulthood, after the epiphyseal closure, bone length does not change but bone width increases; this is called acromegaly (Fig. 34-4). This form of hyperpituitarism results in a prominent jaw, enlargement of the nose, and unusual thickening of the hands, feet, and skin. Unusual hyperactivity of the pituitary gland is associated with a tumor of the gland. Treatment of acromegaly requires surgical removal of the tumor or its destruction by radiation.

Checkpoint Question
6. How does hypopituitarism differ from hyperpituitarism?

Diabetes Insipidus

Diabetes insipidus results from hyposecretion (deficiency) of antidiuretic hormone (ADH) in the posterior pituitary. Deficient ADH causes the renal tubules to reabsorb water and salts resulting in as much as 5 to 10 liters of urine output a day **(polyuria)**. Clinical symptoms also include **polydipsia** (excessive thirst) as the body's effort to restore fluid balance. The cause is not usually known but may be due to head trauma or tumor formation. Treatment involves correction of the causative factor and the administration of synthetic ADH by injection or by nasal spray for vascular absorption.

Goiter

A dietary deficiency of iodine and certain other thyroid disorders are frequently accompanied by an enlargement of the gland, known as a **goiter**. Simple goiter is caused by insufficient dietary iodine. **Hyperplasia** (increased number of cells) is present, but there is neither inflammation nor malignancy. The condition does not lead to the thyrotoxic conditions associated with other thyroid pathologies. Simple goiter is **endemic**, occurring in areas in which the available supply of iodine in the drinking water and in the soil is low. In the United States, the areas of greatest concern are the Pacific Northwest, the Great Plains, the basin of the St. Lawrence River, and the Great Lakes regions.

In simple goiter there is no clinical syndrome because there is no hyposecretion or hypersecretion of the gland. The gland is essentially normal, capable of manufacturing a normal concentration of hormone if iodine is supplied in the diet. However, the gland may become so enlarged that it compresses the trachea and other structures located in the neck. Under these conditions, the goiter must be surgically removed. Generally, in the early stages of goiter development, supplemental iodine can reverse the glandular enlargement. The value of iodine used prophylactically against goiter is now generally accepted and recommended for all areas low in natural iodine. The most feasible method of administration has been the addition of sodium or potassium iodide to table salt.

Hypothyroidism

Hypothyroidism results from a deficiency of thyroid hormone secretion. It produces a number of symptoms depending on the degree of deficiency and the age at which it occurs.

In very early childhood, thyroid hormone deficiency leads to **cretinism**, a condition characterized by a low basal metabolic rate, slowed or retarded mental and physical development, slow heart rate, poor appetite, and constipation. The face is usually puffy with a characteristic apathetic expression (Fig. 34-5). The skin is dry, coarse, and pale yellow in color. Cretinism follows the incomplete development or congenital ab-

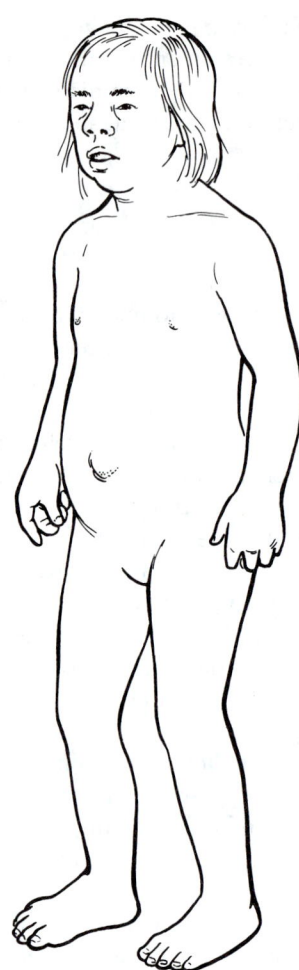

FIGURE 34-5
A patient with cretinism.

In adults, hypothyroidism usually results from atrophy of the thyroid gland. Its progression may lead to **myxedema,** a condition characterized by expressionless, puffy, and pallid face; slowed mental and physical processes; dry, thick skin; and loss of hair and teeth. Sometimes, obesity and an undue sensitivity to cold are other signs. If not corrected, severe myxedema may lead to coma and death. The administration of adequate amounts of thyroid hormone usually results in a dramatic relief of all symptoms within 10 days of the start of treatment. With adequate continuous therapy, symptoms do not return.

If hypothyroidism is mild, a state of hypothyroidism without myxedema may exist. This is characterized chiefly by a lowered metabolic rate of variable degree.

Hyperthyroidism

The most common form of hyperthyroidism (hypersecretion of thyroid hormone) may also be known as Graves' disease (Fig. 34-6). The most characteristic symptoms are **exophthalmic goiter** (abnormal protrusion of the eyeballs accompanied by goiter), nervousness, irritability, purposeless movements, fatigue, loss of weight, increased heart rate, elevated metabolic rate, emotional instability, and increased body temperature with excessive perspiration. A severe form of hyperthyroidism is known as **thyrotoxicosis.** Treatment consists of medications that decrease thyroxine (T_4) secretion or administration of radioactive iodine. When radioactive iodine becomes concentrated in the gland, it depresses glandular activity and decreases the output of pituitary thyrotrophic hormone.

sence of the thyroid gland. It can be treated successfully if thyroid supplements are administered early in infancy. Treatment may be lifelong in the many cases.

In later childhood, thyroid hormone deficiency results in childhood hypothyroidism or juvenile myxedema. This condition differs from cretinism in that it is not apparent as early in development. The severity of the symptoms depends primarily on the degree of thyroid activity and on the age at which the deficiency occurs. In general, the most characteristic symptoms are short, squatty stature; a head proportionately larger than normal for the child's age; a short, thick neck; puffiness and bloating around the face and eyes; a dull expression; dry, flaky skin; and a large tongue accompanied by drooling.

Treatment of childhood myxedema with thyroid supplements gives remarkable results. The outcome, however, depends on the degree of thyroid deficiency, the age at which treatment is begun, and the regularity with which it is continued.

Checkpoint Question

7. *What are the characteristic symptoms of cretinism and Graves' disease?*

Hypoparathyroidism

This deficiency disorder is caused most commonly by accidental removal or injury of the parathyroid glands as a result of surgery on the thyroid. Degenerative disease of the glands may also occur. The symptoms associated with this condition are muscle weakness, irritability, and **tetany**—the most common characteristic. Tetany is an abnormally increased sensitivity of the nervous system to external stimuli, resulting in painful muscle spasms. It requires prompt injection of calcium salts, either intramuscularly or intravenously. Gener-

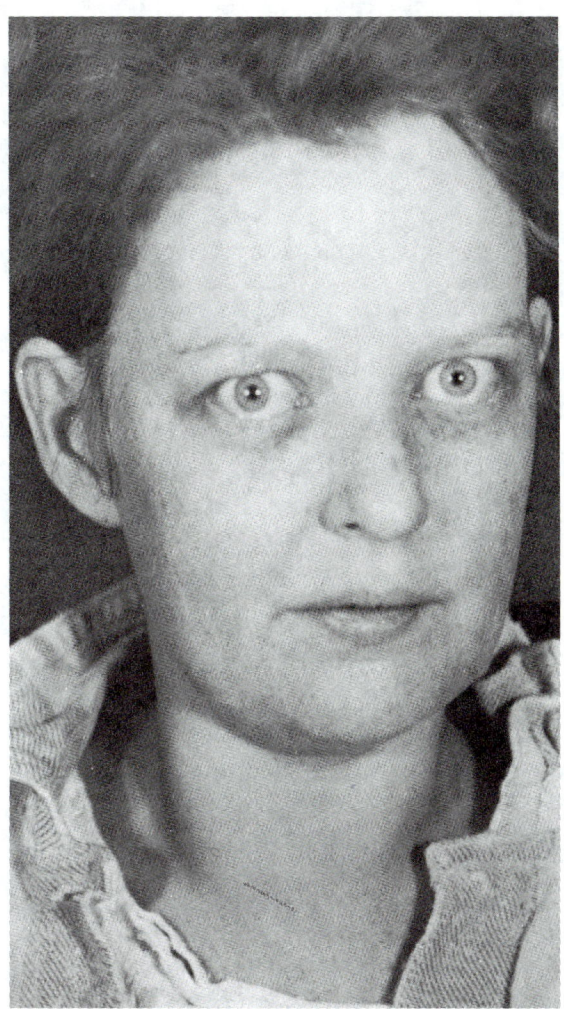

FIGURE 34-6
Woman with Graves' disease. Note the exophthalmos and enlarged thyroid gland.

ally, hypoparathyroidism is treated by administration of calcium lactate.

Hyperparathyroidism

Excess parathyroid hormone (PTH) secretion is called hyperparathyroidism. It is usually due to a tumor of the gland. Hyperparathyroidism causes **hypercalcemia**, an excessive secretion of calcium. As a result, polyuria usually occurs and may be the first and sometimes the only symptom of increased parathyroid activity. Kidney stones may form, and the decalcification of bones that usually occurs causes pain, deformities, and spontaneous fractures. The long bones and ribs may soften and bend. Occasionally, alterations in muscular function occur, including weakness and decreased response to stimulation.

Treatment of hyperparathyroidism usually involves surgical removal of the parathyroid tumor. After the surgery, the parathyroid deficiency that usually occurs requires calcium and vitamin D supplements.

Thymic Abnormalities

Pathology of the thymus gland is usually congenital. There is usually accompanying hypocalcemia with facial dysplasia, cardiac abnormalities, and early death. The only cure at this time is fetal thymic transplant.

Hypoadrenocorticalism

Degeneration of the adrenal cortex resulting in hypoadrenocorticalism (adrenal deficiency) is called **Addison's disease.** The symptoms of Addison's disease are skin hyperpigmentation, appetite loss, weight loss, weakness, hypotension, and anemia. Sodium loss due to decreased renal reabsorption occurs. Chloride and bicarbonate are lost, and potassium is retained. Changes in the ion concentration of the circulation cause water loss from the blood and the tissue spaces, resulting in severe dehydration and hemoconcentration. Addison's disease is treated with high doses of hydrocortisone.

What If?

A patient with Addison's disease is prescribed a course of hydrocortisone. What if you must assess the patient's understanding of the potential long-term effects of this medication?

Long-term cortisone therapy has many adverse effects, including increased risk for the development of cataracts and osteoporosis. The patient also is at high risk for developing secondary infection and must take care to minimize exposure to infectious diseases. Ensure that the patient has a clear understanding of dietary needs because long-term therapy may result in hypocalcemia, hypokalemia, and hypernatremia. Also assess the patient's understanding of signs and symptoms of gastric ulcers; steroid therapy is contraindicated for patients with existing gastric ulcers. Additionally, the patient should be cautioned against abruptly stopping this medication, but instead should follow the physician's orders to taper the dosage until the treatment has run its course.

Hyperadrenocorticalism

Hyperadrenocorticalism may be caused by hyperplasia of the adrenal cortex resulting from increased production of corticotropin (ACTH) from the pituitary, or by tumors of the cortex. Hyperadrenocorticalism is known as Cushing's syndrome. Excessive cortisol promotes fat deposits in the trunk of the body, with the extremities remaining thin. The skin is fragile and thin, and healing after injuries is slow. Osteoporosis is accelerated. The face is characteristically rounded. Cushing's syndrome may also be present in patients who are receiving corticosteroids for medical reasons. These patients may include transplant recipients and patients with severe asthma or rheumatoid arthritis. Treatment for hyperadrenocorticalism requires removal of the cause of the hypersecretion, which could be either a pituitary or an adrenal tumor.

Diabetes Mellitus

In the pancreas, dysfunction of the islets of Langerhans results in diabetes mellitus, a disorder of carbohydrate metabolism. It is characterized by hyperglycemia and **glycosuria** (glucose in the urine) resulting from inadequate insulin production or utilization.

The exact cause of diabetes mellitus is unknown, but it arises from failure of the beta cells in the islets of Langerhans to secrete adequate insulin. Some cases of diabetes mellitus can be attributed to a genetic predisposition, but it may also result from a deficiency of beta cells caused by inflammation, pancreatic cancer, or surgery. It is also thought to be an autoimmune disorder perhaps triggered by a virus.

There are two types of diabetes mellitus—type I: insulin-dependent diabetes mellitus (IDDM); and type II: non–insulin-dependent diabetes mellitus (NIDDM).

Type I occurs most often in children and young adults. Onset of type I is abrupt, with symptoms such as polyuria, polydipsia, **polyphagia** (abnormal hunger), weight loss, and **ketoacidosis**—acidosis accompanied by an accumulation of **ketones** (end products of fat metabolism) in the body. Insulin must be administered parenterally to control type I diabetes.

Type II occurs most often in adults over age 40. Onset of type II is gradual, with symptoms such as polyuria, polydipsia, **pruritus** (severe itching), and peripheral neuropathy. In this condition, insulin is produced but cannot exert its effect on cells because of a deficiency of insulin receptors on cell membranes. Risk factors are obesity and a family history of diabetes.

Control of type II diabetes may not require insulin. The patient is usually placed on a well-balanced diet, adequate in all basic essentials: carbohydrates, pro-

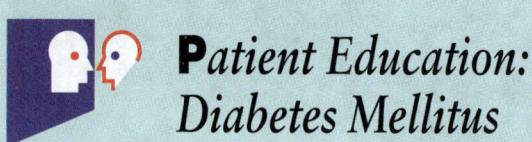

Patient Education: Diabetes Mellitus

All patients with diabetes mellitus should understand:

- the need for good hygiene (opportunistic diseases are attracted to the high levels of sugar in the body)
- dietary management (calorie intake must be regulated)
- proper foot care (peripheral circulation is poor and injuries or lesions heal slowly)
- proper dosage administration of insulin or an oral agent (inaccuracies may result in shock or coma)
- proper disposal of insulin syringes (state laws regulate hazardous waste disposal)
- how to correctly test the blood by a capillary puncture finger stick or the urine for glucose or ketones (insulin is sometimes calibrated by the results of patient self-testing)
- signs and symptoms of insulin shock and diabetic ketoacidosis, and the procedure to follow if symptoms occur

Without insulin, the patient's blood glucose levels will remain high and glucose will be lost in the urine. More water will be lost as well, resulting in polyuria and polydipsia. Ensure that patients recognize that although diabetes can be controlled, the long-term effects of hyperglycemia produce vascular changes. The capillary walls thicken and the exchange of gases and nutrients diminishes. The effects of these circulatory changes can be seen in the retina, the kidneys, and the skin, particularly the feet. Uncontrolled diabetes can lead to blindness, dry gangrene, and severe kidney damage. Atherosclerosis is also common in non–insulin-dependent diabetes mellitus.

There are various support groups for diabetics. The American Diabetes Association has a broad selection of printed materials to help diabetic patients adjust to life-style changes. Type I diabetic individuals may need a support group to learn to incorporate medical compliance into their lives with as little disruption as possible.

teins, fats, vitamins, minerals, and fluids. Obese patients must be placed on a diet that will enable them to lose weight. Controlling diabetes is difficult in an obese person. When the patient is given an adequate diet and glucose still appears in the urine, insulin may be required. Oral drugs that enable insulin to react with the remaining cell membrane receptors have been used successfully in middle-aged and older patients.

As the medical assistant, you must help patients understand their disease by instructing them about possible complications and treatments available.

Checkpoint Question

8. How would you describe the difference between diabetes mellitus and diabetes insipidus?

Diabetic Ketoacidosis

Ketoacidosis is a serious problem for patients with IDDM. When glucose cannot be used for energy, the body turns to fats and proteins, which the liver converts to ketones. Ketones accumulate in the blood because the cells cannot use them rapidly; as these organic acids build up, they lower the pH of the blood. The kidneys will excrete excess ketones, but in doing so will excrete more water. This excess excretion of water will lead to dehydration, worsening the acidosis.

The administration of insulin is necessary to permit the use of glucose for energy. Intravenous fluids are used to restore blood volume to normal. If left untreated, ketoacidosis will progress to coma and death.

Checkpoint Question

9. In diabetic ketoacidosis, what happens when the kidneys excrete excess ketones?

Diabetic Coma and Insulin Shock

Diabetic coma results from lack of insulin. This condition causes metabolic changes with excess production of ketone bodies. Insulin shock occurs from an overdose or overproduction of insulin. This results in blood sugar levels well below normal. Skipping a meal without adjusting insulin levels will also result in insulin shock. Table 34-3 provides a comparison of these two disorders.

Gonadal Abnormalities

Pathologies of the gonads occur in malignancies, in pituitary malfunctions, and in genetic anomalies. Sexual dysfunction is the usual result in cases of nonmalignant gonadal pathology. Specific disorders of the gonads are discussed in Chapter 40, Caring for Patients With Disorders of the Male Reproductive System, and Chapter

Table 34-3
Comparison of Diabetic Coma and Insulin Shock

	Diabetic Coma	Insulin Shock
Onset	Gradual	Sudden
Skin	Flushed, dry	Pale, moist
Tongue	Dry or furred	Moist
Breath	Smell of acetone	Not present
Thirst	Intense	Absent
Respiration	Deep	Shallow
Vomiting	Common	Rare
Pulse	Rapid, feeble	Rapid, bounding
Urine	Glucose and acetone present	No glucose or acetone
Blood glucose	Elevated (>200 mg/dL)	Subnormal (20–50 mg/dL)
Blood pressure	Low	Normal
Abdominal pain	Common, often acute	Absent

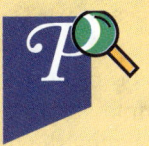

Focus on the Patient: Monitoring Elderly Diabetic Patients

Frail, elderly diabetic patients who live alone require special attention. These patients are at high risk for insulin shock or coma. They may tend to measure their insulin incorrectly due to poor vision, may forget to take their insulin, or may forget to eat after taking their insulin.

Assess each patient's ability with each office visit because conditions may deteriorate between scheduled visits. For example, ask the patient what time of day insulin is taken, how much is taken, how it is administered, when food is eaten, and how often blood sugar levels are checked. To determine the patient's ability to self-administer insulin, ask the patient to demonstrate how medications are drawn up. Look at the amount of medication in the syringe; it is not uncommon to see errors.

Home health nurses may be able to help monitor compliance. Often, home health services will prefill and label syringes for patients for each day until the next visit. Some forms of insulin can be administered in special syringes that allow only a preset amount of insulin to be injected. Diabetic patients are perfect candidates for Lifeline boxes to be installed in the home. Check with your local hospital or pharmacy for your community resources.

41, Caring for Patients With Obstetric and Gynecologic Disorders.

COMMON LABORATORY TESTS AND DIAGNOSTIC PROCEDURES AND THE MEDICAL ASSISTANT'S ROLE

Through various laboratory tests and diagnostic procedures, the physician can identify endocrine disorders so that treatment may be initiated.

Tests of blood and urine can be used to measure hormone levels (Table 34-4). For example, a glucose tolerance test (GTT) measures the glucose levels in a blood sample from a fasting patient and in specimens taken at intervals of 30 minutes, 1 hour, 2 hours, and 3 hours after the ingestion of a measured dose of glucose. Delayed return of blood glucose to normal levels indicates diabetes mellitus.

Urinary hormone excretion can be measured using a 24-hour urine sample. (Because of fluctuations in hormonal activity, STAT specimens or one-time specimens may not contain the substances necessary for a diagnosis of the presenting condition.)

As the medical assistant, you may be responsible for obtaining the blood and urine samples necessary for these two tests and for actually performing the procedures. Chapter 44, Urinalysis, includes the procedure for obtaining a 24-hour urine specimen and performing various urine tests. Chapter 45, Phlebotomy, explains the procedure for obtaining a blood specimen. Chapter 48, Clinical Chemistry, discusses the steps for performing a GTT.

Table 34-4
Serum Tests for Diagnosing Endocrine Disorders

Serum tests for	Help Diagnose Disorders of the
Follicle-stimulating hormone (FSH), growth hormone (GH), thyroid-stimulating hormone (TSH), luteinizing hormone (LH), and prolactin	Anterior pituitary
T_3, T_4	Thyroid
Calcium, parathyroid hormone (PTH)	Parathyroids
Corticoids	Adrenal cortex
Glucose, insulin	Pancreas
Estradiol	Ovaries

Table 34-5
Thyroid Hormone Levels in Abnormal Conditions

	T_3	T_4	TSH
Hyperthyroidism			
Hyperthyroidism or thyrotoxicosis	↑	↓	Normal/↑/↓
Graves' disease	↑	↑	Normal/↑/↓
Hypothyroidism			
Cretinism	↓	↓	Normal/↓
Endemic goiter	Normal/↑	Normal/↓	Normal/↑
Myxedema	↓	↓	↑

↓, *decreased hormone levels;* ↑, *increased hormone levels;* T_3, *triiodethyronine;* T_4, *thyroxine.*

Thyroid function tests (TFT) measure the levels of thyroxine (T_4), triiodothyronine (T_3), and thyroid-stimulating hormone (TSH) in the blood. Table 34-5 shows thyroid hormone levels for several abnormal conditions. During a thyroid scan, a radioactive compound is administered and localizes in the thyroid gland. The gland is then visualized with a scanner device to detect tumors or nodules. Radioactive iodine uptake is a procedure in which iodine is administered orally and its absorption into the thyroid gland is measured as evidence of thyroid function.

Radioimmunoassay (RAI) measures hormone levels in plasma by introducing radioactive substances into the body. The test is based on the ability of antibodies to bind specifically to radioactively labeled hormone molecules and to nonradioactive molecules.

Computed tomography (CT) scans provide transverse views of the pituitary and other endocrine glands and are used in the diagnosis of pathologic conditions. Ultrasonography is used to identify pancreatic, adrenal, and thyroid masses.

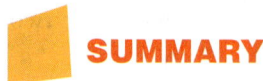

SUMMARY

Through the secretion of chemical messengers called hormones, the endocrine system helps regulate body processes. Endocrine glands include the pituitary, thyroid, parathyroids, thymus, adrenals, pancreas, and gonads. Alterations in hormone secretion by any of these glands—either hyposecretion (deficiency) or hypersecretion (excess)—result in various disorders that can affect systemic functioning.

CRITICAL THINKING CHALLENGES

1. While performing a complete physical examination, the physician will palpate the patient's neck. Identify the gland that is located here, then explain why the physician would palpate it.
2. Your patient has recently been diagnosed with asthma and will need to use an inhaler. Considering the sympathomimetic effects of epinephrine. What symptoms might you expect the patient to exhibit?

ANSWERS TO CHECKPOINT QUESTIONS

1. The anterior lobe of the pituitary is responsible for most of the body's hormonal control. The posterior lobe stores two hormones that are produced in the hypothalamus.
2. The thyroid gland produces calcitonin, a hormone that inhibits the release of calcium and phosphates from the bones to the blood, thereby decreasing the amount of calcium in the circulation.
3. In the kidneys, PTH promotes the renal excretion of phosphate by decreasing reabsorption, thereby causing the serum phosphorous levels to decrease. In bone tissue, PTH causes bone cells to break down through increased osteoclastic activity.
4. The adrenal medulla has only one function: to secrete epinephrine and norepinephrine in response to sympathetic nervous system stimulation. In contrast, the adrenal cortex affects nearly all body systems and is essential for life.
5. Hypoglycemia (low blood glucose level) stimulates the secretion of glucagon, which raises the blood glucose level and makes energy stores available for metabolic needs.

6. Hypopituitarism is an undersecretion of the anterior pituitary hormones; hyperpituitarism is marked by excess secretion of growth hormone.
7. Cretinism is characterized by low basal metabolic rate, slowed or retarded mental and physical development, slow heart rate, poor appetite, and constipation. In Graves' disease, the most characteristic symptoms are exophthalmic goiter, nervousness, irritability, purposeless movements, fatigue, weight loss, increased heart rate, elevated metabolic rate, emotional instability, and increased body temperature.
8. Diabetes mellitus involves dysfunction of the islets of Langerhans in the pancreas and is a metabolic disorder. Diabetes insipidus involves dysfunction of ADH in the posterior pituitary.
9. When the kidneys excrete excess ketones, more water also is excreted. This excess excretion of water will lead to dehydration, worsening the acidosis.

SUGGESTIONS FOR FURTHER READING

Burke, S. (1992). *Human Anatomy in Health and Disease* (3rd ed.). Albany, NY: Delmar.

Memmler, R., Cohen, B., & Wood, D. (1996). *The Human Body in Health and Disease* (8th ed.) Philadelphia: Lippincott-Raven Publishers.

(1992). *Professional Guide to Diseases* (4th ed). Springhouse, PA: Springhouse.

Memmler, R. L., Cohen, B. J., and Wood, D. L. (1992). *Structure and Function of the Human Body*, 5th ed. Philadelphia: J. B. Lippincott.

Porth, C. M. (1994). *Pathophysiology: Concepts of Altered Health States*, 4th ed. Philadelphia: J. B. Lippincott.

Rosdahl, C. B. (1995). *Textbook of Basic Nursing*, 6th ed. Philadelphia: J. B. Lippincott.

Caring for Patients With Cardiovascular Disorders

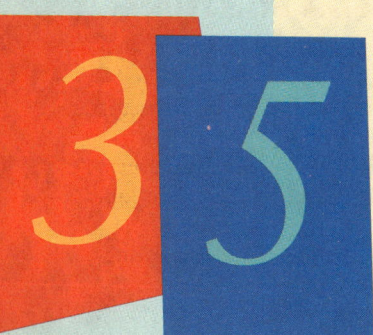

Chapter Outline

Structure and Function of the Cardiovascular System
- Heart
- Blood Vessels
- Blood
- Circulation
- Conduction System

Common Cardiovascular Disorders
- Atherosclerotic Coronary Heart Disease or Coronary Artery Disease
- Arterial Occlusive Disease
- Myocardial Infarction
- Hypertension
- Valvular Heart Disease
- Aortic Stenosis
- Congestive Heart Failure
- Cardiac Arrhythmia
- Varicose Veins
- Stasis Ulcers
- Venous Thrombosis and Pulmonary Embolism
- Cerebrovascular Accident
- Carditis
- Aneurysm
- Anemia

Common Diagnostic Procedures and the Medical Assistant's Role
- Cardiovascular Examination
- Electrocardiogram
- Procedure: Performing a 12-Lead Electrocardiogram
- Procedure: Mounting the Electrocardiogram Strip for Reading
- Holter Monitor

Procedure: Applying a Holter Monitor
- Chest X-ray or Chest Roentgenogram
- Cardiac Stress Testing
- Echocardiography
- Cardiac Catheterization
- Coronary Arteriography

Summary

Critical Thinking Challenges

Answers to Checkpoint Questions

Suggestions for Further Reading

DACUM Components

1.3 Practice within the scope of education, training, and personal capabilities
1.6 Conduct oneself in a courteous and diplomatic manner
2.2 Treat all patients with empathy and impartiality
4.5 Prepare and maintain examination and treatment area
4.7 Prepare patients for procedures
4.8 Assist physician with examinations and treatments
4.11 Perform selected tests that assist with diagnosis and treatment
5.1 Document accurately
7.3 Teach patients methods of health promotion and disease prevention

Chapter Competencies

Learning Objectives

Upon successfully completing this chapter, you will be able to:

1. Spell and define the Key Terms.
2. Understand the basic structure and function of the cardiovascular system.
3. Trace a drop of blood through the circulatory system.
4. Describe the blood components and state their functions.
5. Trace the conduction of an electrical impulse through the heart.
6. List and describe common cardiovascular disorders.
7. Identify and explain common cardiovascular procedures and tests.
8. Describe the role and responsibilities of a medical assistant during a cardiovascular examination.
9. Explain the information recorded on a basic 12-lead electrocardiogram.
10. Explain the purpose for a Holter monitor.

Performance Objectives

Upon successfully completing this chapter, you will be able to:

1. Perform a basic 12-lead electrocardiogram (Procedure 35-1).
2. Mount an electrocardiogram strip for reading (Procedure 35-2).
3. Apply a Holter monitor for a 24-hour test (Procedure 35-3).

Key Terms

(See Glossary for definitions.)

aneurysm	epicardium
angina pectoris	leads
artifacts	mediastinum
atria	myocardium
atrioventricular (AV) node	pericardium
bundle of His	Purkinje fibers
depolarization	repolarization
dextrocardia	sinoatrial (SA) node
endocardium	ventricles

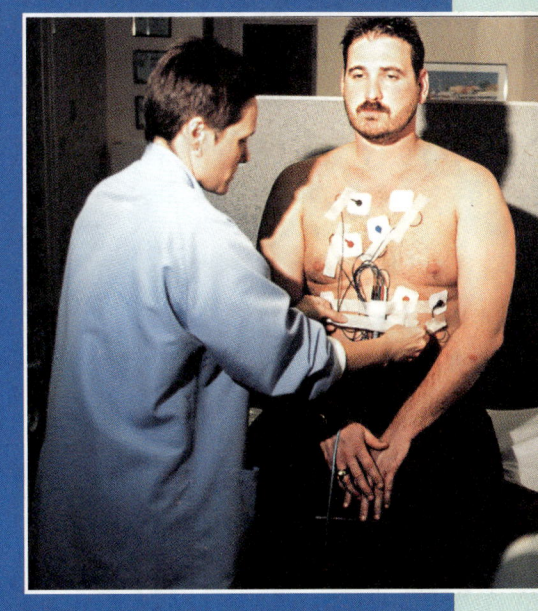

Cardiovascular disease is a major cause of illness and death in today's society. Because medical assistants often work with patients who have cardiovascular disorders that require frequent monitoring through the physician's office, you must understand the cardiovascular system, associated disorders, and the common tests and procedures that are ordered for diagnosis and treatment. This chapter will help you to understand cardiovascular function and dysfunction. It will also help you to work independently and confidently in performing a 12-lead electrocardiogram and applying a Holter monitor.

➤ STRUCTURE AND FUNCTION OF THE CARDIOVASCULAR SYSTEM

Heart

The heart is a hollow, muscular organ that by rhythmic contractions pumps oxygen-rich blood throughout the body to oxygenate and nourish the tissues and return wastes to the points of elimination. It is located between the lungs in the part of the thoracic cavity known as the **mediastinum**. It is triangular, with the tip, or apex, extending toward the left in the chest cavity and resting on the diaphragm. The bulk of the heart is located behind the sternum and extends from the second rib to the fifth intercostal space distally. The heart itself weighs less than 1 lb (about 250–350 g) and is approximately the size of a closed fist (Fig. 35-1).

The heart is enclosed within a double sac of serous membrane called the **pericardium**. The pericardium has two layers: a fibrous layer and a serous layer. The fibrous layer, which is composed of tough, white connective tissue, protects the heart and anchors it to surrounding structures such as the diaphragm, sternum, and great vessels issuing from the heart base. The serous layer, which lines the fibrous layer, is composed of serous membrane and connective tissue. Between the serous and the fibrous layers is serous fluid that cushions and protects the heart.

The serous layer turns downward at the heart base and continues over the heart surface as the vis-

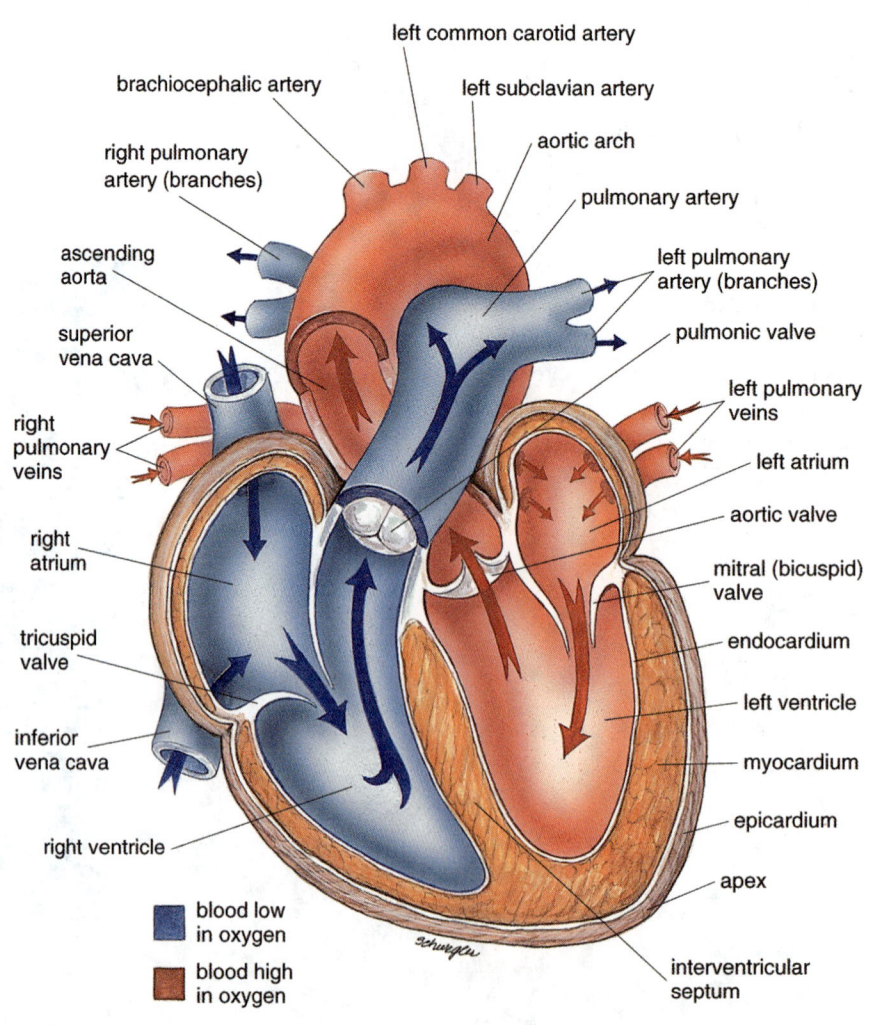

FIGURE 35-1
Heart and great vessels.

ceral pericardium, also called the **epicardium**. The epicardium is an essential part of the heart wall; it adheres closely and forms the outermost layer of the heart wall.

The **myocardium** (middle layer) is composed of cardiac muscle and forms the bulk of the heart. It is this layer that actually contracts. Within the myocardium, the branching cardiac muscles are bonded to each other by connective tissue fibers and arranged in spiral or circular bundles. The bundles link all parts of the heart together. The connective fibers form a dense network, called the fibrous skeleton or the skeleton of the heart. This network reinforces the heart internally. The **endocardium** or innermost part of the heart wall lines the heart chamber and covers the connective tissue skeleton of the heart valves.

The inner portion of the heart is made up of four chambers. Two upper chambers, the right and left **atria**, receive the blood pumped into the heart. The two lower chambers, the right and left **ventricles**, are the pumping chambers (see Fig. 35-1).

Blood Vessels

Arteries, capillaries, and veins are the three major types of blood vessels that form the transportation path of the blood in the cardiovascular system (Fig. 35-2).

Arteries (Fig. 35-3) transport blood away from the heart by the pumping action of the ventricles. Arterial blood leaves the heart for the periphery by way of the aorta and is under relatively high pressure. Arteries have thick walls to withstand this pressure. Blood is transported by the initial pumping action of the heart and then by an inner muscular wall in the arteries that helps maintain the blood flow. Blood flows through the arteries, which become progressively smaller and divide into small arteries called arterioles. These arterioles feed into the capillary beds of the body organs and tissues (Fig. 35-4).

Capillaries provide contact with tissue cells and interstitial fluid to directly serve cellular needs. The exchange of oxygen, nutrients, and waste products occurs in the capillary beds.

From the tiny capillaries, blood then flows into small *veins* called venules, which merge into larger veins for the return of the blood to the heart. The blood return is aided by skeletal muscle contractions and by valves within the veins that prevent the backflow of blood and keep it moving in the direction of the heart. The large veins combine into the largest vein at the heart entrance called the vena cava, which returns the blood to the heart. Although the walls of the veins increase in thickness as the vessels increase in size, they are never as thick as the walls of arteries Fig. 35-5).

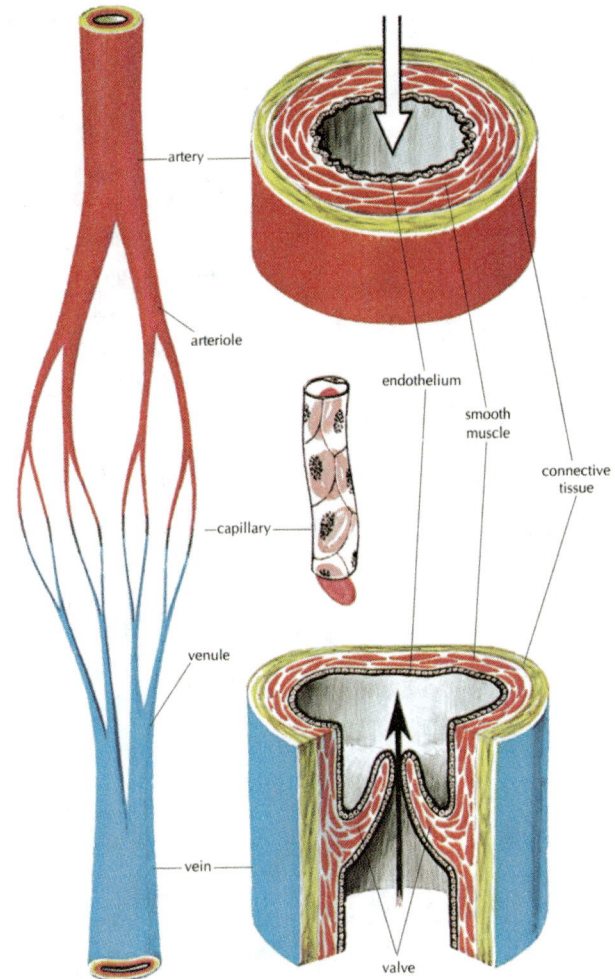

FIGURE 35-2
Sections of blood vessels showing the thick arterial walls and the thin walls of veins and capillaries are illustrated. Venous valves also are shown. The arrows indicate the direction of blood flow.

   **Checkpoint Question**
1. *Where does the exchange of nutrients and oxygen occur?*

Blood

Blood consists of erythrocytes (red blood cells), leukocytes (white blood cells), and thrombocytes (platelets) suspended in plasma. A 150-lb. adult has about 5 to 6 quarts of blood.

Cells are formed in the red marrow of long bones and in the centers of smaller bones. All of the formed elements of blood develop from stem cells called *hemocytoblasts*. As the body signals the need for a certain type of cell, the available stem cells differentiate into

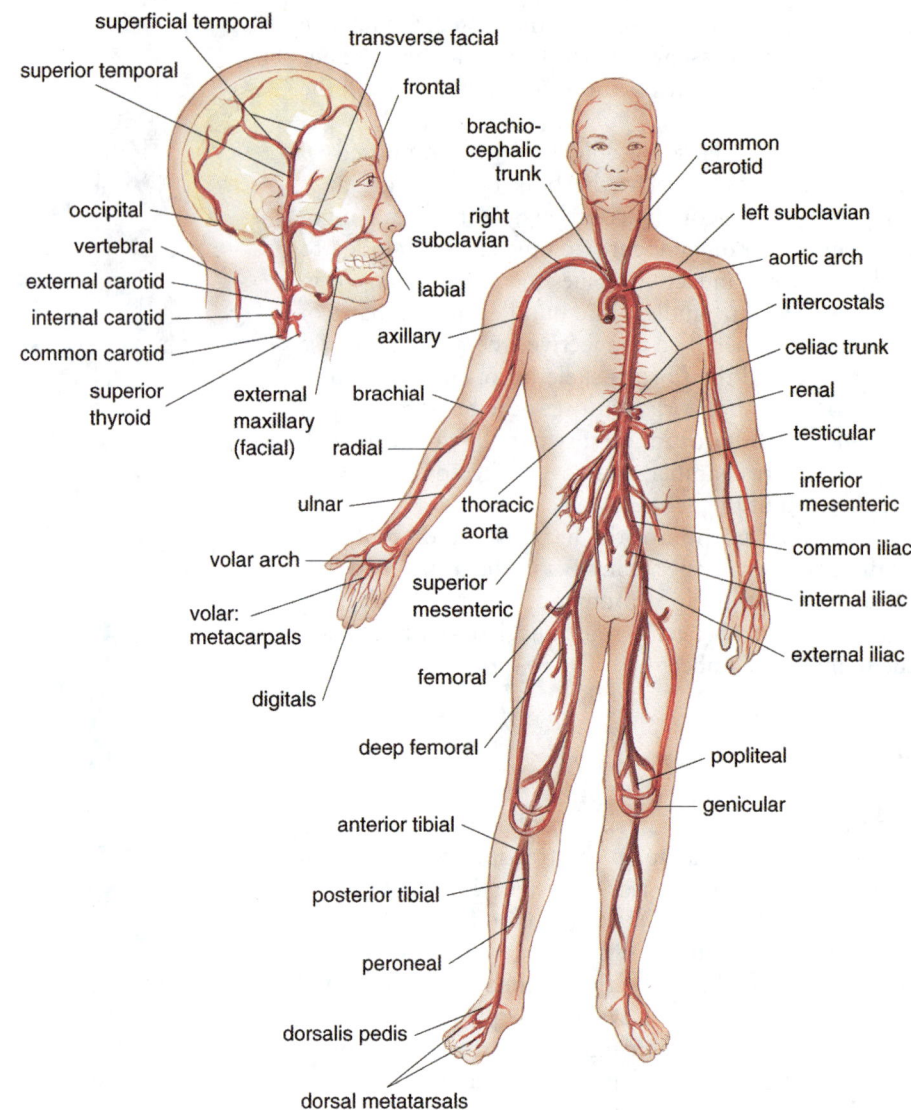

FIGURE 35-3
Principal arteries.

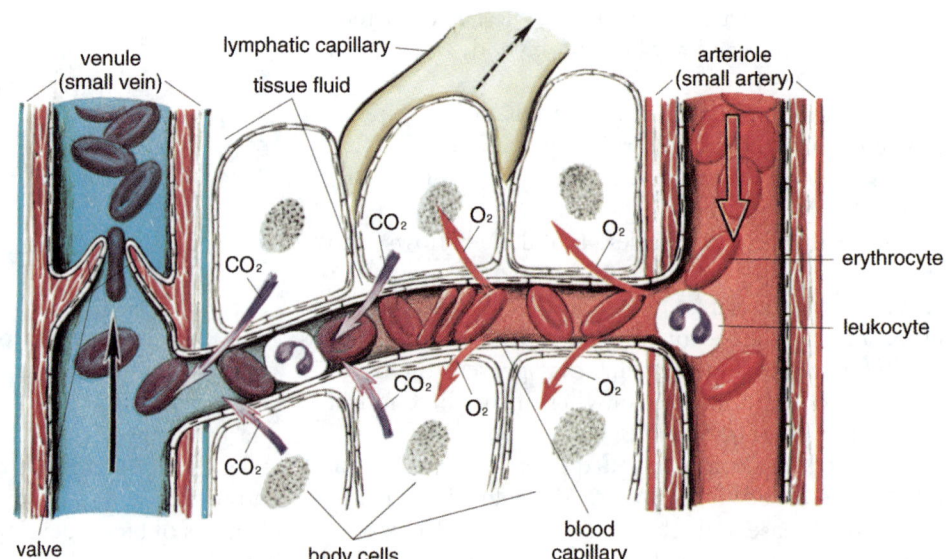

FIGURE 35-4
Diagram showing the connection between the small blood vessels through capillaries. Note the lymph capillary, a part of tissue drainage.

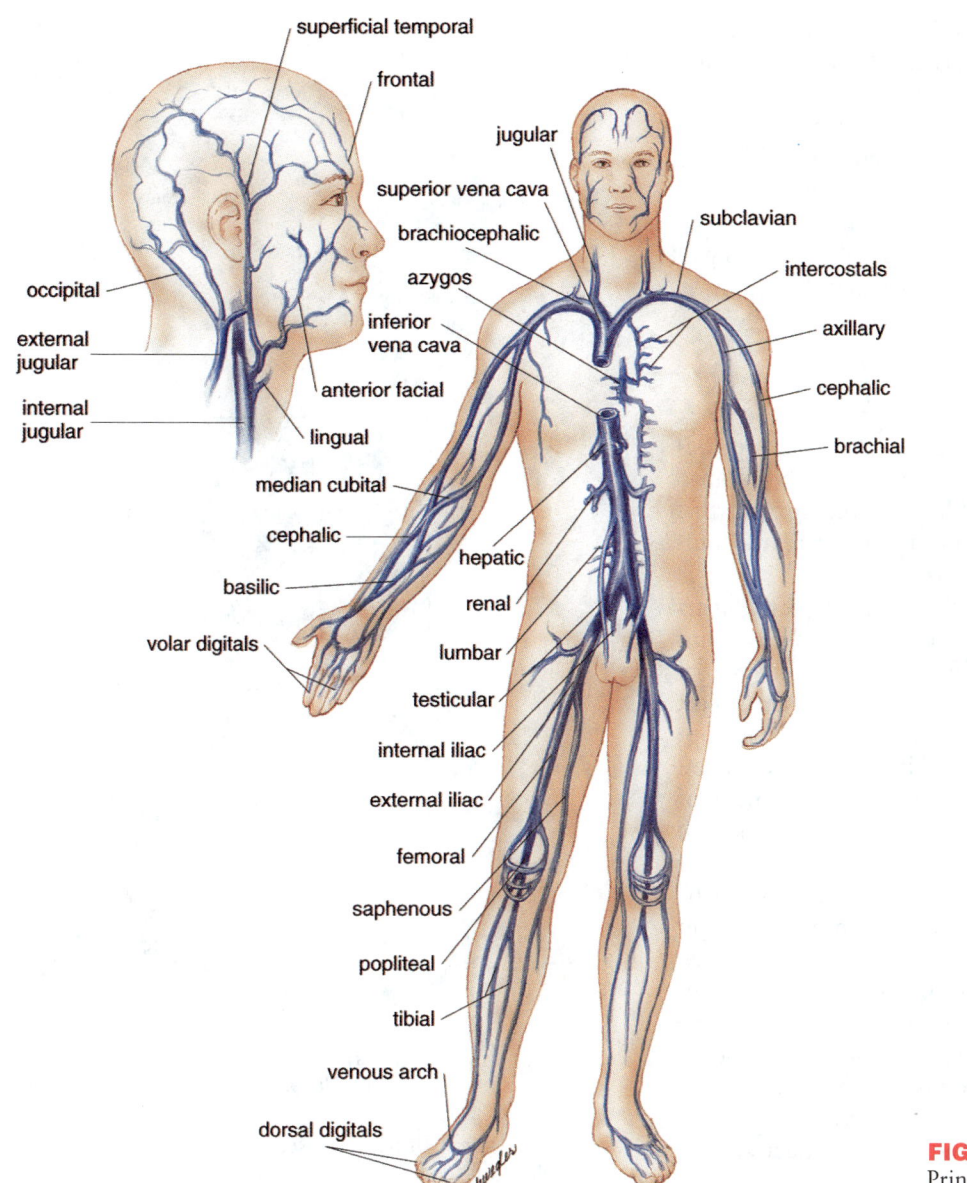

superficial temporal
frontal
jugular
superior vena cava
brachiocephalic
azygos
inferior vena cava
anterior facial
lingual
occipital
external jugular
internal jugular
median cubital
cephalic
basilic
volar digitals
subclavian
intercostals
axillary
cephalic
brachial
hepatic
renal
lumbar
testicular
internal iliac
external iliac
femoral
saphenous
popliteal
tibial
venous arch
dorsal digitals

FIGURE 35-5
Principal veins.

the needed cell. If infection is present, more stem cells become leukocytes; if the number of red blood cells is low, more cells differentiate into erythrocytes. (See Chap. 46, Hematology, for further discussion and illustrations of blood components.)

Plasma accounts for about 55% of the blood, and about 90% of plasma is water. The other components vary because of the plasma functions but remain a fairly constant mix of protein, salts, oxygen, nutrients, wastes, and hormones.

Erythrocytes, or red blood cells, are the most numerous and are specialized for packaging hemoglobin, an iron-containing protein, for transporting oxygen to the cells. As the red cell matures, the nucleus disintegrates to allow more room for oxygen transport. Without a nucleus, the red blood cell is unable to reproduce

itself and dies within a short time, usually about 120 days. Dead red blood cells are filtered by the liver and the spleen. The iron content is recycled to the marrow where it is used for new cells. The waste products of dead red blood cells become bile and give feces their characteristic color.

Leukocytes, or white blood cells, are much larger than erythrocytes and are designed to fight infection. They come in various sizes and shapes, use the bloodstream for transport to tissues, and may live for years in the tissues as they wait to be needed.

There are two types of leukocytes: granulocytes and agranulocytes. Granulocytes contain granules within the cytoplasm, agranulocytes do not. Granulocytes are named for the dyes that will stain the granules within the cytoplasm. This concept is discussed in

Chap. 43, Microbiology. Table 35-1 lists types of white blood cells and their functions. (See Chap. 46, Hematology, for more information).

Thrombocytes (platelets) are fragments of megakaryocytes, the portion of the stem cell that is used for platelet formation rather than a red or white blood cell. Platelets are important in clot formation. The numbers and significance of all types of blood cells will be discussed in detail in Chap. 46, Hematology.

Circulation

The heart is actually two pumps and, although physically joined, each pump controls the flow of blood into one of the two loops of the blood's circulatory paths. The two routes that blood must travel are the pulmonary and the systemic circuits (Fig. 35-6).

In the pulmonary circuit, the right side of the heart receives deoxygenated blood from the vena cava into the right atrium and sends it by way of the right ventricle and pulmonary arteries to the lungs. In the lungs, blood is reoxygenated and returned to the left side of the heart. The oxygen-rich blood is pumped by the left ventricle into the systemic circuit. The equivalent of about 4000 to 5000 gallons of blood is pumped through this circuit each day.

Each pump consists of a receiving chamber (the right and left atria) and an ejection chamber (the right and left ventricles). The ventricles must develop enough pressure to drive the blood through the entire circuit and back to the proper receiving chamber. Because there is more resistance in the systemic circuit to move blood through, a greater force is required. Therefore, the left ventricle and the larger systemic arteries have thicker walls than the right ventricle and the pulmonary artery.

Blood flows through the heart in one direction—from the atria (receiving chambers) to the ventricles (ejection chambers) and out of the great arteries leav-

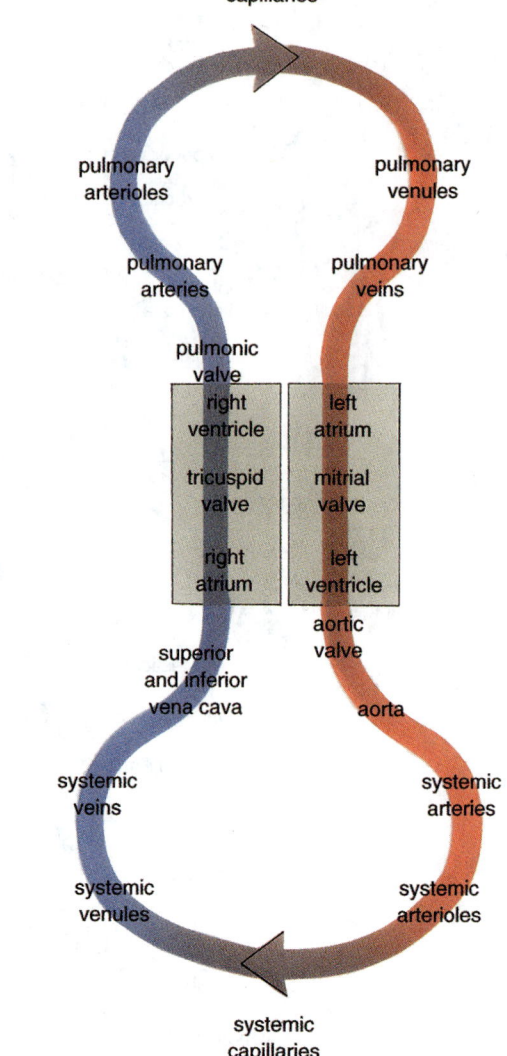

FIGURE 35-6
Blood vessels constitute a closed system for the flow of blood. Note that changes in oxygen content occur as blood flows through the capillaries.

ing the base of the heart. The forward path of circulation is enforced by four heart valves that prevent the backflow of blood. There are two atrioventricular (AV) and two semilunar valves (Fig. 35-7).

The two AV valves are located at the junction of the atrial and ventricular chambers of the heart and prevent the backflow of blood into the atria when the ventricles are contracting. The right AV valve, or tricuspid valve, has three flexible valve flaps or cusps. The left AV valve has two valve flaps or cusps and is called the bicuspid valve or mitral valve.

When the heart is relaxed, the AV valve flaps hang limply into the ventricular chambers below; blood flows into the atria and then through the open AV valves into the ventricles. When the ventricles begin to

Table 35-1
Types of White Blood Cells

Granulocytes	• Neutrophils: increased in bacterial infections
	• Eosinophils: increased in parasitic infections and allergies
	• Basophils: thought to play a role in clot production
Agranulocytes	• Monocytes: enter the tissue to become macrophages
	• Lymphocytes: increased in the immune response

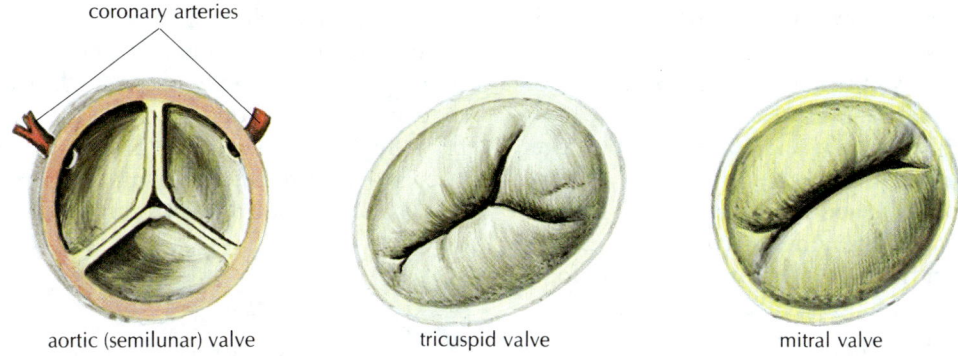

coronary arteries

aortic (semilunar) valve   tricuspid valve   mitral valve

FIGURE 35-7
Valves of the heart, seen from above, in the closed position.

contract, compressing the blood in their chambers, the blood is forced superiorly against the valve flaps, causing their edges to meet and close the valve. The chordae tendineae and the papillary muscles anchor the valve flaps and help them to remain in their closed position.

The two semilunar valves guard the bases of the large arteries leading from the heart and prevent backflow of blood into the ventricles. The aortic semilunar valve is at the junction of the aorta and the left ventricle and prevents the blood in the aorta from flowing back into the left ventricle. The pulmonary semilunar valve protects the opening between the right ventricle and the pulmonary artery.

Each semilunar valve is similar in structure. Their mechanism of action differs from that of the AV valves. When the ventricles are at their peak of contraction, the semilunar valves are forced open and the cusps flatten against the arterial walls as the blood flows past them. When the ventricles relax, the blood (no longer propelled forward by the pressure of the ventricular contraction) begins to flow backward toward the heart, fills the cusps, and closes the valve.

The blood supply to the heart is provided by the coronary arteries. They arise from the aorta, just above the aortic semilunar valve, and encircle the heart, passing to the right and to the left in an indentation known as the atrioventricular groove, marking the junction between the atria and the ventricles. Blood from the coronary circulation is returned to the heart by the right and left coronary veins, which empty into the coronary sinus, then into the right atrium (Fig. 35-8).

Checkpoint Question
2. How many chambers are in the heart? What are the upper chambers called? The lower chambers?

Conduction System

The pumping action of the heart is regulated by the electrical activity of the cardiac muscle cells in the myocardium. These impulses follow a specific path-

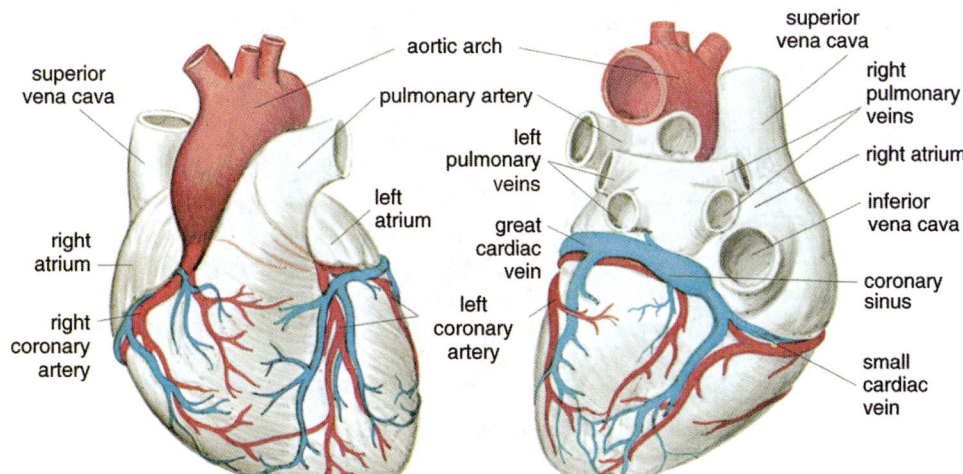

aortic arch

superior
vena cava

pulmonary artery

superior
vena cava

right
pulmonary
veins

left
pulmonary
veins

right atrium

left
atrium

inferior
vena cava

right
atrium

great
cardiac
vein

left
coronary
artery

coronary
sinus

right
coronary
artery

small
cardiac
vein

FIGURE 35-8
Coronary arteries and cardiac veins. (*Left*) Anterior view. (*Right*) Posterior view.

way known as the conduction system of the heart (Fig. 35-9).

The components of the conduction system are the sinoatrial (SA) node, the atrioventricular (AV) node, the bundle of His, the right and left bundle branches, and the Purkinje fibers.

The **sinoatrial (SA) node** is referred to as the pacemaker of the heart. This node, a group of specialized cells, is located in the right atrial wall, just inferior to the entrance of the inferior vena cava. The cells depolarize (send an impulse) spontaneously at a rate of 70 to 80 times per minute. The SA node initiates each **depolarization** wave that travels across the heart causing the heart to contract (or beat). It sets the pace for the heart as a whole. Its characteristic rhythm is called the normal sinus rhythm.

From the SA node, the depolarization wave spreads across both atria causing them to contract, and reaches the **atrioventricular (AV) node**, located in the inferior portion of the interatrial septum. This action takes approximately 0.04 second. The impulse is delayed a moment at the AV node, approximately 0.1 second, which allows the atria to complete their contraction. It then passes rapidly into and through the AV **bundle of His** (specialized cardiac muscle fibers) and the bundle branches in the interventricular septum and continues to the **Purkinje fibers**, which penetrate the ventricular myocardium causing the ventricles to contract. The pumping action of the heart depends on the proper sequence of events in this transmission (Box 35-1).

The normal rhythm may be altered by extrinsic factors that initiate sympathetic nervous system activation (eg, when the body needs the heart to beat faster to deliver more blood to meet the demands of the fright-flight-fight syndrome). During times of normal circulatory need, the parasympathetic nervous system allows the SA node to control the pace of the heart.

> **Checkpoint Question**
> *3. What are the five components of the conduction system? Which component is the pacemaker?*

COMMON CARDIOVASCULAR DISORDERS

The life-styles and diets of the American public contribute to the increase in premature death by cardiovascular causes, making heart disease the leading cause of death in the United States.

Symptoms of cardiovascular disorders can include:

- Chest pain
- Dyspnea
- Fatigue
- Diaphoresis
- Nausea and vomiting with chest pain
- Irregular heartbeat

Other less obvious symptoms might include:

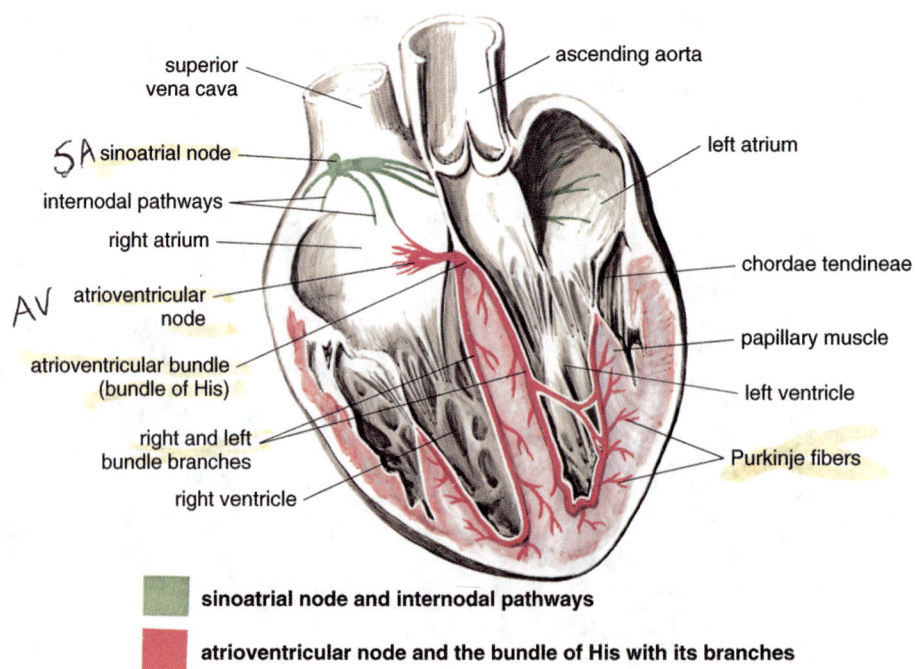

FIGURE 35-9
Conduction system of the heart.

sinoatrial node and internodal pathways

atrioventricular node and the bundle of His with its branches

BOX 35-1 Artificial Pacemakers

When a patient's conduction system can no longer maintain normal sinus rhythm without assistance, an electrical source can be implanted to assist or to replace the sinoatrial node function. Artificial pacemakers are surgically implanted either between the chest wall and the rib cage or within the chest cavity. They are battery operated and usually are manufactured to retain their charge for up to 20 years. They may be permanent or temporary and may work constantly to ensure electrical activity or may be calibrated to override the sinoatrial node only when the heart slows below a certain rate.

Pacemaker programming is frequently conducted by transtelephone monitoring, using a special remote surveillance device. At any properly outfitted site, such as a long-term care facility, remote health care center, or physician's office, the patient will insert moistened fingertips (usually bilateral index fingers) into the devices connected to a telephone modem. A tone is transmitted to a receiving system at a centrally located pacemaker clinic. The pacemaker rate and function are obtained and evaluated by a cardiologist at the receiving site.

If battery function is failing and replacement is not possible or advisable, batteries can be recharged transdermally. A charging unit is placed over the implantation site and plugged into an ordinary electrical outlet. The power cell is then recharged through the skin with no discomfort to the patient.

Focus on the Patient: Handling Cardiovascular Complaints

A patient reporting cardiovascular symptoms typically will have a high level of anxiety. You must be aware of and attentive to the patient's needs and concerns. It is vital that you listen carefully to complaints and provide accurate data related to the duration and type of symptoms experienced by the patient. This attention to detail is especially important during telephone calls, when decisions must be made regarding directions for evaluation or treatment of the presenting problem. The information you obtain assists the physician in determining if immediate attention is necessary.

- Changes in peripheral circulation, such as aching in the extremities
- Edema
- Skin ulcers that do not heal
- Pain that increases with ambulation and decreases during rest
- Changes in skin color and symptoms associated with inflammation

Below are descriptions of cardiovascular disorders that you may frequently see in the medical office.

Atherosclerotic Coronary Heart Disease or Coronary Artery Disease

Diseases of the coronary arteries are caused initially by the collection of fatty plaques and other material inside the walls of the coronary arteries. These plaques narrow the lumen (opening) of the arteries and constrict normal blood flow through the arteries that serve the heart. The plaques are rougher than the walls of a normal artery and may cause a thrombus to form (Fig. 35-10).

Common symptoms of atherosclerotic coronary heart disease are:

- **Angina pectoris** (pain radiating to the arm, jaw, shoulder, back, or neck, usually felt on exertion and relieved by rest)
- A pressure or fullness in the chest, felt more severely during exertion and relieved by rest
- Syncope (fainting)
- Edema

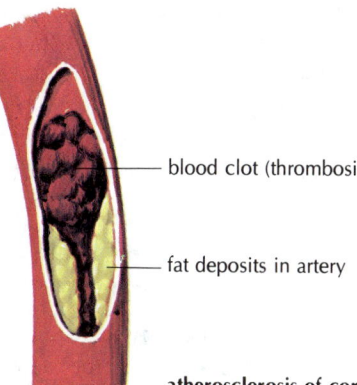

blood clot (thrombosis)

fat deposits in artery

atherosclerosis of coronary artery

FIGURE 35-10
Development of coronary thrombosis.

- Unexplained cough, generally without respiratory symptoms
- Hemoptysis (coughing up blood from the respiratory tract)
- Excessive fatigue

Predisposing conditions for coronary artery disease (CAD) include either a high intake of cholesterol or saturated fats or a familial hypercholesterolemia. A history of high cholesterol and triglyceride levels, cigarette smoking, diabetes mellitus, or hypertension is also likely to precede CAD. It may be controlled by a diet low in cholesterol and saturated fats, exercise, maintaining normal body weight, blood pressure control, and not smoking. If these methods are not successful, medication may be necessary. Atherosclerosis contributes to many other cardiovascular diseases.

Checkpoint Question
4. What are four predisposing factors for heart disease?

Arterial Occlusive Disease

This disease is caused by an obstruction or narrowing of an arterial lumen in areas other than the coronary arteries. Occlusions may occur in any artery and may be acute or chronic. They are caused by atherosclerotic plaques that may remain stationary as a thrombus or break away to become an embolus.

Signs and symptoms usually indicate ischemia to a part, such as pain or numbness, loss of normal blood flow, or loss of palpatory pulse. Diagnosis is made by arteriography to locate the occlusion and evaluate the degree of obstruction. Doppler ultrasonography is a noninvasive but less diagnostic method of evaluating peripheral circulation for occlusion.

Treatment for mild chronic occlusions require a life-style change to reverse atherosclerotic formations. If the condition is moderately severe, drug therapy may be initiated. If the occlusion is severe, the clot may be removed by embolectomy using various and constantly improving methods of treatment. If the clot cannot be removed, a bypass graft may be performed.

Myocardial Infarction

Death of the heart muscle, called myocardial infarction (MI), occurs when the coronary artery becomes totally occluded (blocked), usually by atherosclerotic plaques or by an embolism. An MI may occur suddenly, without prior symptoms, or in patients with diagnosed ath-

erosclerotic coronary heart disease. Studies by the American Heart Association reveal that in the United States alone, approximately 1,500,000 people develop MIs annually, with approximately 500,000 deaths or one-fourth of all deaths attributed to the killer disease.

Symptoms of myocardial infarction may be similar to those felt during angina pectoris, but this disorder is distinguished by pain that lasts longer than 20 to 30 minutes and is unrelieved by rest or nitroglycerin (Box 35-2). Other symptoms may include nausea, diaphoresis, weakness, vomiting, or abdominal cramps. The patient may complain of a viselike grip around the chest wall. The skin is cool and clammy and pale, and there may be a feeling of impending doom. Some patients only experience nonspecific symptoms of indigestion and do not seek medical attention. In 20% of patients, and particularly in diabetic patients, the MI may be silent, diagnosed only by routine electrocardiography (ECG) and later blood work when complications develop. It is imperative not to ignore or dismiss complaints by patients with

Patient Education: Nitroglycerin

A medication commonly prescribed for cardiac patients is nitroglycerin, a vasodilator. Vasodilators open the lumen of vessels, resulting in increased blood supply to the heart muscle. Patient education should include the following instructions:

- Keep the medication in the dark bottle supplied by the pharmacy because nitroglycerin can become deactivated in sunlight.
- Be alert for any side effects, such as lightheadedness, syncope, and hypotension.
- Be aware the nitroglycerin may be prescribed as either tablets or a spray, to use on an as-needed basis. (The spray is often easier for patients with poor dexterity or with poor eyesight.) The usual administration guidelines are for three doses at 5-minute intervals. If pain persists, call emergency medical services. Check with the physician for dosage instructions. (Nitroglycerin can also be prescribed as a skin patch, to be used on a daily basis to maintain vasodilation.)
- Check the expiration date of the medication frequently and always have an adequate supply available.
- Ensure that the medication is kept out of the reach of children.

BOX 35-2 Is It Angina or MI?

The pain felt with angina and myocardial infarction is brought about by myocardial anoxia, which is caused by an increased need for oxygen to the heart muscle due to exertion, stress, or temperature extremes of heat or cold. Typically, angina may be relieved by rest or nitroglycerin. However, pain from a myocardial infarction will not be relieved by these measures. Below is a brief comparison of these two disorders:

	Angina	Myocardial Infarction
Description	Moderate pressure felt deeply in the chest; a squeezing, suffocating feeling	Severe deep pressure not relieved by reducing stressors; a crushing pressure
Onset	Pain may occur gradually or suddenly and subsides quickly, usually in less than 30 minutes. It can be relieved by reducing the stressors, by rest, and by nitroglycerin protocol.	Pain occurs suddenly and remains even after stressors are reduced or relieved. Pain will not be relieved by nitroglycerin, which may be given up to three times, one dose every 5 minutes for a total of three doses in 15 minutes.
Location	Mid-anterior chest, usually diffuse, radiates to the back, neck, arms, jaw, and epigastric area	Mid-anterior chest with the same radiating patterns
Signs and Symptoms	Dyspnea, nausea, signs of indigestion (eg, burping), profuse sweating	Nausea and vomiting, fear, diaphoresis, pounding heart, palpitations (possible)

Any patient who calls the medical office complaining of chest pain must be examined immediately. The office should have an established protocol for handling these calls. The physician will need to be consulted to decide if the patient should be directed to the nearest emergency room, if emergency medical services should be dispatched, or if the patient should come directly to the office. This is not a decision that medical assistants should make.

---

symptoms of MI because this is a life-threatening condition. If the patient is found to have coronary occlusion, surgery may be performed before MI occurs or afterward to prevent further damage (Box 35-3).

Hypertension

Patients with a resting systolic blood pressure above 140 mm Hg (millimeters of mercury) and a diastolic pressure above 90 mm Hg are said to be hypertensive. Hypertension cannot be diagnosed on the basis of one blood pressure measurement alone. A physician will often require several readings before making the diagnosis of hypertension.

Hypertension is a major cause of stroke and renal failure and is a major consequence of atherosclerosis anywhere in the circulatory system. The long-term effects of hypertension cause weakening of the arteries and enlargement of the left ventricle, which results from overwork as the ventricle works harder to overcome the higher pressure in the arteries. The disease itself frequently produces no symptoms. The cause usually is unknown, but a correlation between hyper-

**BOX
35-3 Corrective Cardiac Surgery**

The least traumatic form of cardiac surgery is the *percutaneous transluminal coronary angioplasty (PCTA)*. A double-lumen catheter with a balloon surrounding the upper portion is inserted into a vessel in the groin or axilla. This catheter is threaded into the coronary vessels by watching a fluoroscopic screen as the procedure is performed. When the occlusion is found, the balloon is inflated to press the atherosclerotic plaque against the arterial walls and relieve the occlusion. Lasers may be used to remove the plaque. Springs or mesh (called a stent) may be inserted and left in place within the vessel to maintain patency. This procedure is less invasive than bypass surgery, but occasionally the artery will rebuild plaque at the site or the stent may fill with plaque and support occlusion.

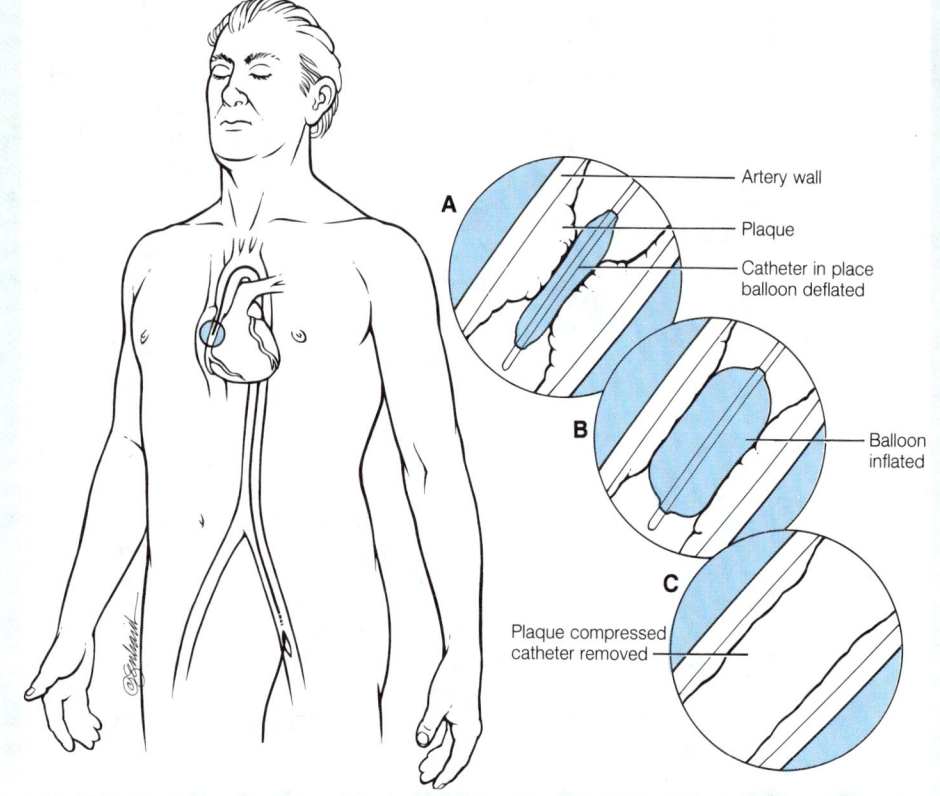

Percutaneous transluminal coronary angioplasty. (*A*) A balloon-tipped catheter is passed into the affected coronary artery and placed within the atherosclerotic lesion. (*B*) The balloon is then rapidly inflated and deflated with controlled pressure. (*C*) After the plaque is cracked, the catheter is removed, allowing improved blood flow through the vessel.

Artery wall
Plaque
Catheter in place balloon deflated
Balloon inflated
Plaque compressed catheter removed

Coronary artery bypass graft (CABG) surgery is performed by grafting a piece of vessel from another part of the body to the area beyond the occlusion and to the ascending aorta, providing a patent passage for the blood supply. The surgery requires a still field of surgery, so the heart must be stopped and the patient supported by a cardiopulmonary bypass machine for the length of the operation. The saphenous vein may be used if multiple bypasses will be performed, or the internal mammary artery will be used if the surgery is not extensive. Hospitalization may be as long as 5 to 7 days. As many 20% of patients will develop a repeat thrombus within 1 year.

tension and an elevated cholesterol level has been shown. Hypertension can strike anyone, regardless of age, race, sex, or ethnic origin.

Some high blood pressure (usually mild or borderline) may be controlled with a low-sodium diet, an ex-

ercise program, or weight reduction if needed. If hypertension cannot be controlled by these measures, a diuretic medication may be prescribed. Diuretics reduce the amount of sodium in the body, which in turn reduces the total fluid volume. The decrease in fluid volume reduces strain on the heart and blood vessels. Patients with high blood pressure should be advised to eliminate stressors in their lives, to limit the intake of alcohol, to stop smoking, and to lower their levels of cholesterol and triglycerides.

It should be emphasized to hypertensive patients that medication should be taken as prescribed. Often patients feel that because their blood pressure has reached a manageable level, they do not need to continue the prescribed medication. Explain that the medication is the cause of the lowered pressure and that discontinuing the treatment will jeopardize recovery.

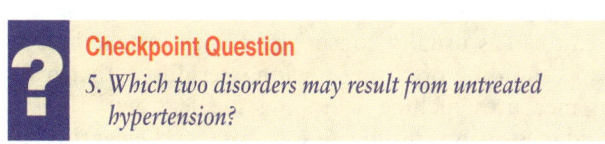

Checkpoint Question

5. Which two disorders may result from untreated hypertension?

Valvular Heart Disease

Disease of the heart valves is an acquired or congenital abnormality of any of the four cardiac valves. It is characterized by stenosis and obstructed blood flow or by valvular degeneration and backflow of the blood against the course of the circulatory pathway. Isolated stenosis and regurgitation of one or more valves may also be present, although the left heart valves are more often involved.

Congenital heart disease is present at birth in approximately 8 to 10/1000 live neonates. The most common diseases in this category are atrial septal defect (ASD), ventricular septal defect (VSD), patent ductus arteriosus (PDA), coarctation of the aorta, pulmonic stenosis, bicuspid aortic valve, mitral valve prolapse, and tetralogy of Fallot.

Rheumatic heart disease, an acquired valvular disease, presents clinically as a generalized inflammatory disease occurring 10 to 21 days after an upper respiratory infection caused by group A β-hemolytic streptococci. It is characterized by inflammatory lesions of the connective tissues, particularly in the heart, joints, and subcutaneous tissues. The heart valves are damaged by an abnormal response of the immune system caused by the turbulence of the bacterially infected blood. This damage results in a systolic murmur. The disease usually attacks young people between the ages of 5 and 15.

Since the 1940s, when there were an estimated 200,000 to 250,000 cases of rheumatic fever per year in the United States, incidence has dropped significantly. Today, rheumatic heart disease is considered rare in North America and Western Europe. The decline is due to improved health care and the availability of antimicrobial agents.

Mitral stenosis is most commonly a manifestation of rheumatic heart disease. Congenital forms of mitral stenosis may occur but are rare. Stenosis occurs when the mitral valve leaflet cusps fuse and thicken, resulting in an abnormally narrow valve. In addition, scarring of the free margins of the anterior and posterior leaflets occurs with shortening and thickening of the chordae tendineae. This may contribute to mitral regurgitation, which is a backflow of blood from the left ventricle into the left atrium across the mitral valve. Patients with mitral stenosis present with symptoms of dyspnea and their ability to exert themselves physically may be limited. Pulmonary edema may also develop.

Treatment of valvular disease depends on the type and severity of the abnormality. Severe cases may require medication, sodium-restricted diets, and prophylactic antibiotics before surgery or dental work. If medication is not successful, replacement valves may be necessary.

Aortic Stenosis

Aortic stenosis results from the narrowing of the aortic valve leaflets. Because blood cannot easily pass out of the left ventricle into the aorta, the ventricle has to work harder to pump blood through the narrow opening. This causes a turbulence of the blood as it flows past the stricture and is heard as a systolic murmur. If aortic stenosis progresses, the valve will become inflexible, reducing the opening of the valve to a small slit. Symptoms seen with aortic stenosis include angina, syncope, and heart failure. Treatment may require dilatation of the aortic arch or, in severe cases, replacement of the stenosed area.

Congestive Heart Failure

Congestive heart failure (CHF) is a condition in which the heart is unable to pump a sufficient blood volume through the body to meet the metabolic needs of the tissues (called forward failure) or cannot distend sufficiently during diastole, leading to cardiac and pulmonary congestion (called backward failure). Coronary artery disease, myocardial disease, valvular heart disease, and hypertension are among of the causes of CHF.

As a result of impaired cardiac function, pressure increases in the atria. Symptoms include reduced exercise tolerance and ventricular arrhythmias. Patients with CHF have a shortened life expectancy. CHF affects about 3 million Americans or about 1% of the population. It is one of the most common hospital discharge diagnoses for patients over the age of 65, and each year approximately 400,000 people develop CHF.

Cardiac Arrhythmia

Cardiac arrhythmia or dysrhythmia is an abnormal heart rhythm. It may occur as a primary disorder or as a secondary response to a systemic problem. It may also be a reaction to a drug toxicity or an electrolyte imbalance.

The sinoatrial (SA) node is considered the pacemaker of the heart. If the SA node is damaged, or a blockage occurs in the conduction pathway, the heart will beat too slowly to meet the body's demands. This type of arrhythmia is called bradycardia, which is a heart rate less than 60 beats/min.

More serious arrhythmias occur when the ventricles beat too fast, a condition known as ventricular tachycardia (VT). VT occurs when some of the electrical signals originate in the ventricles, rather than in the SA node. Once the ventricles begin to beat at a very rapid rate, less blood is pumped out of the heart with each contraction. This occurs because the heart's chambers do not have time to adequately fill with blood before the next contraction begins. Because less blood is being pumped into the circulation, less oxygen is being carried to the tissues. This lack of adequate blood and oxygen may cause dizziness, unconsciousness, or even cardiac arrest. Ventricular fibrillation is a medical emergency that occurs when the heart is quivering rather than contracting in an organized fashion. Very little blood is pumped out of the heart and the blood pressure may fall to 0. A patient in ventricular fibrillation will become unconscious and die very quickly unless an electrical shock with a cardiac defibrillator is administered immediately to restore normal cardiac electrical activity.

What If?

What if your patient asks you to explain a defibrillator?

A defibrillator is used to correct ventricular fibrillation. Defibrillators work by releasing an electrical current that is aimed at the conduction system in the heart. The goal of the defibrillator is to restore a normal rhythm in the heart. The current is released into the body by placing two paddles on the anterior aspect of the chest wall and delivering a preset number of joules (a electrical current measurement). Defibrillators are used in hospitals, ambulatory care centers, physician's offices, and ambulances. Special training is needed to operate this machine. Patients may have surgically "implanted defibrillators" in the chest wall. The implant releases "shocks" as needed to keep the heart rhythm regular.

Varicose Veins

Varicosities, the most common circulatory disease of the lower extremities, occur when the superficial veins of the legs become swollen and distended. Eventually the valves fail to close properly, allowing blood to pool and stretch the walls of the veins. People who sit or stand for long periods without moving or contracting their leg muscles are predisposed to developing varicose veins. A hereditary weakness in the vein walls is also a predisposing factor. Varicosities may also be secondary to deep-vein thrombosis. Symptoms of varicose veins are swelling, aching, or a feeling of heaviness in the legs. Varicosities may also be totally asymptomatic. Treatment is usually conservative with instructions to avoid standing or sitting for long periods. Other helpful measures include wrapping the legs with Elastic bandages, using sturdy support hose, and elevating the legs for specified periods. Surgery to remove the vein is usually the last approach. Newer treatment techniques involve the injection of a sclerosing agent into small varicose vein segments but is not suggested for large areas.

Stasis Ulcers

Peripheral vascular occlusion leads to stasis ulcers. Signs and symptoms include deep red discolorations, itching, pitting edema, and large areas of scaling skin leading to fissures and ulcers. Diagnosis is obvious by observation of the peripheral venous insufficiency but may be confirmed by Doppler ultrasonography. Treatment is directed at prevention by weight reduction, support stockings, and elevation of the affected limbs. If ulcers develop, measures to aid healing are instituted such as wet dressings and pressure dressings.

 **Checkpoint Question**

6. What disease occurs when the superficial veins in the legs become swollen and distended?

Venous Thrombosis and Pulmonary Embolism

Deep-vein thrombosis and pulmonary embolism are common cardiovascular illnesses, accounting for thousands of hospitalizations annually. Risk factors are either primary (inherited), which include the sickling diseases and hemolytic anemias, or secondary (acquired), which include long-term immobility, chronic pulmonary disease, thrombophlebitis, varicosities, and defibrillation after cardiac arrest. Oral contraceptives have been implicated in young women with none of the usual predisposing factors.

Symptoms include dyspnea, syncope, lightheadness, or severe pleuritic chest pain. Testing for venous thrombosis or pulmonary embolism requires a chest x-ray or an electrocardiogram. Doppler studies are also used to diagnose deep-vein thrombosis. If the diagnosis is still uncertain, a lung scan and a pulmonary arteriogram may be ordered. Depending on severity, treatment may include bed rest with elevation of the affected extremity, anticoagulant therapy, or surgery.

Cerebrovascular Accident

Cerebrovascular accidents (CVAs), sometimes called strokes, result when damage occurs to the blood vessels in the brain. The damage blocks the circulation, resulting in ischemia (lack of oxygen) to that part of the brain. Death of the brain tissue will occur without adequate oxygen. A common cause of CVA is blockage of the cerebral artery by a thrombus or embolus. Hemorrhage is another common cause. Atherosclerotic heart disease and hypertension also contribute to CVAs. CVAs are the most common nervous system disorder in the elderly and one of the leading causes of death in the United States.

If a CVA occurs on the right side of the brain, the left side of the body is affected and vice versa. Patients who suffer CVAs usually exhibit varying degrees of weakness or paralysis of one side of the body, with possible involvement of language and comprehension. Symptoms vary according to which artery and which part of the brain is affected. CVAs are fatal when vital centers of the brain are damaged. Treatment involves rehabilitation of these deficiencies after recovery from the acute phase. Therapy includes occupational and physical rehabilitation. Support may be offered to the patient in the form of counseling and a strong post-CVA support group.

Transient ischemic attacks (TIAs), or "mini-strokes," should be considered a warning sign for a major CVA. TIAs signal that small areas of the brain are without oxygen for short periods of time. The symptoms will vary, as those of a true stroke, according to the arteries affected, but will usually include:

- Mild numbness or tingling in the face or a limb
- Difficulty swallowing
- Coughing and choking
- Slurred speech
- Unilateral visual disturbances
- Dizziness

As many as 50% to 80% of patients who exhibit symptoms of TIAs will progress to a stroke. The signs of a major stroke may begin as a TIA but will progress to loss of consciousness, hyperpnea (deep, gasping breaths), anisocoria (unequal pupils), and hemiplegia (unilateral paralysis).

Carditis

Inflammation may affect any of the layers of the heart muscle and, although other factors may be cited, it is usually the result of a systemic infection.

Pericarditis

Pericarditis is caused by pathogens, neoplasias, autoimmunity (as in lupus erythematosus and rheumatoid arthritis), certain chemicals, radiation, and uremia. It may be acute or chronic.

Signs and symptoms include a sharp pain in the same locations expected with a myocardial infarction with the exception that pain increases on inspiration and on lying down, but decreases on sitting up and leaning forward. Dyspnea, tachycardia, neck venous distention, pallor, and hypertension are warning signs that serous fluid is compressing the heart and interfering with cardiac function.

Diagnosis is made by eliminating the other disorders with similar presenting signs and symptoms. There will be a characteristic pericardial rubbing sound caused by friction within the sac as the heart contracts and relaxes. Chronic pericarditis may not produce the rubbing sound. White blood cell counts, erythrocyte sedimentation rates, and cardiac enzymes may or may not be elevated. Cardiocentesis will aid in diagnosis if the causative agent is a pathogen. An electrocardiogram (ECG) or echocardiogram may show changes consistent with effusion.

Treatment involves relieving the symptoms and correcting the underlying cause. Treatment during recovery is usually directed toward pain relief and reducing inflammation.

Myocarditis

Myocarditis may be chronic or acute and may be diffused through the heart muscle or may be localized at a focal point. Causes include radiation, chemicals, or infections such as a virus, bacteria, parasites, or helminths.

Signs and symptoms of early acute episodes are usually nonspecific such as fatigue, fever, and mild chest pain. Chronic cases may lead to heart failure with cardiomegaly, arrhythmias, and valvulitis.

Diagnosis is made by patient history, which usually reveals a recent upper respiratory infection with fever. On auscultation, a murmur may be heard and arrhythmias are usually present during acute episodes.

Myocarditis has no conclusive laboratory studies although cardiac enzymes may be elevated and ECG tracings may be atypical. If bacteria are suspected, stool or throat cultures may identify the pathogen.

Treatment includes antibiotics if a pathogen has been identified. Recovery is usually good and is frequently spontaneous. Supportive care during resolution hastens a return to health.

Endocarditis

Endocarditis may be chronic or acute and is caused by a systemic bacterial or fungal invasion. The lining of the heart and its valves may gather clusters of platelets, fibrin, and white blood cells to trap the pathogens. These clusters are called vegetations and may break away to become emboli that travel to the spleen, kidneys, lungs, or nervous system. These formations may also cause scarring of the valves and erosion of the chordae tendinea with resulting valvular reflux.

Signs and symptoms are general to many infectious disorders and include fatigue, low-grade fever, joint pain, and anorexia. Auscultation may reveal a murmur during febrile episodes. If the vegetations become emboli, evidence of occlusion will be seen wherever the clot lodges, such as central nervous system signs of ischemia or an infarction, or signs of a pulmonary infraction.

Diagnosis requires a blood culture to identify the causative agent. Treatment is directed toward eliminating the infecting organism.

Checkpoint Question

7. How does the pain in pericarditis differ from pain with a myocardial infarction?

Aneurysm

Weakened vessel walls are predisposed to abnormal dilatation. Dilatation in the form of an **aneurysm** may occur in any vessel, but arteries are most often affected. Because of the high pressure so close to the heart, the aorta is the most common site. The normal elastic vessel wall develops a ballooning effect in many different forms, all of them dangerous:

- A *dissecting aneurysm* tears the inner walls of the artery and allows blood to leak into the lining of the vessel; the wall will eventually die and tear.
- A *sacculated aneurysm* balloons from the wall into a sac, which may burst.

- A *berry aneurysm* is usually a congenital defect in a cerebral vessel.

Causes of aneurysms include trauma, hypertension, atherosclerosis, certain fungal infections, syphilis, and congenital defects. Symptoms include pain or pressure at the site. An abdominal aneurysm may be asymptomatic; the pain becomes sharp and tearing if it bursts. Death may occur quickly if the tear is not repaired. If an aneurysm is suggested by the presence of pain or discovered on a routine physical examination, diagnosis is confirmed by an arteriogram, or an aortogram, computed tomography scan, or magnetic resonance imaging. Surgical resection is the only option.

Anemia

Deficiencies in hemoglobin or in the numbers of red blood cells are called anemia. Anemia is not considered a disease but a symptom of an underlying disorder. Anemia can result from:

- Blood loss due to hemorrhage or slow internal bleeding
- A diet low in iron or a malabsorption condition (nutritional anemia)
- Suppressed or diseased marrow, resulting in decreased blood cell formation (aplastic anemia)
- Vitamin B_{12} deficiency (pernicious anemia)
- Genetic abnormalities (sickle cell anemia [Fig. 35-11] or thalassemia)
- Destruction of functioning red blood cells by various means such as liver or spleen dysfunction or toxins (hemolytic anemia)

Symptoms may include cardiovascular alterations, anorexia and weight loss, dyspnea on exertion, and fatigue. Laboratory tests reveal decreased hemoglobin and hematocrit levels.

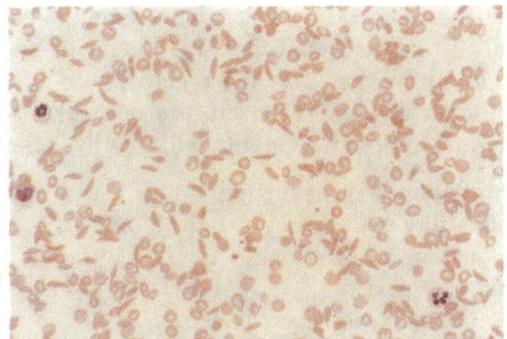
FIGURE 35-11
Abnormal red cells showing sickled cells.

Treatment of anemia must address the cause. Nutritional or malabsorption anemias respond to diets rich in iron, iron supplements, folic acid, or ascorbic acid and replacement of vitamin B_{12}, if these substances are deficient. If anemia is due to blood loss, the cause must be found and corrected and blood volume restored. If erythrocytes are destroyed by premature hemolysis, the cause must be found and corrected. Aplastic anemia may require marrow transplant or supportive therapy. Genetic abnormalities cannot be corrected at this time.

➤ COMMON DIAGNOSTIC PROCEDURES AND THE MEDICAL ASSISTANT'S ROLE

Testing for cardiovascular disorders is either noninvasive, which does not require entering the body or puncturing the skin, or invasive, which requires entering the body cavity by use of either a tube, needle, or other device. Depending on the patient's symptoms, testing may be basic (eg, auscultation of the heart and chest cavity done during the physical examination) or intensive and extensive. For instance, a simple chest x-ray or 12-lead electrocardiogram (ECG) may give the cardiologist (a physician who specializes in the treatment of heart disease) enough information to make the proper diagnosis. Sometimes, however, the initial findings may indicate the need for more sophisticated procedures (eg, cardiac catheterization). The most commonly performed cardiovascular tests are discussed below and summarized in Table 35-2.

Cardiovascular Examination

The cardiovascular examination is the most basic, noninvasive procedure. When preparing a patient for cardiovascular examination, you are responsible for obtaining vital information (Box 35-4). Data collected may include an accurate weight (without shoes), blood pressure in one or both arms (depending on physician preference), resting apical pulse when indicated, respirations, and temperature. (See Chap. 20, Medical History and Patient Assessment, and Chap. 21, Anthropometric Measurements and Vital Signs, for a more detailed discussion.) You may also be responsible for obtaining a complete list of the patient's medications and current dosage, including over-the-counter drugs.

The physician or cardiologist usually begins the examination with a review of the patient's history and reason for the office visit. The physician also reviews vitals signs and medications, noting allergies to med-

---

BOX 35-4   Obtaining a Cardiovascular Patient's History: Key Questions to Ask

By asking the following questions, you can elicit important information from a patient with cardiovascular problems.

- Why are you seeing the cardiologist today?
- What symptoms have you been having?
- How long have you been experiencing the pain, discomfort, distress, or unusual sensation? (Patients may not associate chest discomfort as a cardiac symptom.)
- Where is the pain located? Does it stay in one place or does it radiate in any direction?
- Rate the pain on a scale of 1 to 10.
- Is the pain associated with any other symptoms such as shortness of breath, nausea, weakness, sweating, dizziness?
- If you have been experiencing shortness of breath, does it restrict any of your activities or require you to sleep on additional pillows at night?
- Are you a smoker?
- Do you drink alcoholic beverages?
- Have you noticed any additional problems?

As you proceed with the interview, keep in mind that patients with cardiovascular problems are usually understandably anxious and concerned. They may bring with them family members who also are concerned or anxious. It is your responsibility to help ease apprehension and to offer reassurance and support when appropriate.

---

ications and other substances or, if no allergies are present, noting NKA (no known allergies). A brief social history may be taken, noting risk factors for cardiovascular disorders such as smoking, drinking, family history of heart disease, or hypercholesterolemia. The physician then examines the eyes, ears, nose, throat, neck, lungs, heart, and extremities. The circulatory system is examined by use of inspection, palpation, percussion, and auscultation (see Chap. 22, Physical Examination, for more information).

The physician uses visual inspection to evaluate the general appearance of the body, noting the circulation to extremities, configuration of the chest, facial expression, color, respiratory patterns, jugular venous distention (JVD), circumoral cyanosis, clubbed nails, and so on.

Table 35-2
Common Cardiovascular Tests

Diagnostic Test	Description	Indications
Chest x-ray or chest roentgenogram	Noninvasive diagnostic tool using high-energy electromagnetic waves	Used to detect and follow the advancement of cardiovascular and other diseases and to evaluate the patient's response to therapy. Posterior and lateral views are generally used to assess normal radiographic findings.
12-lead electrocardiogram (ECG)	Graphic recording of the electrical activity of the heart from different angles, using leads uniquely placed on the chest and extremities	May be done to obtain a baseline during a physical examination or in acute situations as seen in patients with myocardial infarctions. Also used to eliminate or complete a potential diagnosis in patients with cardiovascular symptoms.
Holter monitor	Continuous cardiac monitoring of heart rhythm via a portable device worn by patients for 12, 24, or 48 h.	Used for patients with symptoms of rhythm disturbances not shown on ECGs or during physical examinations. Holter monitors are also used to show effectiveness of antiarrhythmic drugs or proper pacemaker function.
Cardiac stress test	ECG recording of heart rhythm while patient is exercising on a graded treadmill or stationary bicycle.	May be ordered with or without isotopes to help diagnose patients with known or suspected heart problems. Stress testing may also be used to obtain a baseline in healthy adults who are at high risk for cardiovascular disease or in patients starting an exercise program.
Echocardiogram (also kown as echo)	Ultrasound of the heart using harmless sound waves generated from a small device known as a transducer.	Used to diagnose adults and pediatric patients with suspected or known valvular disease. Also used in diagnosing the severity of heart failure and cardiomyopathy. May be indicated in patients with trauma to diagnose injury to the heart or in situations involving possible harvest of the heart for transplant.
Cardiac catheterization	Common nonsurgical procedure involving insertion of a catheter into the heart	Used to help diagnose or determine severity of heart disease. Often indicated after a preliminary stress test or echocardiogram reveals an abnormality or indications of a heart problem.
Coronary arteriography	Injection of a contrast medium into the coronrary arteries, allowing visualization	Used to assess congenital or acquired heart disease and to assess damage after myocardial infarction.

Cardiovascular Examination

The cardiovascular examination is the most basic, noninvasive procedure. When preparing a patient for cardiovascular examination, you are responsible for obtaining vital information (Box 35-4). Data collected may include an accurate weight (without shoes), blood pressure in one or both arms (depending on physician preference), resting apical pulse when indicated, respirations, and temperature. (See Chap. 20, Medical History and Patient Assessment, and Chap. 21, Anthropometric Measurements and Vital Signs, for a more detailed discussion.) You may also be responsible for obtaining a complete list of the patient's medications and current dosage, including over-the-counter drugs.

The physician or cardiologist usually begins the examination with a review of the patient's history and reason for the office visit. The physician also reviews vitals signs and medications, noting allergies to medications and other substances or, if no allergies are present, noting NKA (no known allergies). A brief social history may be taken, noting risk factors for cardiovascular disorders such as smoking, drinking, family history of heart disease, or hypercholesterolemia. The physician then examines the eyes, ears, nose,

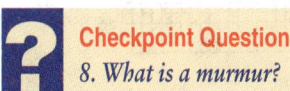

Checkpoint Question
8. What is a murmur?

throat, neck, lungs, heart, and extremities. The circulatory system is examined by use of inspection, palpation, percussion, and auscultation (see Chap. 22, Physical Examination, for more information).

The physician uses visual inspection to evaluate the general appearance of the body, noting the circulation to extremities, configuration of the chest, facial expression, color, respiratory patterns, jugular venous distention (JVD), circumoral cyanosis, clubbed nails, and so on.

Palpation is used to detect vibrations produced by the cardiac cycle. Thrills may be felt over the cardiac area in some diseases of the circulatory system. Palpation of peripheral pulses evaluates the efficiency of the circulatory pathways.

Percussion helps to determine the areas of dullness outlining the heart and aids the physician in the diagnosis of cardiac enlargement.

By auscultating with a stethoscope, the physician can evaluate the sounds made by blood coursing through the heart, the carotid arteries, or the peripheral vessels. During auscultation, abnormal heart sounds (bruits or murmurs) may be detected (Box 35-5).

After completing the examination of the heart, the physician examines the abdomen. Then the neurologic system is reviewed. Lastly, in no specific order, a review of the peripheral vascular system is performed. The physician then makes recommendations and comments.

During the examination, your role is to provide proper gowning and physical support as necessary (see Chap. 22, Physical Examination, for more information). After the examination, the physician may order an electrocardiogram (ECG). Depending on the size of the clinic, this test may be performed either by a technician in the ECG department or by a medical assistant (see below).

Electrocardiogram

One of the most valuable diagnostic tools for the cardiologist is the electrocardiogram, known by the acronym ECG or EKG. The ECG is the graphic record of the electrical current as it progresses through the heart. Patients with symptoms of chest heaviness or pain, or jaw or arm pain, or those with feelings of skipped heartbeats may undergo an ECG to eliminate or complete a potential diagnosis. Combinations of electrodes called **leads** are placed on the patient's limbs and in the precordium (the area anterior to the heart) to measure the electrical impulses. ECGs are used to assist in diagnosing ischemia, delays in impulse conduction, hypertrophy of the chambers, and arrhythmias. They are not considered reliable for predicting an impending myocardial infarction.

ECG Paper

The ECG tracing is printed on graph paper at a standard speed of 25 mm/s (millimeters per second), with a 0.1 mV (millivolt) electric impulse. The ECG graph paper, although it appears white, is either blue or black with a white, heat-labile coating. A graph is printed over the white coating. The stylus of the ECG machine is heated to melt the white coating, exposing the dark background to record the movement of the stylus. The ECG paper is affected by pressure as well as heat and should be handled carefully to prevent extraneous markings. Newer ECG machines have controlled stylus temperatures; older machines may require adjustment of the temperature. If the stylus is

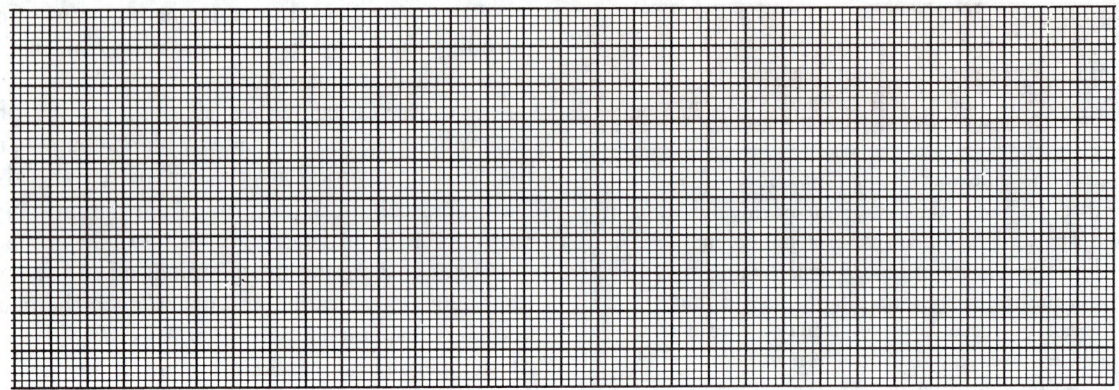

A   On standard ECG paper, each small block is 1 millimeter by 1 millimeter. The large blocks are 5 millimeters by 5 millimeters. (actual size)

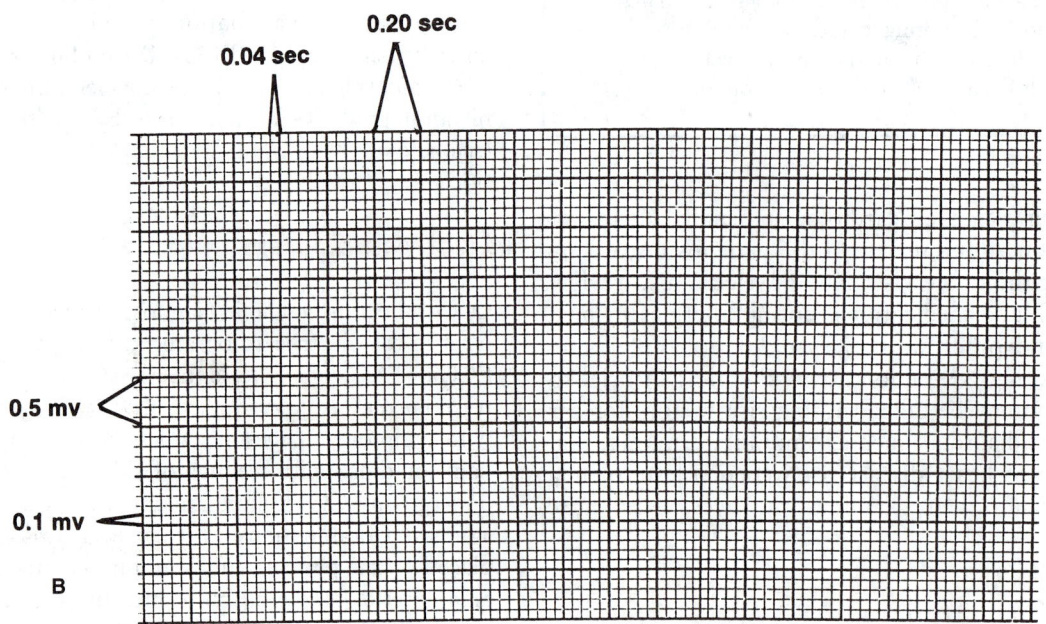

0.04 sec

0.20 sec

0.5 mv

0.1 mv

B

FIGURE 35-12
Electrocardiogram (ECG) graph paper. (A) Each small square is 1 mm × 1 mm. Each fifth line is marked darker to make a cube of 5 mm × 5 mm. (B) Time in seconds. Each small square is .04 second in duration and each large square is .20 second in duration. Five large squares = 1 second (5 × .20).

ECG Leads

Over the years, a standard system of electrode placement has evolved and a nomenclature has been developed for the recordings made from different electrode combinations. Each combination is known as a lead. Each lead records the electrical impulse through the heart from a different angle. The standard ECG has 12 leads that produce a three-dimensional record of the impulse wave.

There are four wires with connectors labeled for the patient limbs (Box 35-6). The four limb electrodes should be positioned away from bony areas and onto more muscular areas such as the calves, outer thighs, and above the elbow. The leads may be placed in any position on the patient's limbs for recording, but the best results are obtained by proper placement. Adjustments may be necessary for amputees, patients who have had limb surgery, or trauma patients.

The right leg electrode is the grounding lead to reduce alternating current (AC) interference. It keeps the average voltage of the patient the same as that of the recording instrument and is the "referencing" electrode. The first three combinations derived from the other three limb electrodes are standard bipolar limb leads or Einthoven leads. These leads also allow a frontal visualization of the heart's electrical activity from side to side. Figure 35-14 shows 12-lead ECG electrode placement.

PR Interval. The time from the beginning of the P wave to the beginning of the QRS complex is called the *PR interval*. This time interval represents depolarization of the atria and the spread of the depolarization wave up to and including the AV node.

PR Segment. The PR segment represents the period of time between the P wave and the QRS complex.

ST Segment. The distance between the QRS complex and the T wave from the point where the QRS complex ends (J-point) to the onset of the ascending limb of the T wave is called the *ST segment*. On the ECG, this segment is a sensitive indicator of myocardial ischemia or injury.

QT Interval. The time from the beginning of the QRS complex to the end of the T wave is called the *QT interval*. This interval represents both ventricular depolarization and repolarization.

Ventricular Activation Time. The time from the beginning of the QRS complex to the peak of the R wave is called the *ventricular activation time* and represents the time necessary for the depolarization wave to travel from the inner surface of the heart (endocardium) to the outer surface of the heart (epicardium).

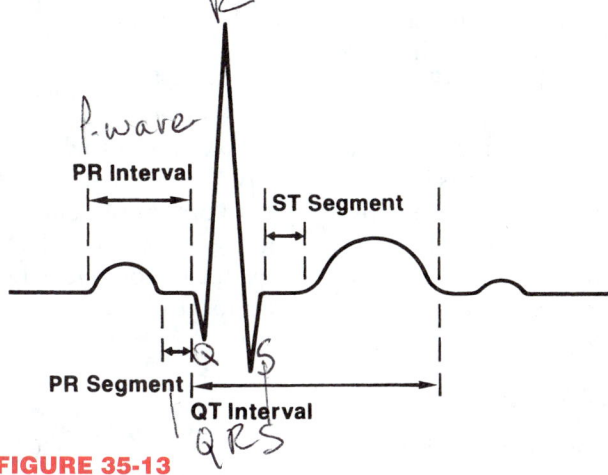

FIGURE 35-13
Intervals and segments.

Each lead provides a specific measurement:

- Lead I measures the difference in electrical potential between the right arm (RA) to left arm (LA).
- Lead II measures the difference in electrical potential between the right arm (RA) and the left leg (LL).

> **BOX 35-6** **Abbreviations Used in Performing ECGs**
>
> RA—right arm
> LA—left arm
> LL—left leg
> RL—right leg
> V_1–V_6—chest lead
> aVR—augmented voltage right arm
> aVL—augmented voltage left arm
> aVF—augmented voltage left foot or leg

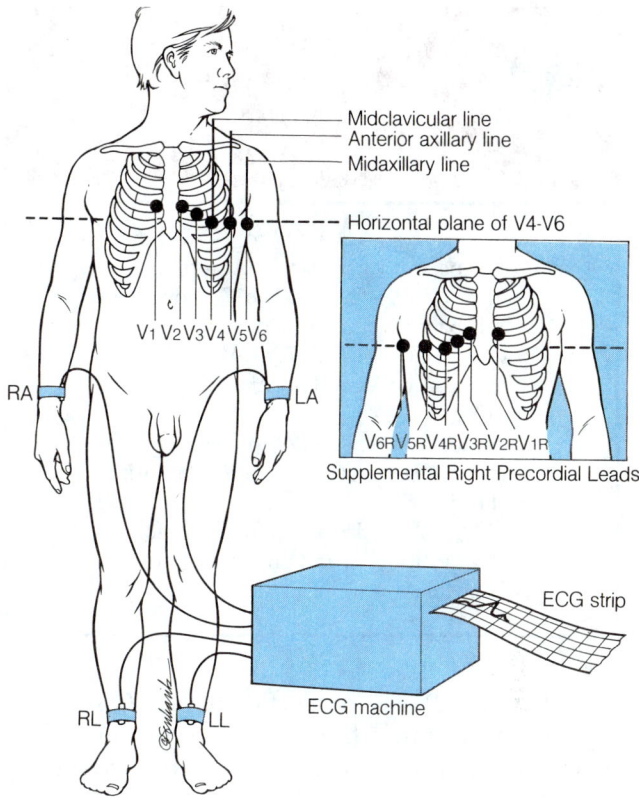

FIGURE 35-14
Twelve-lead ECG-electrode placement.

- Lead III measures the difference in electrical potential between the left arm (LA) and the left leg (LL).

Using the same three electrodes, measurements can be made of the signal between one electrode and the average of the remaining two. These second three combinations are the augmented unipolar limb leads and allow visualization from a frontal view top to bottom:

- Lead aVR = (LL + LA) to RA measures the potential at the right arm.
- Lead aVL = (LL + RA) to LA measures the potential at the left arm.
- Lead aVF = (RA + LA) to LL measures the potential at the left foot (see Fig. 35-14).

To take a closer look at the heart, electrodes are placed directly on the chest wall. The limb electrodes must remain attached to the patient. Six chest positions are universally defined. Positioning of these electrodes must be precise to record the chest leads accurately. These leads show the comparison of the chest electrode potential to the average of the three limb electrodes and are called the unipolar precordial (chest) leads (Box 35-7).

All electrodes must connect to the wires of the ECG machine. Specific codes are used to mark each

BOX 35-7 Positioning of Unipolar Precordial (Chest) Leads

- Lead V_1 = (RA + LA + LL) to V_1: Fourth intercostal space at right margin of sternum
- Lead V_2 = (RA + LA + LL) to V_2: Fourth intercostal space at left margin of sternum
- Lead V_3 = (RA + LA + LL) to V_3: Midway between position V_2 and position V_4
- Lead V_4 = (RA + LA + LL) to V_4: Fifth intercostal space at junction of mid-clavicular line
- Lead V_5 = (RA + LA + LL) to V_5: At horizontal level of position V_4 at left anterior axillary line
- Lead V_6 = (RA + LA + LL) to V_6: At horizontal level of position V_4 and position V_5 at mid-axillary line.

lead (Table 35-3). The production of the ECG recording onto paper varies from one ECG machine to another, but the principle and technique are universal.

Checkpoint Question

9. *Which three waves represent a cardiac cycle on an ECG?*

Preparing for the ECG

Many offices are equipped with ECG machines that are designed to interpret the readings as they are recorded. These machines will also alert you on the printout if any of the various attachments are not in the correct order or are placed incorrectly. Most offices now use three-channel machines that automatically progress from one lead to the next and mark each lead on the graph paper as it moves through the standard order of recording. Some offices still use older machines that must be advanced by hand and marked with standardized lead indicators. You must become familiar with the particular machine used where you work by reading the manuals provided by the manufacturer and by asking questions to clarify points of concern.

The area in which an ECG is recorded should be comfortable, warm, and private. Lighting should be indirect and restful. A small pillow or cushion should be placed under the patient's head and perhaps also under the knees and shoulders to provide comfort. Tables should be long and wide enough to support the patient's body and limbs comfortably.

To calm and comfort a frightened patient, give friendly smiles, offer assistance when needed, and provide reassurance that the ECG is harmless. A frightened patient is not as likely to be compliant with instructions and may interfere with the quality of the recording by moving about or actually trembling in fear. Procedures 35-1 and 35-2 describe the steps for performing a 12-lead ECG and mounting the strip for reading.

ECG Interpretation

Interpretation of the standard 12-lead ECG is done by the physician, who takes the following elements into consideration:

- Rate: how fast the heart is beating
- Rhythm: regularity of recurring amplitudes and intervals

text continues on page 680

Table 35-3 Coding ECG Leads

Lead	Code	Lead	Code
I	.	V_1	-.
II	..	V_2	-..
III	...	V_3	-...
aVR	-	V_4	-....
aVL	--	V_5	-.....
aVF	---	V_6	-......

Charting Example

| 09/08/98 | 1330 | 12-lead ECG done. Patient tolerated procedure well. No complaints of chest pain during the ECG. ECG mounted and given to Dr. Bruno to evaluate. Patient was discharged by Dr. Bruno.———— Aisha Perez, CMA |

Procedure 35-1

Performing a 12-Lead Electrocardiogram

Equipment/Supplies

- equipment for measuring vital signs
- ECG machine
- ECG paper
- coupling gel or pads
- electrodes
- gown or cape
- razor (if necessary)
- comfortable table

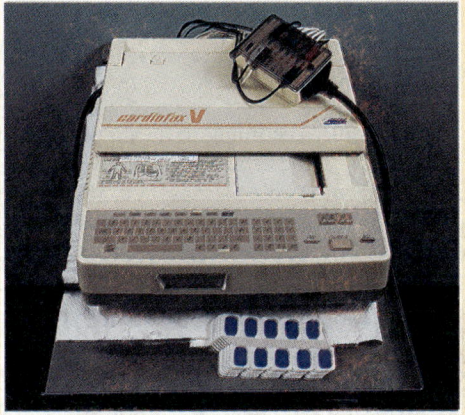

ECG machine.

Steps	Purpose
1. Wash your hands.	1. Handwashing aids infection control.
2. Assemble the equipment.	2. This ensures that all supplies are available.
3. Greet and identify the patient. Explain the procedure, noting that the machine will pick up tremors or muscle movement and instructing the patient to lie still for the usually brief duration of the test. Ask for and answer any questions.	3. This avoids errors in treatment and helps gain patient compliance and ease anxiety.
4. Before beginning the ECG, record the patient's data base: name, age, sex, height, weight, vital signs, symptoms, and medications. Note the time and date of the recording.	4. This information is needed for proper diagnosis.
5. Note any preparation required for the test. Generally, no preparation is needed. However, the physician may request that the patient exercise for a prescribed period of time before the test to record changes brought about by physical stress. Also, skin preparation (eg, slight skin abrading or shaving) may be necessary for patients with extreme cases of excessively dry or oily skin, or for those with coarse arm or chest hair.	5. The physician may want the patient to exercise beforehand so the test can record changes brought about by physical stress. Skin preparation ensures properly attached leads and helps avoid improper readings and lost time repeating the test.
6. Instruct the patient to disrobe above the waist and provide a gown for privacy. Nylons or tights should be removed also.	6. Clothing may interfere with the proper placement of leads.
7. Position the patient comfortably in a supine position with pillows as needed for comfort. Drape for warmth and privacy.	7. If the patient is uncomfortable, too cool or improperly draped, movement is likely, resulting in artifacts (see Table 35-4).
8. Check the machine for safety of grounding. Position it with the power cord away from the patient. Turn the machine on to warm the stylus.	8. With cord away from the patient, electrical current artifacts are less likely. The warmth of the stylus melts the white coated surface of the ECG paper, exposing the dark background to record the movement of the stylus.

(continued)

Steps	Purpose
9. Apply the electrodes according to the manufacturer's directions. Some offices still use metal electrodes attached with rubber straps, but most are now using disposable electrodes that adhere to the skin without straps. Follow the instructions for	9. An electrolyte-conducting gel transmits electrical impulses from the skin to the electrodes. Unequal amounts on electrodes will lead to artifacts. If

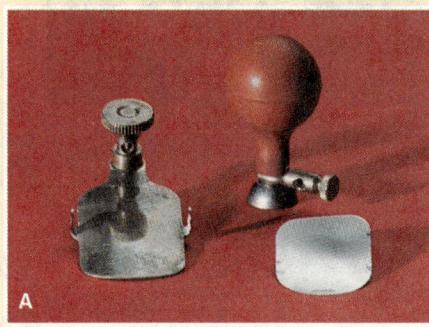

Step 9: (From left to right) A metal electrode, a welch cup, a disposable adhesive electrode.

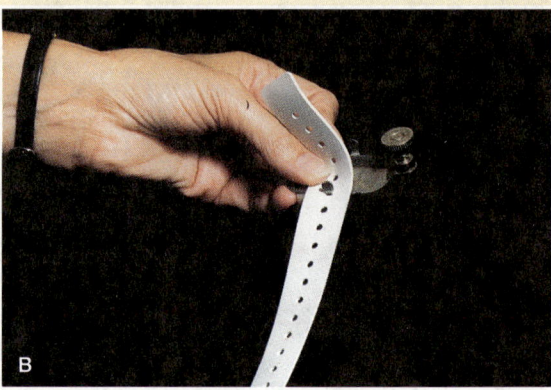

Step 9B: Flexible, stretchy straps are applied to the prongs of the metal electrode.

the particular machine you are using. Be aware that disposable electrodes will have electrolyte gel already applied equally and adequately. If metal disks are used, apply a small amount of the gel to the electrode, or use a pad impregnated with elec-

leads are not snug against the skin, an improper reading will result.

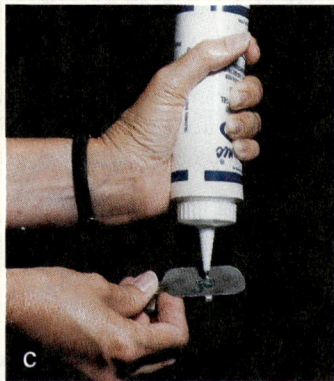

Step 9C: If metal disks are used, apply gel evenly and equally to all disks.

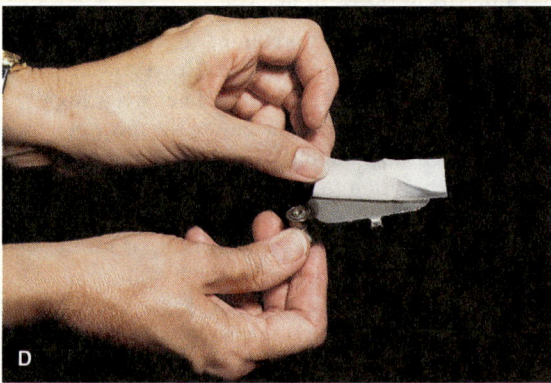

Step 9D: A pad impregnated with electrolyte gel may be used.

trolyte gel. Rub the gel into the skin using the side of the electrode to slightly redden the skin for increased conduction. Apply rubber straps snugly to the limbs.

(continued)

Procedure 35-1

Performing a 12-Lead Electrocardiogram *(continued)*

Steps	Purpose
10. Place electrodes on the fleshy, muscular parts of the upper arms and lower legs. The attachments will point to the hands and feet of the patient.	10. Conduction will be impaired if attachments are placed on bony prominences. Attachments pointing toward the lower portion of the patient's body will offer better connections and follow the patient's contours.
11. If using Welch electrode cups for the chest leads, apply a small amount of electrolyte gel, compress the bulb to create a suction, press it against the patient's chest at first position, V_1, and release the bulb. Some chest leads may be attached with a rubber strap around the patient's chest, and others may be weighted with a metal strip.	
12. Connect the leads securely. They will be coded RA, LA, LL, RL, and C-V. Some are color coded. Untangle the leads before applying to decrease electrical artifacts. Each lead must lie unencumbered along the contours of the patient's body to decrease the incidence of artifacts. Double check the placement.	12. Improperly placed leads will result in time lost to an inaccurate reading and retesting.
13. Plug in the cable and arrange it along the side of the patient on the table.	13. This placement will decrease pressure and tugging on the lead attachments.
14. Center the stylus and press the standardization button (STD). Set on RUN 25. The mark should be 2×10 mm, or two small squares wide by ten small squares high. Adjust appropriately within those parameters. Check at this time for artifacts.	14. The standardization mark documents accuracy of operation and provides a reference point for reading impulses.

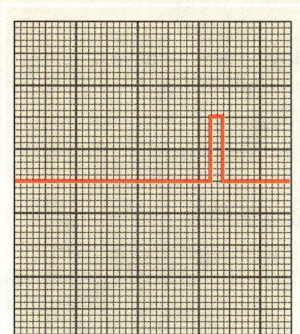

Normal Standard
Standardization mark
is 10 mm high

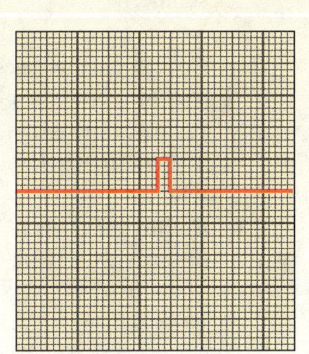

One-Half Standard
Standardization mark
is 5 mm high

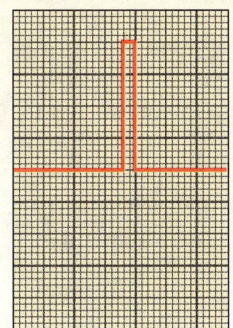

Double Standard
Standardization mark
is 20 mm high

Step 14: Standardization marks.

(continued)

Procedure 35-1

Performing a 12-Lead Electrocardiogram (continued)

Steps	Purpose
15. Center the stylus on the paper and run 8–10 inches of leads I, II, III. If the R wave is too large for the reading, reduce the standardization to 1/2. If the reading is too small to be accurately read, increase the standardization × 2. If you must move the stylus from the position of the standardization mark, make another mark for reference. If any of the leads are not properly attached, it will be apparent at this time.	
16. If the leads were accurately placed and the stylus was appropriately centered for correct readings of leads I, II, III, then proceed manually to aVR, aVL, and aVF, if the machine does not progress automatically. Check the standardization each time a progression is made.	
17. Switch to V_1 through V_6 for 5–6 inches of paper. If the instrument is not automatic, you will need to mark each lead as it is run (see Table 35-3 for standard marks).	17. The physician will need these markings to identify the leads that are being recorded for interpretation.
18. If the machine does not progress automatically, and chest leads must be manually moved to the next position, turn off the machine before disconnecting the leads and restandardize each time.	18. If the leads are removed from the patient or from an electrode, the stylus will thrash across the paper. Each time the machine is turned off, or leads moved, the machine must be restandardized.
19. Turn off and unplug the machine at the completion of the reading.	
20. Remove the electrodes and clean the patient's skin. Assist the patient from the table and help with dressing, as needed.	20. Some patients may become dizzy from lying supine.
21. Thank the patient and give appropriate instructions.	21. Courtesy encourages the patient to have a positive attitude about the physician's office.
22. Carefully roll the ECG strip. Do not use clips to secure the roll.	22. Creases and clips may remove some of the coating and mar or mark the surface, obscuring the reading.
23. Store the equipment by carefully coiling the leads. Clean the electrodes with kitchen cleanser if reusable.	23. Coiling the leads reduces tangling and damage to the wires. Cleaning the electrodes will prevent build up of electrolyte gel, which would cause artifacts.

- Axis: position of the heart and direction of depolarization
- Hypertrophy: size of the heart
- Ischemia: decrease in the blood supply to an area
- Infarction: death of heart muscle resulting in loss of function

Under usual diagnostic conditions, the 12-lead ECG demonstrates sufficient data. As the medical assistant,

you are responsible for obtaining an ECG that is of good quality without avoidable **artifacts**. An artifact is the appearance of an abnormal signal that does not reflect electrical activity of the heart during the cardiac cycle. It can be attributed to patient movement, mechanical problems with the ECG machine, or improper technique. Table 35-4 describes three types of artifacts and how to prevent them. To avoid artifacts due to improper technique, review and practice the procedure. It is your responsibil-

Procedure 35-2   Mounting the ECG Strip for Reading

Equipment/Supplies

- physician-preferred mounting device
- clean, flat surface
- scissors

Steps	Purpose
1. Label the mounting paper with the patient's data.	1. This information is important for interpretation of the reading.
2. Unroll the strip on a clean, flat surface and identify the area of lead I with the standardization mark. Cut this strip with scissors to the length preferred by the physician.	2. A soiled strip may be illegible. The standardization mark will be used as a reference. Physicians have set opinions regarding the proper length for various types of readings.
3. If the mounting device has protective sleeves, carefully open the sleeve as far as possible and insert the strip. If the mounting papers have adhesive strips and clear plastic covers, use care to prevent marring the surface of the strip.	3. A scratch may mar the surface and make it unreadable.
4. Repeat the procedure until all of the leads are in their proper places on the sheet.	
5. File the report in the area the physician has designated for reports pending review.	

ity to feel comfortable with the ECG and to ensure good technical quality and attain the proper ECG tracing.

Sometimes the physician may request a rhythm strip along with the ECG. A rhythm strip is a long strip of QRS complexes of a certain lead, or combinations of leads; it may be used to define certain cardiac arrhythmias. The physician may also request that chest electrodes be positioned on the right side of the chest, instead of the left, for cases of true **dextrocardia** (right-sided heart placement) or in pediatric patients (the heart of a young child is not angled as sharply to the left as an adult's).

Holter Monitor

In many instances, cardiac problems will not be apparent during a brief ECG. For diagnosis of intermittent cardiac arrhythmias and dysfunctions, a monitor that records for at least a 24-hour period is used. The Holter monitor is small and portable and can be worn comfortably for long periods of time without interfering with daily activities. It may be set to record continuously, or it may be programmed to record when the patient presses a record button at the onset of symptoms. This

is also known as an incident or event button. As part of this test, the patient must also keep a diary of daily activities (Box 35-8). Frequently, the medical assistant will be responsible for applying the monitor and instructing the patient in its purpose and use (Procedure 35-3).

Not all Holter monitors record on graph paper. Newer, less bulky Holter monitors have computer memory and print the reading at the end of testing. The physician will receive the computerized synopsis of the diary and the cardiac events for the testing period.

A 30-day event monitor is designed for use during a longer period than is possible with the Holter monitor. Two leads are used rather than six and the machine is very small and light. The recorder must be activated whenever symptoms are perceived by the patient and will not record unless the marker is pressed (Fig. 35-15).

Chest X-ray or Chest Roentgenogram

A chest x-ray provides valuable basic information about the anatomic location and gross structures of the heart, great vessels, and lungs. Chest x-rays aid in the evaluation of such cardiovascular disorders as congestive heart failure and pericardial effusions.

Table 35-4
Types of Artifacts

Artifact	Possible Causes	How to Prevent Problems
Wandering baseline	• Electrodes are too tight or too loose	• Apply electrodes properly.

WANDERING BASELINE

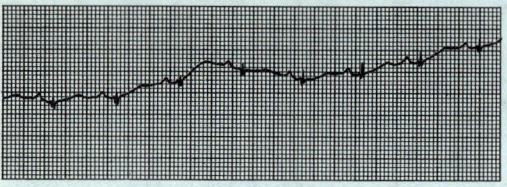

Artifact	Possible Causes	How to Prevent Problems
Muscle or somatic artifact	• Electrolyte gel may have built up on electrodes • Patient's skin may not have been cleaned of oil, lotion, or excess hair • Patient cannot remain still due to involuntary tremors or fear	• Thoroughly remove old gel before applying new gel. • Prepare the patient's skin before performing the test. • Reassure the patient about the test and stress the need to keep still, but be aware that patients with diseases that cause tremors may not be able to remain motionless.

SOMATIC MUSCLE TREMOR

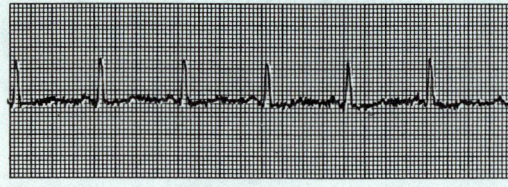

Artifact	Possible Causes	How to Prevent Problems
Alternating current artifact	• Improperly grounded ECG machine	• Check cables to ensure the machine is properly grounded before beginning the test.

AC INTERFERENCE

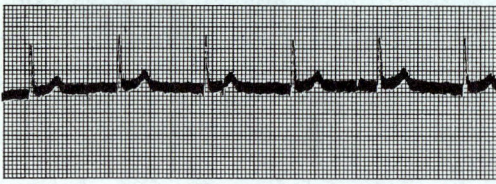

Artifact	Possible Causes	How to Prevent Problems
	• Electrical interference in the room	• Move the patient to an area that is free of interference or unplug any appliances in the immediate area for the duration of the test. If possible, set aside one room that is completely free of electrical appliances other than the ECG machine.
	• Dangling lead wires	• Arrange the leads along the contours of the patient's body and neatly support them on the table.

BOX 35-8

Patient Diary for Holter Monitoring

A patient with a Holter monitor must keep a diary of daily activities. When symptoms are experienced, the patient depresses an incident (or event) button on the machine, then records in the diary the activity that caused the incident and the resulting symptoms. At intervals, the patient also records daily activities such as working quietly at a desk, driving a car, eating a meal, watching television, or sleeping. All activities must be noted, including elimination, sexual intercourse, anger, laughter, and so on. Some monitors are equipped with small tape recorders so the patient can keep an audio diary instead of a written one.

Cardiac Stress Test

To measure the body's response to increased demands made on the myocardium, the physician may request a cardiac stress test. This is usually done on a treadmill, but it may also be done on a stationary bicycle (Fig. 35-16). The patient will be attached to an ECG monitor for a constant tracing. The medical assistant should never perform a cardiac stress test without the physician on site. The test is performed according to the physician's orders, and the ECG strip is mounted for the patient's record. Based on a positive or negative reading, this test may indicate the need for further cardiac testing.

In some instances, the physician may order a thallium scan to be performed with the stress test. Thallium 201, an isotope, is administered intravenously and localizes in the myocardium. A scintigraphy machine produces two-dimensional images of radioactivity in the tissues of the myocardium, instantly showing areas of decreased perfusion or "cold spots." These areas are diagnostic for occlusion of coronary arteries when a regular ECG or stress test may not be as exact. This is frequently the test of choice for patients who are unable to perform a standard stress test.

Checkpoint Question

10. What is the purpose of a cardiac stress test?

Echocardiography

An echocardiogram, or echo, uses harmless sound waves generated from a small device called a transducer. These waves travel through the cardiac chambers, walls, and valves and are then transmitted back

text continues on page 686

Charting Example

11/28/98	1400
	S: "I need my Holter monitor hooked up."
	O: Holter monitor ordered. Skin on the chest was shaved and the 5 electrodes were attached. A defatting agent was used to ensure adhesion. Baseline ECG done.
	A: Application of Holter monitor
	P: Oral and written instructions for maintenance and care of Holter monitor given. Instructions for diary completion given to patient. Scheduled to return in 24 hours for Holter removal. Patient verbalized understanding of all instructions. ————
	———————— Robert Steele, CMA

Procedure 35-3   Applying a Holter Monitor

Equipment/Supplies

- monitor
- fresh batteries
- roll of blank tape
- carrying case with strap
- electrodes
- skin swabs
- gauze
- razor (as needed)
- patient diary

Steps	Purpose
1. Assemble the equipment.	1. Fresh batteries and a whole roll of monitor tape will avoid battery failure and prevent the patient from running out of tape during the test.
2. Greet and identify the patient. Explain the procedure. Remind the patient that it is important to carry out all normal activities for the duration of the test.	2. Identifying the patient helps avoid errors in treatment. Explanations help gain patient compliance and ease anxiety. Avoiding a normal routine will not allow the physician to identify areas of concern.
3. Explain the purpose for the incident diary, emphasizing the need for the patient to carry it at all times during the test.	
4. Prepare the patient's skin for electrode attachment. Provide privacy and have the patient sit down. Expose the chest, then shave the areas of attachment as needed. Clean with the approved de-fatting agent to remove skin oils. Abrade the area with the gauze.	4. The chest must be exposed for proper placement of the electrodes. Shaving and abrading will improve adherence of the adhesive on the electrodes.
5. Apply the five special Holter electrodes at the specified sites: a. the right manubrium border b. the left manubrium border c. the right sternal border at the fifth rib level d. the fifth rib at the anterior axillary line e. the right lower rib cage over the cartilage as a ground lead. To do this, expose the adhesive backing of the electrodes and follow manufacturer's instructions to attach firmly. Check for security of attachment.	5. Products will vary, but all will require moist electrolyte and secure adhesive to ensure a full 24 hours of operation.

(continued)

<table>
<tr><td>**Procedure**
35-3</td><td>**Applying a Holter Monitor** (continued)</td></tr>
</table>

Steps

Purpose

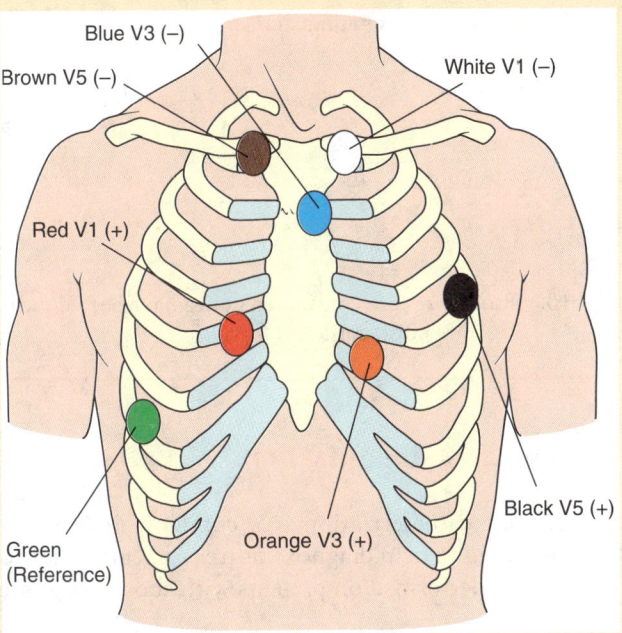

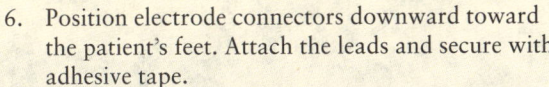

Step 5: Sites for Holter electrodes.

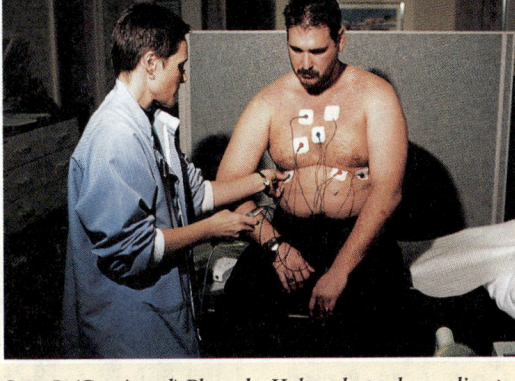

Step 5: (Continued) Place the Holter electrodes as directed by the manufacturer.

6. Position electrode connectors downward toward the patient's feet. Attach the leads and secure with adhesive tape.

6. The addition of adhesive tape over the connections will help ensure that the leads to not work loose during the day.

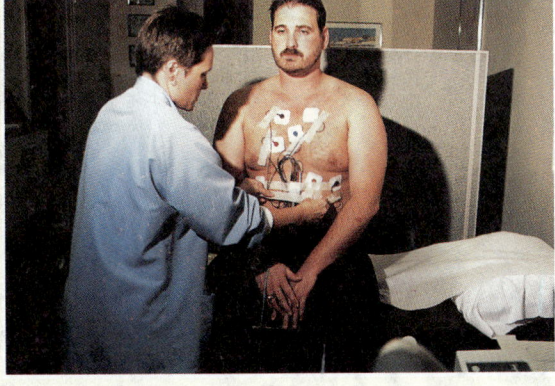

Step 6: Securely tape each electrode. Tape the lead wires to the patient's body.

7. Connect the cable and run a baseline ECG by hooking the Holter to the ECG with the cable hookup.

7. Do this to check for accurate function of the Holter.

(continued)

Procedure 35-3 Applying a Holter Monitor (continued)

Steps	Purpose
8. Assist the patient to redress carefully with the cable extending through the garment opening. Clothing that buttons down the front is more convenient.	8. This prevents pulling and strain on the leads.
9. Plug the cable into the recorder and mark the diary. If needed, explain the purpose of the diary to the patient again. Give instructions for a return appointment to evaluate the recording and the diary.	
10. Record the procedure in the patient's chart.	10. Procedures are considered not to have been done if they are not recorded.

to a screen where they can be viewed and interpreted. Echocardiograms help the physician to diagnose adult and pediatric patients with suspected or known valvular disease. Echoes also aid in diagnosing the severity of heart failure and cardiomyopathy, using the measurement of the ejection fraction of the heart. In addition, this test can be used to detect injuries to the heart in patients with trauma or in situations involving possible harvest of the heart for transplant after a fatal accident.

Cardiac Catheterization

Cardiac catheterization is a common invasive procedure used to help diagnose or treat a heart condition. It may be performed on patients with shortness of breath,

FIGURE 35-15
Monitors. (*Left*) A 30-day event monitor. (*Right*) A 24-hour Holter monitor.

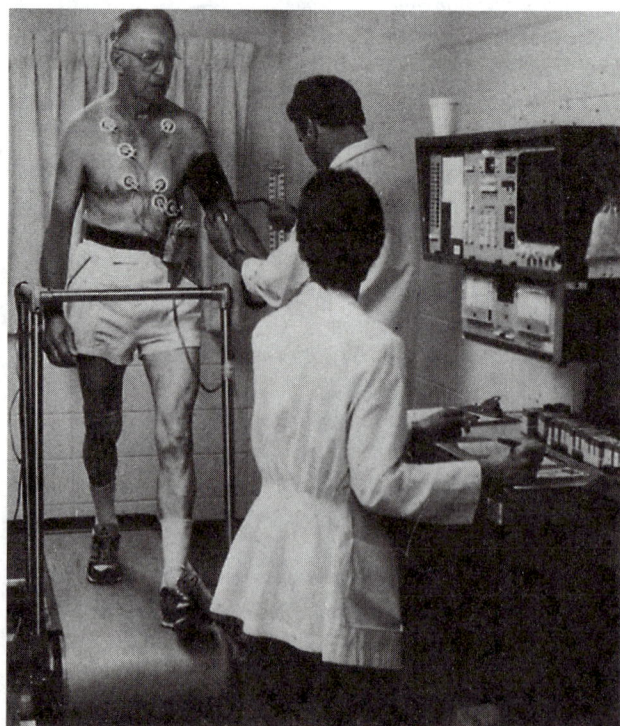

FIGURE 35-16
Walking a treadmill that moves at a progressively faster pace while the heart's activity is recorded, is a way of determining the heart's ability to adapt to increased work during exercise. (Courtesy of Borgess Medical Center, Kalamazoo, MI.)

angina, dizziness, palpitations, fluttering in the chest, rapid heartbeat, and other cardiovascular symptoms to determine the severity of the problem. It is often indicated after a cardiac stress test or echocardiogram reveals an abnormality.

The cardiologist inserts a flexible tube called a catheter into a blood vessel in either the arm or groin, then guides it gently toward the heart. When the catheter is in place, contrast medium is injected, allowing the heart's chambers, valves, great vessels, and coronary arteries to be visualized. If atherosclerotic plaques are found at this time, angioplasty may be performed (see Box 35-3).

Coronary Arteriography

This invasive procedure involves injecting a contrast medium into the coronary arteries located on the outer surface of the heart, allowing visualization of any lesions that may be present. It provides enough data for an accurate assessment of possible congenital or acquired heart disease. It also is frequently used to assess heart damage after myocardial infarction.

 ## SUMMARY

The circulatory system is a closed transport system kept in motion by the force of the heartbeat. The double pump called the heart propels blood through the four chambers of the heart, through the lungs and through the circulatory pathways. Nutrients are delivered to cells, cellular wastes are picked up and deposited at exit sites, hormones are directed to target cells, and disease-fighting mechanisms are transported to areas of concern. Malfunction in any part of the system interferes with the overall function.

Your responsibility for the cardiac patient includes obtaining a complete patient history, assisting with the physical examination, performing or assisting with diagnostic testing, and providing patient support.

 ## CRITICAL THINKING CHALLENGES

1. Draw a diagram of the heart. Draw a cardiac cycle as seen by the ECG. Connect the ECG waves to the appropriate areas of the heart. How would you explain an ECG to a patient? How would you assist the patient in relaxing for this procedure?
2. Compare and contrast the signs and symptoms of a cerebrovascular accident and a transient ischemic attack. Make a list of questions that you would ask a patient to determine if he or she is having a stroke. What kind of help would a patient need at home after experiencing a stroke?

3. Explain anemia and identify the symptoms seen with it. Why does anemia cause these symptoms? What dietary instructions should be given to a patient with iron deficiency anemia?

 ## ANSWERS TO CHECKPOINT QUESTIONS

1. The exchange of nutrients and oxygen occurs in the capillary beds.
2. There are four chambers in the heart. The upper chambers are the atria; the lower chambers are the ventricles.
3. The five components of the conduction system are: sinoatrial node, atrioventricular node, bundle of His, right and left bundle branches, and the Purkinje fibers. The sinoatrial node is the pacemaker.
4. Four predisposing factors for heart disease are history of elevated cholesterol, smoking, diabetes mellitus, and hypertension.
5. Stroke and renal failure may result from untreated hypertension.
6. Varicose veins occur when the superficial veins in the legs become swollen and distended.
7. With pericarditis, pain increases with inspiration and movement; pain in a myocardial infarction will not change with patient positioning.
8. A murmur is an abnormal heart sound.
9. P, QRS, and T waves represent a cardiac cycle on an ECG.
10. A cardiac stress tests measures the response of the myocardium to increased demands for oxygen.

 ## SUGGESTIONS FOR FURTHER READING

Akhtar, M. (1994). *Examination of the Heart—The Electrocardiogram.* Dallas, TX: American Heart Association.

Canobbio, M. M. (1990). *Cardiovascular Disorders—Mosby's Clinical Nursing Series.* St. Louis: C. V. Mosby.

Catalano, J. T. (1993). *Guide to ECG Analysis.* Philadelphia: J. B. Lippincott.

Davis, D. (1992). *How to Quickly and Accurately Master ECG Interpretation.* Philadelphia: J. B. Lippincott.

Kloner, R. A. (1995). *The Guide to Cardiology,* 3rd ed. LeJacq Communications.

Memmler, R. L., Cohen, B. J., & Wood, D. L. (1996). *The Human Body in Health and Disease,* 8th ed. Philadelphia: Lippincott-Raven.

(1992). *Professional Guide to Diseases,* 4th ed. Springhouse, PA: Springhouse.

Smeltzer, S., & Bare, B. (1996). *Brunner and Suddarth's Textbook of Medical-Surgical Nursing,* 8th ed. Philadelphia: Lippincott-Raven.

Thaler, M. S. (1995). *The Only EKG Book You'll Ever Need,* 2nd ed. Philadelphia: J. B. Lippincott.

Caring for Patients With Immune Disorders

Chapter Outline

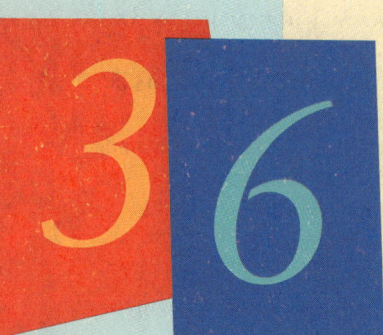

Structure and Function of the Lymphatic System
    Lymph
    Lymph Vessels
    Lymph Nodes and Nodules
    Tonsils
    Spleen
    Thymus
Common Lymphatic Disorders
    Lymphangitis
    Elephantiasis
    Lymphadenitis
    Mononucleosis
    Splenomegaly
    Hodgkin's Disease
    Lymphosarcoma
Functions of the Immune System

    Nonspecific Defenses
    Antigens and Antibodies
    Specific Defenses
    Types of Immunity
Common Immune Disorders
    Allergies
    Autoimmunity
    Immunodeficiency Diseases
Common Diagnostic Procedures and the Medical Assistant's Role
    Allergy Testing
    Laboratory Testing for Human Immunodeficiency Virus (HIV)
Summary
Critical Thinking Challenges
Answers to Checkpoint Questions
Suggestions for Further Reading

DACUM Components

1.3   Practice within the scope of education, training, and personal capabilities
2.2   Treat all patients with empathy and impartiality
4.1   Apply principles of aseptic technique and infection control
4.7   Assist physician with examinations and treatments
7.3   Teach patients methods of health promotion and disease prevention

Chapter Competencies

Learning Objectives

Upon successfully completing this chapter, you will be able to:

1. Spell and define the Key Terms.
2. Describe the circulation of the lymph fluid through the lymphatic system from the capillaries to the return of fluid to the circulatory system.
3. State the location and functions of the lymph nodes and nodules.
4. Explain the role of the thymus in immunity.
5. State the location and functions of the spleen.
6. List and describe disorders of the lymphatic and immune systems.
7. Identify laboratory tests and clinical procedures related to the lymphatic and immune systems.
8. Describe what is meant by the term immunity.
9. Describe and compare the types of immunity.
10. Describe the function of T cells and B cells in immunity.
11. Explain what a vaccine is and identify some of the common vaccines in use today.
12. Define HIV and AIDS.
13. Explain the methods of transmission and the impact of HIV and AIDS on the body.

Key Terms

(See Glossary for definitions.)

acquired immuno-
   deficiency
   syndrome (AIDS)
allergy
antibodies
antigen
antihistamine
attenuated
B cells
complement
didanosine (formerly
   dideoxyinosine, ddI)

ELISA
histamine
immune globulins
interferon
Kaposi's sarcoma
macrophage
opportunistic infection
phagocyte
phagocytosis
retrovirus
septicemia
T cells

titer
toxoid
vaccine
Western blot
zalcitabine
   (formerly
   dideoxycyti-
   dine, ddC)
zidovudine
   (formerly
   azidothymi-
   dine, AZT)

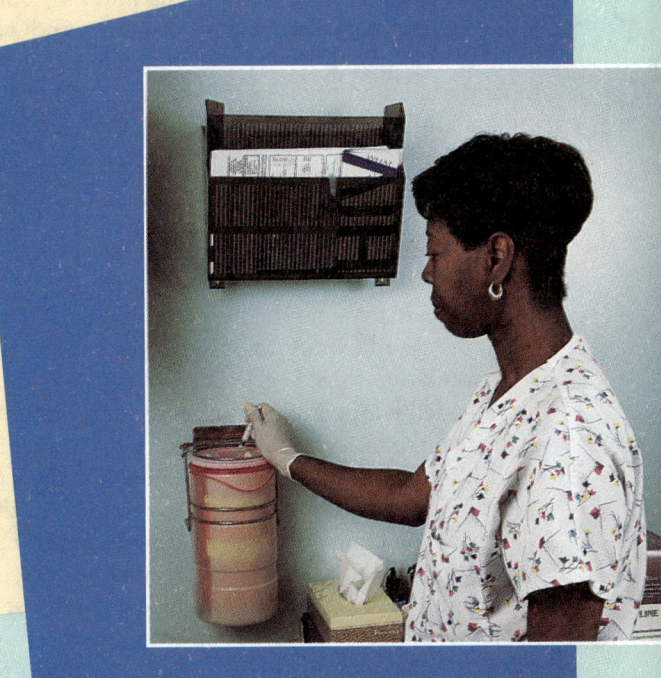

Our environment contains a large variety of infectious agents such as viruses, bacteria, fungi, and parasites. Any of these agents can cause pathologic damage, and if they are allowed to multiply unchecked, they may eventually kill their host. In a normal individual with an intact immune system, the majority of infections are of limited duration and rarely result in permanent damage. The lymphatic system and certain specifically designed blood cells make up the immune system and are responsible for protecting us from the pathogens in our environment. The lymphatic system is considered part of the circulatory system, and although its functions are different from those of the circulatory system, all of the functions of both systems are interdependent.

➤ STRUCTURE AND FUNCTION OF THE LYMPHATIC SYSTEM

Lymph

Clear, watery fluid filtered from the blood in the capillaries exchanges with fluid found in the interstitial spaces. Most of this fluid is reabsorbed by osmosis back into the blood in the capillaries. Some tissue fluid, however, remains in interstitial spaces and must be returned to the blood by the lymphatic system. As soon as the tissue fluid enters the lymphatic system through a lymphatic capillary, it is referred to as lymph. Lymph is similar to plasma and may contain a few erythrocytes, electrolytes, proteins, and variable numbers of lymphocytes, the white blood cells that function in immunity. The milky, fatty fluid brought to the system by the lymphatic vessels that surround the intestines is called chyle.

Lymph Vessels

The lymphatic system is a network of vessels to convey the excess fluid from the tissue spaces back to the general circulation (Fig. 36-1). These vessels begin as fine, blind-ended lymphatic capillaries made from one layer of flat epithelial cells. The capillaries act as wicks to absorb and filter fluid from around the cells. They do not join corresponding veins and arteries, like the capillaries of the circulatory system, but begin in pools of tissue fluid and join with larger lymphatic vessels.

Lymph vessels have thicker walls than those of the lymph capillaries. Like veins, lymph vessels contain valves so that lymph flows in one direction—toward the thoracic cavity. Lymphatic vessels include superficial and deep sets. The superficial vessels are immediately below the skin, often accompanying the superficial veins. The deep vessels are usually larger and accompany the deep veins. Lymphatic vessels carry lymph away from the regional nodes, eventually draining it into one of two terminal vessels: the right lymphatic duct or the thoracic duct.

The right lymphatic duct receives lymph from the right side of the head, neck, and thorax, as well as from the right upper extremity and empties into the right subclavian vein. The rest of the body is drained by the thoracic duct, which receives lymph from all parts of the body except those above the diaphragm on the right side. The thoracic duct empties into the left subclavian vein. Both ducts are separated from the general circulation by semilunar valves that prevent blood from entering the lymphatic system and prevent the backflow of lymph.

Lymphatic vessels are usually named according to their locations. For example, those in the breast are called mammary lymphatic vessels, those in the thigh are called femoral lymphatic vessels, and those in the leg are called tibial lymphatic vessels. The vessels that drain fatty chyle from the intestinal area are called lacteals because of the milky appearance of the fluid from this area.

Lymph Nodes and Nodules

Collections of stationary lymphatic tissue are called lymph nodes and nodules.

Lymph nodes (Fig. 36-2), sometimes incorrectly called lymph glands, are located along the path of the lymphatic vessels (Table 36-1). Afferent vessels bring fluid in; efferent vessels carry it away. Lymph nodes are designed to filter the lymph once it is drained from the tissues. They are rounded masses of lymph tissue varying in size from a pinhead to about 1 inch and occur from one or two to hundreds at a site. Inside the nodes are masses of lymphatic tissue with spaces designated for the production of lymphocytes and partitioned into compartments that bring the lymph fluid into contact with **macrophages**, cells that are responsible for **phagocytosis** of pathogens. Phagocytosis is the process by which cells engulf and digest microorganisms.

Lymph nodules are small masses of lymphatic tissue found just beneath the epithelium of all mucous membranes of the respiratory, digestive, urinary, and reproductive tracts. They bring macrophages and lymphocytes as close as possible to these barrier surfaces.

Checkpoint Question

1. What is the purpose of the lymphatic vessel system and the lymph nodes?

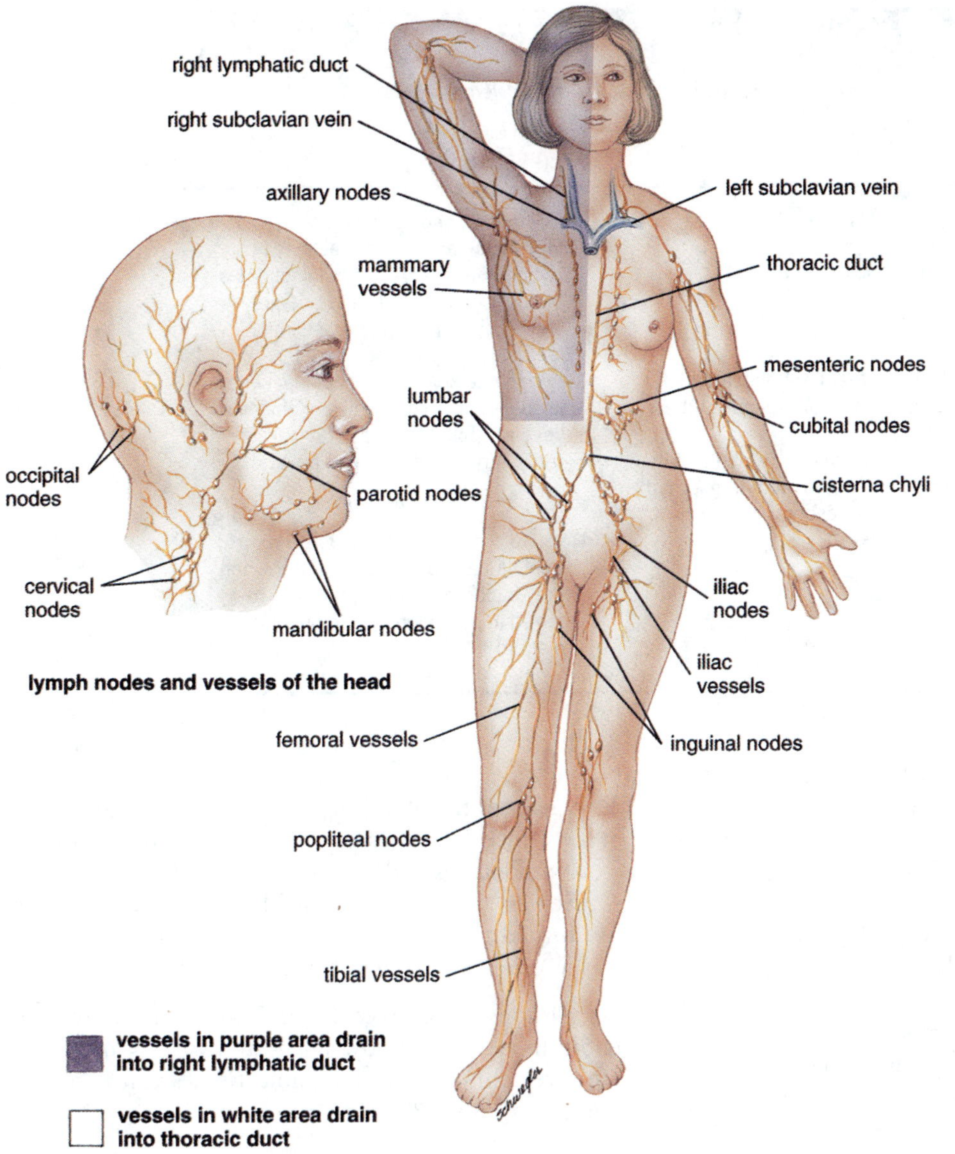

right lymphatic duct

right subclavian vein

axillary nodes

mammary vessels

left subclavian vein

thoracic duct

mesenteric nodes

cubital nodes

lumbar nodes

cisterna chyli

occipital nodes

parotid nodes

iliac nodes

cervical nodes

iliac vessels

mandibular nodes

lymph nodes and vessels of the head

femoral vessels

inguinal nodes

popliteal nodes

tibial vessels

■ **vessels in purple area drain into right lymphatic duct**

□ **vessels in white area drain into thoracic duct**

FIGURE 36-1
The lymphatic system.

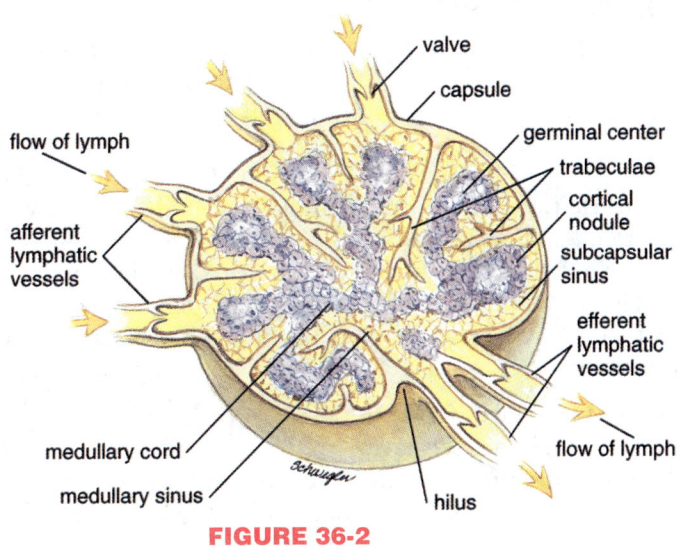

valve

capsule

germinal center

flow of lymph

trabeculae

cortical nodule

afferent lymphatic vessels

subcapsular sinus

efferent lymphatic vessels

medullary cord

medullary sinus

flow of lymph

hilus

FIGURE 36-2
Structure of a lymph node.

Table 36-1
Important Lymph Nodes, Locations, and Immune Responses

Nodes	Location	Immune Response
Cervical	Neck	Become enlarged during upper respiratory, facial, and scalp infections
Axillary	Axillae (armpits)	May become enlarged after infections of the upper extremities and breasts; cancer cells from the breasts often metastasize to axillary nodes
Tracheobronchial	Near the trachea and the larger bronchial tubes	May become solid masses of blackened tissue in patients who live or work in severely polluted areas
Mesenteric	Between the layers of the peritoneum that form the mesentery	Filter lymph from the abdominal and pelvic organs
Inguinal	Groin	Receive drainage from the lower extremities and external genitalia; when they become enlarged, they are referred to as buboes (as in bubonic plague)

Tonsils

Tonsils are the lymph nodules of the pharynx. The palatine tonsils are located on each side of the soft palate at the oropharynx. Pharyngeal tonsils are commonly referred to as adenoids and are located in the nasopharyngeal space on the back wall of the upper pharynx. The lingual tonsils are located at the base of the tongue. Any or all of these tonsils may become so loaded with bacteria (tonsillitis) that their removal is necessary. However, because the tonsils appear to function in immunity during early childhood, efforts are made to remove them only if absolutely necessary. (See Chap. 37, The Respiratory System, for a discussion of tonsillitis.)

Spleen

The spleen is located in the upper left quadrant of the abdominal cavity, just below the diaphragm and behind the stomach. The lower rib cage protects the spleen from physical trauma. The spleen contains lymphoid tissue designed to filter blood.

The spleen has several functions:

1. Destroys old red blood cells. As hemoglobin from the red blood cells is broken down, iron is salvaged and liberated into the bloodstream for reuse by the body.

2. Cleanses the blood by filtration and phagocytosis.
3. Produces all types of blood cells before birth and lymphocytes and monocytes in adulthood.
4. Serves as a reservoir for blood, which can be returned to the bloodstream in case of hemorrhage or other emergency.

Although the spleen is the largest mass of lymphoid tissue in the body, splenectomy is not ordinarily life-threatening; other lymphoid tissues can take over the spleen's function.

Thymus

The thymus is located in the upper thorax above the heart and behind the sternum. The thymus is thought to play a key role in the development of the immune system before birth and during the first few months of infancy. Certain lymphocytes (T cells) mature in the thymus gland before they can perform their functions in the immune system (see below). Usually by the age of 2 years, the immune system matures and becomes fully functional. By adolescence, the thymus undergoes involution and is replaced with adipose and connective tissue. It is insignificant in the adult.

All of the lymphoid tissues:

- Remove impurities such as carbon particles, certain cancer cells, pathogenic organisms, and dead blood cells through filtration and phagocytosis.

- Process lymphocytes. Some of these lymphocytes produce **antibodies**, which are substances in the blood that aid in combating infection; other lymphocytes attack foreign substances directly. This is explained later in this chapter.

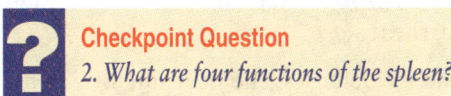

Checkpoint Question
2. What are four functions of the spleen?

➤ COMMON LYMPHATIC DISORDERS

Any disease of the lymphatic system is referred to as lymphadenopathy. Listed below are several of the more common diseases affecting the organs of the lymph system.

Lymphangitis

Lymphangitis is an inflammation of the lymphatic vessels. Red streaks may be seen extending along an extremity following the course of a lymph vessel, usually beginning in the region of an infected or neglected injury. If the infection is not treated by antibiotics, the lymph nodes may not be able to stop a serious infection and may allow pathogens to enter the bloodstream, causing **septicemia**, or blood poisoning. Streptococci are often the invading organisms in these infections. The disease is usually treated with antibiotics such as streptomycin.

Elephantiasis

Elephantiasis is characterized by enormous swelling of the legs and, in men, the scrotum. It is caused by small worms called filariae. These parasites, which are carried by insects such as flies and mosquitoes, invade the tissue as embryos then grow in the lymph channels, thus blocking the flow of lymph. The excessive swelling may cause affected individuals to become incapacitated. Elephantiasis is common in certain parts of Asia and the Pacific Islands. Diagnosis of filariasis can sometimes be made by observing the microfilariae in wet mounts or in Wright-stained smears of blood. There is no known cure.

Elephantiasis without an infectious process is sometimes seen as the result of metastasis into lymph nodes that block the return of fluid and cause swelling in the limb distal to the nodes.

Lymphadenitis

Lymphadenitis is an inflammatory condition that commonly results from an infection (eg, measles, septic sore throat, scarlet fever, diphtheria, common cold) or sometimes cancer. Symptoms include enlarged, tender lymph nodes. This enlargement is caused by increased drainage of bacteria or toxins from the infection into the nodes. The infection's site of origin can often be determined by the location of the affected node. For example, enlarged inguinal lymph nodes typically result from infections of the external genitalia; enlarged axillary nodes are caused by infections in the upper extremities or breast cancer. Treatment is directed at eliminating the primary infection.

Mononucleosis

Mononucleosis is caused by the Epstein-Barr virus and affects the entire lymphatic system. Symptoms include fatigue, asthenia (weakness), sore throat, and enlarged tender nodes in the cervical region and sometimes in the axillary and inguinal regions. Mononucleosis is usually transmitted by direct oral contact and primarily affects young adults. The diagnosis is usually made by blood test. The presence of more than 10% atypical T lymphocytes in the blood, and a total white blood cell count of 15,000 to 20,000 cells/mm are further signs of the disease. Recovery usually takes 4 to 8 weeks. As with any virus, treatment is symptomatic and palliative.

What If?
What if a mother voices concern over her teenage daughter's diagnosis of mononucleosis?

The mother may be concerned because mononucleosis has sometimes been referred to as the "kissing" disease. However, it is important to note that the virus is spread through contact with contaminated saliva, which can occur through other activities besides kissing (eg, sharing drinking cups).

Splenomegaly

Splenomegaly is an enlargement of the spleen. It is often associated with the destruction of blood cells and accompanies acute infections and diseases, including scarlet fever, typhus fever, typhoid fever, and syphilis.

It is considered a sign of disease rather than a distinct disease process.

Hodgkin's Disease

Hodgkin's disease is a malignancy characterized by lymphadenopathy, splenomegaly, fever, weakness, anorexia, and weight loss. It can originate in any lymphoid tissue but usually begins in the lymph nodes of the supraclavicular, high cervical, or mediastinal areas. It commonly affects young men. The diagnosis is often made by identifying a malignant cell (Reed-Sternberg cell) in the lymph nodes. If the disease is localized, the treatment of choice is radiotherapy using high-dose radiation. If the disease is more widespread, chemotherapy is given alone or in combination with radiotherapy. There is a high probability of cure with available treatments.

Lymphosarcoma

Lymphosarcoma, a malignant disease affecting lymphoid tissue, usually leads quickly to death. There is no known cause, but it is more common in men than in women. Symptoms include swelling of the affected nodes, usually painless, progressing to weight loss, fatigue, and malaise. Currently, the only cure is early surgery with radiotherapy. Diagnosis of lymphosarcoma is made by biopsy.

Checkpoint Question
3. In lymphadenitis, why do the lymph nodes become enlarged and tender?

➤ FUNCTIONS OF THE IMMUNE SYSTEM

The body is protected from the microorganisms around it by two types of defenses. These defenses can work against any invading pathogen (nonspecific defenses), or they may work against only a particular pathogen (specific defenses).

Nonspecific Defenses

The body's first line of protection involves the barrier defenses (as noted in Chap. 19, Asepsis and Infection Control). These can be mechanical or chemical in nature and include:

- Intact skin
- Respiratory barriers (eg, nostril hairs, cilia, and mucus)
- Enzymes of the digestive tract and acidity of the genitourinary tract
- Tears (which are slightly bactericidal)
- Protective reflexes (eg, coughing, sneezing, vomiting, and diarrhea)

After the barrier defenses, the next line of defense includes phagocytosis. When pathogenic organisms are found in the body by its immune surveillance system, phagocytes (cells that ingest and destroy microorganisms) are called to the site to ingest the pathogens. The phagocytes release proteins that attract other immune cells and cause a local inflammatory process. Macrophages from local tissue and from the bloodstream move in to clear away the dead cells and debris as the infection subsides.

When bacteria or viruses enter the body in sufficient numbers and overcome these phagocytic cells, the next line of defense consists of lymphocytes known as natural killer cells, which can destroy invading microorganisms.

Fever is another of the body's nonspecific defenses. Certain pathogens affect the heat-regulating mechanism of the hypothalamus causing it to reset itself higher that normal for the patient. Most pathogens prefer a body temperature of 97° to 100°F and find a higher temperature inhospitable for replication.

Inflammation is the body's effort to protect itself by limiting the effect of the disease process. Blood vessels in the area dilate, increasing the blood flow to the area and bringing with it extra phagocytes, oxygen, nutrients, and immunoglobulins. This increase in blood flow causes the skin to appear red. Vasodilation opens the walls of the capillaries allowing plasma fluid to escape causing edema (swelling). The edema presses against the nerve endings in the skin causing discomfort. Extra blood to the area causes the skin to feel warm to the touch.

Interferon, another nonspecific defense, is produced by cells infected with viruses. Viruses must be inside a living cell to reproduce, and although interferon cannot prevent the entry of viruses into cells, it does block the reproduction of infected cells. When this happens, viruses cannot replicate themselves and therefore the disease will not spread. Interferon is thought to be the self-limiting factor of many viral diseases and certain tumor cells (Box 36-1).

Antigens and Antibodies

Antigens are chemical markers that identify cells. Human cells have their own antigens that identify all the cells in an individual as "self" (autoantigen). When

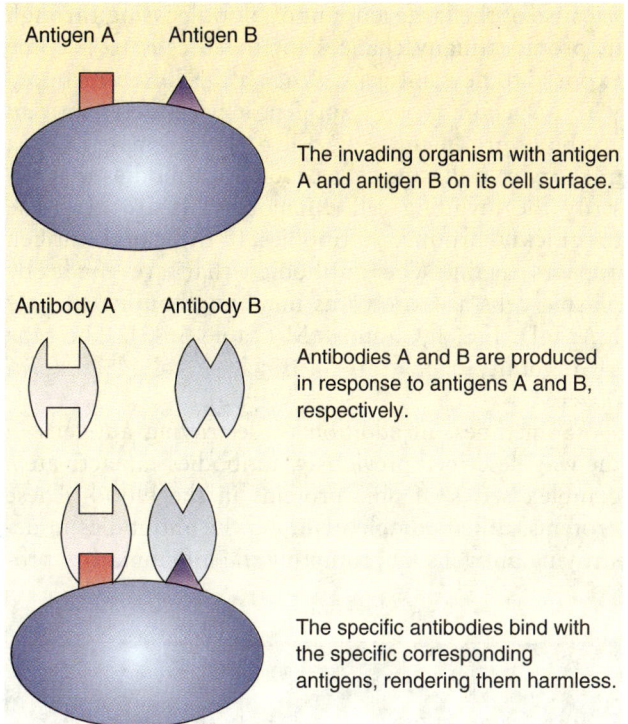

Antigen A   Antigen B

The invading organism with antigen A and antigen B on its cell surface.

Antibody A   Antibody B

Antibodies A and B are produced in response to antigens A and B, respectively.

The specific antibodies bind with the specific corresponding antigens, rendering them harmless.

FIGURE 36-3
Antibody specificity. Antibodies are produced by B-cell lymphocytes to bind with specific antigens.

BOX 36-1   Types of Interferon

There are three types of human interferon: alpha (α), beta (β), and gamma (γ). These were first produced in amounts sufficient for clinical research in the 1970s. At that time, there was hope that interferon would be an effective anticancer therapy, but results proved disappointing. Alpha interferon is effective, however, in the treatment of a rare form of leukemia called hairy cell leukemia, and has been approved for use in cases of genital warts and Kaposi's sarcoma.

Studies have shown that alpha interferon may be useful in the treatment of AIDS. When given in small doses and in combination with zidovudine (AZT), alpha interferon seems to block the reproduction of HIV, the virus that causes AIDS. This might be useful in people who are infected with HIV but who have no symptoms and might slow the progress of the infection.

antigens are foreign, or other than "self," they must be recognized as such during immune surveillance and destroyed. Bacteria, viruses, fungi, protozoa, malignant cells, and organ transplants are all foreign antigens that activate immune responses.

Antibodies, also called **immune globulins** or gamma globulins, are proteins produced by plasma cells in response to foreign antigens. Antibodies do not themselves destroy foreign antigens, but rather become attached to such antigens to label them for destruction. Each antibody produced is specific for only one antigen. It is estimated that as many as one million different antigen-specific antibodies can be produced (Fig. 36-3).

Several laboratory tests involving antibodies are useful in confirming a diagnosis, as described in Table 36-2.

Specific Defenses

Immunity is the body's specific defense against invading pathogens. Two types of lymphocytes—B cells and T cells—play a major role in immunity.

B Cells

B cells are lymphoid stem cells from the bone marrow that migrate to and become mature antigen-specific cells in the spleen and lymph nodes. Many immature B cells are found in the spleen, which,

Table 36-2
Antibody-Specific Laboratory Tests

Test	Purpose
Complement Fixation Test	Measures the severity of an infection and helps indicate the extent and effectiveness of antigen–antibody reactions occurring in the body.
Antibody Titer	Measures the amount of a specific antibody in the blood. If in several weeks there is an increase in the antibody level, the infection is identified as a current one.
Fluorescent Antibody Test	Antibodies are stained or marked by a fluorescent material, permitting rapid diagnosis of various kinds of infections.

because of the large amount of blood passing through it, provides many chances for the B cells to become exposed to new antigens. When a B cell is confronted with a specific type of antigen, it transforms into an antibody-producing cell called a plasma cell or a memory cell. Plasma cells produce antibodies that destroy the invading cell. Memory cells are available to quickly produce antibodies if the same antigen appears again. The antibodies that are made by plasma cells are known as immunoglobulins such as IgA, IgD, IgE, IgG, and IgM (Table 36-3). The type of immunity dependent on B cells is called *humoral immunity*.

Sometimes, in addition to destroying antigens in the way described previously, antibodies can activate a complex series of nine proteins in the blood. These proteins, called **complement**, aid the antibodies in destroying antigens by prompting the inflammatory process. They are responsible for the components of inflammation such as promoting vasodilation, attracting white blood cells to the area, destroying antigens, and preventing the spread of bacteria.

T Cells

T cells are lymphoid cells from the bone marrow that migrate to the thymus gland, where they develop into mature differentiated lymphocytes that circulate between blood and lymph. T cells are antigen specific, meaning that each one responds usually to only one antigen.

A type of immunity called *cell-mediated immunity* is dependent on T lymphocytes. If a T cell encounters an antigen, usually brought to it by a macrophage that has ingested it, the T cell has the ability to multiply rapidly and, in some instances, destroy the antigen, such as cancer cells, viruses, fungi, or bacteria. T cells also, unfortunately, react to beneficial foreign tissues, such as skin grafts and transplanted organs.

Activated T-helper cells secrete interleukin, a chemical that stimulates B cells and other T lymphocytes to destroy the invading antigen. T-helper cells also stimulate the production of interferon. Two other types of T cells are cytotoxic (killer) T cells and suppressor T cells. Cytotoxic T cells are directly responsible for the destruction of cells bearing antigens, such as tumor cells and tissue transplanted from an organ donor as noted above. Suppressor T cells regulate the amount of antibody produced by inhibiting the activity of B cells once the need for their production is no longer present.

Table 36-3
Immunoglobulins

Immunoglobulin	Properties/Functions
IgA	Found in exocrine secretions, such as milk, tears, mucous secretions Probably a protective device for mucosa
IgD	Plasma preparation from persons with a high concentration of Rh antibodies Given to an Rh-negative mother soon after delivery of an Rh-positive infant to prevent hemolytic disease of the newborn in subsequent pregnancies
IgE	Found in the mast cells of the respiratory and gastrointestinal tracts Important in allergic responses Elevated in the presence of an allergic response
IgG	Main immunoglobulin in human serum Produces antibodies for various pathogens Elevated in the presence of infection Activates complement to complete the immune response Frequently given to provide immediate, but temporary, immunity
IgM	Formed in the early stages of almost all immune reactions Controls the ABO blood group antibodies Helps to stimulate the production of complement

---

Checkpoint Question

4. *What are antigens? What does the body form in response to foreign antigens?*

Types of Immunity

Genetic Immunity

Genetic, or natural, immunity does not involve antibodies. Genetic immunity is programmed in the DNA. Some individuals are born with a natural, inherent immunity to certain diseases. Some pathogens invade certain host species but not others; this is called species immunity. For example, infections such as measles, scarlet fever, diphtheria, and influenza do not affect animals in contact with humans who have these illnesses. In the same way, many animal infections do not affect humans in contact with the animals that have these disorders (eg, chicken cholera, distemper).

Acquired Immunity

Acquired immunity involves antibodies. It may be natural or artificial and may be acquired either passively or actively.

- *Passive acquired natural immunity* is acquired from another source, such as transplacentally from mother to fetus or through breast milk to a nursing infant from a mother who has immune factors.
- *Passive acquired artificial immunity* is acquired through the injection of gamma globulins after presumed exposure. Gamma globulins are NOT **vaccines**. (A vaccine is a suspension of infectious agents given to establish resistance to an infectious disease.) Gamma globulins do not stimulate immune mechanisms but provide immediate antibody protection. Passive acquired artificial immunity is always temporary, lasting a few weeks to a

Table 36-4
Gamma Globulins

Globulin	Function
Tetanus immune globulin	Prevents tetanus in patients not currently immunized
Immune serum globulin	May prevent infectious hepatitis
Immune globulin Rh_0 (concentrated human antibody)	Prevents the formation of antibodies against the Rh factor in an Rh-negative mother after the birth of an Rh-positive fetus
Rabies antiserum (from humans or horses)	Used to treat victims of rabid animal bites

Table 36-5
The Importance of Vaccines

Disease	Vaccine
Pertussis	Protects against whooping cough; is given in conjunction with diphtheria toxoid and tetanus toxoid, all in one mixture referred to as DPT
Hepatitis B	Protects high-risk individuals, such as health care workers and ambulance personnel; now administered to infants as part of routine immunization
Measles, mumps, and rubella (MMR)	Protects against all three viruses; although each vaccine can be administered separately, immunity is conferred just as effectively with the triple vaccine. This vaccine should not be administered before 15 months of age
Influenza	Given annually to high-risk groups but has limited effectiveness in influenza epidemics because of the new strains of the virus that develop periodically
Haemophilus B (HiB)	Produces an immunity to *Haemophilus influenzae* and prevents *Haemophilus* B influenza meningitis; administered routinely during pediatric immunizations
Poliomyelitis	Usually given in live oral form, except in instances when a member of the patient's family is receiving immunosuppressive medication or is on antineoplastic (cancer) drugs; such individuals are at risk from the shedding of live poliovirus in the stool that occurs for several weeks after the administration of the oral polio form

Without vaccines, infant mortality in the United States would be high and death from childhood diseases would occur much more frequently. In certain parts of the world, however, this is still the case. Many developing countries still cannot afford extensive vaccination programs for their children. Although some of the diseases listed below may rarely be seen in general practice today, many still pose significant threats to the lives of millions of people throughout the world.

few months. Some examples of gamma globulins are noted in Table 36-4.

- *Active acquired natural immunity* is acquired through contracting a specific disease with production of antibodies and memory cells. Memory cells survive in the body for a long time and are ready to respond immediately when they encounter that same antigen again.
- *Active acquired artificial immunity* is acquired through administration of a vaccine, which stimulates production of antibodies and memory cells to prevent specific diseases. A vaccine contains an antigen to which the immune system will respond just as it would to the actual pathogen. Vaccines take the place of the first exposure to a disease. Types of vaccines are described in Table 36-5.

Vaccines can be made with organisms killed by heat or with live organisms. If live organisms are used, they must be nonvirulent for humans, or the organisms must be treated in the laboratory to weaken them. An organism weakened for use in vaccines is described as **attenuated**. A third type of vaccine is made from a form of the toxin produced by a disease organism. The toxin is altered with heat or chemicals to reduce its harmfulness, but it can still function as an antigen to induce immunity. Such an altered toxin is called a **toxoid**.

"Booster" shots are administered at intervals to maintain a high level (**titer**) of antibodies in the blood. In some cases, active immunity acquired by artificial means does not last a lifetime, making it necessary to "boost" the body's production of antibodies against a specific disease.

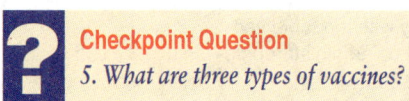

Checkpoint Question
5. What are three types of vaccines?

➤ COMMON IMMUNE DISORDERS

Allergies

An **allergy** is a hypersensitivity reaction (exaggerated response) to a particular foreign antigen, called an allergen. The reactions may be as mild as seasonal rhinitis (hay fever) or as severe as anaphylaxis (a total system collapse). Allergens include plant pollens, foods, chemicals, antibiotics, and mold spores. They may be inhaled, ingested, injected, or absorbed into the skin. Because of the complexity of the antibody response, the first contact builds the memory cells that will wait for the next contact with the allergen to produce a reaction.

In sensitive individuals, the antigen–antibody reaction may cause the release of excessive amounts of **histamine**, a substance found normally in the body in response to injured cells. The histamine causes an inflammatory reaction including vasodilation, increased capillary permeability resulting in edema. It may also cause contraction of involuntary muscles, particularly those in the bronchial tree. **Antihistamines** (medications that oppose the action of histamine) are sometimes effective in reducing the allergic reaction.

Autoimmunity

Normally the body is able to recognize those proteins that belong to its "self" and only produces antibodies when "foreign" proteins invade. Autoimmune diseases are conditions in which the body fails to recognize its own proteins and produces antibodies that will destroy its own cells and tissues. Some examples of autoimmune diseases include rheumatoid arthritis, chronic

BOX 36-2 History of AIDS

No other disease has ever generated such negative stereotyping as AIDS. Once thought of as a male homosexual disease, AIDS is now identified as a disease that can affect everyone. In fact, from 1990 to 1995, the number of reported AIDS cases among men who have sex with men fell from 55% to 42%, but the number of AIDS cases among heterosexuals increased from 6% to 11%.

AIDS was first diagnosed in the early 1980s. The Centers for Disease Control and Prevention (CDC) began officially recording cases of AIDS in 1981, but not by the name AIDS. (At that time, it was called "Gay Related Immune Deficiency.") In 1982, the CDC designated a new condition called AIDS and began formal surveillance.

In 1984, French researchers isolated what is now known as the human immunodeficiency virus (HIV); they called it lymphadenopathy-associated virus (LAV). At the same time, U.S. researchers isolated the same virus; they called it human T-cell lymphotropic virus type III (HTLV-III). The virus was officially called HIV in 1985.

As of December 1995, the CDC recorded 513,486 cases of AIDS in the United States. (This number included all cases starting from June 1981.) The CDC estimates that over 1 million individuals in the U.S. are currently infected with HIV.

thyroiditis, lupus erythematosus, and pernicious anemia. Diabetes mellitus, colitis, and multiple sclerosis are thought to be caused by autoimmune processes. At this time there is no cure for autoimmunity.

Immunodeficiency Diseases

Failure of any of the components of the immune system will result in an immune deficiency. This may be genetic and may be apparent soon after birth or it may be acquired as the result of a disease process. The deficiency may involve any part of the immune system and will vary in its severity.

Infantile Hypogammaglobulinemia

Infantile hypogammaglobulinemia, an inherited disorder, is passed by a carrier mother usually to a son. The immunoglobulins and B cells may be either absent or deficient, but the T cells are usually not affected. Infants with this disorder may retain transplacental immunity for several months but will then exhibit chronic, devastating infections. Diagnosis requires testing for immunoglobulins after about 9 months when inherited immunity is no longer a factor. Treatment involves injections

and transfusions of immunoglobulins. Prognosis is mixed and depends on the severity of the deficiency.

Acquired Immunodeficiency Syndrome (AIDS)

Acquired immunodeficiency syndrome (AIDS) is an example of an infectious disease that overwhelms the body's immune system. The human immunodeficiency virus (HIV) is the pathogen that causes AIDS by destroying T-helper cells and suppressing the body's cell-mediated immune response. HIV is a **retrovirus**, which means that it enters the cell, infiltrates the cell's RNA, and transfers its own DNA to the cell's DNA by means of an enzyme called transcriptase. The change in DNA prevents the affected cell from functioning normally; it can only function to nourish and incubate more HIV. The patient is predisposed to life-threatening infections and malignancies. Box 36-2 provides a brief overview of the history of AIDS.

The infectious diseases associated with AIDS are called **opportunistic infections** because HIV lowers resistance and allows opportunity for infection by bacteria, parasites, and abnormal cell development that are usually contained by normal defenses. Table 36-6 lists a number of opportunistic infections associated with AIDS.

Table 36-6
Opportunistic Infections Associated with AIDS

Infection	Description
Candidiasis	Yeast-like fungus that overgrows, causing infections of the mouth (thrush), respiratory tract, and skin
Cryptococcus	Yeast-like fungus causing lung, brain, and blood infections
Cryptosporidiosis	One-celled parasitic infection of the gastrointestinal tract, causing diarrhea, fever, and weight loss
Cytomegalovirus (CMV)	Virus causing colitis, pneumonitis, and retinitis
Herpes simplex	Viral infection causing small, painful blisters on the skin of the lips, nose, or genitalia
Histoplasmosis	Fungal infection from inhalation of dust contaminated with *Histoplasma capsulatum;* causes fever, chills, and lung infections
Mycobacterium avium-intracellulare	Bacterial disease with fever, malaise, night sweats, anorexia, diarrhea, weight loss, and lung and blood infections
Pneumocystis carinii pneumonia (PCP)	One-celled organism causing lung infection with fever, cough, chest pain, and sputum production
Toxoplasmosis	Parasitic infection involving the brain, lungs, and other organs and causing fever, chills, visual disturbances, confusion, hemiparesis, and seizures

Although a direct result of HIV infection, AIDS is a combination of several disease processes. Alone, none is considered to be specific to AIDS, but each of the signs and symptoms carries a reason for serious concern. Box 36-3 describes some of the signs and symptoms frequently associated with AIDS.

The incubation period for HIV infection can range from a few months to several years. An infected person may unknowingly spread HIV to others before any symptoms appear. HIV is not spread by casual contact. Transmission of HIV most often occurs through an exchange of blood or body fluids that may result from sexual contact, sharing contaminated needles, transfusions of contaminated blood, or accidental injury from sharp instruments used in invasive procedures. It also may be spread transplacentally from an infected mother to her infant.

A person with HIV may experience the following stages as the infection progresses to AIDS.

1. Acute infectious stage, with generally mild flulike symptoms
2. Latent period, without symptoms
3. Complaints of weight loss, lymphadenopathy, fever, diarrhea, anorexia, fatigue, and skin rashes
4. Onset of immunodeficiency disorders such as Kaposi's sarcoma and *Pneumocystis carinii* pneumonia (possibly the initial stages of full-blown AIDS)

Patients who are HIV positive are treated prophylactically based on laboratory data. One parameter

---

BOX 36-3 Signs and Symptoms Frequently Associated With AIDS

Malignancies: One of the malignancies associated with HIV is called **Kaposi's sarcoma**, a cancer arising from the lining cells of capillaries. Kaposi's sarcoma produces bluish red nodules on the skin, particularly on the lower limbs. Cancer of the lymph nodes, called lymphoma, is also associated with HIV infection.

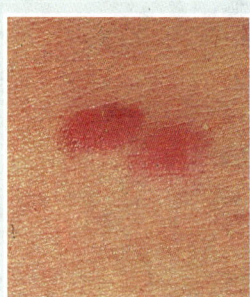 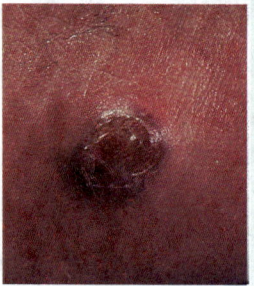

Periods of severe fatigue: Even though everyone experiences periods of some fatigue, these periods should not be prolonged or unexplained. Periods of extreme fatigue that last for more than several weeks should be considered a warning sign.

Sudden, unexplained weight loss: As a general rule, an unexplained weight loss of 10 lb. or more in less than 60 days should be cause for concern.

Night sweats or fever: Drenching night sweats and chills with fever often occur with AIDS as well as with tuberculosis and other serious illnesses.

Diarrhea: Diarrhea that persists for more than a week is common among AIDS patients.

Bruising or bleeding: The blood of an HIV-positive person has an unusually delayed clotting time. The HIV-positive patient will have a tendency to bleed or bruise easily; even minor injuries can result in severe bruising. The mucous membranes may bleed with no evidence or history of trauma or injury.

Coughing, shortness of breath, and other respiratory symptoms: Pneumocystis carinii pneumonia is a type of pneumonia associated closely with HIV infection. It begins as a cough, either dry or productive. If the patient is HIV positive, the cough will persist for weeks and lead to severe shortness of breath. The persistent cough may be accompanied by chills, fever, tightness in the chest, increased pulse, and increased respirations. *Pneumocystis carinii* pneumonia is considered to be the most frequent life-threatening opportunistic infection in persons with HIV.

Persistent generalized lymphadenopathy: When a person has AIDS, the lymph system is unable to process the infections associated with the disease. The lymph glands and nodes become enlarged in an effort to control the disease. Lymphadenopathy is manifested as enlarged, hard, painful nodes in various parts of the body.

Oral thrush: Candida albicans thrives in the suppressed immune system. Although AIDS patients frequently present with thrush, esophageal thrush is the most significant indicator of HIV infection. A condition called hairy leukoplakia often is observed in HIV-positive patients. This symptom presents as lesions on each side of the tongue with grayish white patchy discolorations.

Neurologic problems: Patients who are HIV positive often experience a variety of nervous system disorders including headaches, stiff neck, generalized pain, and weakness or numbness of the extremities. They have also experienced depression, delusions, hallucinations, paranoia, and dementia.

Patient Education: AIDS Prevention

When providing instructions about AIDS prevention, explain to your patient that it is safest, of course, to abstain from sex. However, if that is not feasible, instruct your patient to have sex only with a partner who is known not to be infected, who has sex with no one but the patient, and who does not use needles or syringes. Also tell the patient to use a latex condom and a spermicide if it is not known whether the sexual partner is infected.

Generally, instruct patients to:

- Avoid contact with another person's blood, body fluids, semen, or vaginal secretions.
- Avoid sharing needles or syringes, or any objects that come in contact with blood or body fluids.
- Avoid using alcohol or drugs. Use of these substances can hinder clear thinking and lead to unwise decision making.

---

that is continuously monitored is the CD4 count. The CD4 is a surface molecule on the T cell. When HIV enters the body, it attaches to these molecules and destroys them, causing the CD4 count to fall. Treatment begins as the CD4 count falls, whether or not the patient has symptoms. As the CD4 count falls further, prophylactic antibiotic therapy may be started. Three primary drugs are used to treat HIV and AIDS: **zidovudine (formerly azidothymidine [AZT]), zalcitadine and didanosine (formerly dideoxysine [ddI] and dideoxycytidime [ddC]).** These drugs work by blocking the growth of the virus after it enters the T cell. D4T, a new medication in the final stages of research trials, works by preventing the virus from entering the T cell. It is important to note that although these medications can help the patient, they also have significant side effects. Therefore, the physician will continuously monitor T-cell counts and other laboratory values.

As a medical assistant, you must be knowledgeable about AIDS, especially its transmission, both for your own protection and for the protection of your patients. In accordance with new guidelines issued by the Centers for Disease Control and Prevention (CDC), you must follow Standard Precautions when caring for all patients, regardless of their known or suspected infection status. (See Chap. 19, Asepsis and Infection Control, for a detailed discussion of Standard Precautions.)

A good understanding of this disease and methods for preventing its transmission will help prevent misinformation, rumor, apathy, and fear (Box 36-4). Additionally, obtaining an accurate medical history from patients at risk for HIV or AIDS is important. Table 36-7 offers some suggestions for interview questions.

Besides being informed about AIDS, you must also be aware of AIDS patients' need for compassion. Patients are sometimes abandoned by family and friends and shunned at work. You and other health care workers may provide the only personal contacts these individuals may have on a regular basis. You will need to foster a caring attitude that puts aside prejudices and value judgments. Special care should be given to individuals with organic brain damage who will need instructions and treatment information.

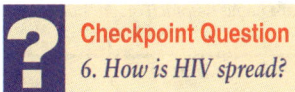

Checkpoint Question
6. How is HIV spread?

BOX 36-4   AIDS Facts

1. AIDS is caused by a virus called HIV.
2. People infected with HIV may look and feel healthy long before symptoms appear.
3. When symptoms do appear, they vary from person to person.
4. Most people who are HIV positive or who have AIDS became infected by having sex or sharing needles with someone who was infected.
5. You cannot "catch" HIV as you do a cold or the flu.
6. It is impossible for a donor to get HIV from giving blood or plasma.
7. The chances of contracting AIDS from a blood transfusion in the United States are now very low.
8. There are reliable blood tests for HIV.
9. So far, there is no vaccine for HIV or a cure for AIDS.
10. You can protect yourself from the virus by observing Standard Precautions.
11. Latex condoms can help prevent the spread of HIV.
12. People with HIV and AIDS need you to show them love and understanding.

Table 36-7
Obtaining an Accurate History from a Patient at Risk for HIV or AIDS

Instead of asking . . .	Ask . . .	Rationale
Do you have sex with prostitutes?	Have you ever paid for sexual activities?	Some patients may not admit to using a prostitute, but may acknowledge paying for sexual favors.
Do you do IV drugs?	Do you do skin popping? Steroid injections?	Some patients do not perceive skin popping or steroid injections as IV drug use.
Do you practice safe sex?	What method of safe sex do you use? Do you use a condom? Do you reuse condoms?	Some patients perceive using birth control as practicing safe sex; birth control offers no protection against HIV.
Are you a homosexual?	What is your sexual preference? Do you have sex with members of your same sex?	Some patients may not perceive themselves as homosexuals or do not want to be labeled.

A patient who is at risk for HIV or AIDS may be reluctant to provide you with an accurate social history. Here are some helpful hints for obtaining an accurate history.

➤ COMMON DIAGNOSTIC PROCEDURES AND THE MEDICAL ASSISTANT'S ROLE

Allergy Testing

As a medical assistant, your responsibility for allergy testing will vary with the practice. However, it will probably include obtaining a careful history of allergic episodes, setting up the allergens as ordered by the physician, and following up with patient education. Because of the potential for anaphylaxis, the administration of the test is usually done by the physician or a trained technician. An emergency setup must be close at hand during the complete process.

As noted in Chapter 30, Caring for Patients with Integumentary Disorders, allergy skin testing methods include scratch tests, intradermal injections, and patch tests. Diagnosis for the scratch, intradermal, and patch will be made by comparing the response to the specific allergen with a control substance administered in the same manner. Reactions are usually graded according to comparison with guides supplied by the manufacturers of the allergens.

Laboratory blood tests, which are more expensive and invasive, test for specific antibodies in the blood, usually ingestants. You may be responsible for collection and transportation of blood specimens.

Laboratory Testing for Human Immunodeficiency Virus (HIV)

ELISA, or enzyme-linked immunosorbent assay, is used to screen blood for antibodies to the AIDS virus. A pos-

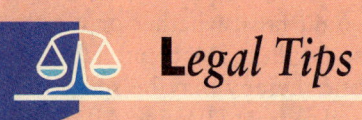

Legal Tips

Testing for HIV has many legal implications. The laws vary from state to state, but they generally hold that:

- Patients must sign an informed consent form before being tested.
- Pre- and posttest counseling (usually by a state-approved HIV counselor) is required, regardless of the test results.
- Results cannot be given over the telephone. Most laws have specific standards that state who, when, and how results can be given.
- Utmost care must be given to ensure patient confidentiality. Most laboratory settings will use a patient coding system rather than the patient's name on the requisition slip to ensure privacy.
- Laboratories that test for HIV must be approved by the state for this testing.

itive result indicates probable exposure to the virus and the possibility that the virus is in the blood. Since false-positive results can occur with the ELISA test, the Western blot test is used to confirm positive findings and is considered to be diagnostic. Your responsibility in this testing is usually confined to collecting the specimen by phlebotomy and routing it to the proper laboratory.

SUMMARY

An intact immune system is our best protection against constant exposure to microorganisms that are potentially dangerous to our health. The medical setting is understandably especially high risk for transmission of pathogens. An understanding of the interaction of our natural defenses and proper Standard Precautions as outlined by CDC will prevent the spread of the multitude of microorganisms that are endemic to the medical profession.

CRITICAL THINKING CHALLENGES

1. Your patient has been diagnosed with breast cancer. Why would it be important to biopsy lymph nodes in the axillary area?
2. Why might the removal of lymph vessels from a region, such as the axillary area, cause edema of the area drained by those nodes? How might you help your patient understand this concept?
3. The mother of your pediatric patient questions the need for booster shots for her son. How would you impress on her the importance of immunization boosters? Explain in terms that a lay person would understand.

ANSWERS TO CHECKPOINT QUESTIONS

1. The lymphatic vessels return excess fluid from the tissues back to circulation. The lymph nodes filter the lymph once it is drained from the tissues.
2. The spleen destroys old red blood cells, cleanses the blood, produces blood cells, and serves as a reservoir for blood.

3. Lymphadenitis usually results from an infection. The enlarged lymph nodes are caused by increased drainage of bacteria or toxins from the infection into the nodes.
4. Antigens are chemical markers that identify cells. Foreign antigens must be destroyed. The body forms antibodies that attach to these antigens, marking them for destruction.
5. Three types of vaccines are live, attenuated, and altered toxin (toxoid).
6. HIV is transmitted through an exchange of blood or body fluids that may result from sexual contact, sharing contaminated needles, transfusions, or accidental injury from sharp instruments used in invasive procedures. It also can be transmitted transplacentally from infected mother to infant.

SUGGESTIONS FOR FURTHER READING

American Red Cross. (1992). *HIV and AIDS*.

Blood Borne Pathogens, OSHA Inst. 29CFR 1910.1030.

Bullock, B. L., Rosendahl, P. P. (1992). *Pathophysiology*, 3rd ed. Philadelphia: J. B. Lippincott.

Centers for Disease Control and Prevention. (199). Recommendations for prevention of HIV transmission in the health care setting. *MMWR*

Fischbach, F. (1992). *A Manual of Laboratory and Diagnostic Tests*, 4th ed. Philadelphia: Lippincott-Raven Publishers.

Fischbach, F. (1995). *Quick Reference for Laboratory and Diagnostic Tests*. Philadelphia: Lippincott-Raven Publishers.

Hamann, B. (1994). *Disease: Identification, Prevention and Control*. St. Louis: Mosby-Yearbook.

Memmler, R., Cohen, B., & Wood, D. (1996). *The Human Body in Health and Disease*, 8th ed. Philadelphia: Lippincott-Raven Publishers.

Porth, C. M. (1994). *Pathophysiology: Concepts of Altered Health States*, 4th ed. Philadelphia: Lippincott-Raven Publishers.

Professional Guide to Diseases, 4th ed. (1992). Springhouse, PA: Springhouse Corporation.

Staines, N., Brostoff, J., & James, K. (1993). *Introducing Immunology*. London: Mosby-Yearbook.

Caring for Patients With Respiratory Disorders

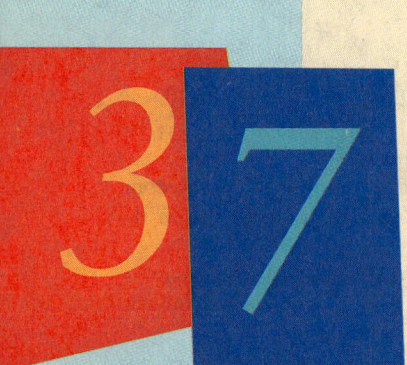

Chapter Outline

Structure and Function of the Respiratory System
Organs of the Respiratory System
  Airways
  Lungs
Ventilation
  Inspiration
  Expiration
Respiration
  External Respiration
  Internal Respiration
Defense Mechanisms of the Respiratory System
Common Respiratory Disorders
  Upper Respiratory Disorders
  Lower Respiratory Disorders
  Common Cancers

Common Diagnostic Procedures and the Medical Assistant's Role
  Physical Examination of the Respiratory System
  Throat Culture
Procedure: Collecting a Specimen for a Throat Culture
  Sputum Culture or Cytology
Procedure: Collecting a Sputum Specimen
  Chest X-rays
  Bronchoscopy
  Pulmonary Function Tests
  Arterial Blood Gases
Summary
Critical Thinking Challenges
Answers to Checkpoint Questions
Suggestions for Further Reading

DACUM Components

1.3 Practice within the scope of education, training, and personal capabilities
1.6 Conduct oneself in a courteous and diplomatic manner
2.2 Treat all patients with empathy and impartiality
4.1 Apply principles of aseptic technique and infection control
4.7 Prepare patients for procedures
4.10 Collect and process specimens
5.1 Document accurately

Chapter Competencies

Learning Objectives

Upon successfully completing this chapter, you will be able to:

1. Spell and define the Key Terms.
2. List and explain the primary functions of the respiratory system.
3. Label a diagram of the organs of the respiratory system.
4. List and discuss the function of each part of the airways, from the nares to the alveoli.
5. Discuss the structure and function of the lungs.
6. Explain the process of ventilation in relation to Boyle's law.
7. Discuss and explain the processes of external and internal respiration.
8. List the primary defense mechanisms of the respiratory system.
9. List and describe disorders of the respiratory system.
10. Identify and explain diagnostic procedures of the respiratory system and state the medical assistant's responsibilities where applicable.
11. Describe the physician's examination of the respiratory system and state the medical assistant's responsibilities in assisting with this procedure.

Performance Objectives

Upon successfully completing this chapter, you will be able to:

1. Collect a specimen for throat culture (Procedure 37-1).
2. Collect a sputum specimen for culture or cytologic examination (Procedure 37-2).

Key Terms

(See Glossary for definitions.)

alveolar-capillary membrane	dyspnea	respiration
aspiration	endotracheal tube	status asthmaticus
atelectasis	epiglottis	stoma
carina	eustachian tubes	thoracentesis
cilia	hemoptysis	tonsils
chronic obstructive pulmonary disease (COPD)	iatrogenic	tracheostomy
	laryngectomy	tracheotomy
	mediastinum	turbinates
diaphragmatic excursion	palliative	
	pleura	

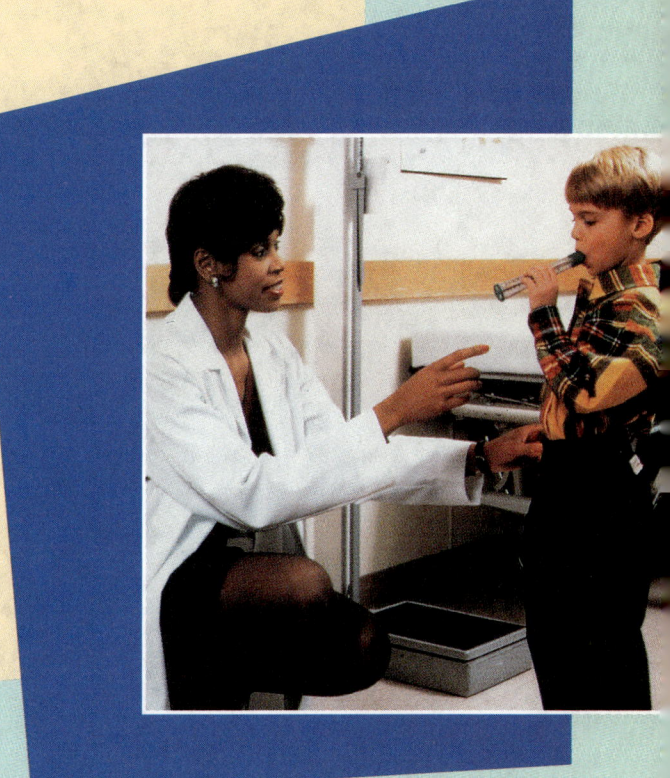

The respiratory system provides the body with the oxygen that every cell needs to perform its designated function. It also eliminates from the body one of the waste products of cellular metabolism, carbon dioxide. The respiratory system works closely with the cardiovascular system in performing this function. Oxygen is carried by the blood, which is pumped by the heart through the blood vessels to reach every cell. When a cell is deprived of oxygen for a period of time, it dies. The processes involved in getting oxygen to the cells include ventilation and **respiration** (gas exchange), which can be external and internal. These processes are discussed later in this chapter.

➤ STRUCTURE AND FUNCTION OF THE RESPIRATORY SYSTEM

Figure 37-1 shows the major organs of the respiratory system. These include the nose, sinuses, mouth, pharynx (the mouth and pharynx are shared with the digestive system), larynx, trachea, airways, and the lungs. The mouth, nose, pharynx, larynx, trachea, and conducting airways serve simply as a passageway for fresh air that is warmed and filtered to enter the lungs and for exhaled air, rich in carbon dioxide, to leave the body. Within the lungs, the exchange of gases occurs between the lung fields and the blood. These processes are described in more detail below.

The major function of the respiratory system is to supply oxygen to the bloodstream for delivery to the cells and to eliminate carbon dioxide from the body. The respiratory system also eliminates water from the body. In addition, parts of the system are involved in the sense of smell and in speech.

Checkpoint Question
1. What are the functions of the respiratory system?

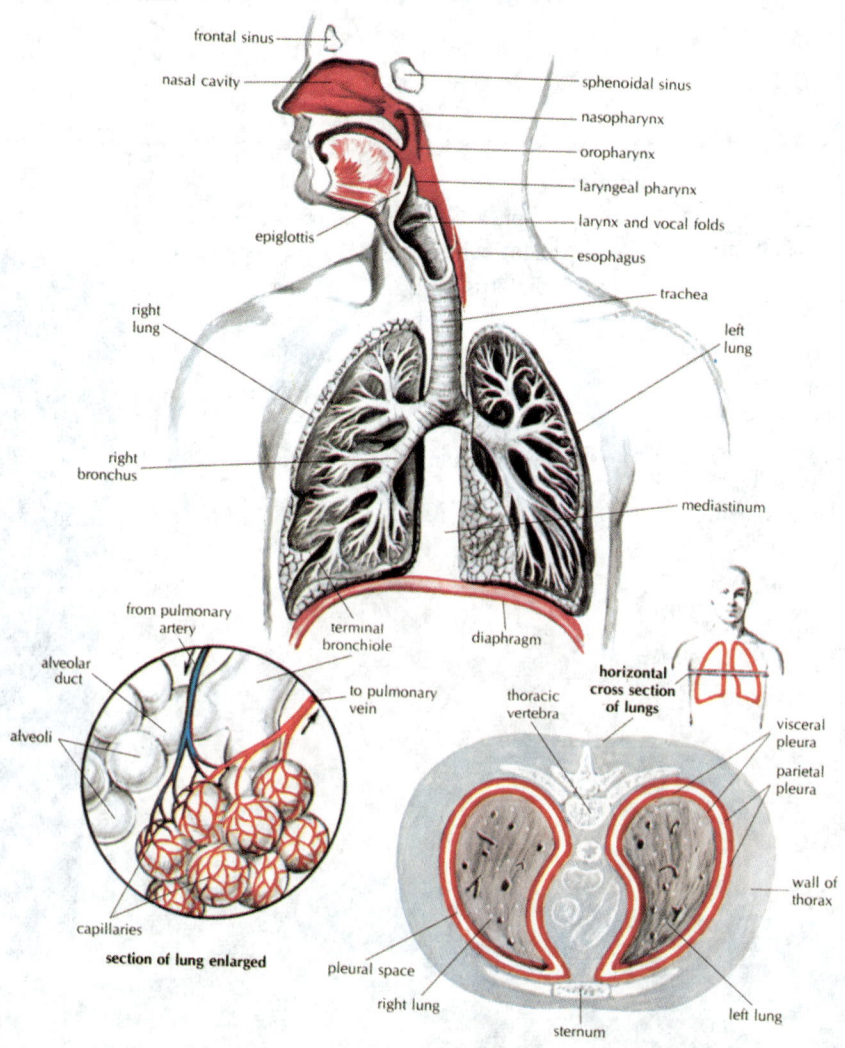

FIGURE 37-1
The respiratory system.

➤ ORGANS OF THE RESPIRATORY SYSTEM

Airways

Using the illustration of the respiratory system (see Fig. 37-1), follow the path of the air as it enters and passes the structures on its way to the lung fields. The mechanism of air movement is discussed later.

Nose

Usually, air enters the body through the nose. The external nose is formed by bone and cartilage and has two openings in its anterior surface called nares or nostrils. As the air enters, it is filtered by hairs within the nasal cavity. The walls of the nasal cavity contain bony projections called **turbinates**, which increase the surface area and whirl the air around to allow it to be warmed and humidified by the mucous membranes that line the cavity.

Paranasal Sinuses

The paranasal sinuses are hollow cavities in the bones around the nose, which are lined with mucous membrane (Fig. 37-2). There are four pairs of paranasal sinuses (Table 37-1). The paranasal sinuses have several functions including providing mucus that drains through a duct to the nasal cavity, acting as a resonating chamber for speech, and lightening the bones of the skull. The sinus ducts are somewhat narrow and, if

they swell shut because of infection, can cause pain and pressure in the areas around the eyes, nose, cheeks, and forehead. The paranasal sinuses do not conduct air to the lungs but are important accessory structures.

Mouth

The structures of the mouth are discussed in detail in Chapter 38, Caring for Patients with Gastrointestinal Disorders, and therefore are not included here. The mouth provides an alternate passageway for air if the nose is blocked for some reason. Some people breathe through their mouths out of habit.

Pharynx

The pharynx (throat) serves the dual purpose of providing a passageway for food and drink to the digestive tract via the esophagus and air to the respiratory tract via the larynx. It can be divided into three sections: the nasopharynx (posterior to the nasal cavity), the oropharynx (posterior to the oral cavity), and the laryngopharynx (the most inferior section).

The pharynx contains several important structures. The eustachian tubes, which connect the nasopharynx with the middle ear, allow the pressure between the atmosphere and the area between the eardrum and the inner ear to equalize. These tubes also provide a route for infection to spread from the throat to the middle ear. These infections are more common in young children whose eustachian tubes are more horizontal than those of adults. Also within the phar-

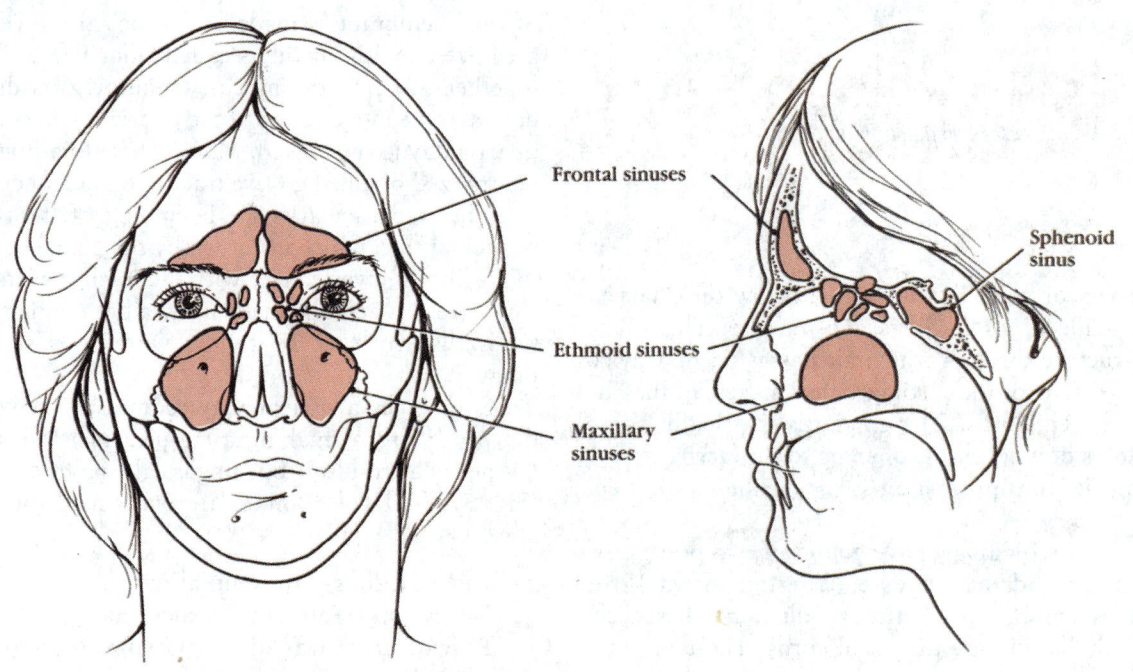

FIGURE 37-2
Location of paranasal sinuses.

Table 37-1 Paranasal Sinuses	
Name	**Location**
Frontal	Located just above the brow ridge on each side of the nasal bridge
Sphenoid	Within the sphenoid bone at the base of the skull, between the occipital and ethmoid bones in front and the parietal and temporal around its sides
Ethmoid	Within the spongy bone that forms the roof of the nasal cavity and part of the floor of the skull
Maxillary	Paired sinuses within the bones that form the floor of the orbits and the sides of the nasal cavities

ynx are three sets of **tonsils** (lymphoid tissue). These include:

- Pharyngeal tonsils (also known as adenoids)
- Palatine tonsils (at the back of the oral cavity; ones commonly referred to as tonsils)
- Lingual tonsils (at the base of the tongue)

The tonsils are made of lymphoid tissue and are designed to prevent infection from spreading to the lower respiratory tract. If the tonsils are overwhelmed by the virulence of the infection they are trying to contain, they also may become a site of infection, especially in children.

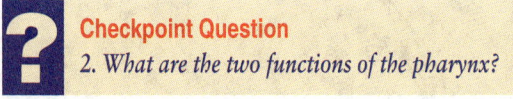

? Checkpoint Question
2. What are the two functions of the pharynx?

Larynx

The larynx or voice box is located below the pharynx and is made up of cartilage and muscles. This is the next structure through which air passes on its way to the lungs. One of the cartilages that makes up the larynx is the **epiglottis**. The epiglottis is a leaflike flap that closes down over the opening to the larynx during swallowing, thus preventing solids or liquids from entering the airway.

Besides providing a passage for air and preventing aspiration (solids or liquids entering the airway), the larynx is important in the production of speech. Within the larynx are the vocal cords. These are tendons that are tightly stretched across the opening of

the airway in the shape of a V. They can vibrate like the strings of a violin, producing sound as air passes over them. The pitch of the sound produced is regulated by tightening the vocal cords (for a higher pitch) or relaxing them (for a lower pitch). The loudness of the sounds produced is regulated by how fast or hard air is forced through the vocal cords.

Another of the large cartilages of the larynx is the thyroid cartilage or Adam's apple. This cartilage can be felt moving up and down while swallowing. This is due to the movement of the epiglottis as it closes over the larynx.

Trachea

The trachea (sometimes referred to as the windpipe) is a tube that extends from the larynx in the neck down into the chest. The trachea conducts air down to the bronchi that then take it into the lungs. It is about 1 inch wide and 5 inches long and is anterior to the esophagus. It is rigid on three sides due to the presence of many C-shaped cartilage rings that are placed with the open end of the C facing posteriorly, toward the esophagus. The rings are connected to each other by bits of soft tissue to allow the neck to bend in all directions. The front of the trachea is rigid so that the airway will stay open, even when the neck is struck or bumped. The back is more flexible to allow a large bolus of food to pass down the esophagus without catching.

The trachea is lined with a mucous membrane containing special cells and glands that produce mucus. This mucus is designed to trap any dust or other particles inhaled on its sticky surface. The innermost layer of this membrane is made up of specialized cells that are covered with tiny hairs called **cilia**. These cilia beat together to cause the mucus, containing its dust and debris, to be moved toward the pharynx where about a quart a day is swallowed. Many inhaled pathogens are neutralized by the digestive tract in this manner.

The trachea marks the beginning of the tracheobronchial tree, which is known by this name because it looks like an inverted tree with the trachea as its trunk. This "tree" is actually made up of a branching series of tubes that conduct air to the working parts of the lungs.

Sometimes a patient may require a **tracheotomy**, the procedure of making a surgical incision into the trachea. The resulting opening is called a **tracheostomy** (Fig. 37-3). Tracheotomies are performed for various reasons:

- Facilitate long-term ventilation
- Relieve upper airway obstruction
- Provide an airway after a **laryngectomy** (removal of the larynx) has been performed

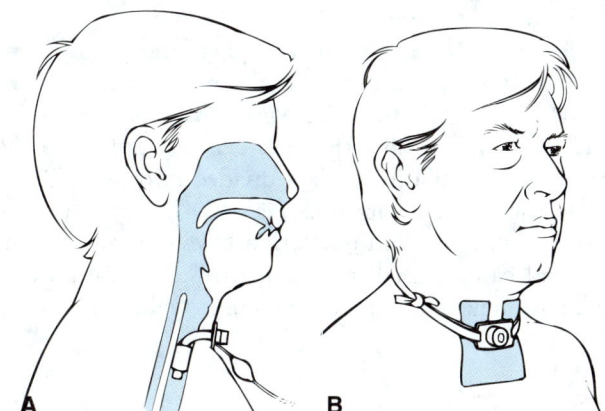

FIGURE 37-3
Pictured are a sagittal view (**A**) and a frontal view (**B**) of a tracheostomy tube in place.

- Facilitate suctioning in a patient who is unable to cough effectively
- Decrease "dead space ventilation" in patients with **chronic obstructive pulmonary disease (COPD)**, a progressive disorder of diminished respiratory capacity

Tracheostomies may be temporary or permanent, and the patient may or may not have a tracheostomy tube in the **stoma**, or opening. The area around a tracheostomy needs to be kept very clean and tracheostomy tubes need to be changed or cleaned regularly.

Checkpoint Question
3. How are inhaled particles trapped in the trachea and then neutralized?

Bronchi and Bronchioles

The trachea splits at about the level of the second ribs into two large tubes called the right and left mainstem bronchi. These bronchi enter the right and left lungs and continue to branch again and again, with the tubes getting narrower each time they branch. The larger tubes are called bronchi and contain smooth muscle and some cartilage. As the tubes get smaller, the cartilage diminishes but they still have the smooth muscle. When something irritates the airways, this smooth muscle constricts, narrowing the opening to prevent the irritant from traveling any further in the airway. This is the same type of constriction (bronchoconstriction) that is partly responsible for asthma attacks.

The airways branch approximately 27 times. When the tubes reach about 1 mm or less in diameter,

they are called bronchioles. Bronchioles also have smooth muscle in their walls and conduct air down to the tiny grapelike sacs called alveoli.

Alveoli

Alveoli are tiny sacs whose thin walls are only one cell thick. They are covered with thin-walled capillaries and are the site of gas exchange in the lungs. Oxygen diffuses through the wall of the alveolus (singular) into the blood, and carbon dioxide diffuses out of the blood into the alveolus where it can be exhaled. The bulk of the lung tissue is made up of these little air sacs, which gives the lungs their spongelike appearance. There are approximately 300 million alveoli in the lungs of an adult. Their shape makes them specialized to provide as much area as possible for gas exchange. If all the alveoli in a pair of lungs were flattened out, they would cover a tennis court!

The alveoli also contain specialized cells that produce a substance called surfactant, which lines the alveoli and keeps them from collapsing with every expiration. Premature infants frequently lack surfactant in their lungs. This is the major cause of the respiratory distress syndrome often seen in these infants.

Checkpoint Question
4. After air enters the nose, what other structures must it pass through before oxygen can be diffused into the blood?

Lungs

The lungs are large, spongy organs located in the chest or thoracic cavity. They are somewhat cone shaped, with the broad base of each cone resting on the diaphragm (the dome-shaped muscle that separates the thoracic and abdominal cavities) and the apex (point) extending up above the clavicles. The heart is nestled between the lungs, in a cavity called the **mediastinum**.

The right lung is broader and thicker than the left, due to the presence of the liver below the diaphragm on the right side. This causes the right diaphragm to be somewhat higher than the left. The right lung is divided into three lobes or sections; the left lung has only two lobes. Each lobe of the lung is separate from the other and is attached by a separate bronchus to the tracheobronchial tree. If one lobe of the lung is severely damaged or diseased (eg, with cancer), it can be surgically removed without affecting the other lobes.

The lungs are enclosed in a serous membrane called the **pleura**. The visceral pleura covers the surface of the lungs; the parietal pleura lines the internal surface of the chest cavity and the top of the diaphragm. These two membranes normally are stuck together with a thin layer of fluid between them, just as two flat pieces of glass will stick together if there is a layer of water between them. (Try this with two glass slides. There is a negative pressure between the slides that makes them stick together.) These two membranes are important in the process of ventilation.

➤ VENTILATION

Ventilation is the movement of gases from the atmosphere to the alveoli and from the alveoli back into the atmosphere. The path these gases take as they move through the upper airways and lungs has been discussed above, but what makes these gases move? To understand the forces that cause this movement of gas, it is necessary to understand one of the basic physical laws governing gas, Boyle's law.

Boyle's law states that when gases are kept at the same temperature, if the volume holding the gas is increased, the pressure of the gas will decrease. Conversely, if the volume is decreased, the pressure will increase. Consider how this law can be applied to the process of ventilation as it is divided into two phases, inspiration and expiration (Fig. 37-4). Note that the terms inspiration and inhalation have the same meaning and can be used interchangeably. Expiration and exhalation have the same meaning as well.

Inspiration

Inspiration involves the movement of air from the atmosphere into the lungs. In the medulla of the brain stem is a respiratory center, which periodically sends a signal by way of the nerves to the muscles of inspiration as the level of carbon dioxide builds up in the blood. The major muscle of inspiration is the diaphragm, which is innervated by the phrenic nerve. When the diaphragm gets a signal from the respiratory

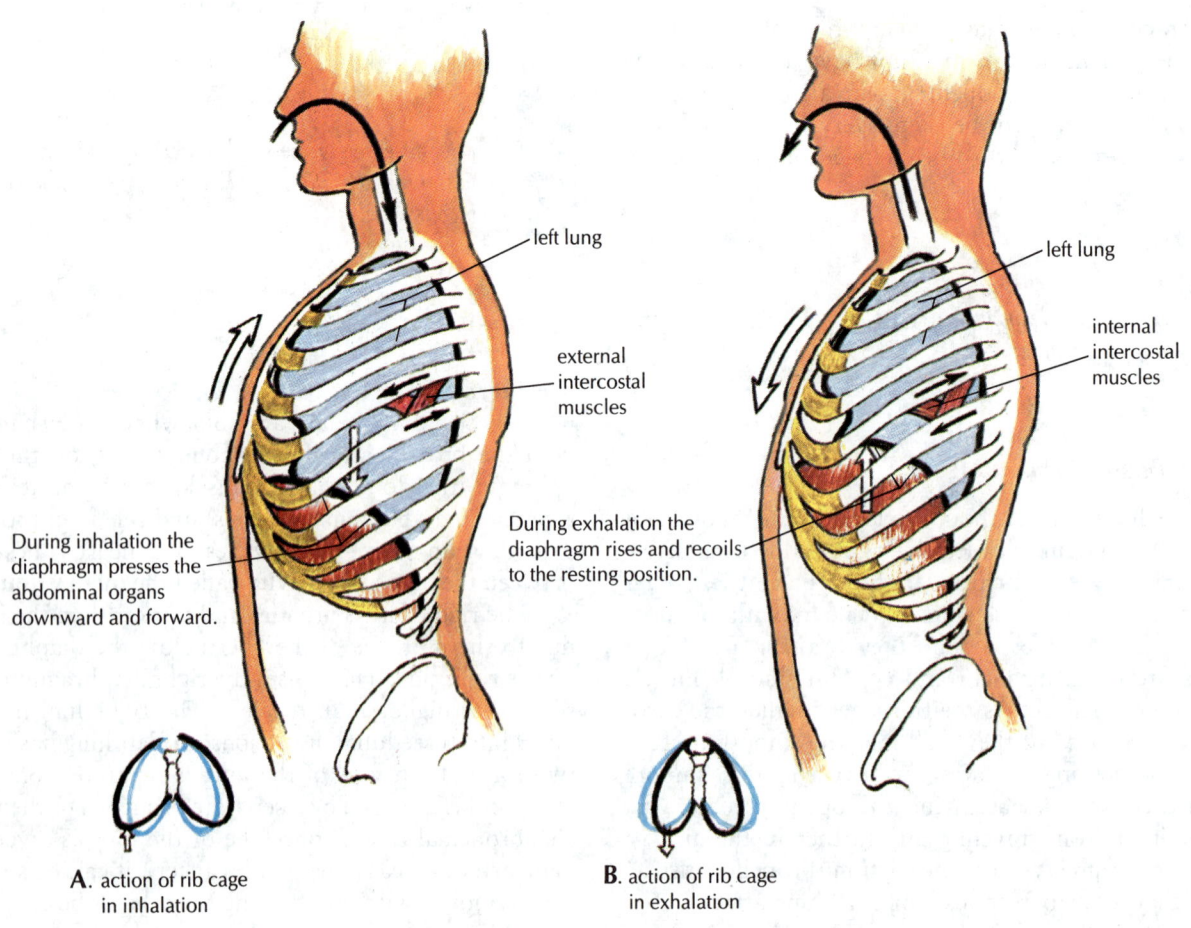

left lung

external intercostal muscles

left lung

internal intercostal muscles

During inhalation the diaphragm presses the abdominal organs downward and forward.

During exhalation the diaphragm rises and recoils to the resting position.

A. action of rib cage in inhalation

B. action of rib cage in exhalation

FIGURE 37-4
Diagram showing (**A**) inhalation and (**B**) exhalation.

center, it contracts, which causes it to flatten out and pull downward. At the same time, the external intercostal muscles (located between the ribs) also contract, causing the ribs to move outward. Both of these movements enlarge the chest cavity. Because the lungs are "stuck" to the chest wall and diaphragm by the forces between the visceral and parietal pleura, as the chest expands, the lungs expand as well. Thus, the volume in the lungs increases and (according to Boyle's law), the pressure within the lungs decreases.

Remember that the alveoli are directly connected to the atmosphere by the tracheobronchial tree and the upper airways. Thus, when the pressure drops in the lungs, the pressure in the atmosphere is higher than the pressure in the alveoli. Gases will always flow from higher to lower pressures, thus gas flows from the atmosphere into the lungs until the pressures within the lungs equal the atmospheric pressure. The more the muscles of inspiration (the diaphragm and external intercostals) are contracted, the more air will flow in and the deeper the breath will be.

Notice that inspiration is an active process; in other words, energy is used to produce the contraction of the inspiratory muscles. In situations where the diaphragm and external intercostals are unable to meet the ventilatory needs of the body, accessory muscles of inspiration may be called on to try to expand the chest cavity even more. This can occur when someone with normal lungs is trying to breathe very rapidly and deeply, or when someone has a respiratory disease and is unable to move enough air with the diaphragm and external intercostals alone.

Expiration

The process of expiration, or movement of gas out of the lungs into the atmosphere, is normally a passive process. This means that no muscles must be contracted to remove the air from the lungs, so no energy is used. When inspiration has ended, the diaphragm and external intercostals automatically relax and the chest wall and diaphragm recoil to their resting position. As they do this, the volume within the lungs is decreased, which (again according to Boyle's law) causes the gas pressure within the lungs to increase. The pressure of the gas within the lungs becomes higher than that in the atmosphere, and, once again, gas flows from higher to lower pressure until the pressures are equalized. When the pressure within the lungs is equal to that in the atmosphere, expiration stops.

Expiration is normally a passive process. However, when someone with normal lungs wishes to forcefully exhale, or when someone has a disease that makes it difficult to get air out of the lungs, such as asthma

or emphysema, accessory muscles of expiration may be used.

Checkpoint Question
5. How would you contrast the processes of inspiration and expiration?

➤ RESPIRATION

External Respiration

External respiration is the exchange of gases between the alveoli and the pulmonary capillaries within the lungs. The wall of the alveolus is only one cell thick, as are the walls of the capillaries that surround the alveoli. The respiratory gases (oxygen and carbon dioxide) must pass through the **alveolar-capillary membrane** (Fig. 37-5). This membrane is only about 0.5 μm thick to make it easy for these gases to pass through.

The blood entering the pulmonary capillaries is high in carbon dioxide and low in oxygen. The alveolus contains a good deal of oxygen and small amounts of carbon dioxide. As the blood passes through the pulmonary capillaries, oxygen diffuses from the alveolus into the blood and carbon dioxide diffuses from the blood into the alveolus. When the lungs are not diseased, equilibration is complete—that is, the blood leaving the pulmonary capillary has the same oxygen pressure and carbon dioxide pressure as the alveolus it just passed.

Certain respiratory and cardiac diseases can interfere with the process of external respiration by thickening the alveolar capillary membrane, thus interfering with diffusion (as seen in pulmonary edema), by decreasing the surface area available for external respiration (as seen in emphysema), or by decreasing the amount of oxygen that reaches the alveolus (as seen in pneumonia). These diseases are discussed later in this chapter.

Internal Respiration

Internal respiration is the exchange of gases between the systemic capillaries, located throughout the body, and the cells of the body. Every cell in the body is located near enough to a capillary so that internal respiration may occur. In internal respiration, oxygen in the systemic capillaries diffuses out of the blood and into the cells to fuel the cell's work. Carbon dioxide, a waste product of cellular metabolism, diffuses out of the cell and into the blood of the systemic capillaries. The blood from the sys-

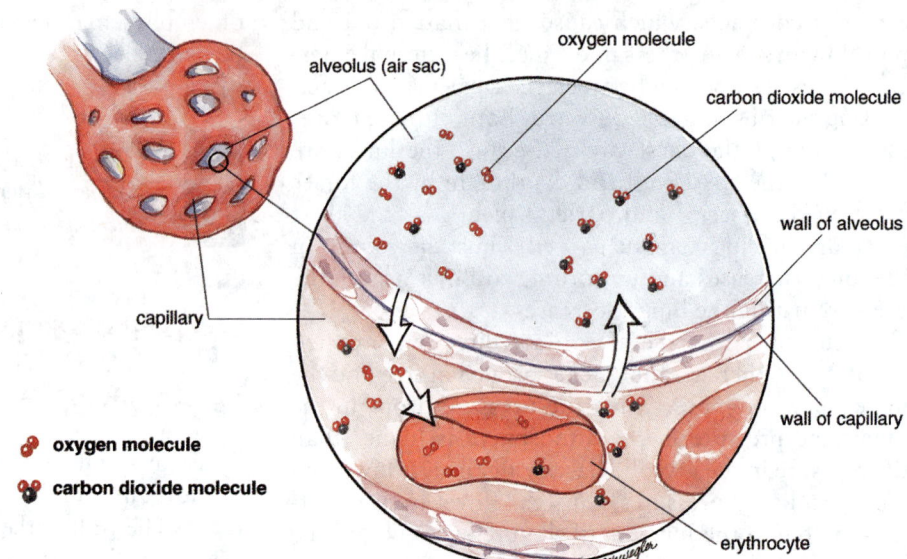

FIGURE 37-5
Diagram showing the diffusion of gas molecules through the cell membranes and throughout the capillary blood and air in the alveolus.

temic capillaries enters the venous system, returns to the right side of the heart, and is circulated through the lungs where external respiration occurs again.

➤ DEFENSE MECHANISMS OF THE RESPIRATORY SYSTEM

The respiratory system has a series of defense mechanisms designed to protect it from disease. Remember that the upper airways, tracheobronchial tree, and al-

veoli are all directly connected to the atmosphere, which can contain dust, pathogenic bacteria and viruses, and other irritants.

Table 37-2 summarizes the major defense mechanisms of the respiratory system. Without these defenses, infections and other diseases of these organs would be more common than they already are. Diseases of the respiratory system can occur when defenses are overwhelmed by cigarette smoking (Box 37-1), air pollution, infectious organisms, or other irritants.

Table 37-2
Defenses of the Respiratory System

Defense	*Function*
Hairs (vibrissae) at entrance to nose	Filter large dust particles from air
Mucous membranes in nose	Trap dust and other particles, adds moisture
Turbinates in nose	Whirl air around to increase warming, humidifying and filtering
Epiglottis	Closes over airway to prevent aspiration of liquids and solids
Airway reflexes	Trigger a cough when irritation occurs to pharynx, larynx, trachea, or **carina** (ridgelike structure) to help clear airway
Mucous membranes of trachea and airways	Trap particles of dust and debris in air
Airway smooth muscle	Constricts when irritation occurs to prevent entry of foreign substances
Macrophage in alveoli (type III cells)	Phagocytize ("eat") bacteria or other foreign cells or debris that reach the respiratory zone
Tonsils (palatine, pharyngeal, lingual)	Act as filters for air moving through passageways to protect against bacterial invasion; aid in the formation of white blood cells

Effects of Smoking on the Airways

Cigarette smoking has many harmful effects on the body. The normal functioning of the mucous membrane lining the trachea and other airways is described in the text. Smoke from a cigarette irritates the airways and causes the membrane to produce more mucus. This increased production of mucus, as well as the increase in dust and debris that collects in the mucus, slows down the clearing process. The smoke anesthetizes the cilia so they stop waving the debris away. Over time, large amounts of thick, sticky mucus are retained in the lungs, blackening the lung tissue and sealing the alveolar sacs. This thick, tarry mucus causes the patient to cough frequently (especially in the mornings) and to be prone to bronchitis (both acute and chronic).

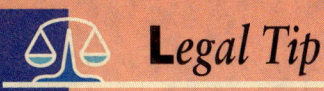

Legal Tip

A patient calls the office at 4:45 PM complaining of a sore throat. Scheduled appointments are running 1 to 2 hours behind. Because it is the middle of the flu season, you assume that the patient has a viral sore throat and can be seen in the morning. During the night, the patient's throat closes due to the infection and obstructs his airway. The patient is rushed to the hospital and is pronounced brain dead from anoxia. After his death, an autopsy shows the patient had a tonsillar abscess. Could you be sued? Yes! As a medical assistant, you cannot presume to diagnose medical conditions. Only the physician can make a diagnosis. Many symptoms may seem minor but may be warning signs of a more serious condition. Always follow your office policy regarding telephone advice. Document all phone conversations and bring them to the physician's attention.

➤ COMMON RESPIRATORY DISORDERS

Because it is open to the atmosphere, the respiratory system is susceptible to diseases. These diseases can be divided into diseases of the upper respiratory tract and those of the lower respiratory tract. Cancers of the respiratory system are discussed separately. Table 37-3 describes respiratory disorders that commonly affect pediatric patients.

Upper Respiratory Disorders

The most common problems associated with the upper respiratory tract are caused by infectious organisms or allergic reactions that produce inflammation.

Acute Rhinitis

Acute rhinitis is an inflammation of the mucous membranes of the nose. It produces sneezing, nasal discharge, swelling of the mucous membranes (which may make it difficult to breathe through the nose), and tearing of the eyes. If the problem is an infection, it is usually caused by a virus and is called a "common cold." It may also be caused by allergens, in which case it is called "hay fever." Treatment is symptomatic rather than curative and usually includes over-the-counter medication, rest, and fluids.

Sinusitis

Sinusitis is inflammation of the mucous membrane of the sinuses. It can produce pain and pressure over the upper facial area, headache, and fever. The problem may be acute or chronic and treatment may include symptomatic over-the-counter remedies as well as antibiotics (for bacterial infection), heat application, irrigation, and, occasionally, surgery.

Pharyngitis/Tonsillitis

Inflammation of the epithelial tissues of the throat or of the tonsils produces similar symptoms of sore throat and difficulty swallowing. Throat examination will reveal red, swollen tissues and possibly pustules on the tonsils or in the throat. The medical assistant may be asked to obtain a throat culture from these patients. Treatment of sore throat may include antibiotics (especially if the throat culture reveals streptococcal infection), gargles, and analgesics. Tonsillitis may be treated with antibiotics or, if the problem is chronic, the tonsils may be surgically removed. This procedure usually includes removal of the pharyngeal tonsils (adenoids) and the palatine tonsils.

Laryngitis

Inflammation of the larynx can result from an infection, irritation (as from cigarette smoke), or from

Table 37-3
Common Pediatric Respiratory Disorders

Disorder	Description
Infant respiratory distress syndrome (IRDS)	IRDS occurs in premature infants in whom the lungs have not fully developed. The alveolar-capillary membrane is thickened and mature surfactant is insufficient to keep the alveoli open. These infants often need assistance with their breathing for several days to a week, until the lungs mature.
Bronchopulmonary dysplasia (BPD)	This disease is seen in infants who have suffered from IRDS and still require assisted ventilation after a week. It is thought to be caused by the treatment (high pressures of ventilation and high oxygen concentrations) and is therefore an **iatrogenic** (resulting from medical treatment) disease. The infant's lungs are damaged and require prolonged treatment with ventilation, oxygen, or medication. Some children have residual damage from this disease; others outgrow all signs and symptoms.
Bronchiolitis	This disorder is characterized by inflammation of the bronchioles, wheezing, and congestion. It is most serious in children under 6 months old although it is commonly seen in children up to 3 years old. The most common causative virus is respiratory syncytial virus (RSV). Very young infants and those with other respiratory or cardiac problems often require hospitalization and even mechanical ventilation.
Croup (laryngotracheobronchitis)	Croup is a disease seen primarily in children 3 months to 3 years of age. It is caused by a viral infection of the larynx, resulting in swelling and narrowing of the airway. This causes difficulty in breathing, characterized by a high-pitched crowing wheeze (stridor) on inspiration and a sharp barking cough. Treatment may include hospitalization, mist tents, and medications to decrease the swelling.
Epiglottitis	Swelling of the epiglottis may present similarly to croup but is usually more serious and may be life-threatening if it progresses to complete obstruction of the airway. It occurs most frequently in children aged 2–6 years, although it can be seen in all age groups. It is caused by a bacterial infection, usually *Haemophilus influenzae.* A child with epiglottitis must be treated in the hospital. The first priority is establishing an airway, usually by inserting an **endotracheal tube** (tube in the trachea).
Cystic fibrosis	Cystic fibrosis is an inherited disease that affects the exocrine glands of the body, changing their secretions and causing mucus to be extremely thick and sticky. Although it affects several areas of the body, the most serious complications of cystic fibrosis are usually respiratory. Children with this disease are prone to repeated respiratory infections because of the difficulty in clearing the mucus from their airways. Many new treatments are being developed for this disease and much exciting research into prevention and cure is ongoing.

overuse of the voice. The result is hoarseness, a cough, and difficulty speaking. Laryngitis may be treated with antibiotics if it is thought to be caused by a bacterial infection, but more often it is left to resolve on its own. The patient is told to rest the voice and speak as little as possible. Cool mist humidifiers may be helpful in soothing the throat.

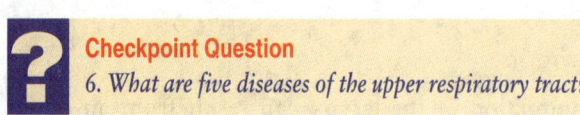

Checkpoint Question
6. *What are five diseases of the upper respiratory tract?*

Lower Respiratory Disorders

Diseases of the lower respiratory tract may be acute (sudden in onset with relatively short duration) or chronic (progressing over time or appearing frequently). Acute diseases of the lower respiratory tract include bronchitis and pneumonia. Chronic diseases include asthma, chronic bronchitis, and emphysema. The latter two diseases are usually grouped together as chronic obstructive pulmonary disease (COPD). Because most patients with COPD have elements of both emphysema and chronic bronchitis, these are discussed together.

Bronchitis

Bronchitis is an inflammation of the mucous membranes of the bronchi, which causes an increased production of mucus. This inflammation can be produced by infection or irritation of the mucous membrane. The most prominent symptom of bronchitis is a productive cough. If infection is present, the sputum produced may change color from the normal white or clear to yellow, green, gray, or tan. The medical assistant may be asked to obtain a sterile sputum specimen for culture and sensitivity from these patients. Treatment generally includes antibiotics (if bacterial infection is suspected), smoking cessation, and rest and fluids. Cough suppressants may be prescribed, especially for nighttime use, but their use is controversial because of the need to clear secretions from the airways. Retained secretions can become infected and lead to pneumonia.

Pneumonia

Pneumonia is an infection in the working areas of the lungs, or alveoli, that prevents effective gas exchange (external respiration) in the affected area. It may be bacterial or viral in origin. Diagnostic testing usually includes a sputum specimen and a chest x-ray. Bacterial pneumonias tend to be more sudden and severe in onset, presenting with fever, cough, chills, and **dyspnea** (difficulty breathing). They also tend to be localized to one lobe or area of the lung.

Treatment primarily involves appropriate antibiotics, bed rest, and symptomatic medications. Bacterial pneumonias often require hospitalization for administration of intravenous antibiotics and oxygen, especially in elderly or debilitated patients. Viral pneumonia is usually more gradual in onset but can be just as serious; antibiotics are generally ineffective. Viral pneumonia tends to be spread throughout the lung fields, instead of localized, and may present with fever and a hacking cough. Treatment may include bed rest or hospitalization.

Checkpoint Question

7. What are the characteristic symptoms of bacterial and viral pneumonia?

Asthma

Asthma is a reversible inflammatory process involving primarily the small airways. It is manifested by constriction of the smooth muscle lining the airways (bronchospasm), increased mucus production with a productive cough, and swelling of the mucous membranes of the airways. All three of these manifestations narrow the airways, which makes it difficult to move air into and out of the lungs.

The person having an asthma attack may present with dyspnea, coughing, wheezing, and, in a severe attack, cyanosis (bluish discoloration of the skin caused by lack of oxygen). Patients with asthma usually have periods when they are experiencing an attack (exacerbations) and other periods when they are relatively symptom free (remissions). Attacks may be brought on by allergens in the environment, irritants, infection, psychological stress, rapid breathing, cold air, or unknown causes. Many medications are available to treat asthma, but it is important that they be used properly.

A peak flowmeter may be used by an individual patient to assess his or her breathing daily and to determine what medication regime to use that day (Fig. 37-6). To use the peak flowmeter, the patient blows as hard as possible into the device during a period when breathing is at its best to establish a "personal best." The physician then devises a medication protocol based on this information.

A patient who is having an asthma attack that does not respond to medications is said to be in **status asthmaticus.** Because such asthma attacks can be fatal, the patient needs to be taken to a hospital immediately. In recent years, with increased levels of air pollution, the mortality rate from asthma has been increasing despite new and improved diagnostic techniques and medications.

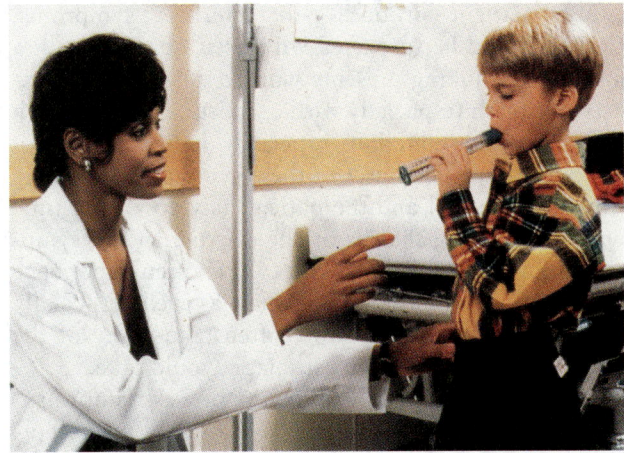

FIGURE 37-6
Using a peak flowmeter (Courtesy of Monaghan Medical Corporation, Plattsburgh, PA).

Chronic Obstructive Pulmonary Disease (COPD)

Both chronic bronchitis and emphysema are most commonly caused by cigarette smoking. Thus, patients who have smoked over a long period of time often exhibit signs and symptoms of both of these disorders.

Chronic bronchitis is a chronic inflammation and swelling of the airways, with excessive mucus production, obstruction of the bronchi, and trapping of air behind mucous plugs, which causes alveoli to become overinflated. During inspiration, as the chest expands, the airways are stretched open and air enters the alveoli. However, during expiration, as the chest closes down, the airways also close and the air is trapped and cannot be exhaled. This produces alveoli that are stretched and overinflated. Chronic bronchitis is not usually an infectious process, but instead is produced by chronic irritation of the airways by cigarette smoke or other pollutants. However, because of the increased sputum produced and the difficulty these patients have in clearing their sputum, they are prone to develop respiratory infections.

Emphysema is a disease process affecting primarily the alveoli themselves. Remember that normally alveoli exist in small clusters like bunches of grapes. In emphysema, the walls of the alveoli become stretched and break down. The pulmonary capillaries also break down and the tiny airways leading to each grapelike cluster weaken and collapse. The end result of this is that there is much less surface area for gas exchange and, once again, air is trapped in the enlarged "sacs" that were once clusters of tiny alveoli.

The combination of these two diseases in the COPD patient produces characteristic symptoms. **COPD should be suspected whenever a patient with a history of smoking presents with complaints of shortness of breath (especially with exercise), chronic cough and sputum production (especially in the morning), and wheezing.** The onset of these symptoms is usually slow and gradual and the patient may go a long time without realizing that he or she is experiencing symptoms of a disease. People with COPD often experience some of the symptoms of asthma as well, especially bronchospasm, and therefore often take many of the same medications that an asthmatic would take.

Once a patient has COPD, the process is not usually reversible. Many patients have a hard time accepting that fact and insist that their physician must be able to provide a "cure." Although the disease is not curable, the progression of COPD can be slowed and the quality of life for the patient may be improved sig-

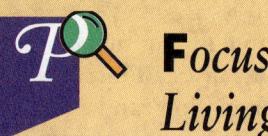

Focus on the Patient: Living With COPD

To help improve the quality of life, encourage a patient with COPD to follow these suggestions:

1. If you have not already done it, QUIT SMOKING! Even if you have permanent damage to your lungs, their deterioration will slow if you stop smoking now.
2. Have the current flu vaccine each fall and be sure to get a pneumococcal pneumonia vaccine.
3. Avoid being out in crowds whenever possible, especially in the winter when colds and influenza are prevalent. If you live in an area with high air pollution, you may want to wear a respiratory mask outside on days when the pollution level is high.
4. When you breathe, inspire through your nose, then exhale slowly through pursed lips. Do not puff your cheeks or blow—allow your expiration to be passive.
5. Use your abdominal muscles instead of your shoulder and neck muscles to help you breathe. On inspiration, allow your abdominal muscles to relax and your abdominal wall to move outward to give the diaphragm room to move downward. On expiration, tighten your abdominal muscles to push upward on your diaphragm and help get a more complete expiration.
6. Drink a lot of fluids all day long (unless your physician has limited your fluid intake). Water is the best fluid. Avoid drinking too many caffeinated drinks or alcohol. Good fluid intake is the best way to keep the mucus in your airways thinned so that it is easier to cough up.
7. Follow a healthy, balanced diet.
8. Avoid doing difficult physical tasks (eg, vacuuming or mowing the lawn) all in one day. If you must do these chores, do them in short periods spaced throughout the day, with frequent rest periods.
9. Organize your home to minimize the amount of standing, reaching, and lifting you have to do. For example, put a high stool in your kitchen. Keep frequently used items at waist level (on the counter), rather than in high or low cabinets. Have a rolling basket in your home that you can push around to take items (such as laundry) from one room to another.

nificantly through thorough patient education about the disease, a supervised exercise regimen, proper use of medications, good nutrition, home oxygen therapy, and so on.

Many patients with severe COPD or end-stage lung cancer are discharged from the hospital with oxygen to use in the home. Most surgical supply companies and pharmacies can arrange to have oxygen therapy equipment delivered to the home. The oxygen is usually supplied by a machine called a concentrator, which runs on electricity. The concentrator separates oxygen out of room air. Attached to the cylinder is a flowmeter that indicates the amount of oxygen being delivered. The patient should be instructed to leave the oxygen at the setting prescribed by the physician. In some cases, too much oxygen can be toxic. A cannula (plastic tube with pronged openings that fit into the nares) will be attached to the flowmeter and will deliver the oxygen. The company supplying the oxygen should instruct the patient regarding safe home oxygen administration. In addition, the supplier should be available 24 hours a day for emergency oxygen maintenance.

Common Cancers

Laryngeal Cancer

Cancer of the larynx is seen most commonly in heavy smokers and alcoholics. The presenting symptoms are usually hoarseness for longer than 3 weeks, a "lump" in the throat, or pain and burning in the throat when drinking citrus juice or hot liquid. The patient with laryngeal cancer may be treated with radiation or surgery or both. Surgery usually involves removal of the larynx and formation of a permanent tracheostomy stoma. Patients who have had a laryngectomy are unable to speak normally, but they can be trained to speak using esophageal speech or a prosthetic device.

Lung Cancer

Lung cancer is one of the most common causes of death in both men and women. Cigarette smoking is believed to be the most common cause; 80% of lung cancer patients are smokers. Prognosis is generally poor for patients with lung cancer, with only 8% of men and 12% of women surviving for 5 years. One of the reasons for this is that symptoms tend to present rather late in the disease when it has already had a chance to spread. Also, many of the symptoms are nonspecific and are seen in most heavy smokers. These symptoms include chronic cough, wheezing, dyspnea, **hemoptysis** (coughing up blood), and chest pain.

Diagnosis is made by chest x-ray, sputum cytology, bronchoscopy, biopsy, or **thoracentesis** (surgical puncture and drainage of the thoracic cavity). Treatment is generally **palliative** (giving relief but not cure) and usually includes some combination of surgery, radiation, and chemotherapy. These treatments may improve the patient's prognosis and prolong survival.

➤ COMMON DIAGNOSTIC PROCEDURES AND THE MEDICAL ASSISTANT'S ROLE

Many different studies, procedures, and examinations are performed to detect and diagnose the previously mentioned disorders as well as other respiratory problems. Some of these studies can be performed in the physician's office, whereas others need to be done in the hospital.

Physical Examination of the Respiratory System

You may be responsible for preparing the patient for an examination of the respiratory system by the physician or you may assist in the examination. It is important to maintain a calm, reassuring attitude while you prepare the patient for the examination. If the physician is performing a chest assessment, the patient will have to remove all clothing from the waist up and put on a gown.

Upper Airway Examination

When the physician examines the nose, ears, and throat of the patient, you may be required to prepare the equipment for the examination. Because the ears open into the pharynx through the eustachian tubes, they are usually assessed as part of the upper airway examination. An otoscope is the instrument used for this examination and must be prepared with the correct size earpiece (speculum) for the patient. The nose and sinuses are then assessed, using a nasal speculum, followed by a visual inspection of the throat, using a tongue depressor and small light. The physician will also palpate the lymph nodes in the neck as well as the other neck structures that relate to the upper airway.

Lower Airway Examination (Chest Examination)

The traditional examination of the chest consists of four parts: inspection, palpation, percussion, and auscultation. Each is briefly described below. To allow the physician to perform this examination, the patient should be sitting up and all clothing should be removed from the waist up, except for a hospital gown for female patients. You may be asked to help adjust the gown to allow the physician adequate access to all areas of the chest and back.

INSPECTION

This part of the examination consists of a visual inspection of the chest and the patient's respiratory pattern (Table 37-4). During inspection, the physician looks for abnormal shape of the thorax, use of accessory muscles for ventilation, surgical scars, cyanosis, or any other visual signs of previous or current respiratory disease.

PALPATION

In the palpation segment of the examination, the physician uses his or her hands to feel the patient's throat for lumps, areas of tenderness, and location of the trachea. The patient may be asked to say "99" while the physician feels the chest wall in different places to assess the vibrations produced. Solid masses (such as tumors) or fluids (as in pneumonia) will produce an increase in vibrations, whereas increased air (as seen in emphysema) will produce a decrease in vibrations.

PERCUSSION

Percussion is performed by placing a finger or fingers on the chest and striking it with the fingers of the other hand. During percussion, the physician listens for the sound produced to determine if it is a normal (resonant) sound, like that produced by a drum; dull or flat, which would be seen in consolidation of pulmonary tissue as in **atelectasis** (collapse of alveoli), pneumonia, or tumor; or hyperresonant (more hollow in sound), which would be seen in emphysema. The physician may also use percussion to assess **diaphragmatic excursion**, or how far the diaphragm moves during a deep inspiration.

AUSCULTATION

Auscultation involves listening to the patient's lungs with a stethoscope. The physician will systematically listen to each side of the chest in each area to compare the sounds bilaterally. The patient should breathe somewhat deeply, with an open mouth and the head turned away from the physician's face. Make sure the patient does not breathe too rapidly to avoid hyperventilation, which could cause dizziness. During auscultation, the physician listens for abnormal or adventitious sounds such as crackles and wheezes, which could indicate a disease process (Table 37-5). The physician may also wish to assess vocal sounds and may ask the patient to say "e," "1, 2, 3," or "99" while auscultating.

Checkpoint Question
9. What are the four parts of the chest examination?

Throat Culture

A throat culture is done in cases of suspected pharyngitis or tonsillitis to help determine what microorganism is causing the problem. The patient's throat is gently swabbed with a sterile culture stick to obtain the specimen (Procedure 37-1).

Sputum Culture or Cytology

Sputum cultures are obtained to aid with diagnosis and treatment decisions in patients with suspected pneumonia, tuberculosis, or other infectious diseases of the lower airway. A microbiology laboratory will culture and incubate the specimen to identify any pathogenic microorganisms. Sputum is obtained for cytology to search for abnormal cells that might indicate cancer or

---

Table 37-4
Abnormal Respiratory Patterns

Pattern	Description
Apnea	No respirations
Bradypnea	Slow respirations
Cheyne-Stokes	Rhythmic cycles of dyspnea or hyperpnea subsiding gradually into periods of apnea
Dyspnea	Difficult or labored respirations
Hypopnea	Shallow respirations
Hyperpnea	Deep respirations
Kussmaul	Fast and deep respirations
Orthopnea	Inability to breathe in other than a sitting or standing position
Tachypnea	Fast respirations

Table 37-5
Abnormal Breath Sounds

Breath Sound	Description
Bubbling	Gurgling sounds as the air passes moist secretions in the airways
Crackles (rales)	Crackling sound, usually inspiratory, as air passes moist secretions in the airways. Fine to medium crackles indicate secretions in the small airways and alveoli. Medium to coarse crackles indicate secretions in the larger airways.
Friction rub	Dry, rubbing or grating sound; may indicate pericarditis or pleuritis
Rhonchi	Low-pitched, continuous sound as air moves past thick mucus or narrowed air passages
Stertorous	Snoring sound on inspiration or expiration; indicates a partial airway obstruction
Stridor	Shrill, harsh inspiratory sound; indicates a laryngeal obstruction
Wheeze	High-pitched musical sound, either inspiratory or expiratory; indicates partial airway obstruction

a precancerous condition of the lung or airway. In either case, it is important to obtain a specimen that has been coughed up and expectorated from the lower airways, with minimal contamination by oral and pharyngeal secretions. The patient must be asked to cough deeply and the specimen is collected in a sterile container (Procedure 37-2).

Sputum collection for suspected cancer or for tuberculosis may be required for three consecutive mornings. The specimens should be brought to the office as soon as possible to avoid deterioration of the material.

Most diagnostic specimens are obtained early in the morning when the greatest volume of secretion has had a chance to accumulate. If this is not possible, specimens may also be collected after respiratory treatments or therapy.

It is vitally important that the patient understand that the specimen must be collected from the lung fields and not from the mouth. The difference between saliva and sputum may need to be explained on the patient's level of understanding. Before the collection, encourage the patient to increase fluid intake to decrease the viscosity of the secretions. The patient may be weak from illness and thick mucus will be hard to bring up, causing the patient to be even more exhausted. A cool mist humidifier may help also.

Chest X-rays

Chest x-rays can help in the diagnosis of a large variety of pulmonary problems, including pneumonia, lung cancer, emphysema, pulmonary edema, and many others. When performed in a radiology department, usually two views are ordered: a posterior to anterior view and a lateral view. This gives the radiologist a more three-dimensional perspective of the chest. X-rays may also be taken of the sinuses in cases of sinusitis.

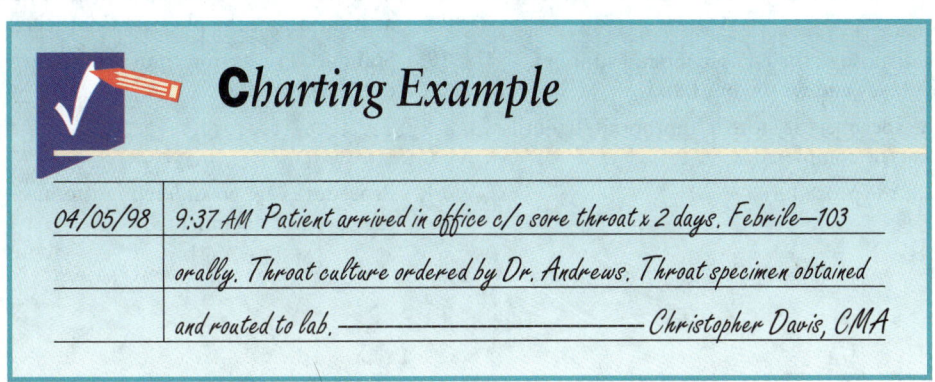

Charting Example

04/05/98	9:37 AM Patient arrived in office c/o sore throat x 2 days. Febrile—103 orally. Throat culture ordered by Dr. Andrews. Throat specimen obtained and routed to lab. —————————— Christopher Davis, CMA

Procedure 37-1   Collecting a Specimen for a Throat Culture

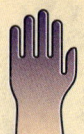

Equipment/Supplies

- tongue blade
- sterile specimen container
- sterile swab (if one is not supplied with the specimen container)
- gloves
- completed laboratory request slip

Steps	Purpose
1. Wash your hands.	1. Handwashing aids infection control.
2. Assemble the equipment and supplies.	2. Doing this ensures that all of the materials are available.
3. Put on gloves.	3. Standard Precautions must be followed.
4. Greet and identify the patient. Explain the procedure.	4. Identifying the patient avoids errors in treatment. Explanations help to gain patient compliance and ease anxiety.
5. Have the patient sit with a light source directed at the throat.	5. Good visibility is vital to collection from the areas of concern.
6. Carefully remove the sterile swab from the container.	
7. Have the patient say "AHHH" as you press on the midpoint of the tongue with the tongue depressor.	7. Saying "AHHH" raises the uvula out of the way and will decrease the urge to gag. If the depressor is placed too far forward, it will not be effective; if it is placed too far back, it will gag the patient unnecessarily.
8. Swab the areas of concern on the mucous membranes, especially the tonsillar area, the crypts, and the posterior pharynx. Turn the swab to expose all of its surfaces. Avoid touching areas other than those suspected of infection.	8. Pathogens must be collected from sites of concern with a twisting motion for maximum collection. Touching other areas will alter the substances on the swab.
9. Maintain the tongue depressor position while withdrawing the swab.	9. Keeping the tongue down will avoid contaminating the swab unnecessarily.
10. Follow the instructions on the specimen container for transferring the swab. Some require that the wooden swab stick be broken after dropping into the culture; others may have a special swab that is contained within the cap and is secured when the container is sealed.	10. Improper handling of the specimen will alter the results.
11. Thank the patient and give appropriate instructions.	11. Courtesy encourages the patient to have a positive attitude about the physician's office.
12. Properly dispose of the equipment and supplies. Remove gloves and wash your hands.	12. Standard Precautions must be followed throughout the procedure.
13. Route the specimen or store it appropriately until routing can be completed.	
14. Document the procedure.	14. Procedures are considered not to have been done if they are not documented.

Procedure 37-2

Collecting a Sputum Specimen

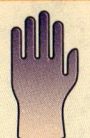

Equipment/Supplies

- labeled sterile specimen container
- cover bag
- gloves
- face shield and impervious gown (if you will be assisting the patient with sputum collection)

Steps	Purpose
1. Wash your hands.	1. Handwashing aids infection control.
2. Assemble the equipment.	2. Doing this ensures that all of the materials are available.
3. Greet and identify the patient. Explain the procedure.	3. Identifying the patient avoids errors. Explanations will help gain patient compliance and ease anxiety.
4. Put on gloves and, if necessary, face shield and impervious gown.	4. Standard Precautions must be followed when handling blood and body fluids. If the patient will be coughing in your presence, a face shield and impervious gown provide protection.
5. Have the patient brush the teeth or rinse the mouth well.	5. Food particles will contaminate the specimen.
6. Have the patient cough deeply, using the abdominal muscles as well as the accessory muscles to bring secretions from the lung fields and not just the upper airways.	6. The specimen needs to reflect the pathogens at the lower levels rather than from the upper throat.
7. Have the patient expectorate directly into the specimen container without touching the inside and without getting sputum on the sides of the container. About 5–10 mL is usually needed.	7. Touching the inside will contaminate the container. Sputum on the outside of the container is potentially hazardous.
8. Handle the specimen observing standard precautions. Cap the container immediately and drop it into the cover container.	8. The specimen is potentially hazardous. Capping it immediately will eliminate the danger of spreading microorganisms, and covering it will contain microorganisms that may have settled on the outside of the container.
9. Assist the patient to rinse the mouth after collecting the specimen.	9. The procedure may be upsetting to some patients. Some patients may become nauseated during the procedure.
10. Thank the patient and give appropriate instructions.	10. Courtesy encourages the patient to have a positive attitude about the physician's office.
11. Properly care for or dispose of equipment and supplies. Clean the work area. Remove gloves, gown, and face shield and wash your hands.	11. Standard Precautions must be followed throughout the procedure.
12. Process the specimen immediately, or within 2 hours, to avoid compromising the studies.	12. The pathogens may either proliferate, causing overgrowth, or die, causing a false-negative result.
13. Document the procedure.	13. Procedures are considered not to have been done if they are not documented.

Charting Example

01/03/99	10:30 AM
	S: "I have an awful cough."
	O: 80-year-old COPD patient. Complaining of dyspnea x 3 days and
	a productive cough. Sputum greenish yellow in color. Crackles in
	left lower lung field. Febrile—102 orally.
	A: Productive cough
	P: 1. Sputum specimen obtained.
	2. Specimen sent to laboratory.
	3. Patient education done regarding the need to stop smoking.
	Patient instructed on the need to use tissues to cover nose and
	mouth when coughing. Patient verbalized understanding of all
	teachings.
	4. Dr. White ordered CXR. Patient given directions to x-ray
	department. ——————————— Jackie Shapiro, CMA

Bronchoscopy

Bronchoscopy is an endoscopic procedure in which a lighted scope is inserted into the trachea and large airways for direct visualization. Bronchoscopy can be used for many diagnostic purposes such as obtaining sputum specimens, obtaining tissue for biopsy, removing foreign objects, or visually assessing airway changes. It can also be used therapeutically, for example, to clear out mucous plugs or remove foreign bodies. Bronchoscopy is an invasive procedure and written consent must be obtained from the patient.

Pulmonary Function Tests

Pulmonary function tests are done using a spirometer that measures the amount of air a patient can move in and out and how fast he or she can process it. The patient breathes into a mouthpiece and performs several different breathing maneuvers that are explained by the technician performing the test. By measuring the patient's airflow and comparing the results with predicted values for each patient's height, weight, age, and gender, valuable information can be obtained concerning whether the patient has mild, moderate, or severe obstructive or restrictive lung disease.

Arterial Blood Gases

Arterial blood gases (ABGs) measure the pH and pressures of oxygen and carbon dioxide in arterial blood. They can tell the physician whether the lungs are adequately exchanging gases. ABGs can also give information about metabolic acid–base problems such as diabetic ketoacidosis. Drawing blood from an artery takes special training and is not considered a medical assisting procedure. The site most commonly used is the radial artery in the wrist. Instead of visualizing the vessel as is commonly done in phlebotomy (drawing blood from a vein), the pulse is palpated and the needle is inserted where the pulse is felt. Due to the higher pressures in an artery, after arterial puncture the site must be held tightly with sterile gauze for at least 5 minutes or until all signs of bleeding stop.

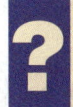

Checkpoint Question

10. What are seven ways the physician can obtain information to help diagnose respiratory disorders?

SUMMARY

The respiratory system provides the body with oxygen—the essential ingredient required for cell metabolism. Without oxygen, cells quickly cease to function and die. The respiratory system also eliminates from the body the buildup of carbon dioxide, a chemical that causes acidosis. Because it is open to the atmosphere, the respiratory system is susceptible to infection and irritant injury. You can play an important role in helping the patient to maintain healthy lungs as well as in diagnosing and treating respiratory disease.

CRITICAL THINKING CHALLENGES

1. Describe the structures of the nose. Why do you think it is better to inhale through the nose than through the mouth?
2. Mr. Gardner, age 55, has been diagnosed with COPD and has many questions about his condition. Identify the characteristics of COPD. How would you explain this disease to Mr. Gardner? Develop educational materials on COPD that can be given to all patients with this disorder.

ANSWERS TO CHECKPOINT QUESTIONS

1. The respiratory system supplies oxygen to the blood, eliminates carbon dioxide, assists with the sense of smell, and assists with speech.
2. Functions of the pharynx include passage of food into the digestive tract and passage of air into the respiratory tract.
3. Special cells and glands in the trachea produce mucus, which traps any inhaled particles on its sticky surface. Tiny hairs called cilia beat together to move the mucus toward the pharynx, where it is swallowed. Once in the digestive tract, pathogens in the mucus are neutralized.

4. After air enters the nose, it must pass through the pharynx, larynx, trachea, bronchi, bronchioles, and alveoli.
5. Five upper respiratory tract disorders are rhinitis, sinusitis, pharyngitis, tonsillitis, and laryngitis.
6. Inspiration is the process by which air is drawn into the lungs from the atmosphere; it is an active process (requires energy). Expiration involves the movement of gas out of the lungs and into the atmosphere; normally, it is a passive process (requires no energy).
7. The onset of bacterial pneumonia is usually sudden and severe; symptoms include fever, cough, chills, and dyspnea. This type of pneumonia is typically localized. In contrast, the onset of viral pneumonia is usually gradual; symptoms include fever and a hacking cough. Unlike bacterial pneumonia, viral pneumonia tends to be spread throughout the lung fields.
8. Six factors that may trigger an asthma attack are environmental allergens, irritants, infections, stress, cold air, or rapid breathing.
9. Four parts of the chest examination are inspection, percussion, palpation, and auscultation.
10. Seven methods for diagnosing respiratory disorders include physical examination, throat culture, sputum culture, chest x-ray, bronchoscopy, pulmonary function tests, and arterial blood gases.

SUGGESTIONS FOR FURTHER READING

Burton, G. G., Hodgkin, J. E., & Ward, J. J. (1991). *Respiratory Care: A Guide to Clinical Practice.* Philadelphia: J. B. Lippincott.

Des Jardins, T. (1993). *Cardiopulmonary Anatomy and Physiology.* Albany, NY: Delmar.

Hodgkin, J. E., Connors, G. L., Bell, C. W. *Pulmonary Rehabilitation: Guidelines to Success.* Philadelphia: J. B. Lippincott.

Miller, B. F., & Keane, C. B. (1992). *Encyclopedia of Medicine, Nursing and Allied Health,* 5th ed. Philadelphia: W. B. Saunders.

(1992). *Professional Guide to Diseases,* 4th ed. Springhouse, PA: Springhouse.

Whitaker, K. (1992). *Comprehensive Perinatal and Pediatric Respiratory Care.* Albany, NY: Delmar.

Caring for Patients With Gastrointestinal Disorders

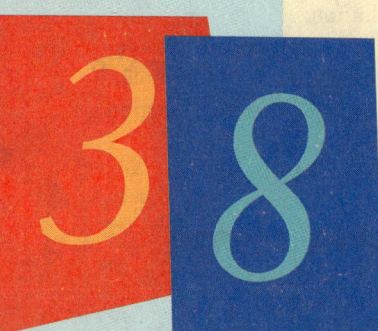

Chapter Outline

Structure and Function of the Gastrointestinal System
    Construction of the Transport System
    Digestion
    Metabolism
Organs of the Gastrointestinal System
    Mouth
    Oropharynx
    Esophagus
    Stomach
    Small Intestine
    Large Intestine
Accessory Organs
    Liver
    Gallbladder
    Pancreas
Common Gastrointestinal Disorders
    Mouth Disorders
    Esophageal Disorders
    Stomach Disorders
    Intestinal Disorders

    Colon Disorders
    Functional Disorders
    Liver Disorders
    Gallbladder Disorders
    Pancreatic Disorders
Common Diagnostic Procedures and the Medical Assistant's Role
    History and Assessment
    Blood Tests
    Radiologic Studies
    Endoscopic Examinations
Procedure: Preparing the Patient for Colon Procedures
    Stool Specimens
Procedure: Collecting a Stool Specimen
    Screening for Occult Blood
Procedure: Testing Stool for Occult Blood
Summary
Critical Thinking Challenges
Answers to Checkpoint Questions
Suggestions for Further Reading

DACUM Components

1.3   Practice within the scope of education, training, and personal capabilities
1.6   Conduct oneself in a courteous and diplomatic manner
2.2   Treat all patients with empathy and impartiality
4.1   Apply principles of aseptic technique and infection control
4.5   Prepare and maintain examination and treatment area
4.7   Prepare patients for procedures
4.8   Assist physician with examinations and treatments
4.10 Collect and process specimens
4.11 Perform selected tests that assist with diagnosis and treatment
4.12 Screen and follow up patient test results
5.1   Document accurately
7.3   Teach patients methods of health promotion and disease prevention

Chapter Competencies

Learning Objectives

Upon successfully completing this chapter, you will be able to:

1. Spell and define the Key Terms.
2. Describe the action of anabolism and catabolism.
3. Describe the process of digestion.
4. List and describe the structure of the digestive system.
5. List and locate the primary and accessory organs of the gastrointestinal system.
6. Describe the function of the primary and accessory organs of the gastrointestinal system.
7. List and describe disorders of the gastrointestinal system.
8. Identify and explain the purpose of diagnostic procedures of the gastrointestinal system.

Performance Objectives

Upon successfully completing this chapter, you will be able to:

1. Prepare a patient for procedures pertaining to the colon (Procedure 38-1).
2. Collect a stool specimen (Procedure 38-2).
3. Perform testing on stools for occult blood (Procedure 38-3).

Key Terms

(See Glossary for definitions.)

ascites	gingiva	metabolism
bolus	guaiac	obstipation
chyle	hematemesis	papilla (pl. papillae)
chyme	hepatomegaly	papillae lingua
deciduous	hepatotoxic	peristalsis
defecation	hiatus	reflux
deglutition	insufflator	rugae
dentin	malocclusion	turgor
emulsify	mastication	villus (pl. villi)
enzyme	melena	

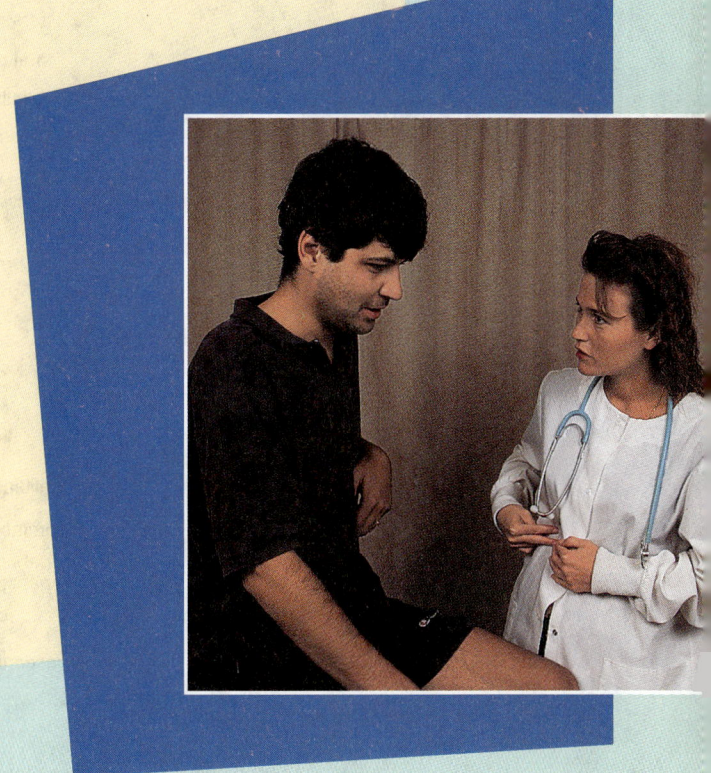

The gastrointestinal (GI) system, or tract, is responsible for the ingestion, digestion, transportation, and elimination of the food we eat. Nutrients are broken down by the action of digestive **enzymes** (proteins that start a chemical reaction) into units that can be absorbed through the walls of the GI system into the circulatory and lymphatic systems. The nutrients are transported to the cells to supply fuel for all metabolic processes. The solid waste products are eliminated as feces.

➤ STRUCTURE AND FUNCTION OF THE GASTROINTESTINAL SYSTEM

The GI system of organs includes the mouth, oropharynx, esophagus, stomach, small intestine, and large intestine. Accessory organs include the liver, the gallbladder, and the pancreas (Fig. 38-1).

Construction of the Transport System

The entire GI tract is lined with mucous membranes from the lips to the anus. The properties of the membrane change at intervals to accommodate the digestive action at that point. For instance, the gastric mucosa is able to withstand the hydrochloric acid (HCl) present for digestion but the esophagus, just above the stomach, can be seriously damaged by this same acid. Little absorption occurs within the stomach because of its protective membranes, but just beyond the stomach, the membranes of the small intestines are designed for great absorption of nutrients and fluids and become progressively less resistant to digestive enzymes through their length.

Most of the length of the GI tract beyond the mouth consists of four layers.

1. The inner mucosa keeps the **bolus** (mass) of food moving. It is composed of epithelium throughout its length. It changes characteristics from the relatively smooth inner surface of the mouth and esophagus to the velvety **villi** (tiny projections) of the intestines.

2. The submucosa is highly vascular with a strong nerve supply.

3. The smooth muscle layer has an inner circular lumen to dilate and constrict and an outer longitudinal layer that shortens with contractions. The food is pushed along by squeezing the inner lumen and shortening the outer layer in rhythmic waves of

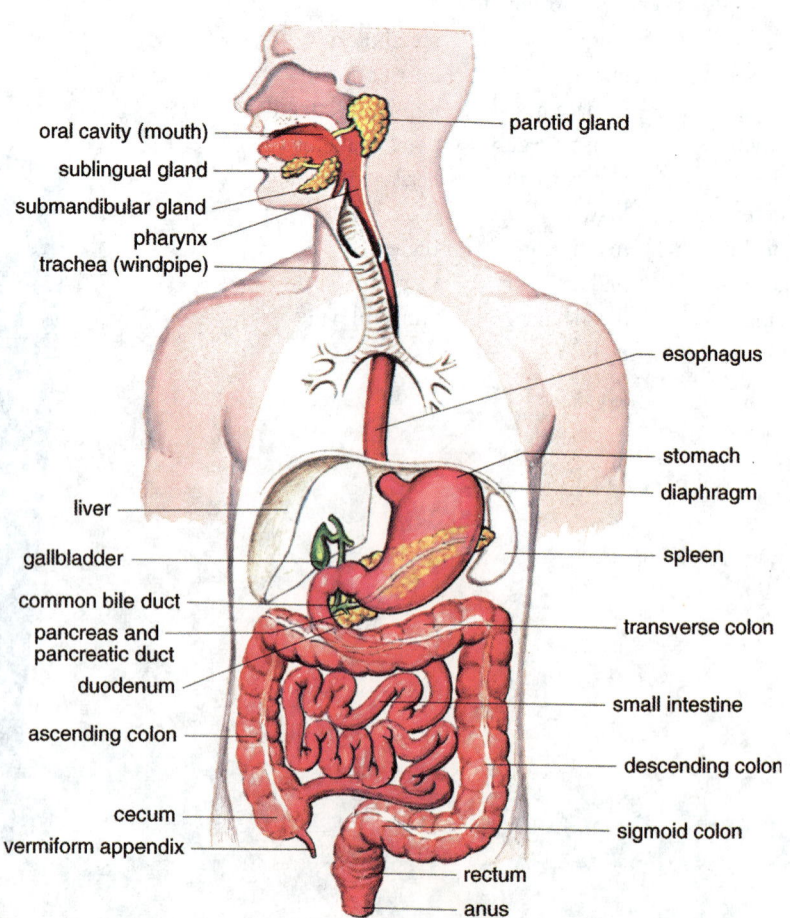

FIGURE 38-1
The gastrointestinal system.

peristalsis. This movement continues to break the bolus into segments and mix it with enzymes to hasten the digestive breakdown.

4. The outer wall connects the tract to the peritoneum, which supports, insulates, and cushions the organs within its highly vascular connective tissue (Fig. 38-2).

Digestion

Digestion starts in the mouth with the intake, or ingestion, of food. The teeth and tongue break the food into small pieces and mix it with saliva for swallowing. Saliva begins the process of digestion by breaking down some of the carbohydrates into sugars. Food flows through the esophagus by peristalsis and enters the stomach to be mixed with the gastric enzymes (Table 38-1). Wavelike motions of the stomach press this thick liquid, called **chyme**, through the pyloric sphincter into the duodenum. Bile from the liver and gallbladder and pancreatic enzymes continue to break the food into molecules that can be absorbed through the lining of the small intestines into the bloodstream and lymph system. Liquid portions of the chyme are reabsorbed in the large intestines and the solid waste is eliminated as feces.

Checkpoint Question
1. *What is peristalsis and how does it aid digestion?*

Metabolism

Food is broken down into usable units by a process of physical and chemical changes called metabolism. There are two phases of metabolism: anabolism and catabolism. As part of the anabolic or constructive phase, digested nutrients are converted into units that can be absorbed and used by the cells for growth, repair, and each cell's specific functions. As part of the catabolic or destructive phase, these chemical units are broken down to release the energy stored within the compounds.

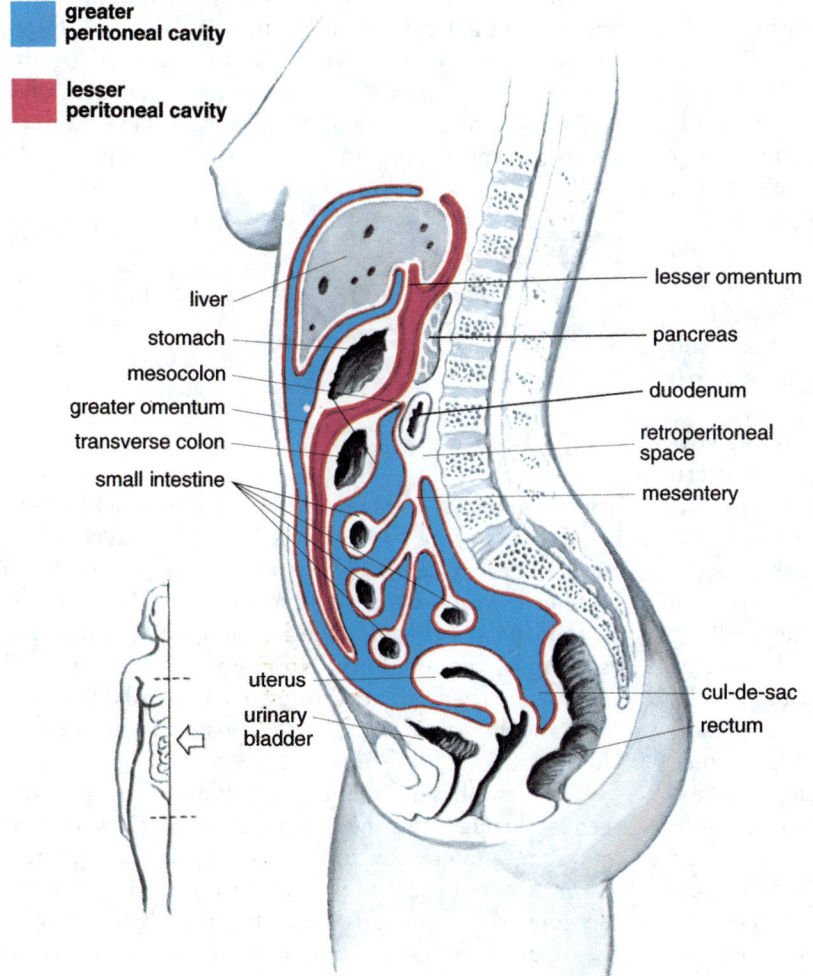

greater peritoneal cavity

lesser peritoneal cavity

liver
stomach
mesocolon
greater omentum
transverse colon
small intestine

lesser omentum
pancreas
duodenum
retroperitoneal space
mesentery

uterus
urinary bladder

cul-de-sac
rectum

FIGURE 38-2
Diagram of the abdominal cavity showing the peritoneum.

Table 38-1
Digestive Enzymes

Enzyme	Source	Action Target
Amylase	Salivary glands and pancreas	Starch
Hydrochloric acid	Gastric glands	Protein, sucrose, collagen
Pepsin	Gastric glands	Protein
Bile	Liver (stored in gallbladder)	Fats
Trypsin	Pancreas	Protein
Lipase	Pancreas	Fats
Lactose	Duodenal mucosa	Glucose
Maltase	Intestinal villi	Maltose (sugar)

➤ ORGANS OF THE GASTROINTESTINAL SYSTEM

Mouth

The oral cavity begins at the lips, which help to move the food into the mouth during ingestion and aid in speech formation. The cheeks are formed by the buccal muscles and aid in pushing the food from side to side for more efficient chewing. The tongue is composed of skeletal muscle and covered with mucous membranes. Within the mucous membranes of the tongue are several sizes and shapes of **papillae**, or taste buds, called **papillae lingua**. They provide friction for the food and are part of the sensory system that provides us with the sense of taste. The tongue moves the food back and forth to aid in chewing and helps mix the food particles with saliva for swallowing.

The palate consists of the mucous membrane-covered palatine bone anteriorly and soft tissue posteriorly. When the bolus of food reaches the pharynx, the soft palate rises, lifting the uvula, and closes the nasopharynx to keep food from entering the nasal cavity.

The teeth break the food into manageable pieces in a process called **mastication**, or chewing. The teeth are fixed in the **gingiva**, or gums, with a root below the gum line, firmly attached in the mandible and maxilla. They are composed internally of **dentin**, which surrounds the inner pulp and lies just below the enamel, and covered with enamel above the gum line. The exposed portion is called the crown. The 20 **deciduous** teeth (baby teeth) begin to erupt at about 6 months. As the roots are absorbed, these teeth are shed; 36 permanent teeth begin to replace the deciduous teeth by about age 6. The replacement teeth consist of central

and lateral incisors for cutting, canines for tearing and grasping, and premolars and molars for grinding.

The salivary glands secrete saliva to moisten the ground food particles and bind them for swallowing. The three main pairs of salivary glands are:

- *parotid*, just below and in front of the ears; ducts open into the cheeks
- *submandibular*, in the floor of the mouth; ducts open near the frenulum
- *sublingual*, under the tongue with several small ducts

Saliva is usually neutral (6.5–7.5 pH) to protect the teeth. Its production is easily affected by olfactory stimuli, emotions, visual impulses, and even by memories. Digestion begins with saliva production and the breakdown of some of the carbohydrates into sugars.

Oropharynx

The oropharynx, or throat, is common to both the GI and respiratory systems. Just above the oropharynx is the nasopharynx, posterior to the nasal cavity. Just below the oropharynx is the laryngopharynx, which opens into the larynx and the trachea. When the bolus of food is ready to be swallowed, it is lifted by the tongue and moved to the oropharynx, a process called deglutition, or swallowing. Smooth muscles and peristalsis transport it to and through the esophagus.

Checkpoint Question
2. *What is the difference between mastication and deglutition?*

Esophagus

The esophagus is located behind the trachea (see Chap. 37, Caring for Patients With Disorders of the Respiratory System). Except during the act of swallowing, the esophagus remains closed. When a bolus of food passes through the laryngopharynx into the esophagus, the epiglottis closes over the larynx and seals the airway. The esophagus expands into the thin, membranous area at the posterior of the tracheal cartilages.

The esophagus is about 10 inches long and descends through the mediastinum, penetrates the diaphragm, and empties into the stomach. No digestive action occurs in the esophagus. The cardiac sphincter separates the esophagus from the stomach at the **hiatus** (opening or gap). The esophagus is not protected from the stomach's digestive enzymes and can be damaged if acids **reflux** (flow backward) through the cardiac sphincter.

Stomach

The stomach is a J-shaped muscular pouch located under the diaphragm in the left upper quadrant and extends to the inner curve of the underside of the liver. The stomach has a three-tiered muscular structure consisting of circular, longitudinal, and oblique smooth muscle. The function of the muscle layers of the stomach is to churn the food and mix it with gastric enzymes. The inner layers are composed of a mucosa and submucosa layer to protect the underlying muscular structure from the acids necessary for digestion (Fig. 38-3).

The stomach is divided into four main regions:

1. Cardiac region (the upper curve of the stomach near the heart)
2. Fundus (balloons above the cardiac region)
3. Body (middle or main portion)
4. Antrum or pylorus (narrows to the pyloric sphincter)

The pyloric sphincter guards the opening between the stomach and the first portion of the small bowel.

The cells that make up the inner lining of the stomach produce hydrochloric acid (HCl) to help dissolve the food and kill ingested bacteria. The pH of HCl is approximately 2. The presence of HCl stimulates the production of pepsin from cells in the mucous membrane lining of the stomach walls. The mixing, churning action of the muscular walls of the stomach aid the enzymes in liquefying the food into chyme. The chyme is then pressed in small amounts through the pyloric sphincter and passes into the small intestine.

Very few substances are absorbed through the gastric mucosa. These substances may include limited amounts of water, alcohol, and certain drugs. Food that is absorbed through the stomach walls has been ingested as simple molecules such as the simple sugars.

When the stomach is empty, it folds into **rugae** to allow for expansion. The stomach can hold about one quart of food or liquid and completes its part of the digestive process in about 3 to 4 hours.

Small Intestine

The small intestine is the longest portion of the GI system and is divided into three sections: duodenum, jejunum, ileum. The divisions of these sections are marked only by microscopic structural differences. The total small bowel can stretch to 23 to 26 feet long. The final stages of digestion occur in the small intestine.

The upper section, the *duodenum,* is about 12 inches long. It is located in front of the kidney and just below the liver. It is connected to the gallbladder for bile and to the pancreas for enzymes to begin the digestion of the chyme pressed from the stomach. Bile breaks down the fats into small globules that can be digested. The pancreatic enzymes break down carbohydrates, fats, and proteins. The middle section, the *jejunum,* is the longest section, measuring about 6 to 8 feet. Digestion and absorption continue throughout its length and are completed in the *ileum,* the remaining 1- to 2-foot section.

The entire inner surface of the small intestine has a soft, velvety covering of villi that slow the chyme and increase the surface area for greater absorption (Fig. 38-4). Each projection of villi is also covered with microvilli, which further increase the opportunities for absorption. Most of the digestion occurs in the duodenum by the action of the bile and pancreatic enzymes; absorption occurs further into the jejunum and ileum. Passage through the small intestine usually takes from 3 to 10 hours, with peristalsis pushing the food slowly through. The bowel sounds that can be heard are produced by the relaxation and contraction of the intestinal walls against the mass of food as it moves toward the large intestine.

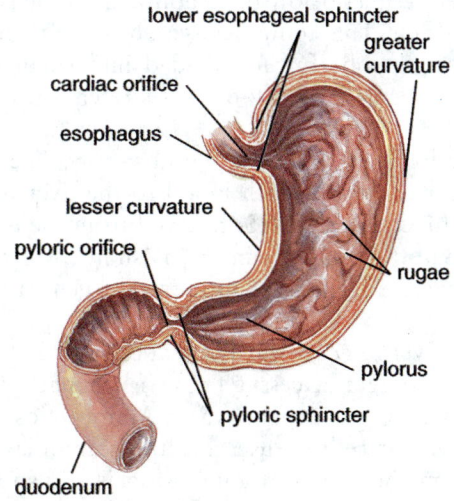

lower esophageal sphincter
greater curvature
cardiac orifice
esophagus
lesser curvature
pyloric orifice
rugae
pylorus
pyloric sphincter
duodenum

FIGURE 38-3
Longitudinal section of the stomach and a portion of the duodenum showing the interior.

Checkpoint Question
3. What are the three sections of the small intestine? In which sections do digestion and absorption occur?

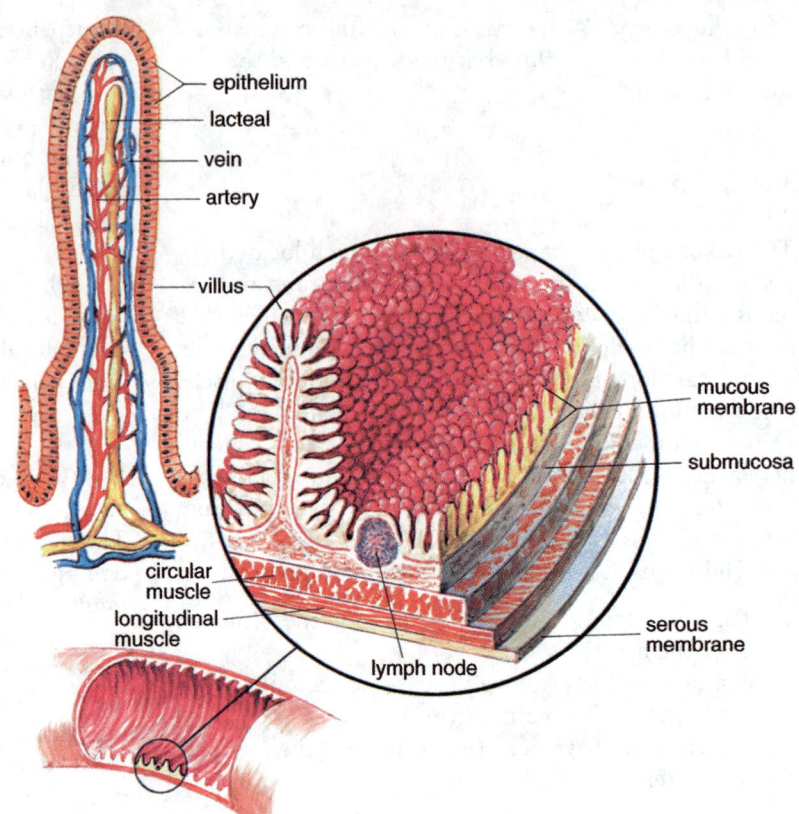

FIGURE 38-4
Diagram of the wall of the small intestine showing numerous villi. At the left is an enlarged drawing of a single villus.

Large Intestine

The ileocecal valve divides the ileum from the first part of the large intestine, called the *cecum*. The large intestine stores the digested material while fluids are reabsorbed into the bloodstream and the indigestible particles are passed along for elimination. The large intestine is about 6 to 8 feet long.

From the cecum in the right lower quadrant, the intestine rises as the ascending colon toward the liver in the right upper quadrant. It turns at the hepatic flexure and crosses the abdominal cavity toward the left upper quadrant as the transverse colon. At the gastric flexure, it turns downward toward the left lower quadrant as the descending colon. In the extreme lower left quadrant, it turns toward the midline as the sigmoid colon and joins the rectum. The rectum ends at the anus.

Little is absorbed in the colon except water, minerals, and certain vitamins. A normally present bacteria, *Escherichia coli*, synthesizes vitamin K and some of the B-complex vitamins and devours the last of the nutrients. As the undigested material fills the sigmoid colon and rectum and presses against the inner rectal sphincter, the urge to defecate builds. Expelling the feces (the products of digestion) is called defecation.

ACCESSORY ORGANS

The accessory organs of the gastrointestinal system include the liver, gallbladder, and pancreas (Fig. 38-5).

Liver

The liver lies just below the diaphragm in the right upper quadrant. This complex organ has two main lobes, a large right lobe further divided into smaller partitions and a smaller left lobe that stretches toward the top of the stomach.

The liver has a double blood supply. The hepatic artery carries oxygen-rich blood to the liver to maintain its functions. Blood is received from the intestinal vessels into the portal vein and is shunted to the liver to be processed before rerouting to the general circulation.

The liver removes glucose and converts it to glycogen for storage. Excess glucose is changed to fatty acids, carbon dioxide, and water. Amino acids are broken down for cellular use, and the ammonia that results from the chemical conversion is transported as urea to the kidneys for elimination. The liver manufactures and metabolizes many of the proteins, fats, and

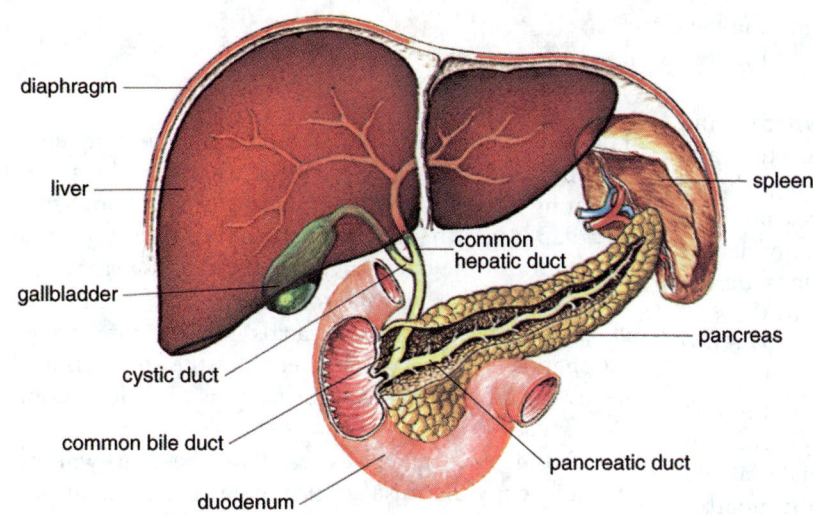

diaphragm

liver

gallbladder

cystic duct

common bile duct

duodenum

common
hepatic duct

spleen

pancreas

pancreatic duct

FIGURE 38-5
Accessory organs of digestion.

carbohydrates used by the body. It removes and stores vitamins A, D, B_{12}, K, and the mineral iron. The liver destroys old red blood cells and manufactures bile to **emulsify** (disperse) fats for digestion. Special phagocytic cells, called Kupffer cells, remove toxins, bacteria, and foreign agents to clean the blood before returning it to the heart by way of the hepatic veins.

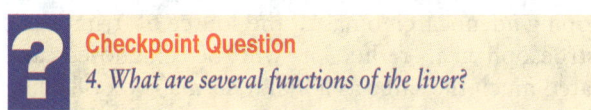

Checkpoint Question
4. What are several functions of the liver?

Gallbladder

The liver constantly manufactures the enzyme bile even though bile is only needed during digestion. Bile flows from the liver through the cystic duct to the gallbladder for storage until needed. As chyme leaves the stomach in small 5- to 15-mL portions, bile is added to the mixture to break the fat particles into globules that can be absorbed through the intestinal walls into the lymph system. This milky, fatty substance is called **chyle** and is carried to the thoracic lymphatic duct and added to the general circulation.

Pancreas

The pancreas is a large, long organ that stretches behind the stomach from the duodenum to the spleen. It has several functions, such as filtering old red blood cells for the lymphatic system and storing blood for emergencies. It

functions in both the endocrine and the exocrine systems. As an endocrine gland, the pancreas secretes insulin and glucagon from the islets of Langerhans to regulate blood sugar levels. As an exocrine gland, it excretes pancreatic enzymes for the digestion of fats, proteins, and carbohydrates. The pancreatic enzymes are very alkaline to counteract the acidity of the gastric enzymes as they pass through the duodenum. The pancreas empties into the duodenum through a duct that it shares with the gallbladder called the common bile duct.

➤ COMMON GASTROINTESTINAL DISORDERS

Mouth Disorders

Caries

Dental caries (tooth decay) is the most widespread disease of the oral cavity. Bacteria allowed to remain on the tooth surfaces erode the enamel and allow infection to reach the inner portions of the tooth. There are many reasons for a susceptibility to tooth decay. These include diet, hygiene, **malocclusion** (abnormal contact between the teeth), and the prenatal diet. The treatment includes a proper diet low in sugars, good oral hygiene as prescribed by the dentist, and frequent professional dental care.

Stomatitis

The most common disease of the mouth tissues is stomatitis or inflammation of the oral mucosa. It may be caused by a virus or a bacteria. The two most common forms are herpetic stomatitis, caused by the herpes simplex virus, and candidiasis, caused by the fungus *Candida albicans*.

Herpes simplex is usually self-limiting after the initial exposure to the virus. The exposure is usually hand to mouth, mouth to mouth, or by vector (eg, shared drinking glasses or eating utensils). It presents as a painful sore in the mouth or on the lips. The virus lies dormant for long periods with exacerbations during periods of illness, stress, and overexposure to the sun. There is no cure; palliative measures relieve discomfort until the ulcers heal.

Candida albicans, formerly called *Monilia albicans*, is an opportunistic yeast or fungus. It is always present in the mouth but is kept in check by other normal oral bacteria. When the normal bacterial balance in the mouth is altered, *C. albicans* organisms multiply. Broad-spectrum antibiotics kill many different bacteria, upsetting the balance and allowing the opportunistic organisms to grow without control. In babies, the disease is call thrush. It occurs because milk has changed the pH in the mouth, establishing a more favorable environment for the growth of the *C. albicans*. Oral treatments with antifungal agents are usually effective at relieving the disorder.

When *Candida* spreads to the esophagus, it is usually caused by a breakdown in the immune system, as seen in immunosuppression.

Gingivitis

Gingivitis is inflammation of the gingiva or gums. It may lead to periodontitis and destruction of the support structures of the teeth. In Americans, more teeth are lost to gum disease than to tooth decay. Good oral hygiene and frequent dental care will prevent premature loss of teeth. Vincent's angina is a severe form of gum infection with systemic symptoms. It is usually treated by antibiotics.

Oral Cancers

Oral cancers are common, especially among individuals who use tobacco products. The constant irritation of the tobacco causes white spots or patches, called leukoplakia, to form on the oral mucosa, particularly the lips and tongue. These lesions frequently become malignant and are treated by surgery or chemical agents. Cancer of the lips usually responds well to radiation or surgery. Cancer of the margins of the tongue metastasize quickly and are hard to treat.

? Checkpoint Question
5. What are four common mouth disorders?

Esophageal Disorders

Hiatal Hernia

Hiatal hernia is a common condition that frequently affects people over age 40. Weight gain can be a contributing factor. A hiatal hernia is caused by a defect in the diaphragm that allows a portion of the stomach to slide up into the chest cavity. Normally, the stomach's cardiac sphincter and the tone of the diaphragm muscle prevent reflux of gastric acids into the unprotected esophagus. This barrier loss enables the stomach acid to invade the esophagus, causing considerable discomfort (Fig. 38-6).

Diagnosis is made by chest x-ray, barium swallow, or endoscopy. Because surgically corrected hiatal hernias frequently recur, medical treatment is usually the first choice. This includes diet modification (eg, small frequent meals with no food at least 2 hours before bedtime), antacid treatments, weight loss, elevating the head of the bed, and drug therapy to increase the tone of the cardiac sphincter.

Constant exposure to gastric acid from a hiatal hernia or gastroesophageal reflux can lead to esophagitis, a condition that resembles abraded skin along the lining of the esophagus. Constant irritation of the lining of the esophagus may lead to malignancy. This condition is called Barrett's esophagus. Patients with Barrett's esophagus have a 30% to 40% chance of developing adenocarcinomas. If the source of irritation is gastroesophageal reflux, it will be diagnosed and treated much the same as a hiatal hernia (Box 38-1).

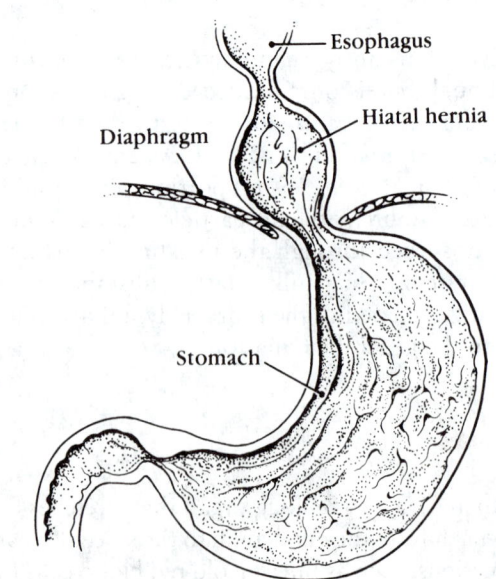

FIGURE 38-6
Location and appearance of hiatal hernia.

BOX 38-1 Avoiding Gastric Reflux

1. Avoid spicy foods and chocolate, especially in the evening.
2. Limit caffeine.
3. Maintain optimum weight.
4. Avoid overeating.
5. Wait 1 hour after meals before exercising.
6. Do not eat just before going to bed.
7. Do not lie down just after eating.
8. Stop smoking.
9. Raise the head of the bed with blocks, bricks, or stacks of books.
10. See the physician if symptoms persist.

Esophageal Varices

Varicose veins of the esophagus result from pressure within the esophageal veins. This is common with cirrhosis of the liver because the damaged liver structure impedes the drainage of the portal vein. Hemorrhage is the most common and dangerous possibility. Pressure tubes are applied in the esophagus as an emergency procedure. Endoscopic procedures, such as chemical sclerosis, are the treatment of choice when the patient is able to tolerate the procedure.

Esophageal Cancer

Cancer of the esophagus is most common among older men and is usually fatal. Gastric reflux, smoking, and alcohol use are predisposing factors.

The malignancy narrows the lumen of the esophagus and causes dysphagia. As the mass enlarges, swallowing solid food may become extremely painful. Vomiting and weight loss will occur as the symptoms progress. This cancer usually spreads to the mediastinal organs. A barium swallow fluoroscopy will outline the lesion and esophagoscopy with biopsy will confirm the diagnosis. If the disease is localized, surgical resection is the treatment of choice. Radiation and chemotherapy are also used. No treatment has proven satisfactory and survival rates are very low.

Checkpoint Question

6. What is hiatal hernia and how can it affect the esophagus?

Stomach Disorders

Gastritis

Gastritis is an inflammation of the stomach lining. The most common causes are irritants, such as alcohol, and the excessive intake of aspirin and nonsteroidal anti-inflammatory drugs (NSAIDs). The organism *Helicobacter pylori* is also frequently implicated. The ingestion or presence of any sufficiently irritating substance can erode the mucosal lining and cause inflammation. The condition may be acute or chronic.

Gastritis can cause significant oozing of blood and may result in a positive test for occult (hidden) blood. In elderly patients, sufficient blood loss can cause anemia. Symptoms include GI bleeding, epigastric discomfort, nausea, and vomiting. Diagnosis usually includes gastroscopy. Treatment usually involves eliminating the irritant and restoring the proper gastric acidity. Chronic atrophic gastritis is seen frequently with types of severe anemia. Vitamin B_{12} must be given by injection to combat the anemia.

Ulcers

Ulcers are sloughed tissues that leave erosions or sores. Within the GI tract, these erosions can expose small blood vessels and produce bleeding and pain. The exposure of subsurface areas of the gastric mucosa to hydrochloric acid (HCl) causes pain that is intensified by the action of peristalsis. The acids flow in abundance through the pylorus and may also erode the duodenum. The bleeding ranges from oozing to massive, life-threatening hemorrhage. Slight seepage can be detected by a test for occult blood. Heavier bleeding will lead to **melena** (black, tarry stools) or a "coffee-ground" appearance in **hematemesis** (vomiting blood). **Ulcers in the GI tract may perforate into the abdominal cavity with life-threatening consequences.** Ulcerative conditions may progress to malignancies.

Peptic or gastric ulcers are frequently caused by the use of salicylates, NSAIDs, and alcohol. **It has recently been discovered that many gastric ulcers are caused by a chronic *H. pylori* infection.**

Helicobacter pylori is a bacteria presumed to enter the body either by the fecal/oral route or the oral/oral route. It resides in the mucous lining of the stomach and through its metabolism secretes enzymes that attack the mucous membrane. A small tissue sample is obtained by endoscopy and placed on a gel that will indicate if *H. pylori* is present.

Helicobacter pylori is treated with antibiotics, antifungal agents, and bismuth subsalicylate. The prescribed treatment for ulcers caused by hyperacidity involves limiting the production of hydrogen by the gastric cells to neutralize the acid in the stomach. The gastric acids produced by the stomach are under nerve and hormonal control and are increased in stressful situations. Severing the vagus nerve (vagotomy) reduces the secretion of HCl. Pyloroplasty to open the lumen of the pyloric sphincter eases gastric emptying to reduce the gastric load and also reduces the length of mucosal exposure to the gastric enzymes.

Pyloric Stenosis

Pyloric stenosis occurs when an abnormally narrow pylorus delays or obstructs the emptying of the gastric contents. Vomiting (sometimes projectile) occurs as peristalsis pushes against the stricture. There is no known cause. A pyloroplasty relaxes the lumen (see Fig. 38-3).

Gastric Cancer

Gastric cancer has no known cause although smoking, high alcohol intake, and genetic predisposition have been implicated. Populations consuming foods high in preservatives, such as smoking, pickling, and salting, have a high incidence of gastric cancer.

Gastric cancer spreads rapidly to the adjacent organs and throughout the peritoneal cavity. Symptoms include chronic indigestion, weight loss, anorexia, anemia, and fatigue. The patient may have hematemesis with bright blood or "coffee-ground" vomitus with dark blood. There may also be dark, bloody stools.

Diagnosis requires an upper GI series with fluoroscopy and fiberoptic gastroscopy. The extent of the disease can be determined by computed tomography (CT) scans and by biopsy of the suspected metastatic sites. Surgery to remove the lesion may range from a subtotal gastric resection to a total gastrectomy. If the cancer has metastasized, other organs may be removed and radiation and chemotherapy may be necessary.

Intestinal Disorders

Gastroenteritis

Gastroenteritis is the inflammation of the stomach, small intestine, or colon. It can include one organ or all three. It is caused by ingesting food or water that contains bacteria, viruses, parasites, or irritating agents. It can be provoked by food allergies or a reaction to medication, such as antibiotics. Symptoms include abdominal pain and cramping, nausea, vomiting, and diarrhea; sometimes fever is present.

Gastroenteritis is usually self-limiting, but in the elderly, young children, or persons with diabetes mellitus, the dehydration that can accompany the diarrhea

---

What If?

What if your pediatric patient's mother complains that her baby vomits everything he eats?

If the vomiting is projectile, the child might have pyloric stenosis. This disorder is usually seen in infants and young children from several days to several months of age. Diagnosis is usually made by parental history, physical examination, and radiologic examination. The physician is often able to palpate an olive-shaped lump in the right upper quadrant while the child is in a supine position. Surgery (pyloroplasty) is the treatment. Although pyloric stenosis is not an emergency, surgery is usually scheduled promptly to prevent dehydration. Educate the parents about the disorder, reassure them, and offer supportive counseling.

---

and vomiting could be life-threatening. Bacteria and parasites are treated with medication if the condition persists. Fluids and electrolytes are restored intravenously as needed.

Duodenal Ulcers

Ulcers formed in the duodenum are caused by the highly corrosive gastric acid. Unlike the stomach, the pH of the duodenum is more alkaline and the mucosa is not as well protected as the gastric mucosa. The lining of the duodenum may tolerate bile, but it does not tolerate concentrated gastric juices. When the food material passes through the pylorus and brings with it excessive acid, an ulcer forms.

Treatment for duodenal ulcers involves lowering the stomach acid by reducing the gastric acidity and limiting the irritating factors. If these measures are not successful, surgery is an option. If left untreated, ulcers both in the stomach and the duodenum may perforate or may progress to cancer.

Malabsorption Syndromes

Malabsorption syndromes prevent absorption of certain substances through the walls of the small intestines. Fat is a common substance at risk. Stools associated with fat malabsorption will be frothy and pale. Because fat is necessary for the metabolism of vitamins A, D, E, and K, patients with this disorder require supplemental vitamin therapy. Celiac sprue is a malabsorption syndrome with an intolerance of gluten. Gluten is a protein found in wheat and wheat by-products. Celiac sprue can develop at any stage of life and many times presents with diarrhea high in fat. The treatment is usually a gluten-free diet. The cause of sprue is not known but it runs in families, so a genetic factor may be involved.

Malabsorption syndromes are treated by addressing the suspected causes and replacing the substances at risk.

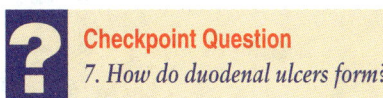

Checkpoint Question
7. How do duodenal ulcers form?

Colon Disorders

Crohn's Disease

Crohn's disease is an inflammation of the bowel, ranging from very mild to severe and debilitating. The cause of Crohn's disease is unclear; it is thought to be an autoimmune disorder with a possible genetic link. Crohn's disease can affect the small bowel and the colon but is more common in the area of the ileocecal valve. The bowel walls become inflamed and the lymph nodes become enlarged; this in turn leads to edema of the bowel wall. When the lining of the bowel is swollen, the fluid from the intestinal contents cannot be absorbed, causing diarrhea and cramping, and may lead to more irritation and bleeding.

Each episode of inflammation causes scarring. The scarring may lead to narrowing of the colon causing an obstruction of the bowel. Bowel obstruction, no matter what its cause, can be life-threatening and is a medical emergency. Laboratory tests reveal an increase in white blood cells (WBCs) and the erythrocyte sedimentation rate (ESR). A barium enema (BE or BaE) shows strictures alternating with normal bowel (the "string sign"). Sigmoidoscopy and colonoscopy show patchy areas of inflammation.

The treatment is symptomatic and involves restoration of electrolytes, administration of corticosteroids for the inflammation, rest, and a low-fiber diet. Surgery is performed for perforation or hemorrhage. If the situation is severe, a colectomy with an ileostomy may be performed (Fig. 38-7).

Ulcerative Colitis

Ulcerative colitis is a chronic inflammatory disease of the lining of the colon. It occurs most often in young women, but may occur at any age and may affect men also. The cause is not known but is thought to be an abnormal GI immune reaction to foods or microorganisms. Like Crohn's disease, it can be mild or severe.

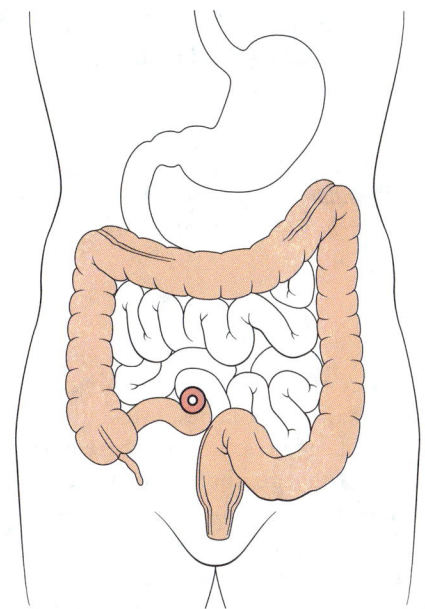

FIGURE 38-7
An ileostomy.

The tissue that lines the colon becomes congested and edematous and sloughs off, leading to ulcers and bloody diarrhea. Sometimes pus and mucus are present in the diarrhea. Malabsorption of fluids causes weakness, anorexia, and nausea and vomiting. Scarring can occur as the ulcers heal. The colon may produce pseudopolyps, which can be precancerous. Diagnosis may be made by sigmoidoscopy, which shows a fragile mucosa with inflammation or by BE, which will show areas of edema and ulceration. Biopsy confirms the diagnosis. Colonoscopy will evaluate strictures caused by scarring and assess the risk of cancer.

Treatment requires controlling the inflammation and preventing debilitating loss of fluids and nutrients. If the disease is severe, corticosteroids will relieve the inflammation. Surgery is a last resort and usually involves a proctocolectomy with an ileostomy (see Fig. 38-7).

Irritable Bowel Syndrome

Patients with irritable bower syndrome (IBS) frequently complain of bouts of constipation alternating with diarrhea. Although it presents with symptoms resembling mild Crohn's disease or ulcerative colitis it usually does not result in weight loss and the prognosis is good. It can be debilitating because there is no warning for the bouts of diarrhea. It has a range of symptoms from mild to severe. Women are more likely than men to experience spastic colon. Its origin is thought to be psychogenic but food irritants may precipitate an attack. Diagnosis requires a careful history, both physical and emotional. Other diseases are ruled out by testing. Treatment requires stress management and identifying the offending food irritants.

Checkpoint Question

8. *Which inflammatory bowel disorder can lead to life-threatening bowel obstruction? How?*

Diverticulosis

Diverticulosis results from the thinning of the bowel wall causing small out-pouches. It usually occurs in the sigmoid colon but may occur anywhere in the GI tract. The cause has been attributed to a diet deficient in roughage. Diverticulosis becomes serious when the bowel wall becomes so thin that it exposes veins and arteries. When nicked by a piece of stool, bleeding can occur. The bleeding can be so severe that surgery is required to stop the hemorrhage.

Diverticulosis may progress to diverticulitis or inflammation of these areas of weakness in the bowel wall. The inflammation is usually caused by fecal material becoming lodged in the thin pockets. The symptoms are fever and abdominal pain. As the bowel becomes swollen and distended, the diseased areas may rupture, exposing the peritoneum to fecal material and resulting in peritonitis. The pouches usually show on BE or other radiologic studies.

During the acute phase, treatment includes a bland diet and stool softeners. When the initial inflammation has subsided, a high-fiber diet is ordered.

Polyps

Colon polyps are masses of mucous membrane tissue. Polyps are usually slow growing but over a period of years may become cancerous. They may be discovered by a BE or during a colonoscopy performed to evaluate a change in bowel habits or after occult blood is found in the stool. If the polyps are discovered at an early stage and removed, cancer of the colon can be prevented. Cancer of the colon may invade the muscle of the bowel and metastasize through the lymph system to other organs.

Hemorrhoids

Hemorrhoids are dilated veins (varicosities) in the rectum. They may be external or internal. Internal hemorrhoids may become enlarged and may bleed during defecation. External hemorrhoids may become very painful and itchy and may also bleed. The bleeding may range from a stain on the toilet paper to massive hemorrhage. The blood will be bright red rather than the darker blood expected from sites higher in the GI tract. External hemorrhoids are obvious on inspection. Internal hemorrhoids are diagnosed by anoscopy or proctoscopy. Hemorrhoids are caused by poor muscle tone, poor dietary habits, and constipation.

Treatment involves regulating the diet to control constipation, providing local pain relief, using stool softeners, administering chemical sclerosing agents, and surgical ligation.

Colorectal Cancers

Cancer of the colon and rectum usually spread slowly with good survival rates with early diagnosis and treatment. The cause is unknown, but its incidence has been linked to diets high in animal fats and low in fiber. It is commonly seen in patients with a history of ulcerative colitis or colorectal polyps (Fig. 38-8).

Early signs are vague pains with occasional bloody stools. Later signs depend on the section of the colon involved and the degree of metastasis. These signs usually include anemia, weakness, diarrhea or **obstipation** (extreme constipation), anorexia, and weight loss. Many rectal cancers are discovered by a digital examination or an anoscopy. Sigmoidoscopy or colonoscopy are suggested to determine the extent of involvement. Barium enema (BE) with contrast air will aid in diagnosis. Laboratory tests include **guaiac** (reagent) tests, such as the Hemoccult, which test for occult blood in the stool. Surgery to remove the affected area is the treatment of choice and is usually followed by chemotherapy and radiation.

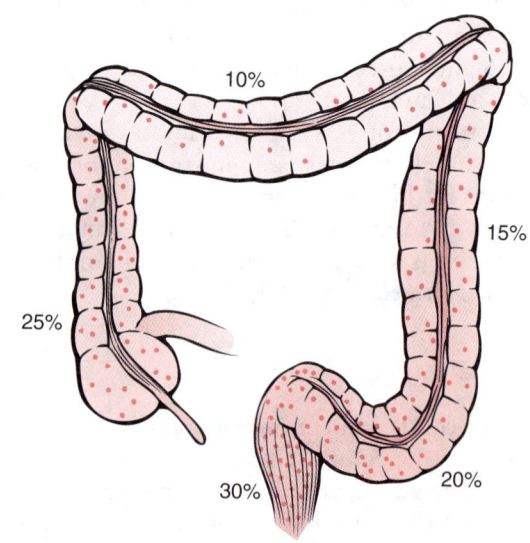

FIGURE 38-8
Percentage distribution of cancer sites in the colon and rectum.

Functional Disorders

Constipation

When the lower colon is full of fecal material, nerve endings send impulses to the brain that in turn tell the pelvic and rectal muscles to expel the accumulated material. If the nerve endings have been injured or paralyzed, these impulses are not transmitted. Most constipation is caused by poor bowel habits, low-fiber diets, and inadequate fluid intake. The solid material stays in the colon too long and becomes progressively dryer and harder. The normal interval between bowel movements varies with the individual. Infrequent but easy-to-pass stools are not considered constipation. The quality of the stool is more important than the quantity.

Constipation that is not attributed to poor dietary and bowel habits may be due to spasticity of the intestinal walls. The walls clamp against the stool and will not allow it to pass. Several intestinal disorders result in spasticity and constipation. The underlying cause must be treated.

Atonic or flaccid constipation is the opposite and is considered a lazy colon. The causes include poor dietary habits, low fluid intake, lack of exercise, chronic laxative use, and reliance on enemas. Reversing the causes will usually correct the situation in time.

Diarrhea

Normal peristalsis allows the products of digestion to move at a speed that allows fluid reabsorption. When the fluid contents of the bowel are rushed through, as in diarrhea, the water and minerals are not reabsorbed into the system. Infections (bacterial or viral) or GI irritants cause the smooth muscles and the mucous membranes to work to flush out the bowel as quickly as possible. The treatment for diarrhea includes medication to slow peristalsis, a bland diet, and increased fluids. Diarrhea is usually self-limiting. Any significant or prolonged changes in bowel habits should be evaluated by a physician.

Gas

Bacterial decomposition of proteins in the digestive process produces gas that can lead to abdominal discomfort. Gas causes a feeling of fullness that can be expelled by erupting the gas from the stomach through the mouth (eructation) or from the intestines through the rectum (flatulence). The causes include an intolerance of milk products, swallowing air, chewing gum, eating gas-producing or fatty foods, or slow emptying of the stomach and bowels. The problem can usually be relieved by avoiding the offending foods. Various

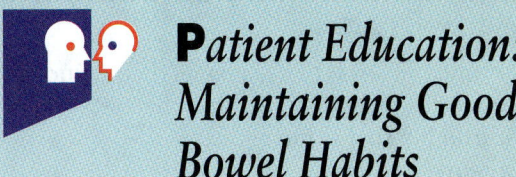

Patient Education: Maintaining Good Bowel Habits

By following the guidelines below, patients can avoid problems of elimination.

1. Eat a wide variety of foods, especially fresh fruits, vegetables, and whole grains. Limit intake of highly processed foods.
2. Drink eight glasses of water a day to help keep the stools moist and easy to pass and to hydrate the tissues.
3. Participate in some form of exercise daily. Even a walk around the block will aid muscle tone and help prevent a sluggish metabolism.
4. Make time for bowel movements when the stimulus is felt. Avoiding or delaying defecation will result in loss of moisture from the stool and may make the bowel insensitive to the stimulus.
5. Avoid laxative or enema use. Frequent use may result in a "lazy bowel."
6. Recognize that the frequency of bowel elimination is an individual characteristic. If stools are passed only several times a week but are soft formed and passed with little effort, there should be no concern about constipation. However, constipation may be a problem if stools are passed daily but are hard, dry, and difficult to pass.

over-the-counter preparations and prescription medications can be used if the problem persists.

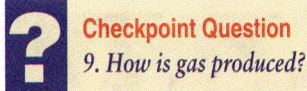

Checkpoint Question
9. How is gas produced?

Liver Disorders

Liver disorders are assessed by observing the cardinal signs of liver dysfunction: jaundice, **ascites** (fluid accumulation in the peritoneal cavity) and **hepatomegaly** (liver enlargement). It is vital to obtain a complete medical history from an individual with suspected liver disorder; focus particularly on the history of prior jaundice, anemia, splenectomy, past alcohol use, travel to third-world countries, blood transfusions, use of **hepatotoxic** medications (drugs that are damaging to the liver), or controlled substance abuse. Diagnostic tests for liver disorders include:

- liver function tests (LFT), a panel that includes levels of bilirubin, alkaline phosphatase, albumin, prothrombin times, and cholesterol
- x-rays and barium studies
- radioisotope liver scans
- biopsy
- percutaneous peritoneoscopy
- surgical laparotomy

Hepatitis

Hepatitis is an inflammatory process that causes liver destruction and necrosis. Its cause can be viral, bacterial, or toxic.

Five types of viral hepatitis exist. Table 38-2 summarizes the detailed descriptions of each type listed below:

- *Hepatitis A (HAV)*, the most common type of viral hepatitis, is also known as infectious hepatitis. HAV is spread through fecal/oral contamination, from contaminated food and water, or from seafood high in coliform bacteria. It is highly contagious and will spread through closely confined communities. The prognosis for recovery is good.
- *Hepatitis B (HBV)*, also known as serum hepatitis, can be transmitted by contaminated sera and other body fluids. The disease may be so severe that death results. Use of standard precautions will prevent its spread. Hepatitis B vaccine is recommended for health care workers at high risk for contact with individuals infected with HBV or with the blood or body fluids from these persons.
- *Hepatitis C (HCV)*, also known as non-A, non-B hepatitis, can be transmitted via blood transfu-

sion or percutaneous contamination. It frequently progresses to chronic hepatitis. As with HBV, use of standard precautions will prevent its spread.
- *Hepatitis D (HDV)* occurs only in patients who have had HBV; it cannot survive without the hepatitis B virus.
- *Hepatitis E (HEV)* is spread through fecal/oral routes or through dirty water. It is self-limiting.

For all types of viral hepatitis, the symptoms may include fatigue, joint pain, flulike symptoms with fever, jaundice, dark urine, and light stools. Complications include impaired liver function, chronic hepatitis, liver cancer, and death.

Diagnosis is made through medical history (eg, past transfusions or exposure to hepatotoxic drugs or chemicals), blood work for hepatitis antibodies, and liver function studies. There is no cure at this time except rest and supportive diet. Interferon-A studies are currently in clinical trials to assist the immune system in responding to viral forms of hepatitis. Standard precautions must be observed to protect caregivers and health care workers from viral hepatitis.

Toxic hepatitis may result from exposure to chemical toxicants or hepatotoxic substances, including certain medications and alcohol. If the offending toxicant is eliminated early enough, the prognosis for recovery is good. The symptoms of toxic hepatitis resemble viral hepatitis, and the diagnosis is similar. A liver biopsy may identify underlying pathology.

Checkpoint Question

10. How does the cause of viral hepatitis differ from that of toxic hepatitis?

Cirrhosis or Fibrosis

Cirrhosis is a chronic inflammatory disease characterized by destruction of liver cells and the formation of fibers throughout the liver, altering its function and efficiency. It occurs most often in men. Causes include a history of alcoholism, prolonged biliary obstruction, or posthepatitis sequela.

In the early stages of cirrhosis, symptoms include vague GI discomfort. In the late stages, diminished respiratory efficiency occurs as ascites force the abdominal contents against the diaphragm. Bleeding tendencies result from the loss of clotting factors formed in the liver. Dermal pruritus (itching), jaundice, and hepatomegaly are usually present. Diagnosis is made by liver biopsy, liver scan, and blood work. Treatment includes removing the cause of the damage (such as abstinence from alcohol), a good diet, vitamin supplements, and supportive care.

Table 38-2
Types of Viral Hepatitis

Type of Virus	Mode(s) of Transmission	Precautions
HAV	Fecal/oral route	Handwashing
HBV	Sera and body fluids	Standard Precautions HBV vaccine
HCV	Blood transfusions Percutaneous contamination	Standard Precautions
HDV	Co-infector of HBV	Standard Precautions HBV vaccine
HEV	Fecal/oral route	Handwashing Standard Precautions

Liver Cancer

The liver is rarely a primary site for cancer but is frequently the target site for metastasis. It is more common in men and is rapidly fatal. There is no known cause, but primary liver cancers are thought to be due to exposure to carcinogens. Patients who have cirrhosis or who have hepatitis B are more likely than the general population to develop liver cancer.

Patients usually complain of weight loss, weakness, and right upper quadrant pain. Jaundice may be present in the early stages and will definitely develop as the disease progresses. Diagnosis is confirmed by biopsy, liver function tests, and computed tomography (CT) scan or magnetic resonance imaging (MRI). If the lesion is small and localized, resection is possible. Chemotherapy may be used in some instances. If there is no metastasis, transplantation may be a possibility.

Gallbladder Disorders

Cholelithiasis and Cholecystitis

Cholelithiasis is the formation of gallstones (Fig. 38-9). Gallstones are made of cholesterol and bilirubin. When the peristaltic action of the gallbladder is sluggish and the bile is allowed to pool in the sac, fluid is absorbed leaving the solids to concentrate and solidify into stones. Cholecystitis is an acute or chronic inflammation of the gallbladder, usually resulting from an impacted stone in the duct.

Cholecystitis or cholelithiasis usually cause pain as peristalsis presses bile against the blockage, especially after a fatty meal. Acute right upper quadrant pain may radiate to the shoulders, back, or chest. Later in the illness, jaundice may appear. Treatment requires removal of the stones, usually by endoscopic laparotomy. Diet modification may prevent recurrence.

Choledocholithiasis is a stone lodged in the duct system. Cholangitis is an infection of the bile ducts.

Signs and symptoms of any gallbladder disorder include pain, indigestion, nausea, and an intolerance for fatty foods. Tests to determine the cause include cholecystography after the ingestion of a radiopaque dye, percutaneous transhepatic cholangiography, endoscopic retrograde cholangiopancreatography (ERCP), and duodenal endoscopy. Noninvasive procedures include ultrasound and CT scans. Flat plate x-rays are not especially accurate for evaluating gallbladder disorders.

Gallbladder Cancer

Cancer of the gallbladder is rare and difficult to diagnose. It is usually discovered during gallbladder series to diagnose cholelithiasis. It is more common in older women and is rapidly fatal. The cause is not known, but theory suggests that cholelithiasis is a predisposing factor. The signs and symptoms are indistinguishable from cholecystitis: right upper quadrant pain, nausea and vomiting, weight loss, and anorexia. However, cholecystitis pain is usually sporadic and pain due to malignancy is usually chronic and severe. The gallbladder may be palpable and jaundice may be present. Diagnosis includes liver function tests, CT scan, MRI, and cholecystography. Cholecystectomy is the treatment, but survival rates are low.

Checkpoint Question
11. What is cholelithiasis and how does it occur?

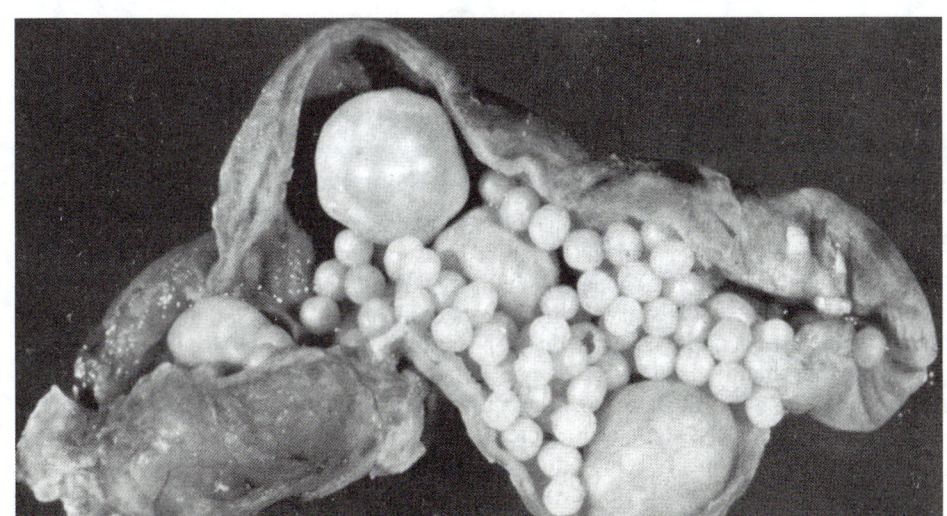

FIGURE 38-9
Multiple gallstones in a gallbladder. (Courtesy of National Institute of Diabetes and Digestive and Kidney Diseases.)

Pancreatic Disorders

Pancreatitis

Pancreatitis is an inflammation of the pancreas that may be related to alcoholism, trauma, gastric ulcer, and biliary tract disease. Symptoms include vomiting and steady epigastric pain radiating to the spine; signs of progressive disease include abdominal rigidity and decreased bowel activity. Complications include diabetes mellitus, hemorrhage, shock, coma, and death as the digestive enzymes cause the organ to digest itself. Diagnostic blood work will show an increase in serum amylase and glucose levels. Ultrasound and CT scans are useful in diagnosing the disorder. Treatment includes pain relief and medication to reduce pancreatic secretions while the organ recovers.

Pancreatic Cancer

One of the deadliest malignancies is pancreatic cancer. Most patients die within a year of diagnosis. There is no definitive cause but it occurs most often in middle-aged African American men who smoke, have diets high in fats and proteins, or who are exposed to industrial chemicals for long periods of time.

Patients complain of weight loss, back and abdominal pain, and diarrhea. They are frequently jaundiced. Diagnosis is made by laparoscopic biopsy, CT scan, MRI, endoscopic retrograde cholangiopancreatography (ERCP), and pancreatic enzyme studies. Pancreatotomy is an operative option; chemotherapy and radiation therapy are used also but the survival rate is very low with current therapies.

➤ COMMON DIAGNOSTIC PROCEDURES AND THE MEDICAL ASSISTANT'S ROLE

History and Assessment

Before beginning any client's care, an adequate history must be obtained. The patient presenting with GI concerns will be assessed for signs (eg, vomiting) and symptoms (eg, nausea). From that base, the physician will determine the direction of the diagnostic testing to rule out or to confirm possible diagnoses. The history must include occupation, family history, recent travel to third-world countries, and current medications. You may be required to assist the patient in completing a checklist of concerns, which might include heartburn, GI bleeding, weight gain or loss, social history of alcohol use, and laxative and enema use.

The physician will assess skin **turgor** (tension), jaundice, edema, bruising, breath odor, size and shape of the abdomen, presence and quality of bowel sounds and will palpate the abdominal contents.

Blood Tests

Blood work may include hemoglobin or hematocrit to assess possible anemia as the result of GI bleeding. White blood cell (WBC) counts can help detect the presence of infection. The erythrocyte sedimentation rate (ESR) is used to assess inflammatory processes. (See Chap. 46, Hematology, for a detailed discussion of these specific tests.)

Radiologic Studies

Radiologic studies of the stomach and bowels consist of instilling barium, a radiopaque substance, to outline the organs. Barium swallows are used to test for abnormal narrowing or masses in the esophagus. Fluoroscopy will be used to watch the chalky liquid as it fills the esophagus.

The upper GI (UGI) will show abnormal constrictions, masses, and obstruction in the esophagus, stomach, and duodenum. This examination requires that the client have nothing by mouth (NPO) after midnight. A small bowel series is an extension of the UGI that visualizes the barium flowing through the small intestines.

A barium enema (BE) provides an outline of the colon. It can reveal a blockage, cancerous growth, polyps, and diverticula. A BE requires that the colon be empty of stool. Box 38-2 outlines the standard patient preparation for a BE.

Flat plate x-rays of the abdomen may be ordered without contrast media but are not as diagnostic as contrast x-rays.

Endoscopic Examinations

The definitive test for the hollow organs of the GI system is an endoscopy examination. Fiberoptic technology has enabled physicians to pass soft, flexible tubes down the esophagus into the stomach and small bowel or up into the colon for direct visualization of these organs. Supplemental laboratory specimens can be obtained, such as tissues biopsies, samples for gastric analysis, fluids to check for bacteria, bile for crystals, and cells for cytology to diagnose malignancies.

Endoscopic examinations also are used to diagnose biliary disorders. ERCP is used to visualize the esophagus, the stomach, the proximal duodenum, and the pancreas. Dye is injected directly into the ducts of the gallbladder and the pancreas to establish patency and function.

Anoscopy involves inserting a metal or plastic instrument into the rectal canal for visual inspection of the anus and the rectum and to obtain swabs for cultures. The sigmoidoscopy examination is a visualization of the sigmoid colon using either a rigid sigmoidoscope or the more widely accepted flexible fiberoptic sigmoidoscope.

The rigid sigmoidoscope is about 10 inches (25 cm) long. This instrument is supplied as reusable metal or disposable plastic and is calibrated in centimeters. An obturator in the lumen allows the instrument to be inserted with minimal discomfort. The lens at the end is magnified for closer observation of the intestinal mucosa and can be moved aside to allow the physician to swab, suction, or biopsy the mucosa. The handle contains the light source. The scope may be equipped with a hand bulb **insufflator** (a device for blowing air, gases, or powders into a cavity) or a powered source of air to expand the walls of the colon for easier visualization to diagnose hemorrhoids, polyps, and diverticula.

The flexible fiberoptic sigmoidoscope is rapidly gaining favor. It offers better visualization and is more acceptable and less uncomfortable to patients. The scope is very thin, can bend and maneuver curves, and can be inserted much farther than the rigid scope (Fig. 38-10). The instrument is supplied as 35 cm (about 14 inches) or 65 cm (about 26 inches). The electrical source of the instrument usually includes an insufflator and suction in addition to the light source. Though smaller than the rigid scope, it also can be used to obtain samples and cultures.

Some physicians prefer that the bowel be as free of feces as possible and may order a light, low-residue meal the evening before the endoscopic examination. An evening laxative maybe also ordered to be followed by a cleansing enema in the morning before the procedure. A light breakfast may be allowed. Other physicians, however, prefer to view the mucosa as it normally appears without preparation. Most medical offices will note the preferred preparation in a policy and procedure manual (Procedure 38-1).

Checkpoint Question

12. *What does anoscopy involve and how does it differ from sigmoidoscopy?*

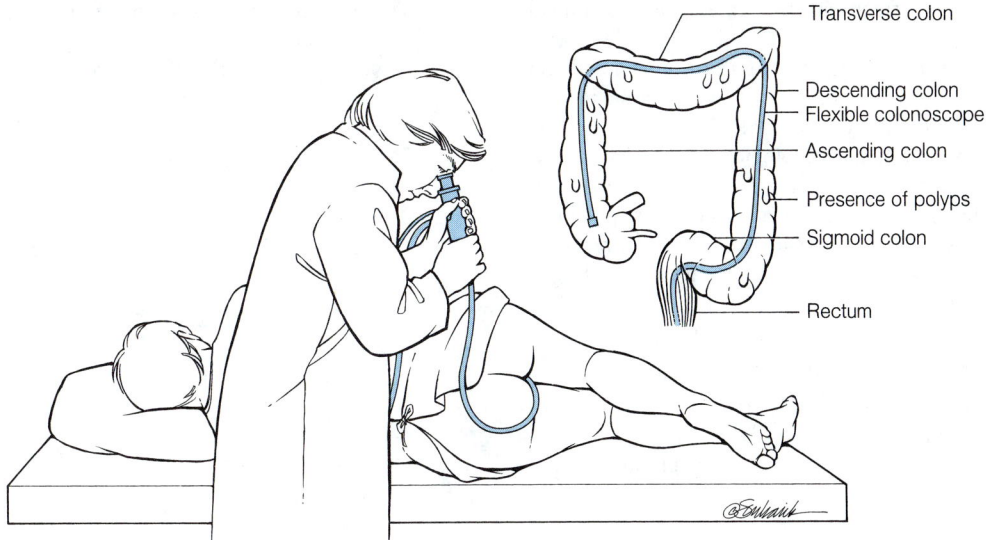

FIGURE 38-10
Colonoscopy. Flexible scope passes through rectum and sigmoid colon into the descending, transverse, and ascending colon.

Procedure 38-1   Preparing the Patient for Colon Procedures

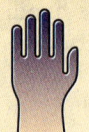

Equipment/Supplies

- appropriate instrument (flexible or rigid sigmoidoscope, anoscope, or proctoscope)
- water-soluble lubricant
- fenestrated drape or gown
- cotton swabs
- suction source (if not part of the scope)
- biopsy forceps
- specimen container with preservative
- completed laboratory requests
- personal wipes
- equipment for assessing vital signs
- gloves

Steps	Purpose
1. Wash your hands.	1. Handwashing aids infection control.
2. Assemble the equipment.	2. This ensures that all of the materials are available.
3. Check the illumination of the light source. Turn off the power to avoid a build up of heat.	
4. Greet and identify the patient. Explain the procedure. The patient will feel pressure and may have the urge to defecate. Tell the patient that the pressure is from the instrument and that the feeling will ease. The patient may also experience gas pressure when air is insufflated. *Note:* Some patients are ordered a mild sedative before the procedure.	4. Identifying the patient prevents errors in treatment. Explaining the procedure helps ease anxiety and ensure compliance.
5. Instruct the patient to empty the bladder.	5. Pressure from the instrument may injure a full bladder. Urine in the bladder may increase discomfort.
6. Assess the vital signs and record.	6. Colon examination procedures may cause cardiac arrhythmias and a change in blood pressure in some patients. Baseline vital signs will allow you to detect variations from the patient's normal signs.
7. Have the patient undress from the waist down, or undress completely and put on a gown.	
8. Assist the patient onto the table. If the instrument of choice is an anoscope or a fiberoptic device, Sims' position or a left-lying position is most comfortable for the patient. If a rigid instrument is used, the patient will assume a knee-chest position or be placed on a proctologic table that supports the patient in a knee-chest position. *Note:* Do not ask the patient to assume the knee-chest position until the physician is ready to begin. The position is difficult to maintain and the patient may become faint.	8. The suggested positions reposition the abdominal contents into the abdominal cavity rather than the pelvis to facilitate the procedure.
9. When the patient is in position, drape properly. A fenestrated drape is usually used.	
10. Continually monitor the patient's response and offer reassurance during the examination. Instruct the patient to breathe slowly through pursed lips to aid in relaxation.	

(continued)

Procedure 38-1

Preparing the Patient for Colon Procedures (continued)

Steps	Purpose
11. Assist the physician as needed with lubricants, instruments, power sources, swabs, biopsy equipment, and specimen containers.	
12. Following the procedure, assist the patient into a comfortable position and allow a rest period. Offer personal cleaning wipes and assist with cleaning as needed. Monitor the vital signs before allowing the patient to stand. Assist the patient from the table and remain close at hand to avoid falls.	12. A drop in blood pressure on standing is common after any of these procedures and may cause fainting.
13. Have the patient dress.	
14. Thank the patient and give appropriate instructions.	14. Courtesy encourages the patient to have a positive attitude about the physician's office.
15. Clean the room. Route the specimens to the proper laboratory. Clean or dispose of the supplies and equipment as appropriate and wash your hands.	
16. Document the procedure.	16. Procedures are considered not to have been done if they are not recorded.

Stool Specimens

As a part of the routine examination for patients over a certain age, many physicians order a stool specimen to test for occult blood. Stool specimens to test for ova and parasites are ordered if an infestation is suspected. Stool specimens also are collected to test for bile, fat, pus, or mucus (Box 38-3). Standard Precautions must be followed when collecting stool specimens for any purpose.

As a medical assistant, you may be responsible for instructing the patient in the procedure, or you may assist in the collection of a stool specimen. A stool specimen may be collected in the office in situations in which the patient may not understand directions for appropriate collection or if test results require a fresh specimen. Appointments for stool specimens should be scheduled early in the morning. Most people move their bowels shortly after awakening; delaying the appointment may cause the patient discomfort or may result in loss of the specimen. Some specimens may be collected and transported in containers with preservatives. All specimens should be transported as quickly as possible. Procedure 38-2 describes the specific steps for collecting a stool specimen.

Charting Example

05/31/99	12:45 PM Patient was escorted
	into examination room. P-100 regular,
	BP 120/85. Patient was instructed to
	empty bladder and put on patient gown.
	Patient was assisted onto examination
	table. Colon examination done by Dr.
	Jacobs. Patient tolerated colonoscopy
	procedure well and was d/c by Dr.
	Jacobs. ————Sam Clay, CMA

> ## BOX 38-3   Special Stool Examinations
>
> Follow the tips below when collecting stool specimens to test for pinworms or parasites, or to obtain a swab for culture. Keep in mind that Standard Precautions must be followed.
>
> - *Pinworms:* Schedule the appointment very early in the morning, preferably before a bowel movement or bath. Pinworms tend to leave the rectum and lay eggs around the anus during the night. Use clear adhesive tape to press against the perineal area. Remove it quickly and place it sticky side down on a glass slide for the physician's inspection.
> - *Parasites:* Caution the patient not to use a laxative or enema before the test to avoid destroying the evidence of parasites. If the stool contains blood or mucus, include as much as possible in the specimen container, because these substances are most likely to contain the suspected organism.
> - *Stool culture:* A sterile cotton-tipped swab is passed into the rectal canal beyond the sphincter and rotated carefully. Place it into the appropriate culture container or process as directed for smear preparation (see Chap. 43, Microbiology, for specific procedure).

Screening for Occult Blood

Testing stool for occult blood using a test pack or kit is convenient, quick and easy, and readily acceptable to most patients. This method is used widely for screening purposes to identify disorders that cause GI bleeding: hemorrhoids, polyps, diverticula, ulcers, or cancers. Most physicians routinely screen patients over age 50 for occult blood. Testing may be done for younger patients if the history suggests a need. Testing for the presence of occult blood will not diagnose the cause, but will alert the physician to the need for further testing.

Several pharmaceutical companies manufacture test packs or kits to detect fecal occult blood. Smith-Kline Diagnostics supplies three methods: Hemoccult I, a simple slide for a single, simple test; Hemoccult II, with three test areas for collection from separate sites from three separate stools if intermittent bleeding is suspected; Hemoccult Tape, for quick testing during rectal examinations.

These tests use the guaiac reagent to indicate the presence of blood. Developers are added to the combination of stool and guaiac to turn the test site an indicated color. Laboratory quality control monitors are supplied on each test pack. Read the package inserts to be familiar with the procedure. Store packs, reagents, and developers properly. Follow the directions for the exact amount of reagent or developer to add and the specific period of time to elapse before reading the results (Fig. 38–11).

Negative Smears*

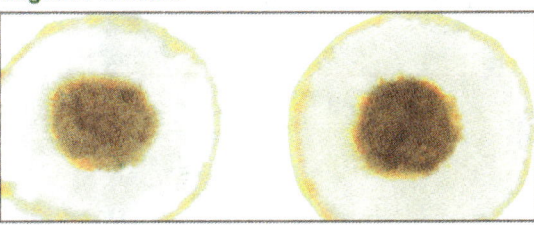

Negative and Positive Smears*

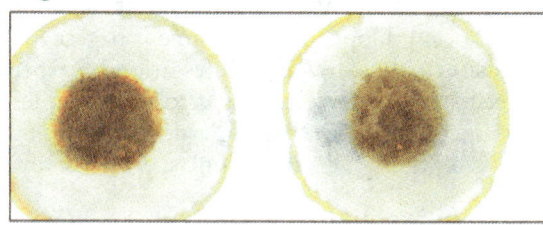

Positive Smears*

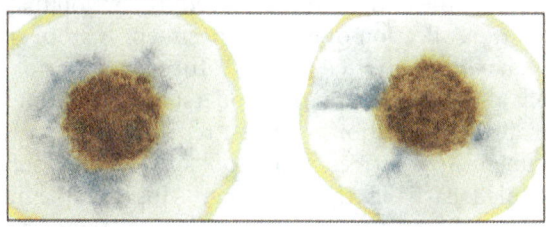

FIGURE 38-11

Test results for fecal occult blood using the Hemoccult routine screening test. Two samples from the specimen are included on each slide. No detectable blue on or at the edge of the smears indicates the test is negative for occult blood. Any trace of blue on or at the edge of one or more of the smears indicates the test is positive for occult blood. (Courtesy of SmithKline Diagnostics, Inc.)

Procedure 38-2

Collecting a Stool Specimen

Equipment/Supplies

- stool specimen container (usually waxed cardboard or plastic to avoid the transfer of pathogens through a moist container)
- wooden spatulas or tongue blades
- bedpan with cover or toilet collection container (popularly called a "nun's cap" or "Mexican hat") with cover
- personal wipes for the patient
- gloves

Steps	Purpose
1. Wash your hands.	1. Handwashing aids infection control.
2. Assemble the equipment.	2. This ensures that all of the materials are available.
3. Greet and identify the patient. Explain the procedure. Tell the patient to defecate in the bedpan or toilet collection container, not the toilet. The patient must void separately. Make sure the patient discards toilet tissue in the toilet and not in the bedpan or collection container.	3. Identifying the patient prevents errors in treatment. Explaining the procedure helps ease anxiety and ensure compliance. Water, urine, or toilet tissue mixed with the stool may interfere with test results.
4. Put on gloves and obtain the bedpan or collection container from the patient.	4. Standard Precautions must be followed when handling stool.
5. Using a tongue blade or wooden spatula, remove small portions of the stool from the bedpan or collection container. Take the specimens from the first and final portions of the stool. Transfer the stool to the specimen container. Do not allow feces to soil the outer surface of the specimen container.	5. The first and last portions of the stool usually contain concentrations of the substances most often required for testing.
6. Discard the supplies in biohazard containers.	
7. Cap the specimen quickly and tightly.	7. This prevents loss of moisture, which may alter the results.
8. Assist the patient with cleaning the rectal area. Have the patient wash hands.	8. This provides comfort and aids infection control.
9. Thank the patient and provide appropriate instructions.	9. Courtesy encourages the patient to have a positive attitude about the physician's office.
10. Clean, disinfect, and store or properly dispose of the bedpan or collection container. Remove gloves and wash hands after handling the specimen and supplies.	10. Standard Precautions must be followed throughout the procedure.
11. Label the specimen and attach the laboratory requests.	
12. Store the specimen as directed. Some require refrigeration, others are kept at room temperature, and some must be incubated. Check the office policy and procedure manual for recommendations for storage and routing of all specimens.	
13. Document the procedure and the time it was performed, the description of the stool, and the routing procedure.	13. Procedures are considered not to have been done if they are not recorded.

BOX 38-4   Simple Screening for Occult Blood

The simplest way to screen for occult blood is the test tape. This method is commonly used by the physician during a routine physical examination. A measure of the tape is removed from the dispenser and held by the medical assistant. After the physician has completed the digital rectal examination with the gloved hand, the gloved finger is swiped across the tape to make a smear of the contents of the rectal canal. Developer is dropped onto the opposite side of the tape and the results are read in 60 seconds.

Charting Example

06/13/98	1500	Patient was instructed to collect a stool specimen in a specimen container. Stool was obtained and tested for occult blood. Test results were positive. Dr. Franklyn was alerted to the findings. ——Paula Jones, CMA

Procedure 38-3   Testing for Occult Blood

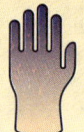

Equipment/Supplies
- patient's labeled specimen pack
- developers or reagents
- gloves

Steps	Purpose
1. Identify the patient's pack or the specimen from the physician. Depending on the method of testing, the specimen may be tested as quickly as 3 to 5 minutes after collection or up to 14 days if properly stored.	1. Proper identification prevents errors.
2. Wash hands and put on gloves.	2. Standard Precautions must be followed when handling stool.
3. Open the test window on the back of the pack and apply the testing reagent or developer. Read the color change in the specified time frame, usually 60 seconds. Apply developers as directed onto the control monitor section of the pack. Wait the specified time.	3. This ensures accurate results.
4. Properly dispose of the pack, gloves, and supplies. Wash your hands.	4. Standard Precautions must be followed throughout the procedure.
5. Record the procedure.	5. Procedures are considered not to have been done if they are not recorded.

Avoid having the patient collect a specimen during menses or when there is obvious rectal bleeding. Patients are usually cautioned to avoid certain foods or medications that may interfere with testing. Red meat and certain vegetables and fruits (especially those high in vitamin C) interfere with test results. Aspirin and NSAIDs are usually avoided for a week before testing.

The physician may perform a quick test during a

routine physical examination (Box 38-4). Or the patient may take the test kit home to perform the more extensive testing and bring in or mail the completed pack (Procedure 38-3).

SUMMARY

The body's cells require nutrients from food to function properly. The organs of the GI system are responsible for ingestion, digestion, transportation, and elimination of food. Through the process of metabolism, food is broken down into usable energy units. Various disorders can interfere with the essential processes of the GI system. Diagnostic procedures such as colon examinations and stool testing can help the physician detect abnormalities in GI functioning.

CRITICAL THINKING CHALLENGES

1. Review the patient preparations needed for an upper GI series and a barium enema. Create a patient education handout that includes:
   • a description of the procedure
   • a list of reasons for the procedure
   • preparations required to ensure reliable test results
   (Hint: Review Chap. 27, Diagnostic Imaging.)
2. Trace a bolus of food through the GI tract. Describe the metabolic process occurring at each step. (Review Chap. 32, Caring for Patients With Disorders of the Nervous System.) How does the autonomic nervous system affect the process of digestion?
3. Many endoscopic examinations require the patient to be in an uncomfortable and embarrassing position. How can you help alleviate the stress and anxiety that a patient may experience?

ANSWERS TO CHECKPOINT QUESTIONS

1. Peristalsis is rhythmic waves of smooth muscle contractions that move food from the esophagus into the stomach. The motion helps break the food bolus into pieces and mix it with digestive enzymes to accelerate digestion.
2. Mastication is the process of chewing. Deglutition is the process of swallowing.
3. The small intestine is divided into the duodenum, jejunum, and ileum. Most of the digestion occurs in the duodenum by the action of the bile and pancreatic enzymes. Absorption occurs further into the jejunum and ileum.
4. The liver is responsible for glucose and glycogen metabolism and storage; breakdown of amino acids; manufacture and metabolism of protein, fats, and carbohydrates; storage of vitamins and minerals; destruction of old red blood cells; manufacture of bile; and removal of toxins.

5. Four common mouth disorders are caries, stomatitis, gingivitis, and oral cancer.
6. A hiatal hernia is caused by a defect in the diaphragm that lets part of the stomach slide up into the chest cavity. The stomach's cardiac sphincter and the diaphragmatic muscle tone normally prevent gastric acid reflux into the esophagus. Hiatal hernia permits the stomach acid to invade the esophagus, causing irritation.
7. Because the lining of the duodenum cannot tolerate concentrated gastric juices, ulcers form when food material containing excessive gastric acid passes through the pylorus.
8. Crohn's disease can lead to bowel obstruction. With each episode of inflammation, the scarring that occurs may lead to narrowing of the colon, which may cause an obstruction.
9. Gas is produced from the bacterial decomposition of proteins during digestion.
10. Viral hepatitis is caused by a virus; toxic hepatitis results from toxic reactions to chemical toxicants, certain medications, or alcohol.
11. Cholelithiasis is the formation of stones in the gallbladder. It occurs when slowed peristalsis allows bile to pool in the sac; fluid is absorbed and the solids are left to concentrate and solidify into stones.
12. Anoscopy involves the insertion of an instrument into the rectal canal for visualization of the anus and rectum and to obtain swabs for culture. Sigmoidoscopy involves visualization of the sigmoid colon using either a rigid or flexible sigmoidoscope.

SUGGESTIONS FOR FURTHER READING

Bates, B., Bickley, L. S., Hockelman, R. A. (1995). *A Guide to Physical Examination and History Taking*, 6th ed. Philadelphia: Lippincott-Raven.

Bullock, B. L., Rosendahl, P. P. (1992). *Pathophysiology*, 3rd ed. Philadelphia: Lippincott-Raven.

Fischbach, F. (1992). *A Manual of Laboratory and Diagnostic Tests*, 4th ed. Philadelphia: Lippincott-Raven.

Fischbach, F. (1995). *Quick Reference for Common Laboratory and Diagnostic Tests*. Philadelphia: Lippincott-Raven.

Memmler, R. L., Cohen, B. J., & Wood, D. L. (1996). *The Human Body in Health and Disease*, 8th ed. Philadelphia: Lippincott-Raven.

(1992). *Professional Guide to Diseases*, 4th ed. Springhouse, PA: Springhouse.

Porth, C. M. (1994). *Pathophysiology: Concepts of Altered Health States*, 4th ed. Philadelphia: Lippincott-Raven.

Smeltzer, S. C., & Bare, B. G. (1996). *Brunner and Suddarth's Textbook of Medical and Surgical Nursing*, 8th ed. Philadelphia: Lippincott-Raven.

Timby, B. K., & Lewis, L. W. (1992). *Fundamental Skills and Concepts in Patient Care*, 5th ed. Philadelphia: J. B. Lippincott.

Caring for Patients With Urinary Disorders

Chapter Outline

Structure and Function of the Urinary System
    Formation and Transportation of Metabolic Wastes
    Excretion of Wastes
    Maintaining Fluid Balance
    Regulation of pH Balance
    Maintenance of Blood Pressure
    Production of Erythropoietin
    Metabolism and Retention of Calcium and Vitamin D
Organs of the Urinary System
    Kidneys
    Ureters
    Urinary Bladder
    Urethra
The Voiding Reflex
Common Urinary Disorders
    Renal Failure

    Glomerulonephritis
    Calculi
    Pyelonephritis
    Hydronephrosis
    Cystitis
    Urethritis
    Tumors
Common Diagnostic Studies and the Medical Assistant's Role
    Urine Tests
    Blood Tests
    Cystoscopy or Cystourethroscopy
    Intravenous Pyelogram (IVP)
    Retrograde Pyelogram
    Ultrasound
Summary
Critical Thinking Challenges
Answers to Checkpoint Questions
Suggestions for Further Reading

DACUM Components

1.3   Practice within the scope of education, training, and personal capabilities
1.6   Conduct oneself in a courteous and diplomatic manner
2.2   Treat all patients with empathy and impartiality
4.1   Apply principles of aseptic technique
4.7   Prepare patients for procedures
4.8   Assist with examinations and treatments
7.3   Teach patients methods of health promotion and disease prevention

Chapter Competencies

Learning Objectives

Upon successfully completing this chapter, you will be able to:

1. Spell and define the Key Terms.
2. List and describe the primary functions of the urinary system.
3. Label a diagram of the organs of the urinary system.
4. Describe the gross and microscopic anatomy of the kidney.
5. Differentiate between the structures within a nephron and give the functions of each.
6. Identify and describe the functions of the organs of the urinary system below the level of the kidney.
7. Describe the way that wastes are formed and transported to the urinary system.
8. Name other systems involved in the excretion of wastes and the types of wastes usually managed by those systems.
9. Trace a drop of liquid waste in the bloodstream through the urinary system to its eventual elimination as urine.
10. List and describe disorders of the urinary system.
11. Identify and explain diagnostic procedures of the urinary system and the medical assistant's responsibilities.

Key Terms

(See Glossary for definitions.)

angiotensin
anuria
blood urea nitrogen (BUN)
calyces (singular, calyx)
catheterization
convoluted tubules
cystoscopy
dialysis
enuresis
erythropoietin
filtration
glomerulus
hematuria
incontinence
intravenous pyelogram (IVP)
lithotripsy
loop of Henle
micturition
nephron
nephrostomy
nitrogenous
nocturia
oliguria
pH
proteinuria
pyuria
renal cortex
renal medulla
renal pelvis
renal pyramids
renin
retrograde pyelogram
retroperitoneal
specific gravity
staghorn
trigone
urea
uremic frost
ureterostomy
ureters
urethra
uric acid
urinalysis

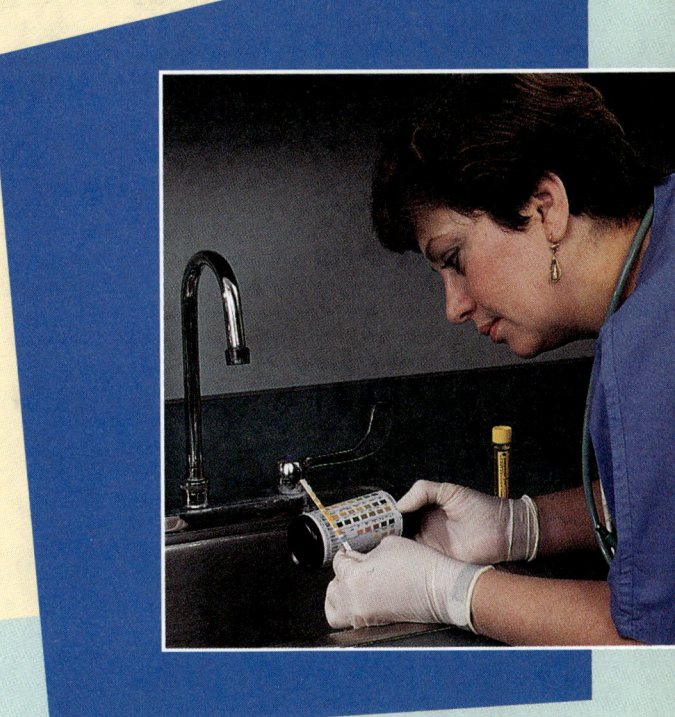

Nutrients and substances required for metabolism create waste products that must be eliminated from the body. Several systems are responsible for helping to prevent a build up of the end-products of metabolism. Solid waste, water, bile, and some salts are eliminated by the gastrointestinal system. Products of respiration, such as carbon dioxide and water, are excreted by the respiratory system. Even the integumentary system is responsible for its share of excretion of water, salts, and some nitrogen in the form of perspiration. The body rids itself of liquid wastes by way of the urinary system. The urinary system also regulates fluid volume, electrolytes, red blood cell production, blood pressure, and pH (acid–base) balance.

➤ STRUCTURE AND FUNCTION OF THE URINARY SYSTEM

The urinary system consists of six distinct organs: two kidneys, two **ureters**, the bladder, and the **urethra** (Fig. 39-1). The kidneys remove the products of cellular metabolism from the bloodstream and aid in homeostasis. The ureters are a pair of tubes that transport the urine from the kidneys. The bladder is a hollow sac that holds the urine until **micturition** (voiding or urination). The urethra is a tube that transports the urine to the outside of the body.

The urinary system is involved in multiple functions to maintain the homeostasis of the body. In cooperation with chemoreceptors throughout the body, various functions turn on and off as indicated by rising and falling levels of those substances necessary for the maintenance of life.

Formation and Transportation of Metabolic Wastes

As the body uses the available nutrients for metabolism, wastes accumulate at the cellular level. Initially, the breakdown of amino acids, the building blocks of protein, yields ammonia, which is then converted to **urea**, the final product of protein metabolism. In addition, the breakdown of nucleic acids, found in all cells, is somewhat similar to urea and is also excreted by the urinary system as **uric acid**, a by-product of protein metabolism. Creatinine, a by-product of the catabolism of creatine in muscle activity, is the third major waste product eliminated by the urinary system.

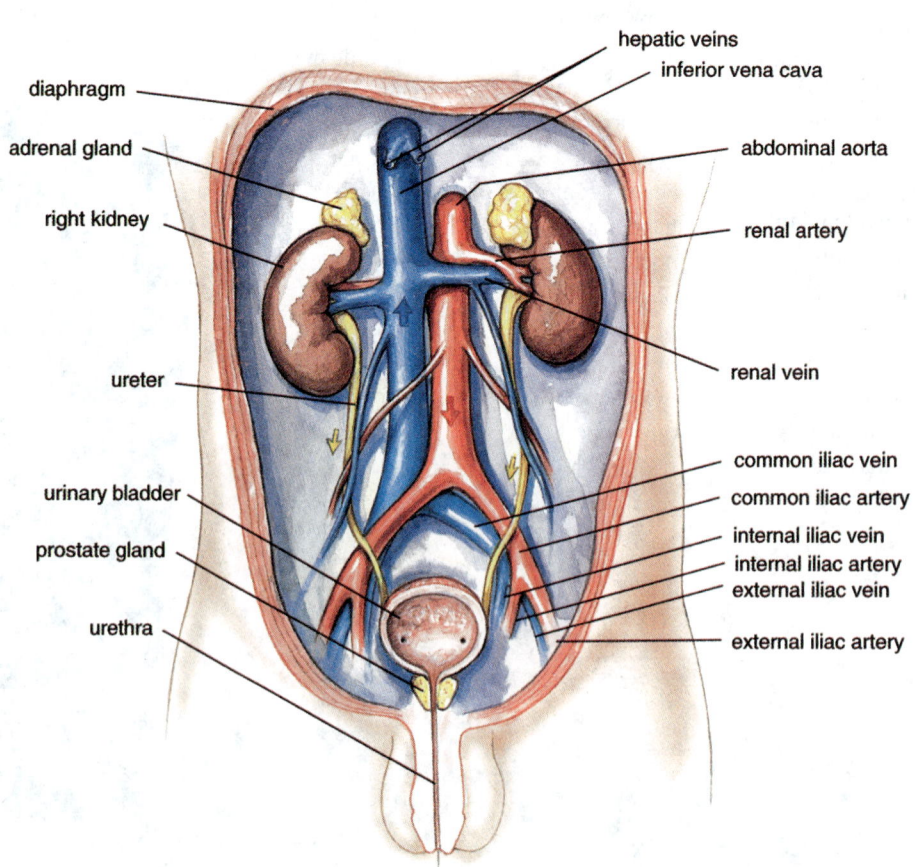

FIGURE 39-1
Urinary system, with blood vessels.

These wastes are filtered from the blood by the liver and are transported to the kidney by the renal arteries, which are short branches of the abdominal aorta. The cleansed blood leaves the kidney by way of small vessels that connect with the renal vein, which empties into the vena cava for recirculation through the bloodstream.

Excretion of Wastes

The capillary system of the kidney is specially designed to retain or reabsorb substances needed for normal blood levels and to eliminate substances in abundance or no longer needed. As these levels fluctuate, the kidneys receive signals to excrete more or less of these substances as indicated. Waste products are generally small enough to fit between the walls of the renal capillary cells. They are squeezed out to be filtered into the waste water that will become urine. Protein, fats, blood cells, and other components coursing through the kidneys are generally too large to fit between the walls of the capillaries unless there is an imbalance of these substances or an impairment of the **filtration** system. (Filtration involves removal of particles from a solution by passing the solution through a membrane.) Some toxins and expendable salts are also excreted by the kidneys. Metallic salts, such as lead and mercury, can be detected in the urine in cases of poisoning.

Checkpoint Question
1. What are the main products of metabolism that are filtered by the kidneys?

Maintaining Fluid Balance

When the volume of blood decreases because of fluid loss or inadequate fluid intake, levels of dissolved salts in the blood increase, causing a change in the osmotic pressure of the blood. Chemoreceptors in the brain and several large vessels signal the posterior lobe of the pituitary to release antidiuretic hormone (ADH). ADH in turn passes the signal to the distal **convoluted tubules** (the twisted portion of the nephron connecting the glomerulus to the collecting tubules) and collecting ducts of the kidneys to allow more water to be reabsorbed into the bloodstream, thereby increasing the fluid level of the blood. Conversely, when too much fluid is circulating, blood becomes diluted, causing sensors in the brain and large vessels to decrease the ADH levels, reducing the amount of water reabsorbed by the filtering system so that urine production is increased and fluid balance is restored.

Regulation of pH Balance

Cell metabolism produces acids that must be excreted by the body to maintain a fairly constant blood pH of about 7.4. The ingestion of bases, such as too many antacids, will alter the pH of the blood. If the sensitive monitoring devices throughout the body detect levels of acid that are becoming dangerously high, extra hydrogen ions are combined with either ammonia or phosphates in the distal tubules to be excreted in the urine. If these sensors detect acid levels too low and base levels too high, the distal tubules hold back hydrogen ions to increase the blood acid level to normal limits.

Maintenance of Blood Pressure

When oxygen levels in the kidney are low because of a decrease in blood pressure that slows blood flow to the vessels of the kidneys, the hormone **renin** is released to activate the production of **angiotensin**, a powerful vasoconstrictor. Vasoconstriction causes blood pressure to rise, which in turn signals the adrenal cortex to release aldosterone to retain the sodium and water flowing through the kidney. This increases the blood volume and raises the blood pressure to increase the blood and oxygen flow through the sensors in the kidneys. When the kidneys are satisfied by the increase in oxygen levels, the whole process is reversed.

Production of Erythropoietin

If oxygen levels are low because of decreased production of oxygen-bearing red blood cells rather than decreased blood pressure, the kidneys release the hormone **erythropoietin** to act on the red bone marrow to increase the production of red blood cells.

Metabolism and Retention of Calcium and Vitamin D

In conjunction with the parathyroid hormone, the kidneys regulate the blood levels of calcium. This is done by activating vitamin D molecules, which control the mechanism by which calcium is absorbed by the intestines.

Checkpoint Question
2. How does the pituitary affect fluid balance?

➤ ORGANS OF THE URINARY SYSTEM

Kidneys

The kidneys excrete wastes and aid in the maintenance of homeostasis. They are located in the **retroperitoneal** area, near the back body wall at about thoracic 12 to lumbar 3. They are just below the diaphragm and are protected by the lower rib cage. The left kidney is slightly higher than the right because of the position of the liver. Encased in a capsule of renal fat, the kidneys are held in position by renal fascia. They are reddish brown, bean-shaped, fist-sized, and approximately 4 inches by 2 inches by 1 inch. The inner curve has a notch called the hilus where nerves and the blood and lymph vessels enter and exit and the renal pelves (singular, pelvis) are attached. An adrenal gland covers the top of each kidney (see Fig. 39-1).

The kidneys are surrounded by heavy fibrous connective tissue called the renal capsule. There is an outer **renal cortex** and an inner **renal medulla.** The renal cortex is the shell that surrounds the medulla and is made up of the microscopic **nephron** units that do most of the work for the kidney (see the section "Nephrons," below). The renal medulla contains the conical structures, called **renal pyramids**, that collect the urine from the nephrons for transport to the **renal pelvis** (Fig. 39-2).

The renal pelvis is a funnel-shaped collecting basin formed from a dozen or more minor calyces embedded in the medulla. The minor **calyces** (cuplike collecting structures) empty into several major calyces (singular, calyx). The distal end of the renal pelvis is continuous with its ureter.

Nephrons

Each kidney is composed of about one million nephrons (Fig. 39-3), each consisting of a renal corpuscle and a renal tubule. The renal corpuscle is made up of a twisted mass of capillaries, called the **glomerulus**, surrounded by a double-walled, funnel-shaped structure called Bowman's capsule. The renal tubule is an extension of Bowman's capsule that twists and turns on its way to transport the filtrate that will become urine.

The purpose of the nephron is to filter the blood through the corpuscle and produce a filtrate to be passed on to the renal tubule. As the body works to maintain its balance, substances needed for homeostasis are returned by reabsorption to the circulatory system by the mechanisms described above. Waste products and excess water are passed on to the collecting tubules and eliminated as urine.

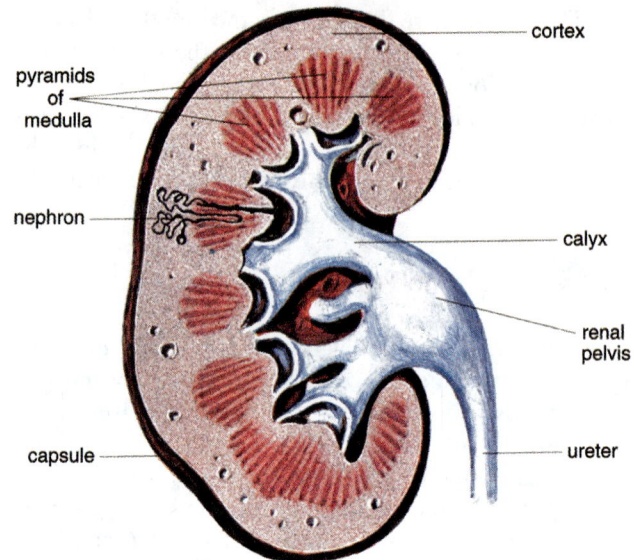

FIGURE 39-2
Longitudinal section through the kidney showing its internal structure and a much enlarged diagram of a nephron. There are more than one million nephrons in each kidney.

Urine Formation

Blood is brought to the kidney by the renal arteries that arise from the abdominal aorta. In a 24-hour period, 160 to 180 liters (about 45 gallons) of filtrate pass through the kidneys to become approximately 1 to 1.5 liters (about 1–1.5 quarts) of urine. The rest of the filtrate returns to the circulation. About 25% of the cardiac output from each heartbeat goes to and through the kidneys. About every 4 minutes, all of the blood in the body is filtered by the kidneys and sent back to the heart as clean blood. Follow a drop of fluid as it becomes a drop of urine on the illustration of a nephron.

Blood enters the renal corpuscle, where filtration begins, by way of a wide-diameter renal arteriole. This initial vessel is called an afferent arteriole. Once within Bowman's capsule, the afferent arteriole branches to become the glomerulus, a dense network of capillaries, which are compressed by the walls of the surrounding chamber. The efferent arteriole exiting Bowman's capsule has a smaller diameter than the afferent, or entering, arteriole. This change in the exiting diameter plus the small size of the glomerular capillaries raises the pressure within these capillaries. The backup of pressure forces the fluid from the blood through the capillary walls, rather like squeezing a sponge. Blood components are generally too large to pass between the capillary cells, but salts (such as electrolytes), glucose, and other small dissolved molecules are pressed out with the plasma.

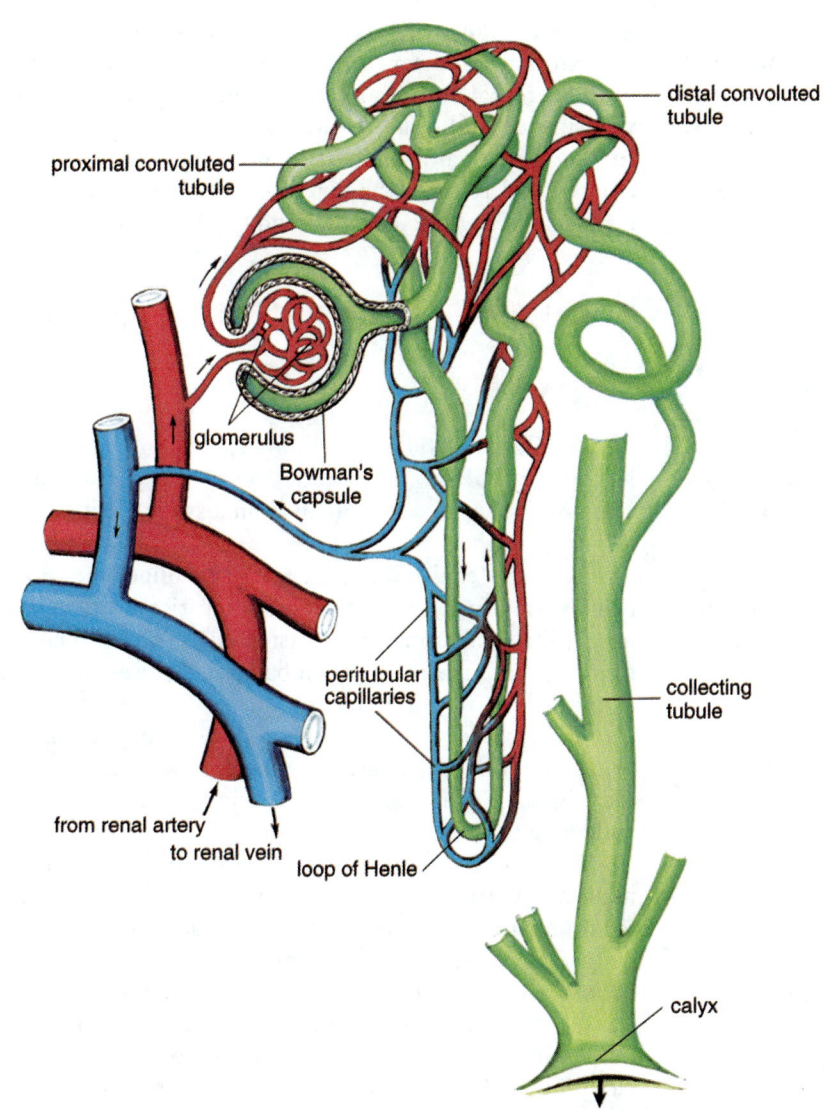

FIGURE 39-3
Simplified diagram of a nephron.

From the collecting basin of Bowman's capsule, the filtrate begins a twisting, turning journey through the proximal convoluted tubule. This tubule eventually descends to become the **loop of Henle**, a much narrower and straighter tube. At this point, more plasma and wastes are pressed out to enter the tissue fluid of the nephron. By the process of filtration, some of this fluid that has been pressed out will be reabsorbed by the distal convoluted tubule as it widens just past the loop of Henle and begins to twist and turn toward the collecting tubule. Some of the fluid will be reabsorbed by the peritubular capillaries. These capillaries are extensions of the efferent arteriole that has been winding its way around the various portions of the tubular system and is most dense at the loop of Henle. These will become renal venules that will drain into the renal veins to take the filtered blood away from the kidney and back to general circulation.

If all of the checks and balances of the mechanisms that make up homeostasis are in place and the body does not require that the nephron reabsorb the filtrate, it will make its way through the collecting tubule to the minor calyx, the major calyx, the renal pelvis, the ureter, the bladder, and the urethra and will be voided.

 Checkpoint Question
3. What is the glomerulus and where is it located?

Ureters

The ureters are two long, slender tubes reaching from the kidney basin, or renal pelvis, through the lower posterior portion of the bladder (see Fig. 39-1). They are about 10 to 13 inches long and are lined with epithelial cells that are continuous with the kidney and the bladder. They contract rhythmically with peristalsis triggered by the presence of urine in the renal pelvis. The entry of the ureters into the bladder is covered by a flaplike fold of mucous membrane, which acts as a valve to prevent reflux when the bladder is full.

Urinary Bladder

The bladder is a temporary urine storage and collecting sac below the parietal peritoneum and behind the pubis (see Fig. 39-1). When it is full, it may rise above the pubis into the abdominal cavity. It is highly expandable although the urge to urinate is usually felt when it contains about 5 ounces. Discomfort is usually triggered when it contains about 10 ounces.

The inner layer is mucous membrane, which becomes rugae when the bladder is empty. The outer layers are very elastic and are interlaced in many directions.

The inferior and posterior portion of the bladder, in an area formed as a triangle by the openings of the ureters and the urethra, is called the **trigone.** This area does not expand when the bladder is filled.

Urethra

The urethra is a tube that reaches from the bladder to the outside of the body (see Fig. 39-1). In the female, the tube is about 1½ inches long. It passes anteriorly from the bladder, behind the symphysis pubis, and terminates between the labia minora, anterior to the vaginal meatus and posterior to the clitoris. In the male, the urethra is part of both the urinary and reproductive systems. It is about 8 inches long and is S shaped. It passes from the bladder through the prostate gland just below the bladder and is joined by various ducts arising from the reproductive system. The urethra exists at the tip of the penis.

Checkpoint Question

4. *What is the difference between the ureters and the urethra?*

➤ THE VOIDING REFLEX

When the bladder begins to fill with urine, stretch receptors transmit the signal to the sacral section of the spinal cord, which will release the internal sphincter at the base of the bladder. If timing is not appropriate, it is possible to override the impulse to void by inhibiting the external sphincter through control by nerve centers in the cerebral cortex and midbrain. The urge to void will subside and return in waves. If the timing is right to void, the parasympathetic nervous system takes control and releases the external sphincter. The bladder muscles begin to contract and urine is expelled.

➤ COMMON URINARY DISORDERS

Renal Failure

Renal failure is a sudden drop in kidney function manifested by inability of the kidney to excrete wastes, concentrate urine, and aid in homeostatic electrolyte conservation.

In acute renal failure, there will be **oliguria** (scant urine formation) and a corresponding rise in **nitrogenous** (nitrogen-containing) wastes in the blood, dehydration, and an electrolyte imbalance. Causes include a grave loss of fluid due to burns or hemorrhage, trauma, toxic injury to the kidney (as in nephrotoxic drugs or poisons), acute pyelonephritis or glomerulonephritis, or an obstruction beyond the level of the collecting tubules.

Chronic renal failure is a gradual loss of the nephrons with a corresponding inability of the kidney to complete its functions. It may result from other disease processes, such as lupus erythematosus, diabetic neuropathy, radiation, or renal tuberculosis. There will be general weakness, edema of the lungs and the tissues in general, and neurologic symptoms such as clouding or dullness progressing to seizures and coma. If **dialysis** (removal of urine wastes) is not performed, the patient will likely exhibit pale or white crystals on the skin called **uremic frost.** This is formed by the urea and waste products as they exit the skin.

Treatment for both acute and chronic renal failure may involve dialysis (Box 39-1). Chronic failure frequently involves other systems as well as the urinary system and will require treatment to reflect the level of involvement.

Glomerulonephritis

Glomerulonephritis is an inflammation of the glomerulus of the kidney. Symptoms range from very mild edema, **proteinuria, hematuria,** and oliguria to complete renal failure. It is common in children several weeks after a streptococcal infection as the strep antibodies attack and injure the glomeruli. It may be chronic in adults with scarring and hardening of the glomeruli and eventual renal failure. Symptoms of the

BOX 39-1 Renal Dialysis

Patients whose kidneys are not functioning will need the assistance of dialysis to remove nitrogenous waste products and excess fluid from the body. Dialysis dependence may be short term in acute illness or long term in end-stage renal disease (ESRD). In the absence of functional nephrons, wastes must be filtered through membranes other than those in the renal tissues. Two methods are currently used for dialysis. These are hemodialysis and peritoneal dialysis.

Hemodialysis

Toxins are removed from the blood by routing the patient's blood through a dialysis machine containing synthetic filters and a dialysate (a substance used to balance the electrolyte concentration in the blood). The machine can be regulated to remove or retain substances as needed for the individual patient.

The patient's circulatory system must be accessed as many as three times a week for 3–4 hours. Therefore, most patients will receive a surgically created fistula (an opening or passage) or a graft between an artery and a vein to make entry easier for the patient.

Hemodialysis is confining and life changing. Maintaining employment is difficult. Many complications such as nausea and vomiting, chest pains, cramping, seizures, and air embolus are possible complications with hemodialysis.

Peritoneal Dialysis

The peritoneal membranes can also be used to filter wastes. An appropriately balanced dialysate is administered through a catheter into the abdominal cavity, then allowed to flow out into a collecting bag, bringing with it the wastes and excess fluid that must be removed. Patients who have had extensive abdominal surgery with disruption of the peritoneal membranes are not good candidates for peritoneal dialysis. Systemic inflammatory disease and immunosuppression are also contraindications for this method.

Peritoneal dialysis allows the patient the freedom to move about and continue a more normal life-style than hemodialysis. However, the presence of an abdominal catheter may result in an altered body image leading to depression. The access to the peritoneal cavity as a source of infection is always a consideration.

Neither of these methods is a cure for the underlying renal dysfunction but both can prolong life almost indefinitely if properly performed.

---

chronic form include proteinuria (excessive protein in the urine), casts in the urine, and hematuria (bloody urine). Treatment is usually symptomatic. If infection is involved, antibiotics will be prescribed.

Calculi

Calculi are stonelike formations. These may be found anywhere in the urinary system and may range from a sandlike consistency to **staghorn** structures that fill the renal pelvis and assume the shape of the calyces, or huge stones that fill the bladder. Stones seem more likely to form if the urine is alkaline; acidity will frequently discourage this formation. Symptoms vary with the size and the location of the stone. Hematuria

may be present if the rough edges abrade the mucous membrane of the system. The patient will have flank pain if the stone lodges in a ureter.

Treatment may not be needed if the stones are small enough to flush with increased fluid intake. Large stones may require surgery or **lithotripsy** (crushing the stone in situ, usually using ultrasound). In either case, the chemistry of the stones will need to be evaluated for the forming components, and the patient's diet will need to be adjusted to prevent recurrence (Box 39-2).

Checkpoint Question
5. What are calculi and when are they more likely to form?

BOX 39-2 Diagnosing and Treating Calculi: A Case Study

Clark Watkins, a 45-year-old white man, presents with severe right flank pain radiating to the suprapubic and inguinal regions. He has a fever of 100.3°F, nausea, and some vomiting. His urinalysis shows gross and microscopic hematuria and calcium crystal casts; it is clear of pyuria and white blood cells.

Dr. Brown performs an in-office ultrasonography and the results are suggestive of calculi. He then orders an intravenous pyelogram (IVP) for further study to rule out appendicitis, cholecystitis, and a gastrointestinal ulcer. The IVP reveals sand-to-gravel calculi precluding the need for lithotripsy, surgery, or transurethral manipulation.

Your role in this case is to provide patient education. Demonstrate to Mr. Watkins the procedure for straining his urine through the filter of Dr. Brown's choice. Provide him with an appropriate receptacle to save the solid material for Dr. Brown to analyze. (See Chap. 44, Urinalysis, for a detailed description of the procedure.) Mr. Watkins' diet will be altered to reflect the composition of the stones. Referral forms may be completed for him to consult with a dietitian, or he may be given diet lists after counseling by Dr. Brown.

Encourage Mr. Watkins to increase his fluid intake to flush the stones and to ambulate to assist peristalsis. Urge him to drink fruit juices, especially cranberry juice, in addition to water, and discourage caffeine drinks. He may need an antiemetic if nausea and vomiting interfere with fluid intake. Caution him to watch for signs of infection and obstruction such as those outlined under the sections "Calculi" and "Pyelonephritis."

Pyelonephritis

Pyelonephritis is an inflammation of the renal pelvis and the body of the kidney. It usually results from an infection ascending the ureters and may be acute or chronic. Symptoms include those of any infection, such as chills and fever, nausea and vomiting, but with the addition of flank pain and **pyuria** (pus in the urine).

Medication to acidify the urine, making the system less hospitable to bacteria, may be the treatment of choice. In addition, antibiotics may also be prescribed.

Hydronephrosis

Hydronephrosis is a distention of the renal pelvis and calyces from an obstruction that causes a backup of urine. The symptoms include flank pain, hematuria, pyuria, fever, and chills.

To restore the flow of urine, the stricture must be removed. If it is not possible to restore the flow to the bladder, it may be necessary to perform a **nephrostomy** (opening into the kidney) or **ureterostomy** (opening into a ureter).

Cystitis

Cystitis is inflammation of the bladder. Because of the short length of the urethra, cystitis is far more common in women than in men. Symptoms begin with frequency, dysuria, and urgency, and progress to chills, fever, nausea and vomiting, and flank pain.

Identification of the organism will precede the decision for treatment, which usually involves antibiotics. Educating the patient about personal hygiene is also important to prevent recurrence.

Urethritis

Urethritis is inflammation of the urethra. This may be a prelude to simple cystitis, or it may be symptomatic of a sexually transmitted disease such as gonorrhea or nongonococcal urethritis. The treatment for cystitis, noted above, is also effective for urethritis.

What If?
What if a mother brings her 5-year-old daughter to the office with complaints of burning on urination? What questions might you ask? How might you educate the mother and child?

First, ask if the child urinates when she feels the urge or if she holds her urine for long periods. Some young girls are inclined to hold their urine long past the time to void, setting up a perfect situation for bacterial growth. Caution the child to void when the need arises, making sure to use terms she can understand. Next, ask the mother if she uses bubble bath in the child's bath water. Young girls have a very short urethra and are prone to urethritis if they bathe in water with certain types of bubble bath. Finally, explain that the child must learn to wipe from front to back when cleaning herself to avoid urinary tract infections.

Patient Education: Urinary Tract Health

Frequently it will be your responsibility as the medical assistant to educate the patient in everyday habits that will ensure good general health. Encourage patients presenting with urinary system symptoms to follow the suggestions below to avoid problems in the future.

FOR ALL PATIENTS

- Ensure adequate fluid intake, which helps remove waste products from the fluid compartments. There is wisdom in the "old wives' tale" advising 8 glasses of water a day. Tissues will be well hydrated, feces will be softer, and infections will be less likely in the lower urinary system.
- Empty your bladder when you feel the need. Urine held for periods beyond comfort will cause bladder stress and irritation. Allowing urine to stagnate in the bladder increases the risk of infection.
- Keep in mind that cranberry juice and vitamin C help acidify the urine and make the urinary system less attractive to bacteria.

ESPECIALLY FOR WOMEN

- Avoid using perfumed products in the perineal area. The female urinary meatus is very short and prone to irritation. Urethral infections quickly become bladder infections without proper precautions.
- Avoid tight-fitting lower garments, especially nylon underwear. Loose-fitting cotton underwear will absorb moisture and allow for an air flow, making both bladder and vaginal infections less likely.
- Wipe carefully from front to back after using the toilet, particularly after defecating. Wash with soap and water and rinse well if infections are a recurrent problem.
- If you are prone to urinary tract infections, void immediately after intercourse to free the area of bacteria that might have intruded into the urethra. Avoid tub baths, particularly bubble baths; showers will be less likely to contribute to infections.

Table 39-1
Symptoms of Urinary Tract Disorders and Possible Causes

Symptom	Possible Cause(s)
Anuria (lack of urine production)	Renal failure, acute nephritis, metal poisoning (lead, mercury), complete obstruction of the urinary tract
Burning during voiding	Urethritis
Burning during and after voiding	Cystitis
Dribbling	Prostatic hypertrophy, infection, neurogenic bladder
Dysuria	Infection
Edema	Renal failure, nephrosis
Enuresis (bed wetting)	Normal to age 3; thereafter, it is functional or symptomatic of disease
Frequency	Infection, diabetes
Hematuria	Diseases of the glomeruli, trauma, neoplasms, calculi
Hesitancy	Prostatic hypertrophy
Incontinence (inability to control elimination)	Infections, uterine prolapse, nerve damage, neoplasms, senility, neurogenic bladder
Stress incontinence	Impaired sphincter control
Nocturia (voiding at night)	Infection, prostatic hypertrophy, pressure (eg, pregnancy), diabetes, inability to concentrate urine
Oliguria	Acute nephritis, heart disease, dehydration, inadequate intake, fever, obstructions, renal insufficiency, neoplasms
Polyuria	Diabetes mellitus, diabetes insipidus, neurologic diseases, diuretics, increased fluid intake
Proteinuria	Diseases of the glomeruli, infection, nephrotic syndrome, diseases of protein metabolism
Pyuria	Infection
Renal colic	Calculi
Urgency	Infection, diseases of the prostate

Tumors

The urinary system may be the primary or the secondary site for tumors. Tumors are more common in the bladder but may also occur in the kidney. Symptoms will vary but usually include hematuria and an unexplained abdominal mass. Treatment, which will be dictated by the extent and type of tumor, may include surgery, chemotherapy, radiation, or a combination of these.

Table 39-1 summarizes the symptoms of urinary tract disorders and their possible causes.

Checkpoint Question

6. Why are women more likely than men to experience cystitis?

➤ COMMON DIAGNOSTIC STUDIES AND THE MEDICAL ASSISTANT'S ROLE

Urine Tests

The single most important step in diagnosing urinary system diseases begins with the examination of the patient's urine, or urinalysis. This should be performed routinely on all patients but particularly on those presenting with urinary system symptoms. Tests should always be on fresh urine specimens and on the first morning specimen when a more concentrated specimen is needed. Tests performed on the obtained urine may involve a chemical evaluation, **specific gravity** (relative density), microscopic examination, and cultures (see Chap. 44, Urinalysis, for more detailed information).

If infection is suspected, it may be necessary to obtain either a clean-catch, midstream urine specimen or a specimen obtained through **catheterization**, which involves introducing a tube into the bladder to remove urine. The physician is more likely to choose the first procedure, rather than catheterization, because there is far less chance of introducing bladder infection and there is no patient discomfort involved. (Box 39-3 presents information about catheterization.) With proper precautions, there is little chance that surface contaminants will interfere with diagnostic procedures ordered for the urine. You may be responsible for collecting the urine in some cases (see Chap. 44, Urinalysis, for the procedure for obtaining a clean-catch, midstream urine specimen.) However, the patient is generally instructed to do this in the restroom alone.

Blood Tests

Serum levels of uric acid, **blood urea nitrogen (BUN)**, or creatinine may be indicated in some disease processes. It will likely be your responsibility to draw the blood and process it on site or direct it to the proper testing facility. (See Chap. 45, Phlebotomy, and Chap. 46, Hematology, for more information.)

BOX 39-3 Principles of Catheterization

Catheterization is a last resort in most cases in the medical office. Even under the most aseptic conditions, the possibility of introducing infection into the urinary system exists. However, some patients will require catheterization when there is no other alternative. For example, catheterization is required when:

- It is impossible to obtain a clean-catch, midstream specimen for urinalysis
- Intake and output must be measured accurately (these patients will usually be hospitalized)
- Other methods of bladder retraining have failed and the patient is incontinent and in danger of decubiti formation (this may be avoided with good skin care)
- The residual urine must be measured
- Medication must be instilled into the bladder

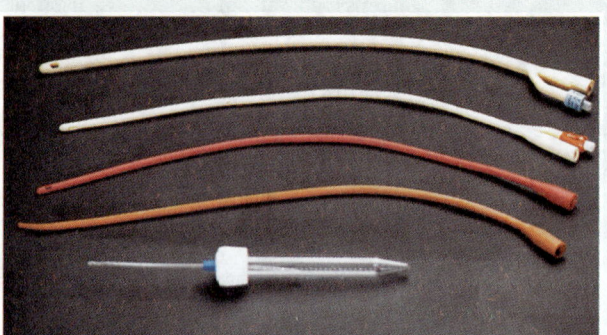

Types of catheters. From the top: #24 Foley catheter, #16 Foley catheter, #16 straight catheter, coudé catheter, self-contained catheterized specimen collection unit.

(continued)

BOX 39-3 Principles of Catheterization *(Continued)*

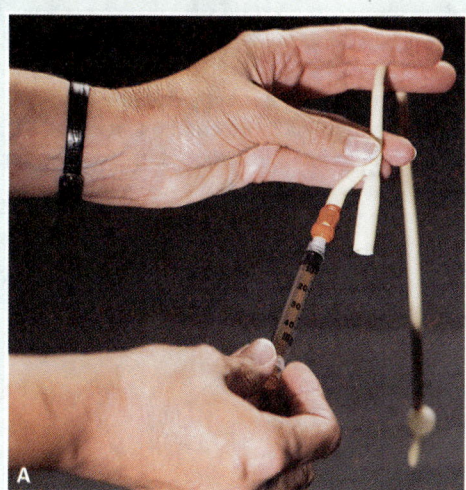

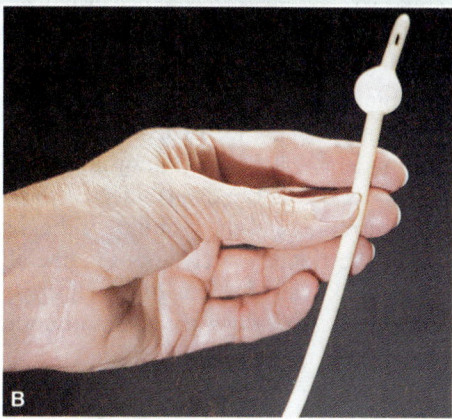

(A) Sterile water is inserted into the indicated lumen to inflate the balloon of the catheter. (B) When the balloon is inflated, the catheter will remain within the bladder.

You must be precepted by your physician for the first few times that you attempt to catheterize and thereafter must be authorized by the physician to perform the procedure.

The catheter types and sizes will vary. They may be plastic or rubber and occasionally metal or woven silk. The catheters may be straight, to use immediately and remove, or retention (usually called a Foley catheter) to inflate and leave in. If the patient has prostatic hypertrophy, the physician may use a coudé, which is slightly curved and a bit stiffer than the others mentioned, making it easier to advance beyond the obstructing prostate.

Catheters are sized from 8–10 for children and 14–20 for adults. Larger catheters are also available. The retention, or Foley, catheter is a double-lumen tube with a second, smaller tube inside with a balloon near the tip to inflate to hold in place within the bladder. Many sterile disposable kits with a wide array of options are available; many contain everything needed to perform a successful catheterization. It will likely be the responsibility of the medical assistant to order these kits and to set them up for the physician before the procedure.

Some states do not allow medical assistants to perform urinary catheterization. If your state allows catheterization, you will need to observe catheterization several times before attempting it without supervision.

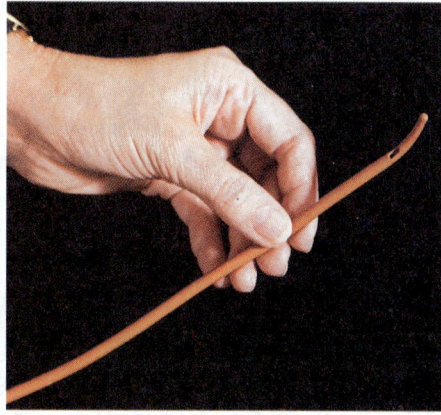

The coudé is firm and slightly curved for easier insertion past prostatic hypertrophy.

Cystoscopy or Cystourethroscopy

Cystoscopy is direct visualization of the bladder and the urethra with a lighted instrument called a cystoscope. Cystoscopy allows the physician to diagnose many diseases common to the lower urinary tract. You may be responsible for providing preoperative instruc-tion, as outlined by the physician, to the patient. This will probably include instructing the patient to increase fluid intake pre- and postoperatively and alerting the patient to the probability of some hematuria. Be sure to caution patients to report gross hematuria. These procedures are usually done under local anesthesia but may require hospitalization and general anesthesia.

Intravenous Pyelogram (IVP)

An *intravenous pyelogram* (IVP) is an x-ray examination of the kidneys and urinary tract requiring the injection of a radiopaque dye into the circulatory system. The dye will be filtered by the kidneys to enhance visualization of the renal structures. The patient will be required to cleanse the bowels with a laxative the night before the test and to administer an enema the morning of the procedure to prevent the presence of feces from obscuring the film. The patient will be NPO (nothing by mouth) for at least 8 hours before the dye is injected to increase the blood concentration and the visibility of the dye. The patient must be questioned closely about iodine allergies and may require a skin test for sensitivity. Fluids must be increased after the test to flush the dye and counteract dehydration from the preliminary cleansing.

Retrograde Pyelogram

A **retrograde pyelogram** is similar to the IVP except that dye is not injected intravenously but is introduced through a catheter inserted into the ureters through a cystoscope. This test is commonly used when the IVP procedure is contraindicated because of poor kidney function.

Ultrasound

Similar to other uses of ultrasound, this noninvasive use of sound waves will show the presence of stones and obstructions and the tissue involved. No special preparation is required other than explanation to the patient.

Checkpoint Question

7. How does a retrograde pyelogram differ from an intravenous pyelogram?

SUMMARY

The urinary system performs many vital functions in the maintenance of a homeostatic internal environment. It is responsible for the regulation of fluid volume, electrolyte levels, and the acid–base balance of all body fluid. The system works in cooperation with the liver in the detoxification of blood and eliminates wastes through urine formation and excretion. Blood pressure and red blood cell production are functions of the urinary system involving the circulatory and the skeletal systems. Working with all other systems, the urinary system is one of the keys to a state of whole body wellness that is the prime objective of the medical profession.

CRITICAL THINKING CHALLENGES

1. Analyze how a breakdown in any body system will affect the urinary system. What would happen if the liver is in failure? How would severe anemia, heart failure, or bone marrow suppression affect the kidney? Describe the effects.
2. What do you think has happened if the capillary walls allow the escape of large components such as red blood cells, white blood cells, or protein? Justify your response.
3. What is a neutral pH? Why are ammonia and phosphates good transportation devices for hydrogen ions?
4. Differentiate between hemodialysis and peritoneal dialysis. Why are some patients poor risks for peritoneal dialysis?

ANSWERS TO CHECKPOINT QUESTIONS

1. The kidney filters urea, uric acid, and creatinine.
2. The pituitary secretes antidiuretic hormone (ADH), which helps regulate the amount of urine produced, thereby maintaining fluid balance.
3. The glomerulus is the twisted mass of capillaries located within Bowman's capsule.
4. The ureters are a pair of tubes that transport urine from the kidneys to the bladder. The urethra is a tube that transports urine from the bladder to outside the body.
5. Calculi are stonelike formations that are more likely to form when the urine is alkaline.
6. In women, the urethra is shorter, allowing more bacteria to reach the bladder. Also, the urethra is contained within the labia, a site that can harbor bacteria.
7. With a retrograde pyelogram, dye is introduced through a catheter inserted into the ureters, not injected intravenously.

SUGGESTIONS FOR FURTHER READING

Bullock, B. L., Rosendahl, P. P. (1992). *Pathophysiology*, 3rd ed. Philadelphia: Lippincott-Raven.

Craven, R. F., & Hirnle, C. J. (1996). *Fundamentals of Nursing: Human Health and Function*, 2nd ed. Philadelphia: Lippincott-Raven Publishers.

Memmler, R. L., Cohen, B. J., & Wood, D. L. (1996). *The Human Body in Health and Disease*, 8th ed. Philadelphia: Lippincott-Raven Publishers.

Porth, C. M. (1994). *Pathophysiology: Concepts of Altered Health States*, 4th ed. Philadelphia: Lippincott-Raven.

Professional Guide to Diseases, 4th ed. (1992). Springhouse, PA: Springhouse Corporation.

Smeltzer, S. C., & Bare, B. G. (1996). *Brunner and Suddarth's Textbook of Medical-Surgical Nursing*, 8th ed. Philadelphia: Lippincott-Raven Publishers.

Taylor, C., Lillis, C. & LeMone, P. (1993). *Fundamentals of Nursing: The Art and Science of Nursing Care*, 2nd ed. Philadelphia: J. B. Lippincott.

Timby, B. K., Lewis, L. W. (1992). *Fundamental Skills and Concepts in Patient Care*, 5th ed. Philadelphia: Lippincott-Raven.

Caring for Patients With Disorders of the Male Reproductive System

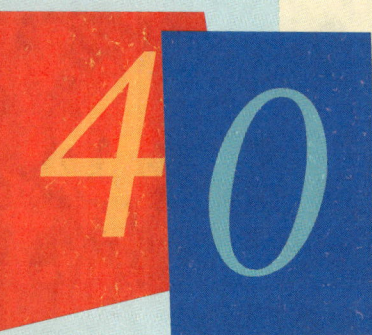

Chapter Outline

Evolution and Differentiation of the Male Reproductive System
Organs of the Male Reproductive System
    Testes
    Epididymis
    Vas Deferens
    Seminal Vesicles
    Prostate
    Cowper's Gland
    Penis
    Spermatozoa
    Composition of Semen
Common Disorders of the Male Reproductive System
    Prostatic Hypertrophy
    Hydrocele
    Cryptorchidism
    Inguinal Hernia
    Infections

    Impotence
    Sexually Transmitted Diseases
    Phimosis
    Infertility
    Testicular Cancer
Common Diagnostic Procedures and the Medical Assistant's Role
    Urinalysis
    Blood Work
    Cultures
    Rectal and Scrotal Examinations
    X-rays
    Cystoscopy
Preparing the Patient for Procedures
    Vasectomy
Summary
Critical Thinking Challenges
Answers to Checkpoint Questions
Suggestions for Further Reading

DACUM Components

1.3   Practice within the scope of education, training, and personal capabilities
1.6   Conduct oneself in a courteous and diplomatic manner
2.2   Treat all patients with empathy and impartiality
4.1   Apply principles of aseptic technique and infection control
4.7   Prepare patients for procedures
4.8   Assist physician with examinations and treatments
7.3   Teach patients methods of health promotion and disease prevention

Chapter Competencies

Learning Objectives

Upon successfully completing this chapter, you will be able to:

1. Spell and define the Key Terms.
2. State the purpose of the male reproductive system.
3. Explain how the male embryo differentiates from the female and how the union of the gametes determines the eventual gender.
4. Describe the descent of the male organs into the pelvic region and the scrotal sac.
5. Name and describe the organs of the male reproductive system.
6. Explain the function of each component of the system.
7. Trace the maturation process of a sperm cell from mitosis to ejaculation.
8. Describe a sperm cell.
9. List the components of semen, their approximate percentages, and their function in the fertilization process.
10. Name and describe common diseases of the male reproductive system, giving their symptoms and possible treatments.
11. List diagnostic procedures the medical assistant may encounter and explain the responsibilities for proper preparation and completion.

Key Terms

(See Glossary for definitions.)

acrosome	meiosis
Bartholin glands	monosaccharide
chancre	nocturia
circumcision	phimosis
corpora cavernosa	prepuce
corpus spongiosum	prostate-specific antigen
flagellum	psychogenic
fructose	smegma
gonads	truss
impotence	urinary frequency
interstitial	

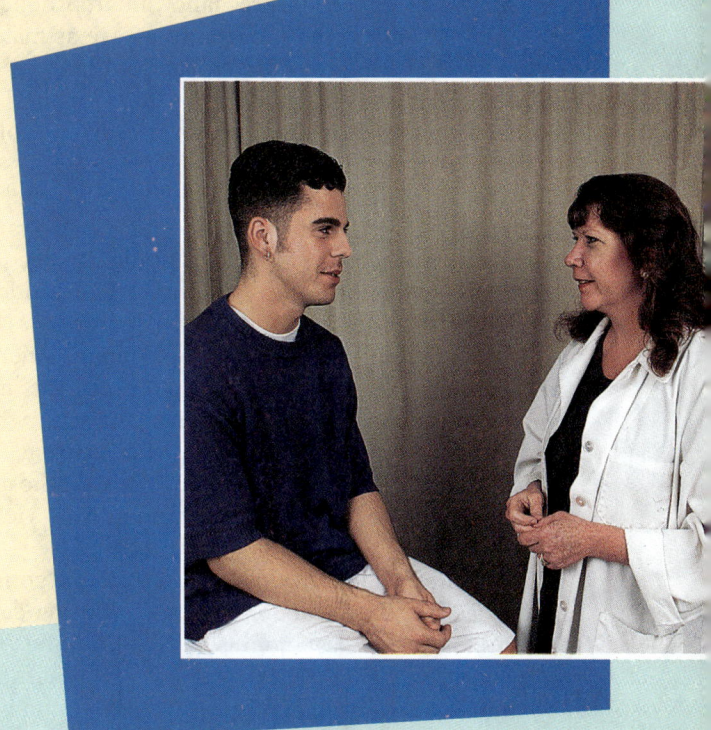

Many lower life forms reproduce without a partner or a sexual contact. The cells simply divide and the primary cell ceases to exist and instead becomes two daughter cells. Higher life forms require sexual reproduction with specialized cells from both parents to perpetuate the characteristics of each in the offspring. The male contributes the spermatozoon and the female contributes the ovum; both are called gametes. These combine to become a zygote, a fertilized egg.

The purpose of the reproductive system in the male is the formation and transportation of gametes necessary for reproduction, the physiology of intercourse, and fertilization of the egg. Cooperation between the hypothalamus, the pituitary glands, and the **gonads** (sex glands) is vital to reproductive success.

Checkpoint Question

1. How does reproduction in higher life forms differ from that of one-celled organisms?

➤ EVOLUTION AND DIFFERENTIATION OF THE MALE REPRODUCTIVE SYSTEM

Every system in the body is identical in the male and female except for components of the reproductive system. By the 12th week of pregnancy, the reproductive organs of the embryo have begun to evolve as male or female. The testes have differentiated within the medulla of the gonad that is common to both the male and female embryo, whereas the ovaries have evolved from the cortex of the gonad.

Early in gestation, the genitalia and internal organs are indistinguishable between male and female. As the embryo becomes a fetus, it gradually becomes clearly defined as one sex or the other and gender is evident by the fourth month. This definition is decided by the presence of the Y chromosome carried by the sperm at the time of conception. If the male gamete carries an X chromosome to the egg, which always brings with it its own X chromosome, the embryo will evolve into a female. A Y chromosome combined with the egg's X chromosome will yield a male.

The testes, which have developed from the gonads, are carried high in the abdominal cavity during development. During the last months of gestation, the testes normally begin to descend through the inguinal canal into the scrotum, bringing with them their supplying nerves and vessels. The canal then closes behind the testes to prevent other organs from protruding through this structure. At this time, all organs of the male reproductive system are in place and include:

- Two testes, contained in an external sac called the scrotum
- Two epididymides (sing. epididymis)
- Two vasa deferentia (sing. vas deferens)
- Two seminal vesicles
- Prostate gland
- Two Cowper's (or bulbourethral) glands
- Penis, containing the urethra, dual-purpose organs serving both the urinary system and the reproductive system (Fig. 40-1)

➤ ORGANS OF THE MALE REPRODUCTIVE SYSTEM

Testes

Located outside of the body between the thighs in a sac called the scrotum, the testes are small, egg-shaped organs about 1½ to 2 inches long by about 1 inch in diameter. In their protective pouch, they are kept at a fairly constant temperature about 2°C lower than the body temperature. To maintain this constant environment, the scrotum contracts and relaxes reflexively to bring it closer to the body for warmth or lower it away if the body is too warm. The scrotum is also rich in blood vessels and sweat glands that aid in keeping the testes at the temperature that is ideal for the production of viable sperm.

Most of the tissue of the testes is made up of tightly coiled seminiferous tubules, which produce the spermatozoa. Between the tubules lie the **interstitial** cells that produce the male hormone testosterone, essential for the maintenance of the reproductive functions and for the development of the masculine secondary sexual characteristics. Testosterone is responsible for the male distribution of hair, deeper voice, larger and heavier bone structure, greater muscle mass, and a generally higher production of red blood cells (possibly due to larger bones).

Checkpoint Question

2. What is the male hormone, where is it formed, and what are its main functions?

Within the testes, spermatogenesis (sperm formation) begins. Spermatogenesis is a continuous process, beginning with a cell containing a full component of 46

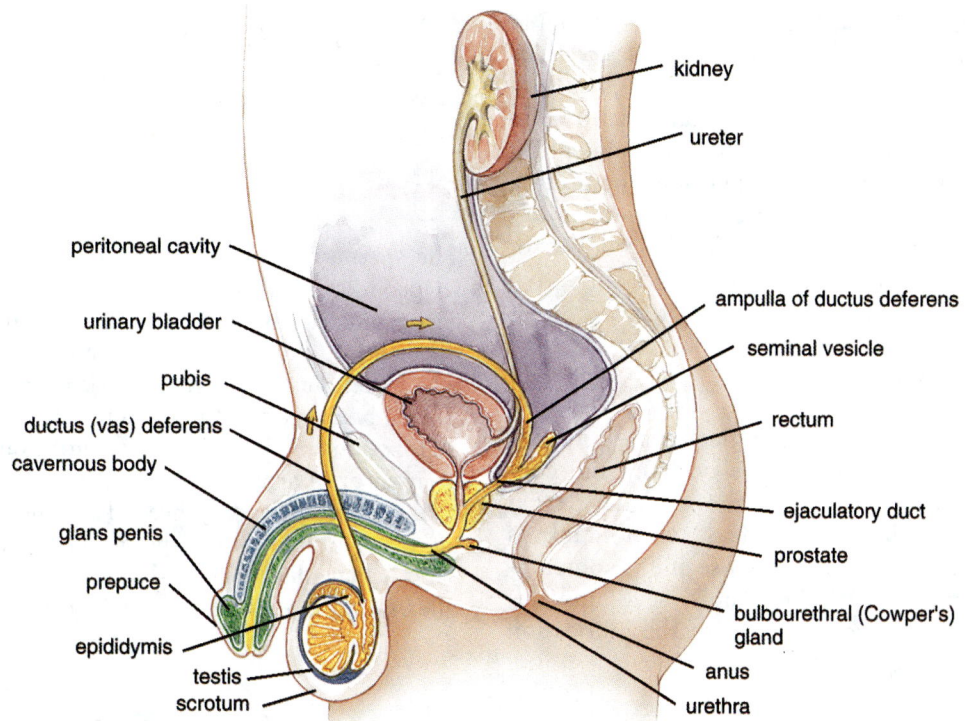

FIGURE 40-1
Male genitourinary system. The arrows indicate the course of sperm cells through the duct system.

chromosomes. This then divides by **meiosis** (cell division specific to sperm and ova), rather than mitosis, and will contain only 23 chromosomes after division. As they mature, the sperm are passed from the seminiferous tubules to the epididymis. As these are passed on, more sperm are in the process of maturation within the various compartments of the system. This process takes 70 to 75 days. However, because excess formation is stored for future use, there is rarely a shortage. Those sperm not used are simply absorbed by the system. The average ejaculate contains 3 to 5 mL of semen, with approximately 120 million sperm per milliliter, all of which will need to be replaced by the supply that has been gradually working its way to full maturity.

Epididymis

Still within the scrotum, each epididymis is a tightly coiled, thin cord that attaches to the ducts of its testes. It wraps around from the top of the testes down the posterior surfaces then turns upward to become the vas deferens. The epididymis serves as a resting place for the sperm as they mature and are slowly moved along by mild peristalsis. Sperm cells gradually become capable of independent movement during this phase of their journey.

Vas Deferens

The vas deferens, or ductus deferens, is continuous with its epididymis at the lower edge of the testes and travels upward through the inguinal canal into the abdominal cavity and curves up and over to the posterior aspect of the urinary bladder. It is primarily an organ of transport.

Seminal Vesicles

Situated just below the posterior bladder, the seminal vesicles are convoluted tubes that connect with the vas deferens and are responsible for producing part of the seminal fluid. The seminal fluid is slightly alkaline and is thought to help neutralize the acid environment in the vagina during ejaculation. It also contains **fructose**, a **monosaccharide** (simple sugar), and several nutrients to provide an energy source for the sperm. This fluid is the largest component of semen.

Prostate

The prostate completely encircles the urethra at the base of the bladder and is about 1½ inches across and about 1 inch thick. This gland includes a passageway for the seminal vesicles and the vas deferens to join at the ejaculatory duct. The prostate produces secretions that add to the volume of semen. This fluid is also alkaline to aid the fluid from the seminal vesicles in altering the vaginal pH for a less hostile environment for sperm. The prostate empties its fluid into the urethra through many small ducts during the smooth muscle contractions of ejaculation along with the products of the vas deferens and seminal vesicles.

Cowper's Glands

The Cowper's, or bulbourethral glands, are mucous-producing organs lying on the pelvic floor and connecting with the urethra below the prostate. Sexual stimulation causes this fluid to release to act mainly as a lubricant. It has little other purpose and is comparable to the female's **Bartholin glands**, small mucous glands that actually produce most of the lubrication needed during intercourse.

Penis

The penis is common to both the urinary and the reproductive systems. It contains three columns of cavernous, spongelike erectile tissue. There are two **corpora cavernosa** (erectile bodies) along each side of the penis. The **corpus spongiosum**, which contains the urethra, is at the lower surface. It is attached with ligaments to the pubic arch. At the distal end is a cone-shaped surface called the glans penis containing the urinary meatus. The glans is normally covered with a fold of loose skin called the **prepuce** or the foreskin. This is frequently removed during infancy as a religious ritual or as an aid to hygiene in a procedure called **circumcision**, which is surgical removal of the prepuce.

During sexual stimulation, nerve impulses cause the arteries supplying the penis to enlarge. This in turn fills the cavernous spaces with blood and compresses the venous spaces, impeding the outflow of blood. The penis elongates and becomes firm, creating an organ capable of vaginal penetration. With sufficient stimulation of the glans penis, sexual satisfaction results in an orgasm. Peristaltic contractions begin throughout the reproductive system, resulting in emission, emptying each of the transporting tubes and storage compartments in turn, and ejaculation, expelling the combined contents with great force. After this event, engorgement subsides with a decrease in the pressure within the supplying arteries, allowing the cavernous spaces to empty and reducing the pressure on the venous outflow.

Checkpoint Question
3. What happens during the sequence of ejaculation?

Spermatozoa

The spermatozoon (pl. spermatozoa) is a small cell, shaped like a tadpole, with an oval head containing 23 chromosomes within the nucleus (Fig. 40-2). At the tip of the head, like a cap, is an area called the **acrosome**, which contains an enzyme that is capable of penetrating the barrier wall of the ovum. The body of the spermatozoon is made up of a concentration of mitochondria wrapped around just under the head, providing a ready source of energy needed for the high degree of motility required for the sperm to reach its destination.

The **flagellum** (pl. flagella) is a long, whiplike, fiber-filled tail. It is an extension of the cell wall with a store

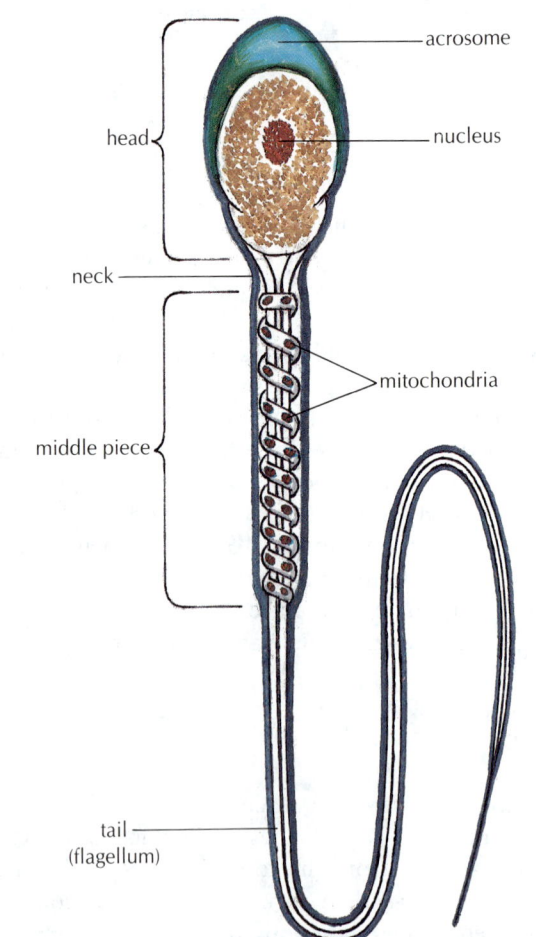

FIGURE 40-2
Diagram of a human spermatozoon showing major structural features. (Chaffee EE, Lytle IM: Basic Physiology and Anatomy, 4th ed, p. 549. Philadelphia, JB Lippincott, 1980)

of adenosine triphosphate (ATP) for energy. Only one cell will succeed in fertilizing the egg, but an abundance of spermatozoa is needed to help that one cell dissolve the barrier wall of the ovum. All others will usually die within a few hours, but some may live up to 3 days.

Composition of Semen

The accessory organs of the male reproductive system provide the secretions necessary for support and transport of the spermatozoa. The thick, white ejaculate is only about 1% to 5% spermatozoa, even though the 3 to 5 mL contains as many as 120 million sperm per milliliter. The primary contributing organ is the prostate, making up to 60% of the fluid. The seminal vesicles add about 30% and the bulbourethral glands about 5%.

Checkpoint Question

4. How would you describe a sperm cell and its motility? Why must there be so many per ejaculate?

➤ COMMON DISORDERS OF THE MALE REPRODUCTIVE SYSTEM

The male reproductive system is so inextricably linked to the urinary system that diseases affecting one frequently affect the other. Listed below are several of the diseases that are most likely to be encountered in the medical office.

Prostatic Hypertrophy

As most men reach their middle years, the prostate begins to enlarge (hypertrophy); this disorder may be benign or malignant. The benign form of the disease has no known cause, but it is presumed to be the result of decreasing hormonal levels. The malignant form of hypertrophy is the second most common form of cancer in men, either as a primary or secondary site.

Presenting symptoms are usually the same for both forms of the disease. Complaints might include a weak urinary stream, a feeling of urgency but with a hesitant start to the stream, dribbling, **nocturia** (excessive urination at night), and **urinary frequency** (frequent urge to urinate). Because the enlarged prostate compresses the internal urinary sphincter, residual urine frequently causes stagnation and urinary tract infections. Symptoms of the malignant form are late in appearing and are usually a sign that the disease is firmly entrenched.

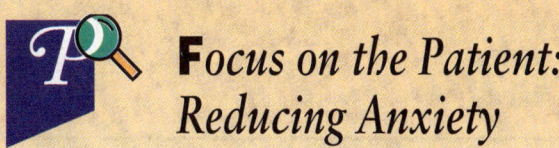

Focus on the Patient: Reducing Anxiety

A variety of diseases that affect the male reproductive system will produce anxiety and tension for the patient. The following tips can help ease stressful situations.

- Provide privacy by closing the examining room door when obtaining the patient history.
- Maintain a nonjudgmental manner when asking questions regarding sexual partners or lifestyle behaviors.
- Always knock on the examining room door before entering.
- Allow the patient to change into the examination gown in private.
- Supply a drape for the patient to cover himself while he is on the examining table.
- Uncover only the area being examined; keep the patient draped during all other aspects of the examination.
- Have all of the equipment ready for the physician to prevent delays while the patient is in an uncomfortable and exposed position.

Treatment in the early stages of the benign form are not usually aggressive, addressing the symptoms until such a time as the enlargement requires surgery. Surgery for either form will vary in the approach to the organ (Box 40-1). If cancer is present, radiation may be required to halt metastasis. A radical resection of the perineum may be required to remove the testes to reduce the production of testosterone, which seems to feed malignancies in this area.

Many patients with prostatic hypertrophy have other diseases common to the aging process and will need to be evaluated to determine which type of treatment will be most beneficial without compromising fragile health. It is vitally important that all men, especially those over age 40, realize the importance of the digital rectal examination (DRE) performed during routine yearly physical examination. The DRE is the easiest and quickest way for the physician to check for prostatic hypertrophy. Although further testing will always be done for a suspiciously enlarged prostate, the physician will be alerted to malignancy by the consistency of the gland. Malignant hypertrophy is generally more firm than simple benign hypertrophy and may present in the early stages as prostatic nodules.

Surgical Intervention for Prostatic Hypertrophy

Transurethral Resection

A type of cystoscope with an electrocautery wire cutting loop, called a resectoscope, is inserted through the urethra and rotated through the prostate to remove pieces of the gland. The pieces are washed out with irrigating fluid. There is no abdominal incision, making this a safer alternative for the high-risk patient. The whole organ is not usually removed in this surgery; therefore the obstruction frequently returns and strictures are likely to develop. This is not a choice for malignancies.

Suprapubic Prostatectomy

Performed from the abdomen and through the bladder, this procedure allows the surgeon to peel out the whole organ through a wide surgical field and to check the bladder for involvement. This approach is the choice for large organs or for malignancies. As in all surgeries, there are postoperative risks, particularly for the elderly. These include pain, hemorrhage, urinary leakage, and prolonged convalescence.

Perineal Resection

An incision between the scrotum and the anus is a short, direct route without interfering with the bladder and is preferred for some large malignancies. It appears to be less traumatic for the very old or infirm. Surgeons find that the field is more restrictive than that for the suprapubic, with less room to maneuver. It is not a good choice for young men because impotence and urinary and fecal incontinence are frequent postoperative complications. Because of the proximity to the anal area, infection is also a risk.

Retropubic

A low abdominal incision that approaches above the pubis but below the bladder avoids trauma to the bladder and thereby allows a shorter convalescence than the suprapubic approach but better removal options than the transurethral. It is a good choice if pathology is limited to the prostate with no bladder involvement that requires attention.

Blood testing is done to determine levels of serum acid phosphatase or **prostate-specific antigen** (PSA). PSA, a normal protein produced by the prostate, is usually elevated in men with prostatic cancer. PSA testing is done frequently as a screening device and is offered by many health departments as a public service. The American Cancer Society recommends a yearly PSA for men over age 50. Abnormal findings on the PSA and DRE are followed by an ultrasound. Definitive diagnosis requires a biopsy.

Checkpoint Question

5. *What happens to the prostate in prostatic hypertrophy and what are the common symptoms of this disorder?*

Hydrocele

Hydrocele, a collection of fluid within the scrotum and around the testes, may be the result of trauma or infection or may simply be due to the aging process (Fig. 40-3). If the condition is extremely uncomfortable, aspiration may be required. If it persists, surgical intervention may be the treatment of choice. In most cases, the fluid is reabsorbed by the body. Hydrocele is common in male infants and will generally gradually subside.

Differentiation between simple hydrocele, hematocele (a collection of blood within the scrotum), a tumor, or a hernia may be accomplished by transillumination, shining a bright light through the structure. The hydrocele will transilluminate easily; hematoceles, tumors, and hernias will obscure the light.

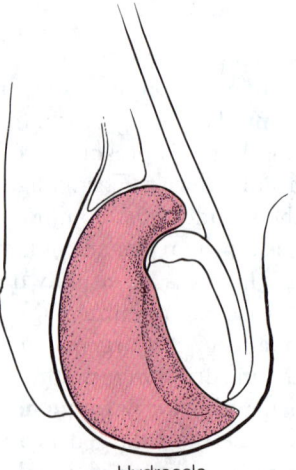

Hydrocele

FIGURE 40-3
A hydrocele.

Cryptorchidism

Cryptorchidism refers to undescended testes (Fig. 40-4). Normally, the testes descend in the male fetus by the eighth month of gestation. In a small percentage of male infants, one or both testes fail to descend by time of delivery. Many of those will descend spontaneously by the end of the first year. Those remaining in the abdomen, the inguinal canal, or at the perineal wall after this time will need to be brought down surgically. If an undescended testis is not surgically corrected (orchiopexy), it will result in sterility of the undescended organ and increases the risk of testicular malignancy. Surgery is usually performed before age 4, preferably by age 1 or 2. The abnormality may increase the risk of inguinal hernia on the affected side if not corrected.

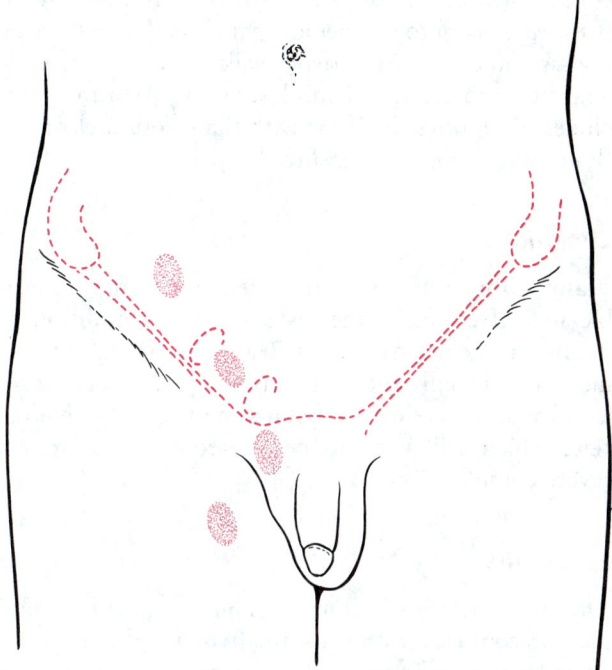

FIGURE 40-4
Possible locations of undescended testicles.

What If?

You are working in a surgeon's office. When the physician informs the mother of a 10-month-old boy that her son needs surgery for cryptorchidism, the mother starts to cry. What if you are asked by the surgeon to comfort her?

The most important thing that you can do is to be supportive of the mother's feelings and to encourage her to verbalize these feelings. Never minimize the surgery or say anything like "It is a very simple operation" or "I know he will be just fine." Encourage the mother to ask questions regarding the surgery and relay these questions to the surgeon. Ask open-ended questions to elicit her concerns. Allow the mother to use the telephone to call friends and family. Offer tissues as needed. If the child senses the mother's anxiety, encourage her to hold and reassure her son.

Diagnosis is made in the early stages by having the patient bear down and cough while the physician inserts a finger into a pouch made by the scrotum up into the external and internal inguinal rings. Pressure against the finger indicates a weakness in this area. In later stages, visual examination will reveal an obvious swelling as loops of the bowel descend into the inguinal area.

Treatment will depend on the patient's physical condition. Elderly or infirm patients will benefit from a **truss**, a pressure device used to hold the hernia in place if surgery is not an option. Herniorrhaphy will replace the organ and repair the opening. Hernioplasty will not only return the organ and repair the opening but will also reinforce the area with wire or mesh.

Inguinal Hernia

After the descent of the testes, the inguinal canals close with small rings left open at the anterior base of the abdominal wall (the external ring) as a passage for the spermatic cord, which encloses the vas deferens and the vessels and nerves that supply the testes. There is no connection between this area and the abdominal contents because of the fascia that encloses the abdominal organs; however, this area remains a possible site for weakness to occur with age or exceptional exertion. Men are many times more likely than women to suffer this type of hernia.

Infections

Infections of the urinary tract are likely to become infections of the male reproductive system because they share many of the same organs and functions. The most common infections for the male reproductive system are listed below.

Epididymitis

Infection here usually results from an infected prostate or urinary tract. Agents include staphylococci, streptococci, *Escherichia coli, Chlamydia,* or *Neisseria gonorrhoeae.* Symptoms include pain, tenderness, fever, malaise, and a characteristic walk with the legs wide apart to protect the painful scrotum. Treatment includes antibiotics, bed rest with the scrotum elevated, fluids, and palliative measures for pain.

Orchitis

Many of the same organisms listed above are responsible for infections of the testes, with the addition of mumps as a causative agent. The symptoms and treatment are virtually the same. In mumps orchitis, sterility is a prime concern. Orchitis may result in hydrocele, which will need to be treated if it becomes a severe complication.

Prostatitis

Chronic prostatitis is common among the elderly and may be confused with prostatic hypertrophy if the repeated infections cause the organs to fibrose. The causative agents are much like those of other infections of the male reproductive system, with the leading cause being *E. coli.* It is frequently a result of catheterization or cystoscopy. Some pathogens reach the prostate by way of the bloodstream or the lymph system. Symptoms may include inguinal pain, fever, low back and joint pain, burning and dysuria, and urethral discharge. Urine specimens will include blood and pus. Antibiotic treatment is required.

Impotence

Impotence, the inability to either achieve or maintain an erection capable of intercourse, may be psychogenic (psychological) or organic in origin. Psychogenic impotence may be caused by something as simple as exhaustion, anxiety, or depression, and will disappear with a resolution of the situational etiology. Deep-seated psychological problems will require extensive psychotherapy. Organic impotence may be the result of disease in almost any other body system, such as endocrine imbalances, cardiovascular problems, nervous system impairment, or urinary diseases. Organic impotence may also be caused by injuries to the pelvic organs or to medications that impair any of the systems serving the reproductive system.

Diagnosis involves a detailed medical and sexual history with a holistic analysis of life-style and current emotional status. Blood studies and measurements of both penile arterial flow and nerve conduction to this area are usually required.

Treatment will reflect the cause, for example, correction of endocrine imbalances, psychotherapy, or medication adjustment, if any of these are found to be the cause. If none of these are effective, penile implants are available after extensive counseling.

Sexually Transmitted Diseases

Many of the diseases transmitted through sexual contact have serious consequences. The most deadly of these currently is acquired immunodeficiency syndrome (AIDS), which is discussed in Chapter 36, Caring for Patients With Immune Disorders. However, the diseases listed below are no less a problem for the health care system. All sexually transmitted diseases (STDs) must be reported to the local health department.

Chlamydia

Chlamydia infections include urethritis in men, cervicitis in women, and lymphogranuloma venereum (LGV) in both, all caused by the organism *Chlamydia trachomatis.* These infections are the most common STDs in the United States.

Without treatment, men with chlamydia infections may develop epididymitis, prostatitis, and sterility. Transmission is by contact with the mucous membranes of infected persons. The disease may be asymptomatic in men. The primary lesion of LGV, a small vesicle or ulcer, may go unnoticed. In 1 to 4 weeks, lymphadenopathy near the site of infection will occur. Systemic symptoms include flulike myalgia, fever, and chills.

In men, the LGV lymph nodes may become very large and tender and spread to surrounding nodal sites. The nodes may become so enlarged they rupture and form sinus tracts to drain the affected nodes.

As the organism ascends the urethral tract, epididymitis may occur with painful scrotal swelling and penile discharge. Chlamydial prostatitis and urethritis will lead to dysuria, urinary frequency, and urethral discharge.

Diagnosis is made by a swab culture of the site. Aspiration of interstitial fluid is used to diagnose epididymitis or prostatitis. Blood tests will determine antibodies in men with previous exposure. Treatment includes courses of penicillin and tetracycline until the patient tests negative for the disease.

Gonorrhea

Gonorrhea is the second most common of the STDs, with an estimated 2 million cases a year in the United States. It is caused by a gram-negative diplococcus,

N. gonorrhoeae. If left untreated, *N. gonorrhoeae* may ascend the reproductive tract and infect the organs located beyond the penis. Adhesions from the infection may cause sterility and, if it enters the bloodstream, septicemia is a possibility. The symptoms are obvious within a few days to several weeks and exhibit as a purulent discharge from the urethra with pain and burning on urination. Diagnosis is established symptomatically and with a urethral culture. An initial dose of ceftriaxone intramuscularly followed by oral penicillin for 7 days is the treatment of choice. If the disease is penicillin resistant, spectinomycin is prescribed. The patient should be warned that, until the cultures are negative, he is considered infectious.

Syphilis

Syphilis first presents as a **chancre**, or ulcer, on the penis or in the genital area. It is caused by a spirochete that spreads quickly through the bloodstream to become a systemic disease with far-reaching consequences. The disease has three stages:

- Primary, with the presenting chancre that may go totally unnoticed
- Secondary, with variable flu-type symptoms up to 8 weeks after exposure and rashes on the skin and mucous membranes, leading to a latency phase that may last for years
- Tertiary, with systemic involvement that will frequently cause death as the spirochete invades virtually every body system

A battery of efficient and effective tests help to determine the presence of syphilis. Penicillin treatment is effective but must be ongoing with strict follow-up for compliance and cure.

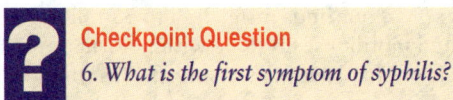

Checkpoint Question
6. What is the first symptom of syphilis?

Herpes Genitalis

Herpes genitalis is commonly caused by the herpesvirus 2, but may mutate with herpesvirus 1, which causes cold sores on the mouth. This disease has reached epidemic proportions and has no known cure. The patient presents with painful vesicles that rupture and leave equally painful ulcers. Lymph nodes are swollen and tender, and flulike symptoms are sometimes reported. Response to the disease is variable,

with symptoms ranging from scarcely noticeable to excruciatingly painful; remissions may last for years or the symptoms may recur with each stressful situation. Diagnosis is symptomatic although tissue cultures may be used for a definitive diagnosis. Acyclovir has been effective as a palliative measure to reduce the severity of the symptoms of herpes genitalis, but it cannot be considered a cure.

Phimosis

Phimosis is a narrowing or tightening of the prepuce (foreskin) that prevents retraction over the glans penis. Uncircumcised males, or those with excessive prepuce covering the glans penis, may find that the skin adheres to the surface of the glans if the accumulation of **smegma** (an oily secretion from small glands under the foreskin) is not regularly washed free and the area of the glans kept clean. As a medical assistant, you may be responsible for educating caregivers of male infants in the proper cleaning techniques at bath time and diaper changes. For both infants and adults, the foreskin should be retracted, the glans washed well and rinsed, and the foreskin returned to its natural position. It may be necessary to use petrolatum on the surface of the glans if it seems to adhere despite these efforts. Adults who experience this may need circumcision.

Infertility

Infertility is the inability to reproduce. Male infertility is easier to diagnose than female infertility. If pregnancy is not achieved after 1 year of regular, unprotected intercourse, infertility tests are initiated. Causes of male infertility include:

- Semen disorders, such as low volume (oligospermia), low motility, abnormal sperm, immature sperm
- Systemic disease, such as diabetes mellitus or renal or hepatic disease
- Sexually transmitted diseases (STDs), such as gonorrhea or herpes
- Testicular disorders, such as cryptorchidism or ductal obstructions
- Sexual dysfunction

A physical examination may reveal many of the above causes. A detailed patient history may direct the diagnosis to a history of prolonged fever, mumps, impaired nutritional status, or genital trauma. The most conclusive laboratory test is a semen analysis. Serum testosterone levels, gonadotrophin assays, and a testicular biopsy may be performed.

If the cause is a correctable anatomic problem, surgery will be performed. Hormonal treatment may correct a diagnosed imbalance and counseling may alleviate psychological dysfunction. If the accepted corrective measures do not result in pregnancy and the woman is fertile, options include artificial insemination or adoption. Box 40-2 presents a case study on infertility.

Testicular Cancer

Testicular cancer accounts for only about 1% of all malignancies, but it involves extremely high metastatic and mortality rates. The cause is unknown, but the factors most often implicated include cryptorchidism, infection, genetics, and endocrine abnormalities. The symptoms are gradual and painless, involving initially only a vague feeling of scrotal heaviness. In fact, the most significant symptom is a painless enlargement of the testes. By the time a patient presents with back or abdominal pain, metastasis has usually occurred.

Testicular self-examination is the best method of early detection and should be performed as a matter of habit for all men. All suspicious areas of thickness or lumps should be reported immediately. Further testing by alpha-fetoprotein and human chorionic gonadotropin blood work will be ordered. A computed tomography (CT) scan is frequently ordered to determine the extent of the malignancy and possible metastasis.

Treatment is usually an orchiectomy through the inguinal approach, with lymph node resection if cancer cells are found in the local nodes. Radiation is added if metastasis is found.

The sequela is sterility if both testes are involved, but sexual function should not be impaired because the testes only provide semen, which is about 1% to 3% of the ejaculate. The other organs of the reproductive system will continue to produce their various secretions. However, the reduction in testosterone produced by the testes usually results in reduced sexual desire.

BOX 40-2 Infertility: A Case Study

Mr. and Mrs. Jones, in their mid-thirties, are waiting in Dr. Brown's office to consult with him regarding their inability to conceive a child. Mrs. Jones recently completed a gynecologic workup that revealed that she has no anatomic or physiologic abnormalities that would interfere with conception. Her gynecologist referred the couple to Dr. Brown for Mr. Jones's evaluation after Mrs. Jones's Huhner test suggested a low sperm count.

Dr. Brown directs Mr. Jones to the interview room for a complete social, sexual, and medical history. Questions in addition to the normal data base and past medical history will concentrate on his early sexual development and puberty, his nutritional status and diet history, history of trauma to the pelvic organs, and questions regarding incidences of high fevers and viral diseases, especially mumps.

Mr. Jones then disrobes for his complete physical examination, including height, weight, urinalysis, and vital signs. Dr. Brown finishes the routine physical with special emphasis on Mr. Jones's testicular, prostatic, and penile health. Mr. Jones's physical is within normal limits, but on closer questioning, he remembers that as a late teenager, he had a mild parotid swelling, high fever, and sore throat, and concurrently or soon after—he is vague regarding the details—he experienced pain and swelling in his scrotum. Neither he nor his mother thought of the two illnesses as connected and never sought medical attention.

Dr. Brown orders a semen analysis and testosterone levels, and a gonadotropin assay for pituitary-gonadal involvement and to rule out endocrine involvement. You will instruct Mr. Jones to submit a semen specimen in a clean, dry, glass container within 2 hours of ejaculation. He should keep this at room temperature and is cautioned to abstain from intercourse for 4 to 5 days before taking the specimen. The remainder of the ordered lab work can be done within that time.

Dr. Brown hopes to find 60 to 100 million sperm per 3 to 5 mL of semen but finds instead 30 to 35 million. The shape and motility seem to be within normal limits. A diagnosis of oligospermia is confirmed as suspected.

Treatment will include instructions regarding what to avoid, such a tight-fitting underwear that will hold the scrotum against the perineum, hot baths, and biking for long periods. Mrs. Jones's ovulation should be timed and intercourse should take place primarily at that time. If these measures are not successful, hormonal therapy might be suggested. Artificial insemination is a possibility, either with Mr. Jones's sperm or that of a donor. Group therapy will help the couple deal with this aspect of their marriage until the situation is resolved.

Patient Education: Testicular Self-examination

The American Cancer Society recommends that all men be taught the fundamentals of self-examination for testicular cancer. It is commonly found between the ages of 15 and 34, at a time when many young men are not yet aware of health concerns. This cancer is highly treatable if found very early, making it imperative that men understand the importance of vigilance.

Men should be taught the signs of testicular cancer in addition to the procedure for the self-examination. They include the following:

- a feeling of heaviness in the scrotal area, generally without pain, although a dull ache may be present
- fluid accumulation in the scrotal sac without a history of injury
- a change in the consistency of the testis or its surrounding sac
- possible breast tenderness

Most physicians recommend that this examination be performed as often as weekly by all men 15 years old and older. The best time is after a warm bath or shower when the scrotal sac is most relaxed. Roll each testicle between the thumb and forefinger and feel for hard lumps or bumps or even a change in the consistency of the scrotal tissue. This procedure should not be hurried and typically takes about 3 minutes.

If there is any cause for concern, any change in the normal texture, size, shape or consistency, an appointment should be made promptly for an examination by the physician. He may order certain x-rays after performing a complete physical examination. Surgery is usually the preferred treatment, possibly in addition to chemotherapy or radiation therapy.

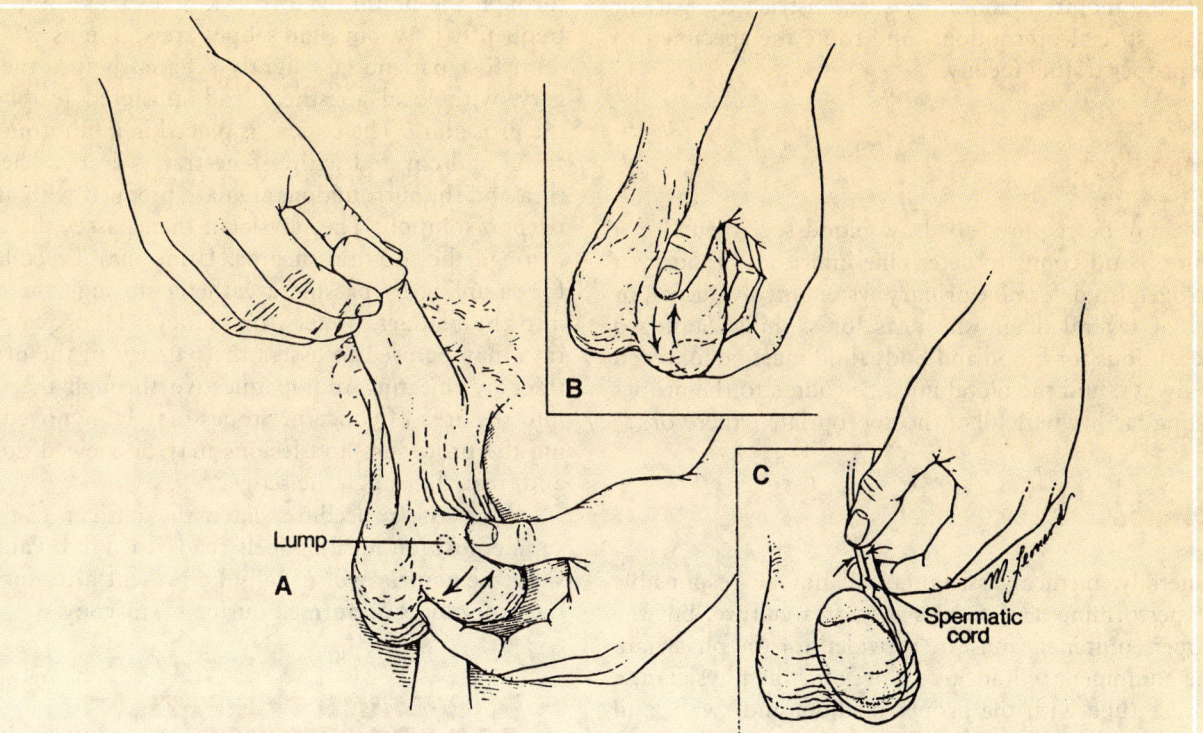

1. Use both hands to palpate the testis; the normal testicle is smooth and uniform in consistency.
2. With the index and middle fingers under the testis and the thumb on top, roll the testis gently in a horizontal plane between the thumb and fingers (A).
3. Feel for any evidence of a small lump or abnormality.
4. Follow the same procedure and palpate upward along the testis (B).
5. Locate the epididymis (C), a cordlike structure on the top and back of the testicle that stores and transports sperm.
6. Repeat the examination for the other testis. It is normal to find that one testis is larger than the other.
7. If you find any evidence of a small, pealike lump consult your physician. It may be due to an infection or a tumor growth.

➤ COMMON DIAGNOSTIC PROCEDURES AND THE MEDICAL ASSISTANT'S ROLE

In addition to the information gathered by diagnostic tests described below, establishing diagnoses for the male reproductive system will often involve a detailed social and sexual history.

Urinalysis

A specifically directed urine workup will differentiate between diseases of the urinary system and of the male reproductive system. They share many of the same symptoms and are difficult to distinguish without the tests that correspond with the presenting symptoms. Cultures and sensitivities are commonly ordered, which will require that you instruct the patient in the proper procedure for a clean-catch, midstream specimen (see Chap. 44, Urinalysis). For all tests, you will need to assemble the proper specimen containers, complete the required laboratory slips, instruct the patient in any special precautions, and route the specimen to the proper testing facility.

Blood Work

You may be required to draw blood specimens for a white blood count to determine infection, blood urea nitrogen (to determine urinary system involvement), or any of several diagnostic tests for syphilis. Standard Precautions for blood and body fluid must be followed as always, and the blood must be routed to the proper testing facility with all of the appropriate paperwork.

Cultures

Generally, medical assistants will not be responsible for performing a urethral swab for a culture, but the proper equipment must be provided for the physician. The equipment will include gloves for the physician, a culture tube with the proper medium and swab, and completed laboratory slips.

Rectal and Scrotal Examinations

You will be required to supply the physician with latex gloves and a water-soluble lubricant and to instruct the patient to disrobe appropriately. The physician will inspect and palpate the scrotum as described for inguinal hernias. To determine if the patient has prostatic hypertrophy, the physician will lubricate a gloved index finger and palpate the patient's prostate rectally for size, shape, and consistency.

X-rays

To confirm diagnoses, the physician may order an intravenous pyelogram (IVP) or computed tomography (CT) scan. These allow the physician to determine the extent of involvement for those disorders that are difficult to differentiate by palpation, inspection, or diagnostic laboratory studies.

Cystoscopy

Physicians diagnose and treat many of the diseases of the male reproductive system and urinary system by cystoscopy. A cystoscope is used to view the interior of the bladder by passing a lighted viewing instrument through the urethra. Fiberoptic scopes are used most frequently now, but rigid scopes are still in use.

Most patients are lightly sedated before the surgery, with local anesthetics administered just before the procedure. The patient is placed in a lithotomy position and covered with a fenestrated drape. The urethra and the surrounding area are prepped with an antiseptic solution. The physician then passes the scope through the urethral meatus. Urine may be collected for sampling by passing a catheter through the scope into the bladder, ureters, or kidneys. Fluoroscopic x-rays may be used to assess the patency of the urinary tract by injecting radiopaque dye through the scope into the area of concern. Stones may be removed during the procedure and lesions may be viewed directly and treated through the scope.

After the procedure, have the patient rest in a supine position until he feels ready to stand. Pain and slight hematuria will usually be present after most of the procedures performed during cystoscopy.

➤ PREPARING THE PATIENT FOR PROCEDURES

Few of the diagnostic procedures involving the male reproductive system will require extensive or involved preparations. Equipment to be assembled will usually only include latex gloves, a water-soluble lubricant, and tissues for the patient's use. Laboratory tests will require the proper specimen containers or tubes and properly completed laboratory slips.

Vasectomy

An increasingly popular form of reproductive control is the vasectomy—bilateral removal of all or a segment of the vas deferens to prevent the passage of sperm from the testes. This procedure is frequently performed in the medical office.

The patient will receive a light preoperative sedative and may be NPO (nothing by mouth). He will be placed in the lithotomy position, covered with a fenestrated drape, and given a local anesthetic. Small incisions are made bilaterally near the scrotal sac. The vas deferens is pulled through the incision, clamped proximally and distally, and the connecting segment is removed. The ducts are replaced and the site is sutured.

Ejaculation and sexual function are not affected by the surgery. The volume of sperm in the ejaculate is so minute that its absence will not be noticed. The sperm that are produced are absorbed by the body. Sterility may not be immediate. The patient is advised to return for sperm counts until the ejaculate is free of sperm. Although vasectomies can be reversed, studies report varied success rates.

SUMMARY

The male reproductive system performs only one major function—reproduction of the species. Disease or dysfunction in this system can have grave psychological as well as physiologic consequences. Major strides are being made in educating the public about maintaining the health of this system to ensure holistic wellness.

CRITICAL THINKING CHALLENGES

1. Review the chapter on the endocrine system. Explain the relationship between the hypothalamus, the pituitary, and the gonads.
2. You are caring for a patient with oligospermia-induced infertility. The physician recommends abstinence for prescribed periods. Why might the physician make this recommendation?
3. Research the available statistics regarding penile cancer rates among circumcised versus uncircumcised men. Compare statistics also for cervical cancer among the wives of both groups. Explain why there might be a difference.
4. Your patient is concerned that if he has a vasectomy, his ejaculate will be noticeably diminished. How would you explain to him why neither he nor his mate will discern any difference?

ANSWERS TO CHECKPOINT QUESTIONS

1. Higher species require a mate or a sexual contact to reproduce. Many lower life forms, such as one-celled organisms, simply divide.
2. The male hormone, testosterone, is produced in the interstitial spaces of the seminiferous tubules. It functions in reproduction and in the development of secondary sexual characteristics.
3. Nerve impulses cause the arteries to enlarge, fill the cavernous spaces, and entrap the venous blood within the penis. The penis enlarges and elongates, peristaltic contractions empty the transfer tubes and storage compartments and result in ejaculation.
4. A sperm cell is a tadpole-shaped cell with a flagellum for motility. It is nourished by the mitochondria wrapped around the flagellum at the base of the cell. Many are required to dissolve the shell around the ovum.
5. The prostate enlarges and closes off the urethra, causing urgency, hesitation, dribbling, weak stream, nocturia, and frequency.
6. The first symptom of syphilis is a chancre at the site of infection.

SUGGESTIONS FOR FURTHER READING

Bates, B., Bickley, L. S., Hockalman, R. A. (1995). *A Guide to Physical Examination and History Taking*, 6th ed. Philadelphia: Lippincott-Raven.

Bullock, B. L., Rosendahl, P. P. (1992). *Pathophysiology*, 3rd ed. Philadelphia: Lippincott-Raven.

Memmler, R. L., Cohen, B. J., & Wood, D. L. (1996). *The Human Body in Health and Disease*, 8th ed. Philadelphia: Lippincott-Raven.

Miller, B. F., & Keane, C. B. (1992). *Encyclopedia and Dictionary of Medicine, Nursing and Allied Health*. Philadelphia: W. B. Saunders.

(1992). *Professional Guide to Diseases*, 4th ed. Springhouse, PA: Springhouse.

Rosdahl, C. B. (1995). *Textbook of Basic Nursing*, 6th ed. Philadelphia: Lippincott-Raven.

Smeltzer, S. C., Bare, B. G. (1992). *Brunner and Suddarth's Textbook of Medical-Surgical Nursing*, 7th ed. Philadelphia: Lippincott-Raven.

Caring for Patients With Gynecologic and Obstetric Disorders

4 1

Chapter Outline

Organs of the Female Reproductive System
    Ovaries
    Fallopian Tubes
    Uterus
    Vagina
    Vulva
    Breasts (Mammary Glands)
The Menstrual Cycle
    Proliferative (Follicular) Phase
    Secretory (Luteal) Phase
    Menstruation
Gynecologic Disorders
    Vulvovaginitis
    Dysfunctional Uterine Bleeding
    Premenstrual Syndrome (PMS)
    Endometriosis
    Uterine Prolapse and Displacement
    Sexually Transmitted Diseases
    Leiomyomas
    Ovarian Cysts
    Gynecologic Cancers
    Infertility
Common Gynecologic Tests and Therapeutic Procedures and the Medical Assistant's Role
    The Gynecologic Examination
    Procedure: Assisting With the Pelvic Examination With Pap Smear
    Colposcopy
    Procedure: Assisting With Colposcopy With Cervical Biopsy
    Culdocentesis
    Hysterosalpingography (HSG)
    Laparoscopy
    Dilatation and Curettage (D & C)
Obstetric Care
    Diagnosis of Pregnancy
    First Prenatal Visit

    Subsequent Prenatal Visits
Obstetric Disorders
    Ectopic Pregnancy
    Hyperemesis Gravidarum
    Abortion
    Pregnancy-Induced Hypertension (PIH)
    Placenta Previa
    Abruptio Placentae
Onset of Labor
Postpartum Care
    First Postpartum Visit
    Postpartum Endometritis
    Postpartum Depression
Common Obstetric Tests and Therapeutic Procedures and the Medical Assistant's Role
    Pregnancy Test
    α-Fetoprotein (AFP)
    Amniocentesis
    Contraction Stress Test
    Nonstress Test
    Doppler Ultrasonography
    Fetal Ultrasonography
Contraception
    Common Methods of Contraception
    Procedure: Assisting With the Insertion of an Intrauterine Device (IUD)
    Procedure: Assisting With the Removal of an Intrauterine Device (IUD)
    Subdermal Hormonal Implants
    Procedure: Assisting With the Insertion of Subdermal Hormonal Implants
Menopause
Summary
Critical Thinking Challenges
Answers to Checkpoint Questions
Suggestions for Further Reading

DACUM Components

1.3	Practice within the scope of education, training, and personal capabilities
1.6	Conduct oneself in a courteous and diplomatic manner
2.2	Treat all patients with empathy and impartiality
2.5	Serve as liaison between physician and others
4.1	Apply principles of aseptic technique and infection control
4.5	Prepare and maintain examination and treatment area
4.6	Interview and take patient history
4.7	Prepare patients for procedures
4.8	Assist physician with examinations and treatments
4.10	Collect and process specimens
5.1	Document accurately
7.3	Teach patients methods of health promotion and disease prevention

Chapter Competencies

Learning Objectives

Upon successfully completing this chapter, you will be able to:

1. Spell and define the Key Terms.
2. Identify and describe the organs of the female reproductive system.
3. Describe the menstrual cycle.
4. Describe menopause.
5. Describe the processes of fertilization, implantation, and gestation.
6. Explain the methods for determining a pregnant patient's estimated date of delivery.
7. Identify and explain fetotoxic and teratogenic factors.
8. Describe the components of prenatal and postpartum patient care.
9. Identify the various methods of contraception.
10. List and describe common gynecologic and obstetric disorders and outline the medical assistant's role as it relates to the disorders.
11. Identify and explain diagnostic tests and therapeutic procedures of the female reproductive system and state the medical assistant's role where applicable.

Performance Objectives

Upon successfully completing this chapter, you will be able to:

1. Assist with performance of a pelvic examination with Pap smear (Procedure 41-1).
2. Assist with performance of a colposcopy with cervical biopsy (Procedure 41-2).
3. Assist with the insertion of an intrauterine device (IUD) (Procedure 41-3).
4. Assist with the removal of an intrauterine device (IUD) (Procedure 41-4).
5. Assist with the insertion of subdermal hormonal implants (Procedure 41-5).
6. Assist with the first prenatal examination.
7. Assist with subsequent prenatal examinations.
8. Assist with the first postnatal examination.

Key Terms

(See Glossary for definitions.)

ablation
abortion
amenorrhea
anovulation
asymptomatic
Braxton Hicks
Chadwick's sign
climacteric period
colpocleisis
colporrhaphy
colposcopy
cul-de-sac
culdocentesis
curettage
cystocele
cytology
dysmenorrhea
dyspareunia
episiotomy
erythematous
etiology

fimbriae
gestation
Goodell's sign
gravid
gravida
gravidity
hirsutism
human chorionic
    gonadotropin (HCG)
hysterosalpingogram
hysteroscopy
idiopathic
intrauterine pregnancy
    (IUP)
introitus
labor
laparoscopy
laparotomy
leukocytosis
lightening
lyse

lochia
menorrhagia
menarche
menses
metrorrhagia
multipara
nulligravida
nullipara
oophorectomy
ovulation
ovum
parity
pessary
polymenorrhea
primigravida
proteinuria
puerperium
pyosalpinx
rectocele
salpingo-oophorectomy

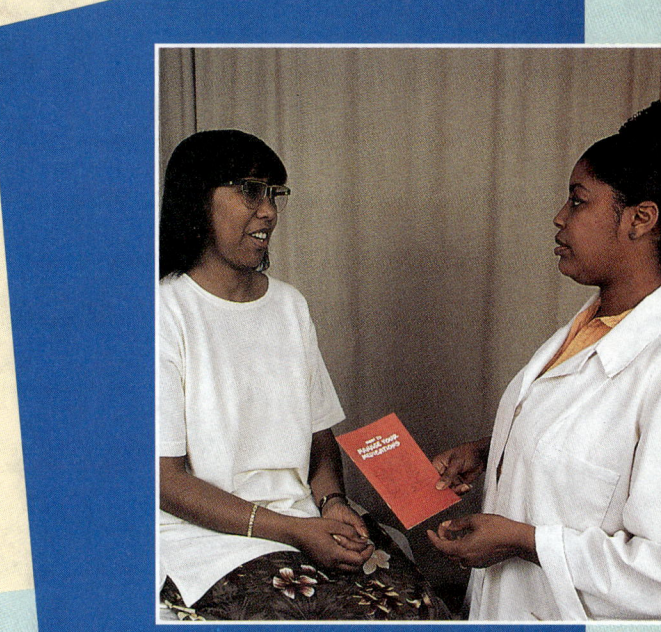

The female reproductive system is responsible for the development and maintenance of secondary sexual characteristics and for sexual reproduction of the species.

Secondary sexual characteristics are developed and maintained by the interaction of the follicle-stimulating hormone (FSH), luteinizing hormone (LH), estrogen, and progesterone. This hormonal interaction brings about the onset of puberty, which is characterized by budding of the breasts, an increase in body fat, growth of pubic and axillary hair, and **menses** (beginning of menstruation).

Sexual reproduction requires the union of specialized sex cells (gametes) from the male and the female. The ovaries produce the female gamete, the **ovum**, which joins with the spermatozoon of the male during fertilization to form a zygote (a fertilized ovum).

Gynecology and obstetrics are the two medical specialties concerned with female sexual and reproductive functions. Gynecology concentrates on the care of female patients with disorders of the reproductive organs. Obstetrics is the branch of medicine that cares for female patients through pregnancy, childbirth, and the postpartum period.

➤ ORGANS OF THE FEMALE REPRODUCTIVE SYSTEM

Ovaries

The primary gonads of the female are the ovaries (Fig. 41-1), which produce ova, the female reproductive cells. The ovaries have an estimated 400,000 follicles present at birth, each containing an undeveloped ovum. Several follicles will begin to grow with each menstrual cycle, but usually only one will develop into a graafian follicle containing a mature ovum. **Ovulation** is the process by which the fully matured ovum ruptures from the graafian follicle and is released from the ovary. (This process is discussed further in the section "The Menstrual Cycle," below.)

Fallopian Tubes

The fallopian tubes, or oviducts, arise from the uterine fundus and extend to just above the ovaries. The fallopian tubes serve as a passageway for the ovum on its way to the uterus and for the sperm in its search for the ovum. At the distal ends of the tubes are many finger-

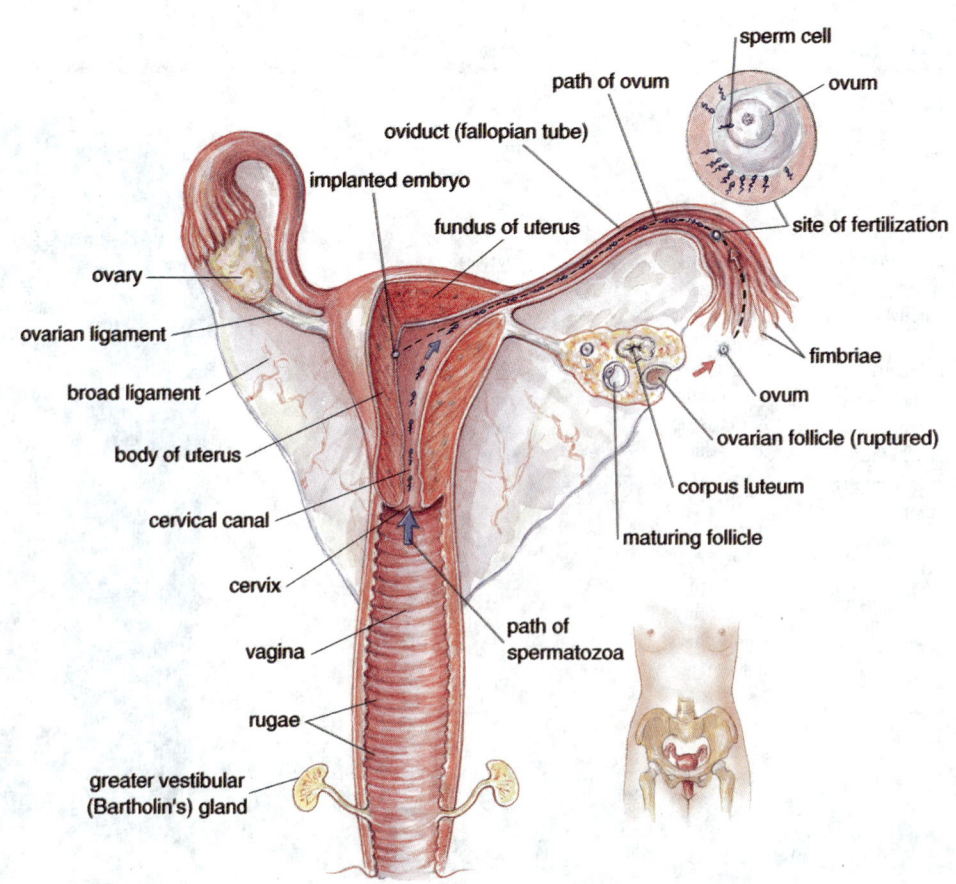

FIGURE 41-1
Female reproductive system.

like extensions called **fimbriae** that wave the released egg toward the duct and pass it to the cilia-lined interior of the tube for transport to the uterus.

Uterus

The uterus is a pear-shaped, muscular organ that is primarily responsible for housing and nourishing the developing fetus from conception to birth. The uterus is made up of three tissue layers:

1. The *endometrium*, the innermost lining, has a rich blood supply and a great ability to regenerate. It is the outermost part of the endometrium that is shed during menstruation.
2. The *myometrium*, the middle, muscular layer, is important in **labor** (the physiologic process necessary for expelling the fetus from the uterus) and delivery of the neonate. The myometrium also contracts during menses to assist in eliminating the necrotic endometrium.
3. The *perimetrium* is a layer of connective tissue that covers the outer walls of the uterus and attaches to the supportive ligaments that secure the uterus in place.

The uterus is actually a tube that has a cervix (neck), body (central portion), and a fundus (see Fig. 41-1). The cervix opens into the vaginal canal; this opening is called the external os. The cervical opening into the uterine cavity is called the internal os. The uterus as a whole may be viewed as a series of ducts because the fallopian tubes, uterine cavity, and the cervix are continuous with one another and are passageways for the functions specific to the female reproductive system.

Vagina

The vagina is a hollow, muscular tube lined with mucous membrane that extends from the cervix to the vulva. Although the vagina canal is generally narrow, the walls are capable of considerable expansion for the birth process.

Vulva

The vulva, or external genitalia, includes the labia majora, labia minora, clitoris, vaginal orifice, Bartholin's glands, Skene's glands, hymen, vestibule, and perineum. Bartholin's glands (one on each side of the vaginal opening) and Skene's glands (just inside the urethral opening) secrete substances that are important in providing lubrication and maintaining the acid–base balance in the vaginal and vulval areas. The clitoris is a small body that is similar to the male penis in that it is made of erectile tissue. It is located in the anterior portion of the labia minora. The labia minora are two small folds of tissue that lie between the labia majora. Between the labia minora is a triangular space called the vestibule that contains the openings of the glands and vaginal orifice, or **introitus**.

From the vestibule to the anus lies the perineum, which is a body of connective tissue that allows for the attachment of muscles and provides for pelvic support. During a vaginal delivery of the fetus, an **episiotomy** (incision of the perineum) may be performed to facilitate the delivery and reduce the risk of a perineal laceration (tear).

Breasts (Mammary Glands)

The breasts are located on the upper anterior portion of the chest and contain 15 to 20 lobes of glandular tissue that are capable of producing milk for nursing an infant (Fig. 41-2). Following delivery, prolactin and oxytocin from the pituitary gland stimulate and maintain the production of milk.

Checkpoint Question

1. *The uterus is composed of what three layers? Briefly explain each.*

► THE MENSTRUAL CYCLE

Menstruation is a normal body process involving the elimination of a bloody discharge from the uterus through the vagina. The age at which a girl begins menses is known as **menarche** and is one of the many signs of puberty. The cessation of menses marks the **climacteric period**, or menopause (see the section "Menopause," below). The menstrual cycle, which is about 28 days in length, involves a series of complex events controlled by hormones secreted by the anterior pituitary gland and the ovaries (Fig. 41-3). It has three phases, which are described below.

Proliferative (Follicular) Phase

During the proliferative phase (days 5–14), the endometrium grows very rapidly, preparing for possible implantation of a fertilized ovum. The anterior pituitary begins secreting follicle-stimulating hormone (FSH), causing several follicles within the ovary to begin development. Although several follicles are grow-

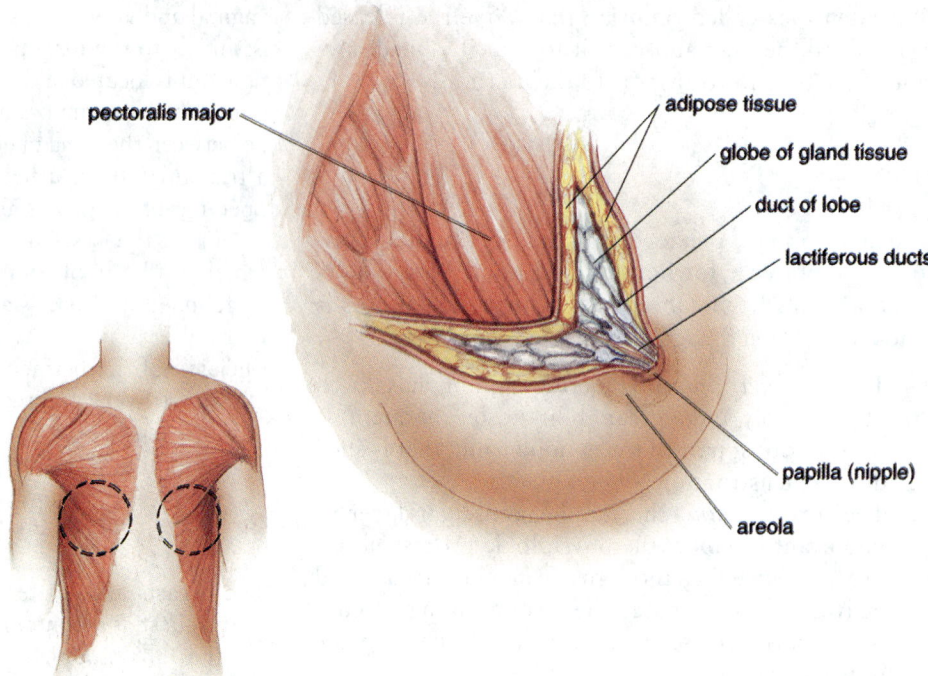

FIGURE 41-2
Section of the breast.

ing, usually only one actually matures into a graafian follicle. The graafian follicle contains the ovum and also secretes estrogen, stimulating the growth of the endometrium.

At the end of the proliferative phase, the graafian follicle bulges against the ovarian wall and eventually ruptures from the ovary, releasing the ovum. This process of ovulation is triggered by the secretion of luteinizing hormone (LH) by the anterior pituitary gland and occurs on about day 15. Once the graafian follicle ruptures, the ovum is pulled into the fallopian tube by the waving action of the fimbriae. The tissue (corpus luteum) left behind begins to secrete progesterone (meaning pro pregnancy), further stimulating endometrial growth.

Ovulation is accompanied by an increase in the basal body temperature after the ovum is released. Some women notice pain, tenderness, or both over the ovary in which ovulation is occurring.

Secretory (Luteal) Phase

The secretory phase (days 15–28) begins immediately after ovulation and is influenced by the progesterone that is produced by the corpus luteum of the ovary. The primary characteristic of the secretory phase is the impact that the progesterone has on the endometrium, which undergoes tremendous growth as it prepares for a possible pregnancy. It becomes very vascular and rich in glycogen, creating an environment that is essential for fetal growth.

If implantation occurs, the corpus luteum will continue to secrete the progesterone until the pregnancy is well established and the placenta takes over the production of the progesterone. The placenta also secretes **human chorionic gonadotropin (HCG)**, which supports the corpus luteum and is the hormone that is detected in the urine and serum of pregnant women. The HCG level is used to confirm suspected pregnancy and to estimate the **gestation,** or the period of time from conception to birth.

If implantation does not occur, then the HCG, which is necessary for the survival of the corpus luteum, is not produced. The corpus luteum will degenerate and without the progesterone there will be thinning of the endometrium with eventual necrosis of the functional layer.

Menstruation

Menstruation itself usually lasts about 5 days (days 1–5). The discharge consists of pieces of the necrotic (dead) endometrium, mucus from the uterine walls, and blood. Often, this phase is accompanied by painful uterine cramps that result from the contractions of the myometrium to assist in eliminating the bloody discharge.

If, however, the ovum unites with the male sperm within 48 hours of ovulation, fertilization occurs. When this happens, the menstrual cycle is interrupted and the endometrium grows and develops, creating an environment that will support the implantation and fetal growth (Box 41-1).

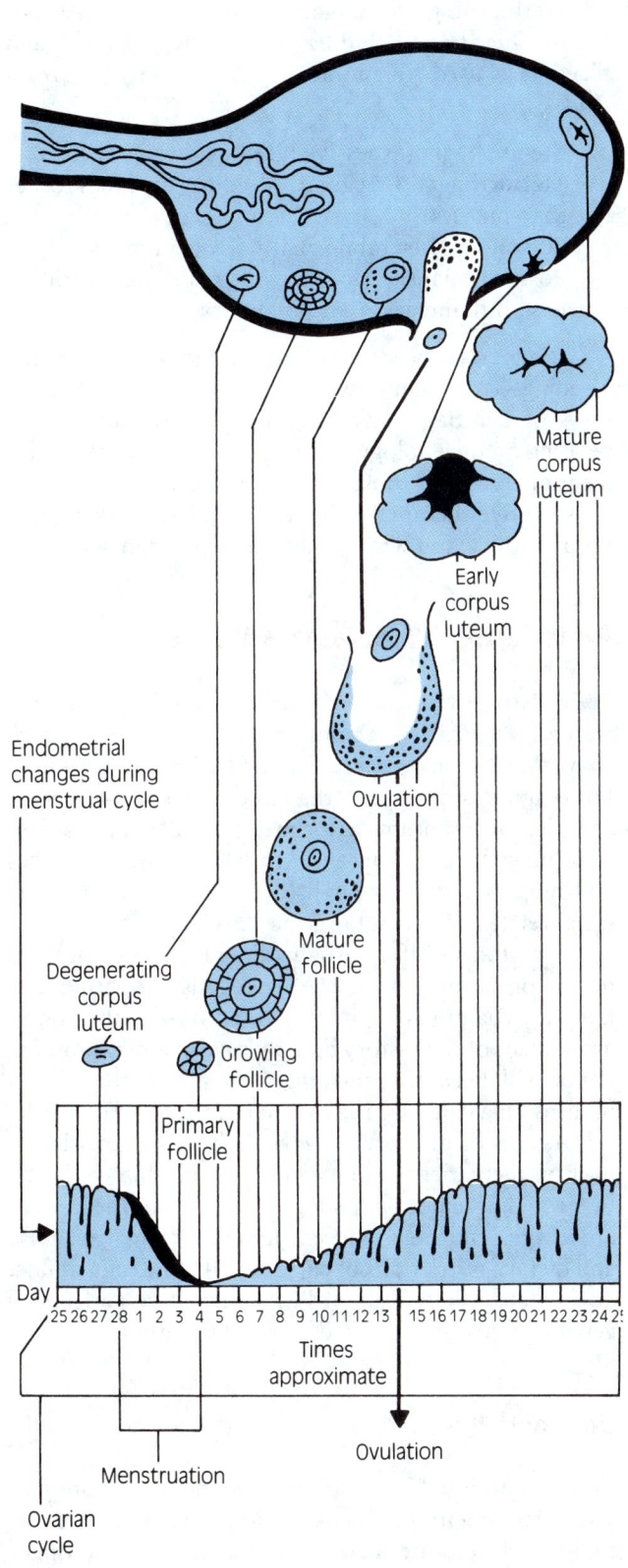

FIGURE 41-3
The menstrual cycle.

BOX 41-1 Fertilization, Implantation, and Gestation

Although only one ovum is needed for conception, many spermatozoa are required to erode the ovum cell membrane to allow the entry of one sperm for fertilization. Fertilization usually occurs in the fallopian tube. At that point, the male and female gametes become a zygote, or fertilized egg. Because sperm and ova each bring to the union 23 chromosomes, the zygote will have 46, or 23 pairs. Sex is determined at this union.

Cell division begins immediately. By the fifth or sixth day, the zygote has traveled by ciliary movement of the fallopian lining to the uterus and implantation begins with the finger-like chorionic villi grasping and burrowing into the endometrium, resulting in a normal **intrauterine pregnancy (IUP)**. Enzymes are secreted by the zygote to help gain access to the endometrial wall, which has been prepared by estrogen and progesterone to receive the egg. Estrogen and progesterone stay high to maintain the endometrium; no more follicles will mature during the pregnancy.

From the second to the eighth week of gestation, the developing offspring is called an embryo. From the eighth week to birth, it is referred to as a fetus. The amniotic sac is formed to protect and hydrate the fetus. The placenta acts as an organ of exchange for nutrients from the mother and wastes from the fetus. The umbilical cord attaches the placenta to the embryo. The average gestation takes between 266 and 280 days, which equals 38 to 40 weeks, or about 10 lunar months or 9 calendar months. (See the section "Obstetric Care.")

The medical assistant should always remind and encourage patients, especially adolescents, to record on a calendar the days of menses. Instruct each patient to note the date of the first day of the last menstrual period (LMP) and to bring the information to the medical office. The regularity of the menstrual cycle is often critical to the physician's assessment of the patient's gynecologic health, the duration of pregnancy and the estimated date of confinement (EDC) or estimated date of delivery (EDD).

Keep in mind that other conditions besides pregnancy (eg, dysfunctional uterine bleeding, leiomyomas) can also alter the normal menstrual cycle. Such conditions are described below.

Checkpoint Question
2. *What is the primary characteristic of the secretory phase of the menstrual cycle?*

➤ GYNECOLOGIC DISORDERS

Vulvovaginitis

Vulvovaginitis is inflammation of the vulva and vagina. It is one of the more common complaints of female patients. Symptoms often include pruritus, burning of the vulva or the vagina (or both), and increased vaginal discharge. On examination, the vulva and vagina are **erythematous** (reddened). The type of discharge often indicates the **etiology** (cause) of the disorder. The most common etiologies include *Candida*, *Trichomonas*, and *Gardnerella vaginitis* (previously known as *Haemophilus vaginalis*). Confirmation of the causative agent is by a microscopic examination of a vaginal smear or by culture of the vaginal discharge. Effective treatment depends on the etiology (Box 41-2).

BOX 41-2 Infectious Agents in Vulvovaginitis

Trichomonas vaginalis: Known as "Trich," this disease is caused by a protozoa and is transmitted through sexual intercourse. The signs are a thin, frothy, greenish or gray discharge with an odor. The symptoms include dysuria with frequency and intense pruritus. Treatment requires that both partners be treated with oral metronidazole.

Candida albicans: Also known as monilia, this fungal disease grows best in the presence of glucose. The signs include a thick, curdlike discharge with white patches on the vaginal walls, usually with no odor. There is usually intense itching. The pathogen is found in the intestines and is more likely to affect the patient during the secretory phase of the menstrual cycle. It is very common during pregnancy and for those on antibiotic therapy. Treatment requires nystatin vaginal suppositories, which may be purchased without a prescription.

Gardnerella vaginitis: A gram-negative bacillus is responsible for this disease. There is a gray discharge with a foul odor. It is treated with metronidazole.

Dysfunctional Uterine Bleeding

Dysfunctional uterine bleeding (DUB), or abnormal uterine bleeding, is defined as abnormal or irregular uterine bleeding including heavy, irregular, or light bleeding caused by an endocrine imbalance. DUB includes:

- **Menorrhagia** (excessive bleeding during menses)
- **Metrorrhagia** (irregular bleeding at times other than menses)
- **Polymenorrhea** (abnormally frequent menses)
- Postmenopausal bleeding not associated with tumor, inflammation, or pregnancy

Diagnosis is based on ruling out other causes for the bleeding. Treatment is with hormones, oral contraceptives, or **curettage** (scraping) of the uterine cavity, depending on the etiology. Hysterectomy may be the treatment of choice for those patients who do not respond to conservative therapy, who are at increased risk of adenocarcinoma, and who do not desire pregnancy.

Premenstrual Syndrome (PMS)

Premenstrual syndrome is characterized by a wide variety of physical, psychological, and behavioral symptoms that occur on a regular, cyclic basis (Box 41-3). For diagnostic purposes, the patient must experience a complex of symptoms associated with PMS, the symptoms must occur during the 7 to 10 days before menses and must be severe enough to interfere with interpersonal relationships and routine activities.

Symptoms of PMS usually diminish a few hours after the onset of menses. The etiology is **idiopathic** (unknown). Diagnosis of PMS is based on the physician's assessment of the history and physical examination. Patients will need to chart their symptoms for several months on a calendar that includes the menstrual cycle.

As a medical assistant, you can have a dramatic impact on the patient's ability to cope with this syndrome by providing emotional support, educating the patient about the syndrome, and encouraging regular exercise and dietary restrictions of caffeine, salt, and animal fats. To minimize the effects of PMS, encourage patients to get adequate rest and avoid stressful situations.

Endometriosis

Endometriosis is a condition of unknown etiology in which endometrial tissue is found growing outside (ectopic) of the uterine cavity in such areas as the fallopian tubes, around the ovaries and uterosacral ligaments,

PMS Symptoms

The hormonal flux associated with the menstrual cycle affects other body systems in addition to the reproductive system. The cascade of events result in a series of symptoms that include:

- Hypoglycemia—A drop in blood sugar results in headaches, nausea, and fatigue and may explain the food cravings many women experience. Increasing carbohydrate intake will ensure a steady blood glucose level.
- Fluid retention—Fluid is retained in all parts of the body with edema, weight gain, mastalgia, sinusitis, backache, and headache. Reducing the inake of salt during this period will alleviate some of the edema.
- Sodium and potassium imbalance—The cyclical fluctuation of these chemotransmitters causes fatigue, irritability, and depression. Dietary forms of these minerals should be encouraged.
- Decreased immunity—At this time, the patient may experience rhinitis and other upper respiratory infections, acne, and herpes outbreaks.

and, in rare cases, in other parts of the abdominal cavity. The patient, who is most often of reproductive age, complains of infertility, **dysmenorrhea** (painful menstruation), pelvic pain, and **dyspareunia** (painful intercourse). The patient's symptoms and physical findings may indicate endometriosis, but the diagnosis and the severity must be confirmed by direct visualization, usually by way of **laparoscopy** (internal examination of the abdominal cavity). Treatment of endometriosis may relieve the pelvic pain but has a less desirable impact on fertility. The type of therapy depends on the age, symptoms, severity, and the patient's desire for pregnancy. Treatment includes hormone and drug therapy to suppress the growth and laparoscopic **ablation** (excision) by laser or cautery to **lyse** (destroy) the adhesions. For patients who have severe symptoms and who do not desire pregnancy, the treatment of choice may be a hysterectomy with bilateral **salpingo-oophorectomy** (excision of both ovaries and fallopian tubes).

? **Checkpoint Question**

3. What are the types of dysfunctional uterine bleeding? Briefly explain each.

Uterine Prolapse and Displacement

Prolapse of the uterus is an abnormal condition in which the uterus droops or protrudes downward into the vagina. Often the condition is accompanied by **cystocele**, **rectocele**, or both. Cystocele is the herniation of the urinary bladder into the vagina; rectocele is the herniation of the rectum into the vagina.

Different methods can be used to describe the degree of prolapse (mild, moderate, severe; grade I, II, III). A commonly used method involves classifying the degree of prolapse:

- First-degree prolapse occurs when the uterus has descended to the level of the vaginal orifice.
- Second-degree prolapse occurs when the uterine cervix protrudes through the vaginal orifice.
- Third-degree prolapse occurs when the entire cervix and uterus protrude beyond the vaginal orifice (Fig. 41-4).

Diagnosis is confirmed by pelvic examination, at which time the degree of prolapse can be determined.

Surgical treatment includes vaginal hysterectomy, **colporrhaphy** (suture of the vagina), and **colpocleisis** (surgery to occlude the vagina). Medical management for patients who are elderly or who are poor risks for surgery include hormone therapy to strengthen the muscular floor of the pelvis and the use of a **pessary**. A pessary is a device that fits around the cervix, usually into the cul-de-sac. The patient inserts the pessary into the vagina to support the uterus.

You will need to educate the patient about the use of a pessary. The pessary should be changed every 2 to 3 months and the patient should be advised to douche about once a week. The patient should be educated

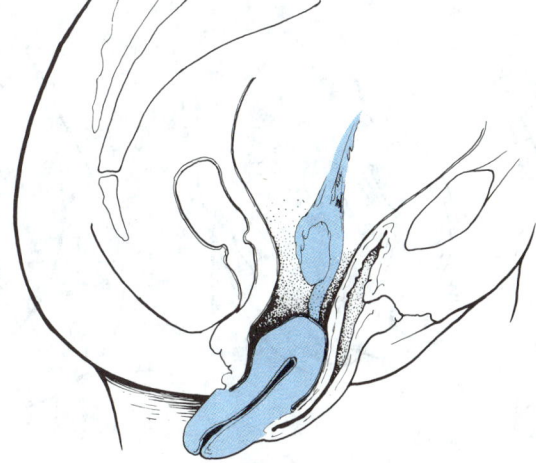

FIGURE 41-4
Complete prolapse of the uterus through the introitus.

about the signs of vaginal infection because the pessary increases the risk of inflammation and infection.

The uterus is normally tilted slightly forward over the bladder with the cervix at a right angle to the direction of the vagina. The uterus is movable, and due to stress on the supporting ligaments, it occasionally tilts from its natural position. This is called uterine displacement (Fig. 41-5).

The symptoms may be simply pressure in the rectal area or against the bladder. The symptoms are not usually severe but are troublesome to the patient. Treatment follows the same protocol as required for uterine prolapse. In some instances, the uterus may simply be stitched back into its original position (hysteropexy).

Sexually Transmitted Diseases

Acquired immunodeficiency syndrome (AIDS), the deadly sexually transmitted disease (STD), is discussed in detail in Chapter 36, Caring for Patients With Immune Disorders. However, it should be noted here that the incidence of AIDS is rising rapidly among young women in the United States.

Chlamydia trachomatis

The STD caused by *C. trachomatis* may be **asymptomatic** (without symptoms) in the female patient or may present with vague, flulike symptoms that are difficult to diagnose without specific reason to suspect the infection. In severe cases, there may be extensive lymph gland involvement known as lymphogranuloma venereum. Chlamydia is one of the leading causes of pelvic inflammatory disease with tubal scar-

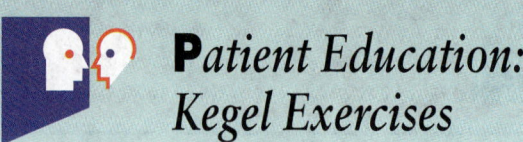

Patient Education: Kegel Exercises

Age, gravity, and childbearing take their toll on the muscles of the perineum. The Kegel exercises can increase the tone of this area. Stronger perineal support will help eliminate stress incontinence and will offer support to the vaginal walls to avoid uterine prolapse.

Explain to the patient that she can practice doing Kegel exercises at any time, standing in the grocery line, waiting at a stop light, sitting in class. Instruct her to tighten the vaginal opening and the buttocks as if she were stopping the flow of urine; this position should be held for about 3 seconds. The patient should work up to doing the exercises as many as 15 to 20 repetitions four or five times a day.

ring and eventual infertility. The disease is treated with doxycycline, tetracycline, or sulfamethoxazole.

Infants born to mothers with chlamydial infection may present with conjunctivitis and an intractable pneumonia. Many infants will spontaneously abort, deliver prematurely, or be stillborn.

Condylomata Acuminata

Condylomata acuminata is a viral infection of the genital area causing the growth of soft, papillary warts that appear in a wide variety of places including the vulva,

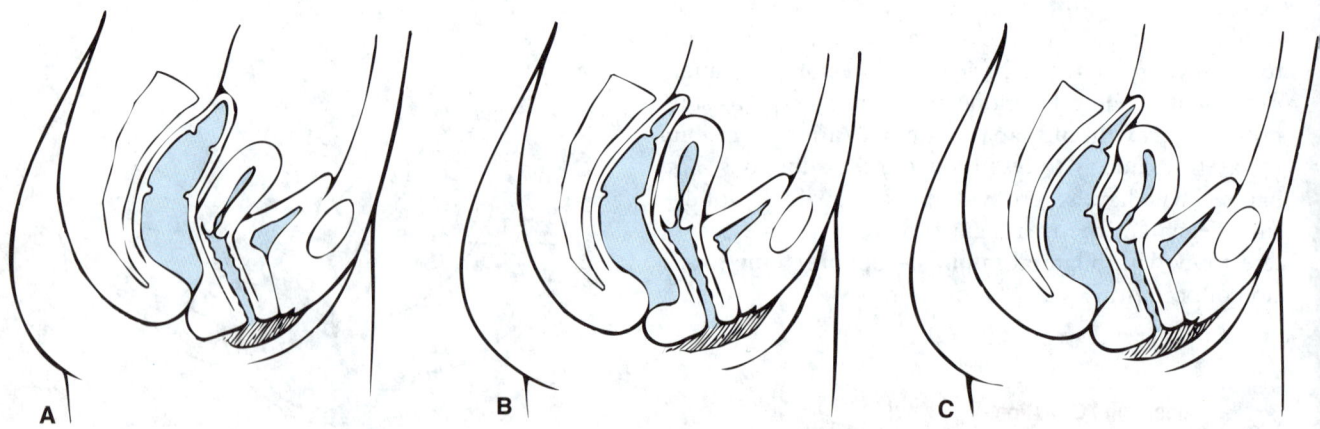

FIGURE 41-5
Retrodisplacements of the uterus. (*A*) The normal position of the uterus detected on palpation. (*B*) In *retroversion* the uterus turns posteriorly as a whole unit. (*C*) In *retroflexion* the fundus bends posteriorly above the cervical end.

vagina, cervix, and perineum. The etiology is human papillomavirus (HPV). The genital warts usually appear about 3 months after exposure. Biopsy of the condyloma is appropriate to rule out the slight possibility of a malignancy. Although HPV is difficult to eradicate, treatment includes cryotherapy or laser ablation (tissue removal) with moderate success. Genital warts have been implicated in an increase in cervical cancer.

Gonorrhea

Gonorrhea is the second most common STD. The symptoms appear in the genitalia 2 to 8 days after exposure. Bartholin's and Skene's glands fill with pus; the infection also may spread to the cervix. The man develops urethritis with large amounts of pus, but the woman may be asymptomatic and unaware of the disease. Gonorrhea responds well to penicillin if detected early; however, penicillin-resistant strains are appearing. The disease may lead to salpingitis with scarring and adhesions or pelvic inflammatory disease (see below).

Infants born to mothers infected with gonorrhea may develop a purulent conjunctivitis with corneal ulcerations that result in blindness. All infants are now treated prophylactically in the newborn nursery.

Syphilis

After AIDS, syphilis is the most serious STD. It is caused by a spirochete, *Treponema pallidum.* Symptoms develop with a chancre (an ulcerated skin lesion) at the primary site of infection several days to several weeks after infection. This chancre may not be noticed and heals fairly quickly. The second phase is expressed by a rash anywhere on the body. The patient is infectious at this stage but can be treated with penicillin. If left untreated, syphilis may lie dormant for years until it exacerbates into the third, or tertiary, phase with cardiovascular damage, central nervous system involvement, and death.

Infants born positive for syphilis by transplacental infection are frequently mentally retarded, deaf, blind, or deformed. Many will spontaneously abort or be stillborn.

Herpes Genitalis

Herpes genitalis is characterized by painful, vesicular lesions in the vaginal, vulvular, or anorectal area. This genital infection usually appears within 3 to 7 days after exposure. The vesicles ulcerate and form necrotic craters that eventually heal in about 10 days. The etiology is herpes simplex virus II (HSV II). The virus is almost always sexually transmitted and is diagnosed by obtaining scrapings for **cytology** (cell study). Patients with herpes genitalis should be advised to avoid sexual contact during episodes of vesiculation because the exudate is highly contagious. Although there is no cure, the condition is somewhat controlled with antiviral agents such as acyclovir.

Infants born vaginally to mothers with active lesions may develop the disease within a few weeks of birth. The virus spreads rapidly to the organs and up to 90% of neonatally infected infants will die.

Salpingitis/Pelvic Inflammatory Disease (PID)

Salpingitis is a bacterial infection of the fallopian tubes that is most often transmitted by sexual intercourse. Young sexually active women, women with multiple sexual partners, and women with intrauterine devices are at increased risk of salpingitis. Numerous microorganisms may cause salpingitis, but the more common etiologies include *Neisseria gonorrhoeae, Chlamydia trachomatis,* genital mycoplasma, and normal flora bacteria.

Salpingitis is sometimes called pelvic inflammatory disease (PID) when the surrounding structures or tissues are inflamed. With PID the infection may be found in areas such as the pelvic peritoneum, uterus, ovaries, and the surrounding tissues. Symptoms include varying degrees of abdominal pain and tenderness, with or without fever, and **leukocytosis** (abnormal increase in the white blood cell count).

Cultures for gonorrhea and tests for chlamydia are essential for the antibiotic therapy. **Culdocentesis** for culture of purulent discharge may be necessary to determine the exact etiology. Culdocentesis involves the surgical puncture and aspiration of fluid from the vaginal cul-de-sac. A laparoscopy may be performed to determine the extent of the infection.

Treatment for mild infections includes antibiotic and analgesic therapy, bed rest, and removal of an intrauterine device, if present. In patients with **pyosalpinx** (pus in the fallopian tubes), tubal obstruction, abscess, and serious inflammation and edema, treatment may involve a hysterectomy with bilateral salpingo-oophorectomy or incision and drainage via **laparotomy** (incision into the abdominal cavity).

Checkpoint Question

4. Which sexually transmitted disease is associated with a female reproductive cancer?

Leiomyomas

Leiomyomas are benign tumors of the uterus, also called fibroids, myomas, or fibromyomas. The tumor may be located in any of the uterine tissue layers:

endometrium, myometrium, or perimetrium. The tumors vary greatly in size. Most patients will be asymptomatic. Large tumors tend to distort the uterus, are palpable, and are more likely to be symptomatic. Symptoms may include abnormal bleeding (menorrhagia, metrorrhagia), pelvic pressure and discomfort, constipation, urinary frequency, and infertility.

A presumptive diagnosis is based on patient symptoms and physician assessment that initially includes bimanual examination and sounding of the uterus. Sounding of the uterus requires the physician to do a pelvic examination and insert a uterine sound into the uterine cavity (see Chap. 23, Instruments and Equipment). Obstruction or resistance can be detected that may be due to the tumor pressing in on the uterine cavity. A differential diagnosis to eliminate other conditions includes ruling out pregnancy by testing for human chorionic gonadotropin (HCG) in the urine or serum, diagnostic curettage or **hysteroscopy** (visual examination of the uterus with magnification) to rule out a malignancy, and ultrasonography of the uterus.

Treatment of leiomyomas depends on the size of the tumors. Small asymptomatic tumors will need to be monitored for excessive growth. Depending on the patient's age and desire for pregnancy, myomectomy or hysterectomy for large tumors or those with symptoms may be indicated.

Ovarian Cysts

There are numerous types of ovarian cysts that are benign, including the functional cysts and polycystic ovaries. Functional ovarian cysts are fairly common and include several types of cysts, one of which is the follicular cyst. This type of cyst is a fluid-filled sac that causes few, if any, problems. The patient is most often asymptomatic unless the cyst is large or if it ruptures or hemorrhages. The functional cysts are usually detected during surgery and treatment is simply puncture or excision.

In contrast, polycystic ovary syndrome (Stein-Leventhal syndrome) is a more troublesome and complex disorder. It affects both ovaries (bilateral) and is most often found in adolescent girls and young women who have numerous symptoms of an endocrine imbalance. The symptoms are manifested as anovulation, irregular menses or **amenorrhea** (no menses), and **hirsutism** (excessive hair growth). Diagnosis is based on pelvic examination, ultrasonography, laparoscopy, or exploratory laparotomy. Treatment is difficult and depends on the patient's symptoms and desire for pregnancy. Management of this disorder includes hormone therapy or oral contraceptives.

Gynecologic Cancers

The malignant tumors affecting the female reproductive system and their characteristics, diagnosis, and treatment are outlined in Table 41-1. For patient education, medical assistants need to be aware of the American Cancer Society's recommendations regarding the frequency of pelvic and breast examinations and Pap smears. The prognosis of all cancers is directly related to early diagnosis and treatment.

Have available and accessible brochures and literature on the various types of cancers. This information can be obtained from the American Cancer Society, which is listed in your local telephone directory.

Cervical and breast cancers have an excellent prognosis when detected and treated early. Medical assistants should instruct patients on breast self-examination to be performed every month (Fig. 41-6).

Also encourage patients to schedule regular annual visits for a complete physical with a thorough pelvic examination that includes the Papanicolaou (Pap) smear. The Pap smear is a screening test for the early detection of cancer (Table 41-2). The procedure for the Pap smear involves scraping cells from the cervix, endocervix, or vagina for microscopic examination (see Procedure 41-1, Assisting With the Pelvic Examination With Pap Smear).

Initially the abnormal growth of the cancerous cells in the cervix is asymptomatic and therefore patients should be encouraged to come regularly for a Pap smear. The Pap smear grades the abnormal growth according to the tissue involvement. Abnormal growth patterns in the epithelium of the cervix is called cervical intraepithelial neoplasia (CIN). The degree of abnormal growth is graded (usually mild, moderate, severe, and carcinoma in situ). **Carcinoma in situ means that the malignant cells have invaded the entire tissue, but have not become invasive to the surrounding structures.** CIN is diagnosed by the Pap smear and further evaluated by **colposcopy** (visualization of the vagina and cervix under magnification) and biopsy.

Infertility

Female infertility is more difficult to diagnose than male infertility. Most testing begins by eliminating the man as the responsible party, then concentrates on the woman. Testing is not usually attempted until 1 year of unprotected intercourse without conception.

The causes may include uterine or cervical abnormalities, tubal occlusion or scarring, a hormonal imbalance that interferes with luteinizing hormone or follicle-stimulating hormone resulting in anovulation or poor ova production, or psychological factors. Diagnosis requires a complete history and physical exami-

Table 41-1
Cancers of the Female Reproductive System

	Warning Signs	Risk Factors	Early Detection	Treatment (Dependent on Involvement)
Breast Cancer	Breast changes: lump, pain, thickening, swelling, tenderness, distortion, retraction, dimpling, scaliness	Over age 40 (risk increases with age), history of breast cancer, early menarche, nulliparity, first birth at late age	Monthly self-examination; mammogram by age 40, every 2 years between ages 40 and 49, and every year after age 50 in asymptomatic women	Lumpectomy, mastectomy, radiation therapy, chemotherapy, hormone manipulation therapy
Cervical Cancer	Often asymptomatic; symptoms, if present, can include irregular bleeding or abnormal vaginal discharge	Intercourse at an early age, multiple sex partners, cigarette smoking, history of certain sexually transmitted diseases such as human papillomavirus	Annual Pap smears for women over age 18 or who are sexually active; after three consecutive normal smears, Pap smears may be done less often at the physician's discretion	Carcinoma in situ: cryotherapy, electrocoagulation, local excision Metastatic cancer: surgery or radiation therapy or both
Endometrial Cancer	Irregular bleeding outside of menses, unusual vaginal discharge, excessive bleeding during menstruation, postmenopausal bleeding	Obesity, early menarche, multiple sex partners, late menopause, history of infertility, **anovulation** (not ovulating), unopposed estrogen or tamoxifen therapy, family history of endometrial cancer	Endometrial biopsy at menopause (for high-risk women)	Precancerous changes: progesterone therapy Diagnosed cancer: surgery or radiation therapy or both
Ovarian Cancer	Often asymptomatic; symptoms, if present, can include abdominal enlargement, vague digestive disorders, discomfort, gas distention	Risk increases with age (especially after age 60), nulliparity, history of breast cancer	Periodic, complete pelvic examination; cancer-related checkup every year after age 40	Surgery, including **oophorectomy** (excision of an ovary), hysterosalpingo-oophorectomy, salpingo-oophorectomy, excision of all intra-abdominal disease; radiation therapy; chemotherapy

nation. An endometrial biopsy will diagnose anovulation, progesterone blood levels may indicate hormonal deficiencies, and a hysterosalpingography will indicate tubal occlusion or uterine abnormalities. Treatment includes identifying and correcting the problem.

Checkpoint Question
5. *What two factors greatly affect the prognosis of all cancers?*

COMMON GYNECOLOGIC TESTS AND THERAPEUTIC PROCEDURES AND THE MEDICAL ASSISTANT'S ROLE

The Gynecologic Examination

As part of the gynecologic examination, the physician will examine the patient's breasts, perform a pelvic examination, and obtain a Pap smear. Because of the risk of contracting infection from body fluids, especially

1

In the shower:

Examine your breasts during bath or shower; hands glide easier over wet skin. Fingers flat, move gently over every part of each breast. Use right hand to examine left breast, left hand for right breast. Check for any lump, hard knot or thickening.

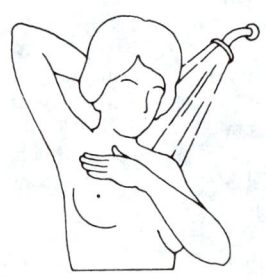

2

Before a mirror:

Inspect your breasts with arms at your sides. Next, raise your arms high overhead. Look for any changes in contour of each breast, a swelling, dimpling of skin or changes in the nipple.

Then, rest palms on hips and press down firmly to flex your chest muscles. Left and right breast will not exactly match—few women's do.

Regular inspection shows what is normal for you and will give you confidence in your examination.

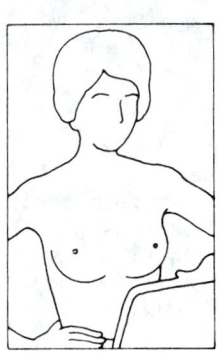

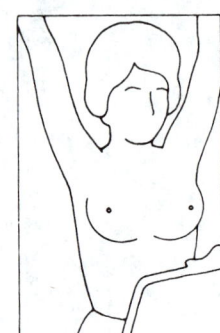

3

Lying down:

To examine your right breast, put a pillow or folded towel under your right shoulder. Place right hand behind your head—this distributes breast tissue more evenly on the chest. With left hand, fingers flat, press gently in small circular motions around an imaginary clock face. Begin at outermost top of your right breast for 12 o'clock, then move to 1 o'clock, and so on around the circle back to 12. A ridge of firm tissue in the lower curve of each breast is normal. Then move in an inch, toward the nipple, keep circling to examine *every part of your breast,* including nipple. This requires at least three more circles. Now slowly repeat procedure on your left breast with a pillow under your left shoulder and left hand behind head. Notice how your breast structure feels.

Finally, squeeze the nipple of each breast gently between thumb and index finger. Any discharge, clear or bloody, should be reported to your doctor immediately.

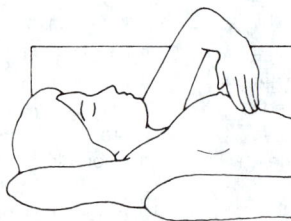

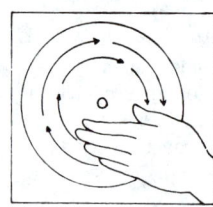

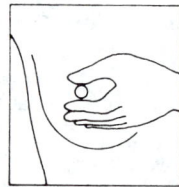

FIGURE 41-6

Following these steps, any woman can perform a breast self-examination. (Courtesy of the American Cancer Society.)

blood, the medical assistant, the physician, and others having direct contact with the patient must observe Standard Precautions and wear protective barriers as appropriate.

Breast Examination

The physician usually begins the examination by examining the breasts with the patient in a sitting position to check for dimpling or size disparity. The patient will then lie back on the table. The physician then systematically palpates all breast tissue, including areas such as the axillae and the tissue up to the clavicle to assess the lymph nodes that lead form the mammary area.

Pelvic Examination With Pap Smear

The purpose of the pelvic examination with Pap smear is to assess the female genitalia and to identify or diag-

Table 41-2
Classifications of Papanicolaou Tests

Class	Characteristics
I	Normal test, no atypical cells
II	Atypical cells but no evidence of malignancy
III	Atypical cells, possible but not conclusive for malignancy
IV	Cells strongly suggestive of malignancy
V	Strong evidence of malignancy

nose any abnormal conditions (Procedure 41-1). When scheduling an appointment for a pelvic examination, instruct the patient not to douche, use vaginal medication, or have sexual intercourse within 24 hours before the examination. If a Pap smear is also to be performed, schedule the appointment for about 1 week after menses.

When preparing for the pelvic examination, ensure that the vaginal speculum is warm and is the correct size for the patient. Warm the speculum by running it under warm water or by storing it on an electric heating pad set on a low setting. Selecting an appropriate vaginal speculum is important to maintain the patient's comfort and to facilitate the examination. Although the patient's age and size are the primary factors, the largest speculum that is comfortable for the patient will provide the best visibility. Two different sizes may be set out to give the physician a choice. Vaginal specula come in pediatric, small, medium, and large sizes; the manufacturers of specula also vary in that some make longer, more narrow specula. A wide variety of sizes should be available in each examination room.

Try to allow plenty of time with the patient to establish rapport, especially with new patients and patients with special needs (young, elderly, adolescents, disabled, distressed). If the procedure is rushed or seems hurried to the patient, it will affect the professional image of the office and the patient's attitude toward the physician and staff.

Although the dorsal lithotomy position provides the best visibility for the physician, the position may be difficult for elderly and some disabled persons to maintain. Elevating the head of the table to 30° may be easier for the patient and also allows the physician to make eye contact. The elevation of the table does not seem to have any disadvantages and often the patient finds the position more comfortable. If elevating the head of the table is not appropriate, then an alternative position, such as Sims', may be necessary. Consult with

Charting Example

05/18/98	0930
	S: "I am here to see Dr. Jacobs for my annual Pap smear."
	O: 37-year-old woman, patient emptied bladder, urine dip negative. Patient was positioned and draped for Dr. Jacobs.
	A: Routine Pap smear
	P: Pap smear sent to laboratory and patient educated regarding the result notification. Patient discharged by Dr. Jacobs.
	———— Kelly Thomas, RMA

What If?

The first Pap smear or gynecologic examination for young women may cause great anxiety. What if an 18-year-old is to have her first Pap smear today? How should you handle the situation?

Bring the patient into the room and encourage her to talk about her feelings. Do not have her change into an examining gown until she has had an opportunity to speak to the physician or practitioner about the procedure. If the patient's mother is present, ask her to follow her daughter's wishes about remaining in the room. (Some young women will want their mothers present and others will not.) You are more likely to be given an accurate sexual history if the mother is not present. The physician will require the presence of another health care worker during the examination; this will give you an opportunity to provide reassurance and patient education.

text continues on page 793

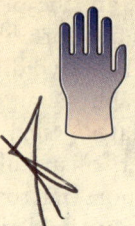

Procedure 41-1   Assisting With a Pelvic Examination With a Pap Smear

Equipment/Supplies

- patient drape
- vaginal speculum, appropriate size
- uterine sponge forceps
- cotton-tipped applicators, long
- water-soluble lubricant
- gloves

- direct lighting
- cleansing tissues or personal wipes
- biohazard barrier devices, as appropriate
- materials for Pap smear—cervical spatula or cervical brush, glass slides, fixative solution (spray or liquid), laboratory request form, identification label

Steps	Purpose
1. Wash your hands.	1. Handwashing aids infection control.
2. Assemble the equipment and supplies.	2. This ensures that everything you need is available.
3. Label and date each slide.	3. Accurate identification of all specimens is critical to an accurate diagnosis.
4. Complete the laboratory request form for Pap smear with essential information, including the date, patient's name, age, first day of last menstrual period, relevant history, physician, and your signature.	4. Complete and accurate patient information is essential to the interpretation of the laboratory report.
5. Greet and identify the patient. Explain the procedure.	5. Identifying the patient prevents errors. Communication will help establish rapport and knowing what to expect will reduce patient apprehension.
6. Ask the patient to empty her bladder and if necessary collect a urine specimen.	6. An empty bladder will make the examination more comfortable for the patient and will help her relax.
7. Provide patient with a drape and ask her to disrobe from the waist down.	7. Providing concise instructions reduces anxiety because the patient knows exactly what is expected.
8. Position the patient in the dorsal lithotomy position with buttocks at the bottom edge of the table.	8. Correct positioning will facilitate the procedure.
9. Adjust the drape to cover the patient's abdomen and knees, exposing the genitalia.	9. Adequately draping the patient will help her relax.
10. Adjust the light over the genitalia for maximum visibility.	10. Good visibility is essential for a thorough examination.
11. Assist the physician with the examination by handing instruments and supplies as needed.	11. Anticipating the physician's needs during the procedure will aid in a more thorough and efficient examination.

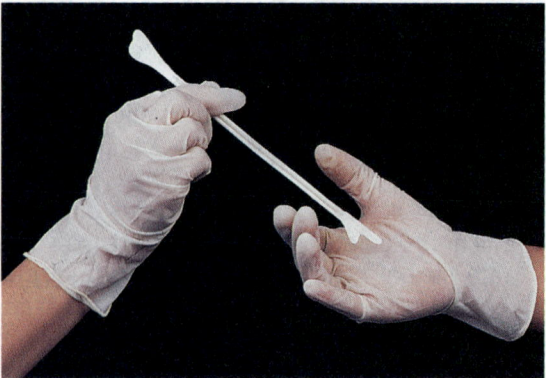

Step 11: Place the spatula firmly in the physician's hand in a functional position.

(continued)

Steps	**Purpose**

12. Hold the microscopic slides while the physician is obtaining and making the smears.

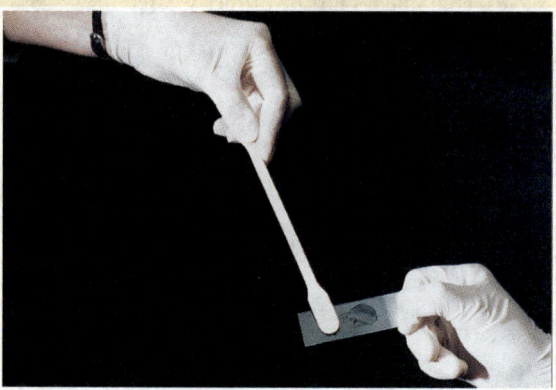

Step 12: Hold the slide by the frosted end to receive the vaginal smear and the endocervical smear.

13. Spray each slide with or immerse each slide in a fixative solution.

14. Explain to the patient that the physician will now remove the vaginal speculum and do a manual examination.

13. When performing a Pap smear, a fixative spray or solution is necessary to preserve the cervical scrapings for cytology.

14. The patient will be more relaxed and cooperative if she is informed of each step.

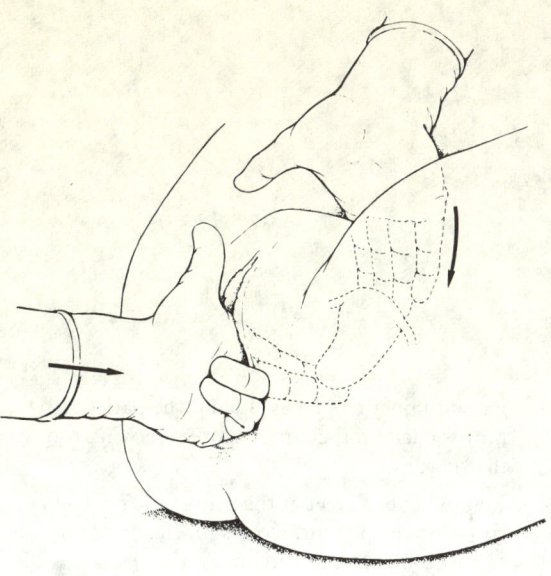

Step 14: Technique for bimanual examination of the pelvis in women.

(continued)

Steps	Purpose
15. Hold a basin for receiving the now contamined vaginal speculum. Place the speculum in a basin of cold water to begin sanitization.	15. All equipment must be properly cared for.

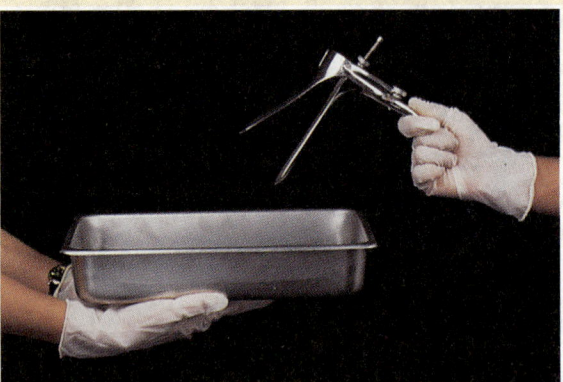

Step 15: Receive the used instruments in a basin to transfer to soaking solution.

Steps	Purpose
16. Apply lubricant across the physician's two fingers.	16. Water-soluble lubricant will help make the manual examination more comfortable.

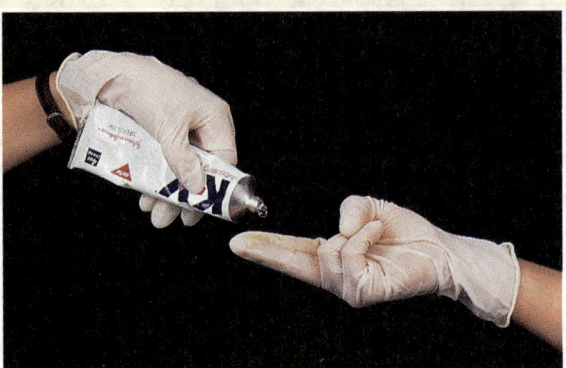

Step 16: Apply about 1–2 inches of water soluble lubricant to the physician's gloved fingers.

Steps	Purpose
17. After completion of the examination, assist the patient in sliding up to the top of the examination table.	17. Patient injury can be avoided if the patient first moves back up the table before removing feet from the stirrups.
18. Assist the patient in removing both feet at the same time from the stirrups. Help the patient to remove excess lubricant by handing her a personal wipe or tissues.	18. Removing both feet at the same time puts less strain on the patient. Excess lubricant can be uncomfortable for the patient.
19. Package the specimen for transport to the laboratory.	19. Special packaging is required for safe transportation or mailing to the laboratory.

(continued)

Procedure 41-1 Assisting With a Pelvic Examination With a Pap Smear *(continued)*

Steps	Purpose
20. Provide for privacy while the patient is dressing.	20. The patient is entitled to respect and privacy.
21. Thank the patient. Reinforce the physician's instructions about follow-up. Address any concerns or questions.	21. Courtesy encourages the patient to have a positive attitude about the physician's office. For quality management, let the patient know when to schedule follow-ups and when and how laboratory results will be obtained.
22. Properly care for or dispose of equipment. Clean the examination room. Wash your hands.	22. Maintaining a sanitary environment prevents the spread of microorganisms.
23. Document your responsibilities during the procedure, such as routing the specimen, patient education, etc.	23. Procedures are considered not to have been done if they are not recorded.

the physician about patient positioning if the lithotomy position is not possible or desirable.

Checkpoint Question

6. *What procedures does the physician perform as part of a complete gynecologic examination?*

Colposcopy

Colposcopy is the visual examination of the vaginal and cervical surfaces with the use of a stereoscopic microscope called the colposcope. It is often performed to evaluate patients with abnormal cell studies; to locate the origin of abnormal cells; to select areas for cervical, endocervical, or endometrial biopsy; to assess tissue with cervical lesions; for an atypical Pap smear; or for follow-up with history of cervical dysplasia or cervical cancer.

If a biopsy is to be done, be sure that a written, informed consent has been obtained. When possible, label specimen containers and complete laboratory request forms before the procedure. The completed forms and labeled containers should be retained in the patient examination room until the specimen is obtained.

Although there is usually very little, if any, bleeding, have available silver nitrate or Monsel's solution, either of which controls bleeding by chemical cautery. The patient preparation for colposcopy with cervical biopsy is similar to that required for the pelvic examination (Procedure 41-2).

Culdocentesis

Culdocentesis is the surgical puncture of the vaginal cul-de-sac and aspiration of fluid from the abdominal cavity. A culdocentesis is often done to diagnose pelvic inflammatory disease or ruptured ectopic pregnancy.

Hysterosalpingography (HSG)

The hysterosalpingography (HSG) is a diagnostic procedure in which the uterus and uterine tubes are radiographed after the injection of a contrast medium. The radiograph is called a **hysterosalpingogram**. The test is

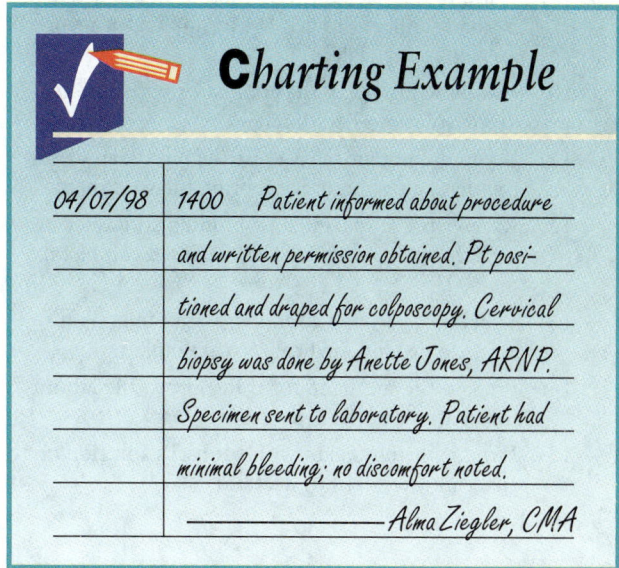

Charting Example

04/07/98	1400	Patient informed about procedure and written permission obtained. Pt positioned and draped for colposcopy. Cervical biopsy was done by Anette Jones, ARNP. Specimen sent to laboratory. Patient had minimal bleeding; no discomfort noted.
		— Alma Ziegler, CMA

Procedure 41-2 — Assisting With Colposcopy With Cervical Biopsy

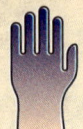

Equipment/Supplies

- setup for pelvic examination
- colposcope
- specimen container with preservative (10% formalin)
- sterile gloves

On the Sterile Field
- long cotton applicators, sterile
- normal saline solution
- 3% acetic acid or vinegar

Sterile Materials for Cervical Biopsy
- biopsy forceps or punch
- uterine curet

- povidone-iodine (Betadine)
- sanitary napkin, mini pad, or tampon
- biohazard barrier devices, as appropriate
- silver nitrate sticks or ferric subsulfate (Monsel's solution)

- uterine dressing forceps
- sterile 4 × 4 gauze
- sterile towel

- endocervical curet
- uterine tenaculum

Steps	Purpose
1. Verify that the patient has signed the consent form.	1. Colposcopy with biopsy is an invasive procedure that requires written consent.
2. Wash your hands.	2. Handwashing aids infection control.
3. Assemble the equipment and supplies.	3. This ensures that everything you need is available.
4. Check the light on the colposcope.	4. Properly functioning equipment is crucial to the quality of the examination.
5. Set up the sterile field.	5. A biopsy is an invasive procedure requiring sterile asepsis.
6. Pour normal saline and acetic acid into their respective sterile containers. Cover the field with a sterile drape.	6. These solutions are critical to the examination of the cervix. The field must be covered to maintain sterility as you prepare the patient.
7. Greet and identify the patient. Explain the procedure. Caution the patient that there may be a sharp cramp at the time of biopsy.	7. Identifying the patient prevents errors. Explaining the procedure helps ease anxiety.
8. Position the patient in the dorsal lithotomy position. *Note: If you are to assist the physician from the sterile field, put on gloves now and assist as follows.*	8. Correct positioning is necessary to properly visualize the cervix.
9. Hand the physician the applicator immersed in normal saline, followed by the applicator immersed in acetic acid.	9. Acetic acid swabbed on the area will improve visualization and aid in identifying suspicious tissue.
10. Hand the physician the applicator with the antiseptic solution (Betadine).	10. An antiseptic solution is used to prevent contaminating the area to be biopsied with pathogens.
11. If you did not glove to assist the physician, from the field, glove before accepting the specimen.	11. The specimen is potentially hazardous; therefore, you must use Standard Precautions.
12. Receive tissue specimen by holding container of 10% formalin in which the specimen can be immersed.	12. For proper preservation, the specimen must be immediately immersed in a preservative.
13. Label the specimen container with the patient's name, date, and medical record number.	13. The specimen must be properly identified.
14. Prepare the specimen for transport to the laboratory/pathology.	14. The specimen must be transported in appropriate packaging.
15. Provide the physician with Monsel's solution or silver nitrate sticks, if necessary.	15. If bleeding occurs, a coagulant may need to be applied.

(continued)

Procedure 41-2   Assisting With Colposcopy With Cervical Biopsy (continued)

Steps	Purpose
16. Explain to the patient that a small amount of bleeding may occur. Have a sanitary pad available.	16. Bleeding with a cervical biopsy is usually minimal and a small sanitary pad should suffice.
17. Thank the patient. Reinforce the physician's instructions.	17. Courtesy encourages the patient to have a positive attitude about the physician's office. Instruct the patient regarding biopsy results and scheduling follow-up visit.
18. Properly care for or dispose of equipment and supplies. Clean the examination room. Wash your hands.	18. This prevents the spread of microorganisms.
19. Document the procedure, including date, time, patient's tolerance and outcome.	19. Procedures are considered not to have been done if they are not recorded.

---

often performed to determine the configuration of the uterus and the patency of the uterine tubes for fertility purposes.

Laparoscopy

Abdominal and pelvic structures can be visualized directly by inserting a lighted scope into the abdominal cavity through a small incision. For better access to the pelvic organs, carbon dioxide or other gas is injected to expand the abdominal walls and intestines away from the organs. Endometriosis, ectopic pregnancies, and tumors are a few of the disorders that may be diagnosed by laparoscopy. This is the method of choice for tubal ligation, the female sterilization procedure. Figure 41-7 illustrates the laparoscopic procedure for tubal ligation covered later in this chapter.

The medical assistant would require extensive training in an outpatient surgical unit to assist with this procedure. In most instances, you are more likely to assist with patient preparation such as signing consents or relaying preoperative and postoperative instructions.

Dilatation and Curettage (D & C)

A D & C may be performed to remove uterine tissue for diagnostic testing, to reduce endometrial tissue, to prevent or treat menorrhagia (excessive menstrual flow), or to remove retained products of conception. The cervical canal will be widened with a uterine sound and the lining will be scraped with a curet (see Chap. 23, Instruments and Equipment). This procedure usually requires anesthesia and will be performed as an inpatient procedure or as an outpatient procedure in a day surgery unit. The patient must sign all preoperative consents, but no specific preoperative preparation is required. The patient will need a perineal pad, light postoperative analgesia and instructions regarding signs of infection, hemorrhage, and follow-up care. Your responsibility will probably be limited to patient preparation and patient education as directed by your physician.

➤ OBSTETRIC CARE

Unlike other physicians, obstetricians are often at the hospital delivering infants during regular office hours. If you are assisting in an obstetric practice, you must use good judgment when pregnant patients present or call with questions and concerns. For instance, you will have to determine if the situation can wait for the physician's return, if another physician should be consulted, if the patient should go to the emergency room, or if you can, with the physician's permission, advise the patient on how to manage the problem. Protocol listed in the policy and procedure manual for action to be taken in specific situations will ensure that, in the physician's absence, safe procedures will be followed for your patients and will protect you and your physician from errors in treatment.

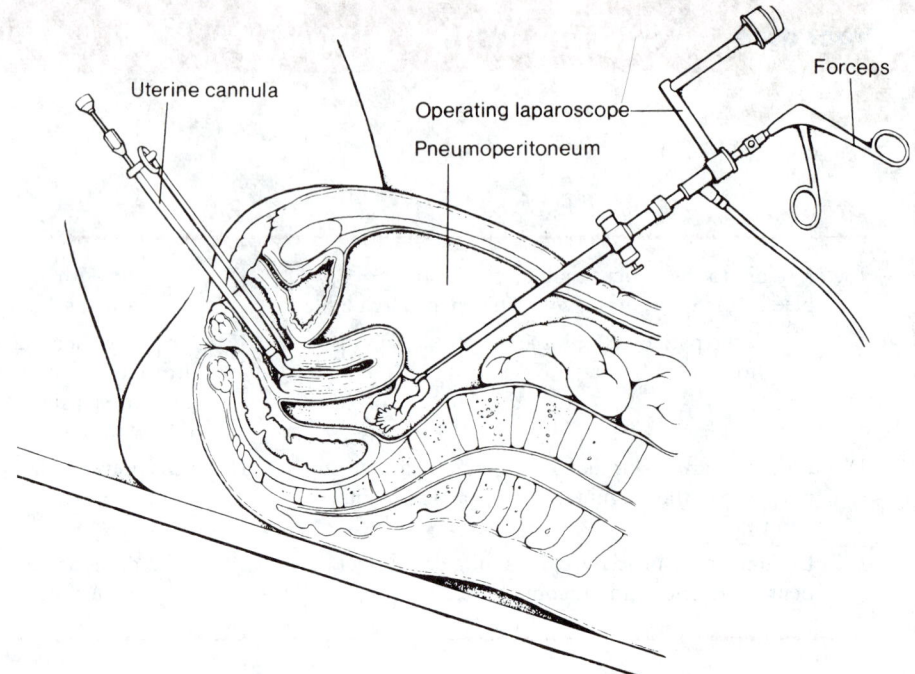

FIGURE 41-7
Laparoscopy. The laparoscope (*right*) is inserted through a small incision in the abdomen. A forceps is inserted through the scope to grasp the fallopian tube. To improve the view, a uterine cannula (*left*) is inserted into the vagina to push the uterus upward. Insufflation of gas creates an air pocket (pneumoperitoneum), and the pelvis is raised (note the angle), which forces the intestines higher in the abdomen.

Diagnosis of Pregnancy

Many patients suspect that they are pregnant (**gravid**) because of the symptoms they are experiencing. However, these early symptoms of pregnancy may be indicative of other disorders, as noted above. Therefore, the early symptoms are called presumptive signs and symptoms of pregnancy, meaning that the pregnancy must still be confirmed by more conclusive diagnostic procedures. The presumptive symptoms include amenorrhea, nausea and vomiting, breast enlargement and tenderness, fatigue, and urinary frequency. Other more probable signs and symptoms of pregnancy include presence of human chorionic gonadotropin (HCG) in the maternal urine or serum, enlargement of the abdomen, changes in the uterus and cervix, and occurrence of **Braxton Hicks** uterine contractions.

Early in pregnancy the patient may notice irregular uterine contractions that occur fairly frequently. These contractions, called Braxton Hicks contractions, do not affect the cervix like the contractions of active labor and are normal for pregnancy. Although the patient may or may not be aware of the contractions, the physician can palpate the contractions during a bimanual examination or by palpating the uterus from the abdomen.

Cervical changes that occur during pregnancy include softening of the cervix (**Goodell's sign**), increased vascularity of the cervix causing the cervix, vulva, and vagina to develop a bluish violet color (**Chadwick's sign**), and formation of a mucous plug. The mucous plug forms in the cervical os and protects the develop-

ing fetus and the amniotic sac from the external environment. With the onset of labor the mucous plug is expelled with a small amount of blood and is often referred to as the "bloody show."

The diagnosis of pregnancy is actually confirmed by the presence of fetal heart tones and fetal movement detected by the physician or the visual image of a fetus on ultrasonography (Table 41-3).

Checkpoint Question

7. Why are presumptive signs and symptoms of pregnancy not considered to be conclusive?

First Prenatal Visit

The pregnant patient's initial prenatal visit is extensive and critical to the ongoing assessment of the pregnancy. A thorough and detailed history of the patient must be obtained (Box 41-4). To elicit the most complete and accurate information, the health history interview should be conducted in a private room where there will be no interruptions.

The first prenatal visit includes the confirmation of pregnancy, complete history and physical, establishment of the estimated date of confinement (EDC) or estimated date of delivery (EDD), assessment of gesta-

Table 41-3
Signs and Symptoms of Pregnancy

Presumptive Signs	Probable Signs	Conclusive Signs
Cessation of menses	HCG present in urine and serum	Presence of fetal heart tones
Nausea and vomiting	Braxton Hicks contractions	Fetal movement detected by the examiner
Breast tenderness	Enlargement of abdomen	Visualization of the fetus
Breast enlargement	Uterine changes	
Quickening or fetal movement felt by the patient	Goodell's sign	
Fatigue	Chadwick's sign	
Urinary frequency		

tional age, identifying risk factors, and patient education. The estimated date of confinement or delivery is a prediction of the "due date," assuming the pregnancy progresses normally (Box 41-5). Normal gestation is 37 to 41 weeks. Infants born before the 37th week are considered to be premature; those born after the 41st week are postmature.

The complete physical examination will include a pelvic examination with Pap smear, pregnancy test, clinical pelvimetry, complete blood count, blood glucose, blood type and Rh factor, antibody screen, urinalysis, serologic tests for syphilis and rubella and hepatitis B virus (HBV) and human immunodeficiency virus (HIV) screen. The medical assistant should reinforce the physician's instructions to the patient and encourage patients to call the office if they have further questions or concerns.

Patients should be instructed to notify the physician or medical assistant if any of the following occur:

- Vaginal bleeding or spotting
- Persistent vomiting
- Fever or chills
- Dysuria
- Abdominal or uterine cramping
- Leaking amniotic fluid
- Altered fetal movement
- Dizziness or blurred vision
- Other problems

Understanding Fetotoxic and Teratogenic Factors

Certain factors can put the developing fetus at risk for problems. Depending on the severity of the factor, fetal development may be so altered as to be incompatible with life; such factors are referred to as *fetotoxic*. Fetuses not spontaneously aborted are stillborn or die soon after birth in the event of fetotoxicity. Certain factors disrupt development, causing abnormalities but not death; these factors are referred to as *terato-*

genic (*terato* is the word root for monster and *genic* means to form or begin). The stage of greatest danger ranges from about the 3rd to the 12th week of devel-

BOX 41-4   Parity Versus Gravidity

The prenatal history must include information regarding previous pregnancies to help predict the outcome of the current pregnancy.

The term **parity** refers to the number of live births and **gravidity** refers to any pregnancy, regardless of its length and outcome. The pregnant, or **gravid**, woman is termed a **gravida**, usually with an indicator of the number, such as **primigravida** (first pregnancy), **secundigravida** (second pregnancy), and so forth to **multigravida** (many pregnancies). A woman who has never been pregnant is a **nulligravida**. The number of live births is also given a prefix indicator, such as **nullipara** (has never borne a living child), **primipara** (first living child), and so forth to **multipara** with many live births.

These numbers are listed for the physician's review as gr (or simply g), p, pret (preterm or premature), and ab (abortion, spontaneous or induced). For example, a woman who is pregnant for the third time, has lost no pregnancies, and carried her previous pregnancies to term is listed:

gr iii, pret 0, ab 0, p ii
(Arabic numbers are acceptable also.)

A woman who is pregnant for the fifth time and who has delivered one set of twins, two single infants, has had no premature infants, and has lost one pregnancy spontaneously would be listed:

gr v, pret 0, ab i, p iv

BOX 41-5 Determining the Estimated Date of Confinement (EDC) or the Expected Date of Delivery (EDD)

The estimated date of confinement (EDC) is frequently referred to as the expected date of delivery (EDD). Because of the negative connotations of "confinement" and because women are no longer "confined" during pregnancy or the postpartum period, terminology for the due date is changing somewhat to reflect current maternity trends. Many methods are used for determining this projected date. Nagele's rule requires a mathematical calculation using the following formula:

The first day of the last menstrual period (LMP) + 7 days − 3 months + 1 year. Example: LMP = May 3, 1996

$$
\begin{array}{cccl}
5 & 3 & 96 & \text{(LMP)} \\
-3 & +7 & +1 & \text{(Nagele's rule)} \\
\hline
2 & 10 & 97 & \text{(EDD)}
\end{array}
$$

A simpler method involves adding 9 months and 7 days to the first day of the LMP. Try that method with the example above.

The third common method is to use one of the various gestational wheels available. Using the inner wheel, line up the first day of the LMP on the outer wheel with the appropriate arrow, and read around the wheel to the indicated milestones in the pregnancy.

Many wheels will indicate the date of conception, times recommended for blood work and other testing, and all will work toward the date that delivery is expected.

More reliable dates are determined by quickening, uterine size and growth, and ultrasound.

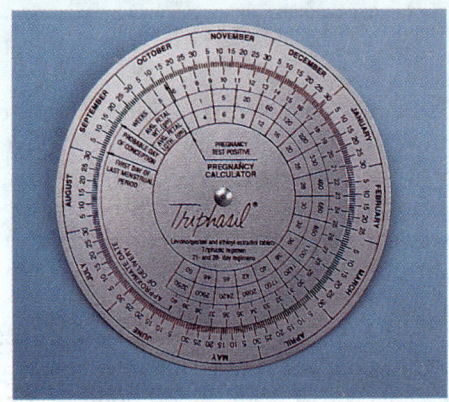

Gestational wheel

opment, a time at which many women are not yet aware they are pregnant.

Advise the pregnant patient against taking any medications or drugs (even over-the-counter preparations) without consulting the physician. The patient also should avoid smoking cigarettes and drinking alcoholic beverages. Evidence indicates that nicotine, alcohol, certain medications (Box 41-6), and other factors (Box 41-7) are harmful to the developing fetus.

Assisting With the First Prenatal Examination

The first prenatal examination is done to establish a detailed baseline of the patient's current physical condition. The examination will be a complete physical examina-

BOX 41-6 Classifying Drugs That May Harm the Developing Fetus

Many of the medications that might be beneficial to the mother may be dangerous to the developing fetus. The Food and Drug Administration has issued a list of categories (A, B, C, D, and X) used for classifying drugs that are dangerous to the fetus. These categories are listed on sources of drug information (eg, the *Physician's Desk Reference*, package inserts) and are based on animal and human research during the development of the drug.

A—Research indicates that there is probably no risk at any point in the pregnancy.

B—Animal research indicates no fetal risk but human studies are not complete.

C—Research on animals show this drug to be a danger. Human studies are inconclusive or no studies are available.

D—There is clear precedence for risk but the drug may be used if there is no substitute.

X—There is clear evidence of risk and the drug should not be used by pregnant women.

BOX 41-7 Other Risk Factors for Fetal Abnormalities

Factors other than medications may result in damage to the fetus. These include inadequate oxygen to the fetus, radiation, and disease processes. The effect on the fetus depends on the degree of exposure and fetal age at the time of exposure. A few of the more commonly encountered risk factors and their effects are listed below.

Risk Factor	Effects
Syphilis	Structural deformities, blindness, deafness, fetal death
Alcohol (fetal alcohol syndrome)	Craniofacial and limb defects, intrauterine growth retardation (IUGR), retarded development
Diethylstilbesterol (DES) (used to prevent threatened spontaneous abortions)	Implicated in reproductive cancers; children of DES mothers may present with ovarian and cervical cancer or testicular cancer
Heavy metals (eg, lead and mercury)	Potentially fetotoxic; both lead and mercury cause physical and mental retardation and a galaxy of related deformities and central nervous system disorders
Toxoplasmosis (protozoal infection spread by cat feces)	Fetotoxic to teratogenic with microcephaly, hydrocephaly, mental and growth retardation
Rubella	Central nervous system involvement, blindness, deafness, cardiac abnormalities
Cytomegalovirus	Fetotoxic to teratogenic with hydrocephaly, mental and growth retardation
Herpes	Infants delivered during active outbreak may develop central nervous system involvement that may lead to neonatal death.

(The last four risk factors, with the addition of "other," form a complex referred to as TORCH. Any of the group may cause many severe pregnancy and fetal difficulties. Testing will be done to evaluate TORCH titers to identify the causative agent.)

---

tion with a pelvic examination including, screening for *Neisseria gonorrhoeae*, chlamydial infection, cervical cancer, syphilis, and tuberculosis.

In addition to what is normally done for a complete physical examination, the first prenatal visit will require:

- Blood work—Venereal Disease Research Laboratory (VDRL), Rapid Plasma Reagin (RPR), or other test for syphilis, complete blood count (CBC) with hematocrit, hemoglobin, white blood cell count with differential, blood type with Rh factor, antibody screen, and other tests as necessary
- Tuberculosis screening—tine test or purified protein derivative (PPD) injection
- Urinalysis—glucose, albumin, and acetone testing

Subsequent Prenatal Visits

If the pregnancy is progressing as expected and without complications (Fig. 41-8), the patient should be scheduled at 12, 16, 20, 24, and 28 weeks of gestation. The patient is usually seen every 2 weeks during the last 2 months and once a week after the 36th week of gestation. Of course, this schedule should be altered according to the patient's condition.

Table 41-4 outlines the specific examination and procedures to be performed during subsequent prenatal visits. This table is useful in preparing the room and patient.

Assisting With Subsequent Prenatal Visits

Subsequent prenatal visits are scheduled to assess the fetal growth and development and the maternal health throughout the pregnancy. As the pregnancy progresses, the patient is always at risk of supine hypotension. Supine hypotension is the result of the fetus resting on the mother's aorta and vena cava when she is flat on her back. The weight of the uterus compresses these major vessels and restricts the blood flow, causing a drop in the maternal blood pressure. The patient may become pale, clammy, and breathless; the fetal heart rate may drop. Immediately turn the patient onto her left side.

To prevent supine hypotension, have the patient rest in an upright position until the physician is ready to examine her. Also try elevating the head of the table about 30° during the examination. If the patient's pregnancy is progressing normally, she may only be required to expose her abdomen to measure the fundal height (Fig. 41-9) and listen for fetal heart sounds. If

Fetal Development*

1st Lunar Month

The embryo is 4 to 5mm in length.

Trophoblasts embed in decidua.

Chorionic villi form.

Foundations for nervous system, genitourinary system, skin, bones, and lungs are formed.

Buds of arms and legs begin to form.

Rudiments of eyes, ears, and nose appear.

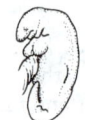

4 weeks

2nd Lunar Month

The fetus is 27 to 31 mm in length and weighs 2 to 4g.

Fetus is markedly bent.

Head is disproportionately large as a result of brain development.

Sex differentiation begins.

Centers of bone begin to ossify.

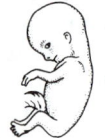

8 weeks

3rd Lunar Month

The fetus average length is 6 to 9 cm, and weight is 45 g.

Fingers and toes are distinct

Placenta is complete.

Fetal circulation is complete.

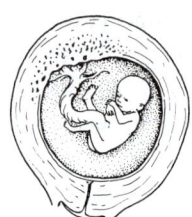

3 months

4th Lunar Month

The fetus is 12 cm in length and weighs 110 g.

Sex is differentiated.

Rudimentary kidneys secrete urine.

Heartbeat is present.

Nasal septum and palate close.

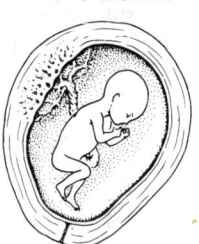

4 months

5th Lunar Month

The fetus is 19 cm in length and weighs approximately 300 g.

Lanugo covers entire body.

Fetal movements are felt by mother.

Heart sounds are perceptible by auscultation.

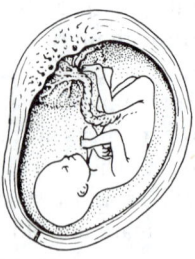

5 months

  * All lengths given are crown to rump.

6th Lunar Month

The fetus is about 23 cm in length and weighs 630 g.

Skin appears wrinkled.

Vernix caseosa appears.

Eyebrows and fingernails develop.

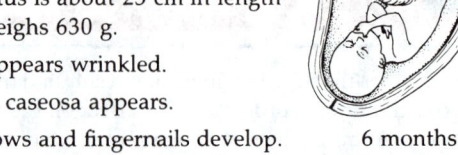

6 months

7th Lunar Month

The fetus is 27 cm in length and weighs about 1100 g.

Skin is red.

Pupillary membrane disappears from eyes.

The fetus has an excellent chance of survival.

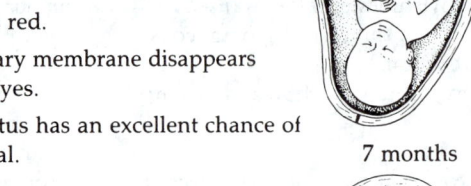

7 months

8th Lunar Month

The fetus is 28 to 30 cm in length and weighs 1.8 kg.

Fetus is viable.

Eyelids open.

Fingerprints are set.

Vigorous fetal movement occurs.

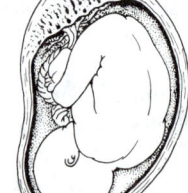

8 months

9th Lunar Month

The fetus' average length is 32 cm; weight is about 2500 g.

Face and body have a loose wrinkled appearance because of subcutaneous fat deposit.

Lanugo disappears.

Amniotic fluid decreases.

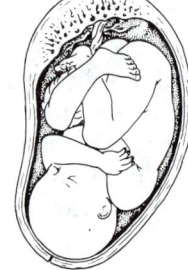

9 months

10th Lunar Month

The average fetus is 36 cm in length and weighs 3000 to 3600 g.

Skin is smooth.

Eyes are uniformly slate colored.

Bones of skull are ossified and nearly together at sutures.

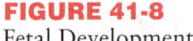

FIGURE 41-8
Fetal Development

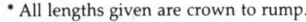

Table 41-4
Schedule of Return Prenatal Visits

First through sixth month—visits once per month
Seventh and eighth months—visits every 2 weeks
Ninth month until delivery—visits once per week

Included in Visit	*When Done*
Weight	Each visit
Blood pressure	Each visit
Fundal height (McDonald's)	Each visit
Fetal heart rate	Each visit
Check for edema	Each visit
Pelvic examination	Middle of ninth month, then weekly as indicated
Other examination	As indicated by symptoms
Inquiry about symptoms, signs, or problems	Each visit
Prenatal education	Each visit
Nutrition and appetite	Each visit
Family and personal adjustment	Each visit
Urinalysis for glucose and albumin	Each visit
Hematocrit and hemoglobin	At 32–34 weeks (more often if anemic)
Urine culture	As indicated by symptoms or signs
Rh titers	If initially negative, twice more during pregnancy; if positive, more often as indicated by titer levels
α-Fetoprotein	At 15–20 weeks
Glucose (blood sugar)	at 24–28 weeks
Ultrasonography	For fetal age, best between 8 and 16 weeks
Other tests	As indicated by symptoms or signs

From Reeder, S. J., Martin, L. L., Koniak, D. (1992). Maternity Nursing, *17th ed., p. 403. Philadelphia: J. B. Lippincott.*

she has had any problems since the last visit, have her disrobe from the waist down.

Checkpoint Question

8. The pregnant patient should be advised to contact the physician when what problems occur?

➤ OBSTETRIC DISORDERS

Ectopic Pregnancy

A gestation in which a fertilized ovum implants somewhere other than in the uterine cavity is an ectopic pregnancy. Usually the implantation of an ectopic pregnancy is in the fallopian tube; this may be referred to as a tubal pregnancy. Other sites include the abdomen, the ovaries, and the cervical os. The patient may present with signs of early pregnancy: breast enlargement or tenderness, nausea, late menses. Pelvic pain, syncope, abdominal symptoms, painful sexual intercourse, and irregular menstrual bleeding present fairly early in the pregnancy. If an ectopic pregnancy is not diagnosed early, there is the potential for rupture of the fallopian tube causing hemorrhage into the abdominal cavity and the possibility of shock and death. Diagnostic procedures include urine or serum human chorionic gonadotropin pregnancy test, ultrasound to determine the location of the pregnancy, laparoscopy to visualize the enlarged tube, and perhaps culdocentesis to confirm abdominal bleeding. Treatment is surgical excision of the ectopic pregnancy by either a laparoscopy or laparotomy.

Hyperemesis Gravidarum

Nausea and vomiting ("morning sickness") are expected during early pregnancy and are treated with small frequent meals, adequate hydration, and pa-

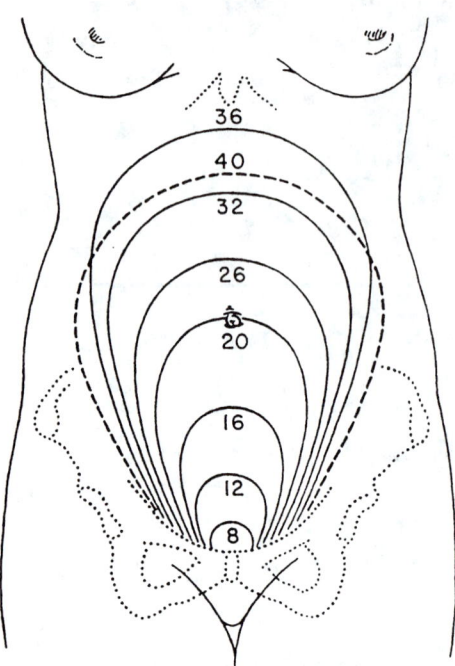

FIGURE 41-9
Height of the fundus at comparable gestational dates varies greatly from patient to patient. Those shown are most common. A convenient rule of thumb is that at five months gestation, the fundus is usually at or slightly above the umbilicus.

tient reassurance. However, if the vomiting becomes unrelenting and leads to dehydration, electrolyte imbalance, and weight loss, then the diagnosis is hyperemesis gravidarum. Occasionally, the patient must be hospitalized. The medical assistant must be prepared to discern between the complaints of morning sickness and the more serious hyperemesis gravidarum.

Abortion

One of the more common disorders of pregnancy is the first trimester **abortion**, also called an early pregnancy loss or miscarriage. Because of early diagnosis of pregnancy, it is now known that the spontaneous abortion occurs with greater frequency than previously thought. Abortions may be either induced or spontaneous. The induced abortion is intentional and is a result of instrumentation. The spontaneous abortion occurs because of fetal or maternal conditions without outside interference in the pregnancy.

A spontaneous abortion is defined as the loss of pregnancy prior to the time that the fetus is viable in extrauterine life or prior to 20 weeks' gestation. You will need to be familiar with the early signs and symptoms of an impending abortion to advise the patient until the physician can be contacted. The patient may be instructed to come into the medical office, go to the emergency room, or remain at home on bed rest until the physician returns the call. The first symptom of the impending abortion is usually bleeding followed by uterine cramps and low back pain. Table 41-5 describes types of abortions and related symptoms.

Pregnancy-Induced Hypertension (PIH)

Hypertension that is directly related to the pregnancy is termed pregnancy-induced hypertension (PIH). There are two types of PIH: preeclampsia and eclampsia.

Preeclampsia

Preeclampsia is characterized by **proteinuria** (protein in the urine), edema of lower extremities, and hypertension occurring after the 20th week of gestation. As the condition progresses the patient may complain of blurred vision, headaches, edema, and vomiting. Medical management includes restricted activities, increased bed rest, sexual abstinence, antihypertensive therapy, and well balanced meals with an increase in proteins and decrease in sodium. Close monitoring of the patient is important and requires scheduling the patient for more frequent office visits. The risk of developing eclampsia increases with the advancing pregnancy.

Eclampsia

Eclampsia is almost always preceded by preeclampsia and its onset is sudden. In eclampsia, the clinical signs of preeclampsia are still present but exaggerated. However, eclampsia is always characterized by seizures that may be followed by coma, hypertensive crisis, and shock. The number and severity of the seizures varies. The progression from preeclampsia to eclampsia constitutes an emergency. Management of eclampsia includes stabilizing the patient and may require that delivery of the fetus be induced.

Placenta Previa

Placenta previa is a condition in which the placenta is implanted either partially or completely over the internal cervical os, making delivery of the fetus before the placenta difficult. During the second or third trimester of pregnancy the patient may have painless,

Table 41-5
Types of Abortions and Related Symptoms

Threatened Abortion	Vaginal bleeding or spotting occurring in early pregnancy that may or may not be associated with mild cramps; closed cervix; the process may abate or result in an abortion.
Inevitable Abortion	The above porcess has progressed such that termination of the pregnancy cannot be prevented; bleeding is moderate to copious; uterine cramping is moderate to severe; the membranes may or may not have ruptured; the cervical canal is dilating.
Incomplete Abortion	Part of the products of conception has been passed, but part (usually the placenta) is retained in the uterus; heavy bleeding usually persists until the retained products of conception have been passed; uterine cramping is severe; the cervix is open, with tissue present.
Complete Abortion	All of the products of conception have been expelled; bleeding is slight; uterine cramping is mild.
Missed Abortion	The fetus dies in utero but is retained; regression in uterine growth and breast changes are present; if 6 weeks or more elapse between fetal death and expulsion, degenerative changes occur, eg, maceration (general softening), mummification (drying up into a leatherlike structure) and, rarely, lithopedion formation (stony material); symptoms, except for amenorrhea, are usually lacking; malaise, headache, and anorexia are occasionally present; hypofibrinogenemia may result; the condition may be discovered because fundal height fails to increase or fetal heart tones are absent.
Habitual Abortion	Spontaneous abortion occurs in successive pregnancies (three or more)
Illegal Abortion	Termination of pregnancy outside of appropriate medical facilities (eg, hospitals or clinics), generally by nonphysician abortionists; the frequency of such abortions is not precisely known but has dropped precipitously in the United States because of legalized abortion; the method may involve ingestion of drugs, such as quinine or castor oil, or the placement of a foreign body, such as a urethral catheter, into the uterus with or without the instillation of toxic substances; severe infection, often with shock and renal failure, may result.

From Reeder, S. J., Martin, L. L., Koniak, D. (1992). Maternity Nursing, 17th ed., p. 774. Philadelphia: J. B. Lippincott.

vaginal bleeding. The vaginal bleeding may be minimal, as in spotting, or it may be profuse. Placenta previa is easily diagnosed by prenatal ultrasound. However, the placenta tends to migrate (move) and the ultrasounds need to be periodic if placenta previa is suspected or diagnosed. Medical management includes bed rest and drug therapy if the patient is preterm. If the patient is near term and if the bleeding is severe and poses a danger to mother or fetus, then delivery of the baby is essential and usually requires a cesarean delivery (Box 41-8).

Abruptio Placentae

The premature separation or detachment of the placenta from the uterus is known as abruptio placentae. Depending on the severity of the separation, symptoms

BOX 41-8 Cesarean Section

In some situations, a normal vaginal delivery is not possible or advisable. These include:

- cephalopelvic disproportion (CPD)—the baby's head is too large for the birth canal
- poor presentation—other than an occipital presentation, such as transverse (the baby lying across the cervix) or breech (a buttocks first presentation)
- failure to progress—inefficient labor or the cervix will not dilate
- infant or maternal distress

In these situations, the infant will be delivered by cesarean section. An incision is made through the abdominal wall into the uterus and the infant is removed. It was once believed that women who had delivered by cesarean must never be allowed to go into labor and deliver vaginally because it was feared that the uterine scar tissue might rupture. Current surgical techniques have lessened that fear and many women now deliver vaginally after a cesarean delivery.

include pain, uterine tenderness, bleeding and signs of impending shock, and fetal distress or even fetal death. If abruptio placentae is confirmed, the baby is usually delivered by cesarean section.

Checkpoint Question

9. What is placenta previa and how is it managed in a preterm patient?

➤ ONSET OF LABOR

Labor is the physiologic process necessary for expelling the fetus from the uterus. About 4 weeks before the onset of labor, **lightening** or dropping indicates that the fetus has descended further into the pelvis and the patient will appear to be carrying the baby lower in the abdomen. The actual onset of labor is characterized by regular uterine contractions that become more intense and more frequent with time. True labor is distinguished from false labor by its effect (dilation and effacement) on the cervix and the increased frequency and intensity of contractions. Another indication of true labor is the appearance of "bloody show," which is the mucous plug from the cervical os. The amniotic sac may break; the patient may call to say that "my bag of water broke."

Whatever signs or symptoms of labor occur, you need to know how to advise the patient. The physician will make the decision to send the patient to the hospital, schedule her to come to the medical office, or to have her stay home and wait. However, you will need to relay the information from patient to physician. Or decisions may need to be made in the physician's absence. A policy and procedure manual must be maintained in the office that includes specific instructions regarding how the physician wants the pregnant patient managed if the physician is not immediately available.

The onset of labor should be discussed with the patient so she knows what to expect and how to manage the situation. Always obtain the patient's medical record when talking with the patient or the physician; the patient's estimated date of delivery and physical condition are critical to the decision-making process.

➤ POSTPARTUM CARE

The postpartum period involves the time frame, known as **puerperium**, from childbirth until the reproductive structures return to normal, referred to as involution, and may take as long as 6 weeks. Once the patient is discharged from the hospital after labor and delivery, her care will be managed at the medical office. Reports received in the medical office from the hospital will contain certain acronyms and abbreviations related to labor and delivery and the postpartum period. The information contained in Box 41-9 will help you become familiar with these special terms.

The appointment time for the first postpartum visit will depend on the type of delivery and the patient's condition when discharged from the hospital. Today, the needs of the postpartum patient may be greater because the length of stay in the hospital is normally short, with some patients discharged within 24 hours. Patients who have no prenatal or postnatal complications or risks will be scheduled for their first postnatal examination within 2 to 4 weeks of delivery.

First Postpartum Visit

At the first postnatal or postpartum visit the physician will perform a complete gynecologic and breast examination. Allow plenty of time for patient counseling regarding her new role as a parent. Many patients will have questions and concerns regarding breast-feeding (Box 41-10), birth control, menstruation, parenting, and so on. Before the physician's examination, the pa-

---

BOX 41-9 Acronyms and Abbreviations Used in Labor and Delivery and the Postpartum Period

Following is a brief list of terms frequently used in the medical record.

AROM	Artificial rupture of membranes
AVD	Assisted vaginal delivery
CPD	Cephalopelvic disproportion
L & D	Labor and delivery
NSVD	Normal spontaneous vaginal delivery
PROM	Premature rupture of membranes
SROM	Spontaneous rupture of membranes
VBAC	Vaginal birth after cesarean

Terms for presentations:

LOA	Left occiput anterior
ROA	Right occiput anterior
LOP	Left occiput posterior
ROP	Right occiput posterior

Fetal descriptors:

AGA	Appropriate for gestational age
LGA	Large for gestational age
SGA	Small for gestational age
LBW	Low birth weight

---

tient's weight and vital signs will need to be determined and a urinalysis, hematocrit, and hemoglobin will be performed.

During the examination, the physician will assess any uterine discharge; **lochia** is usually still present at this stage. Lochia is a discharge from the uterus during puerperium and is composed of mucus, blood, and tissue shed from the uterine cavity:

- Lochia rubra—blood tinged discharge within first 6 days
- Lochia serosa—thin, brownish discharge lasting about 3 to 4 days after the lochia rubra
- Lochia alba—white postpartum discharge that has no evidence of blood

The amount of lochia should diminish considerably during puerperium. The physician should be notified if there is any abnormality of the lochial progression.

Postpartum Endometritis

Endometritis is an infection of the endometrium. In postpartum endometritis, the infection is directly related to puerperium. Usually the patient will complain of low back pain, bleeding, fever, chills, and foul-smelling lochia. Postpartum endometritis is treated with antibiotics.

Postpartum Depression

Postpartum depression occurs fairly frequently and usually within 2 to 3 days after delivery. There are varying degrees of depression and you should always be alert to the more serious form. This discussion is limited to what the patient calls postpartum "blues" or "let down." The patient feels anxious or depressed, cries easily, has difficulty sleeping, or has a loss of appetite. As a medical assistant, you need to

---

BOX 41-10 Breast Feeding

Estrogen and progesterone stimulate the mammary glands and ducts to produce milk. Immediately postpartum, thin white fluid referred to as colostrum is released. It is very high in proteins, antibodies, vitamins, and minerals. Several days postpartum, prolactin from the pituitary stimulates milk production, called lactation. Suckling or nursing stimulates the release of oxytocin to "let down" milk and encourages uterine contractions for involution.

reassure the patient that her feelings are probably due to hormonal changes. Talk with her about her feelings and let her know that the depression is normal and temporary. Encourage the patient to eat well, get adequate rest (including naps), and begin walking short distances daily. Usually the patient feels better just having someone to talk with and knowing that the depression is a normal extension of pregnancy and will subside.

If the patient expresses fear of harming herself or the baby or if she expresses anger regarding the baby, report this to the physician immediately. In some instances, severe parenting problems may be masked by postpartum depression. These cases must be referred to professionals trained to diagnose and treat potentially abusive parenting situations.

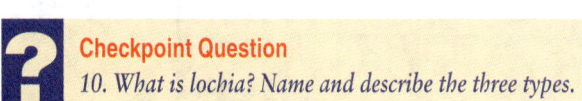

Checkpoint Question

10. What is lochia? Name and describe the three types.

COMMON OBSTETRIC TESTS AND THERAPEUTIC PROCEDURES AND THE MEDICAL ASSISTANT'S ROLE

Pregnancy Test

Many over-the-counter pregnancy tests are available for patients to use at home. If there are questions regarding the results, more reliable tests are available in the obstetrician's office. These are covered in Chapter 47, Serology and Immunohematology.

α-Fetoprotein (AFP)

Levels of AFP are obtained from maternal serum to screen the fetus for possible neural tube defects. Maternal serum AFP levels vary according to numerous factors including gestational age, number of fetuses, and patient weight. The test is used only for screening purposes and not for diagnostic purposes.

Amniocentesis

An amniocentesis is the transabdominal puncture of the amniotic sac and aspiration of amniotic fluid for study. Amniocentesis is usually done for diagnosing genetic problems, estimating gestational age, or assessing the lung maturity of the fetus.

Contraction Stress Test

A contraction stress test (CST) is performed to determine how well the fetus will tolerate uterine contractions. The uterine contractions may be induced by the woman stimulating her nipples (nipple-stimulated CST) or the contractions can be induced by administering oxytocin (oxytocin-stimulated CST) to the patient. In both tests, the fetal heart tones and movement are monitored in relation to the uterine contractions.

Nonstress Test

The nonstress test (NST) is a noninvasive obstetric procedure used to evaluate the fetal heart tones and movement in relation to spontaneous uterine contractions. The NST may be safely performed in the medical office, whereas the CST is usually performed in an outpatient facility or in a labor and delivery unit of the hospital.

Doppler Ultrasonography

Doppler ultrasonography is a noninvasive procedure used to detect fetal heart tones and measure the fetal heart rate. The Doppler, an ultrasonic transducer device, is positioned over the abdomen at a point where fetal heart tones are clearly audible. Dopplers are equipped with earpieces, such as those on a stethoscope that allow only the examiner to hear the sounds, and with an amplifier to broadcast the sound so that it can be heard by the mother and the examiner. The heart rate can be measured in much the same manner as counting a pulse.

Fetal Ultrasonography

An ultrasound of the fetus involves the use of high-frequency sound waves to create an image of internal structures. Fetal ultrasound is performed to assess the size, gestational age, position, and number of fetuses. Some abnormal maternal and fetal conditions such as ectopic pregnancy, placenta previa, neural tube defects, and cardiac defects are diagnosed by ultrasound. The gender of the fetus may be identified; however, this is never a justification for performing an ultrasound.

➤ CONTRACEPTION

Common Methods of Contraception

Numerous methods of contraception (birth control) are available for family planning (Table 41-6). The decision to practice contraception and the selection of the appropriate method involves many factors. The patient's religious, cultural, and personal beliefs as well as the health history, financial situation, and motivation are all important considerations for both the physician and patient.

To reinforce the physician's advice and instructions, the medical assistant must be knowledgeable

---

Table 41-6

Main Methods of Contraception Currently in Use

Method	Description	Advantages	Disadvantages
Surgical			
Vasectomy/tubal ligation	Cutting and tying of tubes carrying gametes	Nearly 100% effective; involves no chemical or mechanical devices	Not usually reversible; rare surgical complications
Hormonal			
Birth control pill	Estrogen and progesterone or progesterone alone taken orally to prevent ovulation	Highly effective; requires no last-minute preparation	Alters physiology; possible serious side effects
Birth control injection	Injection of synthetic progesterone every 3 months to prevent ovulation	Highly effective, lasts for 3–4 months	Alters physiology; possible side effects include menstrual irregularity, amenorrhea
Birth control implants	Devices containing synthetic progesterone implanted under skin prevent ovulation	Highly effective; lasts for 5 years	Alters physiology; possible side effects include menstrual irregularity, amenorrhea; expensive
Barrier			
Male condom	Sheath that fits over erect penis and prevents release of semen	Easily available; does not affect physiology; protects against sexually transmitted disease (STD)	Must be applied just before intercourse, may slip or tear
Female condom	Sheath that fits in vagina, held in place with rings	Easily available; protects against STD	More expensive than male condom; must be applied before intercourse
Diaphragm (with spermicide)	Rubber cap that fits over cervix and prevents entrance of sperm	Does not affect physiology; some protection against STD	Must be inserted before intercourse; requires fitting by physician
Other			
Spermicide	Chemicals used to kill sperm; best when used in combination with a barrier method	Easily available, does not affect physiology; some protection against STD	Local irritation; must be used just before intercourse
Fertility awareness	Abstinence during fertile part of cycles as determined by menstrual history, basal body temperature, or quality of cervical mucus	Does not affect physiology; accepted by certain religions	High failure rate; requires careful record keeping

From Memmler, R. L., Cohen, B. J., Wood, D. L. (1996). The Human Body in Health and Disease, 8th ed., p. 373. Philadelphia: Lippincott-Raven Publishers.

about the various methods, including the indications, risk factors, cost, and effectiveness. Both the physician and medical assistant should be prepared to educate and advise the patient regarding the choice of contraception.

Certain methods of contraception will require the patient to undergo an invasive procedure. These methods and procedures are discussed below.

Intrauterine Device (IUD)

The IUD is a sterile device that is inserted into the uterine cavity to prevent pregnancy. The presence of the device causes a local inflammatory reaction that is possibly toxic to spermatozoa before they reach the ovum. Two IUDs are currently approved for consumer use in the United States, the Progestasert and the Paragard. The IUDs are highly effective (95%) and once inserted the patient need only check the placement. Unless complications develop, the Progestasert can remain in place for 1 year and the Paragard can remain in place for 4 to 8 years. IUDs are only indicated for patients who are in monogamous relationships, are multiparous, and who have no history of pelvic inflammatory diseases.

The insertion of the IUD is recommended during menses because the uterine os will be slightly dilated, which facilitates the procedure. The physician can also be assured that the patient is not pregnant. Furthermore, slight cramping and bleeding, which is to be expected, will not be as alarming to the patient at the time of menses. Some physicians, on the other hand, prefer not to insert IUDs during menses because of increased risk of infection and because growing evidence indicates that the expulsion rate is higher right after menses.

The procedure is invasive; therefore, written, informed consent should be obtained from the patient. Federal regulations mandate that the patient be provided with product information and be counseled about the safety and effectiveness of the IUD. The package insert provides information to the patient on the risks, alternatives, and efficacy of the IUD. Once the patient reads the information and signs it, the documentation should be added to the patient record. A copy should be given to the patient.

Always reinforce the physician's instructions regarding expected and unexpected side effects. There is usually some increase in bleeding and cramping during menses; this usually subsides after the device has been in place for several months. The patient should be advised to notify the office if she misses a period; experiences heavy bleeding, severe cramping, unusual vaginal discharge, or lower abdominal pain; has unexplained fever or chills; or is unable to locate the string or the string feels longer.

Charting Example	
01/08/98	1300	Patient read and signed consent form, positioned in lithotomy, and an IUD was inserted by Dr. Lyons. Patient instructed on procedure for caring for IUD and checking placement. Patient checked placement without trouble. Patient tolerated procedure well, no signs of bleeding. ——— Robin Jones, RMA

When setting up for the procedure, you will need to first prepare for the pelvic examination and assemble materials for the sterile field. To maintain strict sterile technique, the sterile field should be set up just before the procedure. Sterile transfer forceps or sterile gloves should be used while preparing the sterile field. When preparing the antiseptic, note that some physicians may prefer the solution be poured directly onto the 4 × 4 gauze, which remains on top of the packaging as opposed to using sterile containers. If so, do not pour the solution until the physician is ready to cleanse the cervix. (Procedure 43-3)

Removal of an IUD is usually accomplished in patients who do not tolerate the IUD or who desire pregnancy, or in those situations in which the IUD has expired. It is a simple procedure in which the physician grasps the string with a uterine dressing forceps or other instrument and gently retrieves the device (Procedure 41-4). The patient should be prepared for some temporary cramping and slight bleeding.

Checkpoint Question

11. What are the benefits and drawbacks of IUD insertion during menses?

Subdermal Hormone Implants

This form of birth control involves the subdermal implantation of six capsules that contain levonorgestrel (Norplant System), which is a hormone that

<table>
<tr></tr>
</table>

Procedure 41-3

Assisting With the Insertion of an Intrauterine Device

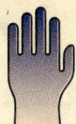

Equipment/Supplies

- setup for pelvic examination
- sanitary pad
- cleansing tissues or personal wipes
- biohazard barrier devices, as appropriate

- sterile gloves for medical assistant or sterile transfer forceps
- scissors

On the Sterile Field
- uterine tenaculum
- uterine sound
- antiseptic solution (Betadine)
- container for solution

- 4 × 4 sterile gauze
- IUD insertion kit
- sterile gloves for physician (possibly at the side)

Steps	Purpose
1. Verify that the patient has signed the consent form.	1. Federal regulations require an informed consent for IUD insertion.
2. Wash your hands.	2. Handwashing aids infection control.
3. Prepare equipment and supplies as needed for the pelvic examination (see Procedure 41-1).	
4. Greet and identify the patient. Explain the procedure.	4. Identifying the patient prevents errors. Understanding what to expect reduces anxiety and enhances patient cooperation.
5. Position and drape the patient in the dorsal lithotomy position, as you would for the pelvic examination.	5. Proper positioning will facilitate the examination.
6. Put on gloves or use sterile transfer forceps. Set up the sterile field using strict sterile technique.	6. An invasive procedure mandates sterile technique to reduce the risk of infection.
7. Pour antiseptic solution into the sterile container on the sterile field.	7. Antiseptic solution, such as Betadine, reduces the risk of infection.
8. Assist the physician as directed with gloving and gowning. Adjust the light source over the genitalia.	8. This facilitates the procedure.
9. Open the IUD insertion kit with sterile technique. Drop it onto the sterile field or allow the physician to grasp it from the opened package. The physician will insert the IUD at this point.	9. Sterile technique must be maintained.
10. Have scissors available for the physician.	10. Scissors are used to trim the string of the IUD so that it extends just beyond the external opening of the cervical os.
11. Assist the patient back up on the table and help her remove her legs from the stirrups.	11. Assisting the patient gives you the opportunity to assess her response to the procedure.
12. Provide the patient with cleansing tissues or personal wipes.	12. These may be used to wipe away any secretions.
13. Instruct the patient on how and when to check for IUD placement.	13. IUD placement must be checked after each menstruation to be sure of correct position.
14. Have the patient check for the placement of the IUD before leaving the office.	14. Patient compliance is increased with understanding of what is expected. If she has difficulty palpating the string in the office, it will be easier to give further instructions now than by phone later.

(continued)

Procedure 41-3   Assisting With the Insertion of an Intrauterine Device *(continued)*

Steps	Purpose
15. Offer the patient a sanitary pad for small amounts of bleeding that may occur.	15. The procedure may cause slight bleeding with uterine cramps.
16. Thank the patient. Reinforce the physician's instructions regarding follow-up and side effects. (If there are no problems, a follow-up visit should be within 4 to 6 weeks.)	16. Courtesy encourages the patient to have a positive attitude about the physician's office.
17. Properly care for or dispose of equipment and supplies. Clean the room. Wash your hands.	17. This prevents the spread of microorganisms.
18. Document the procedure, including date, time, patient tolerance of procedure, and patient education.	18. Procedures are considered not to have been done if they are not recorded.

inhibits ovulation. The implants are usually inserted into the inner surface of the upper arm (Procedure 41-5). Removal of the implants may be necessary because of bleeding, headaches, weight gain, depression, acne, anxiety, nervousness, and breast pain or tenderness.

This is an invasive procedure and therefore requires a written consent. The Norplant System contains a product insert that the patient must read. Ask if she has questions about the implants or the procedure. The procedure for insertion can be performed within a short period of time, usually less than 10 minutes. However, the procedure for removal may take more time because fibrous tissue often forms a capsule around the implants making retrieval more difficult. Occasionally, the devices must be removed by a surgeon. Let the patient know that contraception is achieved within 24 hours of the procedure.

➤ MENOPAUSE

Menopause, or the climacteric period, is the developmental stage during which the ability of the woman to reproduce ceases because of decreasing ovarian func-

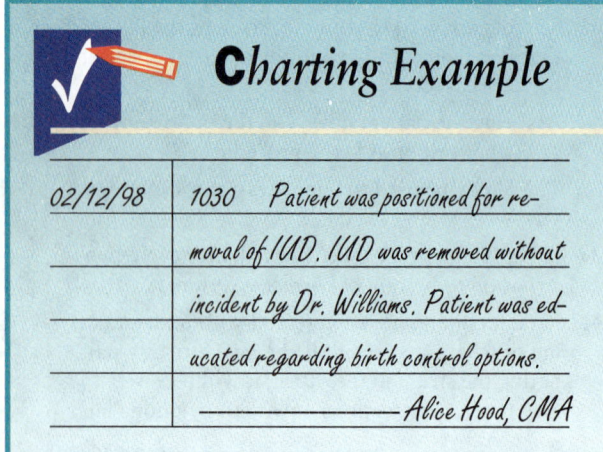

Charting Example

02/12/98	1030	Patient was positioned for removal of IUD. IUD was removed without incident by Dr. Williams. Patient was educated regarding birth control options.
		———— Alice Hood, CMA

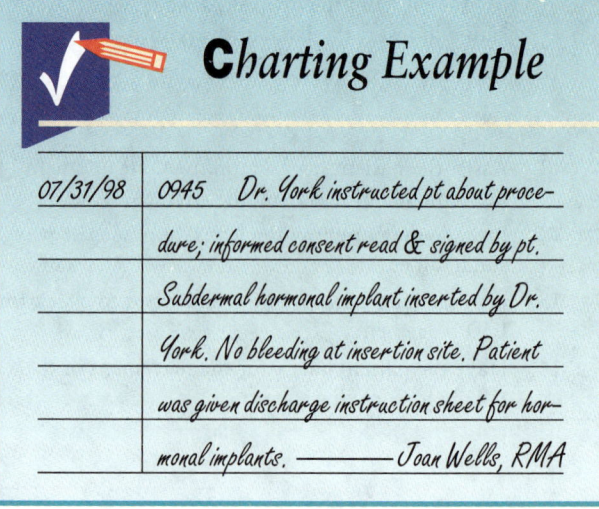

Charting Example

07/31/98	0945	Dr. York instructed pt about procedure; informed consent read & signed by pt. Subdermal hormonal implant inserted by Dr. York. No bleeding at insertion site. Patient was given discharge instruction sheet for hormonal implants. ———— Joan Wells, RMA

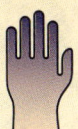

Procedure 41-4   Assisting With Removal of an Intrauterine Device

Equipment/Supplies

- patient drape
- vaginal speculum
- uterine dressing forceps
- gloves
- direct lighting
- cleansing tissues or personal wipes
- sanitary pad or tampon

Steps	Purpose
1. Wash your hands.	1. Handwashing aids infection control.
2. Set up equipment and supplies as for the pelvic examinations (see Procedure 41-1).	
3. Greet and identify the patient. Explain the procedure.	3. Identifying the patient prevents errors. Explaining the procedure helps ease anxiety and ensure compliance.
4. Position the patient in the dorsal lithotomy position.	4. This position makes visualizing the string easier for the physician.
5. Glove and assist the physician as required—adjust the light source, hand the instruments, and receive the contaminated materials on tray or basin.	5. Anticipating each step will facilitate the procedure and increase the confidence of the physician and patient. Standard Precautions must be observed to avoid exposure to hazardous material.
6. Assist the patient back up on the table and remove her legs from the stirrups.	6. Assisting the patient protects her from injury and allows you time to assess her response to the procedure.
7. Offer the patient a sanitary pad or tampon.	7. There may be a small amount of bleeding after IUD removal.
8. Thank the patient. Reinforce the physician's instructions.	8. Courtesy encourages the patient to have a positive attitude about the physician's office.
9. Properly care for or dispose of equipment and supplies. Clean the examination room. Wash your hands.	9. This prevents the spread of microorganisms.
10. Document the procedure, including date, time, patient response and tolerance, and patient education.	10. Procedures are considered not to have been done if they are not recorded.

tion. The climacteric period is characterized by the cessation of the menstrual cycle and usually occurs around 45 to 50 years of age. Perimenopause occurs before menopause and includes changes in the menstrual cycle such as oligomenorrhea, amenorrhea, dysfunctional uterine bleeding, and hot flashes, flushing, or perspiration.

The decrease in circulating estrogen has been implicated in an increase in the risk of atherosclerosis, coronary heart disease, and osteoporosis (brittle bones). Supplementary estrogen (hormonal replacement therapy or HRT) protects against the cardiovascular and skeletal disorders and decreases the menopausal symp-

toms such as hot flashes, depression, and drying of the vaginal mucosa. Estrogen is given alone after a hysterectomy or estrogen and progesterone are given in combination if the woman still has her uterus. In addition to an active exercise program, dietary calcium, and a healthy and moderate life-style, HRT will help menopausal women retain optimum health and vitality. For those with only minor menopausal symptoms, weight-bearing exercises, a healthy diet, and vitamin and mineral supplements have eased the transition through the menopausal stage.

There is inconclusive and conflicting evidence regarding HRT and an increase in the risk of reproduc-

Procedure 41-5 Assisting With the Insertion of Subdermal Hormonal Implants

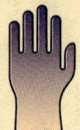

Equipment/Supplies

- Norplant System Kit (completely self contained with all essential materials
- sterile gloves

- sterile towel
- light source
- local anesthetic

Additional Materials on Sterile Field
- antiseptic solution
- sterile container for antiseptic
- sterile syringe (3 or 5 mL)

- sterile needle (1 inch, 23–25 gauge)
- sterile 4 × 4 gauze

Steps	Purpose
1. Verify that the patient signed the consent form. Make sure the patient understands all aspects of the procedure.	1. Invasive procedures require written, informed consent. Patients will be more compliant if they understand the procedure.
2. Wash your hands.	2. Handwashing aids infection control.
3. Position the patient in the supine position.	3. The position should be comfortable for the patient to enhance relaxation and should make insertion easier for the physician.
4. Assemble the equipment and supplies.	4. This ensures that everything you need is available.
5. Set up the sterile field. Pour antiseptic solution. Open and drop gauze, syringe, and needle onto field. Open Norplant system and drop onto field. *Note:* Antiseptic solution can be poured into the sterile container on the field *or* onto 4 x 4 sterile gauze that remain on top of the inside of the packaging. *Note:* The physician may prefer to administer the local anesthetic before gloving. If he prefers to inject after gloving, use the following procedure.	
6. Cleanse top of anesthetic vial with alcohol prep.	6. The use of antiseptic reduces the risk of contamination.
7. Hold anesthetic vial in the physician's preferred position while physician aspirates anesthetic into syringe.	7. Assisting the physician maintains strict sterile technique.
8. Assist the physician as necessary during the implant insertion.	
9. Help the patient into an upright position.	9. Assisting the patient conveys a sincere, caring attitude. Some patients may become dizzy after procedures; assisting may prevent a fall.
10. Thank the patient. Reinforce the physician's instructions.	10. Courtesy encourages the patient to have a positive attitude about the physician's office. Patient understanding of follow-up, side effects, and wound care will enhance compliance to therapy.
11. Properly care for or dispose of equipment and supplies. Clean the room. Wash your hands.	11. This prevents the spread of microorganisms.
12. Document the procedure, including date, time, procedure, patient tolerance, follow-up instructions, and your signature.	12. Procedures are considered not to have been done if they are not recorded.

tive cancers. This concern can be alleviated by regular Pap smears and mammograms.

SUMMARY

Assisting in obstetrics and gynecology is a challenging and fascinating area of medicine. The female reproductive system is highly complex and miraculous when considering the female's ability to bring about dramatic changes in her own growth and development and her ability to produce a healthy newborn. The medical office visit may be an emotional and intimidating experience for the female patient. As a professional medical assistant, you are in a unique position to provide the patient with reassurance and emotional support that may prove to be comforting to the patient and rewarding to you.

CRITICAL THINKING CHALLENGES

1. A multiparous patient who is married and has a history of cigarette smoking desires a highly effective method of contraception. What are her choices for contraception? Explain which choice is best and why.
2. A patient who has a scheduled appointment is complaining of painful blisters in the vaginal and vulvular area. What type of examination would you prepare for? Why?
3. Your patient has both genital herpes and condylomata acuminata. She wants to know if these disorders are contagious and how they can be cured. How would you respond to these questions?

ANSWERS TO CHECKPOINT QUESTIONS

1. The uterus is composed of the endometrium (the inner layer, which has a rich blood supply), the myometrium (the middle, muscular layer), and the perimetrium (connective tissue).
2. The primary characteristic of the secretory phase of the menstrual cycle is the impact of progesterone on the endometrium, which becomes highly vascular and rich in glycogen as it prepares for a possible pregnancy.
3. Dysfunctional uterine bleeding includes menorrhagia (excessive bleeding), metrorrhagia (irregular bleeding), polymenorrhea (abnormally frequent bleeding), and postmenopausal bleeding not associated with tumor, inflammation, or pregnancy.
4. Genital warts have been implicated in an increase in cervical cancer.
5. The prognosis of all cancers is much better with early diagnosis and treatment.

6. As part of a complete gynecologic examination, the physician examines the patient's breasts and performs a pelvic examination with Pap smear.
7. The presumptive signs and symptoms of pregnancy are not conclusive because they may indicate other disorders.
8. The pregnant patient should notify the physician if there is vaginal bleeding or spotting, persistent vomiting, fever or chills, dysuria, or abdominal or uterine cramping, leaking amniotic fluid, altered fetal movement, dizziness, or blurred vision.
9. Placenta previa is a condition in which the placenta is implanted either partly or completely over the internal cervical os. In the preterm patient, the condition is managed with bed rest and drug therapy.
10. Lochia is a discharge from the uterus composed of mucus, blood, and tissue. Types include lochia rubra (blood tinged), lochia serosa (thin, brownish discharge), lochia alba (white discharge with no evidence of blood).
11. During menses, the uterine os will be slightly dilated, facilitating insertion of the IUD. Also, the physician can be certain that the patient is not pregnant. Furthermore, slight cramping and bleeding will not be as alarming to the patient at the time of menses. However, some physicians prefer not to insert IUDs during menses because of increased risk of infection and because growing evidence indicates that the expulsion rate is higher right after menses.

SUGGESTIONS FOR FURTHER READING

Berkow, R., ed. (1992). *The Merck Manual.* Rahway, NJ: Merck Sharp and Dohme Research Laboratories, Division of Merck and Co, Inc.

DeDona, N. A., Marks, M. A. (1996). *Introducing Maternal-Newborn Nursing.* Philadelphia: Lippincott-Raven Publishers.

Glass, R. H., ed. (1993). *Office Gynecology.* Baltimore: Williams & Wilkins.

Nettina, S. M. (1996). *The Lippincott Manual of Nursing Practice,* 6th ed. Philadelphia: Lippincott-Raven Publishers.

Pillitteri, A. (1995). *Maternal and Child-Health Nursing: Care of the Child-Bearing and Child-Rearing Family,* 2nd ed. Philadelphia: Lippincott-Raven Publishers.

Reeder, S. J., Martin, L. L., & Koniak, D. (1992). *Maternity Nursing: Family, Newborn and Women's Health Care,* 17th ed. Philadelphia: J. B. Lippincott.

Rosdahl, C. B. (1995). *Textbook of Basic Nursing,* 6th ed. Philadelphia: J. B. Lippincott.

Scott, J. R., DiSaia, P. J., Hammond, C. B., & Spellacy, W. N. (1994). *Danforth's Obstetrics and Gynecology,* 7th ed. Philadelphia: J. B. Lippincott.

Unit 7

Performing Laboratory Procedures

Piecing together the puzzle of illness requires examining the minute and microscopic components responsible for cellular function. No picture of health or disease is complete without understanding how the body's smallest elements are integral to the total concept of health.

Introduction to the Clinical Laboratory

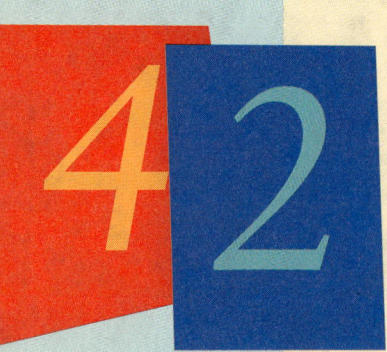

Chapter Outline

Laboratory Types
    Reference Laboratory
    Hospital Laboratory
    Physician's Office Laboratory
Laboratory Departments
    Hematology
    Coagulation
    Clinical Chemistry
    Toxicology
    Urinalysis
    Blood Bank or Immuno-
        hematology
    Serology
    Microbiology
    Pathology
Laboratory Personnel
Physician's Office Laboratory Testing
Laboratory Equipment

    Cell Counters
    Microscope
    Chemistry Analyzers
    Centrifuges
    Refrigerators and Freezers
    Glassware
Laboratory Safety
    Occupational Health and Safety
        Administration
    Important Rules to Follow
Clinical Laboratory Improvement
  Amendments
    Levels of Testing Complexity
    Laboratory Standards
Summary
Critical Thinking Challenges
Answers to Checkpoint Questions
Suggestions for Further Reading

DACUM Components

1.2   Perform within ethical boundaries
4.9   Use quality control
6.2   Operate and maintain facilities and equipment safely

Chapter Competencies

Learning Objectives

Upon successfully completing this chapter, you will be able to:

1. Spell and define the Key Terms.
2. List reasons for laboratory testing.
3. Outline the medical assistant's responsibility in the clinical laboratory.
4. Name the kinds of laboratories available to the medical assistant and the functions of each.
5. List the types of personnel found in laboratories and describe their jobs.
6. Name the types of departments found in most large laboratories and give their purposes.
7. Explain how to use a package insert to determine the procedure for a laboratory test.
8. List the equipment found in most small laboratories and give the purpose of each.
9. List and describe the parts of a microscope.
10. List the safety rules for laboratories.
11. Explain the significance of the CLIA and how to work within its guidelines to ensure quality control.

Performance Objective

Upon successfully completing this chapter, you will be able to:

1. Care for the microscope.

Key Terms

(See Glossary for definitions.)

aerosol
anticoagulant
calibration
capillary action
centrifugal force
Clinical Laboratory Improvement Amendment (CLIA)
material safety data sheet (MSDS)
National Committee for Clinical Laboratory Standards (NCCLS)
normal value
quality control
reagent
specimen

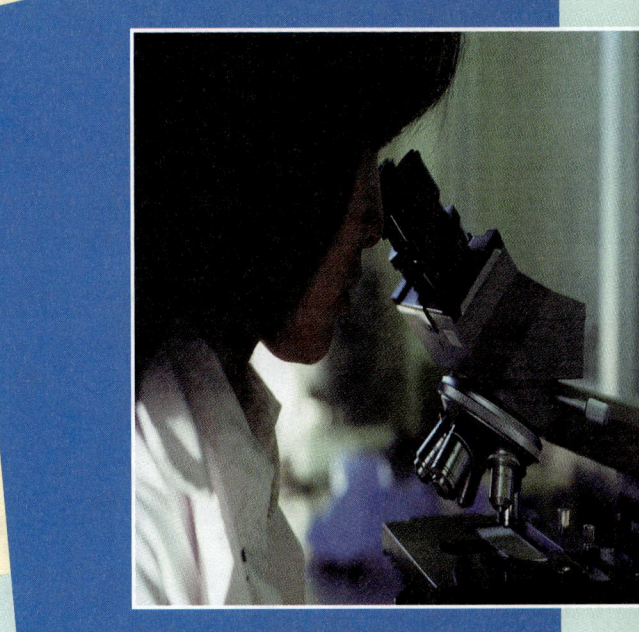

The medical laboratory provides the physician with one of medicine's most powerful diagnostic tools. It can aid the physician in managing medications and in following the progress of patients' diseases. Laboratory personnel analyze blood, urine, and other body samples to identify diseases and disorders. Results of laboratory testing are compared with **normal values** (acceptable ranges) to determine the relative health of body systems or organs. Blood levels of various medications are determined to adjust dosages to therapeutic levels. Bacteria, viruses, parasites, and other microorganisms are identified to begin the treatment process. (See Appendix VII for a list of commonly performed laboratory tests and their normal values.)

Laboratory testing is most commonly used for:

- Diagnosing a disease
- Following the progress of a disease
- Meeting legal requirements (eg, drug testing, a marriage license)
- Monitoring a patient's medication levels
- Determining the levels of essential substances produced by the body
- Identifying the cause of an infection
- Determining a baseline

As a medical assistant, you will play an important role in laboratory analysis—even in instances in which testing is performed at sites other than the medical office. In general, you may be responsible for:

- Educating patients before obtaining laboratory **specimens** (small samples of something used to evaluate the whole)
- Obtaining a quality specimen
- Arranging for appropriate transport if the specimen is to be analyzed at another site
- Performing common laboratory tests in the physician's office and clinics
- Ensuring **quality control** (evaluating proper performance of laboratory testing procedures, supplies, or equipment)
- Maintaining laboratory instruments and equipment

Medical assistants also may control purchasing of laboratory supplies and selection of **reagents**, substances used to produce a reaction in testing situations. In addition, they may be in charge of biohazard safety and waste disposal for their workplace. This chapter outlines the basic information you will need to ensure the quality of the laboratory testing in your facility.

➤ LABORATORY TYPES

There are many kinds of laboratories, but three of the most common types you may encounter include reference, hospital, and physician's office (or clinical) labora-

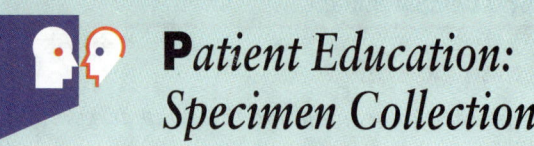

Patient Education: Specimen Collection

At the time of specimen collection, educate the patient about:

- the name of the test (eg, blood cell count)
- the type of specimen required (eg, blood, stool, urine)
- why the test is being performed

Be sure to tell the patient approximately how long it will take for the results to be available and how and by whom the patient will be contacted regarding the results.

Patient education requirements for drawing a human immunodeficiency virus (HIV) test vary from state to state although most require pre- and post-test counseling. Additionally, most states do not allow HIV test results to be given over the telephone.

tories. Hospital and reference laboratories may perform hundreds of different specialized tests and may process thousands of patient samples per day. In contrast, physician's office laboratories (POL) perform only a few types of tests on a limited number of patients.

Reference Laboratory

A reference laboratory is a large facility, similar to a factory, in which thousands of tests of different types are performed each day. A reference laboratory seldom has contact with patients. Instead, it receives specimens from physicians' offices, hospitals, and clinics across the region it serves. Specimens, which are packaged in special transport containers (Fig. 42-1), may be collected for transport by courier, airplane, or mail. Tests are performed in large batches and results and reports are managed by large computer systems. Reference laboratories are not usually responsible for reporting test results to patients. Test results are generally returned to the referring physician who will then relay the results to the patient.

Most employees of reference laboratories have specific job descriptions. *Accessioners* may sort specimens and enter data into computers, which route specimens to various departments to be tested. *Laboratory technicians* and *technologists* perform tests on large automated instruments and equipment and keep records of machine maintenance and quality control. *Customer service personnel* answer telephones to track

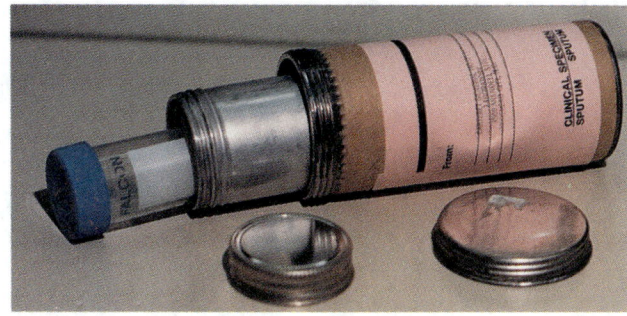

FIGURE 42-1
Transport containers are constructed to maintain the integrity of the transported specimen and to protect those who are responsible for the care and handling of potentially hazardous body fluids and substances.

specimens and report results back to the centers where the specimens were collected. Both accessioning and customer service are areas where medical assistants may be employed in the larger laboratories.

Hospital Laboratory

The hospital laboratory primarily serves patients who are admitted to the hospital. However, it may also serve outpatients to some degree, especially with outpatient surgery allowing for shorter hospital stays. Hospital laboratory workers include *phlebotomists* who collect and process blood samples, *technicians* and *technologists* who perform the tests, and *secretaries* who manage the large volume of test results and other information. Medical assistants are often trained and employed as phlebotomists in laboratories or may serve as the secretary to a laboratory unit.

A hospital laboratory performs batches of common tests on large automated and computerized machines. These batches of samples may help in daily monitoring of patients' cell counts and levels of certain chemicals. Hospital laboratories also respond to STAT requests for immediate results on individual tests. This serves the needs of the emergency room, intensive care units, and surgical center for instant results on patients' conditions.

Most hospital laboratories do not perform every possible type of test. The test menu is usually restricted to those tests that are most commonly requested and those for which results are needed immediately. Samples that require more sophisticated testing are usually sent to reference laboratories. Results from referred or on-site testing are generally available within a short time.

Laboratory Request Forms

Hospital and reference laboratories design forms for requests to suit their individual operations (Fig. 42-2). These forms should be convenient to use, with clear instructions for complete patient and physician identification to avoid errors. Most request forms cover a variety of tests so that a single form can be used for tests in hematology, chemistry, serology, and so on. Many also list the normal values for each test as an instant alert. Box 42-1 lists the information required on all laboratory request forms.

Physician's Office Laboratory

The third common type of laboratory is the physician's office laboratory (POL). There are more of these laboratories than any other type, and they vary greatly in size and quality. POLs generally perform a limited number of low- to moderate-complexity tests (see section "Levels of Testing Complexity," below). Samples for less common or more complex tests may be obtained here but are sent to hospital or reference laboratories for testing.

The most common tests in this type of laboratory are urinalysis, blood cell counts, hemoglobin and hematocrit, and blood glucose or cholesterol levels. In some small laboratories, pregnancy tests and quick screening tests for diseases such as mononucleosis and strep throat are available. Like hospital and reference laboratories, some POLs use forms that list normal adult ranges for various tests (Fig. 42-3).

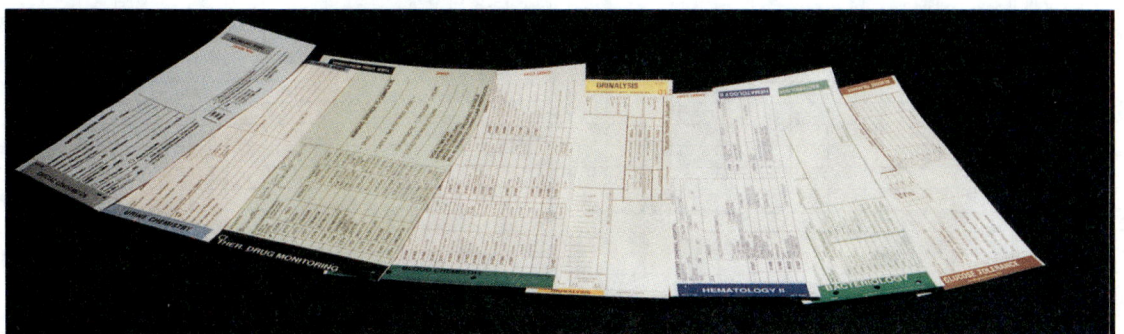

FIGURE 42-2
Laboratory request forms commonly used in a hospital setting.

BOX 42-1 Laboratory Request Forms: Commonly Required Information

- Patient data base. This includes name, address, Social Security number, and the medical office identification number to avoid errors with identical names. Other identifying information may be included.
- Patient birth date and gender. Some test results will vary with age and sex.
- Date and time of collection. Many types of test results will be altered or affected by the passage of time or the time of day the specimen was collected.
- Physician's name and address or identification number (if a contract exists with the office and laboratory). Results may need to be reported immediately; having this information also avoids errors in reporting.
- Checklist of the test(s) to be performed. These may be grouped under one heading as a "profile" (such as a thyroid profile or a liver profile), which will include more than one test to determine the state of health of one organ, or a general health profile, such as a complete blood count (CBC).

Other information that may be required might include the source of the specimen (such as culture swabs for microbiology tests), a list of medications the patient is taking that may alter certain test results (eg, anticoagulants affect prothrombin time), directions for reporting (eg, an immediate need should be marked STAT), and total volume of a 24-hour urine specimen.

FIGURE 42-3

Laboratory data sheet. Note that normal values are provided for the various tests.

LABORATORY DATA SHEET (Patient Identification)

LAB TEST	ADULT NORMAL RANGE
WBC x 10³	4.8-10.8
RBC x 10⁶	M 4.4-6.0 / F 4.2-5.4
Hgb gm	M 13.0-17.0 / F 12.0-16.0
Hct %	M 41-51 / F 37-47
MCV m3	80-96
MCH mmg	27-31
MCHC %	32-36
Polys %	25-62
Band %	0-22
Lymph %	20-53
Mono %	2-12
Eos %	0-2
Sed Rate (West)	M 0-10 mm/hr / F 0-20 mm/hr
Color	amber
Sp. G	1.001-1.035
pH	4.6-8.0
Protein	0
Sugar	0
Ketones	0
Bilirubin	0
Blood	0
WBC	0-5/HPF
RBC	0-3/HPF
Bacteria	0
Vag. Saline	0 trich.
KOH	0 monilia
Uricult	0
Throat	0 Gp. A Strep
G.C.	0

LABORATORY DATA SHEET (Patient Identification)

LAB TEST	ADULT NORMAL RANGE
Gluc. (Random)	
Gluc. (Fasting)	65-110 mg/dl
Gluc. 2 hr. pc.	Less than 120
BUN	10-25 mg/dl
Creatinine	0.7-1.4 mg/dl
Na	135-145 meq/L
K	3.5-5.0 meq/L
Cl	95-105 meq/L
CO_2	24-32 meq/L
Uric A.	2.5-8.0 mg/dl
T. Protein	6.0-8.0 g/dl
Albumin	3.5-5.0 g/dl
Globulin	2.5-3.2 g/dl
A/G	0.9-1.9
Calcium	8.5-11.0 mg/dl
Phos.	2.5-4.5 mg/dl
Chol.	150-300 mg/dl
Trig.	30-200 mg/dl
Alk. Phos.	30-115 U/L
SGOT	7-40 U/L
SGPT	7-40 U/L
LDH	100-225 U/L
T. Bili.	0.2-1.5 mg/dl
D. Bili.	0.2-0.5 mg/dl
Ind. Bili.	0.2-1.0 mg/dl
T_4 RIA	3.8-11.4 meg %
T_3 Uptake	25-35 %
T_7 Index	0.9-3.9 units
TSH	2-10 microunits/ml

A small office laboratory may have only one or two employees who perform all of the duties: collecting samples, performing tests, managing quality control, maintaining instruments, keeping accurate records, and reporting results. In many of these laboratories, medical assistants perform all of these tasks, with a physician monitoring quality control and abnormal results. The chapters in this unit will introduce you to the skills and knowledge necessary to operate a physician's small office laboratory.

> **Checkpoint Question**
>
> **?**
>
> 1. *What is a reference laboratory and how does it differ from a physician's office laboratory? Name and describe the kinds of positions that a medical assistant may hold in a reference laboratory.*

➤ LABORATORY DEPARTMENTS

Most large laboratories are divided into departments. This makes it easier to divide the workload and to group similar kinds of tests together. Small laboratories, such as physician's office laboratories, may have only one department in which all tests are done. Even so, it may be easier to understand the nature of the tests and the information they provide if the basic divisions of laboratory testing are understood.

Below is a list of common laboratory departments, their possible subdivisions, and the kinds of testing performed in each. (See the appropriate chapters in Unit 7 for more specific information about the testing mentioned here.)

Hematology

The hematology department is responsible for studies of the blood. The various types of cells in the blood and the amount or number of each type of cell are determined in this department. Common tests include complete blood count (CBC), hemoglobin (Hgb, Hg) and hematocrit (Hct), white blood cell count (WBC) and differential (diff), and erythrocyte sedimentation rate (ESR).

Coagulation

Often a part of the hematology department, coagulation testing involves evaluating how well the body reacts when blood vessels are injured. The most common tests are prothrombin times (PT), partial prothrombin times (PTT), fibrinogens, and bleeding times. These tests are also used to monitor levels of anticoagulant

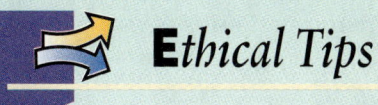

Ethical Tips

While working in a laboratory setting, you will have access to the results of many confidential blood and urine tests, such as tests for human immunodeficiency virus (HIV), drugs, pregnancy, and syphilis. You have an ethical responsibility not to communicate any results to unauthorized persons. Only patients and their physicians are entitled to the results. The only exception is the provision in state laws requiring the reporting of certain test results for public safety.

drugs, such as heparin and Coumadin, during medication therapy. An **anticoagulant** is anything that prevents or delays blood clotting.

Clinical Chemistry

In the clinical chemistry department, chemical substances in blood or serum are measured. These substances may include hormones, enzymes, electrolytes, gases, medicines and drugs, sugars, proteins, fats, and waste products. In large laboratories, chemistry profiles often contain 12 to 20 different chemical analyses. The most common tests in small laboratories are glucose, cholesterol, blood urea nitrogen (BUN), and electrolytes.

Toxicology

Toxicology is often a separate department in the chemistry laboratory. Toxicology testing involves measuring blood levels of both therapeutic drugs and drugs of abuse.

Urinalysis

Urinalysis evaluates both the chemical properties of urine and the types and numbers of cells it contains. A complete urinalysis contains both of these evaluations. Pregnancy tests may also be done in this department. Occasionally, this area is found in either the hematology, chemistry, or microbiology departments.

Blood Bank or Immunohematology

This department is generally found only in hospitals and special blood donor centers. Blood is prepared and stored in the blood bank or immunohematology department for future transfusions.

Serology

Testing in the serology department is based on the reactions of antibodies formed against certain diseases in the presence of proteins called antigens. Recent advances in serology testing have produced quick and accurate tests for diagnosing many diseases, including syphilis, human immunodeficiency virus (HIV), and mononucleosis.

Microbiology

The microbiology department identifies the various microorganisms that cause disease. Through sensitivity testing, microbiology identifies which antibiotics will successfully treat infections grown from patient specimens. Microbiology may include one or more of the following:

- Bacteriology—study of bacteria
- Virology—study of viruses
- Mycology—study of fungi and yeasts
- Parasitology—study of parasitic protozoa and worms

Pathology

The characteristics, causes, and effects of disease are determined in the pathology department by observing the structure and function of the body's cells and tissues. Cellular pathology concentrates on cellular specimens for study and clinical pathology studies disease processes by various laboratory testing procedures.

Histology and Cytology

Although in large institutions these departments may stand alone, they are frequently included as part of the pathology department. Histology is the microscopic study of the composition, organization, and function of tissues. Biopsies are referred to this department. Cytology is the study of the structure, function, pathologies, and biochemical properties of cells. Biopsies are also referred to this department, usually from an aspiration rather than an incisional biopsy. Scrapings, vaginal secretions, sputum, and smears (such as Pap smears) are referred to cytology. Chromosomal studies may also be performed in the cytology department.

Checkpoint Question

2. What departments may be found in a large laboratory? Summarize the testing done in each one.

➤ LABORATORY PERSONNEL

Within the various departments of reference and hospital laboratories, specially trained professionals oversee laboratory operations or perform the diagnostic tests required by physicians. Each professional position requires a particular level of education and training and has specific responsibilities (Box 42-2).

➤ PHYSICIAN'S OFFICE LABORATORY TESTING

Many tests can be performed in an office laboratory that meet the standards set forth by Congress in the 1988 **Clinical Laboratory Improvement Amendments (CLIA)** (see section "Clinical Laboratory Improvement Amendments," below). Most tests performed in the POL fall into one of two general categories: tests performed on a semiautomated machine or tests conducted using a self-contained kit. Tests in either of these categories will vary slightly among manufacturers.

The best source of information for safe and accurate testing is the package insert that is issued with the testing kit or the instrument reagents and quality control instructions specific for various office testing instruments. Box 42-3 outlines the type of information contained in test package inserts. For many kit tests, the package insert is the only information provided to guide the performance of the test and to evaluate the results.

Determining the key or basic information needed for test performance and quality control will make using package inserts a simple and integral part of office laboratory testing. Ask your laboratory procedures instructor for examples of package inserts from pregnancy test kits or serology test kits for practice in obtaining this information.

Checkpoint Question

3. Why are package inserts crucial for safe and accurate testing?

➤ LABORATORY EQUIPMENT

Laboratory equipment and supplies for performing physician's office tests come in hundreds of different types and sizes. It is not necessary to become familiar

BOX 42-2 Laboratory Personnel

- Pathologist: A physician who studies disease processes. Commonly, a pathologist oversees the technical aspects of a laboratory, a histology department, or a blood bank.
- Chief technologist or laboratory manager: A supervisor who manages the day-to-day operations of a laboratory, including staffing, test menu and pricing, purchasing, and quality control.
- Medical technologist: A trained professional with a college degree and advanced training in laboratory science. Medical technologists often supervise laboratory departments.
- Medical laboratory technician: A graduate of a technical program with training in laboratory testing. Technicians may perform tests and may be responsible for collecting and processing specimens as well.

- Phlebotomist: A professional trained to draw blood and to process blood and other samples. Phlebotomists may be technicians, medical assistants, or persons trained specifically in phlebotomy.
- Histologist: A technician trained to process and evaluate tissue samples, such as biopsy or surgical samples.
- Cytologist: A professional trained to examine cells under the microscope and to look for abnormal changes; Pap smears are generally examined by cytologists.
- Accessioner or specimen processor: A professional trained to accept specimens that are received by the laboratory and to centrifuge, separate, or otherwise process the samples to prepare them for testing. In addition, this position usually involves numbering and labeling the specimens and entering specimen information into a computer.

with every possible type of laboratory equipment or supply. However, a few basic pieces are common to most small laboratories. These include:

- Automated cell counter
- Microscope
- Chemistry analyzer
- Centrifuge
- Refrigerator or freezer
- Glassware

BOX 42-3 Understanding Test Package Inserts

Any test package insert will provide the following basic pieces of information.

- Procedure: Explains the test method in numbered steps, usually with illustrations.
- Test principles: Outlines the method required for the test.
- Specimen required: Tells whether the test is done on blood, urine, or other body fluids and what collection method is acceptable.
- Reagents needed (or included): Lists the reagents included in the kit and any other reagents or materials that are necessary to perform the test.
- Quality control: States recommendations for testing procedures to ensure that test results are accurate.
- Expected values: Lists normal values for comparison to results obtained.
- Interferences: Explains any factors that may alter test results or compromise test accuracy.

Cell Counter

A cell counter is used to perform hematology testing on blood specimens. The simplest cell counter is limited to counting red and white blood cells and performing hemoglobin and hematocrit testing. Specimens are inserted one at a time by the technician operating the machine, and results may be printed or may be read from a screen. (See Chap. 46, Hematology, for information on performing a cell count in the medical office.)

Cell counters increase from the basic level of complexity needed for a medical office to huge machines that accept hundreds of specimens from turntables and perform 12 to 15 tests and calculations on each specimen, recording results directly into a computer. Medical assistants would be responsible only for the most basic testing equipment.

Microscope

The microscope is used to identify and count cells and microorganisms in blood and various other body specimens. Learning how to properly use a microscope requires time and patience. Microscopes vary somewhat, but the type most commonly used in the medical office is the compound microscope. This kind of microscope uses a two-lens system in which one system increases the magnification of the other. A light source in combination with the lenses illuminates the objects as they are magnified. Figure 42-4 shows a microscope and its various parts.

The *frame*, which consists of the arm and base, is the basic nonworking structural component of the microscope. The *eyepiece* is located at the top of the instrument for the user's eye. It is marked with its magnification, usually 10×. Many microscopes are binocular (two eyepieces) to reduce eyestrain; these also have adjustments to allow for the individual differences in widths between eyes. For most people, binocular instruments are easier to use than the monocular (one eyepiece) microscope.

The eyepiece is connected by the *body tube*, which directs the visual path from the light source. To bring the object to be viewed into focus, the body tube is raised and lowered by the coarse and fine adjustment knobs. The *coarse adjustment knob* is usually used with the lower powered objective to focus on the object; the *fine adjustment knob* is used with the higher powered objective or the oil immersion lens for the greatest definition.

The *nosepiece* houses the three objective lenses and revolves to bring down the lens required for a specific test. The magnification power of the objectives is referred to as the numerical aperture. The shorter objective, or low power objective, magnifies 10 times for scanning. The higher power magnifies 40 times for closer observation. With the use of oil, the third objective, called the oil immersion lens, magnifies 100 times. If the manufacturer has not identified the lenses, the shorter is the low power and the longest is the oil immersion. In conjunction with the lens in the eyepiece, each total magnification is multiplied by 10; therefore:

- Low power equals 10 × 10 = 100 magnification
- High power equals 10 × 40 = 400 magnification
- Oil immersion equals 10 × 100 = 1000 magnification

The *stage* is the flat surface that holds the slide for viewing. An opening in the solid surface allows illumination of the slide from the power source below. Many stages have clips to hold the slide in place and to move manually as needed. Some stages mechanically adjust the position vertically or horizontally by moving adjustment knobs.

The *condenser* or *substage condenser* concentrates the light rays to focus on the slide. The condenser is adjustable. In the lower position, the light focus is reduced; in the higher position, it is increased.

The *diaphragm* is located in the condenser. It consists of interlocking plates that adjust into a variable-sized opening, or iris, to regulate the amount of light from the source in conjunction with the condenser. The

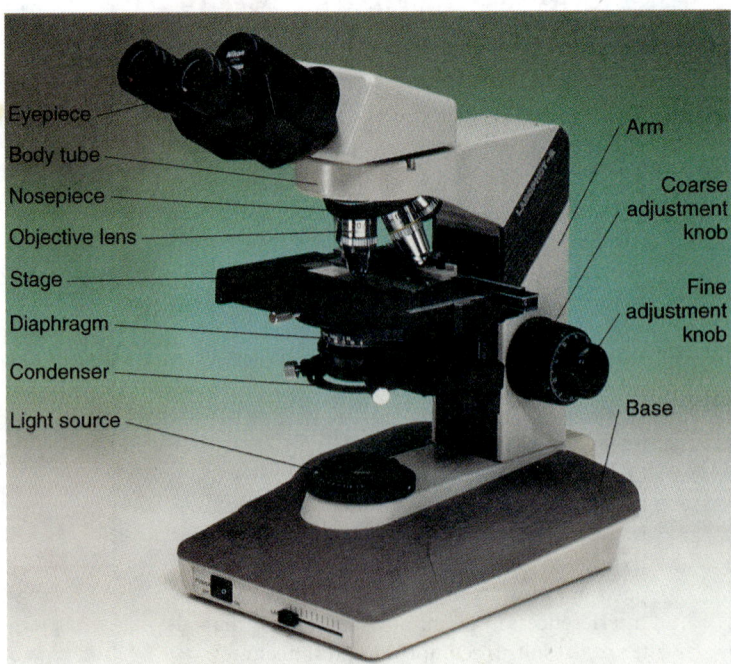

FIGURE 42-4
Basic components of the standard light microscope. (Courtesy of Nikon Inc., Melville, NY.)

BOX 42-4   Caring for the Microscope

1. Clean and service the microscope daily according to the manufacturer's recommendations.
2. To move the microscope, lift it gently by placing one hand under the base and grasping the arm with the other. Set it down gently. Never use the body or eyepieces to transport the instrument.
3. Use lens papers to clean the lens, objectives, and condenser. Never use tissue or gauze. Do not touch the glass areas with your fingers.
4. Use special lens cleaners, according to the manufacturer's recommendation, for build-up of soil.
5. Clean all nonocular areas (stage, base) with a mild soap and water. Rinse and dry thoroughly.
6. Clean the stage with gauze. If it is soiled with oil, use gauze with xylene.
7. To change the bulb for the light source, follow the manufacturer's directions. These usually recommend placing the scope carefully on its side to permit access to the cover plate. Open the plate, cover the bulb with a bulb cover to protect your hand in the event of breakage, and gently twist to release the bulb. Using the bulb cover, reverse the procedure to install a fresh bulb. Keep the light source clean by polishing with lens paper. Keep a supply of bulbs on hand.
8. To store the microscope, turn off the light source. Turn the lowest power objective toward the stage and adjust it downward as close as possible. Unplug the instrument and coil the power cord around the base. Cover with a dust cover designed for this particular microscope and secure it until it is needed again.

more highly magnified the slide must be, the greater the need for light. To visualize all structures on a slide, it is usually necessary to adjust the light source and illumination level by opening and closing the diaphragm during the entire inspection to avoid missing objects visible at variable light levels.

The *light source* is housed within the base and provides the necessary illumination.

Microscopes are delicate and expensive instruments. To ensure that the microscope used in your clinical laboratory is kept in good working order, you must handle it properly and maintain it according to the manufacturer's standards (Box 42-4).

Checkpoint Question
4. How do the three objective lenses of the microscope differ?

Chemistry Analyzers

Like cell counters, chemistry analyzers vary from simple machines that perform very few tests and require manual operation to large complex machines that perform up to 20 tests per sample and are operated by computer.

The most common type of chemistry analyzer found in the physician's office uses a disposable strip, similar to a urine dipstick. The patient's sample is measured onto the strip, and the strip is inserted into the analyzer to be read. Results may be displayed on a screen or may be printed.

Centrifuges

Many kinds of centrifuges are used in laboratories. The centrifuge uses centrifugal force, a spinning motion that exerts force outward, to separate liquids into their component parts. For instance, a whole blood specimen can be placed into a centrifuge and separated into a bottom layer of heavy red blood cells, a tiny middle layer of platelets and white blood cells called the buffy coat (Fig. 42-5), and a top liquid layer that is the lightest of the components. The top layer is serum if the specimen was allowed to clot before centrifuging or plasma if the specimen was anticoagulated and not allowed to clot.

Tubes must always be balanced in the centrifuge. If an uneven number of tubes are to be spun, a tube with water must balance the tube without a counterbalance. Try to place tubes with approximately the same level of liquid in opposing spaces. All tubes must be securely capped. Never start the machine until the lid is locked (many will not start until the lid is securely locked). NEVER open the centrifuge until all motion has stopped, and NEVER stop the spin with your hand. Follow the manufacturer's recommendations for cleaning, oiling, and maintaining the machine. As with all equipment, read the instructions before operating the machine.

Refrigerators and Freezers

Laboratory refrigerators and freezers are similar to those used in the home, but their uses are very different. They are used to store reagents, kits, and patient specimens. The temperature is critical and must be measured and recorded daily. Food should never be

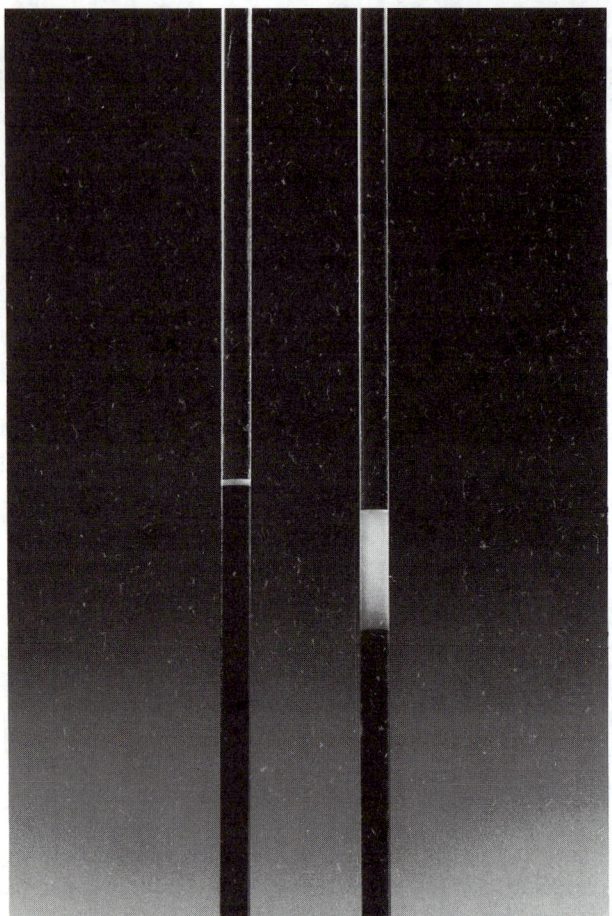

FIGURE 42-5
Comparison of a small (*left*) and large (*right*) buffy coat in hematocrit samples from two patients. Large buffy coat results from increased WBC and platelet counts.

stored in these refrigerators because of the possibility of biohazard contamination.

Glassware

For general purposes, the term glassware also includes the disposable plastic supplies used in many medical offices. As with all other medical supplies, sizes and shapes vary with the purpose. Many forms are named for their inventor or for their use. The term glassware includes the following items:

- Beakers. Containers with wide mouths and straight sides for mixing, holding, or heating liquids. They may be marked with **calibrations** (measurements for size or volume) and are supplied in various sizes.
- Flasks. Containers with narrow necks and a rounded base used for holding or transporting liquids in a laboratory. Most are marked with calibrations. Names include Florence, volumetric, and Erlenmeyer.

- Glass slides and coverslips. Used with the microscope for holding the specimen to be viewed and may or may not be disposable.
- Graduated cylinders. Used for measuring quantities of substances or solutions.
- Petri dishes or plates. Shallow, covered dishes filled with a solidified medium to support the growth of microorganisms for diagnosis.
- Pipettes (pipets). Narrow tubes (glass or plastic) sometimes graduated, open at both ends, used to transport or measure small amounts of liquid. Some pull liquid in by **capillary action**, others by mechanical suction (Fig. 42-6A). Pipettes marked TC (To Contain) are designed to hold a certain volume; those marked TD (To Deliver) are designed to dispense a certain volume. Names include Pasteur, serologic, volumetric, and Mohr (Fig. 42-6B). Box 42-5 describes how to use a pipette.
- Test tubes. Cylindrical containers usually open at one end and rounded or pointed on the other, used for holding laboratory specimens.

Figure 42-7 displays various kinds of glassware. Table 42-1 describes techniques for cleaning glassware used in the laboratory.

➤ LABORATORY SAFETY

Technicians must always be safety conscious when using laboratory equipment. All specimens studied in the laboratory should be considered potentially hazardous and must be treated as such (see Chap. 19, Asepsis and Infection Control). A technician who is aware of the types of hazards presented by the clinical laboratory is much more likely to work safely and avoid injury (Fig. 42-8). A **material safety data sheet (MSDS)** contains a detailed record of all hazardous substances kept within a site.

There are three basic types of hazards in the laboratory:

- Physical hazards (fire, broken glass, liquid spills)
- Chemical hazards (acids, alkalis, chemical fumes)
- Biologic hazards (diseases such as HIV, hepatitis, and tuberculosis)

Methods for handling each of these hazards must be outlined in detail in your facility's policies and procedures manual. Each member of the staff must be familiar with safety protocol to ensure that risks are kept at a minimum.

Employers are responsible for obtaining or developing a protocol for each hazardous agent used on site. This protocol must be bound and kept in a location near the site of use. The protocol must include specific information, which is discussed in Box 42-6.

text continues on page 829

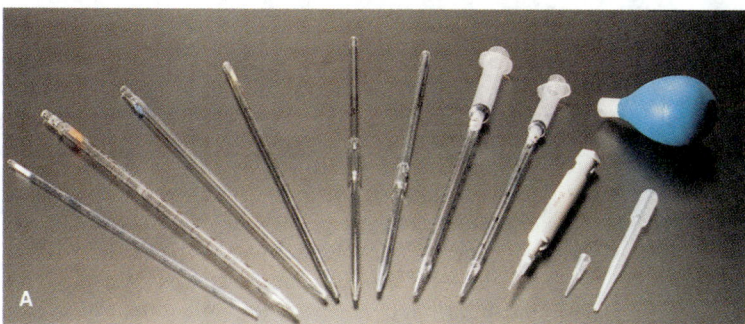

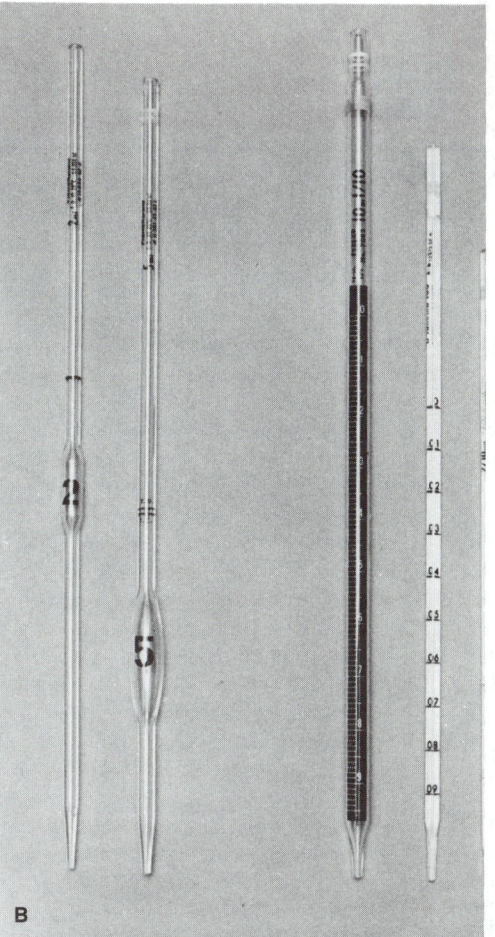

FIGURE 42-6

Assorted pipettes. (*A*) Pipettes on the right have attached or integrated suction. The bulb at top is used for suction with standard pipettes. (*B*) *From left to right:* volumetric pipette, Ostwald-Folin pipette, serologic pipette (10 ml), serologic pipette (1 ml), Mohr pipette.

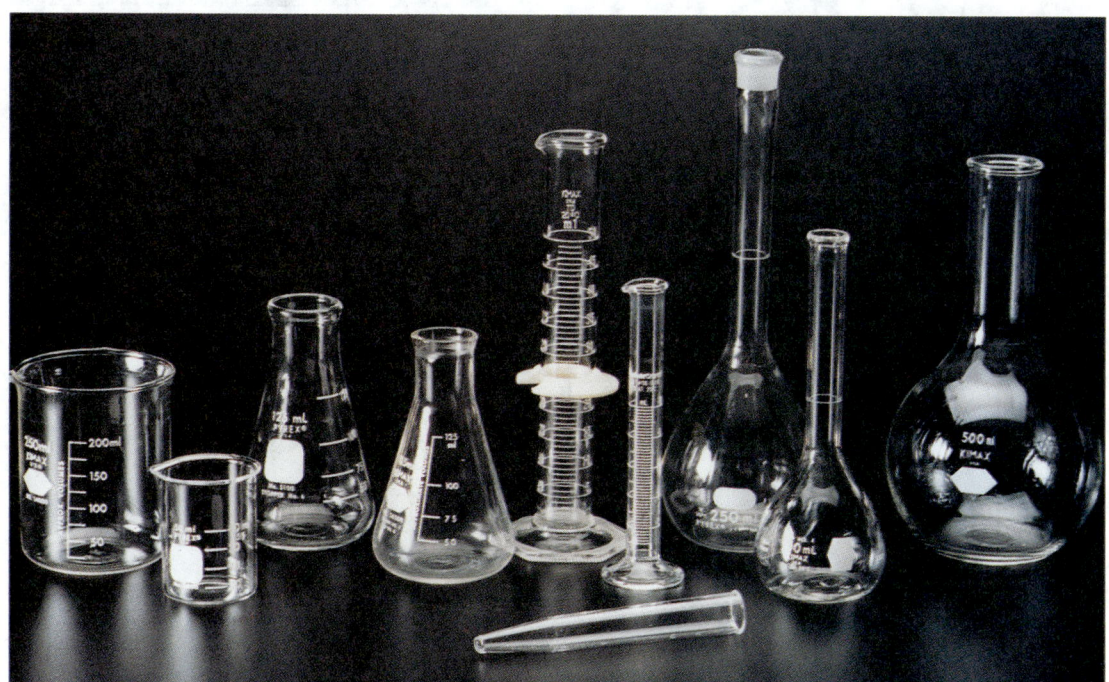

FIGURE 42-7

Glassware. *From left to right:* beakers, Erlenmyer flasks, graduated cylinders, volumetric flasks. *Front:* test tube.

BOX 42-5 How to Use a Pipette

Hold the pipette upright, not at an angle, with the tip slightly under the surface of the liquid. Use a slight suction on the suction apparatus until the meniscus is slightly above the desired level. Maintain the level by holding the finger over the top of the tube or maintaining constant pressure on the mechanical apparatus. Raise the pipette from the liquid and wipe the tip with a tissue. Allow the lowest meniscus curve to reach the desired calibration by releasing a small amount of the liquid into a waste receptacle. With the pipette in a vertical position, place the side of the pipette against the receiving vessel and allow the contents to drain.

Some pipettes, such as the Unopette, are available with premeasured amounts of reagents supplied. The whole unit is discarded in a biohazard receptacle after use. Reusable glass pipettes or the mechanical components of automated pipettes should be cleaned by the manufacturer's instructions. Some may be autoclaved after soaking and rinsing, whereas some require special chemical disinfectants or sterilization.

Serologic/Mohr

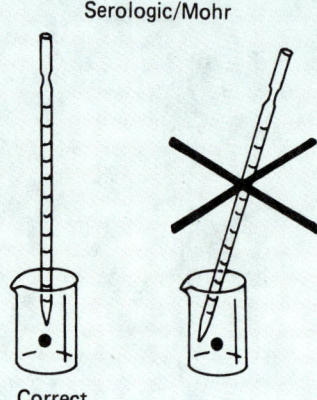

Correct

Volumetric/Ostwald-Folin

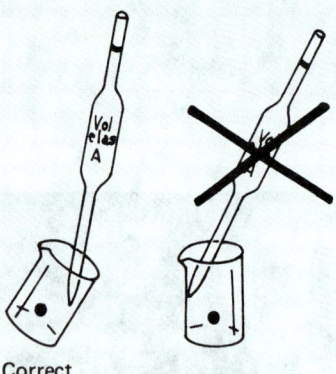

Correct

Correct and incorrect pipette positions.

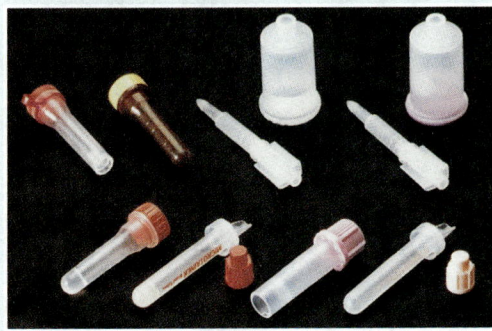

Unopettes are complete units and do not require additional equipment or supplies.

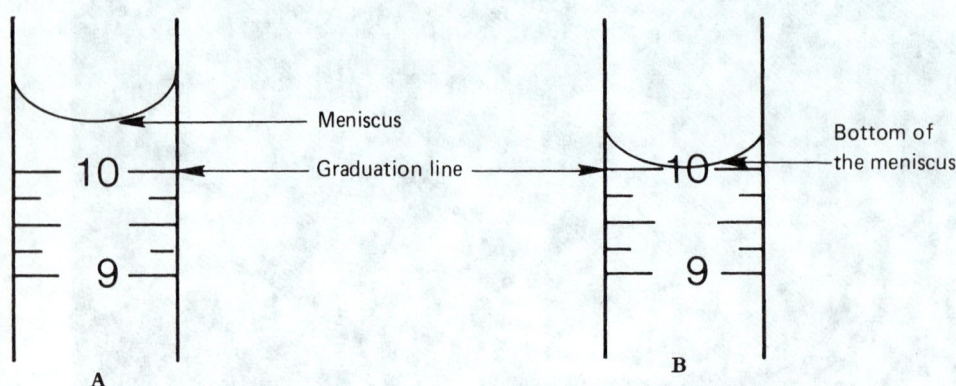

Pipetting technique. (*A*) Meniscus is brought above the desired graduation line. (*B*) Liquid is allowed to drain until the bottom of the meniscus touches the desired calibration mark.

Table 42-1
Cleaning Labware

Glassware "Problem"	Cleaning Technique
General usage (procedure 1 is recommended for routine washing needs)	1. *Dirty* glassware should be immediately placed in a soapy or dilute bleach solution and allowed to soak. Wash using any detergent designed for labware. Rinse with tap water 3 times, followed by 1 rinse with distilled water. Dry in an oven at temperature less than 140°C.
	2. *Acid dichromate.* Dissolve 50 g technical-grade sodium dichromate in 50 mL distilled water. Add this mixture to 500 mL technical-grade concentrated sulfuric acid. This solution is useful until a green color develops. Store in a covered glass jar. Soak glassware overnight and then rinse with dilute ammonia. Rewash glassware according to procedure 1.
	3. *Nitric acid* (20%). Soak for 12–24 h. Wash according to procedure 1.
Blood clots	4. *Sodium hydroxide* (10%). Soak for 12–24 h; then follow routine procedure. Dry micropipets using an acetone rinse.
New pipets (S1 alkaline)	5. *Rinse* with 5% hydrochloric acid or 5% nitric acid. Wash following routine prcedure.
Metal ion determinations	6. *Acid soak* (20% nitric acid), for 12–24 h. Rinse with distilled water 3 to 4 times. Water should be fresh for each rinsing step. Dry.
	7. *Soak* in any organic solvent.
Grease	8. *Dissolve* 100 g potassium hydroxide in 100 mL distilled water. Allow to cool. Add 900 mL commercial-grade 10% ethanol. Not to be used for delicate glassware.
	9. *Contrad 70* (manufactured by Harleco).
	10. *50% Hydrochloric acid.* Rinse with tap water. Wash.
Permanganate stains	11. *Dissolve* 1% ferrous sulfate in 25% sulfuric acid.

(From Bishop, M. L. Duben-Engelkirk, J. L., Fody E. P. (1992). Clinical Chemistry: Principles, Procedures, Correlations, 2nd ed., p. 674. Philadelphia: J. B. Lippincott.)

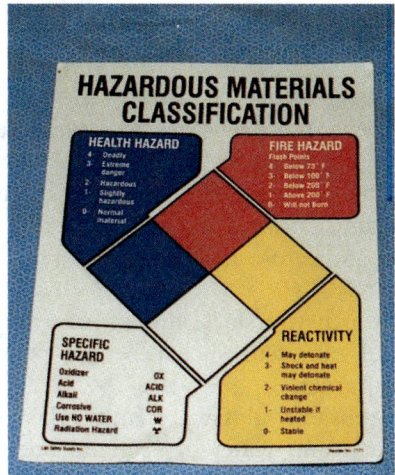

FIGURE 42-8
Hazardous materials classification posters should be prominently displayed in all laboratory areas.

Occupational Health and Safety Administration

The prevention of accidents and the regulation of safety in the workplace is monitored by the Occupational Safety and Health Administration (OSHA) of the United States government. OSHA is involved in monitoring the physical and chemical safety in all workplaces. It has particular standards for the health community because of the additional risk of biologic hazards.

Prevention of disease transmission in a medical facility is often referred to as infection control or biohazard risk management. OSHA requires that all medical employers train their employees in techniques that will protect them from occupational exposure to infectious diseases. Safety manuals must be available or incorporated into the policies and procedures manual to guide employees in correct procedures and emergency protocols.

The OSHA regulations require that all workers who are at risk for exposure to potentially hazardous

Material Safety Data Sheet (MSDS)

An MSDS lists all of the hazardous materials at a particular site. In the laboratory, these can include disinfectants, cleaning compounds, laboratory chemicals, and some office supplies (eg, toners, printing compounds). All of these must be labeled as hazardous, with the contents listed on the label. Protocols for each hazardous agent used on site must be listed on the MSDS and should include the following information:

- Product name and identification. Include all names (trade and generic) by which it may be known.
- Hazardous components. List all hazardous components if the agent contains more than one hazardous ingredient.
- Health hazard data. Note the potential danger that exists for those using the agent.
- Fire and explosive data. If this is a volatile agent, note what precautions are necessary to prevent an accident.
- Spill and disposal procedures. Note how to handle spills and disposal to avoid danger.
- Recommendations for personal protection equipment (PPE). Note whether gloves, gown, face shield, or other equipment should be worn during use of this agent.
- Handling, storage, and transportation precautions. List any special precautions that must be observed.

Any other pertinent information for the protection of the worker should also be included. All of the information necessary to complete the MSDS is available on package inserts, instrument manuals, from the Occupational Health and Safety Administration (OSHA), or from the manufacturer of the chemical.

---

material wear personal protective equipment (PPE) supplied by the employer and readily available for use. PPE includes:

- Gloves
- Gowns
- Aprons
- Face shields
- Goggles
- Glasses with side shields
- Masks
- Lab coats

Workers who are sensitive to allergens such as latex must be supplied with hypoallergenic gloves.

All PPE must be appropriate to the level of exposure (review the use of Standard Precautions in Chap. 19, Asepsis and Infection Control). A medical assistant performing phlebotomy or assisting with the collection of a tissue sample should be considered safe with glove protection. (Be aware that medical assistants working as phlebotomists are required to wear gloves if there is any break in the integument, while training, and when contamination is a risk.) Situations that may result in splashes, splatters, or aerosolization, however, require full coverage including footwear such as shoe covers. (**Aerosol** refers to suspended particles in gas or air.)

According to OSHA requirements, employers also are required to provide immunization against blood-borne pathogens if vaccines are available.

Checkpoint Question

5. What are three hazards found in the laboratory? Give examples of each.

Important Rules to Follow

The rules outlined below are some of the most important safety guidelines followed in all laboratories. You should adhere to them carefully when performing laboratory procedures.

1. Never eat, drink, or smoke in the laboratory area.
2. Wear gloves and appropriate protective barriers whenever contact with blood, body fluids, secretions, excretions, nonintact skin, or mucous membranes is possible. If splatters, splashes, spills, or aerosolization are possible, wear appropriate PPE.
3. Label all specimen containers with biohazard labels.
4. Store all chemicals according to the manufacturer's recommendations. Discard any container with an illegible label.
5. Wash hands frequently for infection control. Hands must always be washed before and after gloving and before and after leaving the laboratory work site.
6. Never touch your face, mouth, or eyes with your gloves or with items such as pens or pencils used in the laboratory.
7. Clean reusable glassware and other containers with soap and water or recommended solutions and dry thoroughly before reuse. Wear gloves to prevent cuts.
8. Avoid inhaling the fumes of any chemicals found in the laboratory.

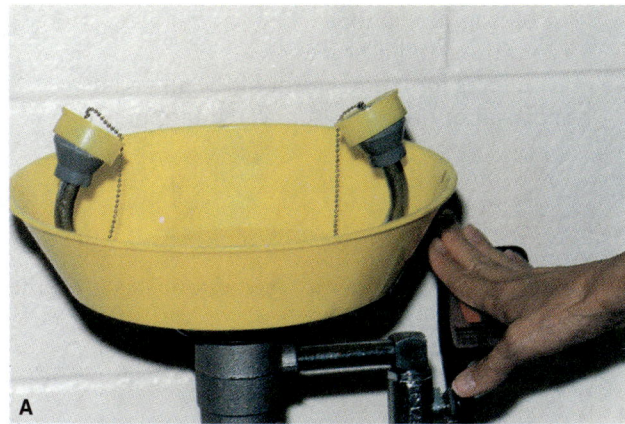

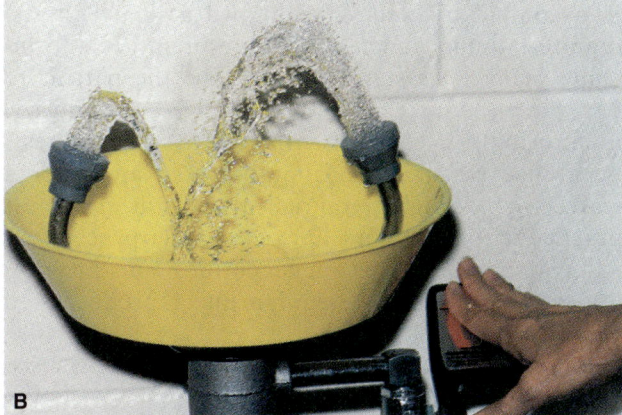

FIGURE 42-9
Eye wash basin. (*A*): Press the lever at the right of the basin. (*B*) The caps are forced from the water source by the stream. Lower your face and eyes into the stream and continue to wash the area until the eyes are clear.

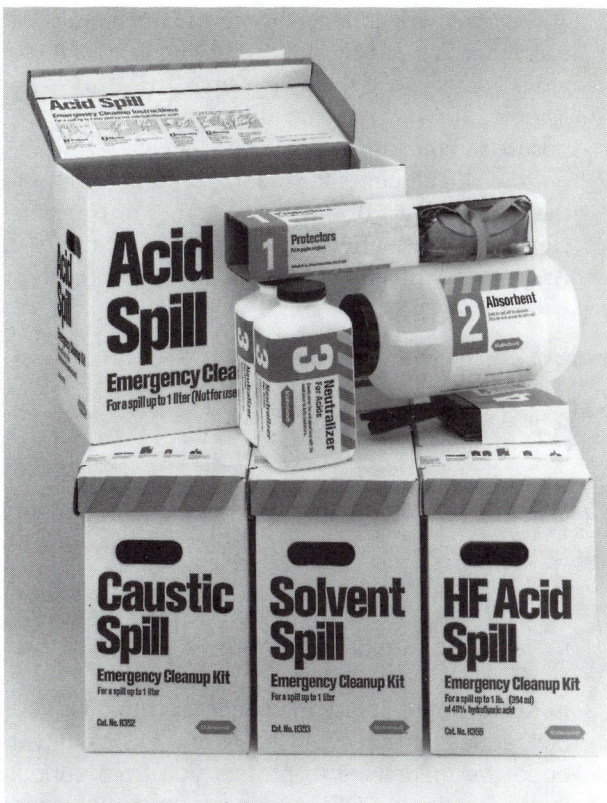

FIGURE 42-10
Spill cleanup kits for safely caring for clinical spills. (Photo courtesy of Scientific Products Division, Baxter Healthcare Corporation)

9. Know the location and operation of all safety equipment such as fire extinguishers, eye washes (Fig. 42-9), and safety showers. Keep fire extinguishers close at hand because many chemicals are flammable.
10. Use safe practices when operating laboratory equipment. Read the manuals and know how to operate the equipment. Avoid contact with damaged electrical equipment.
11. Disinfect all laboratory surfaces concurrently and at the end of the day with a 10% bleach solution or appropriate disinfectant. Never allow clutter to accumulate.
12. Dispose of needles and broken glass in sharps containers. Use biohazard containers for any other contaminated articles.
13. Never mouth pipette; use mechanical pipetters.
14. Use the proper procedure for removing chemical or biologic spills. If the spill is chemical, follow the manufacturer's directions; commercial kits are available for such cleanups (Fig. 42-10). If the spill is biologic:

- Put on gloves.
- Cover the area with disposable material such as paper towels; discard in a biohazard container.
- Flood the area with disinfecting solution, allowing it to sit for 10 to 15 minutes.
- Wipe up the spill.
- Dispose of all waste in a biohazard container.

15. Avoid spills by:

- Pouring carefully (palm the label).
- Pouring at eye level if possible or practical; never pour close to the face.
- Tightly capping all containers immediately after use.

16. Use splatter guards or splash shields in any instance of possible splatter or aerosolization. Spills, splatters, and aerosolization commonly occur when:

- unstoppering blood collection tubes
- transferring blood from a collection syringe to a specimen receptacle
- conducting centrifugation
- preparing smears
- flaming the inoculation loop

17. When removing stoppers, hold the opening away, use gauze around the cap and twist gently. Avoid glove contact with the specimen.
18. Report all work-related injuries or biohazard exposure to your supervisor immediately.
19. Follow all guidelines for Standard Precautions and the requirements of the various types of transmission-based precautions as described in Chapter 19, Asepsis and Infection Control.

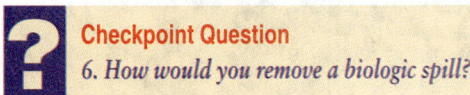

Checkpoint Question
6. How would you remove a biologic spill?

What If?
What if your laboratory is not in compliance with OSHA's safety regulations?

In such a situation, your health and that of your colleagues is placed in jeopardy. OSHA developed the guidelines to protect you from serious injury or death. OSHA can impose significant fines for noncompliance. Continued noncompliance may result in loss of laboratory privileges. In some situations, the physician may not be allowed to file for Medicare compensation. To bring the laboratory back into compliance, any citations issued must be addressed and corrected. OSHA inspectors will then revisit the site and reconsider licensure.

➤ CLINICAL LABORATORY IMPROVEMENT AMENDMENTS

In an effort to standardize and improve the quality of laboratory testing, Congress passed the Clinical Laboratory Improvement Amendments (CLIA) in 1988 to address the issue of regulations governing any facility that performs testing for the diagnosis, prevention, or treatment of disease or for assessment of patients' health status. Standards were developed to cover all laboratory areas from the most complex regional laboratory to the smallest physician office laboratory.

Before the passage of CLIA, physician office laboratories, private clinics, and long-term care facilities were not covered by regulations that govern larger, established laboratories. CLIA was developed by the Department of Health and Human Services (DHHS) and set standards for:

- Laboratory operations
- Application and user fees
- Procedures for enforcement of the amendment
- Approval of programs for accreditation

Levels of Testing Complexity

Three levels of complexity were established for the types of tests performed on site.

Low-Complexity Tests

Low-complexity tests (also known as waiver tests) require minimal judgment or interpretation and include many tests simple enough for the patient to perform at home (eg, dipstick urinalyses and glucose monitoring). If these are the only types of tests performed on site, the laboratory can apply for a waiver of oversight requirements, but it still must practice within the guidelines for proper procedures. All manufacturers' recommendations must be followed for each piece of equipment or product used for testing.

The following are considered low-complexity tests:

- Urine dipstick or reagent tablets
- Fecal occult blood packets
- Ovulation testing in packets with color comparison charts
- Urine pregnancy testing kits using color comparison charts
- Nonautomated erythrocyte sedimentation rate tests such as Wintrobe or Westergren
- Nonautomated copper sulfate testing for hemoglobin
- Centrifuged microhematocrits
- Low-complexity blood glucose determination testing

Moderate-Complexity Tests

Most of the testing performed in large, established laboratories falls under the moderate-complexity heading. Many of the following tests are also performed in a physician's office laboratory if approval has been granted for moderate-complexity testing. These include:

- Urine and throat cultures
- White blood cell counts
- Packaged rapid strep tests
- Automated testing for cholesterol, high density lipoproteins, and triglycerides
- Gram staining
- Helminth testing
- Microscopic urinalysis

High-Complexity Tests

These kinds of tests, which are rarely performed in medical offices, include:

- Advanced cell studies (cytogenetics)
- Cytology (Pap smears)
- Histocompatibility
- Histopathology

If the level of testing to be performed is in question, it must be considered high complexity until its level can be designated by the Health Care Financing Administration (HCFA). HCFA publishes a list of all tests in the moderate-complexity category. States may establish local rules that are more strict than those set by the governing body, but they may not adopt rules less strict.

Laboratory Standards

Laboratories that perform moderate- or high-complexity testing may be inspected in an unannounced visit every year by representatives from HCFA or the Centers for Disease Control and Prevention (CDC) under the direction of the Department of Health and Human Services. As discussed below, they must meet all standards set by CLIA.

Patient Test Management

It must be proven that a system is in place to ensure that the specimens are properly maintained and identified and that the results are accurately recorded and reported. Policies must be written for standards of patient care and employee conduct. Each test performed will be evaluated for safety, reliability, and diagnostic indication for its performance.

Policies and procedures manuals will clearly outline patient preparation, specimen handling, how tests are to be performed, alternatives to the usual testing methods for specific situations, and what to do in the event of questionable testing results.

Quality Control (QC)

The policy and procedure manual must include written directives for each division to ensure that all quality controls for monitoring the accuracy and quality of each test are in place. The protocols established by the manual must include a control sample, management of reagents, and instrument calibration, as explained below.

CONTROL SAMPLE

Manufacturers provide a specimen that is comparable to a human specimen with a known reference

Quality Control Log

Test: ______________________ Control Lot Number: ______________________

Date	Control Value	Performed By	Accept	Reject	Corrective Action Taken

FIGURE 42-11
Quality control log. (From *Physician's Office Laboratory Guidelines, Procedure Manual,* Third Edition. Wayne, PA: NCCLS, 1995, with permission.)

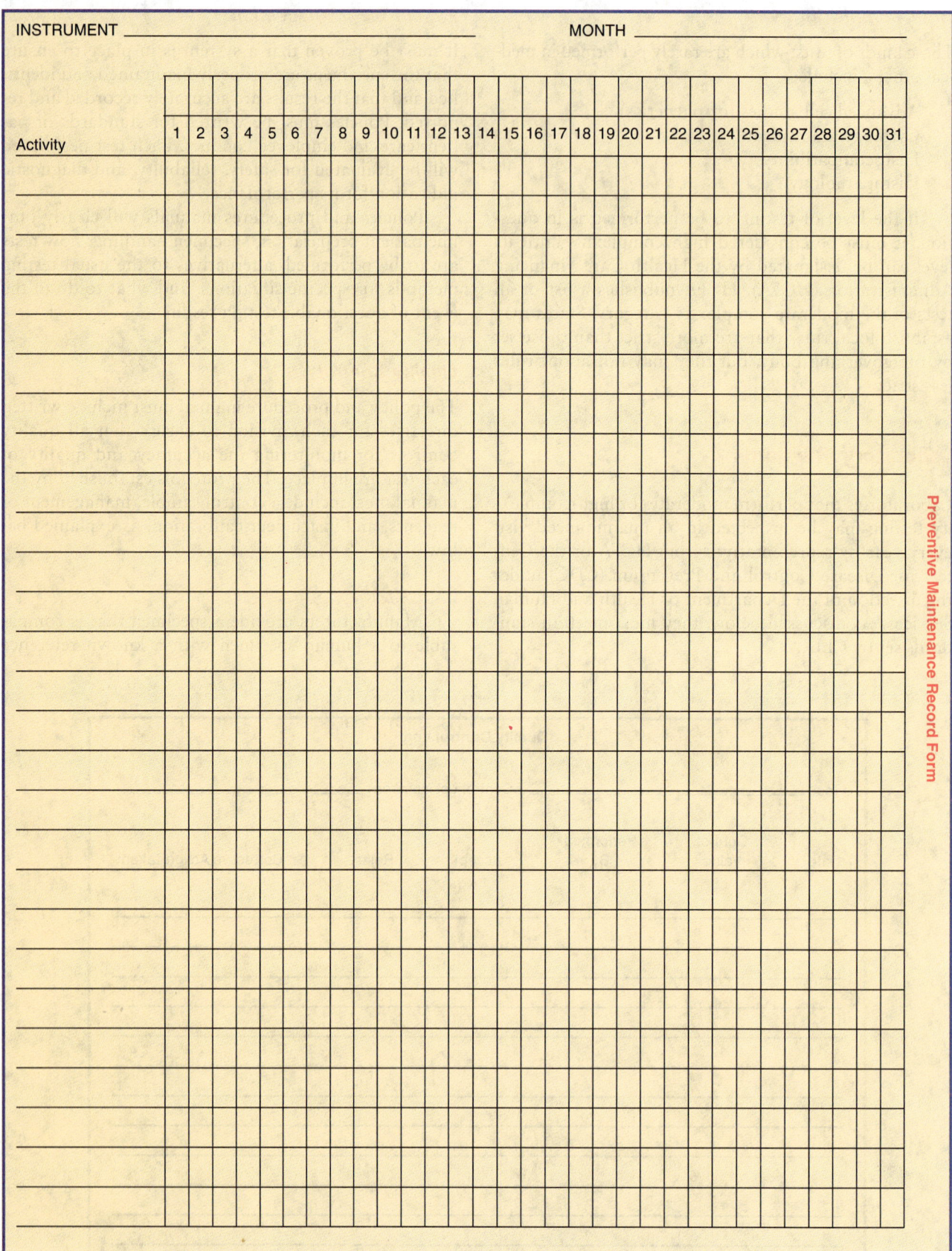

INSTRUMENT _____   MONTH _____

Activity | 1 | 2 | 3 | 4 | 5 | 6 | 7 | 8 | 9 | 10 | 11 | 12 | 13 | 14 | 15 | 16 | 17 | 18 | 19 | 20 | 21 | 22 | 23 | 24 | 25 | 26 | 27 | 28 | 29 | 30 | 31

Preventive Maintenance Record Form

FIGURE 42-12
Preventive maintenance record form. (From *Physician's Office Laboratory Guidelines, Procedure Manual,* Third Edition. Wayne, PA: NCCLS, 1995, with permission.)

range. Testing the control sample at the same time the patient specimen is tested or when a new kit or batch of reagents is received ensures that all testing components are performing as required. Samples should also be performed at the start of each day before testing begins. The performance of these controls must be recorded in the quality control log book.

The **National Committee for Clinical Laboratory Standards (NCCLS)** establishes rules to ensure the safety, standards, and integrity of all testing performed on human specimens. Fig. 42-11 is an example of an NCCLS form on which control sample testing can be recorded.

MANAGEMENT OF REAGENTS

Reagents are chemicals used to produce a reaction in a testing situation. All reagents are given a manufacturer's lot number and expiration date. These must be recorded in a quality control log book with the date received, the date opened, and the initials of the person who opened the package. If the reagent consistently performs inappropriately, the lot number will help the manufacturer identify defects. All supplies and equipment, reagents, and testing components must be labeled with identification, storage requirements, date of preparation or when opened, and expiration date. *Note*: Always store chemicals properly, palm the label when pouring, check the label three times as directed in medication administration, discard expired chemicals, and cap securely when not in use.

INSTRUMENT CALIBRATION

Highly complex laboratory equipment is very sensitive and requires strict operation and maintenance standards. Manufacturers provide maintenance schedules and methods of evaluating performance. Maintenance on equipment and supplies must be documented in the quality control log book; this includes maintenance either by an employee or by a manufacturer's representative. Any corrective action required for equipment or supply malfunction must be documented. Figures 42-12 and 42-13 show sample NCCLS forms on which this information can be recorded.

Instruments are designed to register within a set of standard calibrations. If the specimen test results are

Instrument History Record

Model No.: _____   Instrument: _____

Date Purchased: _____   Serial No.: _____

Manufacturer: _____   Cost: _____

_____   State: _____ Zip: _____

Telephone: _____   Contact Person: _____

Dealer: _____

_____   State: _____ Zip: _____

Telephone: _____   Contact Person: _____

Warranty: _____   Expiration Date: _____

_____

Technical Service Representative: _____

Telephone: _____

Service Record

Date   **Comments**   Who was contacted, action taken

_____

_____

_____

FIGURE 42-13
Instrument history record. (From *Physician's Office Laboratory Guidelines, Procedure Manual,* Third Edition. Wayne, PA: NCCLS, 1995, with permission.)

not within a normal range, the instrument's calibration should be checked by the manufacturer's instructions and the specimen should be retested. If the calibration is correct and the specimen is still outside the normal value, the results are probably correct for this patient. A control specimen tested at the same time and in the same manner as the patient specimen will ensure that proper testing procedures were followed. The flow chart in Figure 42-14 shows how you can evaluate test results for errors.

The manual must state the manufacturer's recommendation for the performance of calibration procedures and supporting documentation must show that controls are performed as directed. Some procedures may require that controls be performed at each testing. Documentation must show the action taken to verify results, what was done when a problem arose, what the solution to the problem was, when the testing equipment was serviced and by whom, and what was done.

Quality Assurance (QA)

The policy and procedure manual should cover recommendations for continuing education for the laboratory personnel and evaluation methods for ensuring worker competence. The qualifications and responsibilities of all laboratory workers are specified by CLIA, giving education and training requirements for all levels of personnel. Employers are responsible for ensuring the educational background of employees, providing opportunities for continuing education, and conducting or providing for proficiency testing. This information must be documented for inspection.

Proficiency Testing (PT)

This requirement allows external evaluation of the laboratory. All laboratories, even those conducting only

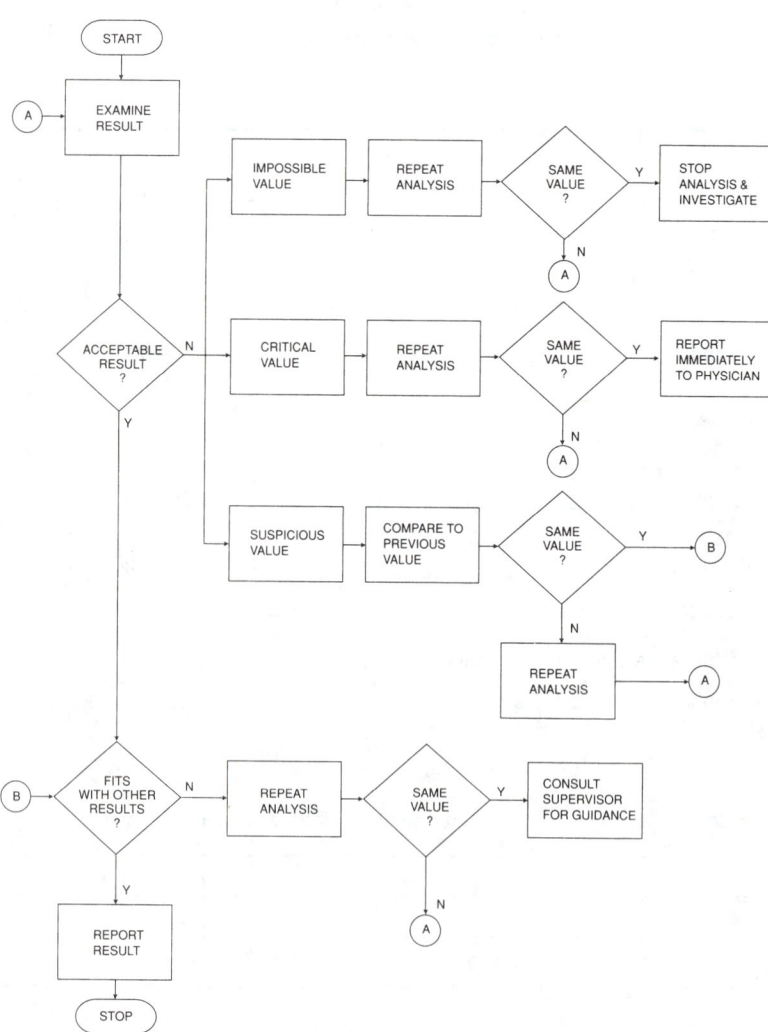

FIGURE 42-14

Flow chart for evaluation of test result for random error: A simple strategy for determining whether individual test result is reasonable and correlates with other results. Y, yes; N, no. Symbols *A* and *B* show interconnection between results of evaluation of repeat testing and where decision-making strategy should resume (*far left*). For example, if an impossible value is obtained, and repeat analysis does not show same value, uppermost horizontal line of chart says that testing procedure should return to symbol *A*, where the steps are begun again with EXAMINE RESULT. (Adapted from Cembrowski GS: Use of patient data for quality control. Clin Lab Med 6:715, 1986)

waiver tests, must participate in three proficiency tests a year and must be available for at least one on-site inspection to continue testing and maintain Medicare eligibility. Three times a year, the laboratory will be shipped specimens prepared by an approved agency. These specimens must be tested by the same procedures used for patient evaluation and the results mailed to the proficiency testing agency.

Quality Control Log Book

To record compliance with CLIA measures, a record must be kept of each control sample and standard test. The log must reflect the date and time of the test, the control or standard results expected, what results were obtained, and the action taken for correction, if any. Documentation must be consistent and a policy must exist for retaining the records for at least 2 years.

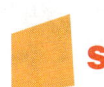

SUMMARY

Although many tests are now referred to reference laboratories, the integrity of any specimen and reliability of any test begins with the proper patient instruction and conscientious collection practices on the part of the medical assistant in the medical office. The laboratory can be a safe, challenging, and pleasant place to work. Laboratory testing can reveal important clues to the causes of disease and the best means of treatment. As a member of the laboratory team, the work that you do will help solve the riddle of disease processes and lead to better health for the patients you serve.

CRITICAL THINKING CHALLENGES

1. Review the laboratory safety rules, then create a poster summarizing these rules for display in the laboratory.
2. Develop a list of all the items that must be documented in the laboratory setting. Design a form that can be used to meet these documentation requirements. Who should complete the form? Where should it be kept? Explain your responses.

ANSWERS TO CHECKPOINT QUESTIONS

1. A reference laboratory is a large facility that serves a particular region, performing hundreds of different specialized tests daily. In contrast, the physician's office laboratory performs only a few kinds of common tests; some specimens may actually be sent to a reference lab-

oratory for testing. Medical assistants working in reference laboratories may be employed as accessioners, sorting specimens and entering data into computers. They may also work as customer service personnel, answering telephones, tracking specimens, and reporting results to the centers from which the specimens were collected.

2. A large laboratory may have the following departments:
   - Hematology—studies blood cells
   - Coagulation—measures clotting time
   - Clinical chemistry—measures chemicals in blood
   - Toxicology—measures drug levels in blood
   - Urinalysis—evaluates chemical properties of urine
   - Blood bank or immunohematology—prepares blood for transfusion
   - Serology—evaluates antibody reaction
   - Microbiology—identifies pathogens
   - Pathology—determines characteristics, causes, and effects of disease

3. Because tests may vary among manufacturers, the package insert is the best source of information on performing the test and evaluating the results.

4. The low power objective lens magnifies objects 10 times and is used for scanning. The high power objective lens magnifies objects 40 times and is used for close observation. The oil immersion lens magnifies objects 100 times for greatest visualization.

5. The three basic types of hazards are physical (eg, fire, broken glass, and liquid spills), chemical (eg, acids, alkalis, and chemical fumes), and biologic (eg, diseases such as HIV, hepatitis, and tuberculosis).

6. To clean up a biologic spill, first put on gloves. Cover the area with disposable material such as paper towels; discard these in an appropriate container. Next, flood the area with disinfecting solution, allowing it to sit for 10 to 15 minutes. Wipe up the spill. Dispose of all waste in a biohazard container.

SUGGESTIONS FOR FURTHER READING

Bishop, M. L., Duben-Englekirk, J. L., & Fody, E. P. (1992). *Clinical Chemistry, Principles, Procedures, Correlations,* 2nd ed. Philadelphia: J. B. Lippincott.

Linn, J. J., & Ringsrud, K. M. (1992). *Basic Techniques in Clinical Laboratory Science,* 3rd ed. St. Louis: C. V. Mosby.

McCall, R. E., & Tankersley, C. M. (1993). *Phlebotomy Essentials.* Philadelphia: J. B. Lippincott.

Walters, N. J., Estridge, B. H., & Reynolds, A. P. (1990). *Basic Medical Laboratory Techniques.* Albany NY: Delmar Publishers.

Microbiology

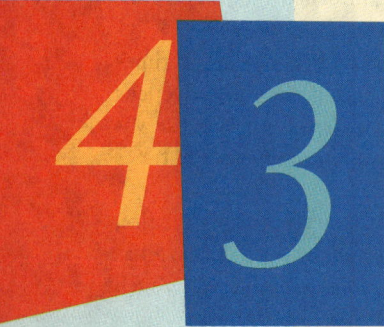

Chapter Outline

Microbiologic Life Forms
  Bacteria
  Rickettsias and Chlamydias
  Fungi
  Viruses
  Protozoa
  Metazoa
Microbiologic Testing: The Medical Assistant's Role
Specimen Collection and Handling
  Types of Specimens
  Types of Culture Media
  Caring for the Media
  Transporting the Specimen
Procedure: Preparing the Specimen for Transport

Microscopic Examination of Microorganisms
  Smears and Slides
Procedure: Preparing a Dry Smear
  Identification by Staining
Procedure: Gram Staining a Smear Slide
  Microbiologic Inoculation
Procedure: Inoculating a Culture
  Sensitivity Testing
  Streptococcal Testing
Summary
Critical Thinking Challenges
Answers to Checkpoint Questions
Suggestions for Further Reading

DACUM Components

1.3 Practice within scope of education, training, and personal capabilities
4.1 Apply principles of aseptic technique and infection control
4.8 Use quality control
4.10 Collect and process specimens
4.11 Perform selected tests that assist with diagnosis and treatment
5.1 Document accurately

Chapter Competencies

Learning Objectives

Upon successfully completing this chapter, you will be able to:

1. Spell and define the Key Terms.
2. List and describe primary bacteria.
3. Identify various bacterial illustrations.
4. Describe the purpose for the formation of spores.
5. Describe the classifications of fungi, Rickettsia, chlamydia, protozoa, and metazoa.
6. State the factors necessary for microbial growth.
7. Describe the medical assistant's responsibilities in microbiological testing.

Performance Objectives

Upon successfully completing this chapter, you will be able to:

1. Properly label and identify specimen for transportation and handling (Procedure 43-1).
2. Prepare a wet mount slide.
3. Prepare a hanging drop slide.
4. Prepare a dry specimen smear (Procedure 43-2).
5. Prepare a specimen with Gram stain (Procedure 43-3).
6. Inoculate a tube of broth medium.
7. Inoculate a culture and conduct sensitivity testing (Procedure 43-4).

Key Terms

(See Glossary for definitions.)

aerobic	diplococci	Rickettsia
anaerobic	flagella	spirochete
agar	mordant	spores
bacteriology	morphology	staphylococci
bacilli (sing. bacillus)	mycology	streptococci
bibulous	nosocomial infection	swab
binary fission	obligate	virology
centesis	parasitology	parasitology
chlamydia	Petri plate	

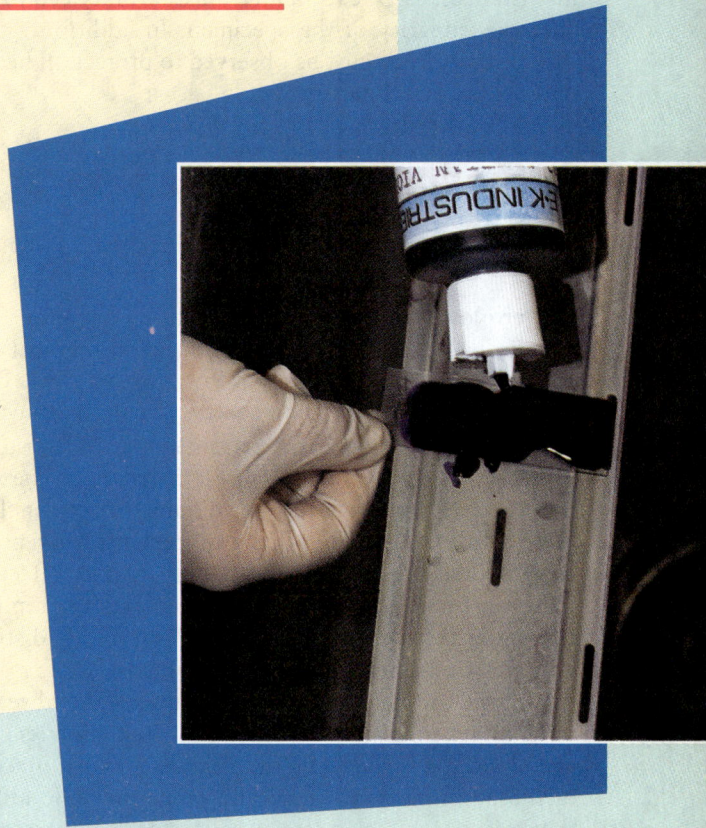

Microbiology is the study of microorganisms too small to be seen without a microscope. Microorganisms exist in the polar ice caps and in the steaming water in hot springs, but the ones most likely to present problems in the health care field are those that thrive at temperatures between 96°F and 101°F in a basically neutral environment. Of course, many normal flora live and thrive on the human body without causing disease. As a medical assistant, you need to be aware of the organisms present around us and their potential for causing disease in order to protect yourself, the physician, patients, and all co-workers from **nosocomial infections** (infections acquired in a medical setting).

Medical microbiology is performed using cultures and smears of the specimens referred to the laboratory. The specimens may be taken from wounds or other areas, such as the throat, vagina, urethra, or skin by using a **swab,** a stick topped with cotton or other absorbent manmade fiber. Specimens may be drawn from the body by **centesis** (surgical puncture) or by venipuncture. Specimens are also excreted from the body as sputum, stool, or urine.

The medical assistant frequently collects specimens or assists the physician with the collection. Medical assistants may collect specimens from wounds or from the throat, but the physician usually collects specimens from the eye, ear, rectum, or reproductive organs. In all instances, aseptic technique must be practiced to ensure the integrity of the specimen. In addition, Standard Precautions must be observed to protect all health care workers and patients.

➤ MICROBIOLOGIC LIFE FORMS

Bacteria

Bacteriology is the science and study of bacteria. Several groups of bacteria are significant in medical microbiology, including the spore-forming bacteria. Bacteria are unicellular (one-celled) simple organisms, each with its own specific characteristics. Bacteria reproduce by **binary fission** (direct division of the cell into 2 equal parts) and do not require a host for their life stages as long as all other requirements for replication are met (see Chapter 19, Asepsis and Infection Control, for information on requirements for replication). Bacteria can be identified by their distinct shapes, or **morphology** (Table 43-1).

Cocci are responsible for many of the diseases transmitted through the population. **Staphylococci** are found on all surfaces of the skin and many mucous membranes. They are generally nonpathogenic unless they reach areas that are usually sterile, where they may cause abscess formation or other forms of infec-

Table 43-1
Categorizing Bacteria

Morphology	Types
Round (spherical)	Cocci
Grapelike clusters	Staphylococci
Chain formations	Streptococci
Paired	Diplococci
Single	Micrococci
Rod-shaped	Bacilli
Somewhat oval	Coccobacilli
End-to-end in chains	Streptobacilli
Spiral-shaped	
Flexible (usually with **flagella**; whiplike extremities that aid movement)	Spirochetes
Rigid	Spirilla
Curved rods (comma-shaped)	Vibrios

tion. **Streptococci** cause sore throats, scarlet fever, rheumatic fever, many pneumonias ,and various skin infections. **Diplococci** cause bacterial meningitis, gonorrhea, and some of the pneumonias.

Bacilli are usually **aerobic** (requiring oxygen to live), may be Gram-positive or negative, and some are spore forming. Diseases caused by bacilli include tetanus, botulism, gas gangrene, tuberculosis, pertussis, Salmonellosis, certain pneumonias, and otitis media.

Spirochetes are long, spiral, flexible organisms classified as spirilla if they are rigid rather than flexible. Spirochetes are responsible for syphilis and Lyme disease; spirilla cause rat bite fever.

Vibrios are curved, comma-shaped bacteria. They are very motile and cause cholera. Figure 43-1 shows the various forms of bacteria.

Bacterial Spore Formation

Some of the microorganisms present in our environment produce **spores** to protect themselves under adverse conditions. The bacterium, usually a bacillus, forms a capsule around itself and enters a resting state that is resistant to most means of asepsis, such as heat or chemicals. When conditions are favorable for reproduction, the spore will revert to its active form and resume its life cycle. Examples include:

- *Clostridium botulinum* (food poisoning)
- *Clostridium tetani* (tetanus)
- *Clostridium perfringens* (gas gangrene)
- *Bacillus anthracis* (anthrax)

Spores are destroyed by autoclaving with the proper components of heat, steam, pressure, and time.

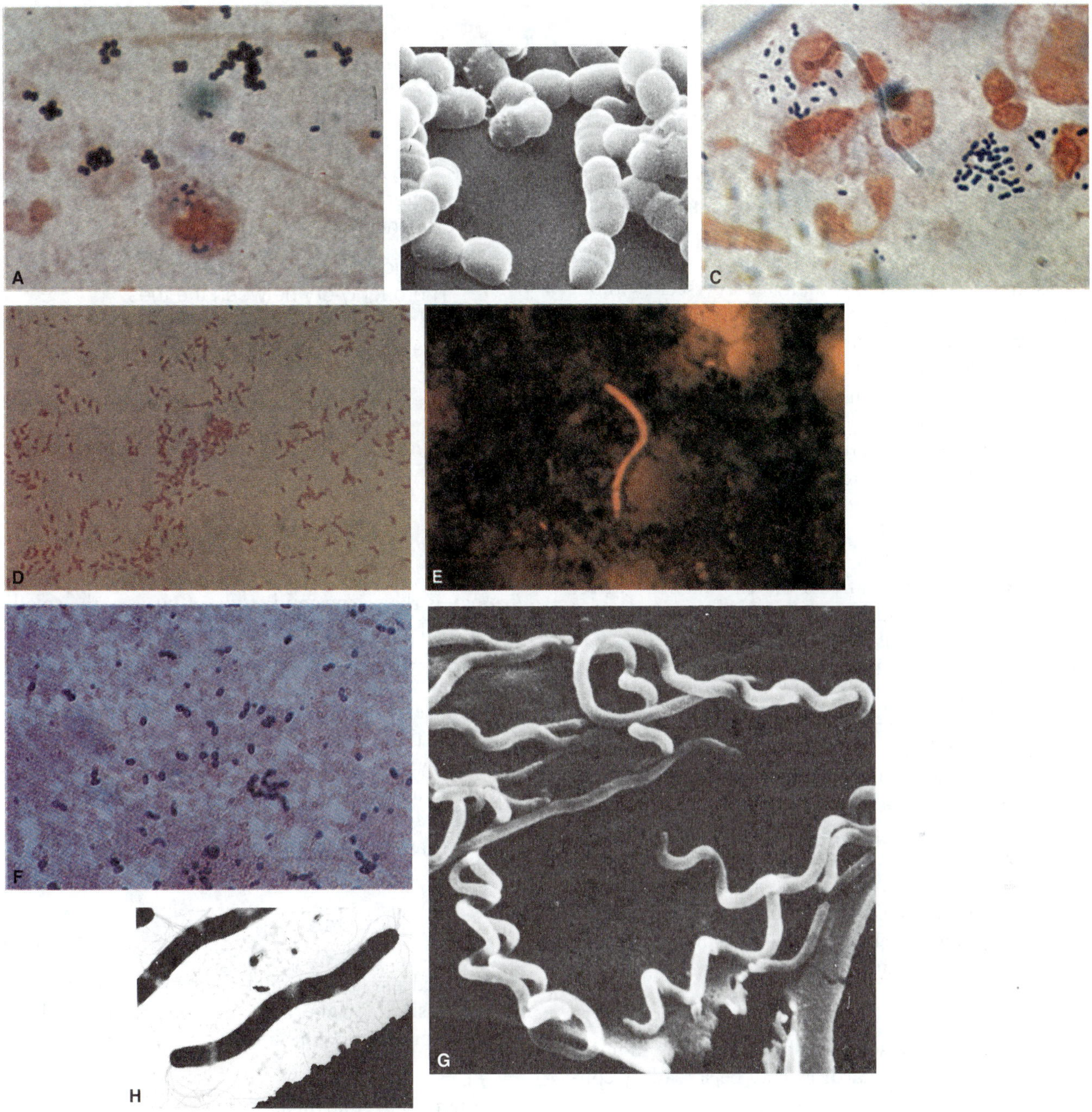

FIGURE 43-1
Forms of bacteria. (*A*) Gram-positive Staphylococcus. (*B*) Streptococcus in short chains. (*C*) Gram-positive diplococci. (*D*) Gram-negative bacilli. (*E*) A long, rod-shaped bacterium. (*F*) Gram-positive, spore-forming bacilli. (*G*) The spirochete *Treponema pallidum* responsible for syphilis. (*H*) *Vibrio*.

(See Chapter 23, Instruments and Equipment, for the autoclave procedure.)

> **Checkpoint Question**
> *1. What are the four main categories of bacteria?*

Rickettsias and Chlamydias

Specialized forms of bacteria that fit in a category of their own are the **Rickettsias** and the **Chlamydias**. Both are smaller than bacteria but larger than viruses. Because they both require a living host for replication and survival, they are referred to as **obligate** intracellular parasites. Rickettsias cause Rocky Mountain spotted fever. The Chlamydias cause trachoma and lymphogranuloma venereum.

Fungi

Mycology is the science and study of fungi. Fungi are small organisms like bacteria, with the potential to produce disease processes in susceptible hosts. Some forms are microscopic but many can be seen without the aid of a microscope. Fungi resemble plants, whereas bacteria appear to resemble one-celled animals. Fungi may be in the form of yeasts or molds in the human body. They are opportunistic, usually becoming pathogenic when the host's normal flora can no longer counterbalance the colony's growth.

Fungal diseases are referred to as mycoses or mycotic infections and include those listed below:

Molds

- Aspergillus—often affects the ear but may affect any organ or surface; may be fatal if widespread
- Blastomycosis—usually asymptomatic but may cause skin ulcers or bone lesions and may spread to the viscera
- Coccidiomycosis—may present with acute flulike respiratory symptoms or may become chronic and infect almost any body part
- Histoplasmosis—spreads through contaminated soil, usually asymptomatic but may lead to pneumonia
- Tinea—cutaneous mycoses (eg, tinea pedis [athlete's foot], tinea corporis [ringworm of the body], tinea capitas [ringworm of the scalp], and tinea unguinum [nail fungus]).

Yeasts

- Candidiasis—causes thrush (skin and mouth), vaginitis, and endocarditis; may be spread by contact (Fig. 43-2).

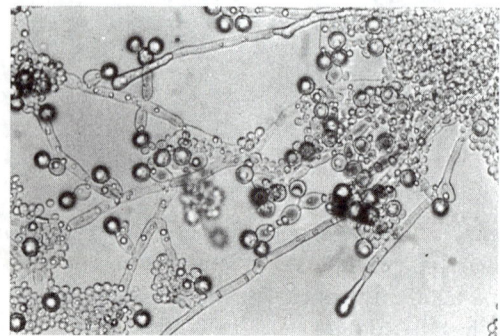

FIGURE 43-2
Fungus—*Candida albicans.*

What If?

What if your patient asks you how to prevent cutaneous mycoses, such as tinea pedis?

Explain to your patient that tinea pedis is a common fungal infection that affects many people. Then offer the following suggestions, which can aid prevention:

- Practice good basic hygiene.
- Thoroughly dry between the toes.
- Do not share footwear.
- Use antifungal powders between the toes and in shoes.
- Wear foot protection when using public showers.

Viruses

Virology is the science and study of viruses, the smallest form of microorganisms. Viruses cause influenza, infectious hepatitis, rabies, polio, and acquired immunodeficiency syndrome (AIDS). They are so small that they can be seen only with a special electron microscope, not the usual microscope found in the medical office. They require a living host for survival and replication and are referred to as obligate intracellular parasites. Because viruses are not susceptible to antibiotics, they are extremely difficult to treat.

Protozoa

Single-celled parasitic animals that may be diagnosed in the **parasitology** laboratory are the protozoa. These microorganisms and conditions they cause include the following:

- Entamoeba—diarrhea, dysentery, and liver and lung disorders
- Giardia—giardiasis, diarrhea, and malabsorption of nutrients
- Trichomonas—trichomoniasis, vaginitis, and urinary tract infection
- Plasmodium—malaria
- Toxoplasma—toxoplasmosis and fetal abnormalities

Metazoa

Metazoa include helminths, nematodes, and arthropods.
The helminth family includes round worms, flat worms, and flukes. Most will survive almost anywhere

Patient Education: Lyme Disease

Deer ticks are a type of arthropod capable of transmitting the spirochete responsible for Lyme disease. The spirochete is called *Borrelia burgdorferi*. When the infected deer tick bites a human, the spirochete enters the body and can produce mild to severe symptoms, including a rash, joint aches, fever, general body aches, and alterations in neurologic and cardiac functioning.

Lyme disease, which has been documented in 47 states, can be prevented with proper education. Instruct patients to avoid tick habitats and to wear shoes and light-colored clothing when working outside in wooded areas. Clothing should be checked for the presence of ticks and washed in hot water with strong soap. Stress the importance of observing for ticks and removing them properly when they are found.

in the human body or may migrate through the body until they find a place to settle. Helminths can cause schistosomiasis, liver fluke infestations, and beef or pork tapeworm infestation.

The nematodes cause roundworm infestations, gastrointestinal obstruction, bronchial damage, pinworm infestation, and trichinosis.

Arthropods include mites, lice, ticks, and fleas. Also included are bees, spiders, wasps, mosquitoes, and scorpions. All may cause injury by their bites or stings but several are also capable of transmitting disease by their bite or sting.

➤ MICROBIOLOGIC TESTING: THE MEDICAL ASSISTANT'S ROLE

The medical assistant's role in microbiologic testing is extensive. Although it varies from office to office and sometimes from state to state, it will include both administrative and clinical responsibilities.

Administrative duties in microbiologic testing include:

- Routing specimens
- Handling and filing reports
- Ensuring patient safety and education
- Billing and insurance filing

Clinical skills require the medical assistant to:

- Collect and process many of the specimens obtained
- Assist the physician and patient as needed
- Maintain Standard Precautions and safety
- Perform terminal cleaning procedures after testing is complete

➤ SPECIMEN COLLECTION AND HANDLING

Laboratory tests are most often performed on specimens that are easily obtained from the body, such as blood, urine, feces, sputum, and other body secretions and fluids. The specimen gives the physician a view of the condition of the system from which the specimen was obtained. For instance, a urine culture will indicate the infectious process at work within the urinary system; a sputum culture will grow the organism responsible for the patient's presenting respiratory symptoms.

As a medical assistant, you may be responsible for collecting most of the specimens obtained in the medical office. To ensure that the laboratory receives a sample that represents the disease process for which the specimen was collected, you must collect the specimen from the appropriate site using the proper method. You also must handle the specimen appropriately so that it will yield accurate diagnostic test results (Box 43-1).

Types of Specimens

Microbiology laboratories work extensively with cultures of the referred biologic specimen. Cultures are colonies of microorganisms that are encouraged to replicate under controlled conditions for the purpose of diagnosing disease. These may be *mixed cultures,* which are used to investigate any or all of the microorganisms found at a site, or *secondary cultures,* which remove from the mixed cultures only those organisms that need to be encouraged to grow for more extensive study. *Pure cultures* contain only one organism and may be a primary or a secondary culture.

Blood is frequently examined in the microbiology laboratory and may be collected by the medical assistant. Care must be taken in any instance of venipuncture, of course, but for the purpose of culture, the specimen must remain uncontaminated for a diagnostic result (see Chapter 45, Phlebotomy). The yellow-stopper tube should be anticoagulated with sodium polyethanol sulfonate unless the pathogen is suspected to be *Neisseria gonorrhoea.* In adults, usually 10 to 20 mL are collected; in children, from 1 to 5 mL.

Sputum is often tested for the diagnosis of respiratory diseases. It should be the first morning specimen

BOX 43-1 Guidelines for Specimen Collection and Handling

- Follow Standard Precautions for specimen collection as outlined by the Centers for Disease Control and Prevention (CDC).
- Review the requirements for collecting and handling the specimen, including the equipment needed, the type of specimen to be collected (exudate, blood, mucus, and so on), the amount required for proper laboratory analysis, and the procedure to be followed for handling and storage.
- Assemble the equipment and supplies. Use only the appropriate specimen container for the sample to be submitted as specified by the medical office or laboratory.
- Ensure the specimen container is sterile to prevent contamination of the specimen by organisms not present at the collection site.
- Examine each container before use to make sure that it is not damaged, the medium is intact and moist, and it is well within the expiration date.
- Label each tube or specimen container with the patient's name and/or identification number, the date, the name or initials of the person collecting the specimen, the source or site of the specimen, and any other information required by the laboratory. Use an indelible pen or permanent marker. Make sure you print legibly, document accurately, and include all pertinent information.

Checkpoint Question

2. What are the differences between mixed cultures, secondary cultures, and pure cultures?

Types of Culture Media

Media support the growth of microorganisms for easier identification. The microorganism will proliferate for easier diagnosis of disease when it has been provided an environment for optimal growth.

Various types of media are prepared with a mixture of substances that nourish pathogens. All of the requirements for replication must exist for the suspected microorganism. Nutrients, moisture, and the proper pH are provided by the medium. The temperature and darkness will be maintained by an incubator and the presence or absence of oxygen will be provided as needed. Some media are solid, some are semisolid, and some are in the form of a liquid or broth.

Media may contain additives to support the growth of specific organisms and inhibit the growth of others; these are referred to as selective media. Nonselective media will grow almost any microorganism introduced to its surface.

Media designed for **anaerobic** bacteria (bacteria that live without oxygen) may contain a tablet that generates carbon dioxide and eliminates oxygen in the closed environment of the medium. Many laboratories use special sealed jars containing a pouch of chemicals that maintain an anaerobic environment. In some instances, the plate may be placed in a jar with a lighted candle. The jar is tightly sealed and the candle will consume the available oxygen and gradually burn itself out. Figure 43-3 displays one type of anaerobic culture set.

Specimens submitted for laboratory study are most frequently cultured on blood **agar**. Blood agar is a solid medium that is prepared by adding 5% sheep's blood to agar, a transparent and colorless substance made from seaweed. The agar congeals the blood and forms a firm surface to support the growth of microorganisms. The firm surface makes it easier to read the culture growth. The blood adds the nourishment required for replication of the microorganisms.

A **Petri plate** is a glass or plastic dish used to hold a solid culture medium such as blood agar. The plate is fitted with a cover to maintain the integrity of the specimen. Petri plates are clear and allow visual examination of a culture as it grows.

A liquid or broth medium is usually provided in a small jar or tube. Many special broth media are supplied with swabs to be used for specimen collection and are enclosed in special envelopes for transporting the specimen.

collected by deep coughing with care that saliva is not also expectorated into the container. You may be responsible for educating the patient regarding the proper procedure for sputum collection. (See Chapter 37, Caring for Patients with Respiratory Disorders.)

Wound specimens may be collected by the medical assistant or the physician. It may be necessary to collect wound specimens from several sites within the wound area. (See Chapter 30, Caring for Patients with Integumentary Disorders.)

Other commonly obtained specimens include throat cultures (see Chapter 37, Caring for Patients with Respiratory Disorders), urine cultures (see Chapter 44, Urinalysis), and stool specimens (see Chapter 38, Caring for Patients with Gastrointestinal Disorders).

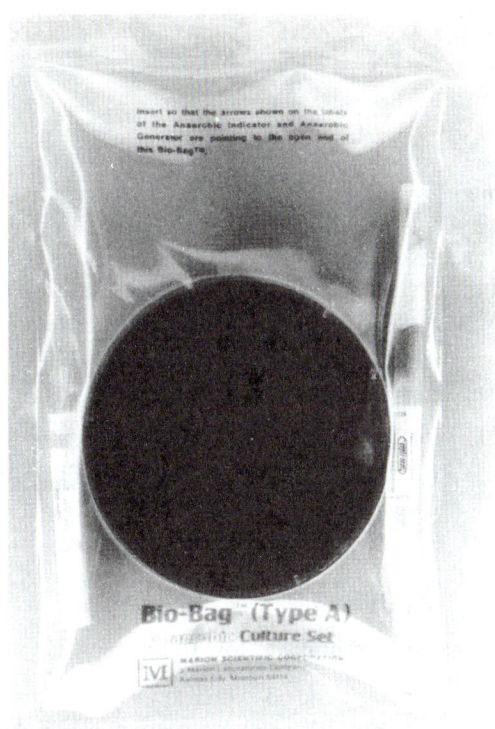

FIGURE 43-3
The Bio-Bag anaerobic culture set (Becton Dickinson Microbiology Systems, Cockeysville, MD). This culture set includes a plate of CDC-anaerobic blood agar contained within an oxygen-impermeable bag. The system contains its own gas-generating kit and cold catalyst.

Caring for the Media

Commercially prepared culture media contained in disposable plastic Petri plates are available for use in medical offices. The plates are supplied in a plastic sleeve and must be stored in the refrigerator with the side containing the medium uppermost (Fig. 43-4). The plates should be stored in the plastic wrapper to keep the media moist. Petri plates stored with the medium downward may form condensation on the lids that will drip onto the surface, making it too moist for an accurate culture. Check the expiration date and the condition of the medium surface before using the plates. Discard any plates that are past the expiration date or any medium that has dried or cracked.

Culture media may also be prepared in the medical office from a commercially available dehydrated form. A culture medium is effective for 72 hours once it has been inoculated with a specimen. Transportation or on-site testing within that time frame is essential.

Agar media must be refrigerated until needed, then warmed to room temperature before use. A cold plate or tube will kill many of the microorganisms that require a warmer temperature for growth. Most physi-

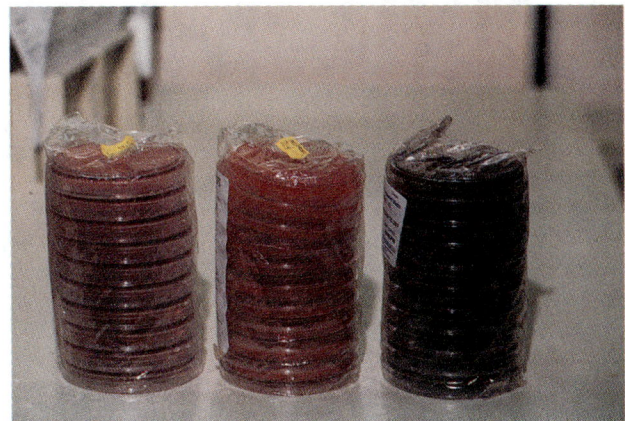

FIGURE 43-4
Solid media is supplied on petri plates wrapped in a plastic sleeve. Petri plates are always stored media side up.

cian's offices will be equipped with an incubator set at about 99°F (37°C) or just about body temperature. Check and record the incubator temperature daily.

Checkpoint Question
3. *Why is it important to store Petri plates with the media side uppermost?*

Transporting the Specimen

Many pathogens are not particularly fragile, but care must be taken to transport or process the specimen as soon as possible to avoid the death of any of the organisms present. The quicker the specimen is processed, the sooner the pathogen can be identified and treatment can begin. Some microorganisms, such as *N. gonorrhoea*, are very fragile and must be cultured under controlled conditions as quickly as possible.

Specimens to be processed in outside or regional laboratories must be placed in transport media such as the Culturette (Marion Scientific Corporation) or Precision Culture CATS (Precision Dynamics Corporation). All directions appropriate to the specimen will be specified by the manufacturer on the packaging. Most of the transport systems are designed to be self-contained and include a plastic tube with a sterile swab and transport medium appropriate for the type of specimen usually collected by this particular system (Fig. 43-5). Most are stored at room temperature. Because transported specimens will be handled by a large laboratory, special care must be taken in filling out all identification slips and information. Procedure 43-1 describes the steps for preparing a specimen for transport.

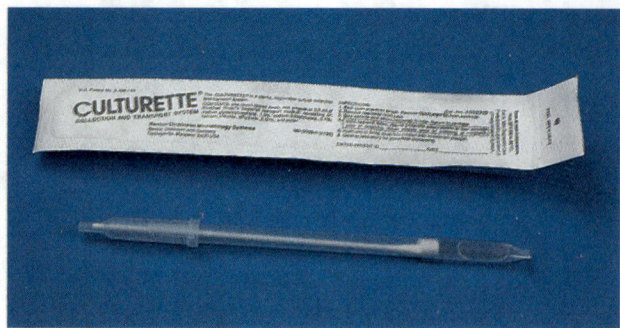

FIGURE 43-5
Transport media.

Properly prepared transport media may be mailed or routed by a courier. The outside laboratory may provide specific mailing or shipping containers, either cardboard or styrofoam, to protect the specimen during transport. A label indicating the presence of a biohazardous biologic specimen is attached to the outside of the container. In many instances, specimens are only collected and transported on days that ensure their arrival during the business week to avoid having them remain in transit until the start of a new week. Delays in testing may cause some of the microorganisms to die or to over-proliferate, possibly compromising the results of the test.

For the most reliable results, laboratory tests should be performed on fresh specimens within 1 hour after collection. When this is not possible, the specimen must be stored properly to preserve the physical and chemical properties necessary for accurate diagnosis. Specimens should never be subjected to extreme temperature changes. Table 43-2 lists general guidelines for handling and storing specimens commonly collected in the medical office.

Charting Example

07/13/99	1300	Wound swab taken from left lower leg. Yellow-green drainage noted. Specimen was labeled and sent via courier to the laboratory.
		— Mark Thomas, RMA

➤ MICROSCOPIC EXAMINATION OF MICROORGANISMS

Smears and Slides

Specimens collected by a swab or spatula from the site of a disease process or by inoculation loop from a primary or secondary culture are frequently spread onto a glass slide to be inspected by microscope in the clinical setting. Sometimes a special treatment with stains or fixatives will be applied to aid in identification. Some pathogens are more easily identified if they are allowed to move freely in what is called a wet mount or a hanging drop slide. These should always be viewed immediately or within 30 minutes of collection.

Wet Mount

To prepare a wet mount, follow these steps:

1. Place a drop of the specimen on a glass slide with sterile saline or 10% potassium hydroxide (KOH).
2. Place a coverslip over the specimen to reduce evaporation.
3. To further decrease evaporation, place petrolatum around the rim of the coverslip (Fig. 43-6).
4. Inspect the slide by microscope using the high power objective with diminished light.

Hanging Drop

This method requires a special slide with a depression in the center. A coverslip edged with petrolatum keeps the specimen from drying out.

1. Place a drop of the specimen in the center of the coverslip with the petrolatum around the edges.
2. Place the depression in the slide over the coverslip with the specimen in the center.
3. Lightly press the slide against the coverslip to seal the edges; this will hold the slide tightly to the coverslip.
4. Invert the slide so that the specimen on the coverslip hangs into the depression on the slide (Fig. 43-7).
5. Inspect the slide arrangement by microscope with the high power objective and diminished light.

If multiple smears are to be made from one culture, the colonies to be observed should be numbered on the back of the Petri plate(s). Number the slides with corresponding numbers with a diamond-tipped pen on the frosted edge of the slide for proper identification of the culture sites (see Procedure 43-2: Preparing a Dry Smear).

Table 43-2

Handling and Storing Commonly Collected Specimens

Specimen	Handling	Storage
Urine	The specimen should be clean-catch midstream with care to avoid contaminating the inside of the container. Do not let the specimen stand for more than 1 hour after collection.	If the urine specimen cannot be tested within 1 hour after collection, it must be refrigerated. An appropriate preservative may be added at the direction of the laboratory; however, preservatives are not usually added to specimens for urine culture.
Blood	Handle the specimen carefully; hemolysis may destroy the microorganisms necessary for diagnosis. Collect the specimen in an anticoagulant tube that is at room temperature. The specimen must remain free of contaminants. Refer to the reference laboratory manual for the proper anticoagulant.	For most blood specimens, refrigerate at 4°C (39°F) to slow changes in the physical and chemical composition of the specimen.
Stool	Collect the specimen in a clean container. To test for ova and parasites, keep the stool warm.	Deliver the specimen to the laboratory immediately. If there is a delay in transporting, mix the stool with preservatives provided or recommended by the laboratory or place it in a transport medium.
Microbiologic specimens	Do not contaminate the swab or the inside of the specimen container by touching either to surfaces other than the site of collection. Protect anaerobic specimens from exposure to air.	Transport the specimen as soon as possible. If transport is not possible, refrigerate the specimen at 4°C (39°F) to maintain its integrity.

Note: Observe Standard Precautions while handling any of these specimens.

Identification by Staining

Staining the microorganisms may help the physician narrow the field of possible pathogens and initiate treatment before a culture has been incubated (see Box 43-2). Most bacteria are colorless and hard to see or to identify without special treatment such as staining.

The Gram stain process was developed by Dr. Hans Gram, a Dutch physician who discovered that certain bacteria (cocci and bacilli) retain crystal violet dye through a process to decolorize the specimen. Those bacteria that retain the purple color are Gram positive. Those that do not are Gram negative and

Charting Example

08/12/99	8:30 AM Specimen taken from nasal cavity and prepared as a dry smear. Gram stain positive. Dr. York read the slide. ——— Tony Diaz, CMA

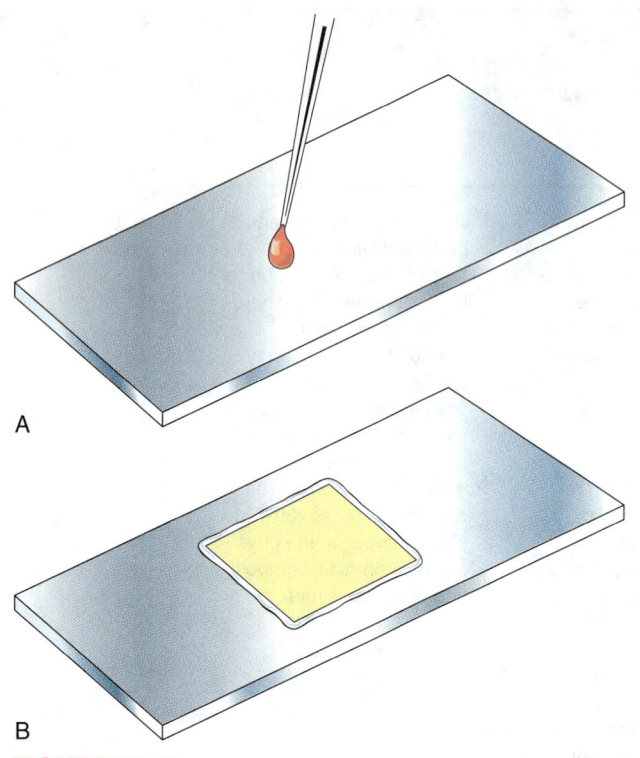

FIGURE 43-6
Wet mount slide preparation. (*A*) A drop of fluid containing the organism is placed on a glass slide. (*B*) The specimen is covered with a coverslip ringed with petroleum jelly.

must be counterstained to be seen under a microscope. The Gram-negative bacteria will retain a pink or red color from the counterstain. Procedure 43-3 details the steps for Gram staining a smear slide.

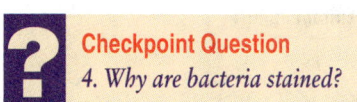
Checkpoint Question
4. Why are bacteria stained?

BOX 43-2 Gram Staining: A Diagnostic Tool

Gram staining provides important diagnostic information. Even before a culture can be incubated, a physician may tentatively diagnose a patient's disease and begin treatment based on the results of Gram staining, the organism's morphology, and the patient's reported symptoms.

Below are some common diseases and their Gram staining results:

Gram Positive	*Gram Negative*
Strep throat	Whooping cough
Scarlet fever	(pertussis)
Diphtheria	*Escherichia coli*
Meningitis	(present in some forms
Tetanus	of cystitis)
Botulism	*Hemophilus influenza*
Certain pneumonias	Certain pneumonias
Gardnerella vaginitis	Gonococcus
Staphylococcal skin	Salmonella
lesions	Shigella
Toxic shock syndrome	Cholera

Microbiologic Inoculation

Microbiologic inoculation refers to the practice of introducing a microorganism into a hospitable environment. To ensure that the specimen is placed on or in the culture medium in the proper manner to encourage maximal growth, the medical assistant will *streak* it with a swab or with an inoculating loop (Fig. 43-8). Broth is considered to be inoculated when the swab is inserted below its surface (Fig. 43-9).

Generally, a swab is used when the specimen is lifted directly from the site to the medium. An inoculating loop is used when lifting a specimen from a culture to inoculate a secondary culture. The specific

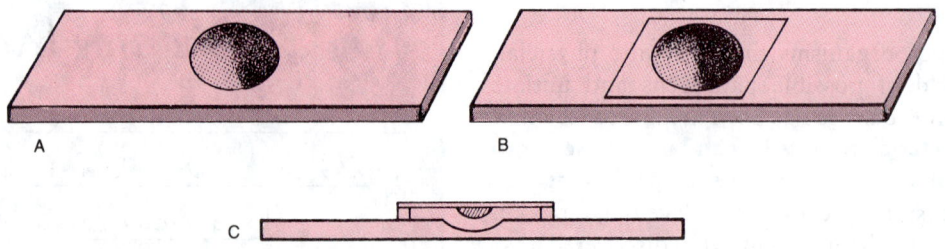

FIGURE 43-7
Hanging drop preparation for study of living bacteria. (*A*) Depression slide. (*B*) Depression slide with coverglass over the depression area. (*C*) Side view of hanging drop preparation, showing the drop of culture hanging from the center of the coverglass above the depression. (Volk WA, Wheeler MF: Basic Microbiology, 5th ed. Philadelphia, JB Lippincott, 1984)

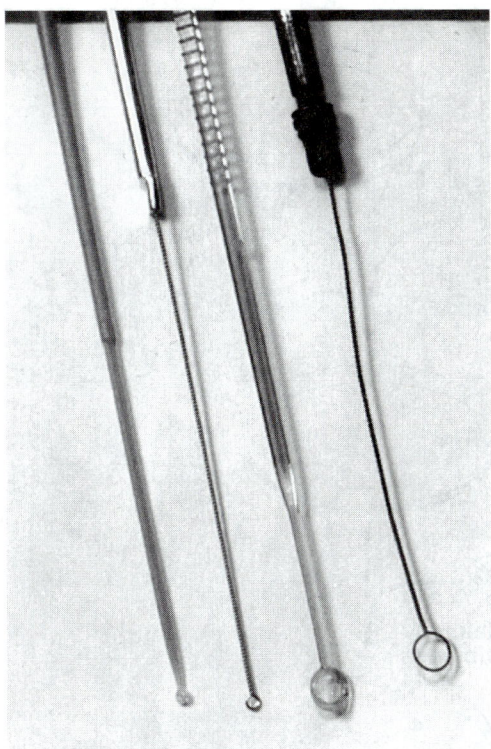

FIGURE 43-8
Bacteriology loops for inoculation and transfer of bacterial cultures. The two loops to the left (plastic and wire construction, respectively) are calibrated to deliver 0.001 mL of fluid for performing semiquantitative colony counts. The plastic and the wire loops to the right are calibrated to deliver 0.01 mL of fluid.

colonies will be lifted from the primary plate and streaked onto the second plate to be re-incubated for further study. Procedure 43-4 describes the steps for culture inoculation.

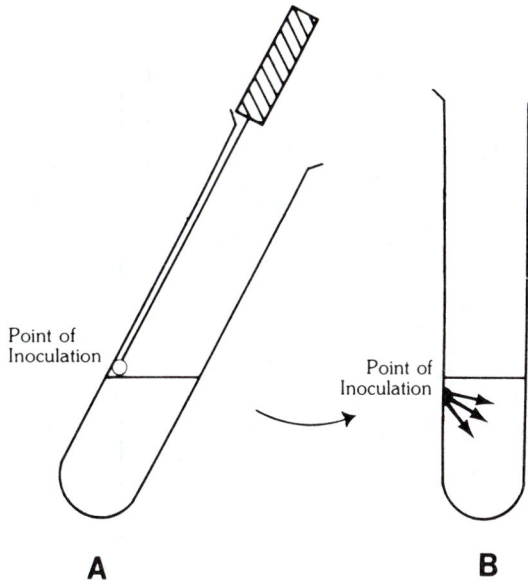

A   B

FIGURE 43-9
Technique for inoculating a tube of broth medium. (*A*) Slant and inoculate the side of the tube as shown. (*B*) Replace the tube upright. This submerges the inoculation site under the surface.

Sensitivity Testing

Once an organism has been identified, its susceptibility to medication must be established. In many cases, pure or secondary cultures are used to avoid confusion of the results. Filter paper disks are impregnated with various antimicrobial agents that will be dropped onto the agar plate after being inoculated with the bacteria and before being incubated. After the plate has been incubated for the prescribed length of time (usually 18-24 hours), it will be inspected for a zone of nongrowth around each disk. Those that exhibit a margin with no bacterial growth indicate that the pathogen is sensitive or susceptible to this medication (Fig. 43-10).

Streptococcal Testing

Streptococcal pharyngitis in children and young adults is one of the most common presenting infections in the medical office. Because of the need for rapid diagnosis to begin appropriate treatment, many kits are available to quickly test for the pathogen group A beta hemolytic streptococcus or *Streptococcus pyogenes*. The results are read in a few minutes while the patient waits. Treatment can begin at once.

Charting Example

12/04/99	0800	Specimen taken from oral cavity. Petri plate was labeled and streaked. Plate placed in incubator. To be read 12/06/99.
		———— Sharon Green, CMA

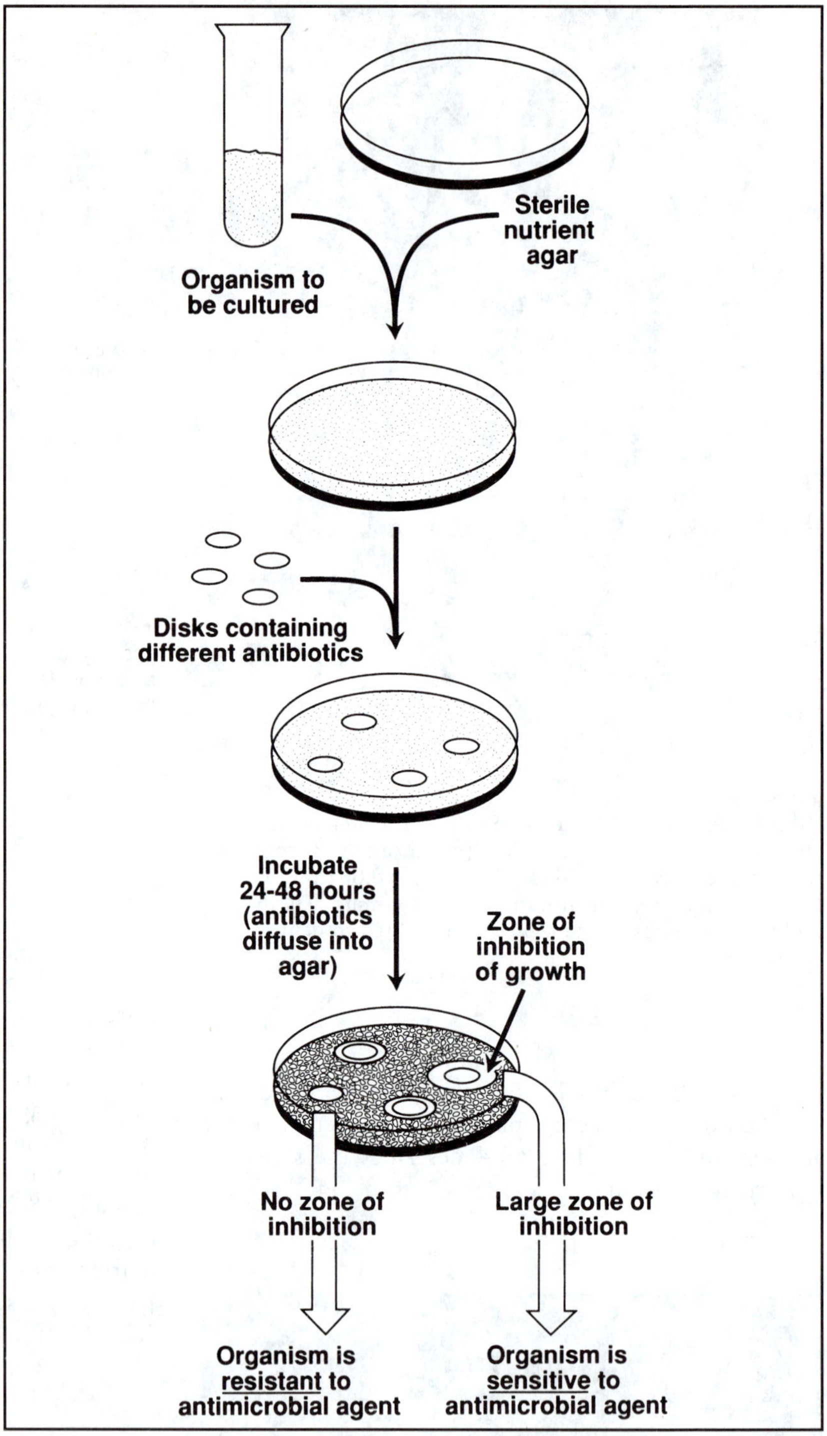

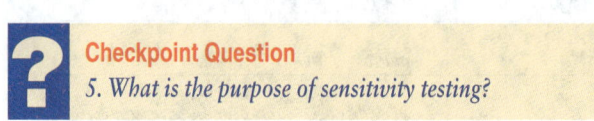

FIGURE 43-10
Disk diffusion method for determining the sensitivity of bacteria to antimicrobial agents.

The theory behind the rapid tests for streptococcus relies on the antigen-antibody reaction that causes a change to occur on the testing material. Quick, easy-to-follow instructions are provided by the manufacturer of the testing equipment chosen by the physician. Quality control measures are included with the testing packages. See Chapter 47 for further discussion of strep testing.

? Checkpoint Question
5. What is the purpose of sensitivity testing?

text continues on page 863

Procedure 43-1 Preparing the Specimen for Transport

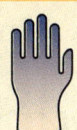

Equipment/Supplies

- appropriate laboratory slip
- specimen container
- specimen
- gloves

Steps	Purpose
1. Assemble the equipment.	1. This ensures that all supplies are available.
2. Complete the laboratory request form.	2. All information must be filled into the appropriate blanks. If information is not applicable or is not available, indicate this on the slip. Do not leave any questions unanswered.
3. Wash hands and put on gloves.	3. Standard Precautions must be observed.
4. Check the expiration date and the condition of the transport medium.	4. Out-of-date media must not be used. If the medium appears to be dried, or looks different than it normally does, do not use it.
5. Peel the envelope away from the transport tube about one-third of the way and remove the tube.	5. Many of the envelopes are used for repackaging the specimen. This will be indicated on the package.
6. Label the tube with the date, the patient's name, the source of the specimen, and initials of the person processing the specimen.	6. The specimen container must be identified to accompany the laboratory slip.
7. Obtain the specimen as directed by the physician or receive the specimen as the collection procedure is performed by the physician.	7. The specimen may be obtained by various methods and from many different sites for transport.
8. Return the swab to the tube and follow the manufacturer's recommendation for immersion into the medium.	8. Instructions vary and are specific to the manufacturer. All instructions must be followed to ensure accurate test results.
9. Remove and dispose of gloves and wash hands.	9. Standard Precautions must be observed throughout the procedure.
10. Package for transport as directed by the manufacturer's recommendations on the packaging. Some specify returning the tube to the peel-apart envelope.	10. The laboratory slip and all components of the transport system must be packaged together to avoid misidentification.
11. Record the procedure.	11. Procedures are considered not to have been done if they are not recorded.
12. Route the specimen.	12. The specimen may be mailed, or a courier may be contacted.

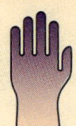

Procedure 43-2

Preparing a Dry Smear

Equipment/Supplies

- specimen
- slide forceps
- sterile swab or inoculating loop
- Bunsen burner
- slide
- gloves
- face shield

Steps	Purpose
1. Wash your hands.	1. Handwashing aids infection control.
2. Assemble the equipment.	2. This ensures that all supplies are available.
3. Label the slide with the patient's name and the date on the frosted edge.	3. Labeling will ensure proper patient identification.
4. Put on gloves and face shield. Hold the edges of the slide between the thumb and index finger. Starting at the right side of the slide and using a rolling motion of the swab or a sweeping motion of the inoculating loop, gently and evenly spread the material from the specimen over the slide. The material should thinly fill the center of the slide within ½ inch of each end.	4. Standard Precautions must be observed. The face shield should be worn to avoid splatters from the inoculating loop. The material should be spread thinly to avoid obscuring the slide with too much material. Rolling ensures that as much of the specimen as possible is deposited on the slide. Sweeping the loop accomplishes the same purpose. Confining the specimen to the area within ½ inch of the edges avoids contaminating the gloves.

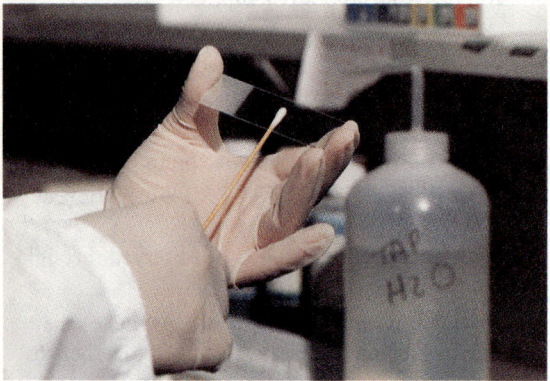

Step 4: Use a rolling motion to deposit the specimen material on the slide.

Steps	Purpose
5. Do not rub the material vigorously over the slide.	5. Doing so may destroy fragile microorganisms.
6. Dispose of the contaminated swab or inoculating loop in a biohazard container. If you are not using a disposable loop, sterilize it as follows: a. Hold the loop in the colorless part of the flame of the Bunsen burner for 10 seconds. b. Raise the loop slowly (to avoid splattering the bacteria) to the blue part of the flame until the loop and its connecting wire glow red.	6. The swab and the loop contain body fluid and are considered hazardous.

(continued)

Procedure 43-2

Preparing a Dry Smear *(continued)*

Steps   **Purpose**

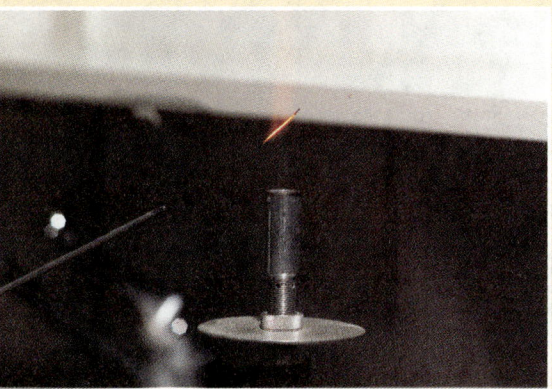

Step 6B: Fire the loop and its connecting wire.

    c. Cool the loop so the heat will not kill the bacteria that must be allowed to grow. Do not wave the loop in the air because doing so may expose it to contamination.

7. Allow the smear to air dry in a flat position for at least ½ hour. Do not wave it about in the air. Heat should not be applied until the specimen has been allowed to dry. Some specimens will require a fixative spray.

8. Hold the dried smear slide with the slide forceps. Pass the slide quickly through the flame of a Bunsen burner three or four times. The slide has been

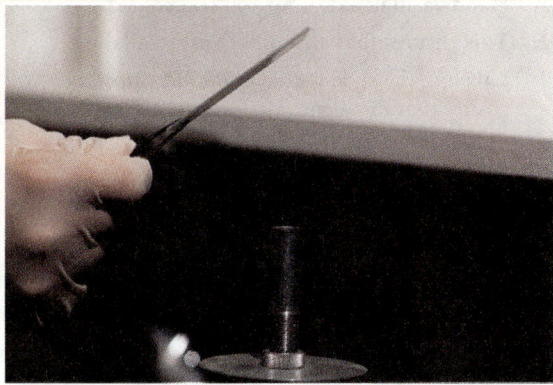

Step 8: Pass the slide through the flame.

fixed properly when the back of the slide feels slightly uncomfortably warm to the back of the gloved hand. It should not feel hot.

7. The cells will dry slowly if allowed to dry at room temperature. Fixatives may be sprayed from a distance of 4 to 6 inches to protect the cells from contaminants or to keep them from becoming dislodged. Heat at this point may destroy the microorganisms.

8. Passing the slide through the heat kills the microorganisms and attaches them firmly to the slide so they do not wash off during the staining process or are not dislodged during the viewing process if they are not to be stained. Excessive heat may distort the specimen cells.

(continued)

Procedure 43-2   Preparing a Dry Smear (continued)

Steps	Purpose
9. Examine the smear under the microscope or stain it according to office policy. In most instances, the physician will examine the slide for confirmation.	
10. Dispose of equipment and supplies in appropriate containers. Remove and dispose of gloves and wash your hands.	10. Standard Precautions must be observed throughout the procedure.
11. Record the procedure.	11. Procedures are considered not to have been done if they are not recorded.

Procedure 43-3   Gram Staining a Smear Slide

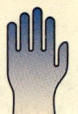

Equipment/Supplies

- crystal violet stain
- Gram's iodine solution
- alcohol-acetone solution
- counterstain (eg, Safranin)
- specimen on a glass slide labeled using a diamond-tipped pen
- Bunsen burner
- slide forceps
- staining rack
- wash bottle with distilled water
- absorbent (**bibulous**) paper pad
- immersion oil
- microscope
- gloves
- stop watch or timer

Steps	Purpose
1. Wash your hands.	1. Handwashing aids infection control.
2. Assemble the equipment.	2. This ensures that all supplies are available.
3. Make sure that the specimen is heat fixed to the labeled slide and that the slide is room temperature before beginning. (See Procedure 43-2: Preparing a Dry Smear.)	3. Labeling the slide with a diamond-tipped pen will ensure that the identification will not wash off during the repeated staining and washing steps of the procedure.
4. Put on gloves.	4. Standard Precautions must be observed. The specimen is a body substance and must be considered hazardous.
5. Place the slide on the staining rack with the smear side upward.	5. The staining rack collects the dye as it runs off the slide for disposal.
6. Flood the smear with crystal violet. Time with the stop watch or timer for 30 to 60 seconds.	6. To stain the bacteria purple.

(continued)

Procedure 43-3

Gram Staining a Smear Slide *(continued)*

Steps	**Purpose**

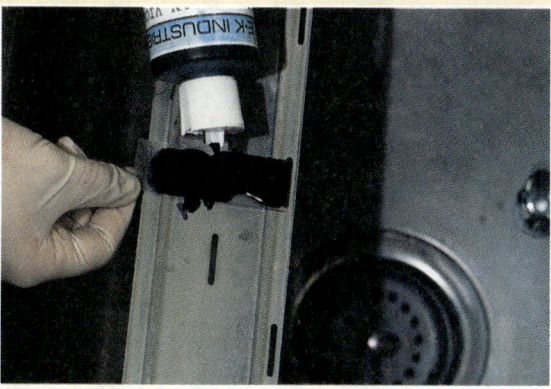

Step 6: Flood the slide with crystal violet.

7. Hold the slide with slide forceps.
   a. Tilt the slide to an angle of about 45° to drain the excess dye.
   b. Rinse the slide with distilled water from the wash bottle for about 5 seconds and drain off the excess water.

7. Washing off the stain stops the coloring process.

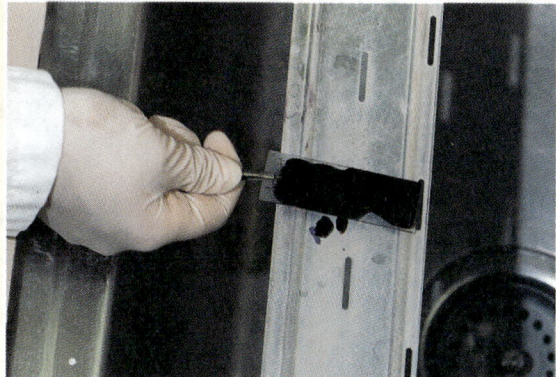

Step 7A: Tilt the slide to drain excess dye.

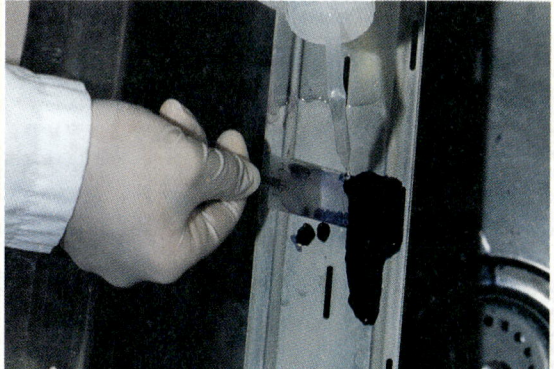

Step 7B: Rinse with water.

(continued)

Procedure 43-3

Gram Staining a Smear Slide *(continued)*

Steps	Purpose
8. Replace the slide on the slide rack. Flood the slide with Gram's iodine solution and time for 60 seconds.	8. The iodine acts as a **mordant** and fixes, or binds, the crystal violet to the Gram-positive bacteria. The stain will be permanent in the receptive Gram-positive cells after being fixed with the iodine solution.

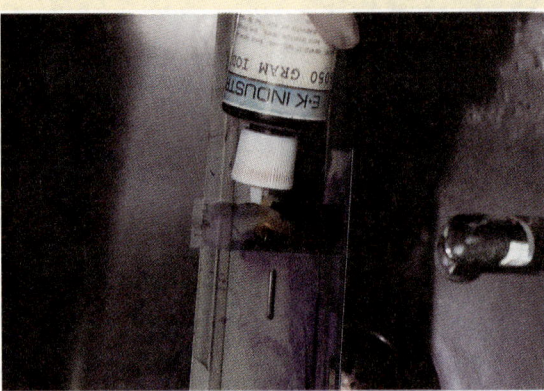

Step 8: Flood with Gram's iodine solution.

9. Using the forceps, tilt the slide at a 45° angle to drain iodine solution. With the slide tilted, rinse the slide with distilled water from the wash bottle for about 5 seconds. Slowly and gently wash with the alcohol-acetone solution until no more purple stain runs off.	9. The alcohol-acetone will remove the crystal violet stain from the Gram-negative bacteria. The Gram-positive bacteria will retain the purple dye. If the process is carried on too long or too vigorously, dye may leech out of the Gram-positive bacteria and lead to incorrect test results.

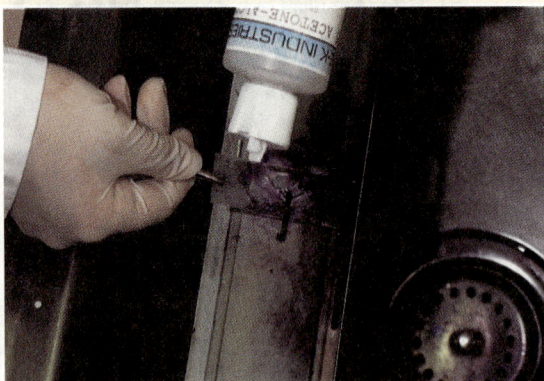

Step 9: Rinse with alcohol-acetone solution until no more purple stain runs off.

(continued)

Procedure 43-3   Gram Staining a Smear Slide *(continued)*

Steps	Purpose
10. Immediately rinse the slide with distilled water for 5 seconds and return the slide to the rack.	10. Rinsing with the wash bottle stops the decolorizing process.

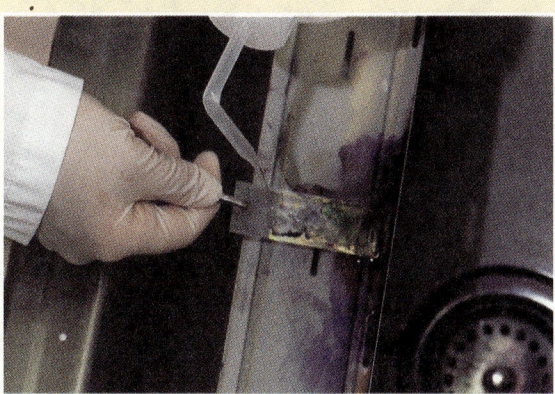

Step 10: Immediately rinse alcohol-acetone solution.

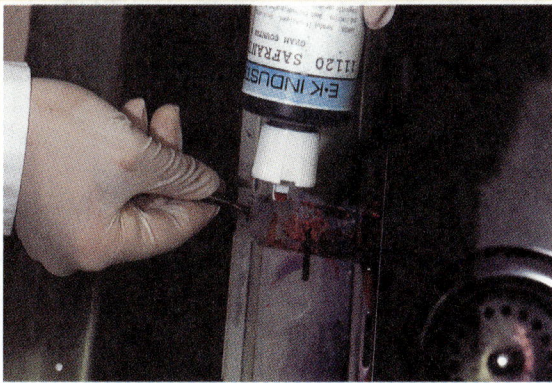

Step 11: Flood with Safranin or counterstain.

Steps	Purpose
11. Flood with the Safranin or suitable counterstain. Time for 30 to 60 seconds.	11. The Gram-negative bacteria will stain pink or red with the counterstain.
12. Drain the excess counterstain from the slide by tilting it at a 45° angle. a. Rinse the slide with the distilled water for 5 seconds to remove the counterstain.	12. Moisture or excess solutions may obscure the slide and hinder identification.

(continued)

Steps

Purpose

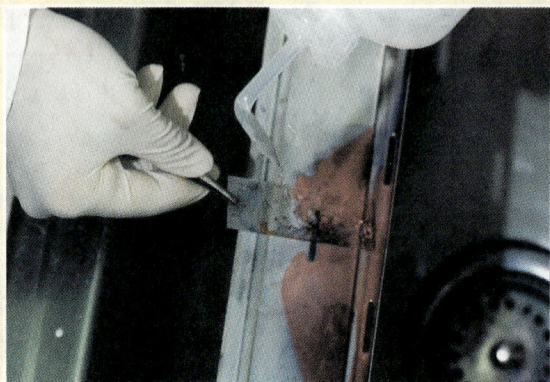

Step 12A: Rinse clear of counterstain.

    b. Gently blot the smear dry using absorbent
        bibulous paper. Take care not to disturb the
        smeared specimen. Wipe the back of the slide
        clear of any solution. It may be placed be-
        tween the pages of a bibulous paper pad and
        gently pressed to remove excess moisture.

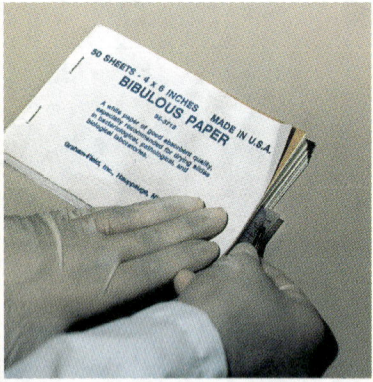

Step 12B: Blot gently with bibulous paper.

13. Inspect, using oil immersion objective lens for
     greatest magnification. The physician will inspect
     the slide.

14. Properly care for or dispose of equipment and sup-
     plies. Clean the work area. Remove gloves and
     wash your hands.

15. Record the procedure.

14. Standard Precautions must be followed through-
     out the procedure.

15. Procedures are considered not to have been done if
     they are not recorded.

Special Precautions: *Results may be misinterpreted if the reagents are defective or near expiration, or if
the timing factors in the staining process are not as directed. The bacteria may overstain or may have
color leeched from the cells if care is not taken to observe the time limits. The results will not be accurate
if the specimen was not heated properly (causing the bacteria to die) or was not incubated long enough
or if the general technique was not performed correctly. Premade smears of known Gram-positive and
Gram-negative organisms are processed with the patient's specimen for quality control.*

Procedure 43-4   Culture Inoculation

Equipment/Supplies

- specimen on a swab or loops
- Bunsen burner
- gloves
- face shield
- labeled Petri dish (the patient's name should be on the side of the plate containing the medium, as it is always placed upward to prevent condensation from dripping onto the culture)

Steps	Purpose
1. Assemble the equipment.	1. This ensures that all supplies are available.
2. Put on gloves and the face shield.	2. Standard Precautions must be observed. The face shield should be worn to avoid splatters from the inoculating loop.
3. Label the plate with the patient's identification and date the plate.	3. Because culture incubation may take 24–72 hours, dating will ensure that the plate is read at the proper time.
4. Remove the Petri plate from the cover (the Petri plate is always stored inverted with the cover downward) and place the cover with the opening upward on the work surface. Do not open the cover unnecessarily.	4. Each time the cover is removed there is the chance of contamination. Placing the cover with the opening upward avoids contamination from the work surface.
5. Using a rolling and sliding motion, streak the specimen swab completely across ½ of the plate starting from the top and working to a midpoint or at the diameter of the plate. Dispose of the	5. The specimen will be spread in gradually thinning colonies of bacteria.

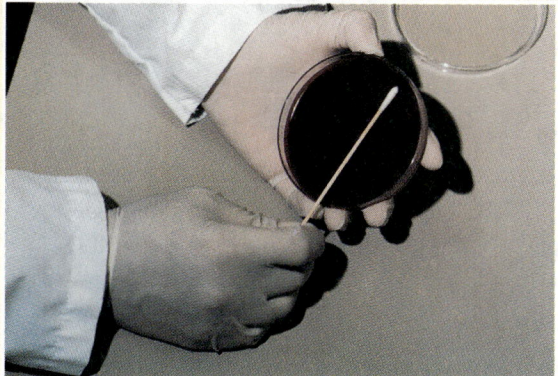

Step 5: Use a rolling, sliding motion to transfer the specimen to the plate.

swab in a biohazard container. If the inoculating loop is used for lifting a secondary culture, streak in the same manner.

(continued)

Procedure 43-4   Culture Inoculation (continued)

Steps	Purpose
6. Dispose of this loop. If your office does not use disposable inoculating loops, sterilize the loop as described in step 6 of Procedure 43-2: Preparing a Dry Smear.	
7. Turn the plate ¼ turn from its previous position. Draw another loop at right angles perpendicular to the specimen by starting at what is now the top of the plate and working to the midpoint of the plate. Do not enter the originally streaked area after the first few sweeps.	7. The loop will draw into the clean surface a bit of the specimen that was streaked in the first part of the procedure.

Step 7: Draw the loop at right angles to the midpoint of the plate.

Steps	Purpose
8. Dispose of this loop. If you are not using a disposable loop, flame loop and allow it to cool again.	8. The loop must be flamed again to avoid contamination from the previous pass.
9. Turn the plate another ¼ turn so that now it is 180 degrees to the original smear. Working in the previous manner, draw the loop at right angles through the most recently streaked area. Again, do not enter the originally streaked area after the first few sweeps. (The accompanying photograph shows *Staphylococcus aureus* on a properly streaked plate.)	9. The loop will pull out gradually thinning bits of the specimen to isolate colonies. Large groups of colonies close together are more difficult to identify than isolated colonies.

(continued)

Culture Inoculation *(continued)*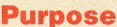

Steps   **Purpose**

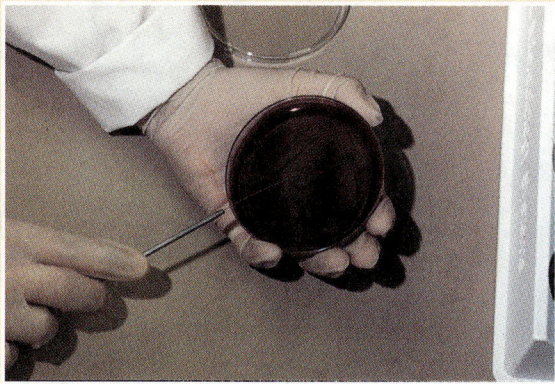

Step 9: Turn the plate another one-quarter turn and streak in the same manner.

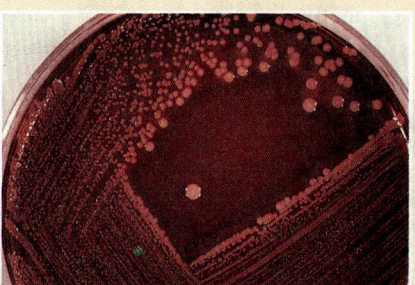

Step 9: (Continued) Pale yellow colonies of Staphylococcus aureus on a properly streaked plate.

10. If the plate is to be used for sensitivity, follow these steps:
    a. Using sterile forceps or an automatic dispenser, place the specified disks on areas of the plate equidistance from each other.

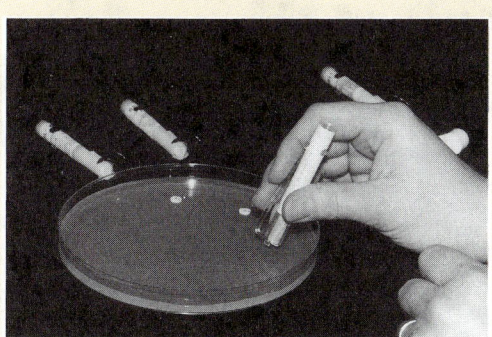

Step 10A: Dispense disks onto streaked plate.

(continued)

Procedure 43-4   Culture Inoculation *(continued)*

Steps	Purpose

Steps

b. Press them gently with the sterilized loop or forceps until good contact is made with the surface of the agar. (The accompanying photograph shows a sensitivity culture with areas of resistance and susceptibility.)

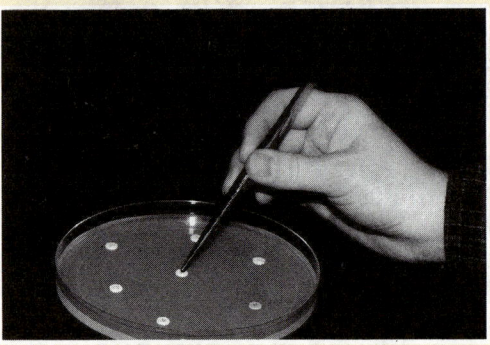

Step 10B: Press Disks firmly into surface.

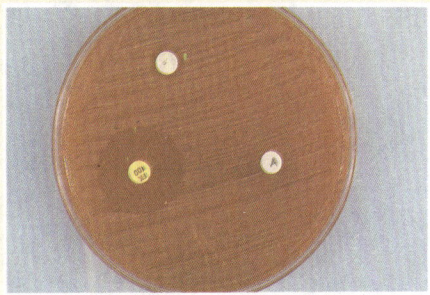

Step 10: (Continued) A sensitivity culture showing area of resistance and areas of susceptibility.

11. Properly care for or dispose of equipment and supplies. Remove gloves and wash your hands.

12. Record the procedure.

13. Incubate for the specified period of time. Read the results and record as directed by office policy.

Purpose

11. Standard Precautions must be followed throughout the procedure.

12. Procedures are considered not to have been done if they are not recorded.

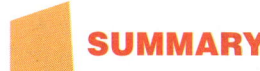

SUMMARY

The identification of disease-producing microorganisms will assist the physician in the treatment of illnesses caused by microbial agents. To do this effectively, the medical assistant may be responsible for collecting, handling, identifying, or transporting biologic specimens.

CRITICAL THINKING CHALLENGES

1. You are asked to give a brief talk to a group of elementary school children on microbiologic life forms. Develop an age-appropriate discussion of this topic. How would you make it possible for the children to correlate the presence of microbacteria with the need to wash their hands?
2. Write a policy that explains how to care for media and how to transport specimens. Be sure to include who can participate in this process.
3. Create a patient education brochure for streptococcal pharyngitis infections. Include information about what it is, how it is transmitted, signs and symptoms, and the testing procedure.

ANSWERS TO CHECKPOINT QUESTIONS

1. The four main categories of bacteria are cocci, bacilli, spirochetes, and vibrios.
2. Mixed cultures are used to investigate any or all of the microorganisms found at a site. Secondary cultures remove from the mixed cultures only those organisms that need to be encouraged to grow for more extensive study. Pure cultures contain only one organism and may be either a primary or a secondary culture.

3. If Petri plates are stored with the medium downward, condensation may form on the lids and drip onto the surface, making it too moist for an accurate culture.
4. Staining bacteria helps the physician narrow the field of possible pathogens and begin treatment before a culture has been incubated. Most bacteria are colorless and hard to see or identify without special treatment such as staining.
5. Sensitivity testing is done to determine which antibiotic effects the bacterial replication.

SUGGESTIONS FOR FURTHER READING

Atkinson, L. Jo. (1992). *Berry and Kohn's Operating Room Technique*, 7th ed. St. Louis, MO: Mosby-Year Book.

Burton, G. R. W. (1992). *Microbiology for the Health Sciences*, 4th ed. Philadelphia: J. B. Lippincott.

Fischbach, F. (1995). *Quick Reference for Common Laboratory Tests*. Philadelphia: J. B. Lippincott.

Fischbach, F. (1992). *Microbiology for the Health Sciences*, 4th ed. Philadelphia: J. B. Lippincott.

Johnson, T. R., & Case, C. L. (1992.) *Laboratory Experiments in Microbiology*, Brief Edition, 3rd ed. Benjamin/Cummings Publishing Company.

Koneman, E. W., et al. (1994). *Introduction to Diagnostic Microbiology*, Philadelphia: J. B. Lippincott.

Koneman, E. W., et al. (1992). *Color Atlas and Textbook of Diagnostic Microbiology*, Philadelphia: J. B. Lippincott.

Hamann, B. (1992). *Disease: Identification, Prevention and Control*, St. Louis: C.V. Mosby.

Memmler, R. L., Cohen, B. J., Wood, D. L. (1996.) *The Human Body in Health and Disease*, 8th ed. Philadelphia: Lippincott-Raven Publishers.

Volk, W. A., et al. (1995). *Essentials of Medical Microbiology*, 5th ed. Philadelphia: J. B. Lippincott.

Urinalysis

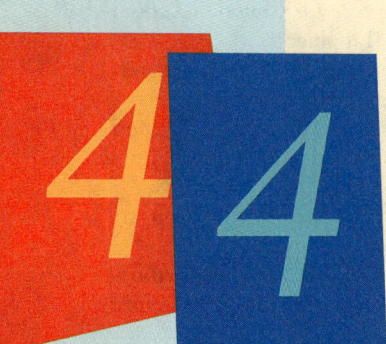

Chapter Outline

Specimen Collection Methods
    Clean-catch Midstream (CCMS)
    Urine Specimen
Procedure: Obtaining a Clean-catch
    Midstream (CCMS) Urine
    Specimen
    Bladder Catheterization
    Suprapubic Aspiration
    24-hour Urine Collection
Procedure: Obtaining a 24-Hour Urine
    Specimen
Physical Properties of Urine
    Color
    Clarity
Procedure: Determining Color and
    Clarity of Urine
    Specific Gravity
Procedure: Determining Specific Gravity
    of Urine Using the Urinometer
Procedure: Determining Specific
    Gravity of Urine Using the
    Refractometer
Chemical Properties of Urine
Procedure: Performing Chemical Reagent
    Strip Analysis
    pH
    Glucose

Procedure: Performing a Copper
    Reduction Test (Clinitest) for
    Glucose
    Ketones
Procedure: Performing Nitroprusside
    Reaction (Acetest) for
    Ketones
    Proteins
Procedure: Performing an Acid
    Precipitation Test for Protein
    Blood
    Bilirubin
Procedure: Performing Diazo Tablet Test
    (Ictotest) for Bilirubin
    Urobilinogen
    Nitrite
    Leukocyte Esterase
Urine Sediment
Procedure: Preparing a Urine Sediment
Procedure: Preparing Urine Sediment for
    a Microscopic Examination
    Structures Found in Urine Sediment
Urine Pregnancy Testing
Summary
Critical Thinking Challenges
Answers to Checkpoint Questions
Suggestions for Further Reading

DACUM Components

1.3   Practice within the scope of education, training, and personal capabilities
4.1   Apply principles of aseptic technique and infection control
4.9   Use quality control
4.10   Collect and process specimens
4.11   Perform selected tests that assist with diagnosis and treatment
5.1   Document accurately
7.2   Instruct patients with special needs

Chapter Competencies

Learning Objectives

Upon successfully completing this chapter, you will be able to:

1. Spell and define the Key Terms.
2. Describe the methods of urine collection.
3. List and explain the physical and chemical properties of urine.
4. State the conditions that can be detected by abnormal urinalysis findings.
5. List and describe the components that can be found in urine sediment.
6. Correlate chemical strip results with sediment findings.

Performance Objectives

Upon successfully completing this chapter, you will be able to:

1. Explain and/or assist a patient in obtaining a clean-catch midstream urine specimen (Procedure 44-1).
2. Explain and/or assist a patient in obtaining a 24-hour urine collection (Procedure 44-2).
3. Determine urine color and clarity (Procedure 44-3).
4. Determine specific gravity by urinometer (Procedure 44-4).
5. Determine specific gravity by refractometer (Procedure 44-5).
6. Accurately interpret chemical reagent strip reactions (Procedure 44-6).
7. Perform copper reduction test (Procedure 44-7).
8. Perform a nitroprusside reaction (Acetest) for ketones (Procedure 44-8).
9. Perform acid precipitation test (Procedure 44-9).
10. Perform diazo tablet test (Ictotest) for bilirubin (Procedure 44-10).
11. Prepare a urine sediment (Procedure 44-11).
12. Prepare a urine sediment for microscopic examination (Procedure 44-12).

Key Terms

(See Glossary for definitions.)

ammonia	hemoglobinuria
bilirubinuria	hydrogen ions
creatinine	lyse
culture	nitroprusside
diazo	particulate matter
electrolyte	phosphates
enumerate	precipitation
Ehrlich units	quantitative
esterase	sulfosalicylic acid
flocculation	urates
galactosuria	

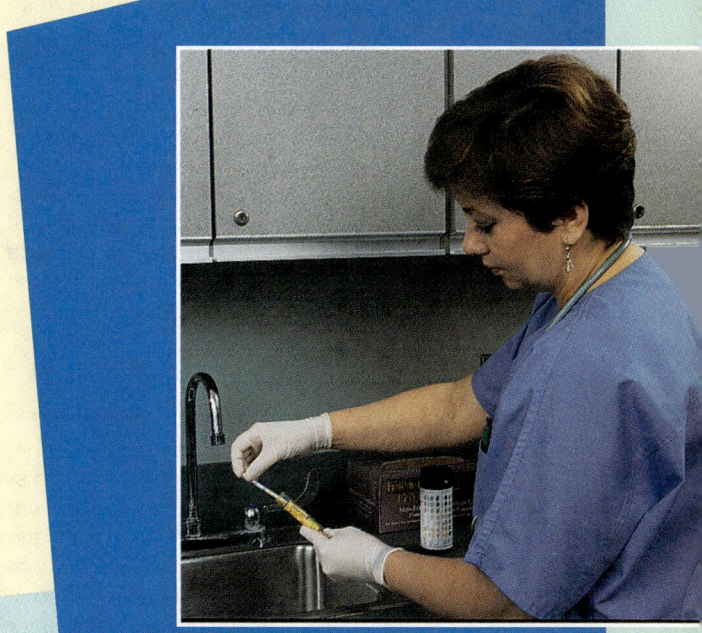

Complete urinalysis involves a physical, chemical, and microscopic examination of urine to assess renal function. Insight into many systemic diseases or conditions can be gained from urinalysis. Diagnosis or assessment of diabetes mellitus, shock, cardiac arrest, malnutrition, preeclampsia, and blood transfusion reactions are several of the disorders that can be detected by an examination of the urine.

Patient Education: Urine Specimen Collection

CLEAN-CATCH MIDSTREAM (CCMS) URINE SPECIMEN

Avoiding contamination during this procedure is vital to obtaining an accurate result. The teaching tips below can help ensure proper collection.
Instruct male patients as follows:

- Do not touch the penis to the inside of the container.
- Properly clean the glans.
- Collect the urine in the middle of the stream.

Instruct female patients as follows:

- Do not allow the labia to close over the meatus.
- Do not let the urine stream run onto the labia or perineum.
- Do not touch the inside of the sterile urine container.

Some facilities give the patients written instructions for the procedure. It is recommended that you assist the patient with this procedure because cleaning and collecting in the middle of the stream can be difficult. See Procedure 44-1 for a complete explanation.

24-HOUR URINE COLLECTION

Instruct the patient to collect *all* voided urine. The results will be inaccurate if any urine is discarded after the test begins. Give the patient several random urine containers to collect the urine, which is then poured into the 24-hour container. Printed instructions are recommended in the event the patient becomes confused after leaving the office. See Procedure 44-2 for a complete explanation.

➤ SPECIMEN COLLECTION METHODS

Proper collection of a urine specimen varies depending on the test to be performed. For a routine urinalysis, a freshly voided specimen is all that is necessary. This is called a "random urine." The patient voids the urine into a clean dry container. Often, however, a sterile specimen must be obtained to diagnose a urinary tract infection (UTI). Detecting the pathologic microorganism may require that a **culture** be performed. A culture is a laboratory process in which microorganisms are grown in a special medium, often for the purpose of identifying a causative agent in an infectious disease. All cultures require an uncontaminated specimen. Results of either a culture or a microscopic examination can be misleading if there is perineal contamination or other bacteria in the urine.

Once the urine is collected, testing should be done within 1 hour. If testing cannot be performed within this time, the specimen requires refrigeration at 4°C–6°C until testing can be performed. If the specimen is not properly refrigerated, alteration of certain chemical and cellular components contained in the urine can occur, causing the specimen to deteriorate. The presence and multiplication of bacteria in an unrefrigerated specimen changes the pH from acidic to alkaline. Glucose present in the urine may be used as a nutrient by the bacteria resulting in a false-negative or lowered glucose result. There are preservatives available that can be used to prevent deterioration if refrigeration is not possible.

The timing of collection may be an important consideration as well. First-morning urine specimens are the most concentrated and are useful for many tests that are more easily read with concentrated components (eg, pregnancy testing). Second-voided specimens are more useful for glucose testing because the urine will be more recently formed than that left in the bladder over night. Random urinalysis is the most common of the specimens required for office testing.

Clean-catch Midstream (CCMS) Urine Specimen

A clean-catch midstream urine is the most commonly ordered random specimen. It is useful when the physician suspects an infection because any bacteria present after a correctly collected CCMS will be from the urinary tract and not from contamination such as the perineal area. This specimen can then be used for a culture if nothing has been allowed to contaminate the urine, such as a pipette or chemical strip. Collection is done after the urinary meatus and surrounding skin has been cleansed. The urine is voided into a sterile container. Be aware that the procedure for obtaining a CCMS urine specimen for males differs from the procedure for females (Procedure 44-1).

Bladder Catheterization

Another method for aseptic urine collection is catheterization. A thin sterile tube (catheter) is placed into the bladder through the urethra. This procedure usually is performed by a physician or nurse. In some instances, medical assistants may be trained by their physicians to perform uncomplicated catheterizations. Bladder catheterization is recommended when the patient is unable to give a urine specimen in a sterile manner using the clean-catch method. (See Chap. 39, Caring for Patients with Urinary Disorders, for more information about catheterization.)

Suprapubic Aspiration

Suprapubic aspiration is the least common method of urine collection. A needle is inserted into the bladder through the skin of the abdominal wall above the symphysis pubis and urine is withdrawn (aspirated). This method is used in rare situations and is performed by a physician.

24-Hour Urine Collection

Because substances such as proteins, **creatinine**, and **electrolytes** are variably excreted during a 24-hour period, a 24-hour collection is a better indicator of values

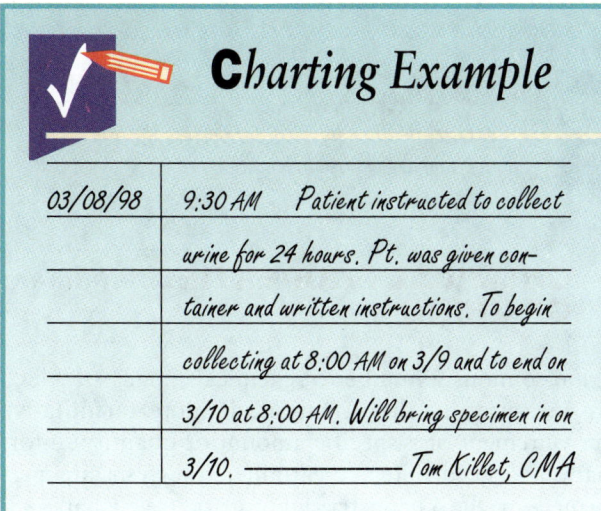

Charting Example

| 03/08/98 | 9:30 AM | Patient instructed to collect urine for 24 hours. Pt. was given container and written instructions. To begin collecting at 8:00 AM on 3/9 and to end on 3/10 at 8:00 AM. Will bring specimen in on 3/10. ————— Tom Killet, CMA |

than a random specimen. (Creatinine is a substance formed from creatine metabolism. Electrolytes are chemical substances dissolved in the blood that have numerous basic functions, such as conducting electrical currents.) To obtain this kind of specimen, the patient collects all voided urine within a 24-hour period (Procedure 44-2).

Checkpoint Question

1. What is the time frame for testing unrefrigerated urine? Why is this important?

► PHYSICAL PROPERTIES OF URINE

The physical properties include the urine's color, appearance (such as clarity or turbidity), specific gravity, and odor (for instance, a diabetic patient's urine may smell sweet and bacteria may give urine a strong odor). Color and clarity are assessed visually and are subjective, meaning the individual performing the testing will determine whether these properties can be considered within the normal range.

Color

Urine color can be affected by many things: diet, drugs, diseases, and the concentration of the urine. The normal color of urine is a pale straw color to dark yellow. The yellow color is due to a urine pigment called urochrome. A pale urine is typically very dilute and is seen after high fluid intake. Likewise a deep, dark yellow can signify a highly concentrated urine, such as when fluids are withheld or the patient is dehydrated.

Clarity

Normal, freshly voided urine is usually clear (transparent). Haziness or turbidity (cloudiness) indicates the presence of some **particulate matter** (material composed of particles). Some alkaline urine may appear turbid owing to the presence of certain chemicals such as **phosphates**, a compound containing phosphorus and oxygen. Some acidic urine may become turbid on standing owing to **precipitation** (settling out) of **urates** (nitrogenous compounds derived from protein use and excreted in the urine). Turbidity caused by either of the above is considered normal. The presence of cells, such as red and white blood cells, bacteria, and other particulate matter, such as mucus, can also cause a urine specimen to become turbid.

Laboratories may vary in terminology used to express clarity or turbidity of urine. However, most agree that when a small amount of turbidity is present so that black lines drawn on white paper can still be seen through the specimen, it is termed hazy. As turbidity increases and these black lines can no longer be seen, it is called cloudy (Procedure 44-3). The three terms most commonly used to describe clarity are clear, hazy, and cloudy. Table 44-1 summarizes the common causes for variations in the color and clarity of urine.

Table 44-1	
Common Causes for Variations in the Color and Clarity of Urine	
Color/Clarity	**Possible Causes**
Yellow-brown or-green brown	Bile in urine (as in jaundice), phenol poisoning (AKA carbolic acid, used as an antimicrobial agent)
Dark yellow or orange	Concentrated urine, low fluid intake, dehydration, inability of kidney to dilute urine, fluorescein (an IV dye), excessive carotene (carotenemia)
Bright orange-red	Pyridium (a urinary tract analgesic)
Red or reddish-brown	Fresh blood (indicating bleeding in the lower urinary tract), porphyrin menstrual contamination (porphyrin binds with iron to form heme), pyrvinium pamoate (Povan) for intestinal worms, sulfonamides (sulfa-based antibiotics)
Brownish-black	Methylene blue medication (commonly used as an antiseptic or in the treatment of a form of anemia)
Black	Melanin (the pigmenting cell)
Grayish or smokey	Hemoglobin or remnants of old red blood cells (indicating bleeding in the upper urinary tract), chyle, prostatic fluid, yeasts
Cloudy	Phosphate precipitation (normal after sitting for a prolonged time), urates (a compound of uric acid), leukocytes, pus, blood, epithelial cells, fat droplets, strict vegetarian diet

Note: *In addition to the causes noted above, foods such as blackberries, rhubarb, beets, and those with red dye are common causes of dark or reddish urine that might resemble hematuria.*

Specific Gravity

The specific gravity reflects the relative concentration of a urine specimen. The weight of the urine is compared with the weight of water. Urine is heavier than water by a small amount. If you were to compare the weight of distilled water to itself, the specific gravity of the water would be 1.000. If salt water were compared with fresh water, its specific gravity would be higher, approximately 1.040, because there are salt particles present that give it more weight. In the same manner, urine (which has particles such as sodium, potassium, chloride, and cells) will be heavier than water. The range of specific gravity for a normal urine specimen is 1.003 to 1.035.

Low specific gravity urines (less than 1.003) are very dilute. As stated previously, this may result from a high fluid intake. Abnormal conditions that produce a dilute urine are diabetes insipidus and kidney infections or inflammations.

High specific gravity urines (those greater than 1.030) are very concentrated. A patient who is dehydrated, perhaps from sweating, vomiting, or diarrhea, may have a more concentrated urine specimen because the body is trying to conserve water. High specific gravities can occur with congestive heart failure and hepatic disease.

Specific gravity can be determined by a variety of methods. The oldest is the urinometer, which requires a relatively large amount of urine (Procedure 44-4). The refractometer requires a drop of urine and is read using a scale (Procedure 44-5). This method uses the principle that light travels slower in liquids with dissolved particles when compared with pure water. The refractometer measures this difference in light velocities. The specific gravity chemical strip also needs a drop of urine and the color change is compared to a chart to determine the value.

Checkpoint Question
2. What are the three physical properties of urine and which two are assessed visually?

➤ CHEMICAL PROPERTIES OF URINE

Urine contains a number of chemicals, many of which are measured in the urinalysis. If more **quantitative** (measurement of a specific amount or quantity) information is needed (eg, creatinine), the tests are performed in the chemistry laboratory (see Chap. 48, Clinical Chemistry). Detecting and measuring urine

Charting Example

07/05/98	7:45 AM Urine specimen collected and
	tested for specific gravity using refrac-
	tometer—results 1.005.
	———— William Bendt, CMA

chemical properties can indicate many conditions. Included in the discussion of each urine chemistry will be the disease processes that might be indicated by abnormal readings.

Many biotechnology companies offer chemical strips that can be dipped into urine (hence the name "dipsticks"). These strips have chemicals imbedded on pads that react with the chemicals in the urine. Each pad will turn certain colors as reactions take place. These colors are then compared with a color chart that is used to interpret the reactions (Procedure 44-6).

Prior to the invention and general use of chemical strips, other methods existed to determine urine chemistries. Some of these are still used as backup methods, or confirmation, for quality control and assurance to check the accuracy of the reagent strips or they may be used in place of some of the more expensive chemical strips. Confirmation of positive chemical strip reactions (eg, bilirubin, protein) are sometimes

Charting Example

12/09/98	4:30 PM Patient instructed in cleans-
	ing procedure and midstream collection
	of urine. Urine specimen collected and
	labeled. Color—straw, Clarity—
	clear, specific gravity tested with
	urinometer—1.020, dipstick was nega-
	tive, pH 7.0. ——— Gene Daggle, RMA

part of laboratory protocol as outlined in the Clinical Laboratory Improvement Amendment (CLIA). (See Chap. 42, Introduction to the Clinical Laboratory, for more information on CLIA.)

pH

The kidneys excrete acids produced during normal metabolic processes. **Hydrogen ions** and **ammonia** are excreted as well. (A hydrogen ion is hydrogen that is missing an electron and therefore readily binds with substances having extra electrons; it is an important constituent of acids. Ammonia is a substance produced by decomposition of organic matter containing nitrogen.) In this manner the kidneys regulate the acid-base balance of the body. Because the body produces more acids than bases, the pH of urine reflects this by being more acidic also.

Expected values for urine pH can range form 5.0 (acidic) to 8.0 (slightly basic). The typical value for a freshly voided urine is 6.0. Neutral is 7.0. Although considered normal, acidic urine is also seen with high-protein diets and uncontrolled diabetes. Alkaline urine (above 7.0) can occur after meals, with vegetarian diets, certain renal diseases, and urinary tract infections. Usually, pH is tested by using the chemical strip reagents designed for this purpose.

Glucose

Glucose is filtered and reabsorbed in the kidneys. If plasma renal threshold levels exceed approximately 175-190 g/dL, not all of the glucose will be reabsorbed and detectable amounts of it will be present in the urine. The amount of glucose in urine corresponds to plasma levels; normal urine will not contain glucose. This corresponds to a plasma level of less than 175 mg/dL. In hyperglycemic states, such as diabetes mellitus, glycosuria (glucose in urine) can occur if plasma levels are greater than 175 mg/dL (Box 44-1). A urine glucose test can be performed as a quick check for a diabetic patient experiencing symptoms.

The copper reduction method (trade name, Clinitest, by Miles Inc.) has been used for many years to detect reducing sugars in urine (Procedure 44-7). This test is used to detect any of the substances that reduce copper (eg, glucose, galactose, and other sugars). It is used also for pediatric patients, aged 2 years or less, to screen for **galactosuria**. (Galactosuria, or increased levels of galactose in the blood and urine, is a condition in newborns lacking an enzyme that metabolizes galactose.) The results of this test may be inaccurate because other sugars and ascorbic acid (vitamin C) can

BOX 44-1 Renal Threshold and Glycosuria

Glucose is absorbed in the proximal convoluted tubule. When blood glucose levels exceed a certain level (175 to 190 mg/dL, depending on the individual), not all of the glucose can be reabsorbed into the bloodstream.

Rarely will a healthy person's blood glucose level exceed this threshold value. Diabetics, however, will pass some glucose in their urine due to high levels in their blood. A frequently used term, "spilling sugar," means that not all of the sugar is reabsorbed and is excreted in the urine.

absence of sufficient carbohydrates, as in starvation, fats are then used and ketones are produced.

In normal urine, ketones are typically too low to be measurable. A positive ketone test indicates that the body is burning more fat than normal. Conditions that can cause an increase in ketones (ketonuria) include starvation and inadequately managed diabetes.

Nitroprusside reactions are used to detect ketones (Procedure 44-8). (Nitroprusside is a nitrogen cyanic compound that reacts with ketones.) This method is used with chemical strips and tablet tests. Many laboratories choose to confirm results with the nitroprusside tablet (brand name: Acetest, Ames Co.).

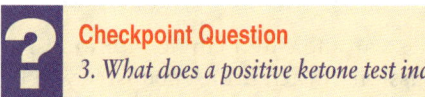

Checkpoint Question
3. What does a positive ketone test indicate?

react with the reagent. The chemical strips are specific for glucose and are preferred for their accuracy; however, the Clinitest tablets may be used as confirmation for chemical reagent strips.

Ketones

Ketones are a group of chemicals that result from fat metabolism. In normal circumstances, energy is derived primarily from carbohydrate metabolism. In the

Proteins

Small quantities of proteins are found in normal urine. Proteinuria (increased amounts of protein in the urine) is an important indicator of renal disease. Chemical strips are usually used to determine the presence of proteins in urine. Other conditions that can cause proteins to appear in urine are strenuous physical exercise, pregnancy, infections, hematuria (blood in urine), pyuria (white cells in urine), and multiple myeloma. Microscopic examination of the urine can help determine what is causing the proteinuria.

Turbidity or precipitation tests are often used to confirm a positive chemical strip reaction (Procedure 44-9). The simplest and most common test involves observing the amount of cloudiness that occurs when equal amounts of urine and **sulfosalicylic acid** (an acid used to test for protein) are added together. The urine used must be centrifuged to remove all particulate matter before adding the acid.

Charting Example

02/09/98	5:45 PM Patient diagnosed IDDM on last visit. Urine specimen collected. Urine tested for glucose with copper reduction method, Clinitest, results 4+. Urine also tested for ketones—results showed large amount. Dr. Wendt notified. ———————Erik Smith, CMA

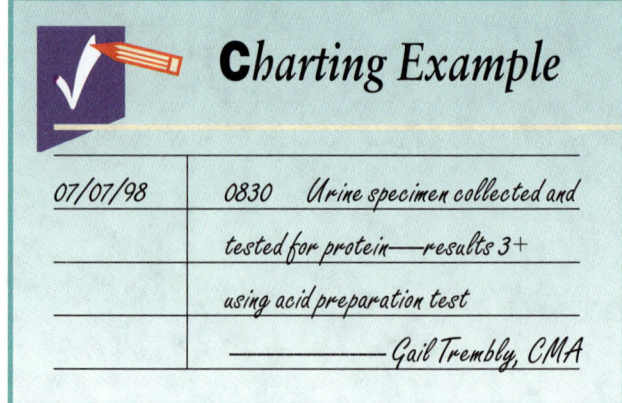

Charting Example

07/07/98	0830 Urine specimen collected and tested for protein—results 3+ using acid preparation test ———————Gail Trembly, CMA

If the amount of protein is negligible and produces a negative reaction with the chemical strip, there should be no cloudiness when the sulfosalicylic acid is added to the urine. When the concentration of urine protein reaches approximately 20 mg/dL, there will be perceptive turbidity. As protein levels increase, so will the degree of turbidity during the reaction with the acid.

Blood

Small numbers of red blood cells occasionally occur in urine. Intact capillaries in the glomerulus usually will not allow the passage of cells into the Bowman's capsule. Hematuria (not due to contamination from menstrual flow) indicates bleeding in the urinary tract that may result from renal disorders, certain neoplasms, urinary tract infection (UTI), or trauma to the urinary tract. Chemical reaction strips are usually used to test for blood in the urine and confirmation is made by microscopic examination.

The chemical strip reacts to hemoglobin, which is the primary constituent of red cells. Free hemoglobin also gives a positive reaction. **Hemoglobinuria** can be seen with transfusion reactions, chemical toxicity, and burns. The strip also reacts to myoglobin, a protein found in muscles. Myoglobin may be released into the bloodstream in crushing injuries and other traumas and then excreted in the urine.

Bilirubin

Bilirubin is formed from the breakdown of hemoglobin. It is processed in the liver before being excreted into the intestines as bile. Urine contains very low levels of bilirubin, reflecting the usual low serum levels. Bilirubinuria (bilirubin in the urine) can be seen with certain liver diseases (eg, hepatitis), biliary tract obstruction, and hemolytic states such as transfusion reactions.

The chemical strip for bilirubin is specifically designed to react to its presence. However, a dark yellow urine can make it difficult to read the reaction because bilirubin is also a yellow pigment. Many laboratories confirm a positive strip by a **diazo** tablet method (brand name: Ictotest, by Miles, Inc.). Diazo is a double nitrogen compound that reacts with bilirubin (Procedure 44-10).

IMPORTANT NOTE: Bilirubin is a highly unstable substance and will break down with prolonged light exposure. Specimens must be shielded from light and processed as soon as possible to avoid deterioration of the specimen.

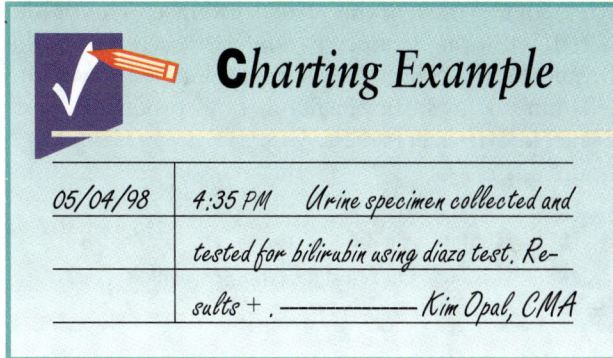

Urobilinogen

When bilirubin is secreted into the intestines in the bile, bacterial action converts it into urobilinogen. Some of this is reabsorbed into the bloodstream and is excreted by the kidneys. The remaining urobilinogen leaves the body in the feces.

Small amounts of urobilinogen are normally found in urine, usually 0.1 to 1.0 **Ehrlich units**/dL (mg/dL). (An Ehrlich unit is a unit of measurement for urobilinogen.) As with bilirubin, increased levels of urobilinogen can be found with conditions that have a high rate of red cell destruction. Also, bowel obstructions cause the feces to remain in the intestines for longer periods, resulting in greater reabsorption of urobilinogen along with the rest of the fluid portion. Urobilinogen levels will rise both in urine and in serum when this occurs. Liver impairment can also lead to increased levels of urobilinogen because some of the urobilinogen that is reabsorbed from the intestinal tract is processed by the liver and re-excreted in the feces. Urobilinogen is tested by chemical reagent strips.

Nitrite

Most types of bacteria that infect the urinary tract have an enzyme that can reduce nitrate to nitrite. This factor is used to assess the presence of bacteria in urine. In the nitrite test, urine is applied to a pad impregnated with nitrates. If bacteria are present, nitrates will be changed into nitrites and the resulting color development can be observed. A positive nitrite test result indicates bacteriuria, which occurs with urinary tract infections.

Leukocyte Esterase

Leukocytes in the urine indicates a urinary tract infection. Phagocytic white cells, such as neutrophils, are called to the kidney to fight the infection. These leukocytes contain an enzyme called **esterase**. This is detected with the leukocyte esterase reaction on the chemical strip. Normal urine may contain a few white cells but not in sufficient numbers to produce a positive leukocyte esterase test.

Checkpoint Question

4. Which two indicators on a dipstick would suggest a urinary tract infection?

➤ URINE SEDIMENT

The microscopic examination of urine can corroborate the findings of the urinalysis and may produce new data of diagnostic value. Cells and other structures are noted and **enumerated** (counted) during a microscopic examination. Microscopic examination of urine is generally considered to be an advanced procedure and is not usually performed by medical assistants.

Urine sediment is prepared by centrifuging urine and saving the button of cells and other particulate matter that collects in the bottom of the tube. This button is resuspended and a drop of this suspension is placed on a slide and viewed with a microscope. Making a sediment concentrates all the structures present in the urine so that it is unlikely that any urine components will be missed (Procedures 44-11 and 44-12).

Many manufacturers have a slide system that is used in conjunction with a centrifuge tube, also made by that company, to examine urine sediments. This provides some standardization of the procedure so that when quantifying the structures seen microscopically, the numbers have meaning with regard to abnormal results. Although glass slides and coverslips may still used by some laboratories, this technique is rarely used and is not recommended.

Charting Example

| 09/03/98 | 1235 | Microscope examination of urine. Results: WBC 8/HPF and RBC casts 1/LPF. |
| | | —Hugh Krent, CMA |

Structures Found in Urine Sediment

The following structures may appear in the urine: red blood cells, white blood cells, bacteria, epithelial cells, crystals, casts, and others. Correlations with chemical properties of the urine are given where appropriate (Fig. 44-1).

Red Blood Cells

The presence of red cells in urine, as stated previously, can indicate a number of conditions including renal damage. A few red cells in every high power field (HPF) is considered normal. Greater than 3 per HPF is abnormal.

When greater than normal numbers of red cells are present in urine sediment, the chemical strip reaction for blood should be positive. Protein may be positive if hemolysis is occurring. A positive chemical strip test for blood with no red cells seen microscopically correlates with various kinds of hemolysis, such as with transfusion reactions and sickle cell crisis (see Chapter 46, Hematolgy, for an explanation of sickling). As stated earlier, myoglobin will cause a positive reaction.

White Blood Cells

Leukocytes in the sediment indicate a urinary tract infection. A finding of 0 to 5 white blood cells per HPF is normal, greater than 5 per HPF is considered abnormal.

The leukocyte esterase test on the chemical strip will be positive when white cells are present in increased numbers. Protein may be positive if some of the white blood cells have **lysed** (broken apart) or if the infection is damaging the renal tubules as in glomerulonephritis.

Bacteria

Bacteria is always present on the surface of the skin but should not be present in the bladder. Normal urine will not contain bacteria if a clean-catch urine specimen is collected properly. Bacteria present in significant amounts (more than trace) is considered an indication of a urinary tract infection.

A positive nitrite test on the chemical strip will correlate with bacteria seen in the sediment. The only bacterium that will not give a nitrite-positive report is *Streptococcus faecalis*. *S. faecalis* causes only 1% of the urinary tract infections.

Epithelial Cells

Epithelial cells cover the skin and organs and line pathways such as the digestive or urinary tracts. Their

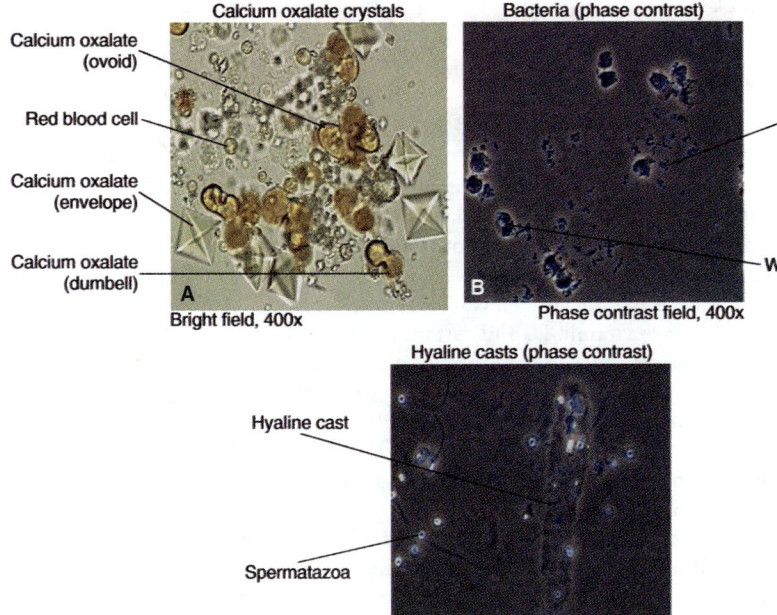

FIGURE 44-1

Structures found in urine sediment. (*A*) This image includes the common forms of calcium exalate crystals. (*B*) Phase microscopy makes bacteria more visible. (*C*) Phase contrast microscopy enhances the visualization of structures with low refractive indices such as hyaline casts. (© University of Washington School of Medicine, Dept. of Laboratory Medicine, Seattle, WA)

shapes vary according to location. Epithelial cells will normally slough off and are found in the urine, but increased amounts can indicate an irritation, such as inflammation somewhere in the urinary system. Three different types of epithelial cells may be found in the urine: squamous, transitional, and renal. Squamous epithelial cells cover external surfaces and are considered a normal finding. Transitional epithelial cells line the bladder and are seen with infections of the lower urinary tract, such as cystitis. Renal epithelial cells line the nephrons and are seen with infections and inflammations of the upper urinary tract.

No chemical test exists for epithelial cells. However, if renal epithelial cells are present, damage to the renal tubules is likely and the protein test may be positive.

Crystals

Crystals are made up of a chemical substance present in the urine in sufficient quantities to form a solid three-dimensional structure that can be seen microscopically. The three most common crystals found in urine sediment—calcium oxalate, uric acid (both of which occur in acidic urine with a pH below 7.0), and triple phosphate (found in alkaline urine, above 7.0)—are not pathologic. Uric acid can, however, be seen with fevers, leukemia, or gout.

Crystals can also contribute to the formation of stones in the urinary tract. Box 44-2 describes urinary tract stone formation and specimen collection.

Casts

Cast formation occurs in the tubules of the nephron. When protein is present in sufficient quantities, it will cement together whatever cells are in the tubule as well; this is a cast. Most casts eventually break free and flow into the urine. The type of cast can indicate certain pathologies. For instance, in pyelonephritis, white cells that are present to combat the infection become trapped in the protein network and form white cell casts. Casts are counted on low power and are reported as a number per LPF (low power field).

 **Checkpoint Question**

5. What are three of the most common crystals found in urine?

Other Structures

Many other structures can be found in the urine sediment. Yeast found in the urine can result from a vaginal contamination of the specimen or may be the causative agent of a urinary tract infection, especially in a diabetic patient. The parasite *Trichomonas vaginalis* is a frequent contaminate from the genital tract of an infected person. Mucus may be present if there is an inflammation in the urinary tract. Mucous threads are usually reported in quantities, such as few, moderate, or many. Spermatozoa may be found when there has been a recent emission.

BOX 44-2 Urinary Tract Stone Formation

Stones are formed in the urinary system by crystals of normally occurring substances such as calcium oxalate, calcium phosphate, and uric acid. Uroliths range in size from minute particles as fine as sand to huge staghorn calculi that fill the renal pelvis and cystoliths that fill the bladder.

Many disorders contribute to the formation of renal calculi. These disorders include hypercalcemia, excessive dietary vitamin D, and certain bone disorders such as leukemia or polycythemia vera. They also may form as a sequela to an ileostomy or a bowel resection.

Patients may present with symptoms ranging from mild discomfort to severe and debilitating pain. Symptoms may include pyelonephritis, cystitis, generalized signs of infection, dysuria, flank pain, hematuria, and pyuria. As stones pass into the ureter, pain may become excruciating.

Diagnosis is confirmed by radiography and blood chemistries. Patient history is important to determining patient predisposition to stone formation.

Patients are instructed to collect a 24-hour urine specimen for measurement of calcium, uric acid, creatinine, sodium, and pH. In many cases, the medical assistant will assist with instructions for collection. Patients with uroliths are usually required to strain the urine before adding it to the collection. Urine may be collected in a bedpan or toilet collection receptacle ("nun's cap" or "Mexican hat"), or it may be voided into a small collection bottle before adding to the 24-hour re-

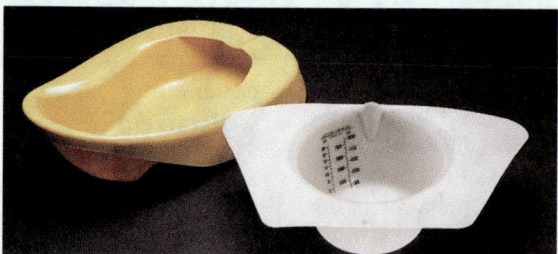

Bedpan (*left*) and toilet collection receptacle ("nun's cap" or "Mexican hat").

ceptacle. In acute onset situations, the patient may bring to the office a specimen collected at home that must be strained at the office. Retain all evidence of solids for analysis.

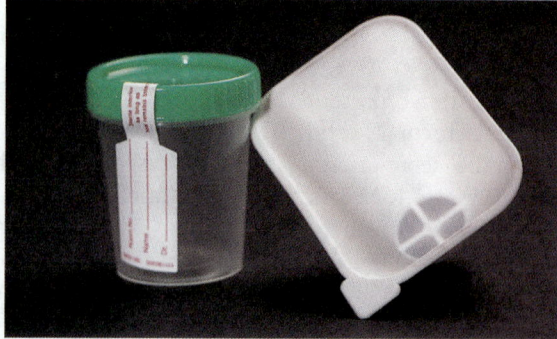

Urine specimen container (*left*) and urine strainer for stone collection.

What if a patient asks you what drugs can be detected in the urine? What would you say?

Many employers are requiring routine drug testing for their employees using urine specimens. Urine specimens are preferred rather than blood tests because they are less expensive and are noninvasive. The following drugs can be detected in the urine: amphetamines, barbiturates, benzodiazepines, cocaine, marijuana, opiates, PCP, and methadone. If you are involved in obtaining urine specimens for drug testing, it is essential that you ensure security of the urine and confidentiality of the results.

➤ URINE PREGNANCY TESTING

Human chorionic gonadotropin (HCG) is a hormone secreted by the developing placenta shortly after conception. Its appearance and rapid rise in concentration in the mother's serum and urine make it an excellent marker for confirming a pregnancy. Many test kits are available that can detect levels as low as 25 mIU/mL. These levels are typically seen within 10 to 12 days after fertilization, often before the first missed period. Most test kits simply require the addition of urine to test and are very easy to use. First-morning urine specimens are the specimen of choice because the urine is most concentrated at that time. Many laboratories will test the specific gravity and will not report a negative pregnancy result if it is below 1.005 because the urine may be too dilute to detect low HCG serum levels.

Procedure 44-1

Obtaining a Clean Catch Midstream (CCMS) Urine Specimen

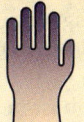

Equipment/Supplies

- sterile cotton balls or appropriate antiseptic wipes
- antiseptic (if using cotton balls)
- sterile water
- sterile urine container labeled with patient's name
- bedpan or urinal (if necessary)
- appropriate biohazard barrier devices (eg, gloves, impervious gown, face shield)

Steps	Purpose
1. Wash your hands. If you are to assist the patient, put on gloves.	1. Handwashing aids infection control. Urine is a body fluid and should be treated as potentially hazardous.
2. Assemble the equipment.	2. This ensures that all supplies are available.
3. Identify the patient and explain the procedure. Ask for and answer any questions.	3. Identifying the patient avoids errors in treatment. Explaining the procedure helps gain patient compliance and ease anxiety.
4. If the patient is to perform the procedure, provide the necessary supplies.	
5. Have the patient perform the procedure. a. *Instruct the male patient to:* (1) Expose the glans penis by retracting the foreskin, then clean the meatus with a cotton ball or wipe soaked in a mild antiseptic or a towelette. The glans should be cleaned in a circular motion away from the meatus. A new wipe should be used for each cleaning sweep.	(1) Antiseptic solutions remove bacteria from the urinary meatus and the surrounding skin. Wiping away from the meatus will remove bacteria from the area; wiping toward the meatus or returning to the area with a used wipe would re-introduce bacteria to the site.

(continued)

Procedure 44-1

Obtaining a Clean Catch Midstream (CCMS) Urine Specimen (continued)

Steps	Purpose
(2) Keeping the foreskin retracted, void the first 30 mL into the toilet or urinal.	(2) Organisms in the lower urethra and at the meatus will be washed away. Collecting the middle of the stream ensures the least contamination with skin bacteria.
(3) Bring the sterile container into the urine stream and collect a sufficient amount (about 30–100 mL). Instruct the patient to avoid touching the inside of the container with the penis.	(3) Touching the inside with the penis may contaminate the specimen.
(4) Finish voiding into the toilet or urinal.	(4) Prostatic fluid may be expressed at the end of the stream and may contaminate the specimen.
b. *Instruct the female patient to:*	
(1) Kneel or squat over a bedpan or toilet bowl. Spread the labia minora widely to expose the meatus. Using cotton balls soaked in a mild antiseptic or wipe, cleanse on either side of the meatus then the meatus itself. Use a wipe or cotton ball only once in a sweep from the anterior to the posterior surfaces, then discard it. Rinse with cotton balls soaked in sterile water in the same manner.	(1) Antiseptic solutions remove bacteria from the urinary meatus. Bringing a cotton ball or wipe back to the surface already cleaned will recontaminate the area. The antiseptic solution must be washed away before the specimen is collected.
(2) Keeping the labia separated, void the first 30 mL into the toilet.	(2) Organisms remaining in the meatus will be washed away.
(3) Bring the sterile container into the urine stream and collect a sufficient amount (about 30–100 mL).	
(4) Finish voiding into the toilet or bedpan.	
6. Recap the filled container and drop it into the outside carry container.	6. The specimen should be transported in a biohazard container for testing.
7. Properly care for or dispose of equipment and supplies. Clean the work area. Remove gloves and wash your hands.	7. Standard Precautions must be followed throughout the procedure.
8. Record the procedure.	8. Procedures are considered not to have been done if they are not recorded.

Obtaining a 24-Hour Urine Specimen

Procedure 44-2

Equipment/Supplies

- one 24-hour container, labeled with the patient's identifying information, possibly with a preservative
- several random urine containers.

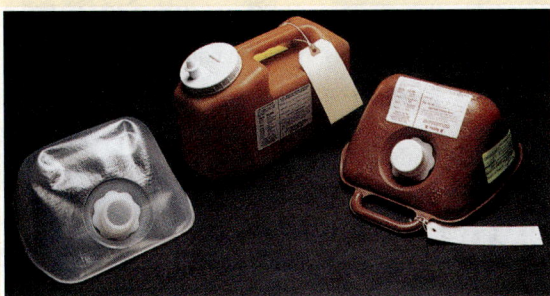

24-hour specimen containers. Each type pictured is used for specific testing procedures.

Steps	**Purpose**
1. Explain to the patient the importance of collecting all of every voiding and adding it to the container with the preservative. Document the patient teaching.	1. The procedure must be explained to the patient's level of understanding to be properly performed.
2. Tell the patient to empty the bladder at 8 AM or a suitable time upon rising. This should be voided normally into the toilet.	2. The urine in the bladder upon arising is considered to be urine from the previous 24-hour period and is not included in this procedure. The next urine to be voided will start the collection.
3. Tell the patient to collect all subsequent urine. Each is poured into the 24-hour container, which is kept refrigerated. (Some preservatives are adequate without refrigeration.)	3. Refrigeration helps maintain the integrity of the urine. Preservatives may be used for certain types of tests.
4. Tell the patient that at 8 AM the next day (or whatever time collection began the previous day) to empty the bladder, collecting this specimen as the last one and adding it to the container. This ends the collection period.	
5. Ensure that the patient transports the specimen properly to the physician's office for testing.	
6. Route the urine to the proper testing facility and record the procedure.	6. Procedures are considered not to have been done if they are not recorded.

Procedure 44-3

Determining Color and Clarity of Urine

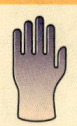

Equipment/Supplies

- urine in a clear glass tube, usually a centrifuge tube
- appropriate biohazard barrier devices (eg, gloves, impervious gown, and face shield)

Steps	**Purpose**
1. Wash your hands.	1. Handwashing aids infection control.
2. Assemble the equipment.	2. This ensures that all supplies are available.
3. Put on gloves, gown, and face shield.	3. You must use Standard Precautions when handling any body fluids.
4. Pour 10–15 mL of urine into the tube.	4. This allows for visual assessment of the urine.
5. In bright light, examine the urine for color. The most common colors are straw (very pale yellow), yellow, dark yellow, and amber (brown-yellow). Other colors include blue, green, red, orange, brown and black.	5. The yellow color is due to urochrome and can range in color intensity depending on urine concentration. (Refer to Table 44-1 for information about other urine colors.)

Step 5: Urine tested for color and appearance (clarity) will be held against a suitable background for observation.

6. Hold the urine tube in front of white paper scored with heavy black lines. Determine how well the lines show through the urine. If seen clearly with no lines obscured, urine is clear. If lines are seen but not well delineated, urine is hazy. If lines cannot be seen at all, urine is cloudy.	6. The lines helps discern urine clarity by providing contrast.
7. Properly care for or dispose of equipment and supplies. Clean the work area. Remove gloves, gown, and face shield and wash your hands.	7. Standard Precautions must be followed throughout the procedure.
8. Record observations of urine color and clarity.	8. Procedures are considered not to have been done if they are not recorded.

Procedure 44-4	Determining Specific Gravity of Urine Using the Urinometer

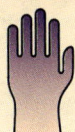

Equipment/Supplies

- urine specimen
- clean glass cylinder
- urinometer
- appropriate biohazard barrier devices (e.g., gloves, impervious gown, face shield)

Steps	Purpose
1. Wash your hands.	1. Handwashing aids infection control.
2. Assemble the equipment.	2. This ensures that all supplies are available.
3. Put on gloves, impervious gown, and face shield.	3. You must use Standard Precautions when handling any body fluid.
4. Fill the glass cylinder 3/4 with well-mixed urine (minimum volume is 15 mL).	4. There must be sufficient urine in the cylinder for the urinometer to float.
5. Gently drop the urinometer into the urine with a spinning motion.	5. This motion ensures that the urinometer is free floating.
6. Read at the meniscus (bottom of the curved surface) of the urine. The urinometer should not touch the sides or bottom of the cylinder. Note results.	6. Fluid forms a curved surface and readings are taken at the bottom of this curve.

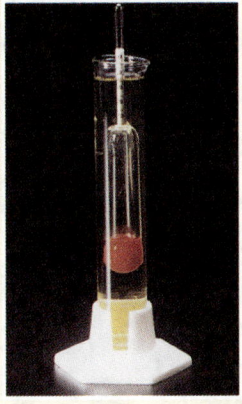

Step 6: Determining specific gravity.

7. Discard urine into proper receptacle. Properly care for or dispose of equipment. Clean work area. Remove gloves, gown, and face shield and wash hands.	7. Standard Precautions must be followed throughout the procedure.
8. Record the results.	8. Procedures are considered not to have been done if they are not recorded.

Note: *Urine should be at room temperature for an accurate reading. If the test is performed on urine that is not at room temperature, specify this when recording the test results. Subtract 0.001 from the reading for every 3° that the specimen temperature is below the urinometer calibration temperature. If urine is over the calibration temperature, add 0.001 for every 3°.*

  Subtract 0.003 for every 1g/100 mL (deciliter—dL) of glucose or protein.

Quality assurance: Fill the cylinder with distilled water and perform the above procedure with the urinometer. The reading should be 1.000. Record the procedure in the appropriate quality control (QC) record.

Procedure 44-5 Determining Specific Gravity of Urine Using the Refractometer

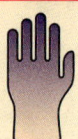

Equipment/Supplies

- urine specimen
- refractometer
- transfer pipette
- appropriate biohazard barrier devices (eg, gloves, impervious gown, face shield)

Steps	Purpose
1. Wash your hands.	1. Handwashing aids infection control.
2. Assemble the equipment.	2. This ensures that all supplies are available.
3. Put on gloves, impervious gown, and face shield.	3. You must use Standard Precautions when handling any body fluids.
4. Clean the surface of the cover and prism with a drop of distilled water and dry with gauze.	4. Particles from previous samples may remain and contaminate the reading.
5. Close the cover and apply 1 drop of urine with the transfer pipette at the notched bottom of the cover so it flows over the entire prism surface.	5. Urine covers the prism to provide the reading.
6. Point the refractometer toward a strong light source and read the specific gravity measurement from the scale at the dividing line between the light and dark contrast.	6. Illumination is needed to read the result.
7. Properly care for or dispose of equipment and supplies. Clean the work area. Remove gloves, gown, and face shield and wash hands.	7. Standard Precautions must be observed throughout the procedure.
8. Record the results.	8. Procedures are considered not to have been done if they are not recorded.

Quality control (QC) assurance: Place a drop of distilled water on the refractometer and read the results. The results should be at 1.000. This must be performed daily and recorded in the appropriate QC record. If the calibration is not at 1.000, set the screen by the manufacturer's recommendation. Check the reading with 5% NaCl; it should read at 1.022, ±0.001.

Procedure 44-6

Performing Chemical Reagent Strip Analysis

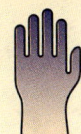

Equipment/Supplies

- urine specimen
- chemical reagent strip
- color chart to interpret reactions
- appropriate biohazard barrier devices (eg, gloves, impervious gown, face shield)

Steps	Purpose
1. Wash your hands.	1. Handwashing aids infection control.
2. Assemble the equipment.	2. This ensures that all supplies are available.
3. Put on gloves, impervious gown, and face shield.	3. You must observe Standard Precautions when handling all body fluids.
4. Mix urine specimen well before testing by gently swirling the urine container with the lid on.	4. Particulate matter may have settled to the bottom.
5. Remove one strip and replace cap. Check the condition and color of the pads on the strip. Check the expiration date of the bottle.	5. The remaining strips may be altered if exposed to air for prolonged periods. If the pads are defective in any way, discard the strip and remove another. If all of the strips are substandard, discard the entire bottle. If the expiration date has passed, discard the bottle.
6. Completely immerse the area of the strip with the reagent pads and remove immediately. Start your stop watch immediately.	6. Some of the chemicals may dissolve out of the pads if immersed for too long. Reactions must be read at specific intervals as directed on the package insert and on the color comparison chart.
7. While removing the strip from the urine, run or gently tap the edge against the rim of the urine container to remove excess urine.	7. Excess urine can cause chemicals to run between the pads causing unreliable results.
8. Compare reagent pad areas to the color chart provided by the manufacturer. The chart must match the lot number of the strips being used. Read the reactions at the times indicated and note the results.	8. Reading the reaction before or after the time indicated by the manufacturer will give unreliable results.
9. Discard the urine and reagent strip in the proper receptacle. Properly care for or dispose of equipment and supplies. Clean the work area. Remove gloves, gown, and face shield and wash hands.	9. Standard Precautions must be observed throughout the procedure.
10. Record the results.	10. Procedures are considered not to have been done if they are not recorded.

(continued)

Procedure 44-6

Performing Chemical Reagent Strip Analysis *(continued)*

Steps   **Purpose**

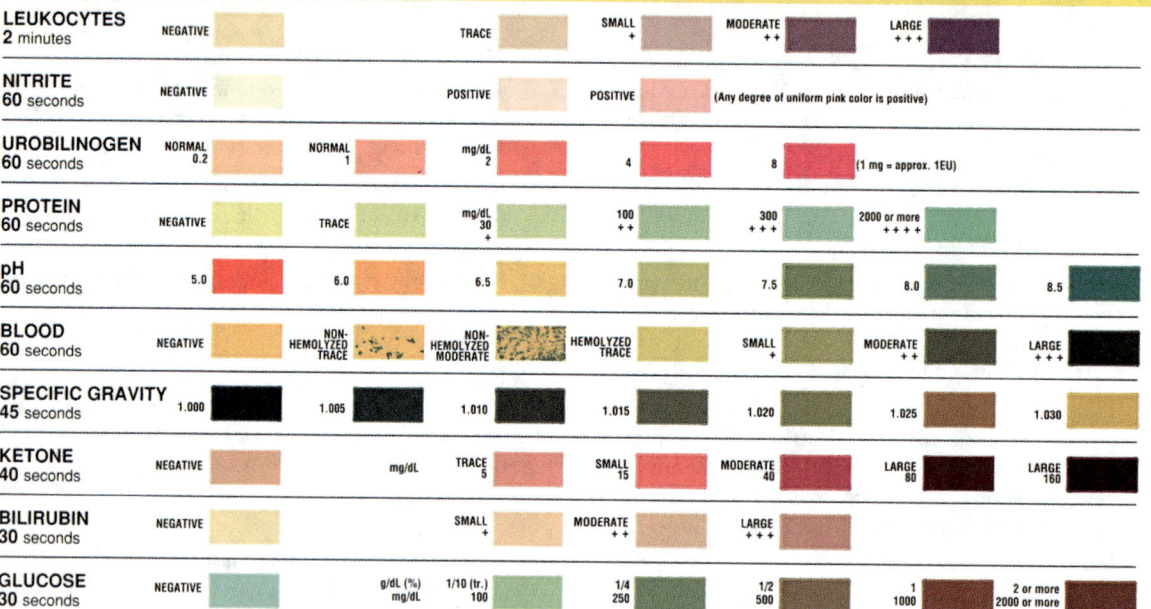

©1995 Bayer Corporation, Diagnostics Division, Tarrytown, NY 10591   6/95   0401123

Step 6: Ames Multistix package insert.

Procedure 44-7 — Performing a Copper Reduction Test (Clinitest) for Glucose

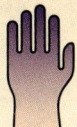

Equipment/Supplies

- urine specimen
- 16 × 125 glass test tube
- transfer pipette
- Clinitest tablet
- color comparison chart
- appropriate biohazard barrier devices (eg, gloves, impervious gown, face shield)

Steps	Purpose
1. Wash your hands.	1. Handwashing aids infection control.
2. Assemble the equipment.	2. This ensures that all supplies are available.
3. Put on gloves, impervious gown, and face shield.	3. You must observe Standard Precautions when handling body fluids.
4. Using a plastic transfer pipette, place 5 drops of urine in a dry glass test tube and add 10 drops of water.	4. The urine must be diluted for proper results. The heat generated may melt plastic test tubes.
5. Add 1 Clinitest tablet into the tube. Drop 1 tablet into the cap of the bottle, then drop the tablet from the cap into the tube.	5. The reaction starts with the addition of the tablet. Do not touch the tablet.
6. Watch as the tablet boils and gently shake the tube 15 seconds after the reaction has stopped.	6. Observe the reaction the entire time so the "pass through" phenomenon will not go unnoticed. Occasionally, the reaction will pass through all of the colors and return to a color that is lower than the actual test results should reflect. "Pass through" occurs when the glucose level is so high that it goes beyond the orange color (colors range from blue to green to orange, with orange indicating the greatest glucose concentration) to give a greenish-brown test result, which may be interpreted as a trace amount of glucose instead of the correct 4+. Use the manufacturer's recommendations for "pass through" interpretation.

(continued)

Procedure 44-7

Performing a Copper Reduction Test for Glucose *(continued)*

Steps	Purpose
7. Compare the color with the chart provided by the manufacturer.	7. Results are interpreted from the color of the reactants when the reaction has stopped. The results will be recorded as trace, 1+, 2+, 3+, 4+.

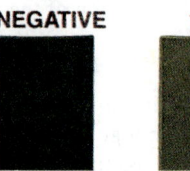 

ames 5-Drop Method Standard Procedure

DIRECTIONS FOR TESTING:

1. Collect urine in clean container. With dropper in upright position, place **5 drops** of urine in test tube. Rinse dropper with water and add 10 drops of water to test tube.

2. Drop one tablet into test tube. Watch while complete boiling reaction takes place. Do not shake test tube during boiling, or for the following 15 seconds after boiling has stopped.
3. At the end of this 15-second waiting period, shake test tube gently to mix contents. Compare

color of liquid to Color Chart below. Ignore sediment that may form in the bottom of the test tube. Ignore changes after the 15-second waiting period.
4. Write down the percent (%) result which appears on the color block that most closely matches the color of the liquid.

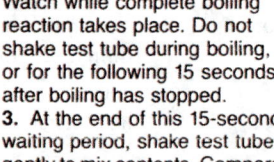
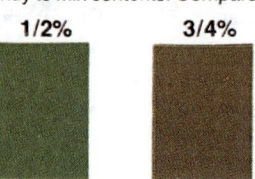
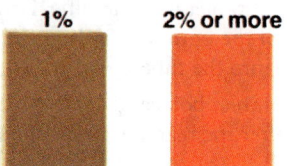

| NEGATIVE | 1/4% | 1/2% | 3/4% | 1% | 2% or more |

Step 7: Ames Clinitest package insert.

8. Discard the tube and the pipette in the proper receptacle. Properly care for equipment and supplies. Clean the work area. Remove gloves and wash hands.	8. Standard Precautions must be observed throughout the procedure.
9. Record the results.	9. Procedures are considered not to have been done if they are not recorded.

Safety note: *The tablets contain a strong alkali and should not be touched by bare skin. Do not touch the bottom of the test tube during or immediately after the test; it will be very hot.*

Testing note: *Patients taking high doses of vitamin C supplements can give positive reactions because ascorbic acid also reduces copper.*

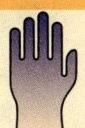

Procedure 44-8

Performing Nitroprusside Reaction (Acetest) for Ketones

Equipment/Supplies

- urine specimen
- white filter paper
- transfer pipette
- Acetest tablet
- color comparison chart
- appropriate biohazard barrier devices (eg, gloves, impervious gown, face shield)

Steps	Purpose
1. Wash your hands.	1. Handwashing aids infection control.
2. Assemble the equipment.	2. This ensures that all supplies are available.
3. Put on gloves, impervious gown, and face shield.	3. You must observe Standard Precautions when handling body fluids.
4. Place 1 Acetest tablet on filter paper by emptying a tablet into the cap and dispensing onto the paper.	4. The tablet should not be touched. The white background of the filter paper allows for contrast.
5. Using a transfer pipette, place 1 drop of well-mixed urine on top of the tablet.	5. When the urine and the tablet meet, the reaction will begin.
6. Wait 30 seconds for the reaction.	6. Nitroprusside reaction will occur if ketones are present.
7. Compare the color of the tablet to the color chart and record the results as negative, trace, small amount, moderate amount, or large amount.	7. Nitroprusside reaction gives a color change of varying degrees of purple if ketones are present. The color correlates to the amount of ketones in the urine.

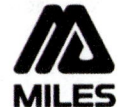

Miles Inc.
Diagnostics Division
Elkhart IN 46515 USA

Colors shown below are for use with ACETEST Reagent Tablets only.

NEGATIVE	SMALL	MODERATE	LARGE

 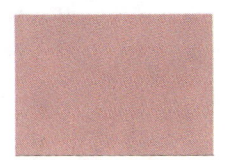  

Step 7: Ames Acetest package insert.

8. Properly care for or dispose of equipment and supplies. Clean the work area. Remove gloves, gown, and face shield and wash hands.	8. Standard Precautions must be maintained throughout the procedure.
9. Record the results.	9. Procedures are considered not to have been done if they are not recorded.

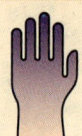

Procedure 44-9   Performing an Acid Precipitation Test for Protein

Equipment/Supplies

- urine specimen
- 3% sulfosalicylic acid (SSA)
- transfer pipette
- clean, clear test tube (preferably glass)
- appropriate biohazard barrier devices (eg, gloves, impervious gown, face shield)

Steps	Purpose
1. Wash your hands.	1. Handwashing aids infection control.
2. Assemble the equipment.	2. This ensures that all supplies are available.
3. Put on gloves, impervious gown, and face shield.	3. You must observe Standard precautions when handling body fluids.
4. Place approximately 3 mL of supernatant urine (the upper portion of centrifuged urine) in a test tube.	4. Particulate matter is no longer in supernatant to add turbidity to the reaction.
5. Add an equal amount of 3% SSA and agitate.	5. The reactants must be mixed together.
6. Let stand 10 minutes and shake again.	6. Allows full reaction to occur.
7. Observe the degree of turbidity: 　Negative: no turbidity 　Trace: slight turbidity 　1+: distinct turbidity 　2+: turbidity with granulation 　3+: turbidity with granulation and **flocculation** (consistency of loose woolly masses) 　4+: clumps of precipitated protein	7. The more protein present, the greater the degree of turbidity. *Note:* The specimen may be matched against a McFarland standard to decrease the degree of subjective interpretation.
8. Properly care for or dispose of equipment and supplies. Clean the work area. Remove gloves, gown, and face shield and wash hands.	8. Standard Precautions must be observed throughout the procedure.
9. Record the results.	9. Procedures are considered not to have been done if they are not recorded.

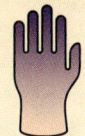

Procedure 44-10

Performing Diazo Tablet Test (Ictotest) for Bilirubin

Equipment/Supplies

- urine specimen
- white mat
- transfer pipette
- diazo tablet
- appropriate biohazard barrier devices (eg, gloves, impervious gown, and face shield).

Steps	**Purpose**
1. Wash your hands.	1. Handwashing aids infection control.
2. Assemble the equipment.	2. This ensures that all supplies are available.
3. Put on gloves, impervious gown, and face shield.	3. You must use Standard Precautions when handling body fluids.
4. Using the transfer pipette, place 10 drops of urine on the white mat provided by manufacturer.	4. Urine is absorbed onto the mat.
5. Place the diazo tablet on top of the mat, add 2 drops of water to the top of the tablet. Allow it to run off of the tablet onto the mat.	5. Chemicals are released from the tablet to react with the urine on the mat.
6. Within 30 seconds, look for a blue or purple color on the mat. Either color indicates a positive result.	6. Diazo reacts with urine containing bilirubin to give this color.

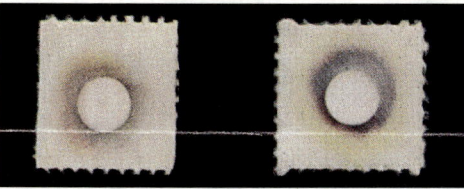

Step 6: Ames Ictotest package insert.

7. Properly care for or dispose of the equipment and supplies. Clean the work area. Remove gloves, gown, and face shield and wash hands.	7. Standard Precautions must be observed throughout the procedure.
8. Record the results.	8. Procedures are considered not to have been done if they are not recorded.

Testing note: *Other compounds may react to give a red or orange color. This is not a positive result.*

Procedure 44-11   Preparing a Urine Sediment

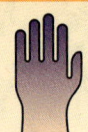

Equipment/Supplies
- urine specimen
- urine centrifuge tubes
- centrifuge
- appropriate biohazard barrier devices (eg, gloves, impervious gown, and face shield)

Steps	Purpose
1. Wash your hands.	1. Handwashing aids infection control.
2. Assemble the equipment.	2. This ensures that all supplies are available.
3. Put on gloves, impervious gown, and face shield.	3. You must observe Standard Precautions when handling body fluids.
4. Pour well-mixed urine into a urine centrifuge tube and cap the tube. Depending on the manufacturer's recommendation, the urine volume will be 10–15 mL.	4. This amount provides sufficient urine to produce adequate sediment.
5. Urine is centrifuged at 15,000 RPM (rotations per minute) for 5 minutes in a typical urine centrifuge. Balance the centrifuge.	5. Centrifugation brings the particulate matter to the bottom of the tube. The tube must be balanced to avoid tube breakage and damage to the centrifuge.
6. Supernatant is decanted (poured off) and is discarded or used for tests such as protein. Depending on the manufacturer's recommendation, the shape of the tube will keep back a small portion of the urine or the pipette with the system holds some of the urine in place. The remaining urine is used to resuspend the sediment for examination.	6. The concentrated sediment is now ready for examination.
7. Properly care for or dispose of equipment and supplies. Remove gloves, gown, and face shield and wash hands unless continuing with microscopic examination.	7. Standard Precautions must be maintained throughout the procedure.

Procedure 44-12   Preparing Urine Sediment for a Microscopic Examination

Equipment/Supplies
- transfer pipette
- sediment slides
- microscope
- appropriate biohazard barrier devices (eg, gloves, impervious gown).

Steps	Purpose
1. Wash your hands.	1. Handwashing aids infection control.
2. Assemble the equipment.	2. This ensures that all supplies are available.
3. Put on gloves and impervious gown.	3. You must observe Standard Precautions when handling body fluids.

(continued)

Preparing Urine Sediment for a Microscopic Examination

Steps	Purpose
4. Thoroughly mix the remaining urine with the sediment at the bottom of the centrifuge tube by squeezing the pipette tube several times.	4. Adequate resuspension of particulate matter is essential.
5. Draw a portion of suspension into the transfer pipette and place 1 drop onto the notched edge of the slide so that fluid fills the compartment.	5. This will transfer the suspension from the tube onto the slide for examination purposes.
6. Place the slide on the microscope stage, turn on the light source, and rotate nosepiece so that the 10× (low power) objective is in place. Using coarse and fine adjustment knobs bring the slide into sharp detail.	6. Focusing the microscope on the slide is accomplished on the lower power lens.
7. Scan the area of slide that contains the specimen. Look for structures such as casts. Ensure an even distribution of the specimen.	7. Scanning for even distribution is a quality control measure. Casts may be missed on high power in later steps.
8. Note that any casts seen are identified using high power objective and enumerated on low power. For example: a cellular cast is noted on low power (10×) and is determined to be a red cell cast under high power (40×). One of these casts is seen in every other field of the low power objective; therefore, report: 0–1 red cell cast/LPF (per low power field).	8. Greater magnification is required to identify the type of cast.
9. Enumerate each of the cell types and other structures using the high power objective. Note the findings.	9. Other structures are reported according to the amount/HPF (per high power field) because the high power lens is used to identify and enumerate.
10. Properly care for or dispose of equipment. Clean the work area. Remove gloves and gown and wash your hands.	10. Standard Precautions must be observed throughout the procedure.
11. Record the results.	11. Procedures are considered not to have been done if they are not recorded.

Note: *Medical assistants are not expected to perform the microscopic examination but may be requested by their physicians to prepare the field to step number 7. If the medical assistant is allowed to examine the field, the remaining steps should be followed.*

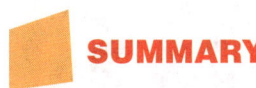

SUMMARY

Identifying abnormalities in urine can aid in diagnosis and management of many diseases and disorders. The medical assistant should notice the correlation between chemical properties analyzed and microscopic examination. Some structures found in urine are not indicated by chemical strip analysis and require that an examination of sediment be performed by the physician or other qualified personnel for final diagnosis.

CRITICAL THINKING CHALLENGES

1. Most laboratories pour off a portion of a urine specimen to test rather than dipping the chemical reagent strip directly into the urine container. Why?
2. Why would burn and trauma patients need a urinalysis? What results would you expect to see and why?

ANSWERS TO CHECKPOINT QUESTIONS

1. Urine should be tested within 1 hour of collection. (If testing cannot be performed within 1 hour, refrigerate the specimen at 4°C–6°C until testing can be performed.) If the urine is not properly refrigerated, the specimen can deteriorate.

2. The three physical properties of urine are color, clarity, and specific gravity. Color and clarity are assessed visually.
3. A positive ketone test indicates that the body is burning more fat than normal.
4. Positive nitrates and leukocytes on a dipstick would suggest a urinary tract infection.
5. Three of the most common crystals found in urine are calcium oxalate, uric acid, and triple phosphate.

SUGGESTIONS FOR FURTHER READING

Bauer, John, & Ackerman, Gelson. (1982.) *Clinical Laboratory Methods*, 9th ed. St. Louis: C.V. Mosby.

Bullock, Barbara L. (1996.) *Pathophysiology: Adaptations and Alterations in Function*, 4th ed. Philadelphia: Lippincott-Raven Publishers.

Fishbach, Frances. (1996.) *A Manual of Laboratory and Diagnostic Tests*, 5th ed. Philadelphia: Lippincott-Raven Publishers.

Graff, Sister Laurine. (1983.) *A Handbook of Routine Urinalysis*. Philadelphia: J.B. Lippincott.

Henry, John. (1984.) *Todd-Sanford-Davidsohn Clinical Diagnosis and Management by Laboratory Methods*, 17th ed. Philadelphia: W.B. Saunders.

Memmler, R.L., Cohen, B.J., & Wood, D.L. (1996.) *The Human Body in Health and Disease*, 8th ed. Philadelphia: Lippincott-Raven Publishers.

Rubin, E., & Farber, J.L. (1994.) *Pathology*, 2nd ed. Philadelphia: J. B. Lippincott.

Phlebotomy

Chapter Outline

Blood Collection Sites
    Capillary Blood
    Venous Blood
    Arterial Blood
General Blood Drawing Equipment
    Blood Drawing Station
    Gloves
    Disinfectants and Antiseptics
    Sterile Gauze Pads
    Bandages
    Needle and Sharps Disposal
        Containers
    Slides
Venipuncture Equipment
    Tourniquets
    Needles
Blood Collection Systems
    Evacuated Tube System
    Syringe System
    Winged Infusion Set
Order of Draw
    Evacuated Tube System
    Syringe System

Skin Puncture (Microcollection)
    Equipment
    Lancets
    Microcollection Tubes
    Microcollection Containers
    Micropipet Dilution Systems
    Filter Paper Devices
    Warming Devices
Patient Preparation
Performing a Venipuncture
Procedure: Obtaining a Blood Specimen
        by Venipuncture
    Complications of Venipuncture
Performing a Skin Puncture
Procedure: Obtaining a Blood Specimen
        by Skin Puncture
    Complications of Skin Puncture
Summary
Critical Thinking Challenges
Answers to Checkpoint Questions
Suggestions for Further Reading

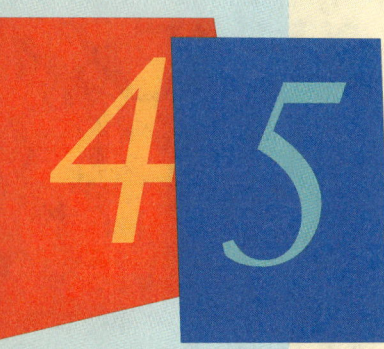

DACUM Components

1.3   Practice within the scope of education, training, and personal capabilities
1.6   Conduct oneself in a courteous and diplomatic manner
4.1   Apply principles of aseptic technique and infection control
4.5   Prepare and maintain examination and treatment area
4.7   Prepare patients for procedures
4.10 Collect and process specimens
4.11 Perform selected tests that assist with diagnosis and treatment
5.1   Document accurately

Chapter Competencies

Learning Objectives

Upon successfully completing this chapter, you will be able to:

1. Define and spell the Key Terms.
2. Identify equipment and supplies used to obtain a routine venous specimen and a routine capillary skin puncture.
3. List the anticoagulants used, the order of draw, and color coding recognized with each type for the collection of blood specimens.
4. Discuss the location and selection of the blood collection sites for capillaries and veins.
5. Explain the importance of correct patient identification and complete specimen and requisition labeling.
6. Describe the steps in preparation of the puncture site for venipuncture and skin puncture.
7. Describe care for a puncture site after blood has been drawn.
8. List precautions to be observed when drawing blood.

Performance Objectives

Upon successfully completing this chapter, you will be able to:

1. Obtain a blood specimen from a patient by venipuncture (Procedure 45-1).
2. Obtain a blood specimen from a patient by skin puncture (Procedure 45-2).
3. Use a butterfly collection system.
4. Use a Unopette system for diluting blood specimens.

Key Terms

(See Glossary for definitions.)

antecubital space
antiseptic
arteriole
cyanotic
edema
gel separator
hemolysis
Luer adapter
palmar
thromboplastin
venule
whorls

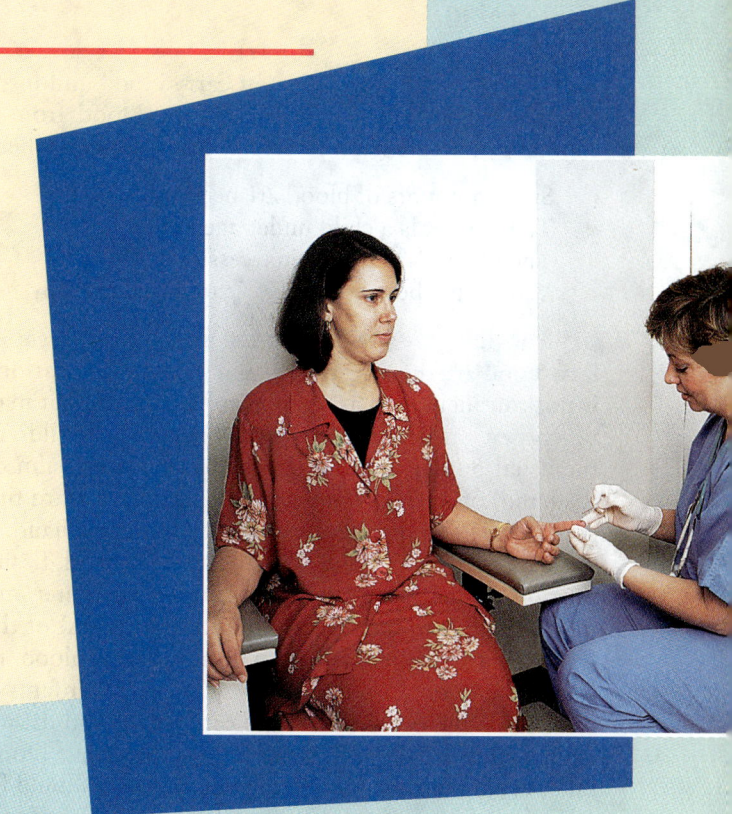

The literal translation of the word phlebotomy means incision into a vein. Phlebotomy is performed today by one of two procedures:

1. *Venipuncture*—involves collecting blood by penetrating a vein with a needle and syringe or other collection apparatus
2. *Skin puncture*—involves collecting blood after puncturing the skin with a lancet or similar puncture device

Most blood collection procedures are performed by the medical assistant or phlebotomist. You will need to study and practice to obtain blood specimens successfully. You also will need to ensure that blood collection is performed in the safest manner possible. Blood is recognized as a hazardous material, so it should be handled with the use of Standard Precautions and appropriate barrier precautions.

➤ BLOOD COLLECTION SITES

The three types of blood vessels are capillaries, veins, and arteries. Blood can be obtained from all three types of vessels. You will routinely use capillaries and veins for collecting blood specimens.

Capillary Blood

Capillaries are small vessels that carry blood and form the link between arterioles to venules. Blood from a capillary puncture (skin puncture) may be taken when:

- Small amounts of blood are needed
- The patient is a child under age 2
- The patient's veins are inaccessible
- Veins must be preserved for parenteral therapy

The puncture sites most often used to obtain capillary blood are the finger, heel, and big toe. The earlobe is not routinely used as a blood collection site but may be chosen on occasion. In adults and older children, the usual puncture site is the **palmar** surface (palm of the hand) of the end segment of the second or third finger (middle or ring finger) of the nondominant hand.

The puncture should be made in the central, fleshy portion of the finger, slightly to the side of center and perpendicular to the **whorls** (spirals and ridges) of the fingerprint. This procedure will allow the blood to form a bead or drop that is easily collected. Infants 3 months of age or younger have capillary blood drawn from a prewarmed heel; older infants may have blood taken from their big toes. Skin puncture sites should be warm, pink, and free of scars, cuts, bruises, **edema** (fluid accumulation), calluses, and rashes.

Venous Blood

Veins carry blood toward the heart after oxygen from the blood has been given to the cells of the body. **Venules** are very small veins that are connected to capillaries. Venules widen as they travel toward the heart and become veins that gradually increase in size until they reach the vena cavae. Most laboratory testing is done on blood drawn from veins because they are easily accessible and can yield larger amounts of blood.

The forearm veins located in the **antecubital space** (the inner surface of the bend of the elbow) are commonly used for venipuncture. The three main veins in this area are the cephalic, median cubital, and the basilic (Fig. 45-1). The primary vein for venipuncture is the median cubital vein. The fingertips should be used to gently press on the vein to determine its direction and to estimate its size and depth. Veins will feel spongy, like an elastic tube. Alternative sites may be indicated if the area is **cyanotic** (bluish skin discoloration caused by lack of oxygen), scarred, bruised, edematous, or burned. Veins on the lower forearm, the back of the hand, or wrist may also be used. Use foot or ankle veins only if the patient has good circulation

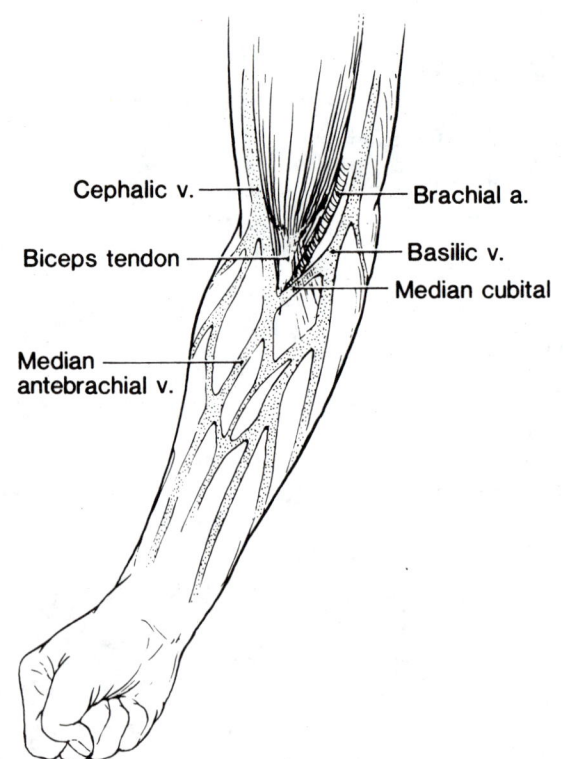

FIGURE 45-1
The venous structure. a = artery; v = vein. (Redrawn from Valaske MD [ed]: So You're Going to Collect a Blood Specimen, rev ed, p 16. College of American Pathologists, Skokie, IL, 1982)

to the legs and permission is received from your supervisor or the physician.

Arterial Blood

Arteries are vessels that carry oxygenated blood away from the heart. Arteries branch into smaller vessels called **arterioles**, which then connect with capillaries. Physicians usually order arterial punctures to assess how well the lungs are functioning. Medical assistants do not usually draw arterial blood but should be aware of artery locations so the arteries will not be entered when performing a venipuncture.

Arterial blood can be suspected if the color of the blood is bright red compared with the darker red color of venous blood. If an artery is entered by mistake, maintain pressure on the site for 5 to 10 minutes or until all bleeding has stopped. If the specimen has already been collected, it may be used for testing. However, the tube, the request, and the laboratory report must be labeled as arterial blood.

Checkpoint Question
1. *What four situations may require capillary puncture?*

➤ GENERAL BLOOD DRAWING EQUIPMENT

Blood Drawing Station

A blood drawing station is equipped for performing phlebotomy procedures on outpatients or patients in medical offices (Fig. 45-2). This station includes a table for supplies close at hand and a chair or bed for the patient. The table should be a convenient height for working with enough space to hold numerous supplies. The chair should be comfortable and have an adjustable armrest with a safety device to lock the armrest in place to prevent the patient from falling out if fainting occurs. A bed or reclining chair should be available for patients with a history of fainting and to perform heel sticks or other procedures on infants and small children.

Gloves

Guidelines from the Centers for Disease Control and Prevention (CDC) and the Occupational Safety and Health Administration (OSHA) require that gloves be worn when performing phlebotomy procedures. A new pair of gloves must be used for each patient and removed when the procedure is finished. Latex, vinyl, or polyethylene nonsterile, disposable gloves are acceptable.

What If?
What if you or your patient are allergic to latex products?

If you are allergic to latex, the Occupational Safety and Health Administration (OSHA) requires your employer to provide other appropriate gloves and supplies for you. If your patient is allergic to latex, you must use products such as gloves and tourniquets made from substances other than latex. Latex is also found in catheters, some elastic bandages, wheelchair tires, disposable diapers, and disposable underpads. Latex is made from the sap of the *Hevea brasliensis* tree. Latex allergies were first identified in 1989 and have resulted in many deaths. The signs of allergic reactions can be minor (redness, rash, itching at the site) or more severe (hives, wheezing, angioedema, and bronchospasm). The signs and symptoms are treated with epinephrine and bronchodilators. Tests are available to determine latex allergies.

Disinfectants and Antiseptics

Disinfectants kill bacteria. They are used on inanimate objects, such as instruments and surfaces. They are not to be used on human skin. Household bleach in a 1:10 solution is commonly used to wipe surfaces and clean

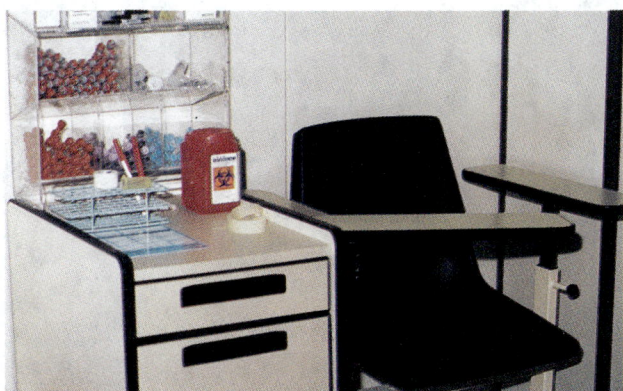

FIGURE 45-2
A well-stocked blood drawing station.

up blood spills in the phlebotomy station. This disinfectant will kill viruses that cause acquired immunodeficiency syndrome (AIDS) and hepatitis.

Antiseptics prevent or inhibit the growth of bacteria. They are safe for use on human skin and are used to clean the skin before skin puncture or venipuncture. The most commonly used antiseptic for routine blood collection is 70% isopropyl alcohol. Another antiseptic frequently used for blood culture collection is povidone iodine.

Sterile Gauze Pads

Sterile 2 × 2 gauze pads are used to hold pressure over the site after skin puncture or venipuncture. Cotton or rayon balls may be used, but these have a tendency to stick to the site and may cause bleeding to start again when pulled from the site.

Bandages

Adhesive bandages are used to cover the site once the bleeding has stopped. If a patient is allergic to adhesive bandages, use paper, cloth, or knitted tape over a folded gauze square. Do not use bandages on infants under 2 years of age because of the danger of aspiration and suffocation.

Needle and Sharps Disposal Containers

Immediately dispose of used needles, lancets, and other sharp objects in puncture-resistant, leakproof, disposable containers referred to as "sharps" containers. These containers are usually marked as "biohazard" and are red or bright orange for easy identification. Needles should not be cut, bent, or broken before disposal. If the needle must be recapped, use the single-handed scoop technique.

Slides

Slides are available either plain or with a frosted end where the patient's name and other information can be written in pencil. Precleaned 1 × 3-inch glass microscope slides are used to make blood films for hematology studies.

Checkpoint Question
2. What are disinfectants and antiseptics used for?

▶ VENIPUNCTURE EQUIPMENT

Venipuncture procedures require the use of the following special equipment.

Tourniquets

The tourniquet constricts the venous flow of blood in the arm and makes the veins more prominent, making them easier to find and penetrate with a needle. The tourniquet is a soft, pliable rubber strip, usually 1 inch wide by 15 to 18 inches long. It can easily be released with one hand, does not cut into the patient's arm, can be easily wiped with a disinfectant to prevent the spread of infection, and is inexpensive enough to be replaced often. Some offices require a fresh tourniquet for each patient.

The tourniquet should be placed 3 to 4 inches above the proposed venipuncture site and secured by using the half-bow. The half-bow makes it easy to remove the tourniquet with just one hand. Velcro-closure, rubber tubing, or a blood pressure cuff may also be used as a tourniquet.

Needles

Sterile, disposable, single-use-only needles are used for venipuncture. They are silicon-coated, which enables them to penetrate the skin smoothly. The end of the needle is cut on a slant or bevel. The bevel allows the needle to penetrate the vein easily and prevents "coring," or the removal of a portion of skin or vein. The long, cylindrical portion of the needle is called the shaft, and the end that connects to the blood-drawing apparatus is called the hub.

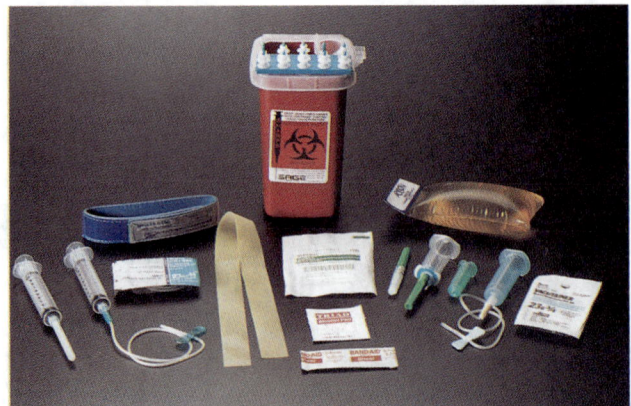
FIGURE 45-3
Equipment and supplies used for phlebotomy.

The gauge of a needle indicates the size of the needle and refers to the lumen or "bore" of the needle. The larger the gauge number, the smaller the actual diameter of the needle (eg, 20 gauge is larger than 25 gauge). Gauge selection depends on the size and condition of the vein.

Figure 45-3 shows the special equipment and supplies used for phlebotomy.

➤ BLOOD COLLECTION SYSTEMS

Two blood collection systems are commonly used for venipuncture. One is the vacuum or evacuated tube system and the other is the syringe system (Fig. 45-4).

Evacuated Tube System

The evacuated tube system consists of a tube holder (adapter) and evacuated tube needle. The tube holder and needle are a unit; neither is able to function without the other. The evacuated tube needle is a double-pointed needle, one end of which is covered with a removable cap. It is this end that, when uncapped, enters the patient. The other end, which may be covered with a rubber sleeve or shield, punctures the blood collection tubes. This needle screws into the threaded end of the holder, and the blood tubes are placed inside the large opening of the holder. The sleeve on the needle prevents blood from leaking into the holder when changing tubes during a multitube draw, as well as when the tube is removed before withdrawing the needle from the vein. These needles are called multisample needles. They come in two lengths: 1 inch and 1½ inches and are available in sizes from 20 to 22 gauge, with 21-gauge needles being the most commonly used for routine venipuncture. Needles come enclosed in sealed, twist-apart covers to ensure sterility.

The holder, sometimes called an adapter, makes the task of collecting the blood sample easier. It has an indentation about ½ inch from the hub. This indentation marks the point where the short, sleeved end of the needle starts to enter the rubber stopper of the tube. If the tube is inserted past this point before entering the vein, the tube will fill with air and it will not be possible to draw a blood sample. There are flanges (extensions) on the sides of the rim of the holder to aid in tube placement and removal.

Evacuated collection tubes contain a vacuum with a rubber stopper sealing the tube. These tubes range in size from 2 to 15 mL. The tubes are sterile to prevent contamination of the specimen and the patient. Evacu-

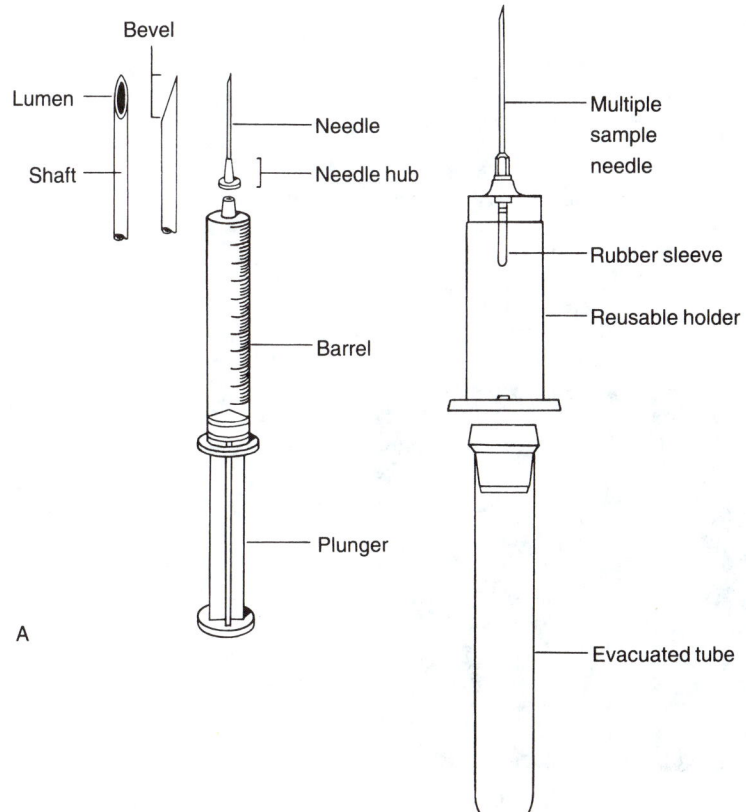

FIGURE 45-4
Blood collection systems. (*A*) Syringe components; (*B*) Components of the evacuated tube collection system.

ated tubes may or may not contain an additive. Blood collected in tubes without additives will clot and separate into serum and cells on centrifugation.

Tube Additives

An additive is any substance (other than the tube coating) that is placed in a tube. Additives have specific functions. Below is a list of the most common additives and their functions:

- Anticoagulants prevent the blood from coagulating or clotting.
- Clot activators enhance coagulation.
- Thixotropic **gel separator**, an inert substance, forms a physical barrier between the cellular portion of a specimen and the serum or plasma portion after the specimen has been centrifuged.

The evacuated tube system uses color-coded stoppers as a means of identifying the additive content of each type of tube (Table 45-1).

Syringe System

Syringes are made of either glass or disposable plastic, varying in volume from 1 to 50 mL. Both types must be sterile for use. The barrel of the syringe is graduated in milliliters. Pulling on the plunger of the syringe creates a vacuum within the barrel. The plunger often sticks and is hard to pull. A technique called "breathing the syringe" makes the plunger easier to move. To do this, before beginning the procedure, pull back the plunger to about halfway the length the barrel, then push the plunger back. This makes the plunger move more smoothly and reduces the tendency to jerk when first pulled after insertion into the vein.

The vacuum created by pulling on the plunger while a needle is in a patient's vein fills the syringe with blood. Pulling the plunger slowly and resting between pulls allows the vein time to refill with blood. Blood specimens collected by syringe must be transferred to evacuated tubes following proper order of draw (see the section "Order of Draw," below).

Table 45-1
Evacuated Tube System: Color Coding

Tube Color	Additive	Laboratory Use
Lavender	Ethylenediaminetetraacetic acid (EDTA)	Hematology testing
Blue	Sodium citrate	Coagulation studies (filled to proper level)
Green	Lithium heparin or sodium heparin	Blood gases and pH; cytogenetics
Gray	Potassium oxalate or sodium fluoride	Glucose testing
Red	None	Serum testing
Red/yellow	Glass particles	Chemistry
Red/gray	Thixotropic gel	Chemistry

Common evacuated tubes for use in phlebotomy

Winged Infusion Set

The butterfly collection system or winged infusion set has a stainless steel beveled needle with attached winged-shaped plastic extensions connected to a 6- to 12-inch length of tubing. The most common butterfly needle sizes are 21 to 23 gauge with ½- to ¾-inch lengths. Butterflies come with attachments to be used with syringes and a special multisample **Luer adapter** (a device for connecting a syringe or evacuated holder to the needle) that allows them to be used in an evacuated tube system (Fig. 45-5). The set is routinely used to collect blood from patients who have difficult or small veins and from pediatric patients. Figure 45-6 shows how to use the butterfly system.

Checkpoint Question
3. What are three chemical substances that may be added to collection tubes? Explain the function of each.

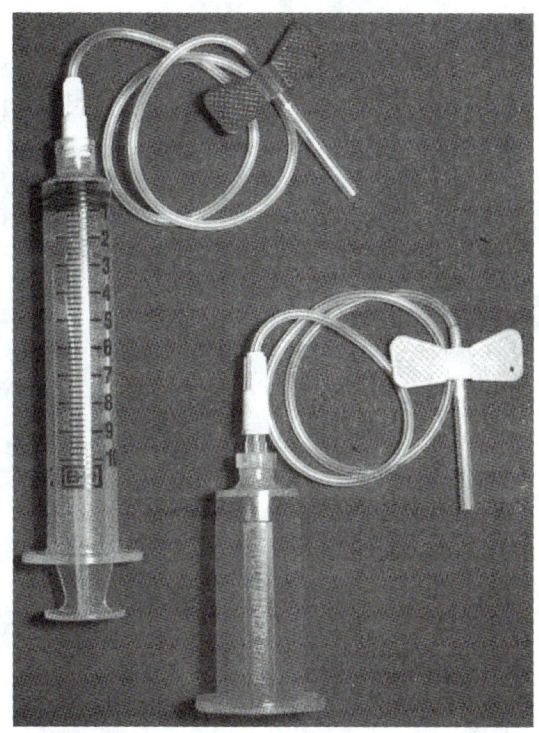

FIGURE 45-5
Winged infusion sets. (*left*) attached to a syringe; (*right*) attached to evacuated tube holder by means of a Luer adapter.

➤ ORDER OF DRAW

Evacuated Tube System

When multiple tubes are to be drawn in the evacuated tube system, the following "order of draw" is recommended to avoid contamination of nonadditive tubes by additive tubes as well as cross-contamination between different types of additive tubes:

1. Blood culture tubes (and other tests requiring sterile specimens)
2. Red stopper or red/gray stopper (nonadditive and gel separator)
3. Light blue stopper (If a light blue-stoppered tube is the first and only tube to be drawn, draw a 5-mL red-stoppered tube first and discard it to eliminate contamination from tissue **thromboplastin**, a substance that aids clotting, picked up during needle penetration.)
4. Green stopper
5. Lavender stopper
6. Gray stopper

Syringe System

The order of draw for this system differs from the evacuated tube system's order of draw. The blood that enters the syringe last is the freshest and will be the first

blood out of the syringe in the transfer process. The clotting process begins the second the blood enters the syringe; therefore, it is important to transfer the blood quickly and fill anticoagulant tubes before serum tubes. The suggested order of draw for syringes is:

1. Blood culture
2. Light blue
3. Lavender
4. Green
5. Gray
6. Red

Checkpoint Question
4. What is the proper order of draw when using the evacuated tube system? Why is this important?

➤ SKIN PUNCTURE (MICROCOLLECTION) EQUIPMENT

Often a blood specimen cannot be obtained by a venipuncture. Microcollection of a sample through a skin puncture can produce a quality specimen. The

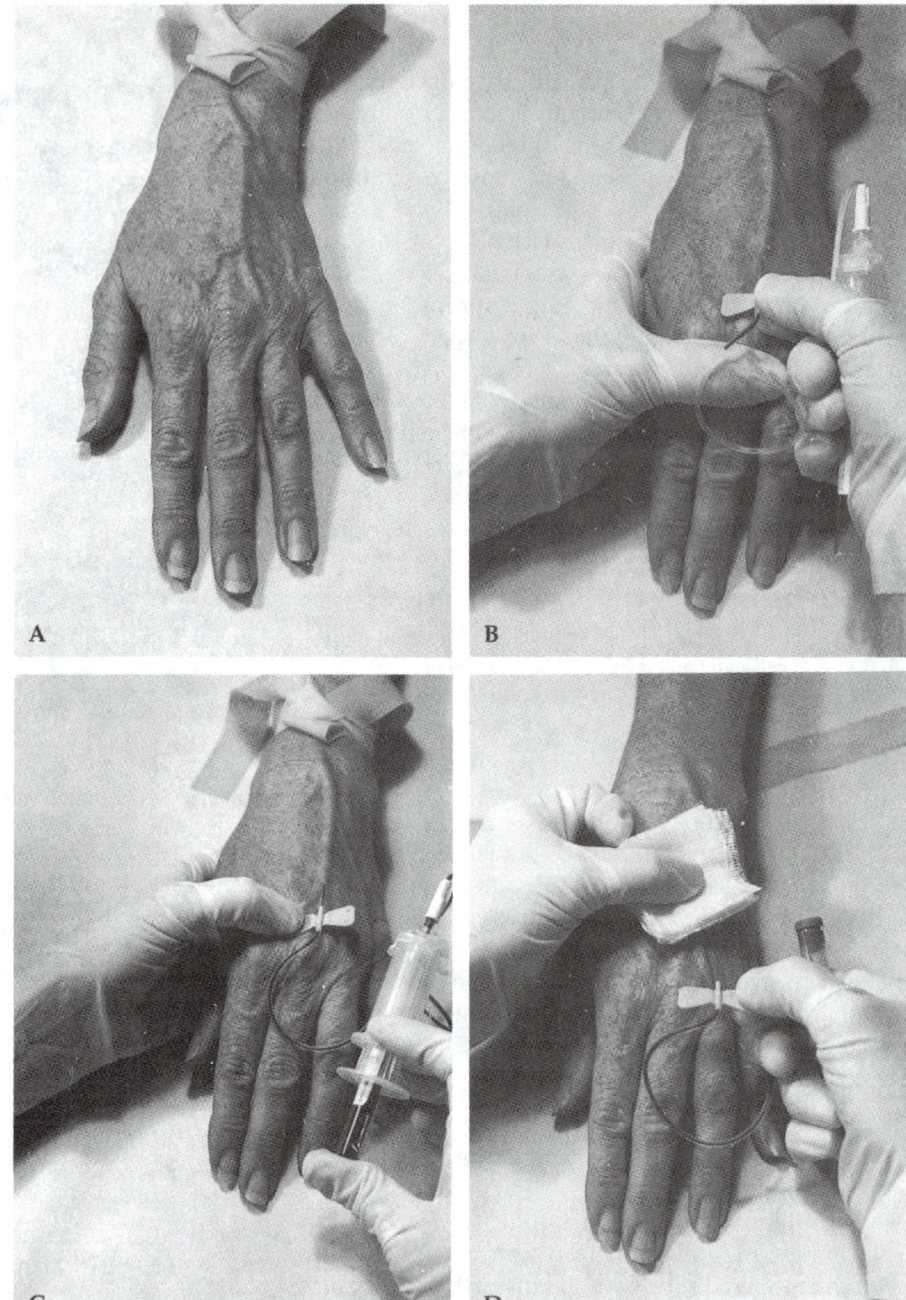

FIGURE 45-6
Procedure for using butterfly in a hand vein. (*A*) Hand with tourniquet in place reveals prominent vein. (*B*) With the skin pulled taught over the knuckles, the needle is inserted into the vein until there is a "flash" of blood in the tubing. (*C*) Using the nondominant hand, a wing of the butterfly is held against the patient's hand to steady the needle while the blood collecting tube is pushed onto the blood collecting needle. (*D*) Once the proper tubes have been drawn, gauze is placed over the vein and the needle is removed.

equipment used to collect the specimen depends on the test being performed.

Lancets

Different sterile disposable lancets are available to pierce the skin for an adequate blood flow. Lancets are now designed to control depth of puncture. You may insert the lancet into a spring-loaded device, or you may hold the blade in your hand and push it into the skin to a selected depth. Automatic puncturing devices are popular. Most consist of a platform and a spring-loaded lancet; the platform controls the tissue penetration depth. Three color-coded platforms are available for use with the automatic lancet device: white (1.8 mm), yellow (2.4 mm), and orange (3.0 mm). The platform and lancet are both disposable. Some devices feature a safety mechanism that inhibits the use of the device unless first reloaded with a new platform and lancet. Figure 45-7 shows lancets and other supplies used for microcollection.

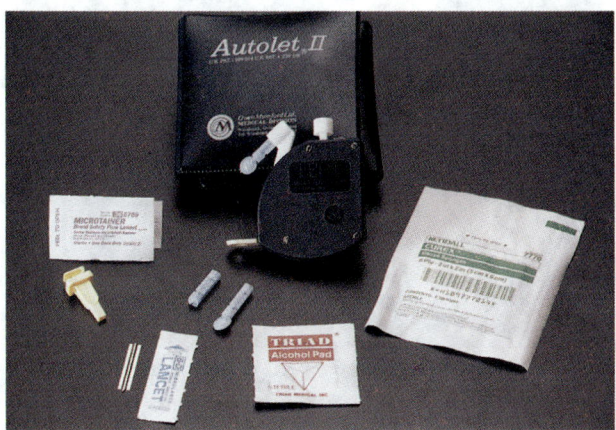

FIGURE 45-7
Microcollection supplies.

These devices should be regularly sanitized and disinfected according to the manufacturer's recommendation. The blades must be sterile; follow the directions for loading the replacement blades and platforms.

Microcollection Tubes

These tubes are narrow-bore glass or plastic disposable capillary tubes used for hematocrit determinations on 50 to 75 µL of blood. Microcollection tubes for collecting serum specimens are plain; those used for hematocrit or other tests requiring plasma may be coated with ammonium heparin. Plain tubes have a blue band on one end of the capillary tube and ammonium heparin-coated tubes have a red band. Clay sealants are used to seal one end of the tubes used in microhematocrit and chemistry determinations (Fig. 45-8).

Microcollection Containers

These microtainers consist of nonsterile, small, round-bottomed plastic tubes and color-coded stoppers that indicate the presence or absence of an additive. The color-coding is identical to blood collection tubes used

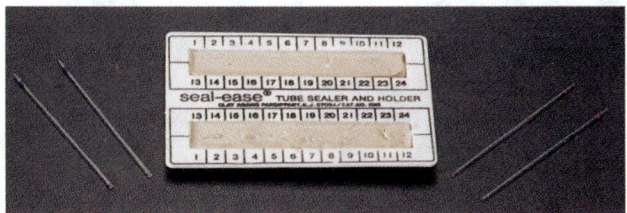

FIGURE 45-8
Microcollection tubes and clay sealant.

in venipuncture. Microtainers are used for filling, measuring, stoppering, centrifuging, and storing all in one container. Samples collected for bilirubin are collected in an amber-colored plastic tube that protects the blood from light.

Micropipet Dilution Systems

The brand name for this type of system is the Unopette, manufactured by Becton Dickinson. Components of this system include a sealed plastic reservoir containing a premeasured amount of reagent or diluent, a disposable self-filling diluting pipette, and a pipette shield for puncturing the reservoir covering before adding the sample. Figure 45-9 shows how to use the Unopette system.

Filter Paper Devices

Another microcollection device is blood collection on filter paper, which is used to test newborns for genetic defects such as hypothyroidism or phenylketonuria. The lateral surface of the newborn's heel is punctured and the blood droplet is absorbed into individual circles on a filter paper card.

Warming Devices

These units can increase blood flow before the skin is punctured. Several heelwarming devices are available; these commercial devices provide a temperature not exceeding 42°C. A diaper or towel may be wet with warm tap water and used to wrap the hand or foot before skin puncture. Do not use water so hot that it might burn the patient.

 Checkpoint Question
5. What are microcollection tubes commonly used for?

➤ PATIENT PREPARATION

Gaining the patient's trust and confidence and putting the patient at ease will help minimize anxiety and divert attention from any discomfort associated with the procedure. To do this, display a cheerful, confident, and pleasant manner, introduce yourself, explain the procedure in simple terms, and communicate effectively with the patient. Ask the patient for preference of sites. Many patients know from experience where it is easi-

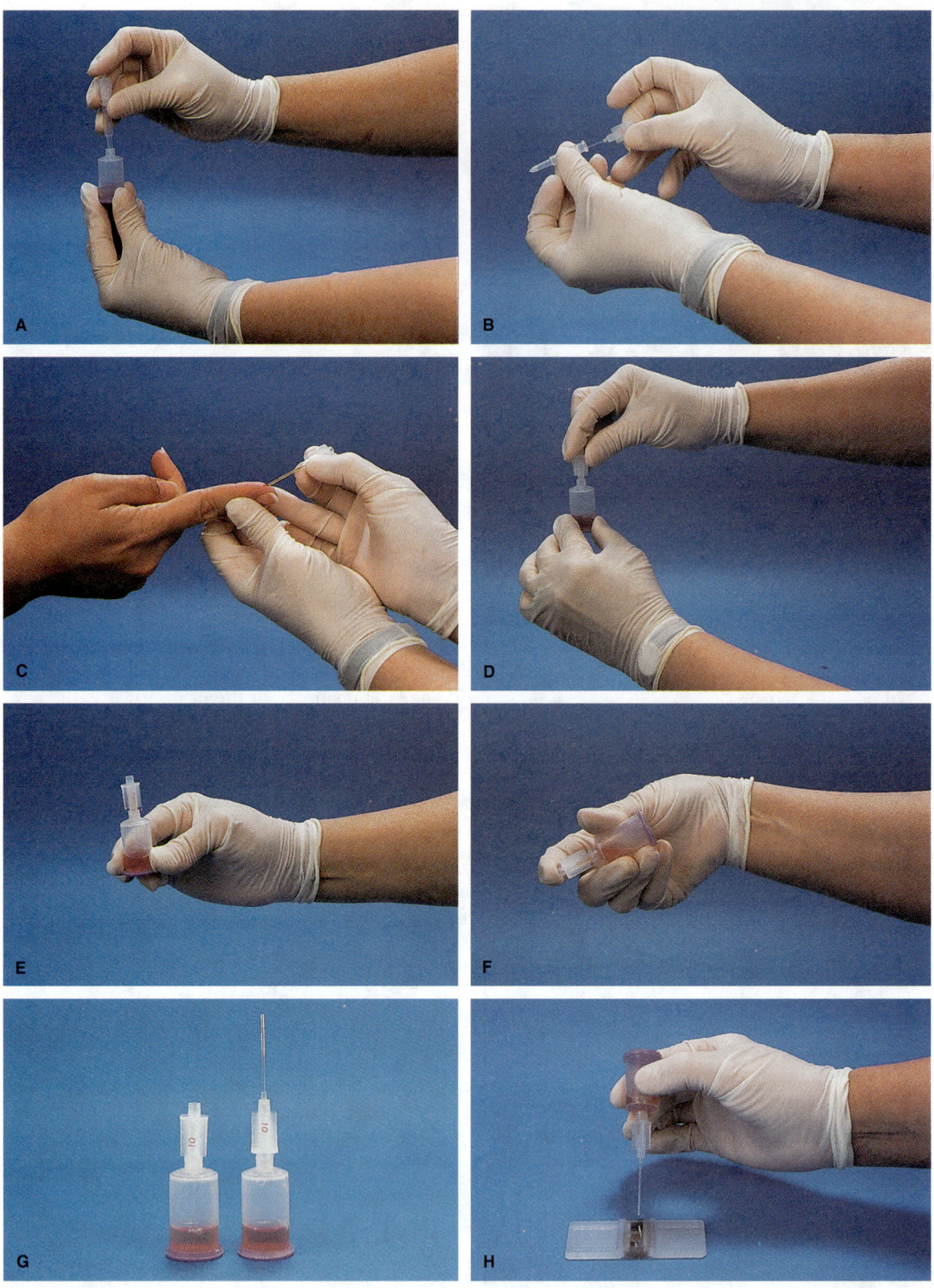

FIGURE 45-9

Steps in the dilution of blood using the Unopette system. (*A*) Puncture diaphragm. (*B*) Remove shield from pipet assembly with a twist. (*C*) Draw sample into pipet from free-flowing skin puncture or tube. Remove excess blood on outside of pipet carefully with a gauze. (*D*) Squeeze reservoir slightly to force out some air. Do not expel liquid. Cover opening of pipet overflow chamber with finger and seat pipet securely in reservoir neck. (*E*) Squeeze reservoir gently two or three times to rinse capillary bore, forcing diluent into, but not out of, overflow chamber. (*F*) Cover opening with finger and gently invert to mix. (*G*) Convert to dropper assembly. Mix well, invert, and expel first few drops of mixture on waste cloth. Maintain pressure on reservoir to avoid air bubbles. (*H*) Charge hemocytometer. (Courtesy Becton Dickinson Vacutainer Systems, Rutherford, NJ.)

est to find an accessible vein. In conjunction with your knowledge and skill, knowing the best site will make the procedure less traumatic. Talk quietly with the patient and progress through the procedure with confidence.

Always believe patients who say they faint during venipuncture. Have these patients lie down during the procedure. This reduces the chance of syncope (fainting), and if fainting does occur, the patient will already be lying down. If the patient is sitting and feels faint, have him or her lower the head between the knees. Never draw blood from a patient who is likely to faint unless the physician is in the office.

One of the most important steps in specimen collection is patient identification. When identifying a patient, ask the patient to state his or her name, date of birth, or any other information to verify identity. After the blood specimen has been collected, the sample must be labeled with the patient's first and last names, an assigned identification number if available, the date and time, and the medical assistant's initials to verify who drew the sample.

➤ PERFORMING A VENIPUNCTURE

The steps for performing a venipuncture (Procedure 45-1) are organized according to the guidelines established by the National Committee for Clinical Laboratory Standards (NCCLS). There may be variations in some methods performed at various clinical settings because of individual technique and specific circumstances.

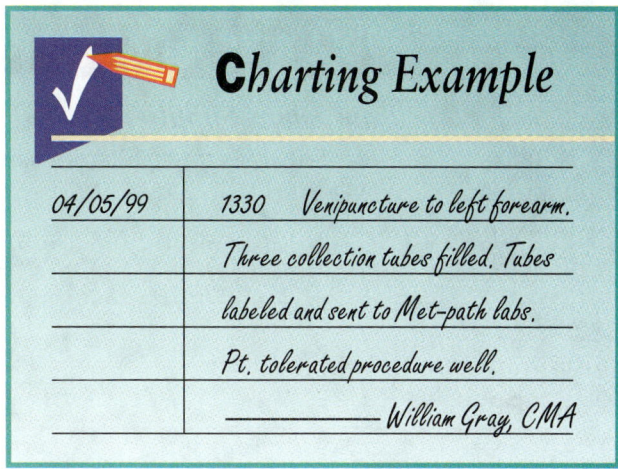

Charting Example

04/05/99	1330 Venipuncture to left forearm.
	Three collection tubes filled. Tubes
	labeled and sent to Met-path labs.
	Pt. tolerated procedure well.
	—————— William Gray, CMA

Complications of Venipuncture

When a blood sample cannot be obtained, you may need to change the position of the needle. Figure 45-10 shows proper and improper needle positions. Rotate the needle half a turn; the bevel of the needle may be against the wall of the vein. If the needle has not penetrated the vein, slowly advance it further into the vein. If the needle has penetrated too far into the vein, pull back a little. The tube being used may not have sufficient vacuum; try another tube before withdrawing. If the vein feels very thick and hard, try for one with more elasticity; this one may roll away. If the patient

text continues on page 913

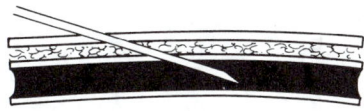

A. Correct insertion technique; blood flows freely into needle.

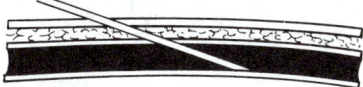

C. Bevel on vein lower wall does not allow blood to flow.

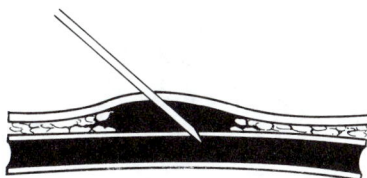

E. Needle partially inserted and causes blood leakage into tissue.

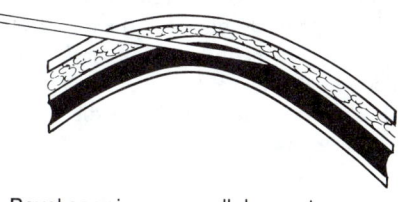

B. Bevel on vein upper wall does not allow blood to flow.

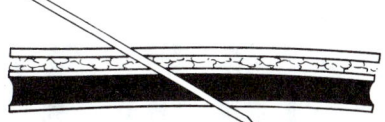

D. Needle inserted too far.

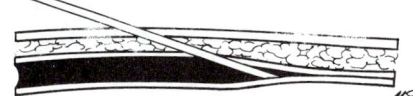

F. Collapsed.

FIGURE 45-10

Proper and improper needle positioning. (A) Proper needle position. (B) Needle bevel against the upper wall of a vein. (C) Needle bevel against or embedded in opposite wall of vein. (D) Needle inserted all the way through a vein. (E) Needle partially inserted into a vein. (F) Needle in collapsed vein.

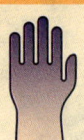

Procedure 45-1

Obtaining a Blood Specimen by Venipuncture

Equipment/Supplies

- needle, syringe, and tube(s) or evacuated tubes
- tourniquet
- sterile gauze pads
- bandages
- needle and adaptor
- sharps container
- 70% alcohol pad or alternate antiseptic
- permanent marker or pen
- appropriate biohazard barriers (eg, gloves, impervious gown, face shield)

Steps	Purpose
1. Check the requisition slip to determine the tests ordered and specimen requirements.	1. This ensures proper specimen collection.
2. Wash your hands.	2. Handwashing aids infection control.
3. Assemble the equipment. Check the expiration date on the tubes.	3. Assembling the equipment ensures that everything you need is available. Expired tubes may no longer have a vacuum; additives may no longer be functional.
4. Greet and identify the patient. Explain the procedure. Ask for and answer any questions.	4. Identifying the patient prevents errors. Explaining the procedure helps ease anxiety and ensure compliance.
5. If a fasting specimen is required, ask the patient the last time food was eaten.	5. For fasting specimens, food should not have been eaten within at least 12 hours.
6. Put on nonsterile latex or vinyl gloves.	6. Standard Precautions must be observed.
7. Break the seal of the needle cover and thread the sleeved needle into the adaptor, using the needle cover as a wrench. Tap the tubes that contain additives to ensure that the additive is dislodged from the stopper and wall of the tube. Insert the tube into the adaptor until the needle slightly enters the stopper. Do not push the top of the tube stopper beyond the indentation mark. If the tube retracts slightly, leave it in the retracted position. If using a syringe, tighten the needle on the hub and breathe the syringe.	7. This ensures proper needle placement, tube positioning, and prevents loss of vacuum in the evacuated tubes or sticking of the plunger in the barrel of the syringe.

(continued)

Steps

Purpose

8. Instruct the patient to sit with a well-supported arm in a downward extended position if possible.
    a. Apply the tourniquet around the patient's arm 3–4 inches above the elbow.

8. Veins in the antecubital fossa are more easily located when the elbow is straight. The tourniquet makes the veins more prominent. Making a fist raises the vessels out of the underlying tissues and muscles.

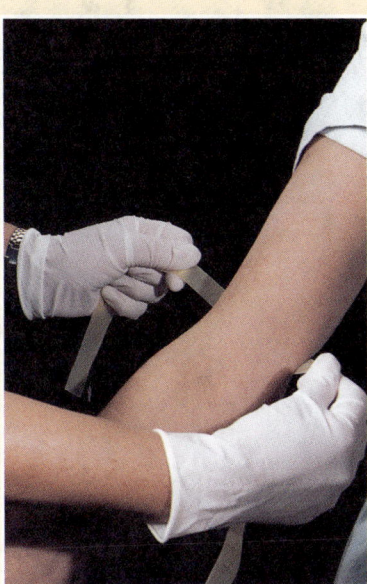

Step 8a: Apply the tourniquet 3–4 inches above the elbow.

    b. Apply the tourniquet snugly, but not too tightly.

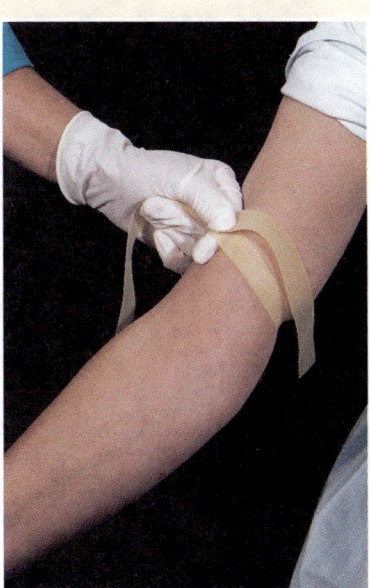

Step 8b: Pull the tourniquet snugly around the arm.

(continued)

Steps	Purpose

c. Secure the tourniquet by using the half-bow.

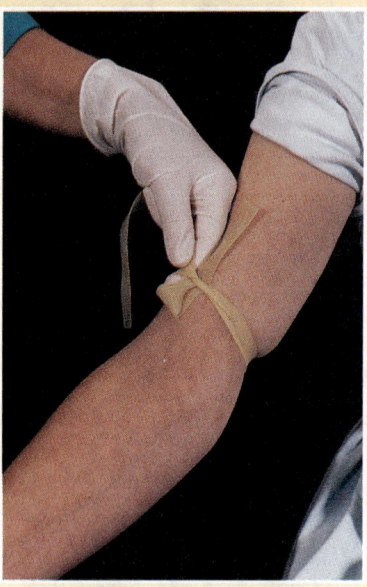

Step 8c: Secure the tourniquet by using the half-bow.

d. Make sure the tails of the tourniquet extend upward to avoid contaminating the venipuncture site.

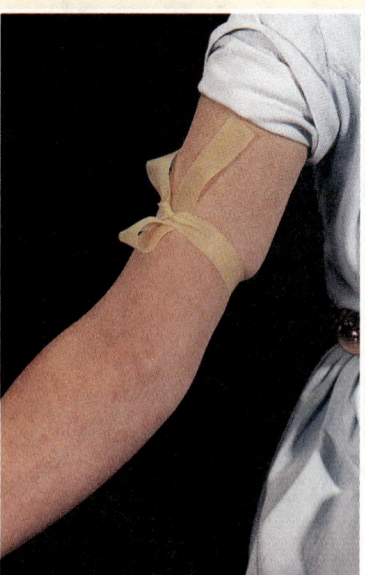

Step 8d: The tourniquet should extend upward.

(continued)

Procedure 45-1

Obtaining a Blood Specimen by Venipuncture *(continued)*

Steps	Purpose
e. Ask the patient to close his hand into a fist, but ask him not to pump his fist.	
9. Select a vein by palpating. Use your gloved index finger to trace the path of the vein and judge its depth.	9. The index finger is most sensitive for palpating.

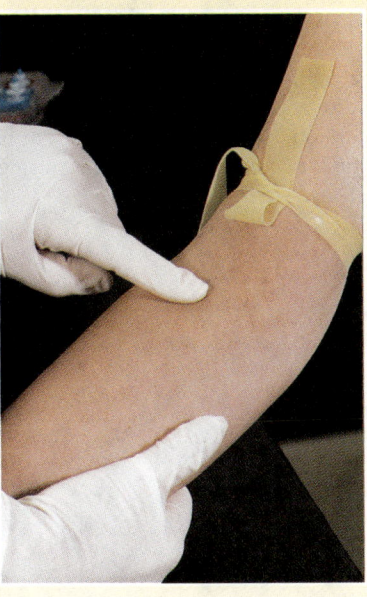

Step 9: Trace the path of the vein.

10. Release the tourniquet after palpating the vein if it has been left on for more than 1 minute.	10. The tourniquet should not be left on for more than 1 minute at a time during the procedure.
11. Cleanse the venipunture site with an alcohol pad starting in the center of puncture site and working outward in a circular motion. Allow the site to dry or dry the site with sterile gauze. Do not touch the area after cleansing.	11. The circular motion helps avoid recontamination of the area. Puncturing a wet area stings and can cause hemolysis of the sample.
12. If blood being drawn for culture will be used in diagnosing septic conditions, make sure the specimen is sterile. To do this, apply alcohol to the area for 2 full minutes. Then apply a 2% iodine solution in ever-widening circles. Never move the wipes back over areas that have been cleaned; use a new wipe for each sweep across the area.	12. Ensuring sterility of the specimen will aid accurate diagnosis.
13. Reapply the tourniquet if it was removed after palpation.	13. If tourniquet time is greater than 1 minute, test results could be altered.

(continued)

Steps	Purpose
14. Remove the needle cover. Hold the syringe or evacuated assembly in your dominant hand. Your thumb should be on top of the adaptor and your fingers underneath. Grasp the patient's arm with the nondominant hand while using your thumb to draw the skin taut over the site and anchor the vein about 1–2 inches below the puncture site.	14. Anchoring the vein allows for easier needle penetration and less pain.
15. With the bevel up, line up the needle with the vein at approximately ¼–½ inch below the site where the vein is to be entered. At a 15°–30° angle, rapidly and smoothly insert the needle through the skin. Remove your nondominant hand and slowly pull back the plunger of the syringe. Or place two fingers on the flanges of the adapter, and with the thumb push the tube onto the needle inside the adapter. When blood flow begins in the tube or syringe, release the tourniquet and allow the patient to release the fist. Allow the syringe or tube(s) to fill to capacity. When blood flow ceases, remove the tube from the adapter by gripping the tube with your nondominant hand and place your thumb against the flange during removal. Twist and gently pull out the tube. Steady the needle in the vein. Try not to pull up or press down on the needle while it is in the vein. Insert any other necessary tubes into adapter and allow to fill to capacity.	15. The sharpest point of the needle is inserted first. Proper tube filling ensures correct ratio of blood to additive. Removal of the tourniquet releases pressure on the vein and helps prevent blood from seeping into adjacent tissues and causing a hematoma.

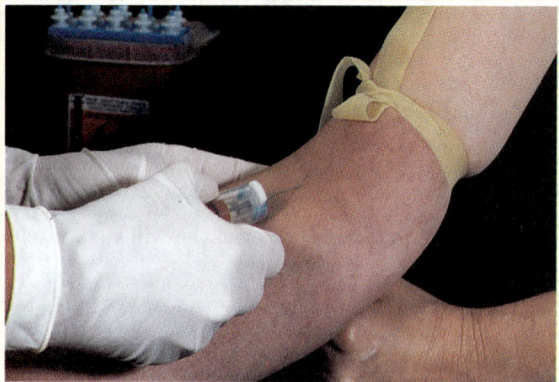

Step 15: Insert the needle at a 15°–30° angle.

(continued)

Procedure 45-1

Obtaining a Blood Specimen by Venipuncture *(continued)*

Steps	**Purpose**
16. Remove the tube from the adapter before removing the needle from the arm. If the tourniquet has not been previously released, do so now.	16. Removing the last tube from the adapter before removing the needle from the vein prevents any excess blood from dripping from the tip of the needle onto the patient. Pressure decreases the amount of blood escaping into the tissues. Bending the arm increases the chance of blood seeping into the subcutaneous tissues.

    a. Place a sterile gauze pad over the puncture site at the time of needle withdrawal. Do not apply any pressure to the site until the needle is completely removed.

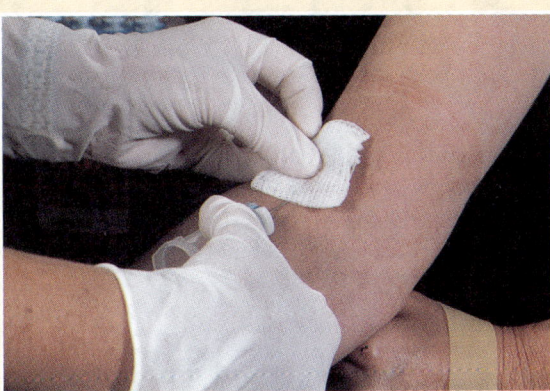

Step 16A: Place a sterile gauze pad over the site.

    b. After the needle is removed, apply pressure or have the patient apply direct pressure for 3–5 minutes. Do not bend the arm at the elbow.

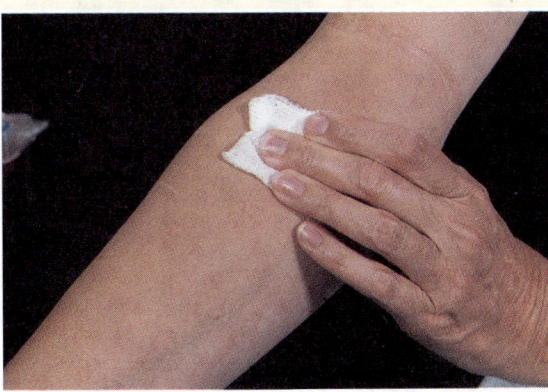

Step 16B: Apply pressure for 3–5 minutes.

(continued)

Procedure 45-1   Obtaining a Blood Specimen by Venipuncture *(continued)*

Steps	**Purpose**
17. Transfer the blood from a syringe into the proper order of draw tubes by inserting the needle through the stopper and allowing the vacuum to fill the tubes. Do not hold the tube when puncturing the stopper and filling the tube; place it in a tube rack and carefully insert the needle through the stopper. If the vacuum tubes contain an anticoagulant, they must be mixed immediately by gently inverting the tube 8–10 times. Do not shake the tube. Label the tubes with the proper information.	17. Mixing anticoagulated tubes prevents clotting of blood. Holding the tube increases the chance of accidental stick. Proper labeling of blood specimens avoids mix-up of samples.
18. Check the puncture site for bleeding. Apply a bandage.	
19. Thank the patient and give appropriate instructions.	19. Courtesy helps the patient have a positive attitude about the procedure and the physician's office.
20. Properly care for or dispose of all equipment and supplies. Clean the work area. Remove gloves and wash your hands.	20. Standard Precautions must be followed throughout the procedure to prevent the spread of microorganisms.

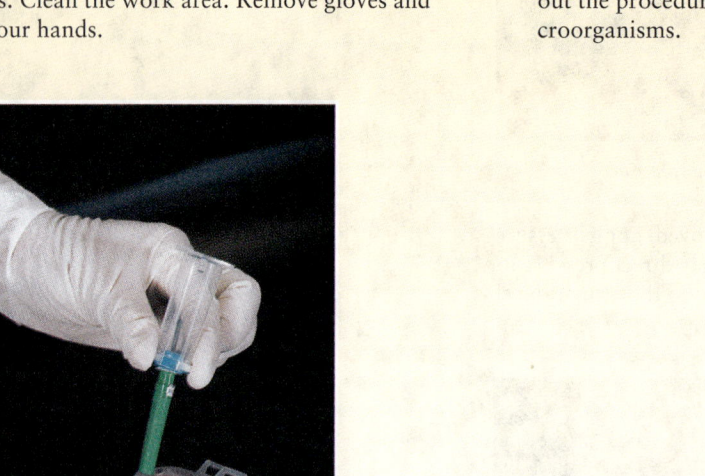

Step 20: Properly care for or dispose of all supplies.

21. Test, transfer, or store the blood specimen according to the medical office policy.	
22. Record the procedure.	22. Procedures are considered not to have been done if they are not recorded.

Table 45-2
Sources of Error in Venipuncture

Errors in Venipuncture Preparation
  Improper patient identification
  Failure to check patient adherence to dietary restrictions
  Failure to calm patient prior to blood collection
  Use of improper equipment and supplies
  Inappropriate method of blood collection
Errors in Venipuncture Procedure
  Failure to dry the site completely after cleansing with alcohol
  Inserting needle bevel side down
  Use of needle that is too small, causing hemolysis of specimen
  Venipuncture in an unacceptable area
  Prolonged tourniquet application
  Wrong order of tube draw
  Failure to mix blood collected in additive-containing tubes immediately
  Pulling back on syringe plunger too forcefully
  Failure to release tourniquet prior to needle withdrawal
Errors after Venipuncture Completion
  Failure to apply pressure immediately to venipuncture site
  Vigorous shaking of anticoagulated blood specimens
  Forcing blood through a syringe needle into tube
  Mislabeling of tubes
  Failure to label appropriate specimens with infectious disease precaution
  Failure to put date, time, and initials on requisition
  Slow transport of specimens to laboratory

(From Lotspeich-Steininger, C. A., Stiene-Martin, E. A., Koepke, J. A. [1992]. Clinical Hematology, *p. 17. Philadelphia: J. B. Lippincott.)*

---

has a history of collapsing veins during evacuated tube draws, try a syringe; you will have a more controlled withdrawal. Never attempt a venipuncture more than twice. If a blood specimen cannot be obtained in two tries, do a microcollection (skin puncture) if possible, or have another person attempt the draw. Table 45-2 lists some common sources of errors in venipuncture that you need to guard against.

➤ PERFORMING A SKIN PUNCTURE

Some veins will not endure a venipuncture. Microcollection of a sample through a skin puncture can provide a medical assistant with a quality specimen with less trauma to the patient (Procedure 45-2).

Complications of Skin Puncture

Several precautions should be observed to produce the most accurate specimen. The greatest concern with microcollection specimens is **hemolysis**, the rupture of erythrocytes with the release of hemoglobin. Do not squeeze or milk the heel or finger to produce a greater

blood flow. Never scrape the microcollection device on the skin surface; only allow the container to touch the drop of blood. You should also be careful to avoid additional sources of errors, which are listed in Table 45-3.

Obtaining a specimen without clots is also a challenge in microcollection. The body's clotting system is activated to stop the bleeding as soon as the skin is punctured. If an ethylenediaminetetraacetic acid (EDTA) specimen is required, this specimen

text continues on page 919

✓ Charting Example

| 02/07/99 | 1500 | Capillary puncture to right ring finger. Blood collected in micro- collection tube. Hct done—42% Robin Jones, RMA |

Procedure 45-2 Obtaining a Blood Specimen by Skin Puncture

Equipment/Supplies

- sterile disposable lancet or automated skin puncture device
- 70% alcohol or alternate antiseptic
- sterile gauze pads
- collection containers (Unopettes, capillary tubes)
- heelwarming device, if needed
- appropriate biohazard barriers (eg, gloves, impervious gown, face shield)

Steps	Purpose
1. Check the requisition slip to determine the tests ordered and specimen requirements.	1. This ensures proper specimen collection.
2. Wash your hands.	2. Handwashing aids infection control.
3. Assemble the equipment.	3. Having the equipment ready will speed the collection process so the blood does not clot before the entire specimen has been collected.
4. Greet and identify the patient. Explain the procedure. Ask for and answer any questions.	4. Identifying the patient prevents errors. Explaining the procedure helps ease anxiety and ensure compliance.
5. Put on nonsterile latex or vinyl gloves.	5. Standard Precautions must be observed.
6. Select the puncture site (the lateral portion of the tip of the middle or ring finger of the nondominant hand, lateral curved surface of the heel, or the great toe of an infant). The puncture should be made in the fleshy, central portion of the second or third finger, slightly to the side of center, and perpendicular to the grooves of the fingerprint. Perform heel puncture only on the plantar surface of the heel, medial to an imaginary line extending from the middle of the great toe to the heel, and lateral to an imaginary line drawn from between the fourth and fifth toes to the heel. Puncture should not exceed 2.4 mm in depth.	6. The ring and middle fingers are less calloused. The lateral part of the tip is the least sensitive part of the finger. A puncture made across the finger prints will produce a large, round drop of blood. In an infant skin puncture, the area and the depth designated reduces the risk of puncturing the bone.

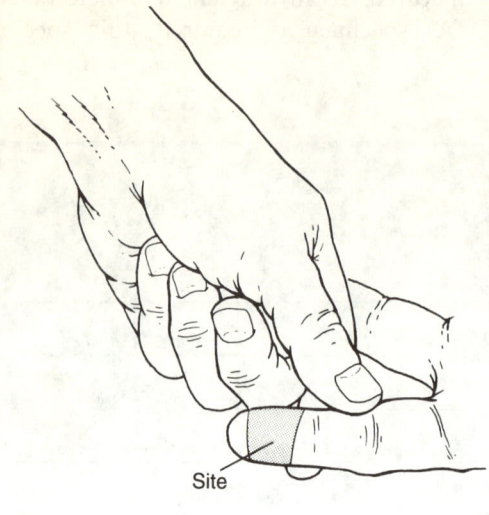

Site

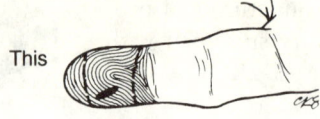

This

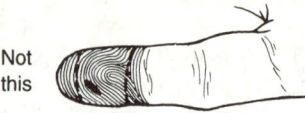

Not this

Step 6: Recommended site and direction of finger puncture.

(continued)

Procedure 45-2   Obtaining a Blood Specimen by Skin Puncture *(continued)*

Steps	Purpose

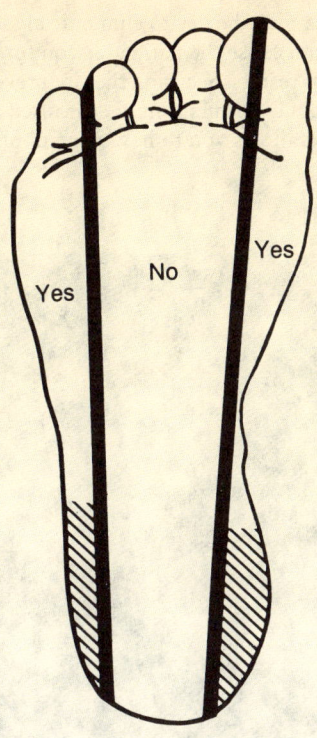

Yes

No

Yes

Yes

Step 6: Acceptable areas for heel-skin punctures on newborns. (Blumfield TA, Turi GK, Blanc WA: Recommended site and depth of newborn heel skin punctures based on anatomical measurements and histopathology. Lancet 1:230–233, 1979)

7. Make sure the site chosen is warm and not cyanotic or edematous. Gently massage the finger from the base to the tip or warm the site for 3 minutes with a warm washcloth or commercial heel warmer.

7. Massaging and warming the area increases the blood flow. Good circulation at the chosen site yields a better blood sample for analysis.

(continued)

Procedure 45-2

Obtaining a Blood Specimen by Skin Puncture (continued)

Steps	Purpose
8. Grasp the finger firmly between your nondominant index finger and the thumb or grasp the infant's heel firmly with the index finger wrapped around the foot and the thumb wrapped around the ankle. Cleanse the ball of the selected finger or heel with 70% isopropyl alcohol and wipe dry with a sterile gauze pad or allow to air dry.	8. The area must be dry to eliminate alcohol residue, which can cause the patient discomfort or interfere with test results. Securing the site prevents the patient from contaminating the cleansed puncture area and allows you to have control of the puncture site.

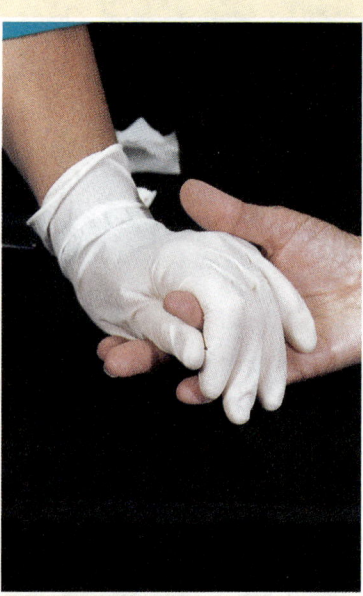

Step 8: Grasp the finger firmly. Cleanse the site with alcohol and dry with a sterile gauze pad.

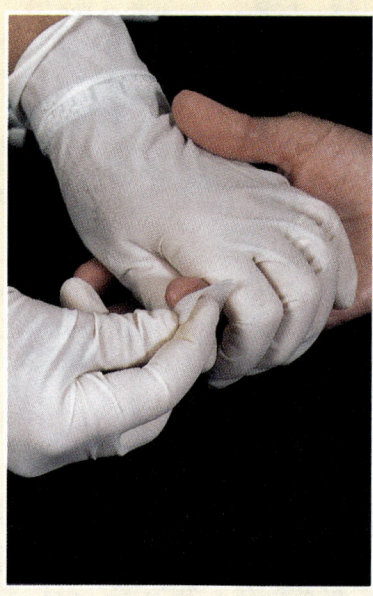

Step 8: Continued

(continued)

Obtaining a Blood Specimen by Skin Puncture (continued)

Steps	Purpose
9. Hold the patient's finger or heel firmly and make a swift, deep puncture. Perform the puncture perpendicular to the whorls of the fingerprint or footprint.	9. The proper puncture will allow the blood to form a rounded drop that can be easily collected.

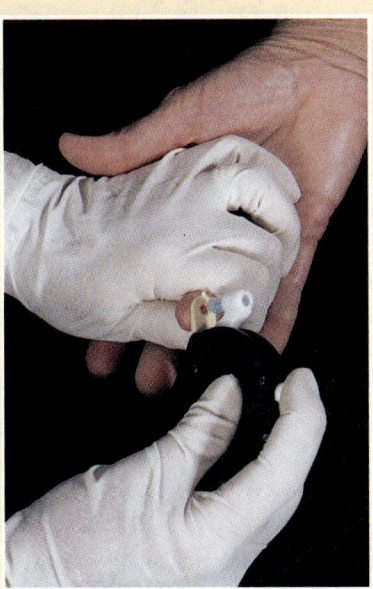

Step 9: The automatic lancet makes a swift, deep puncture.

a. Wipe away the first drop of blood with a sterile dry gauze.	a. The first discarded drop may be contaminated with tissue fluid or alcohol residue.

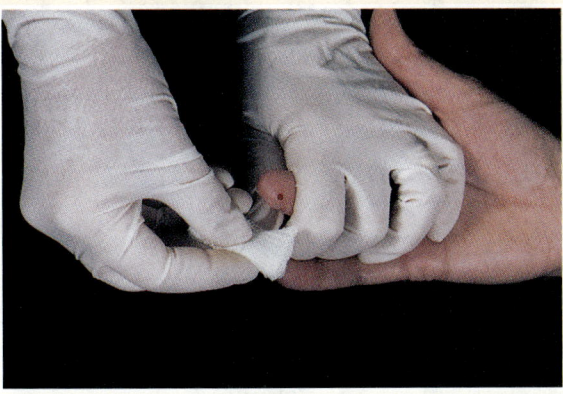

Step 9a: Wipe away the first drop of blood.

b. Apply pressure toward the site but do not "milk" the site.	b. Milking the site will dilute the specimen with tissue fluid.

(continued)

Steps	Purpose
10. Collect the required specimen in the chosen containers or slides. Touch only the tip of the collection device to the drop of blood. Blood flow is encouraged if the puncture site is held in a downward, or dependent, angle and a gentle pressure is applied to the site. Cap microcollection tubes with the caps provided and mix the additives by gently tilting or inverting the tubes 8–10 times.	10. Scraping the collection device on the skin activates platelets and may cause hemolysis. Mixing the specimens prevents clotting. Touching the tube to the site may cause contamination.

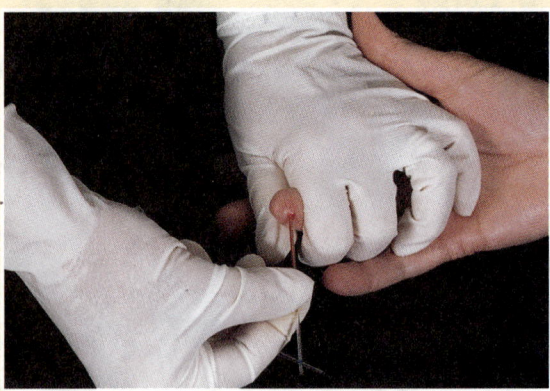

Step 10: Touch only the tip of the collection tube to the drop of blood.

Steps	Purpose
11. When collection is complete, apply pressure to the site with a clean gauze until bleeding stops. Label the containers with the proper information. Do not apply bandages to skin punctures of infants under 2 years of age. Never release a patient until the bleeding has stopped.	11. Proper labeling prevents a mix up of specimens. Younger children may develop a skin irritation from the adhesive bandage. Also, a young child might aspirate the bandage and choke.

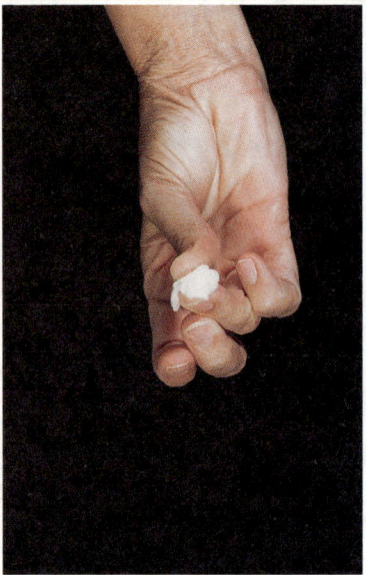

Step 11: Apply pressure with clean gauze.

(continued)

Procedure 45-2: Obtaining a Blood Specimen by Skin Puncture (continued)

Steps	Purpose
12. Thank the patient and give appropriate instructions.	12. Courtesy helps the patient have a positive attitude about the procedure and the physician's office.
13. Properly care for or dispose of equipment and supplies. Clean the work area. Remove gloves and wash your hands.	13. Standard Precautions must be followed throughout the procedure.
14. Test, transfer, or store the blood specimen according to the medical office policy.	
15. Record the procedure.	15. Procedures are considered not to have been done if they are not recorded.

should be drawn first to get an adequate volume of blood before the blood begins to clot. Any other additive specimens are collected next, and clotted specimens are collected last. If the blood has begun to produce microscopic clots while filling the last tube, this is not a problem because clotting is required in this tube.

 Checkpoint Question
6. How should you label the patient's blood sample?

Table 45-3
Sources of Error in Skin Puncture

1. Misidentification of patient
2. Puncturing wrong area of infant heel
3. Puncturing bone in infant heel
4. Puncturing fingers of infants
5. Puncturing wrong area of adult finger
6. Contaminating specimen with alcohol or Betadine
7. Failure to discard first blood drop
8. Excessive massaging of puncture site
9. Collecting air bubbles in pH or blood gas specimen
10. Hemolyzing specimen
11. Failure to seal specimens adequately
12. Failure to chill specimens requiring refrigeration
13. Erroneous specimen labeling
14. Failure to note skin puncture collection
15. Failure to warm site
16. Delaying specimen transport
17. Bruising site as a result of excessive squeezing

(From Bishop, M. L., ed. [1996] Clinical Chemistry, 3rd ed. Philadelphia: Lippincott-Raven Publishers.)

 ## SUMMARY

You must always have a professional attitude and be sympathetic to the fears and anxieties of the patient in all areas of patient care. For many patients, the process of venipuncture is particularly frightening. You will need to provide all of the compassion and understanding that you can to allay their fears. Your skill and knowledge, coupled with a caring approach, will ensure that the patient's experience in phlebotomy is not unpleasant.

The quality of the specimen's test result is only as good as the quality of the specimen obtained. Medical assistants are responsible for collecting specimens properly and testing them accurately. The office laboratory can provide a challenge and opportunity to work with the physician in improving and promoting the health of the patient.

 ## CRITICAL THINKING CHALLENGES

1. How will you help ease patient anxiety about venipuncture? Explain exactly what steps you will take.
2. Review Chapter 49, Pediatric Patients. How would you draw blood on a child? How would you help the child and the parent?
3. Your patient asks you how long you have been drawing blood and if you are "good." How would you respond? Justify your response.

 ## ANSWERS TO CHECKPOINT QUESTIONS

1. Capillary puncture may be required when small amounts of blood are needed, when the patient is under age 2, or when the veins either are inaccessible or must be preserved for parenteral therapy.

2. Disinfectants are used to kill bacteria on equipment and surfaces. Antiseptics are safe for people and are used to clean the skin before skin puncture or venipuncture.

3. Common additives include anticoagulants (prevent the blood from coagulating or clotting); clot activators (enhance coagulation); and thixotropic gel separator (forms a physical barrier between the cellular portion of a specimen and the serum or plasma portion after centrifugation).

4. When using the evacuated tube system, the proper order of draw is blood culture tubes, red or red/gray, light blue, green, lavender, gray. It is important to follow the correct order of draw to avoid contamination between additives.

5. Microcollection tubes are commonly used for hematocrit determinations.

6. You should label the blood sample with the patient's first and last names, an identification number, the date and time, and your initials to verify who drew the sample.

SUGGESTIONS FOR FURTHER READING

Bishop, M. L. (1996). *Clinical Chemistry*, 3rd ed. Philadelphia: Lippincott-Raven Publishers.

Marshall, J. (1993). *Fundamental Skills for the Clinical Laboratory Professional*. Albany, NY: Delmar Publishers.

McCall, R., & Tankersley, C. M. (1993). *Phlebotomy Essentials*. Philadelphia: J. B. Lippincott.

Hematology

Chapter Outline

Formation of Blood Cells
Hematologic Testing
Complete Blood Count
    White Blood Cell (WBC) Count and Differential
Procedure: Performing a Manual WBC Count
Procedure: Making a Peripheral Blood Smear
Procedure: Staining a Peripheral Blood Smear
Procedure: Performing a WBC Differential
    Red Blood Cell (RBC) Count
Procedure: Performing a RBC Count
    Hemoglobin
Procedure: Performing a Hemoglobin Determination
    Hematocrit

Procedure: Performing a Microhematocrit Determination
    Mean Cell Volume
    Mean Cell Hemoglobin and Mean Cell Hemoglobin Concentration
    Platelet Count
Erythrocyte Sedimentation Rate (ESR or SED Rate)
Procedure: Performing a Wintrobe ESR
Coagulation Tests
    Prothrombin Time
    Partial Thromboplastin Time
    Bleeding Time
Procedure: Determining Bleeding Time
Summary
Critical Thinking Challenges
Answers to Checkpoint Questions
Suggestions for Further Reading

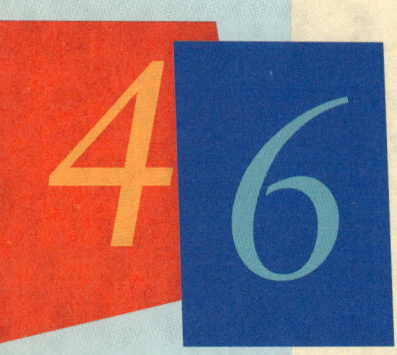

DACUM Components

1.3   Practice within the scope of education, training, and personal capabilities
4.1   Apply principles of aseptic technique and infection control
4.10 Collect and process specimens
4.11 Perform selected tests that assist with diagnosis and treatment
5.1   Document accurately
6.2   Operate and maintain facilities and equipment safely
7.3   Teach patients methods of health promotion and disease prevention

Chapter Competencies

Learning Objectives

Upon successfully completing this chapter, you will be able to:

1. Spell and define the Key Terms.
2. List the indices measured in the complete blood count and their normal ranges.
3. Explain the principle of automated cell counters.
4. State the conditions associated with abnormal complete blood count findings.
5. Explain the functions of the three types of blood cells.
6. Describe the purpose of performing an erythrocyte sedimentation rate.
7. List the leukocytes seen in the blood and their functions.
8. Explain the hemostatic mechanism of the body.
9. List and describe the tests that measure the body's ability to form a fibrin clot.
10. Explain the methodology used to determine the prothrombin time and partial thromboplastin time.

Performance Objectives

Upon successfully completing this chapter, you will be able to:

1. Perform a manual white blood cell count (Procedure 46-1).
2. Make a peripheral blood smear (Procedure 46-2).
3. Stain a peripheral blood smear (Procedure 46-3).
4. Perform a white blood cell differential (Procedure 46-4).
5. Perform a red blood cell count (Procedure 46-5).
6. Perform a hemoglobin determination (Procedure 46-6).
7. Perform a microhematocrit determination (Procedure 46-7).
8. Perform a Wintrobe erythrocyte sedimentation rate (Procedure 46-8).
9. Perform a Westergren erythrocyte sedimentation rate.
10. Determine a bleeding time (Procedure 46-9).

Key Terms

(See Glossary for definitions.)

agranulocytes
anisocytosis
Autolet
coumarin
elliptocytosis
enzyme
erythrocytes
erythropoietin
femtoliter
folate
granulocytes

hematocytometer
    (hemocytometer)
hematopoiesis
hemoglobin C disease
hemolytic anemia
heparin
hyperosmolarity
indices
intravascular
    coagulation
leukocytes

megaloblastic anemia
myelofibrosis
parameters
poikilocytosis
sickle cell anemia
spherocytosis
spicules
thalassemia
thrombocytes
thromboplastin
yolk sac

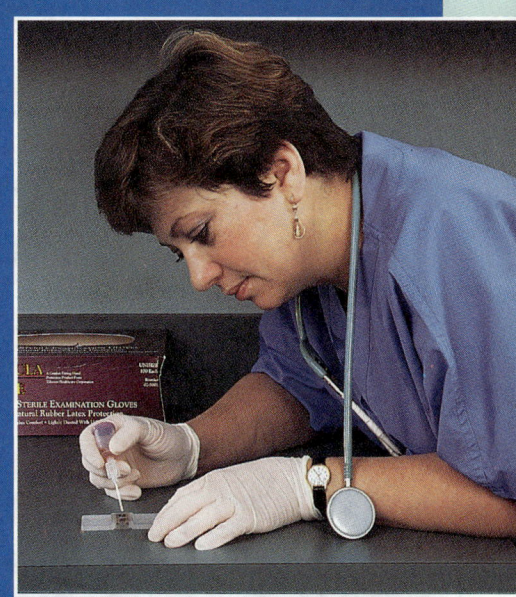

The hematology laboratory analyzes the blood cells, their quantities, and their characteristics for diagnosis and management of many conditions. Anemias, leukemias, and infections are some of the more common disorders detected by hematologic tests.

➤ FORMATION OF BLOOD CELLS

Blood is made up of two parts, including fluid (plasma) and three general types of cells called **erythrocytes** (red blood cells), **leukocytes** (white blood cells), and **thrombocytes** (platelets) (Fig. 46-1A through H).

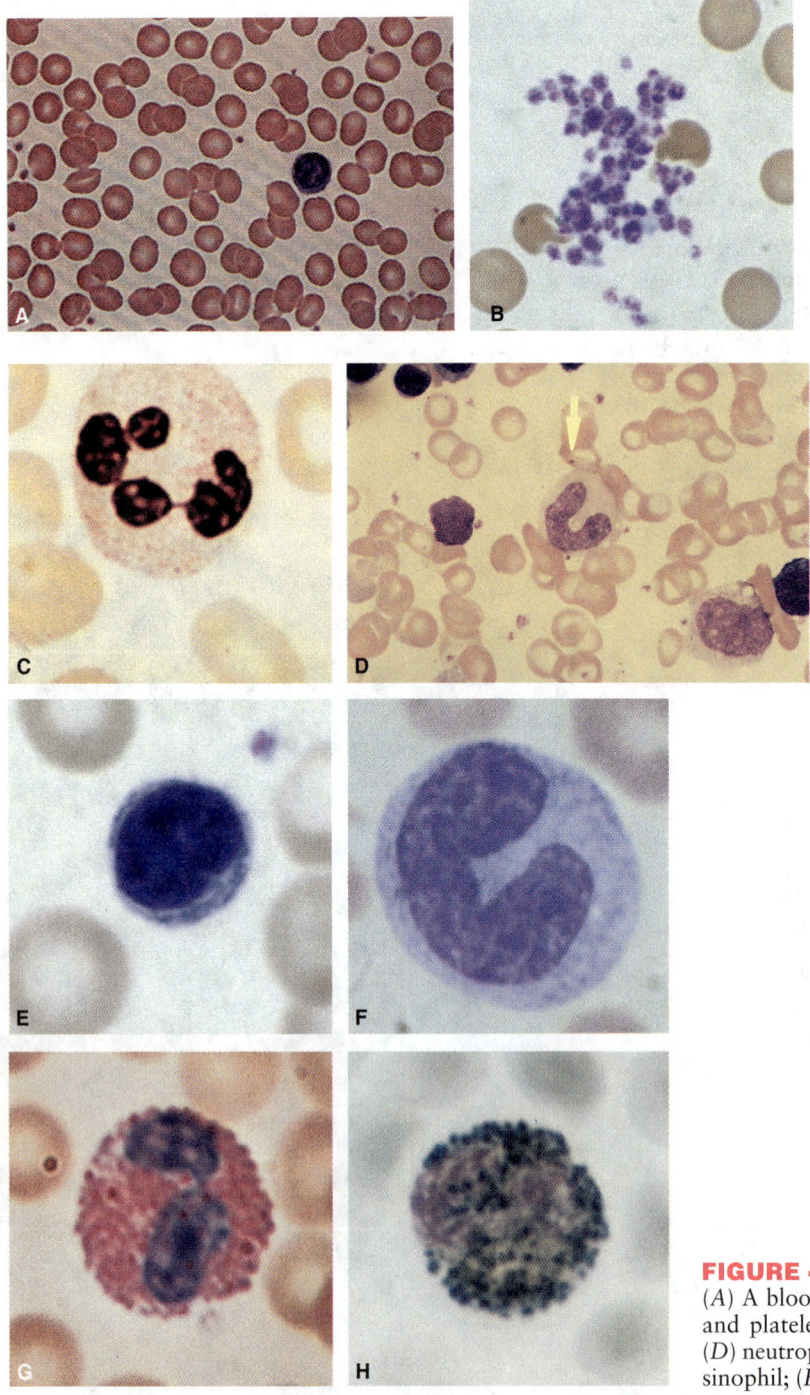

FIGURE 46-1

(A) A blood smear; (B) red blood cells (large, round cells) and platelets (stained purple); (C) segmented neutrophil; (D) neutrophil band; (E) lymphocyte; (F) monocyte; (G) eosinophil; (H) basophil.

Blood cells are formed in the bone marrow. The long bones, skull, pelvis, and sternum are the usual sites for the manufacture of these cells. Alternative sites include the liver and spleen. The **yolk sac** of the developing fetus also produces blood cells. (The yolk sac is the structure that nourishes the embryo until the seventh week, when the placenta takes over.)

Hematopoiesis (blood cell production) starts with very young, immature cells within the marrow that eventually divide and differentiate (acquire distinct or individual characteristics; to mature). These cells become erythrocytes, leukocytes, and thrombocytes according to the body's current needs. Each type of cell has a particular function that is discussed later in this chapter. Hematopoiesis is influenced by hormones and depends on adequate nutrients, such as iron, to produce functional cells. Once these cells have reached maturity, they are released from the bone marrow and travel into the bloodstream.

Checkpoint Question
1. What is hematopoiesis and how is it influenced?

➤ HEMATOLOGIC TESTING

In the hematology laboratory, blood testing is done to detect disease-producing conditions. Common hematologic tests include the complete blood count (CBC), erythrocyte sedimentation rate (ESR or Sed rate), and coagulation tests.

➤ COMPLETE BLOOD COUNT

The complete blood count (CBC) is one of the most frequently ordered tests in the laboratory. It consists of a number of **parameters** (characteristics that are measured), including:

- White blood cell (WBC) count and differential
- Red blood cell (RBC) count
- Hemoglobin (Hgb) determination
- Hematocrit (Hct) determination
- Mean cell volume (MCV)
- Mean corpuscular hemoglobin (MCH) and mean corpuscular hemoglobin concentration (MCHC)
- Platelet count

Most laboratories use the term CBC; a few, however, may use the term hemogram. Each of the blood cells (white, red, and platelets) can be counted using a counting chamber called a **hematocytometer** or a **hemocytometer** (Fig. 46-2). The dilution and diluting fluid used is different for each of the counts. Most lab-

oratories use automated cell counters to determine the CBC parameter values (Box 46-1).

White Blood Cell (WBC) Count and Differential

White blood cells (leukocytes) provide the main line of defense against foreign invaders such as bacteria and viruses. Some types circulate in the peripheral blood and others migrate into tissues and cavities to perform their functions. The normal range for a *white blood cell (WBC) count* is 4300 to 10,800/mm^3. Test results may depend on the method used for testing and normal references will vary in different regions and populations. A patient's WBC count can be determined by using the hematocytometer counting chamber (Procedure 46-1) or an automated cell counter.

Conditions with diminished numbers of leukocytes (leukopenia) can result from several factors, including:

- Chemical toxicity
- Nutritional deficiencies
- Chronic or overwhelming infections
- Certain malignancies

The patient may be vulnerable to infections when the leukopenia is pronounced. Leukocytosis (increased

BOX 46-1 Automated Blood Cell Counters

A number of biotechnology companies have instruments that can count and size the blood cells. Coulter and Technicon are two of these companies. Although each has its own specific method, the main operating principle is similar.

A portion of whole blood (anticoagulated with ethylenediaminetetraaectic acid [EDTA]) is taken in and diluted. These dilutions are moved into counting chambers where they are drawn through tiny holes (apertures). As the cells pass through the holes, either an electrical current, a light beam, or a laser beam is interrupted. The instrument registers the interruption as a cell. It can tell the size of the cell by the length of time the beam is interrupted.

These instruments have become so sophisticated that a white blood cell differential now can be reported accurately. Hemoglobin measurements are performed also. Other parameters such as mean corpuscular hemoglobin are calculated also, adding to the diagnostic value of the complete blood count.

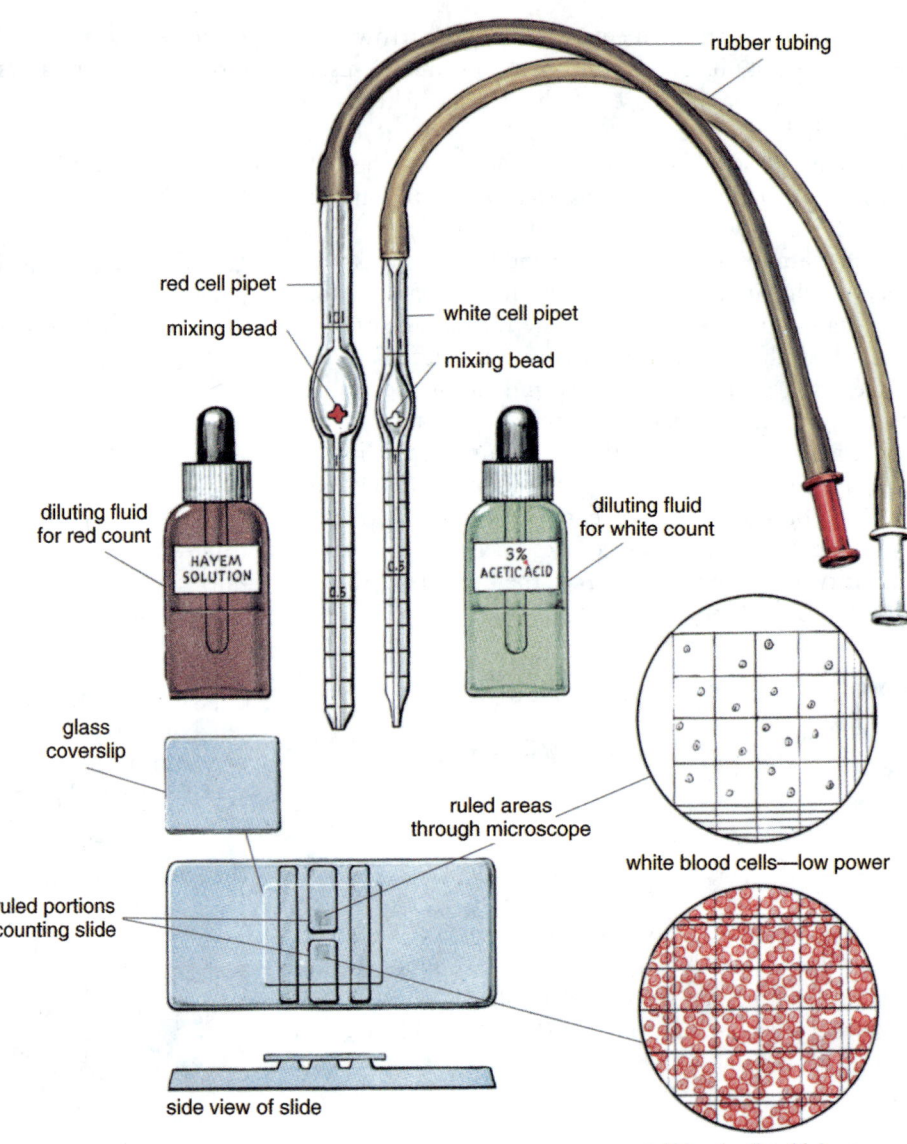

FIGURE 46-2
Equipment and supplies for manual cell counts.

amounts of WBCs) can stem from many sources, such as:

- Infections
- Inflammatory conditions
- Certain drugs
- Injuries to tissues
- Certain malignancies

The *WBC differential* is performed to determine the amounts of various WBC types present in the peripheral blood. These types include:

- Neutrophils (see Fig. 46-1*C* and *D*)
- Lymphocytes (see Fig. 46-1*E*)
- Monocytes (see Fig. 46-1*F*)
- Eosinophils (see Fig. 46-1*G*)
- Basophils (see Fig. 46-1*H*)

Because all of these types of leukocytes are colorless, a drop of blood is smeared on a glass slide and then stained so that they may be seen with a microscope. Once the peripheral blood is stained, 100 WBCs are counted, each tallied as to the type of cell seen, and then reported as percentages (Procedures 46-2, 46-3, and 46-4). These cell types are divided into two categories: the **granulocytes** (so called because of the granules in their cytoplasm that have distinctive staining characteristics) and the **agranulocytes** (meaning their cytoplasm does not contain visibly stained granules).

Checkpoint Question
2. *What is leukopenia and what are four conditions that may cause it?*

Neutrophils

Neutrophils—also called polymorphonuclear neutrophils, PMNs, polys, segmented neutrophils, or segs—are the most abundant leukocyte and are the main granulocyte. Following release from the bone marrow, they circulate in the blood for about 7 hours. They then move into the tissues, where they perform their function. Neutrophils function to defend against foreign invaders by phagocytizing them. The invaders are then destroyed inside the cells with digestive **enzymes** contained within the granules. (Enzymes are substances that speed reactions.) These digestive enzymes eventually cause the neutrophil to die because they are fatal to the cell as well as to all it ingests. The normal range for neutrophils is 50% to 70%; increased numbers are seen with bacterial infections.

When stained, the neutrophil has a light pink cytoplasm. This is due to the many small granules it contains. Its dark purple nucleus is segmented and the typical number of lobes can range from 2 to 5. A hyperseg is one that has more than five lobes or segments. This can indicate a chronic infection or **folate** deficiency. (Folate, a salt of folic acid, is an essential nutrient.) A band (or stab) is a younger, less mature version of the neutrophil. The band's appearance is the same as the more mature counterpart, but its nucleus is not segmented. The normal range for bands is 0% to 5%. Increased amounts of bands (left shift or bandemia) can be an indicator of various acute situations that need more immediate attention.

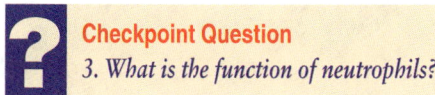

Checkpoint Question
3. What is the function of neutrophils?

Lymphocytes

Lymphocytes (lymphs) are the second most numerous WBC and the main agranulocyte. The main function of lymphocytes is to recognize that a particular cell or particle is foreign to the body and to make antibodies specific to its destruction. The antibodies then coat this foreign mass, resulting in one of two possible outcomes: the phagocytic system is activated to destroy the pathogen, or the complement system (a series of chemicals in the blood) is activated to destroy the cellular invaders by puncturing holes in their membranes. The normal range for lymphocytes is 20% to 35%. Increased numbers, especially atypical ones, can signal a viral infection. The life span of the lymphocyte is generally 3 to 4 days, which is longer than that of the neutrophil. However, some have much longer lives spanning into years or even decades.

In appearance, the lymphocyte is the smallest of the leukocytes. When stained, it has a small round dark purple nucleus. The surrounding cytoplasm is scant and sky blue. Atypical lymphs are larger with more cytoplasm that is either darker or lighter in color.

Monocytes

Monocytes (or monos) are the third most abundant leukocytes. They are agranulocytes. Like neutrophils, monocytes are capable of phagocytizing foreign material. They also aid the lymphocyte in providing the humoral response (destruction of foreign particles by antibodies). Monocytes stay in the bloodstream for about 3 days and then move into tissues.

The monocyte has a nucleus similar to the lymphocyte in that it is rounded and has no lobes. However, it is much larger than the lymph and closer in size to the neutrophil. When stained, the monocyte's cytoplasm is gray blue and has a ground-glass appearance. The normal range for monocytes is 3% to 8%. Monocytosis (increase in monos) is found in inflammatory responses and certain bacterial infections such as syphilis and tuberculosis. Monocytopenia may occur after administration of certain drugs or an overwhelming infection.

Eosinophils

Eosinophils (or eos) are fourth in abundance. Their function is not completely understood. The normal range for eosinophils is 0% to 6% to 7%. They will, however, increase in allergic reactions and some infections (especially parasitic). The eosinophil has a bilobed nucleus with large red granules in the cytoplasm.

Basophils

Basophils (or basos) are the least numerous, representing less than 1% of circulating WBCs. The nucleus is either bi- or trilobed and, on staining, very large dark blue-purple granules are seen in the cytoplasm, making them granulocytes. Basophils appear to be involved in allergic asthma, in contact allergies, and in hypothyroidism and chronic myeloid leukemia.

Checkpoint Question
4. Elevated eosinophils and basophils are both seen with what condition?

Red Blood Cell (RBC) Count

Red blood cells (erythrocytes) are designed to transport gases (mainly oxygen and carbon dioxide) between the lungs and the tissues. Their special structure as a biconcave disk containing hemoglobin enables them to readily exchange gases in the tissues and lung fields. As blood moves through the capillary bed of the lungs, RBCs release carbon dioxide that was picked up at the tissues and then binds oxygen. As the blood leaves the lungs and circulates to the periphery, oxygen is released from the RBCs into the tissues. At the same time, carbon dioxide (the by-product of metabolism) diffuses into the blood and is brought back to the lungs so that it can be removed from the body by exhalation.

Red blood cells are made in the bone marrow along with all other blood cells. Their production is influenced by the hormone **erythropoietin**, which is released mainly from the kidneys. When tissue hypoxia is detected, this hormone migrates to the marrow, which then steps up RBC production (erythropoiesis) and corrects the anemia by releasing more RBCs into the circulation. Other factors can also influence the quality and quantity of erythropoiesis. For example, vitamin B_{12} and folic acid are important substances for the cells to mature properly. Iron is needed for incorporation into the globin molecule to make functional hemoglobin. Initially, erythrocytes have a nucleus, but as they mature the nucleus is pushed out and the color of its cytoplasm changes from blue to red. The mature RBC is a pale red biconcave disk that can squeeze through very small capillaries. The average RBC lives about 120 days.

Measurements of RBCs and associated **indices** (hemoglobin, hematocrit, cell volume, and so on) provide a useful guide in detecting anemia, which can be caused by decreased erythrocyte production (as in iron deficiency), increased RBC destruction (as in hemolytic anemia), or blood loss. The normal range of RBCs for men is 4.6 to 6.2 million/mm³ (per cubic millimeter) and for women, 4.2 to 5.4 million/mm³ (Procedure 46-5).

When performing a differential on a peripheral blood smear, the laboratory technician also notices and comments on the variation in size (**anisocytosis**) and shape (**poikilocytosis**) of the RBCs. Findings such as target cells can indicate liver impairment. Table 46-1 describes some common erythrocyte abnormalities and their associated conditions.

Hemoglobin

Hemoglobin is the functioning unit of the red blood cell. Each hemoglobin molecule contains four protein chains called globins. There are different types of globin chains: A and B are the most common with some F (fetal) in newborns as well as abnormal hemoglobins such as S (sickle) found in persons having sickle cell disease or carrying the sickle trait. Located in the folds of each globin is a heme unit that contains one iron molecule each; the iron can reversibly bind gases such as oxygen and carbon dioxide. The iron also gives RBCs their distinctive red color. There are millions of hemoglobin molecules in each RBC. The normal range for hemoglobin is 13 to 18 g/dL (or g/1000 mL) for men and 12 to 16 g/dL for women. Anemia is detected with a hemoglobin measurement, which is a direct indicator of the body's ability to oxygenate itself (Procedure 46-6).

Hematocrit

The hematocrit is the percentage of red blood cells contained in whole blood. It is expressed as a percentage. For example, a hematocrit of 40% indicates that of the total blood volume, 40% of it consists of RBCs. The remaining 60% is plasma, which includes the WBCs and platelets.

To measure the hematocrit, the blood is centrifuged to pack the RBCs. The percentage is then read. Automated instruments do not measure the hematocrit but rather calculate the hematocrit from the RBC count and mean cell volume (MCV). The purpose for measuring the hematocrit is to detect anemia. The normal range is 45% to 52% for men and 37% to 48% for women (Procedure 46-7).

Patient Education: Iron Deficiency Anemia

Patients who have iron deficiency anemia should be educated regarding proper dietary management. They should be instructed to eat foods high in iron, such as liver, oysters, kidney beans, lean meats, turnips, egg yolks, whole wheat bread, carrots, raisins, and dark greens. Many vitamin supplements with iron are available and can be added to the diet. Patients should be alerted that iron supplements can cause constipation and dark stools.

Checkpoint Question

5. A patient has a hematocrit of 20%. What does this percentage represent?

Table 46-1
Erythrocyte Abnormalities

Abnormality	Associated Conditions
Hypochromasia—diminished hemoglobin in RBCs; appear paler with more area of central pallor	anemias (especially iron deficiency), **thalassemia** (a hemolytic anemia)
Hyperchromasia—increased hemoglobin in RBCs; appear to have less or no area of central pallor	**megaloblastic anemia** (characterized by large, dysfunctional RBCs) hereditary **spherocytosis** (condition in which nearly all the RBCs are spherocytes)
Polychromasia—some RBCs have a blue color	hemolysis, acute blood loss
Microcytosis—RBCs are smaller than usual	iron deficiency anemia, thalassemia
Macrocytosis—RBCs are larger than normal	B_{12} and folate deficiencies, megaloblastic anemias
Elliptocytes/ovalocytes—RBCs are distinctly oval in shape	hereditary **elliptocytosis**, iron deficiency anemia, **myelofibrosis** (disorder in which bone marrow tissue develops in abnormal sites), **sickle cell anemia** (hereditary anemia characterized by the presence of sickle-shaped RBCs)
Target cells—RBCs resemble a target with light and dark rings	liver impairment, anemias, (especially thalassemia), **hemoglobin C disease** (genetic blood disorder)
Schistocytes—RBCs are fragmented	hemolysis, burns, **intravascular coagulation** (clot formation within the vessels)
Spherocytes—RBCs show no area of central pallor	hereditary spherocytosis, hemolytic anemias, burns
Burr cells—RBCs have small, regular **spicules** (sharp points)	artifact as blood dries, **hyperosmolarity** (a condition of increased numbers of dissolved substances in the plasma)

Mean Cell Volume

Because red blood cells can vary in size, mean cell volume (MCV) measures the average size of red blood cells. For example, a patient with a MCV of 85 cubic micrometers or **femtoliters** (one quadrillionth of a liter) may have RBCs that range in size from 75 to 95, but the average would be 85. The MCV can be used as an indicator for anemias caused by the nutritional deficiencies that affect RBC production. The normal range for MCV is 80 to 95 cubic micrometers (or femtoliters).

Microcytosis (MCV < 80) is most commonly caused by iron deficiency. This finding coupled with RBC parameters (RBC count, hemoglobin, and hematocrit) will indicate anemia and lead to a diagnosis of iron deficiency anemia. Likewise, macrocytosis (MCV > 95) may be caused by a deficiency of B_{12} or folic acid. These abnormalities can also result in anemia. Liver disorders may sometimes give increased MCVs.

Mean Cell Hemoglobin and Mean Cell Hemoglobin Concentration

As technology becomes increasingly sophisticated, more measurable parameters are added to the complete blood count. Among the most useful are mean corpuscular hemoglobin (MCH) and mean corpuscular hemoglobin concentration (MCHC). MCH and MCHC indicate relative hemoglobin concentration in the blood; when anemia is present, both measurements

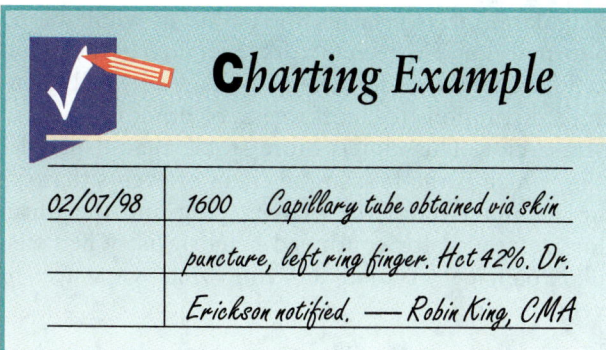

Charting Example

02/07/98	1600	Capillary tube obtained via skin puncture, left ring finger. Hct 42%. Dr. Erickson notified. — Robin King, CMA

Charting Example

05/15/98	1400 Venipuncture to left antecubitus. Hematology results as follows:
	WBC—4880
	WBC diff—neutrophils—60%
	lymphocytes—25%
	monocytes—5%
	eosinophils—8%
	basophils—2%
	RBC—4.6
	Hgb—17
	Hct—50%
	MCV—88
	Platelets—250,000
	ESR—16
	PT—18
	PTT—45
	————Erik Williams, RMA

---

will be decreased. Other conditions may be indicated by these measurements as well.

Both the MCH and MCHC are calculated. The MCH is derived from the ratio of hemoglobin and the number of RBCs present in the specimen. The MCHC is derived from the ratio of hemoglobin and hematocrit.

Platelet Count

Platelets (thrombocytes), like other blood cells, are made in the bone marrow. However, they are not actually cells but cell fragments that adhere to damaged endothelium. Platelets are essential to hemostasis because they not only aid in sealing wounds until a clot can form, but they also help initiate the clotting factors to form the more stable fibrin clot.

The normal range for platelets is 200,000 to 400,000/mm^3. Thrombocytopenia (decreased plate-

lets) can be caused by a variety of conditions and is the most common cause of bleeding disorders. The bleeding usually occurs from many small capillaries. Treatment requires a specific diagnosis of the cause of the thrombocytopenia. Administration of drugs is usually stopped because almost any drug can cause its onset. Thrombocytosis (increased platelets) is typically benign. It can be seen after splenectomies or during inflammatory diseases.

In appearance, platelets are much smaller than RBCs. They stain a light purplish blue, have an irregular shape, and contain no nucleus.

➤ ERYTHROCYTE SEDIMENTATION RATE (ESR OR SED RATE)

The ESR measures the rate at which RBCs settle out in a tube. Anticoagulated blood is placed into a calibrated glass column and then allowed to settle undisturbed for 1 hour. At the end of the hour the distance the RBCs have fallen is measured. This is expressed in millimeters per hour (mm/h). Although there are several different methods for performing the ESR, such as the Wintrobe and the Westergren methods, the principle remains the same. Procedure 46-8 describes the steps for performing a Wintrobe ESR. Figure 46-3 outlines the steps for using the Westergren method.

The normal range for men is 0 to 10 mm/h and for women, 0 to 20 mm/h. Elevations in ESR values are not specific for any disorder; however, they do indicate the presence of either inflammation or any other condition that causes increased or altered proteins in the blood (eg, rheumatoid arthritis). The more rapidly the RBCs fall in the column, the greater the degree of inflammation. Physicians use this as a guideline when monitoring the course of inflammation in rheumatoid arthritis. ESRs can also be elevated with infections and pregnancy.

➤ COAGULATION TESTS

Coagulation tests measure the ability of whole blood to form a clot. Thirteen factors (proteins) in the blood act in sequential order when stimulated by cell membrane disruptions (eg, cuts, tears, or other injuries) to form a clot. This clot is more stable than a platelet plug, which is the first in the chain of events that occur on injury. Both the platelet plug and the fibrin clot are needed for continued hemostasis. When vascular damage occurs, the following sequence of events occurs:

1. *Vasoconstriction.* The vein constricts to reduce blood loss.

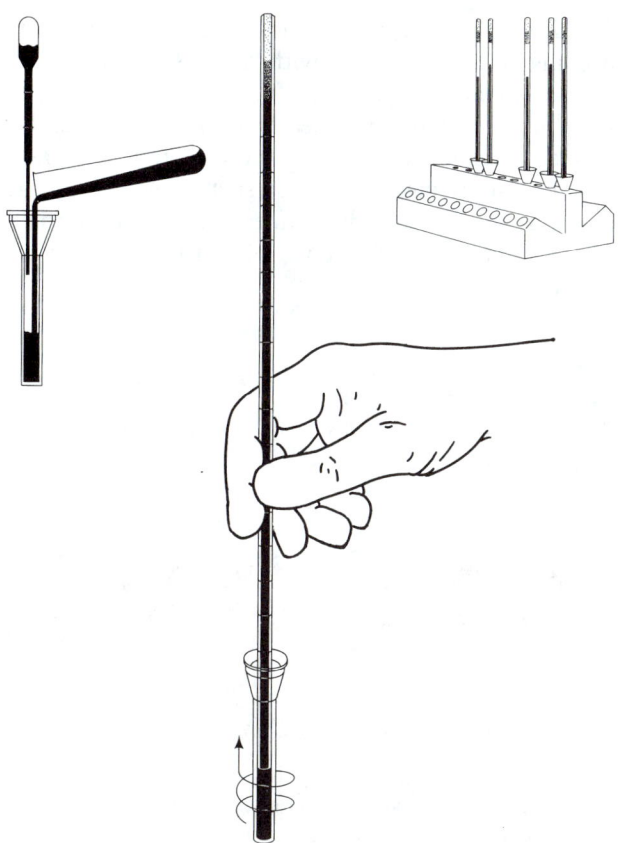

FIGURE 46-3
Westergren Dispette System for erythrocyte sedimentation rate (ESR) determination. (*Left*) After mixing four parts EDTA-anticoagulated whole blood with one part 0.85% saline, mixture is poured into a vial. (*Center*) Dispette is placed in vial using a twisting motion until blood reaches bottom of safety autozeroing plug. (*Right*) Vial and Dispette are placed vertically in a special rack for 60 minutes before reading the ESR. (Courtesy of Ulster Scientific, Inc., Highland, NY)

2. *Platelet plug formation*. The platelets adhere to the wound and form a plug, temporarily slowing the blood flow.
3. *Fibrin clot formation*. When activated, the clotting factors form an insoluble clot at the wound site. (The two most common tests for determining how well a fibrin clot can form are prothrombin time and partial thromboplastin time; see below).
4. *Clot lysis and vascular repair*. Another set of proteins slowly dissolve the fibrin clot as the surrounding endothelial tissue of the blood vessel wall replicates to repair the damage.

Prothrombin Time

The prothrombin time (PT) is a one-stage test in which calcium and **thromboplastin** (a complex substance that starts the clotting process) are added to the patient's plasma. The clotting time is then observed. The normal range is 12 to 15 seconds, but each laboratory establishes its own range. A patient's PT may be prolonged when a deficiency of certain factors exists, such as liver disease or vitamin K deficiency, or as a result of coumarin (anticoagulant) therapy. Current restrictions are in place that do not allow medical assistants to perform the PT test.

What If?
What if your patient is receiving Coumadin (the brand name for coumarin) and does not return for scheduled prothrombin tests? What should you do?

Let the physician know. The physician will determine if a refill prescription for Coumadin will be called in to the pharmacy. Document all phone conversations with the patient, including the date, time, and message given. Also document the patient's responses, using quotes whenever possible. The patient should be educated regarding the dangers of self-medicating Coumadin, such as excessive bleeding with overdose or clotting with underdose. Make sure the patient understands the purpose of the medication and why blood tests are so important. Determine why the patient is refusing to come in for blood work; the reason may be as simple as transportation. Many communities have visiting nurse associations or hospital outreach programs that have staff members who will draw blood for patients in the home.

Partial Thromboplastin Time

The partial thromboplastin time (PTT) is a two-stage test in which partially activated thromboplastin is incubated with the patient's plasma followed by the addition of calcium. The clotting time is then determined. The normal range is 32 to 51 seconds but, again, each laboratory establishes its own range so there may be a slight variation. A PTT may be prolonged in certain factor deficiencies, especially those that cause hemophilia. Heparin (anticoagulant) therapy also will prolong the PTT, so this test is used for monitoring and determining dosages.

Bleeding Time

The bleeding time test is performed to determine the time required for blood to stop flowing from a very small wound. An incision is made on the inside of the forearm with an automated cutting device, such as an

Charting Example

09/15/98	1500	*Bleeding time test done—*
		results 14 minutes. Physician notified.
		—Sam Goldstein, CMA

Autolet, to a depth of 1 mm. Normal bleeding times range from 2 to 6 minutes (Procedure 46-9).

Although it is a rather nonspecific test, prolonged bleeding times can occur with decreased platelets or impaired platelet function. Ingestion of aspirin or other anti-inflammatory medications can also inhibit platelet function. A prolonged bleeding time may indicate the use of medications or such disease states as uremic syndrome. Bleeding times are often performed before surgeries to detect various bleeding problems that can develop.

? Checkpoint Question

6. What are the two most common tests used to determine how well a fibrin clot will form?

Procedure 46-1

Performing a Manual WBC Count

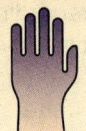

Equipment/Supplies

- white blood cell pipette
- pipette bulb
- diluting fluid (2–3% acetic acid, which lyses red blood cells but not white blood cells)
- hemacytometer
- coverglass
- alcohol
- appropriate biohazard barrier devices (eg, gloves, impervious gown, face shield)

Steps	**Purpose**
1. Wash your hands.	1. Handwashing aids infection control.
2. Assemble the equipment.	2. This ensures that all supplies are available.
3. Greet and identify the patient. Explain the procedure. Ask for and answer any questions.	3. Identifying the patient prevents errors in treatment. Explaining the procedure helps ease anxiety and ensure compliance.
4. Put on gloves, impervious gown, and face shield.	4. Standard Precautions must be observed when handling blood and body fluids.
5. Obtain an EDTA (purple-top tube) blood specimen from the patient following the steps described in Chap. 45, Phlebotomy.	
6. Thoroughly mix the whole blood by inverting at least 60 times before proceeding.	6. Blood tends to separate on standing; not mixing well can cause the count to be inaccurate.
7. Attach pipette bulb to the pipette. Remove the stopper on the patient's blood tube. Place the tip of the pipette just below the surface of the blood. Quickly draw the blood up to the 0.5 mark.	7. If the pipette is placed too far into the blood, the markings will be obscured.

(continued)

Performing a Manual WBC Count *(continued)*

Steps	Purpose

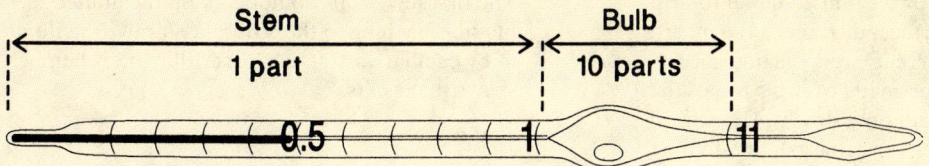

Step 7: Thoma WBC pipette used to dilute specimens for cell counts.

8. Wipe off the pipette with gauze, being careful not to draw it across the tip.

9. Immediately place the pipette into the diluting fluid and draw the fluid up to the 11.0 mark, rotating as this is done.

10. Place the thumb and middle finger on either end of the pipette and shake for 30 seconds. Alternative method: Secure on an automatic shaker and turn on the machine.

11. Place the coverglass over the ruled area of the hemacytometer. Shake the pipette for 2 to 3 minutes. This is not necessary if it was already on the shaker.

8. The gauze will absorb some of the plasma if it comes in contact with the blood.

9. This will give a 1:20 dilution of the blood. This diluting fluid lyses red cells making it easier to count white cells.

10. Shaking facilitates mixing the blood and the diluent.

11. The coverglass provides a site for the fluid. Shaking thoroughly mixes the specimen.

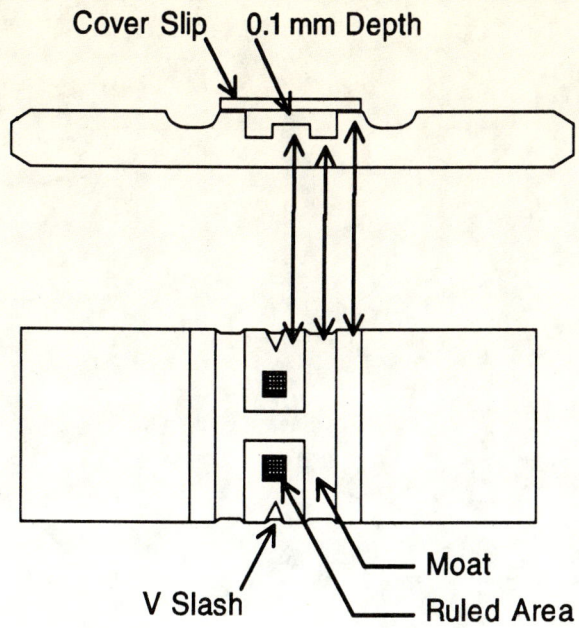

Step 11: The Neubauer hemocytometer.

(continued)

Steps

Purpose

12. Allow several drops of the diluted blood to drip out onto a piece of gauze, then touch the pipette to the coverglass where it meets the floorpiece, keeping the forefinger gently over the top of the pipette so the fluid will flow slowly. Allow the chamber to fill completely (charge), but do not overflow. Repeat this step to charge the other side of the hemacytometer.

13. Allow the cells to settle for several minutes. Remove the face shield.

14. Place the hematocytometer on the microscope stage so that the ruled area can be surveyed with the low-power objective. Focus.

15. Count the areas indicated in the illustration, making sure it is the white cell and not the red cell area of the grid. Include in the count those cells touching the lower and right hand area but not the upper or left.

12. The first few drops do not contain the diluted blood. Touching to the coverglass draws the fluid in by capillary attraction. Overfilling the chamber skews the results.

13. The cells will all settle into the same plane for counting. It would be difficult to use the microscope wearing the face shield.

14. This prepares the hematocytometer for counting.

15. This eliminates confusion and over counting.

(continued)

Steps   **Purpose**

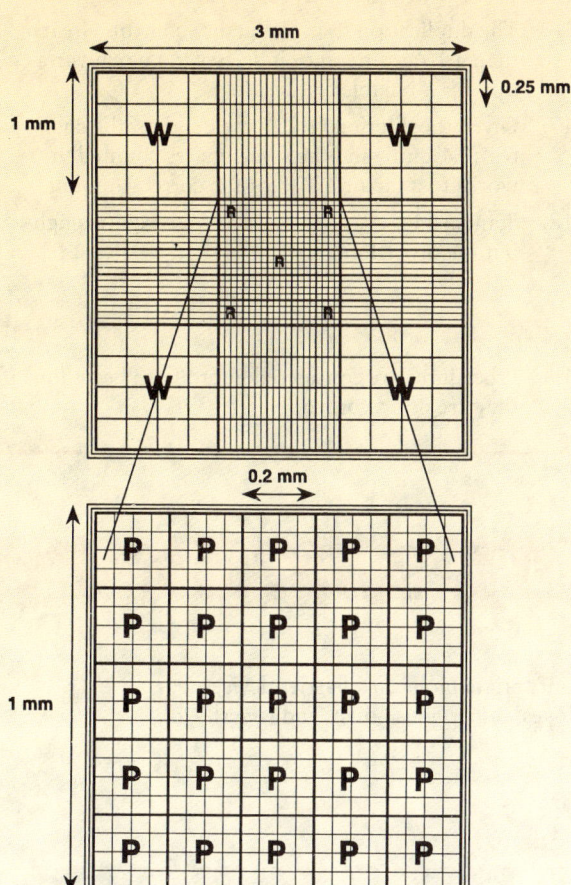

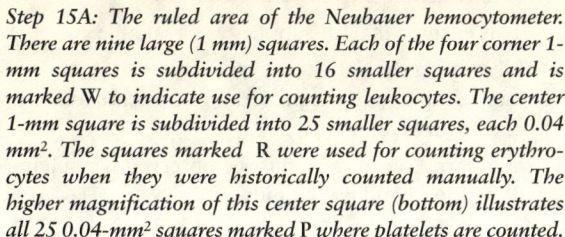

Step 15A: The ruled area of the Neubauer hemocytometer. There are nine large (1 mm) squares. Each of the four corner 1-mm squares is subdivided into 16 smaller squares and is marked W to indicate use for counting leukocytes. The center 1-mm square is subdivided into 25 smaller squares, each 0.04 mm^2. The squares marked R were used for counting erythrocytes when they were historically counted manually. The higher magnification of this center square (bottom) illustrates all 25 0.04-mm^2 squares marked P where platelets are counted.

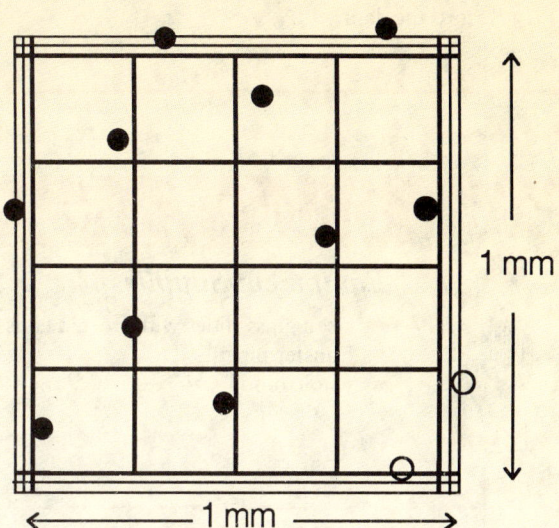

Step 15B: Rules for microscopic counting of leukocytes on the Neubauer hemocytometer. One square millimeter is illustrated. Leukocytes are counted in eight of these 1-mm squares, four on each side of the hemocytometer. Leukocytes that touch the top or left triple boundary lines are counted; those that touch the bottom or right boundaries are not. (Solid circle, cells counted; open circle, cells not counted.)

Procedure 46-1   ## Performing a Manual WBC Count (continued)

Steps	Purpose
16. Count the same area on the opposite side of the hematocytometer. Take the average of the two results if they match within 10% of each other.	16. The duplication tests for quality control. Greater than a 10% difference indicates too much variation for a reliable test result.
17. Multiply this number by 50 for the result.	17. Given the dilution (1:20), the depth of the chamber (0.1 mm), and the four squares counted, it works to a factor of 50 for the correct amount.
18. Clean the hematocytometer and coverglass with 10% bleach solution and wipe dry with lens paper. Place pipette in cleaning solution or discard if disposable. Clean the work area. Remove gloves, gown, and face shield and wash your hands.	18. Standard Precautions must be followed throughout the procedure.
19. Record the data.	19. Procedures are considered not to have been done if they are not recorded.

Procedure 46-2   ## Making a Peripheral Blood Smear

Equipment/Supplies

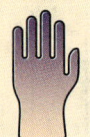

- clean glass slides with frosted ends
- transfer pipette
- whole blood
- appropriate biohazard barrier devices (eg, gloves, impervious gown, and face shield)

Steps	Purpose
1. Wash your hands.	1. Handwashing aids infection control.
2. Assemble the equipment.	2. This ensures that all supplies are available.
3. Greet and identify the patient. Explain the procedure. Ask for and answer any questions.	3. Identifying the patient prevents errors in treatment. Explaining the procedure helps ease anxiety and ensure compliance.
4. Put on gloves, impervious gown, and face shield.	4. Standard Precautions must be observed when handling blood and body fluids.
5. Obtain an EDTA (purple-top tube) blood specimen from the patient, following the steps described in Chap. 45, Phlebotomy.	
6. Label the slide on the frosted area.	6. The slide must be labeled with the patient's name or identification number; the frosted end will retain the markings.

(continued)

Steps   **Purpose**

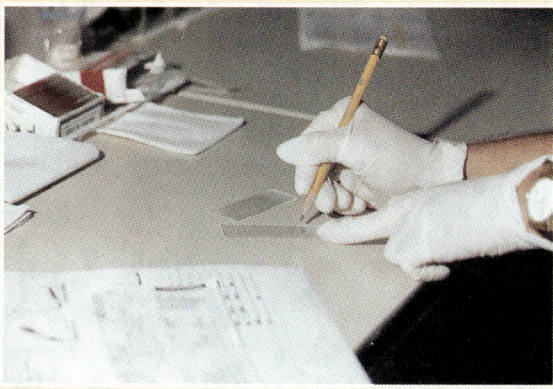

Step 6: Label the frosted end of the slide with the patient's name.

7. Place a drop of blood 1 cm from the frosted end of the slide.

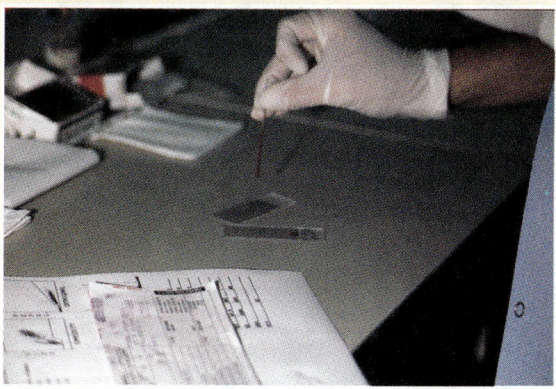

Step 7: Place one drop of blood on the slide.

8. Place slide on flat surface and with the thumb and forefinger of the right hand hold second (spreader) slide against the surface of the first at a 30 degree angle and draw it back against the drop of blood until contact is established. Allow the blood to spread out under the edge and then push the spreader slide at a moderate speed toward the other end of the slide keeping contact between the two slides at all times. Allow the slide to air dry. See the figures for examples of properly and improperly prepared smears.

8. A flat surface allows for smooth movements. A 30° angle allows the blood to be spread out in a thin film for viewing.

(continued)

Procedure 46-2	Making a Peripheral Blood Smear (continued)

Steps	**Purpose**

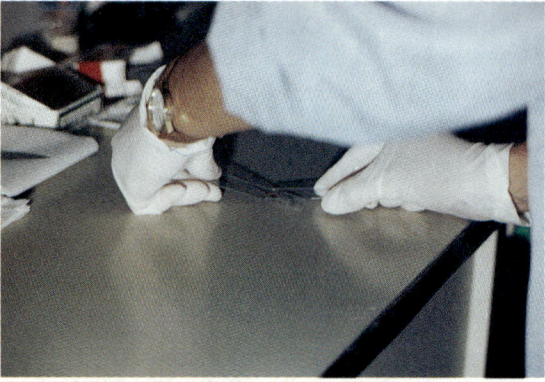

Step 8A: Spread the blood in a thin film across the slide.

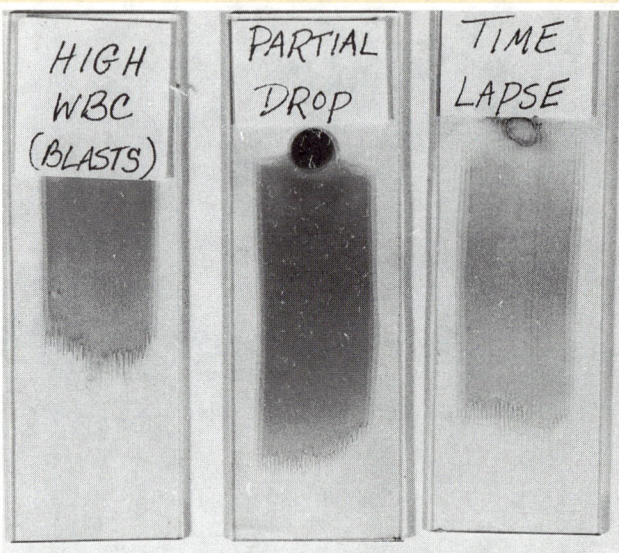

Step 8C: Improperly prepared smears will yield slides that are difficult to read. Slides B and C should be discarded and new slides prepared properly.

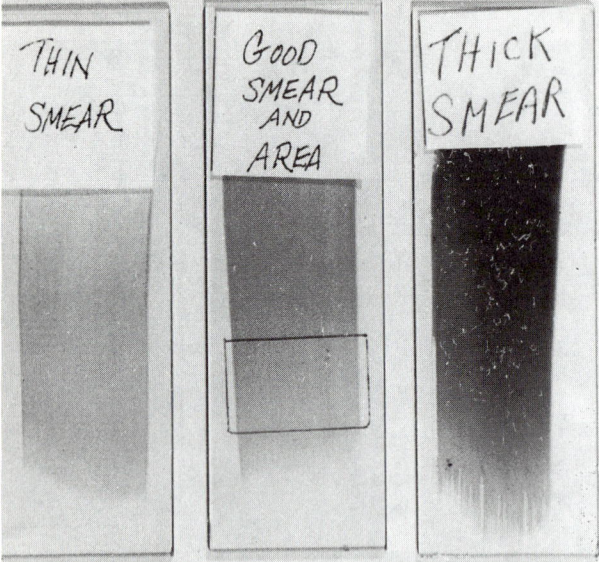

Step 8B: A properly prepared smear will yield a slide that is easy to read.

9. Properly care for or dispose of equipment and supplies. Clean the work area. Remove gloves, gown, and face shield and wash your hands.

10. Record the procedure.

9. Standard Precautions must be followed throughout the procedure.

10. Procedures are considered not to have been done if they are not recorded.

Staining a Peripheral Blood Smear

Procedure 46-3

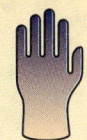

Equipment/Supplies

- staining rack
- Wright's stain
- Giemsa stain
- tweezers
- appropriate biohazard barrier devices (eg, gloves, impervious gown, face shield)

Steps	**Purpose**
1. Wash your hands.	1. Handwashing aids infection control.
2. Assemble the equipment.	2. This ensures that all supplies are available.
3. Put on gloves, impervious gown, and face shield.	3. Standard Precautions must be observed when handling blood and body fluids.
4. Obtain a recently made, dried blood smear.	4. A smear that is more than 2 hours old may deteriorate.
5. Place the slide on a stain rack blood side up.	5. This is where the staining will be done.
6. Flood the slide with Wright's stain. Allow the stain to remain on slide for 3–5 minutes or for the time specified by the manufacturer.	6. Wright's stain contains alcohol to fix blood to the slide as well as to stain the blood cells according to their characteristics.
7. Using tweezers, tilt the slide so that the stain drains off. Apply equal amounts of Giemsa stain and water. A green sheen will appear on the surface. Allow to stain for 5 minutes or the time specified by the manufacturer.	7. This buffers the Wright's stain and provides some added staining.
8. Holding the slide with tweezers, gently rinse the slide off with water. Wipe off the back of the slide with gauze. Stand the slide upright and allow it to dry.	8. This rinses and removes the excess stain for viewing under a microscope.
9. Properly care for or dispose of equipment and supplies. Clean the work area. Remove gloves, gown, and face shield and wash your hands.	9. Standard Precautions must be followed throughout the procedure.

Note: *Some manufacturers provide a simple one-step method that consists of dipping the smear in a staining solution, then rinsing. Directions are provided by the manufacturer for this procedure and will vary with the specific test.*

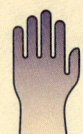

Procedure 46-4

Performing a WBC Differential

Equipment/Supplies

- stained peripheral blood smear
- microscope
- immersion oil
- paper
- recording tabulator
- gloves

Steps	**Purpose**
1. Wash your hands.	1. Handwashing aids infection control.
2. Assemble the equipment.	2. This ensures that all supplies are available.
3. Put on gloves.	3. Standard Precautions must be observed when handling blood and body fluids.
4. Place the stained slide on the microscope stage. Focus on the feathered edge of the smear and scan to ensure an even distribution of cells and proper staining. (See the figure showing a properly prepared smear in Procedure 46-2, Step 8.) Use the low-power objective.	4. Stage mounting sets up the slide to be read. Scanning the slide is a quality control assurance of staining performance.
5. Place a drop of oil on the slide and rotate the oil immersion lens into place. Focus and begin to identify any leukocytes present.	5. Oil is always used with the oil immersion lens. The oil immersion lens allows the greatest magnification and provides a path for the light source.
6. Record on a tally sheet or tabulator the types of white cells found.	6. Tallying the types seen is necessary to record the percentages.
7. Move the stage so that the next field is in view. Identify any white cells in this field and continue to the next field to identify all that are present until 100 white cells have been counted.	7. Many fields must be viewed before 100 cells have been counted. The systematic movement of the stage so that another field comes into view ensures that this is accomplished correctly.
8. Calculate the number of each type of leukocyte as a percentage.	8. Since 100 cells are counted, each represents one percentage point.
9. Properly care for or dispose of equipment and supplies properly. Clean the work area. Remove gloves and wash your hands.	9. Standard Precautions must be followed throughout the procedure.
10. Record the data.	10. Procedures are considered not to have been done if they are not recorded.

Note: *A WBC differential is performed by a trained laboratory technologist. Abnormal cells can appear in the peripheral blood; recognizing them is an important diagnostic procedure that requires specific training.*

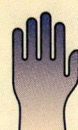

Procedure 46-5

Performing a RBC Count

Equipment/Supplies

- hemacytometer
- cover glass
- diluting pipette for red blood cells
- diluting fluid (0.85% saline or Gower's solution)
- pipette bulb

- alcohol
- microscope
- appropriate biohazard barrier devices (eg, gloves, impervious gown, and face shield)

Steps	Purpose

1–8. Follow steps 1–8 for Procedure 46-1, Performing a Manual WBC Count, but using an RBC pipette.

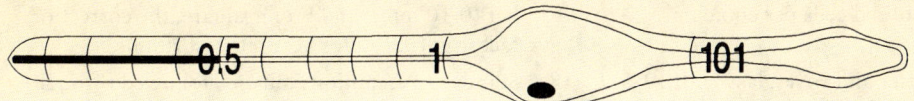

Step 9: Draw the fluid into the RBC pipette up to the 101 mark.

9. Immediately place the pipette into the diluting fluid and draw the fluid into the pipette up to the 101 mark, rotating as the pipette fills.

9. This step must begin immediately so that the blood does not begin to dry in the tip. This will give a 1:200 dilution of the blood.

10. Place thumb and middle finger on either end of the pipette and shake for 30 seconds. Alternative method: Use an automatic shaker.

10. This facilitates mixing the blood with the diluent.

11. Place the coverglass over the ruled area of the hemacytometer. Shake the pipette for 2–3 minutes. This is not necessary if it is already on the shaker.

11. The coverglass provides the area for the fluid for testing. Shaking thoroughly mixes the specimen.

12. Allow several drops of the diluted blood to drip out onto a piece of gauze and then touch the pipette to the coverglass edge where it meets the floor piece (see Fig. 46-1) keeping the forefinger gently over the top of the pipette so the fluid will flow slowly. Allow the chamber to fill (charge) completely, but do not overflow.

12. The first few drops do not contain the diluted blood. Touching the coverglass draws the fluid into the hemacytometer chamber by capillary attraction. This ensures the proper amount of fluid fills the space. Overfilling will skew the results.

13. Allow the cells to settle for several minutes. Remove the face shield.

13. The cells will settle onto the same plane for counting. The face shield must be removed to use the microscope effectively.

14. Place the hemacytometer on the microscope stage so that the ruled area can be surveyed with the low-power objective. Focus.

14. The hemacytometer is in position for counting.

(continued)

Procedure 46-5

Performing a RBC Count (continued)

Steps	Purpose
15. Count the areas indicated in the illustration (see Procedure 46-1). Ignore any cells touching the upper and left-hand side but do count those on the lower and right-hand side.	15. This eliminates confusions and over- or under-counting.
16. Count the same area on the opposite side of the hemacytometer. Take the average of the two counts if they match within 10% of each other.	16. Duplicating the test ensures quality control. Greater than 10% difference indicates too much variation for reliable test results.
17. Multiply this number by 10,000. The answer is reported as the number of red cells per cubic millimeter (/mm³).	17. Given the dilution (1:200), the depth of the chamber (0.10 mm), and ⅕ of a square, the correction factor is 10,000 for accurate test results.
18. Clean the hemacytometer and coverglass with 10% bleach and wipe dry with lens paper. Place the pipette in cleaning solution or discard if disposable. Dispose of or care for any other equipment and supplies appropriately. Clean the work area. Remove gloves and gown and wash your hands.	18. Standard Precautions must be followed throughout the procedure.
19. Record the data.	19. Procedures are considered not to have been done if they are not recorded.

Procedure 46-6

Performing a Hemoglobin Determination

Equipment/Supplies

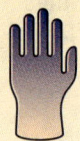

- hemoglobinometer
- applicator sticks
- whole blood
- appropriate biohazard barrier devices (eg, gloves, impervious gown, face shield)

Steps	Purpose
1. Wash your hands.	1. Handwashing aids infection control.
2. Assemble the necessary equipment.	2. This ensures that all supplies are available.
3. Put on gloves, gown, and face shield.	3. Standard Precautions must be observed when handling blood and body fluids.
4. Obtain an EDTA (purple-top tube) blood specimen from the patient, following the steps described in Chap. 45, Phlebotomy.	
5. Place a drop of well mixed whole blood (obtained by venipuncture or skin puncture) on the glass chamber of the hemoglobinometer. Place the coverslip into the holding clip over the chamber and slide into the holding clip.	5. This prepares the sample for the hemoglobin determination.

(continued)

Procedure 46-6 Performing a Hemoglobin Determination *(continued)*

Steps	Purpose
6. At one of the open edges, push the applicator stick into the chamber. Gently move the stick around until the specimen no longer appears cloudy.	6. This lyses the red cells, thereby releasing the hemoglobin.
7. Slide the chamber into the hemoglobinometer. Remove the face shield.	7. The chamber must be inserted into the receiving slot to perform the color comparison reading.
8. With your left hand, hold the meter and press the light button. View the field through the eyepiece. With your right hand, move the dial until both the right and left sides match each other in color intensity. Note the hemoglobin level indicated on the dial.	8. The chamber must be illuminated to compare the colors. Matching fields indicate that the amount of hemoglobin in the sample matches the internal standard.
9. Clean the chamber and work area with 10% bleach solution. Dispose of equipment and supplies appropriately. Remove gloves and gown and wash your hands.	
10. Record the data.	10. Procedures are considered not to have been done if they are not recorded.

Note: *Regarding quality assurance, calibration chambers are included in the hemoglobinometer kit and are used to verify proper functioning of the meter. This procedure may vary according to the instrument used. Some manufacturers offer a digitally read hemoglobin device that is less subjective and is therefore considered more accurate and easier to use.*

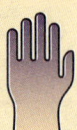

Procedure 46-7   Performing a Microhematocrit Determination

Equipment/Supplies

- microcollection tubes
- sealing clay
- microhematocrit centrifuge
- microhematocrit reading device
- appropriate biohazard barrier devices (eg, gloves, impervious gown, and face shield)

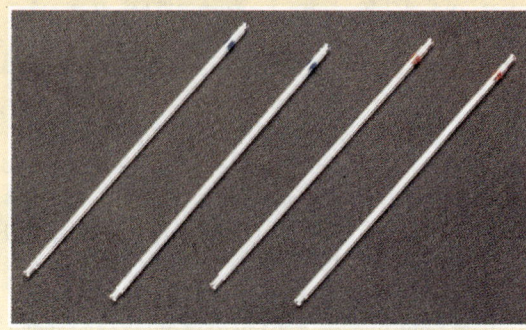

Microcollection tubes

Steps	**Purpose**
1. Wash your hands.	1. Handwashing aids infection control.
2. Assemble the equipment.	2. This ensures that all supplies are available.
3. Put on gloves, gown, and face shield.	3. Standard Precautions must be observed when handling blood and body fluids.
4. Draw blood into the capillary tube by one of two methods: (1) directly from a capillary puncture where the tip of the capillary tube is touched to the blood at the wound and allowed to fill ¾ of the tube or to the indicated mark (see Chap. 45, Phlebotomy); or (2) from a well mixed anticoagulated (EDTA) tube of whole blood where, again, the tip is touched to the blood and allowed to fill ¾ of the tube. Place the forefinger over the top of the tube, wipe excess blood off the sides, and push the bottom into the sealing clay. Draw a second specimen in the same manner.	4. Whole blood from a capillary puncture has not clotted yet and is acceptable. If blood from a tube is not well mixed, the reading is likely to be inaccurate. Holding the finger over the tip stops blood from dripping out the bottom. The clay seals one end of the tube to contain it during centrifugation. A second tube is necessary for duplicate testing as a quality control measure.
5. Place the tubes in the radial grooves of the microhematocrit centrifuge opposite each other. Place the cover on top of the grooved area and tighten by turning the knob clockwise. Close the lid. Spin for 5 minutes.	5. Specimens should always be placed opposite each other to balance the centrifuge. Read the manufacturer's directions for the specific centrifuge used in this facility; 5 minutes is a normal time limit.
6. Remove the tubes from the centrifuge and read the results from the reading device available (instructions are printed on the device). (The accompanying figure shows two methods for determining microhematocrit values.) Results should match within 5% of each other. Take the average and report as a percentage. (*Note*: Some microhematocrit centrifuges have the scale printed within the machine at the radial grooves.)	6. Results greater than 5% variability have been found to offer unreliable results.

(continued)

Steps	Purpose

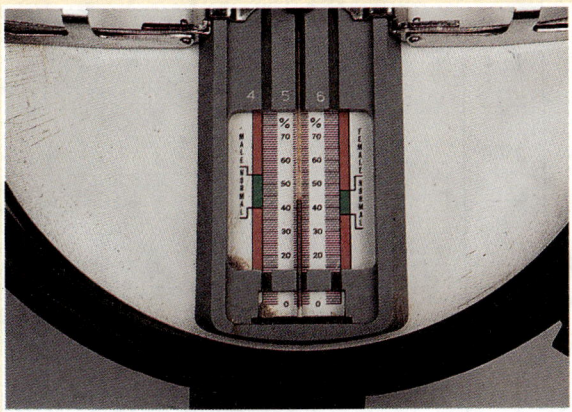

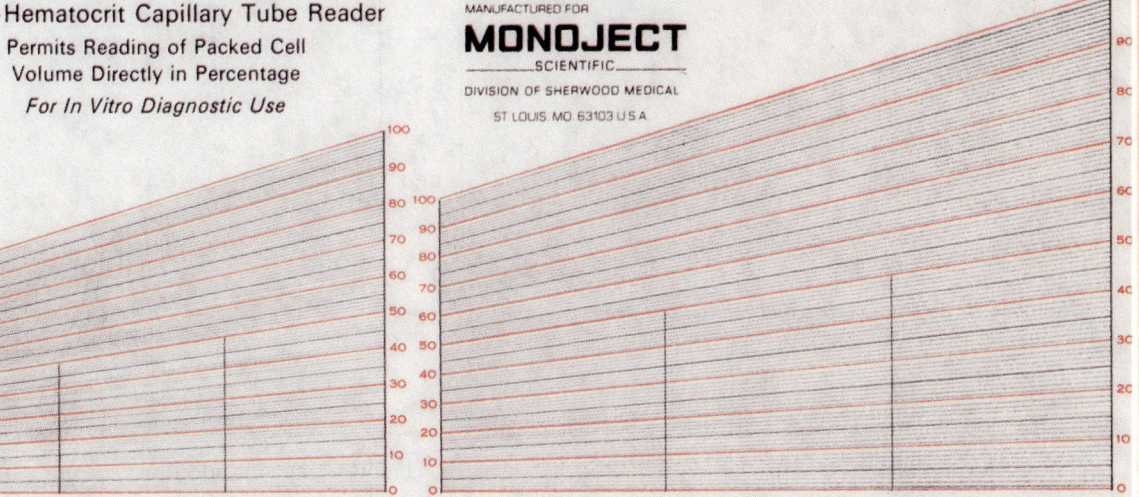

DIRECTIONS FOR USE:
Place the centrifuged Micro-Hematocrit Tube vertically on the chart with the bottom edge of the CRITOCAP just touching the red line below the "0" percent line. The bottom of the column of blood should then be at the "0" percent line. Slide the tube along the chart until the meniscus of the plasma intersects the "100" percent line. The height of the packed red cell column is then read directly as percent cell volume.

HRI
8889-111004   LOT NO   33651

CRITOCAPS™

Micro-Hematocrit Capillary Tube Reader
Permits Reading of Packed Cell
Volume Directly in Percentage
For In Vitro Diagnostic Use

MANUFACTURED FOR
MONOJECT
SCIENTIFIC
DIVISION OF SHERWOOD MEDICAL
ST. LOUIS, MO. 63103 U.S.A.

Step 6: Two methods of determining microhematocrit values.

7. Dispose of the hematocrit tubes in a biohazard container. Properly care for or dispose of other equipment and supplies. Clean the work area. Remove gloves, gown, and face shield and wash your hands.

7. Standard Precautions must be followed throughout the procedure.

8. Record the data.

8. Procedures are considered not to have been done if they are not recorded.

Procedure 46-8

Performing a Wintrobe ESR

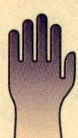

Equipment/Supplies

- anticoagulation tube
- Wintrobe tube
- transfer pipette
- timer
- appropriate biohazard barrier devices (eg, gloves, impervious gown, and face shield)

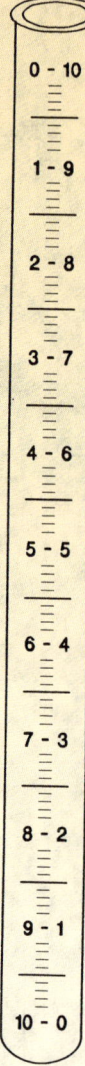

Wintrobe tube for erythrocyte sedimentation rate determination.

Steps	Purpose
1. Wash your hands.	1. Handwashing aids infection control.
2. Assemble the necessary equipment.	2. This ensures that all supplies are available.
3. Put on gloves, impervious gown, and face shield.	3. Standard Precautions must be observed when handling blood and body fluids.
4. Draw blood (see Chap. 45, Phlebotomy) into an EDTA lavender-stoppered anticoagulation tube.	4. The blood must not be allowed to clot; it must be drawn in an anticoagulation tube.

(continued)

Procedure 46-8

Performing a Wintrobe ESR (continued)

Steps	Purpose
5. Fill a graduated Wintrobe tube to the 0 mark with the uncoagulated blood using the provided transfer pipette. Be sure to eliminate any trapped bubbles and fill exactly to the 0 line.	5. Bubbles and incorrect filling with alter the test results.
6. Wait exactly 1 hour; use a timer for accuracy. Keep the tube straight upright and undisturbed during the hour.	6. Never use a shorter time and multiply the answer; less time will give inaccurate results. Tilting or disturbing the tube also will alter the results.
7. Record the level of the top of the red blood cells after 1 hour. Normal results for men are 0–10 mL/h; for women, 0–15 mL/h.	
8. Properly care for or dispose of equipment and supplies. Clean the work area. Remove gloves, gown, and face shield. Wash your hands.	8. Standard Precautions must be followed throughout the procedure.
9. Record the procedure.	9. Procedures are considered not to have been done if they are not recorded.

Procedure 46-9

Determining Bleeding Time

Equipment/Supplies

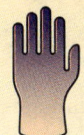

- blood pressure cuff
- Autolet device
- alcohol or antiseptic wipe
- filter paper
- butterfly bandage
- stop watch
- appropriate biohazard barrier devices (eg, gloves, impervious gown, face shield)

Steps	Purpose
1. Wash your hands.	1. Handwashing aids infection control.
2. Assemble the equipment.	2. This ensures that all supplies are available.
3. Greet and identify the patient. Explain the procedure. Ask for and answer any questions.	3. Identifying the patient prevents errors in treatment. Explaining the procedure helps ease anxiety and ensure compliance. Some patients will be nervous before the incision is made; reassure them that the cut is very small and will be barely felt.
4. Put on gloves, impervious gown, and face shield.	4. Standard Precautions must be observed when handling blood or body fluids.
5. Position the patient so that the arm is extended in a manner that is both comfortable and stable.	5. The test requires a moderate length of time and requires that the patient remain still; a comfortable position will help ensure that the patient does not move until the procedure is complete.

(continued)

Procedure 46-9

Determining Bleeding Time (continued)

Steps	Purpose
6. Have the patient turn the palm upward so that the inner aspect of the arm is exposed. Select a site several inches below the antecubital area. The area should be free of lesions and with no visible veins. Clean the site with alcohol or antiseptic wipe.	6. The inner aspect provides a surface relatively free of hair. (Rarely, the patient's arm may need to be shaved at the site). There are no large surface vessels at this site.
7. Apply the pressure cuff and set it at 40 mm Hg for the length of the test. Adjust it as needed throughout the test to maintain the pressure.	7. Placing the pressure cuff on the arm stabilizes the pressure to the arm.
8. Twist the tear-away tab on the Autolet. Make an incision 1 mm in depth on the cleaned skin surface by placing the Autolet bleeding time device on the site and pressing the trigger button on the side. This will spring the blade to make the incision. At the same time, start the stop watch.	8. A 1-mm incision is sufficiently deep to disrupt the surface capillaries but not the underlying veins.
9. At 30-second intervals, bring the filter paper near the edge of the wound to draw off some of the accumulating blood. Avoid touching the wound with the filter paper.	9. Removing the blood from the wound site is essential for observing the slowing of the blood flow. The filter paper *should not* touch the wound because disruption of the platelet plug may occur, resulting in an inaccurate measurement of bleeding time.
10. The test is complete when the blood flow visibly stops. Stop the watch when no more blood is flowing; note the time.	10. When the blood flow stops, this indicates that the platelet plug has formed.
11. Apply a butterfly bandage across the wound to keep it sealed.	11. Butterfly bandages work best to reduce scarring.
12. Thank the patient and give appropriate instructions.	12. Courtesy helps the patient have a positive attitude about the laboratory or physician's office.
13. Properly care for or dispose of all equipment and supplies. Clean the work area. Remove gloves, gown, and face shield and wash your hands.	13. Standard Precautions must be observed throughout the procedure.
14. Record the data.	14. Procedures are considered not to have been done if they are not recorded.

Note: *Low platelet counts and aspirin ingestion will prolong the bleeding time. Each laboratory has a set policy for stopping the test if the flow continues for too long. Most laboratories stop the bleeding test at 15 to 30 minutes. Any testing beyond this point is not needed because it is established that the bleeding time is not normal.*

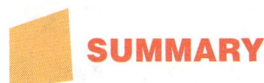

SUMMARY

The hematology laboratory determines blood cell counts and associated properties. Anemias and infections are two conditions that can be diagnosed using the blood count. The complete blood count is the main procedure performed in the hematology laboratory. Other tests, such as coagulation, aid in determining the ability of a patient to maintain hemostasis.

CRITICAL THINKING CHALLENGES

1. A patient was taking a medication that caused him to become neutropenic. To what might he be susceptible?
2. A patient lives at a very high elevation, where there is less oxygen than at sea level. Would you expect her hemoglobin to be greater, lesser, or the same in comparison as if she lived at sea level?
3. A patient with rheumatoid arthritis has an erythrocyte sedimentation rate of 77 mm/h when she has her blood tested at the doctor's office. Two weeks later she returns and now the rate is 31 mm/h. With her condition in mind, would you expect that she is improving or not?

ANSWERS TO CHECKPOINT QUESTIONS

1. Hematopoiesis is the medical term for blood cell production. It is influenced by hormones and depends on adequate nutrients such as iron.

2. Leukopenia is diminished number of leukocytes. It can be caused by chemical toxicity, nutritional deficiencies, overwhelming or chronic infections, and certain malignancies.
3. Neutrophils defend against foreign invaders by phagocytosis.
4. Elevated eosinophils and basophils are both seen with allergic reactions.
5. A hematocrit of 20% indicates that of the total blood volume, 20% of it consists of red blood cells.
6. The two most common tests for determining how well a fibrin clot can form are prothrombin time and partial thromboplastin time.

SUGGESTIONS FOR FURTHER READING

Bullock, B. L. (1996). *Pathophysiology: Adaptations and Alterations in Function*, 4th ed. Philadelphia: Lippincott-Raven.

Fishbach, F. (1996). *A Manual of Laboratory and Diagnostic Tests*, 5th ed. Philadelphia: Lippincott-Raven.

Lotspeich-Steininger, C., Stein-Martin, E. A. & Koepke, J. A. (1992). *Clinical Hematology Principles, Procedures and Correlations*. Philadelphia: J. B. Lippincott.

Rappaport, S. I. (1987). *Introduction to Hematology*, 2nd ed. Philadelphia: J. B. Lippincott.

Rubin E., & Farber J. L. (1994). *Pathology*, 2nd ed. Philadelphia: J. B. Lippincott.

Serology and Immunohematology

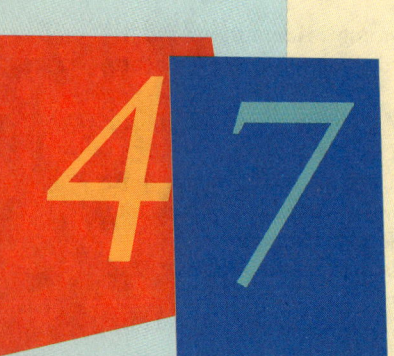

Chapter Outline

Antigens and Antibodies
Serology Test Methods and Principles
    Agglutination Test
    Enzyme Immunoassays
    Chromatographic Assay
Specimen Collection and Handling
    Serum
    Urine
    Other Specimens
Reagent and Kit Storage and Handling
Following Test Procedures
Quality Assurance and Quality Control
    External Controls
    Internal Controls
Serology Tests
    Rheumatoid Factor/Rheumatoid
      Arthritis

Infectious Mononucleosis
C-Reactive Protein
Rubella
Rapid Plasma Reagin Test for
    Syphilis
Pregnancy Test
Group A Streptococcus
Other Serologic Tests
Immunohematology
    Blood Group Antigens
    Blood Group Testing
Blood Supply
Summary
Critical Thinking Challenges
Answers to Checkpoint Questions
Suggestions for Further Reading

DACUM Components

1.3   Practice within the scope of education, training, and personal capabilities
4.1   Apply principles of aseptic technique and infection control
4.9   Use quality control
4.11 Perform selected tests that assist with diagnosis and treatment
7.2   Instruct patients with special needs

Chapter Competencies

Learning Objectives

Upon successfully completing this chapter, you will be able to:

1. Spell and define the Key Terms.
2. List the indications for serologic testing.
3. Describe the antigen–antibody reaction.
4. Name and describe the three most common methods of enhancing the antigen–antibody reaction for testing purposes.
5. List areas to address to ensure quality assurance and quality control in serologic testing.
6. Describe the collection and handling of serum samples, urine samples, and other specimens used for serologic testing.
7. Explain the storage and handling of serologic test kits.
8. List and describe serologic tests most commonly encountered through the medical office.

Performance Objectives

Upon successfully completing this chapter, you will be able to:

1. Perform an agglutination test.
2. Perform an enzyme immunoassay (EIA) test.
3. Perform a chromatographic assay test.

Key Terms

(See Glossary for definitions.)

agglutination
conjugate
donor
hemolysis
immunohematology
sensitivity
serology
specificity
substrate

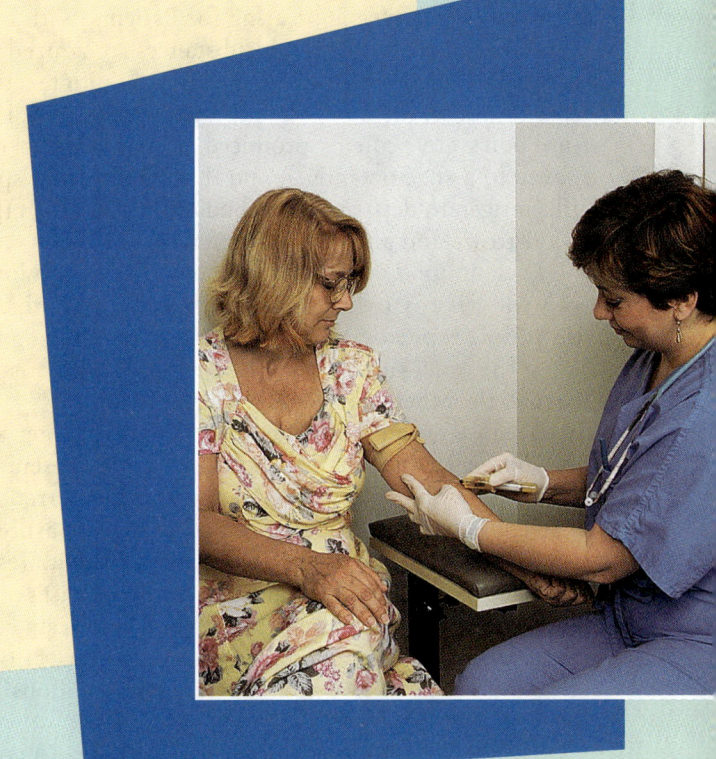

Serology is the study of antigens and antibodies. The term serology refers to the source of most of the samples, the liquid part of blood called serum, produced when whole blood is allowed to clot. Serologic methods are used to:

- Identify bacterial and viral infections (eg, streptococcus, hepatitis A, hepatitis B, human immunodeficiency virus, rubella, and Epstein-Barr virus)
- Diagnose chlamydia infections, syphilis, and Rocky Mountain spotted fever
- Measure substances such as human chorionic gonadotropin (HCG) found in pregnant women, drugs found in the urine, and hormones found in serum

Immunohematology refers to the testing done in the blood bank on red blood cells (RBCs, erythrocytes) and serum to ensure that blood from a **donor** (one who contributes blood) is compatible with a recipient's blood. It involves testing for antigens on the surface of RBCs using reagents containing antibodies called antisera as well as testing for antibodies in the patient's serum using reagent RBCs. These tests are based on the attraction between antigens and antibodies.

All testing described requires the use of Standard Precautions.

➤ ANTIGENS AND ANTIBODIES

As noted in Chapter 36, Caring for Patients With Immune Disorders, antigens are substances recognized as foreign to the body that cause the body to initiate a defense response, including the production of antibodies. Antibodies are proteins produced by the body in response to a specific antigen and that bind to that specific antigen to destroy it. Antibodies float freely in the bloodstream and are found in serum.

Each antibody produced by the body will combine with and destroy (in most instances) only one antigen; this is called specificity. It allows laboratory personnel to test the exact substance desired without interference from all the other substances found in serum.

Because an antibody has a particularly strong attraction for its antigen, little antigen need be present in a sample for the antibody to find it; this is referred to as sensitivity. A test is very sensitive if it can measure a substance even if only a small amount is present. Tests using antigen–antibody reactions as their bases are both very specific and very sensitive. These tests can measure small amounts of a substance and pick it out of a solution such as serum that contains millions of other unrelated substances.

The body's immune system can recognize many different areas or sites on a single antigen and therefore will produce several antibodies that can combine with that one antigen. They will each, however, bind with only that one antigen at different areas or sites of that antigen. For example, the body's immune system produces at least three antibodies to the hepatitis B virus. One is against an antigen found on the surface of the virus; one is against an antigen found in the core or center of the virus; and one is against an antigen named E. These antibodies will combine with different parts of the hepatitis B virus, but will not combine with the hepatitis A or the hepatitis C virus.

An antibody is named by using its specific antigen's name and adding the prefix "anti." If the antigen's name is A, the antibody's name is anti-A. If the antigen is B, the antibody is anti-B. The antibodies mentioned above for the hepatitis B virus are named anti-hepatitis B surface antigen (anti-HBs), anti-hepatitis B core antigen (anti-HBc), and anti-hepatitis B E antigen (anti-HBe).

Checkpoint Question

1. How would you describe a test that is both specific and sensitive?

➤ SEROLOGY TEST METHODS AND PRINCIPLES

In serology, the substance to be tested is identified or the amount present (quantity) is measured using the binding of a specific antibody to its specific antigen. Either the antigen is measured by using a solution containing the antibody (antisera), or the antibody is measured by using a solution containing the antigen. Usually the binding of an antigen and antibody is not visible to the naked eye. The reaction has to be enhanced or enlarged. Methods commonly used to do this include:

- **Agglutination** (clumping) of visible particles such as red blood cells (RBCs) or latex particles
- Enzyme immunoassays (EIA) that produce a color change from colorless to a specific color such as blue or red
- Chromatographic assays in which fluid migration through a membrane leaves a bar of color in a viewing "window"

Other methods include agglutination inhibition and competitive binding assays.

Agglutination Test

Agglutination is a term used to describe the clumping together of particles caused by the binding of antibodies and antigens. For agglutination testing, only two things are necessary:

1. A solution containing the particles (usually RBCs or latex particles)
2. The patient's sample

To perform an agglutination test, follow these steps:

1. Mix together the solution and the patient's sample on a paper card or glass plate.
2. Gently rock the solution and sample back and forth for a few seconds or a few minutes.
3. Observe for agglutination or clumping of particles. If agglutination does not occur, the test solution appears smooth and milky. If agglutination does occur, the test solution appears rough and granular with areas of clumped particles in a clear background.

Both the antigen and antibody will be present in the test mixture formulated for a specific disease. If the suspected disease-causing antigen, or antibodies against the disease, are present in the patient's sample, agglutination will occur. Agglutination is a positive test and indicates that the test substance is present. If no agglutination occurs, the test is negative, indicating that the test substance is absent. Some tests are designed so that agglutination must appear within a specified time period to indicate a positive reaction.

Agglutination tests can be used in two ways:

1. If the specific antigen is on the particle (RBCs or latex), the patient's serum can be tested for the presence of the specific antibody. This method is used to test for infectious mononucleosis, rheumatoid arthritis, syphilis, and rubella.
2. If the manufacturer produces a particle (usually latex) with the antibody attached, the patient's serum or other specimen can be tested for the presence of a specific antigen. This method is used in some tests for streptococci.

Agglutination tests are quick and easy to perform. They are also inexpensive and have a wide range of uses. The procedure for a test must be followed exactly for the results to be accurate (Box 47-1).

Enzyme Immunoassays

Enzyme immunoassays (EIA) often have more steps and more reagents than agglutination tests, but the end point is an easy-to-read color change. Agglutination, particularly if the clumps are small, can be difficult to read. EIA tests usually come with all the necessary reagents packaged together in a kit that also contains any additional components needed for test completion, including:

- A solid surface (plastic test pack, test tube, bead) coated with the first antibody to the antigen to be tested
- A solution containing a **conjugate**, which is a second antibody specific to the antigen to be tested. The conjugate has an enzyme attached (conjugated) to it that will help to initiate the reaction.
- A wash solution used to remove excess conjugate not bound to the antigen or antigen–antibody complex
- A color solution (a **substrate**, or substance that is acted on) that turns from colorless to a specific color in the presence of the enzyme

All that needs to be added is the patient specimen. To perform the EIA test, follow these steps:

1. Remove the plastic test pack and other components from a protective pouch.
2. Add the patient's sample to a specially marked area of the test pack, then add conjugate to that same marked area.
3. Allow time for the first antibody to combine with the antigen and the second antibody (conjugate) to combine to the antigen–antibody complex. The antigen is "sandwiched" between the two antibodies.
4. Rinse the test pack or area one or more times using the wash solution. This removes the excess second antibody (conjugate) not attached to the antigen–antibody complex. The wash removes all the conjugate if no antigen is present in the patient sample.
5. After completing the wash step, add the color solution (substrate) to the test area. If the "sandwich" formed and the conjugate is attached, the color solution will produce a color. If no conjugate is attached, no color will be produced. Color is a positive test and indicates the presence of the antigen in the patient's sample. No color is a negative test and indicates the absence of the antigen in the patient's sample.

BOX 47-1 Tips for Performing Agglutination Testing

1. Start with a clean test slide, one that is free of finger prints and dust.
2. Follow the times exactly.
3. View the test mixture under a direct light source.
4. Mix reagents before using.
5. Mix samples before using.
6. Do not touch reagent droppers to test area.
7. Do not smear one test mixture into another test area.

Tips for Performing Enzyme Immunoassays

1. Follow the times exactly.
2. Add reagents in correct order.
3. Use reagents only with other reagents from the same kit.
4. Use exact amount of reagents stated in directions.
5. Ensure that reagents and samples are at room temperature.
6. Ensure that reagents have not expired.

This test method is often referred to as the sandwich method. Some important tips for obtaining accurate results are listed in Box 47-2.

Chromatographic Assay

Chromatographic assay tests reduce the number of steps involved in an EIA test, but retain the color change end point. These tests are usually more expensive than agglutination tests but are easy to read.

In these tests, fluid flows or migrates through a paper-like membrane combining with reagents embedded in the test pack as the fluid flows. The parts of the test include:

- Test pack
- Patient's sample
- Diluting fluid

To perform the test, follow these steps:

1. Add the patient's sample to a special area of the test pack followed quickly by several drops of the diluting fluid.
2. Allow time for the fluid to flow through the paper membrane.
3. Observe the test pack for the presence of a colored line or bar.

As the fluid flows across a special area containing antibodies, the antigen in the patient's sample attaches to the antibody conjugated to a color substance. This complex continues to migrate across a line or bar containing stationary antibodies. A "sandwich" is formed of stationary antibody–antigen–antibody with color substance producing a line or bar of color. If a color bar develops, the test is positive and the antigen is present in the patient sample. If no color bar develops,

the test is negative and the antigen is absent from the patient sample.

The test packs for some tests already have a horizontal line or bar. Fluid migration containing the antigen produces a vertical line or bar. A positive test is indicated by the presence of a plus or positive (+) sign produced by the two lines. A negative test is indicated by a minus or negative (−) sign produced by the initial single line. Tips to follow in performing these tests are the same as those for EIA tests (see Box 47-2).

Checkpoint Question

2. *What are three serology test methods and how do they indicate the presence of the test substance?*

SPECIMEN COLLECTION AND HANDLING

Whether a patient's result is correct, false, or incorrect depends to a large extent on the quality of each step involved in testing the patient's sample. This starts with the collection of the sample (venipuncture if serum or blood) and ends with the reporting of the result. Mistakes can be made at any step. Each person involved in testing patients' samples must ensure that mistakes are not made and, if they are made, that they are discovered and corrected. This whole process of checking and rechecking to be sure the correct result is reported is called quality assurance. Some of the key areas to address in the assurance of a correctly processed specimen include:

- Specimen collection and handling
- Reagent and kit storage and handling
- Following of test procedures
- Quality assurance and quality control

Serum

Many serology tests require serum. For some tests, plasma or whole blood may be substituted for serum. It is important to use the correct specimen type for a particular test because using the wrong type may result in an incorrect reading.

To obtain serum, collect a red top evacuated tube using standard venipuncture procedure (see Chap. 45, Phlebotomy). A serum-separation or a clot-activator evacuated tube is also acceptable. Immediately label the tube with the patient's name, the date and time, your initials, and any other required information. Because there is no premeasured anticoagulant in a red top tube to be matched by a certain amount of blood, the volume of blood drawn into the tube may vary without affecting the test results. It is not critical that the tube be completely full. There must be enough blood, however, to yield sufficient serum to perform the test and repeat it if necessary.

After obtaining the serum, follow these steps:

1. Allow blood to clot for at least 15 minutes.
2. Invert the tube to be sure the blood has solidified into a firm clot.
3. Allow to stand longer if not clotted.
4. Centrifuge at moderate speed for 10 minutes.

The serum must then be separated from the clot and cells. This can be done by one of three methods:

1. Transfer the serum into a clean test tube using a plastic or glass transfer pipette, label with patient's name and other required information and the word "serum," and cap the tube. Be careful not to stir up the cells and to transfer only clear serum.
2. Use a serum-separation tube. This tube contains gel that migrates between the cells and serum, separating them when the tube is centrifuged.
3. Insert a special plastic tube with a rubber bottom called a serum filter into the already centrifuged tube. The serum filter is pushed through the serum to a level just above the cells. This filter keeps cells from mixing with the serum.

The first method is the best for long-term storage and the only acceptable method if the serum must be frozen. The last two methods are for same-day use only.

If the serum is not tested shortly after separation from cells, it should be stored according to the directions for the test to be performed. For some tests this will be room temperature. For other tests this will be in the refrigerator at 2° to 8°C. For still others this will be in the freezer at −4°C or maybe even −18°C. The proper storage of a sample also depends on when the testing is to be performed. For example, a sample that may be left at room temperature if tested within 8 hours may need to be refrigerated if testing is to be performed in 24 to 48 hours or frozen if not to be tested until the next week or next month.

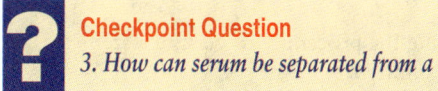

Checkpoint Question
3. How can serum be separated from a clot?

Urine

Urine for serology testing is usually collected by the clean-catch method. (See Chap. 44, Urinalysis, for a description of urine collection methods.) The first voided morning specimen is the most concentrated and so the most suitable sample for measuring an antigen. Mark the specimen container with the patient's name, date and time of collection, and your initials. In general, urine samples should be tested immediately or refrigerated at 2° to 8°C until testing. In some instances, it may be necessary to freeze the sample. If the urine is moderately cloudy or bloody, it should be centrifuged before testing.

Other Specimens

Sometimes an infected area of the body is swabbed to collect bacteria for testing in the laboratory. Swabs that have been collected from the throat, the vaginal area, and occasionally other areas of the body are sent to the laboratory for testing. If both a culture and a serology test are ordered, two swabs should be collected. The swab should be made of cotton or Dacron with a plastic or wooden shaft. Calcium alginate swabs should not be used. A transport medium (solution) such as found in Culturettes is not needed as it is for growing the bacteria. If a medium is used, it should be liquid modified Stuart's medium. A medium that is semisolid or contains charcoal, agar, or gelatin will interfere with serologic tests.

Swab specimens should be tested as soon as possible after collection. Some tests allow for storage up to 8 hours at room temperature or 72 hours refrigerated. The test procedure should be checked for specific specimen storage.

➤ REAGENT AND KIT STORAGE AND HANDLING

For most serology tests, reagents come from the manufacturer packaged in kits. These kits contain all the reagents and often include supplies such as pipettes, tubes, and cups needed to perform tests on a certain number of samples.

The kits must be stored at the temperature recommended on the kit box or package insert (the information sheet that comes inside the kit). Some kits are stored at room temperature and others in the refrigerator. Some kits need to be divided with some reagents stored at room temperature and others in the refrigerator. Still others are stored in the refrigerator until opened and then stored at room temperature. It is important to follow the manufacturer's directions. If the kits are stored improperly, the reagents may deteriorate and false results may be obtained.

Each kit has a lot number and expiration date stamped on the box or package. All reagents with the same lot number were made at the same time in the same manufacturing facility. The expiration date is the day past which the reagents are no longer guaranteed to perform correctly. Reagents from kits with different lot numbers should not be used together. The manufacturer will not guarantee that they will work correctly when components from different lots are mixed.

Reagents should never be used past their expiration date. The date should be written on the kit box when it is received in the laboratory. The date and the initials of the worker who opened the kit should also be written on the box when the kit is opened and used for the first time. Some kits have a new expiration date starting from the day the kit is opened. The package insert that comes in the kit should always be read for details about storing and handling the reagents and supplies.

Checkpoint Question
4. Why is it important to store reagent kits at specified temperatures?

➤ FOLLOWING TEST PROCEDURES

All tests performed in serology should have written procedures. These procedures must be followed each time a patient's sample is tested to ensure correct results. Test procedures typically cover:

- Test principle and clinical use of the test
- Reagents and materials needed to do the test
- Precautions
- Specimen collection and handling
- Controls to be run and how often
- Step-by-step procedure to follow
- Interpretation and reporting of results
- Normal or expected values
- Test limitations

➤ QUALITY ASSURANCE AND QUALITY CONTROL

Reagents do not always function properly even though they are well within the expiration date. Sometimes a reagent is left at room temperature when it should be refrigerated. Sometimes serum or other solutions are accidentally added to a reagent causing it to test or register incorrectly. Kits should be tested periodically for continued reactivity of all reagents. A check needs to be performed each time the reagents are used. Other forms of checks may be performed once a day or only when a new kit is opened. Solutions used to perform some of these checks are called controls.

External Controls

An external control is a solution similar to a patient sample that is tested in the same manner as a patient sample; however, its value or expected result is already known. These controls are often part of the serology kit. In some instances, separate controls can be purchased from the manufacturer.

For most serology tests, positive and negative controls are needed. The positive control should give a positive reaction (agglutination, color, or colored bar). The negative control should give a negative reaction (no agglutination, no color, no colored bar or other specified result). If the controls do not give the expected result, patient results should not be reported and the test should be repeated. If a problem still exists, it should be further investigated (Box 47-3).

Internal Controls

Besides external control solutions, some serology tests also have internal controls that are built into the test packs themselves; such controls monitor that the test procedure is followed correctly and that the reagents are working properly. Sometimes positive and negative test zones exist on each test pack. Sometimes there is only a positive test zone or a test completed zone. These zones are separate from the patient test zone or area. The positive control zone must give a positive color reaction and the negative control zone must give a negative (usually no color) reaction for the test to be valid and patient results to be reported. Do not report patient results if controls do not give proper reactions.

BOX 47-3   Test Troubleshooting Tips

If a serology test using a control is not producing expected results, try:

1. Re-reading the procedure to be sure a step was not omitted.
2. Checking labels of reagents to be sure the correct reagents were added in the correct order.
3. Visually checking reagents for signs of contamination such as cloudiness or color change.
4. Repeating testing with new bottles of control.
5. Repeating testing with new kit or reagents.
6. Calling the manufacturer for assistance.

The positive control zone ensures that the correct reagents have been added in the proper order. The negative control zone ensures there is not a nonspecific reaction of patient sample and test reagents. Problems with internal controls can be investigated in the same manner as used for external controls (see Box 47-3). Positive and negative internal controls do not completely take the place of external control solutions, which should be performed on a daily basis.

➤ SEROLOGY TESTS

Rheumatoid Factor/Rheumatoid Arthritis

Rheumatoid factor is an antibody found in the serum of 70% of people with rheumatoid arthritis. Rheumatoid arthritis is an autoimmune progressive inflammatory disease of the joints causing pain on motion, swelling, stiffness, and subcutaneous nodules near the joints involved. Rheumatoid arthritis can affect people of all ages. Initial occurrence in most cases is between the age of 30 and 50. It is two to three times more common in women than in men.

Testing

The most common tests for rheumatoid factor are based on agglutination of latex particles. The rheumatoid factor in the serum of patients with rheumatoid arthritis causes agglutination of latex particles that are coated with the antigen (immunoglobulin G, IgG). The sample used is serum tested soon after separation from cells or stored at 2° to 8°C for up to 72 hours. External positive and negative controls are run with each batch of patient samples. If agglutination occurs with a patient's undiluted serum, the serum is diluted 1:20 with a diluting fluid and tested with another drop of latex particles. A 1:20 dilution can be obtained by adding 0.1 mL (100 μL) of patient's sample to 1.9 mL of diluting fluid, such as saline or distilled water. If the diluted serum agglutinates with the latex particles, the test is positive for rheumatoid factor. If the serum does not agglutinate on the undiluted or on the diluted serum, the test is negative for rheumatoid factor.

The external controls must give appropriate reactions for the test to be valid and patient results to be reported. That is, the positive control must agglutinate and the negative control must not agglutinate for testing to be valid.

False-Negative and False-Positive Results

Even when the controls react appropriately, laboratory tests are not a perfect indicator of disease. Physicians use test results along with physical examination and patient history to make clinical decisions about disease. Sometimes a negative result occurs even when a patient has a disease. This is called a false-negative result. Because only 70% of patients with rheumatoid arthritis are positive for rheumatoid factor, 30% of patients with rheumatoid arthritis will have a false-negative result.

Sometimes a positive result occurs when the patient does not have the disease. This is called a false-positive result. False positive results sometimes occur in the elderly and in patients with lupus erythematosus, syphilis, or hepatitis.

False-negative and false-positive results can occur because of biologic conditions of patients as the examples above show. They can also be due to technical difficulty with samples or with performing the test. Testing personnel cannot control the biologic conditions, but they can sometimes control the technical conditions. If testing personnel wait too long to read agglutination, a false-positive test result can occur. This can be avoided by following directions carefully. Hemolyzed and lipemic samples (samples with increased fat levels) can give a false-positive result. These samples must be recollected to ensure accurate testing.

Checkpoint Question

5. *What is the difference between a false-negative and a false-positive test result and why do these sometimes occur?*

Infectious Mononucleosis

Infectious mononucleosis is caused by the Epstein-Barr virus. About 50% of exposures reported in medical offices occur before the age of 5 and most of the other 50% occur between the ages of 15 and 24. Children under the age of 5 rarely exhibit symptoms. Adults present with general symptoms such as fatigue, malaise, sore throat, and enlarged lymph nodes. A patient may sometimes exhibit an enlarged spleen or hepatitis. The white blood cell count may be normal, slightly decreased, or slightly increased with atypical lymphocytes visible on blood smears. Infectious mononucleosis is usually self-limiting and most patients fully recover.

Testing

Tests for infectious mononucleosis include agglutination of red blood cells (RBCs) or latex particles, enzyme immunoassays, and chromatographic assays. The substance tested for in each method is heterophil antibodies. These are antibodies produced by a person with infectious mononucleosis that combine with antigens found on the RBCs of other animals such as horses, oxen, and sheep. For most tests, serum, plasma, or whole blood (purple top tube or capillary sample) may be used. Whole blood must be tested as soon as possible. Serum and plasma may be stored in the refrigerator for 2 to 3 days. External or internal controls must give appropriate reactions for testing to be valid and patient results to be reported.

False-Negative and False-Positive Results

False-negative results can occur early in the disease before heterophil antibodies are produced. Only 50% of children under the age of 4 produce heterophil antibodies. The other 50% will give a false-negative reaction. Only 85% to 90% of adults produce heterophil antibodies. False-positive results can be obtained by waiting too long to read agglutination tests.

C-Reactive Protein

The C-reactive protein (CRP) is a test used to detect inflammatory diseases such as bacterial infections, malignant diseases, and autoimmune disorders. It is not a diagnostic test for a particular disease but rather a test for monitoring the inflammatory process. It can be used to monitor the effect of therapy on disease.

Testing

The CRP is an antigen found in serum. Most tests use latex particles coated with antibodies to CRP. Patient serum is tested undiluted and diluted 1:5 (0.1 mL serum and 0.4 mL diluting fluid). Agglutination with either or both the undiluted and diluted serum is considered positive for CRP. If no agglutination occurs in either sample, the test is negative. A positive and negative external control run with each batch of patient samples must give appropriate reactions for the test to be valid and results to be reported.

False-Negative and False-Positive Results

Too much CRP in the serum sample can cause a false-negative result. This is due to antigen excess. The 1:5 dilution of the serum helps avoid this problem. False-positive results can occur from using lipemic or hemolyzed samples.

Rubella

The rubella virus causes a disease also known as German or 3-day measles. Measles occurs most commonly in childhood. Today there is widespread immunization

for rubella. Before immunization, epidemic outbreaks occurred every 6 to 9 years, resulting in stillbirths and birth defects from congenital rubella. In children and adults with measles, the symptoms are mild, low-grade fever and a rash on the face, neck, and trunk. For a fetus of less than 3 months, measles can cause death or birth defects such as bone abnormalities, mental retardation, cataracts, and cardiovascular defects.

Testing

Tests available for rubella include agglutination of RBCs or latex particles, hemagglutination (RBCs) inhibition, and enzyme immunoassays. In latex agglutination tests, particles are coated with rubella antigens. The presence of antibodies in the patient's serum will agglutinate the latex particles. Agglutination is a positive test indicating the patient has immunity to the rubella virus. If there is no agglutination, the serum should be diluted 1:10 with dilution fluid and the diluted serum tested. If both the undiluted and diluted samples show no agglutination, the test is negative for antibodies to the rubella virus. Controls must react appropriately for the test to be valid.

Latex agglutination tests do not distinguish between present and past infections. Enzyme immunoassays are available that determine if the antibodies present belong to the IgG or to the IgM class of immunoglobulins. The IgM class is generally seen in current infections and the IgG class indicates immunity from past infection or vaccination.

False-Negative and False-Positive Results

Very high levels of antibodies can give a false-negative result. Negative serums should be diluted 1:10 and retested. Allowing the test to sit too long before observing for agglutination can cause a false-positive result.

Rapid Plasma Reagin Test for Syphilis

Rapid plasma reagin (RPR) is a screening test for syphilis, a sexually transmitted disease caused by a spirochete bacteria, *Treponema pallidum*. Incidence of the disease declined after World War II, but it has been increasing in recent years. The highest incidence is seen in individuals between the ages of 20 and 24. It can be transmitted from mother to fetus, resulting in congenital syphilis causing notched teeth, nerve deafness, and other symptoms. Syphilis is treated with penicillin. Untreated syphilis is a chronic disease in which the patient demonstrates symptoms at times and is asymptomatic at other times. Untreated syphilis progresses in stages, including primary, secondary, latent, and tertiary.

Testing

Treponema pallidum does not grow in culture; the best test to demonstrate the organism is darkfield microscopy. More frequently the serum is tested for the presence of antibodies and antibody-like substances called reagins. Venereal Disease Research Laboratories (VDRL) and RPR are the most common screening tests for these nonspecific reagins. The microhemagglutination assay for *T. pallidum* (MHA-TP) and fluorescent treponemal antibody absorption test (FTA-ABS) are two confirmatory tests for the organism itself.

The RPR is an agglutination test. The antigen solution contains charcoal to increase visibility of the clumping. Serum is the specimen of choice even though the name implies that plasma is used. One drop of the patient's serum is added to the appropriate circle on a plastic-coated card. One drop of antigen is then added to each circle from a calibrated syringe with a special 18-gauge needle. The card is placed on a mechanical rotator, rotating at 95 to 110 rotations per minute for 8 minutes. The circles are observed for agglutination. Reactive (positive), weakly reactive, and nonreactive (negative) controls are run with each batch of patient samples. They must react appropriately for the test to be valid and patient results to be reported. The rotator is checked each day for the number of rotations per minute, which should average 100/min. The 18-gauge needle is checked periodically for the number of drops it delivers per milliliter of antigen solution, which should be 60 +/− 2.

Agglutination of the antigen solution is considered reactive for the reagin (presumptive positive test for syphilis). Even a weakly reactive agglutination is considered positive or reactive. No agglutination of the antigen solution is considered nonreactive. Determination of titer is performed on any reactive serum. This involves performing a serial dilution to obtain dilutions of the serum of 1:2, 1:4, 1:8, 1:16, and so forth. The diluting of the serum is continued until a diluted specimen gives a nonreactive result (no agglutination). The titer reported is the last dilution showing agglutination. If the last diluted specimen showing agglutination was the 1:8 dilution, the titer would be reported as 1:8. If only the undiluted specimen showed agglutination, the titer would be reported as 1:1. The patient's physician and the health department must be notified of all reactive results for syphilis. Serum should be sent to the state laboratory or reference laboratory for confirmation of a syphilis infection using the MHA-TP or FTA-ABS tests.

False-Negative and False-Positive Results

The RPR is reactive in 80% of cases of primary syphilis, 99% of secondary, and 1% of tertiary. The MHA-TP, in contrast, is reactive in 65% of cases of primary syphilis, 100% of secondary, and 95% of tertiary. A false-negative RPR will be obtained in 20% of primary syphilis cases. A false-negative MHA-TP will be obtained in 35% of primary syphilis cases. A false-positive RPR can be seen in patients with lupus erythematosus, infectious mononucleosis, hepatitis, rheumatoid arthritis, in pregnancy and in the elderly. Improper rotation of specimen can also cause a false-negative result.

Pregnancy Test

The test for pregnancy is based on the detection of the hormone human chorionic gonadotropin (HCG), which is produced by the placenta starting at about 10 days after the fertilization of the ovum by sperm. Modern pregnancy tests can determine pregnancy before the first missed menses. HCG increases during the first 3 months of pregnancy and then decreases to undetectable levels a few days after childbirth. A pregnancy test is frequently used to rule out pregnancy before performing medical procedures that might be harmful to the fetus.

Testing

Tests of HCG include agglutination inhibition (the absence of agglutination), enzyme immunoassay, and chromatographic assay. Many popular test kits are based on the enzyme immunoassay "sandwich" method. Urine or serum is added to the test pack in the test area containing antibodies to HCG. If the kit uses either urine or serum, the serum usually has to be pretreated before testing. Next, the conjugate containing the second antibody attached to an enzyme is added. Time is allowed for the binding of antigen to antibodies. Unbound conjugate–antibody–enzyme is washed off and the color reagent (substrate) is added. Development of color indicates a positive test. No color is a negative test (Fig. 47-1).

Internal positive and negative control areas must react appropriately for results to be valid. Not adding one of the reagents or adding reagents in the wrong order can result in all control and patient test areas appearing negative (no color). Some patients have antibodies to test reagents causing all test areas to appear positive. Either of these patterns indicate an invalid result.

False-Negative and False-Positive Results

A urine specimen that is too dilute can give a false-negative reaction. The first morning urine specimen is the most likely to contain HCG if the patient is pregnant. Certain tumors produce HCG and can cause a false-positive result.

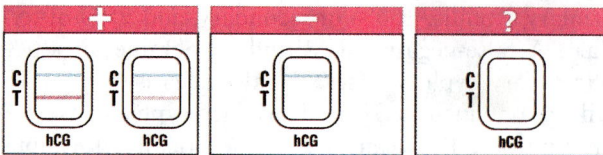

FIGURE 47-1
QuickVue One-Step hcg-urine test (Courtesy of Quidel Corp.)

Group A Streptococcus

Group A streptococcus (*Streptococcus pyogenes*) is one of the most common bacterial causes of sore throat and upper respiratory tract infections. Infections are usually found in school-aged children, especially in winter and spring. These infections can be treated with antibiotics. If not treated, the disease may lead to rheumatic fever and acute glomerulonephritis.

Testing

Group A strep infection can be diagnosed by bacterial culture or serologic tests for the antigenic presence of the bacteria. Serologic tests include agglutination, enzyme immunoassay, and chromatographic assay. The bacteria do not need to be alive for serology tests as they do for culture. Serologic tests are easier and more rapid (5–15 minutes) than culture, which takes 18 to 24 hours; however, culture is considered more sensitive.

The specimen used is a swab of the patient's throat. (See Chap. 37, Caring for Patients With Respiratory Disorders, for a description of performing a throat culture.) The bacterial antigen is extracted from the swab using an acid solution and a nitrite solution. The mixture is then neutralized with a buffer solution. Color indicators are added to these solutions to monitor that correct extraction procedure has been followed. If the color changes described in the procedure do not occur, the extraction process should be repeated using a new specimen (throat swab). The extraction fluid is then filtered before addition to the test. The extracted specimen is tested using one of the methods listed in the section "Serology Test Methods and Principles," above. Internal or external controls must be performed with the patient sample and give appropriate reactions for the test to be valid (Fig. 47-2).

False-Negative and False-Positive Results

If improper technique is used in collecting the throat swab or an inadequate specimen is obtained, a false-negative result can occur. If the test is allowed to stand too long before results are read, a false-positive result can occur. High levels of *Staphylococcus aureus* in the specimen can interfere with the interpretation of results.

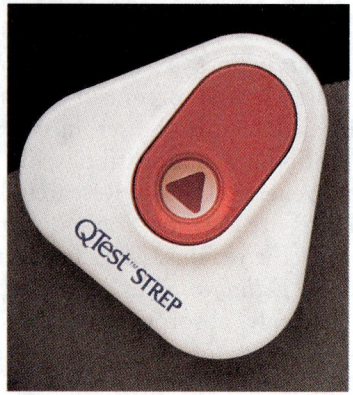

FIGURE 47-2
Qtest Strep test for group A streptococcus. (Courtesy of Becton-Dickinson Primary Care Diagnostics, Sparks, Maryland)

 **Checkpoint Question**
6. What are the benefits and drawbacks of using serology tests versus cultures for group A streptococcus?

Other Serologic Tests

Antinuclear Antibody (ANA)

Normal antibodies react against foreign cells causing their destruction; autoantibodies react against the body's own normal cells, causing their destruction. Antinuclear antibodies react against the nucleus of the body's cells. The antinuclear antibodies are present in the sera of patients with rheumatoid arthritis, systemic lupus erythematosus, progressive systemic sclerosis, and other autoimmune diseases.

Antistreptolysin-O Test (ASOT)

Streptolysin-O is an exotoxin (a poison excreted by an organism) produced by most group A and some C and G streptococci. Stretolysin-O causes **hemolysis** (breakdown) of RBCs and the loss of hemoglobin. ASOT identifies and measures the antibodies produced by the body in response to the presence of the exotoxin (the streptolysin-O). Antistreptolysin antibodies oppose the action of the streptolysin. Streptolysin-O indicates that the exotoxin is inactivated by the presence of oxygen. The antistreptolysin antibodies' presence in serum is used to help diagnose rheumatic fever.

Cold Agglutinins

The sera of patients with atypical pneumonia and certain blood diseases such as hemolytic anemia may contain circulating antibodies that cause RBC agglutination and hemolysis at a less than normal body temperature.

Their presence in the serum may indicate certain viral or mycoplasmic infections. Cold agglutinins are more common in women over the age of 50.

Radioallergosorbent Test (RAST)

The RAST is a radiologic test of the serum capable of measuring and identifying small quantities of immunoglobulin E (IgE). This test is capable of detecting the presence of as many as 45 allergens. Agglutination indicates that an allergic response is present.

➤ IMMUNOHEMATOLOGY

Testing in the blood bank is directed at determining if a donor's blood is suitable for transfusion to a patient (recipient) who needs blood. If the donor's blood is compatible, the patient's immunosurveillance will not immediately recognize it as foreign and the RBCs may circulate in the patient's body for a longer period of time after they are transfused. If the donor's blood is incompatible, the patient's body will immediately recognize the blood as foreign and begin destroying it as soon as it is transfused. This can rapidly lead to death.

Blood Group Antigens

ABO Group

Transfusion compatibility is determined by testing the antigens present on RBCs (patient's and donor's) and the antibodies present in the patient's serum. The main RBC antigens belong to the ABO system. Each person belongs to one of four blood groups: A, B, O, or AB. People, however, are not equally divided among the four groups. Approximately 45% are O, 40% are A, 11% are B, and 4% are AB. Consequently, some blood groups are easier to obtain and some are more in demand than others. The ABO group of each donor and each patient who will need a transfusion is determined as described below under "Testing."

Almost every person's serum contains antibodies to the ABO antigens that he or she lacks. These antibodies occur naturally. Shortly after birth these antibodies are found in serum, even though the person has never received blood. A person in the A group has the A antigen. A person in the B group has the B antigen. A person in the O group lacks both antigens. A person in the AB group has both the A and B antigen. A person in the A group lacks the B antigen and has an antibody to B (anti-B) in serum. Someone who is B lacks the A antigen and has anti-A in serum. One who is O has both anti-A and anti-B in serum. A person who belongs to the AB group has neither antibody in serum.

These antibodies are crucial to safe transfusion of blood to a patient. They are the reason it is unsafe to give B blood to an A patient. An A patient has anti-B in his serum that would bind and destroy the B cells, causing breakdown products that are toxic and can lead to death. The lack of either A or B antigens on O cells makes it the universal donor. This means type O blood may be given to patients no matter what their ABO group. If B blood is unavailable for a patient, O blood can be given safely.

Rh Group

Another group of antigens important to the blood bank is the Rh group. This includes the antigens D, E, C, e, and c. However, D is the most important. The presence of the D antigen is termed Rh positive. The absence of

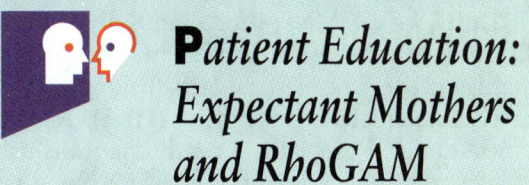

Patient Education: Expectant Mothers and RhoGAM

If you are employed in an obstetrician's office, you will have the opportunity to educate many expectant mothers who are Rh negative regarding the purpose of RhoGAM. Here are some educational pointers:

- Explain what it means to be Rh negative in terms appropriate to the patient's level of understanding.
- Point out that if the Rh factor of the baby's father is either positive or unknown, the baby could be born with Rh-positive blood. Also note that if the Rh factor of the baby's father is negative, there should be no problem.
- Explain that when the baby's Rh-positive blood comes in contact with the mother's Rh-negative blood, she will make antibodies against the baby's blood. In future pregnancies, her antibodies will fight with the fetal blood (if Rh positive), causing severe hemolytic anemia in the fetus.
- Tell the patient that RhoGAM is an immune globulin that prohibits the production of Rh-positive antibodies in the mother. It is given intrapartum and postpartum and will require that a patient consent form be signed.

It is important to note that after a miscarriage or abortion, the Rh-negative mother must receive RhoGAM, unless it is documented that the baby's father was Rh negative.

the D antigen is termed Rh negative. Antibodies to D do not occur naturally. A person lacking the D antigen must be exposed to the D antigen of foreign RBCs to produce antibodies. This can happen if an Rh-negative (D-negative) patient is transfused with Rh-positive (D-positive) blood. This can also happen if an Rh-negative mother is exposed to the Rh-positive cells of her baby before or during childbirth. Rh negative mothers can be prevented from producing antibodies to the Rh (D) antigen by injection of immune-D serum or RhoGAM. This injection prevents the production of antibodies that might destroy the RBCs of a future child, causing hemolytic disease of the newborn (HDN).

Other Blood Groups

Although the ABO and Rh groups are of greatest importance to immunohematology, there are many more significant antigens and antibodies. Some other groups include Duffy, Lewis, MNS, Kidd, and Kell. These are all RBC antigens. White blood cells and platelets also have antigens. Most of these antigens belong to a system called human leukocyte antigens (HLA). Antibodies to these antigens can cause fever during transfusion of RBCs because of the presence of white blood cells (leukocytes). Antibodies to these antigens are also responsible for the rejection of an organ transplant such as kidney, heart, or liver. Most of these antibodies do not occur naturally. A person must be exposed to blood or tissue that is foreign before producing antibodies.

Blood Group Testing

ABO Testing

To test for the ABO group of a patient or blood donor, two reagent antisera are used. One is anti-A. The other is anti-B. The RBCs to be tested are diluted with saline to approximately a 3% solution (3 drops of cells and about 100 drops of saline). One drop of 3% RBCs is mixed with 1 drop anti-A in a glass tube labeled "A." One drop of 3% RBCs is mixed with 1 drop anti-B in another tube labeled "B." The tubes are centrifuged for 15 seconds at low speed. The RBC button on the bottom of the tube is gently resuspended. The solution is examined for agglutination.

The antisera will agglutinate the RBCs if the antigen is present. No agglutination will be observed if the antigen is not present. If a patient's RBCs agglutinate with anti-A but not anti-B, the patient belongs to the A group. If the RBCs agglutinate with anti-B and not with anti-A, the cells belong to the B group (Fig. 47-3). This procedure is called direct or forward typing (Table 47-1).

The serum can be used to verify the ABO group of a patient or blood donor. Reagent "a" group cells and "b" group cells are mixed with serum, centrifuged and examined for agglutination. If a patient is A, serum will contain anti-B only. Agglutination will be observed with the "b" cells. This procedure using serum is called indirect or reverse typing (see Table 47-1).

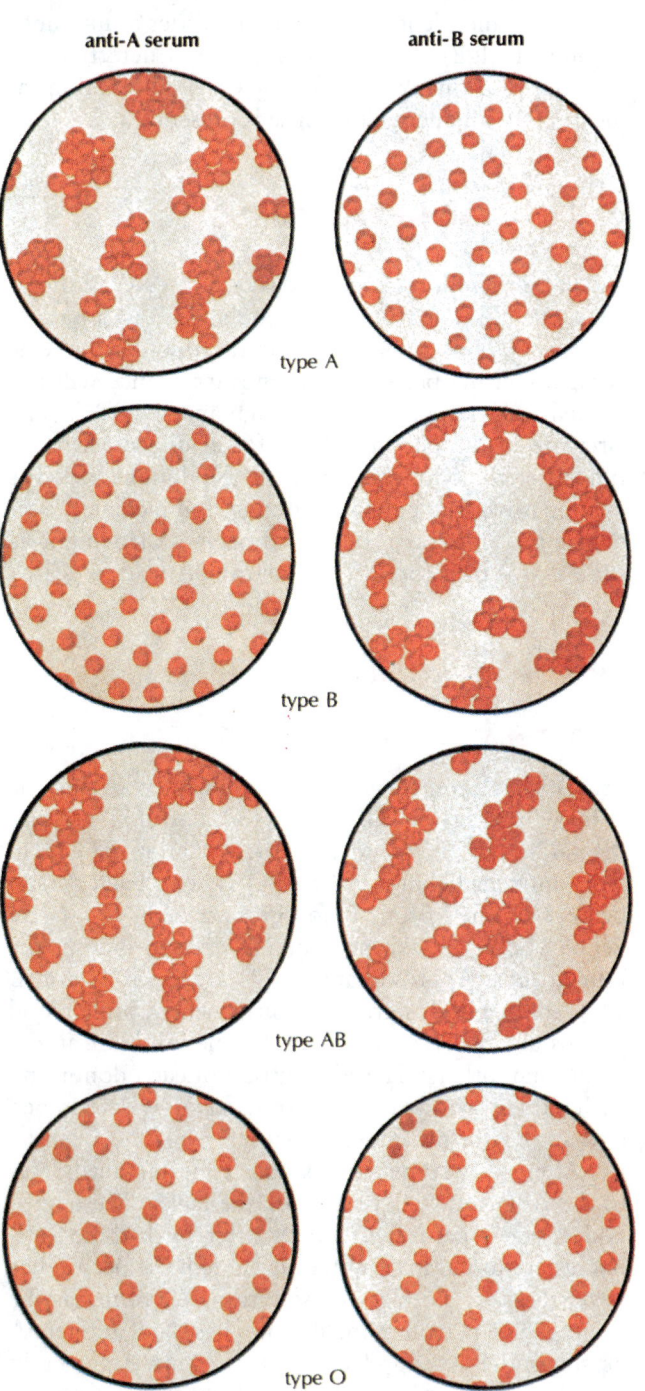

FIGURE 47-3

Blood typing. Red cells in type A blood are agglutinated (clumped) by anti-A serum; those in type B blood are agglutinated by anti-B serum. Type AB blood cells are agglutinated by both sera, and type O blood is not agglutinated by either serum.

Table 47-1
ABO Group Testing Results

| | Reagents | | | | Group |
	anti-A	anti-B	"a" Cells	"b" Cells	
R	+	–	–	+	A
E	–	+	+	–	B
S	–	–	+	+	O
U	+	+	–	–	AB
L					
T					

Rh Testing

Anti-D reagent is used to determine the Rh of RBCs. Add 1 drop of 3% cell suspension and 1 drop anti-D reagent in a test tube labeled "D." Centrifuge for 15 seconds. Resuspend RBC button and observe for agglutination. If agglutination is present, RBCs are Rh positive. If no agglutination is present, RBCs are Rh negative.

Many anti-D reagents require a control. One drop of 3% cell suspension and 1 drop of control reagent are added to a test tube labeled "DC" ("D" control). It is then centrifuged for 15 seconds and resuspended RBCs examined for agglutination. The control should always be negative for the test to be valid. Often in the blood bank, agglutination is graded according to the strength of the clumping. A positive is graded 1+, 2+, 3+, or 4+.

Checkpoint Question

7. *Which ABO blood group is the universal donor? What does this mean?*

➤ BLOOD SUPPLY

Today one of the major problems facing blood banks is obtaining sufficient amounts of safe blood and blood products to meet patient needs. There is a shortage of volunteer donors. The American Red Cross and other agencies collect blood from donors at blood mobiles or sometimes at fixed sites. One donor blood unit containing about 450 mL whole blood can be divided into three products:

1. Packed RBCs, which can be stored at 2° to 8°C for 42 days and used to treat anemia
2. Plasma, which can be frozen for 1 year and used to treat bleeding caused by a lack of coagulation factors such as fibrinogen

3. Platelet concentrates, which can be stored at room temperature for 5 days and used to treat bleeding due to low platelet count or dysfunctional platelets

The American Red Cross tests each donor blood unit for ABO group, Rh type, and unexpected antibodies to RBC antigens. It also tests each unit for infectious agents such as hepatitis, human immunodeficiency virus (HIV), and syphilis. The donors are also asked questions about their medical history to protect the safety of the blood supply.

A patient in an accident, who needs blood quickly, has few options except volunteer donor blood. Patients scheduled for elective surgery, however, have alternatives. Patients who are not anemic may give blood in advance of surgery for themselves. Under the physician's care, they can give up to 6 units starting 6 weeks before surgery. This is called autologous donation. During surgery, blood can be saved and returned to the patient using blood salvage equipment. The patient can ask family and friends to give in the directed donor program. The units are marked for the patient and cannot be given to anyone else. Both the autologous blood units and directed donor blood units are more costly than volunteer donor units. Directed donor units are no safer than volunteer donor units. Patients need to know they have options. The choice is made with the assistance of the physician.

What If?

What if a patient asks you about the criteria for donating blood?

The criteria for donating blood are determined by the American Red Cross based on recommendations from government agencies, the Centers for Disease Control and Prevention (CDC), and through various research projects. In addition, each state has its own laws regulating blood donors. Generally, blood donors must meet the following criteria:

- Age 18 years or older (individuals 17 years of age require a parent's permission; individuals 65 years of age or older require a physician's consent)
- Weight 110 lb or more
- Hemoglobin 12.5 g/dL (women) or 13.5 g/dL (men) or higher values
- Pulse 50 to 110 beats/min
- Blood pressure lower than 180 (systolic)/100 (diastolic)

The donor will also need to complete a brief patient history. The entire procedure will last approximately an hour; the actual blood donation time is about 10 minutes. Blood can be donated every 56 days. Only 1 unit (pint) will be taken at a time. All blood will be tested by the American Red Cross for HIV, hepatitis, and syphilis.

Checkpoint Question

8. What are three products that can be obtained from 1 unit whole blood and what are they used for?

SUMMARY

Testing in serology and other areas of the laboratory use the unique attraction between antigens and antibodies to identify and measure specific substances of interest in diagnosis of disease. The antigen–antibody attraction is both sensitive and specific. Test methods used include agglutination, enzyme immunoassay, chromatographic assay, agglutination inhibition, and competitive binding. For test results to be accurate, care must be taken in all steps leading to obtaining the results. Care in reporting results accurately is the final important step of quality assurance.

Immunohematology is the study of antigens and antibodies associated with RBCs and is used in blood banks to determine the compatibility of a donor's blood with that of a recipient. Major blood group antigens are ABO and Rh. The American Red Cross collects, divides, and tests blood from volunteer donors as well as blood from autologous and directed donors. Blood units can be divided into packed RBCs, frozen plasma, and platelet concentrates. Alternate blood sources include autologous donations, salvage blood systems, and directed donations.

CRITICAL THINKING CHALLENGES

1. You are working for Dr. Mathers, a cardiothoracic surgeon. Dr. Mathers performs many surgeries during which patients experience substantial blood loss, requiring transfusions. Identify the available options for blood transfusions. How would you explain these to a patient facing elective surgery?

2. Your local chapter of the American Red Cross is in great need for volunteer donors. Formulate a plan for encouraging more community members to donate blood. How can you put your plan into action?

ANSWERS TO CHECKPOINT QUESTIONS

1. A test that is specific and sensitive can measure a substance even if only a tiny amount is present (specificity) and it can pick that substance out of a solution containing millions of other related substances (sensitivity).

2. Three serology test methods are agglutination, enzyme immunoassays, and chromatographic assays. Enzyme immunoassays produce a color change and chromatographic assays produce a color bar if the test substance is present. With agglutination tests, clumping of particles (agglutination) occurs if the test substance is present.

3. Serum can be separated from a clot by using a pipette, a serum separation tube, or a serum filter.

4. Improperly stored kits may result in deterioration of the reagents, which may lead to false test results.

5. A false-negative result occurs when a patient tests negative for a disease, even though the disease is present. A false-positive result occurs when a test indicates that a patient has a particular disease, even though the patient is disease free. These results can be caused by technical problems in performing the test or by the patient's biologic condition.

6. Serology tests are easier to perform and provide results more quickly, but cultures are considered to be more sensitive.

7. Type O is the universal donor because it lacks A or B antigens, making it safe to give patients—no matter what their ABO group.

8. A single unit of whole blood can be divided into packed RBCs (used to treat anemia); plasma (used to treat bleeding from a lack of coagulation factors); and platelet concentrates (used to treat bleeding caused by low platelet count or dysfunctional platelets).

SUGGESTIONS FOR FURTHER READING

Barrett, J. T. (1991). *Medical Immunology: Tests and Review*. Philadelphia: F. A. Davis.

Bryant, N. J. (1992). *Laboratory Immunology and Serology*, 3rd ed. Philadelphia: W. B. Saunders.

Fischbach, F. (1992). *A Manual of Laboratory and Diagnostic Tests*, 4th ed. Philadelphia: J. B. Lippincott.

Fischbach, F. (1995). *Quick Reference for Common Laboratory and Diagnostic Tests*. Philadelphia: J. B. Lippincott.

Miller, L. E., (1991). *Manual of Laboratory Immunology*, 2nd ed. Philadelphia: Lea & Febiger.

Quinley, E. D. (1993). *Immunohematology: Principles and Practice*. Philadelphia: J. B. Lippincott.

Sheehan, C. (1990). *Clinical Immunology: Principles and Laboratory Diagnosis*. Philadelphia: J. B. Lippincott.

Turgeon, M. L. (1990). *Immunology and Serology in Laboratory Medicine*. St Louis: Mosby-Year Book.

Clinical Chemistry

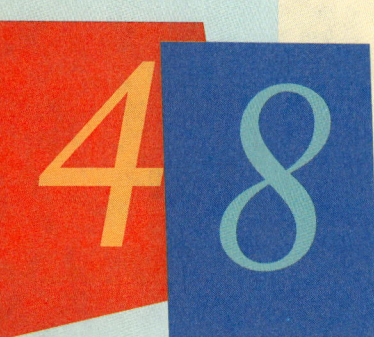

Chapter Outline

Special Instruments and Methods
Renal Function
    Electrolytes
    Nonprotein Nitrogenous Compounds
Liver Function
    Bilirubin
    Enzymes
    Albumin
    Other Tests
Thyroid Function
    Thyroid-Stimulating Hormone
Cardiac Function
    Lactate Dehydrogenase
    Creatine Kinase
Lung Function
    Blood Gases

Pancreatic Function
    Pancreatic Enzymes
    Pancreatic Hormones
Procedure: Determining Blood Glucose Using the Glucometer
Procedure: Glucose Tolerance Testing (GTT)
Lipids and Lipoproteins
    Cholesterol
    Low-Density Lipoprotein
    High-Density Lipoproteins
    Triglycerides
Summary
Critical Thinking Challenges
Answers to Checkpoint Questions
Suggestions for Further Reading

DACUM Components

1.3 Practice within the scope of education, training, and personal capabilities
4.1 Apply principles of aseptic technique and infection control
4.7 Prepare patients for procedures
4.10 Collect and process specimens
4.11 Perform selected tests that assist with diagnosis and treatment
5.1 Document accurately
7.2 Instruct patients with special needs

Chapter Competencies

Learning Objectives

Upon successfully completing this chapter, you will be able to:

1. Spell and define the Key Terms.
2. List the common electrolytes, explain the relationship of electrolytes with fluid and acid–base balance, and identify some conditions in which imbalances may occur.
3. Describe the nonprotein nitrogenous compounds, how they are formed, and name conditions with abnormal values.
4. Describe glucose utilization, regulation, and the purpose of the various glucose tests.
5. Describe the function of cholesterol and associated lipids in the body and their correlation to heart disease.
6. List and describe the substances commonly tested in liver function assessment.
7. Explain thyroid function assessment tests and hormones that regulate and are produced by the thyroid gland.
8. Describe how an assessment for a myocardial infarction is made with laboratory tests.
9. Describe how pancreatitis is diagnosed with laboratory tests.
10. List the components of blood gas analysis and the purpose in determining their levels.

Performance Objectives

Upon successfully completing this chapter, you will be able to:

1. Determine a blood glucose (Procedure 48-1).
2. Perform a glucose tolerance test (GTT) (Procedure 48-2).

Key Terms

(See Glossary for definitions.)

adenosine triphosphate (ATP)
artifactual
azotemia
basal metabolic rate
bicarbonate
bile
biliary obstruction
body fluids
catalyzes

challenge
cortisol
creatine
diuretics
extracellular
gestational diabetes
intracellular
iodine
ion

Krebs's cycle
lipase
lipids
lipoproteins
metabolic acidosis
muscular dystrophies
nitrogenous
pancreatitis
quantification
screening

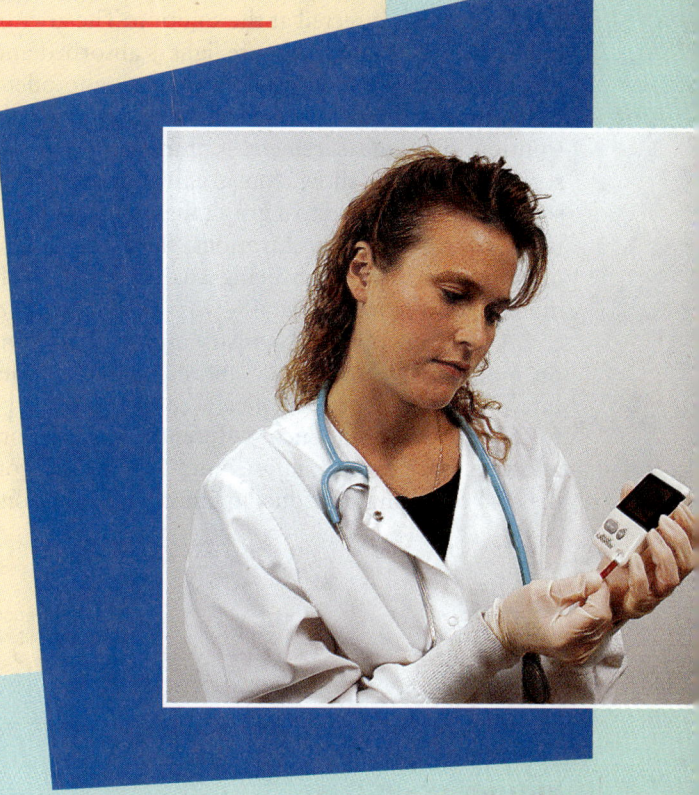

Clinical chemistry involves testing for many of the chemical components found in serum, plasma, blood, and **body fluids** (fluids that accumulate in the body's compartments). The chemical components can be electrically charged atoms called **ions** (K^+, Na^+, Cl^-), *metabolic by-products* (urea, creatinine), *proteins* (albumin, globulin), or *hormones* (testosterone, thyroid stimulating hormone). Determining the amount of these chemicals, or **quantification**, can help the physician to:

- Assess organ function (eg, bilirubin level is an indicator of liver function)
- Gain a better understanding of the patient's overall health status (eg, glucose and cholesterol levels are two chemical tests that can aid in assessing a patient's current level of health)

➤ SPECIAL INSTRUMENTS AND METHODS

A spectrophotometer is one of the earliest chemistry instruments. It is still widely used today for quantifying (determining the concentrations) of various substances in a patient's blood. Certain chemical substances, when reacted with other chemicals, will cause a color formation or a color change. The higher the concentration of the substance, the more intense the color reaction. When this solution is placed in the spectrophotometer, a light source is directed at the solution. The greater the intensity of the color, the more light is absorbed and the less light is allowed to pass through. A photodetector measures the amount of light that passes through the solution. This measurement is translated into an absorbance reading shown on a galvanometer. The absorbance is compared to a graph that contains the readings for all the concentrations, and the unknown quantity in the solution being analyzed can be determined in this manner (Fig. 48-1).

A large portion of chemistry analysis is performed on automated systems that mechanically sample, dilute, or add reagents (chemicals) to the patient's blood for quantifying components. Recently, automation has allowed more rapid analyses and has helped control the cost of testing by reducing human intervention.

Many methods are used to detect and quantify chemical compounds in blood. For example, certain chemicals will produce colors when burned in an instrument called a flame photometer and can be measured during the process. Other compounds will fluoresce (produce visible radiation rays) under certain circumstances, and this method can be used for determining the level or presence of that compound. Substrate (a substance that is acted on by an enzyme) utilization for enzyme levels is another testing method. An example of substrate utilization involves introducing starch into the serum and measuring the length of time for all the starch to be broken down. This can determine the amount of amylase present.

Many office analyzers (also called bench-top analyzers) use the color change principle to determine chemistry levels. Kodak, Baxter, and Miles Diagnostic are a few companies that manufacture bench-top analyzers.

Normal (reference) ranges for all chemistry results will vary from laboratory to laboratory depending on the assay used. The normal ranges that follow in this text may be altered in laboratories because of the use of different substrates, temperatures, and instrumentation.

Checkpoint Question
1. What types of chemical components are tested in the chemistry laboratory? Give examples of each.

➤ RENAL FUNCTION

The kidneys rid the body of waste products and help maintain *fluid balance* and *acid–base balance*. When the kidneys begin to fail, waste products such as urea, ammonia, and creatinine build up in the blood. The patient will become edematous and the delicate acid–base balance will be upset. Abnormal increases or decreases in the substances that affect acid–base balance will seriously compromise health and may cause death. To assess renal function, the physician may order tests for serum measurements of electrolytes, blood urea nitro-

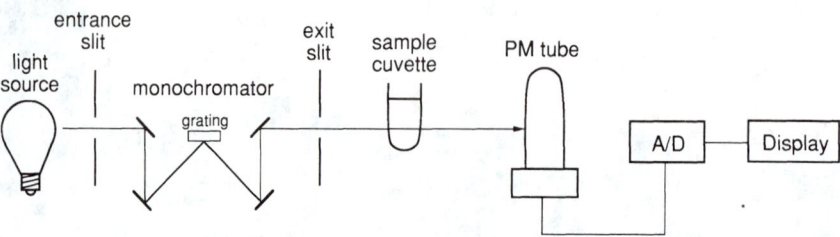

FIGURE 48-1
Single-beam spectrophotometer.

gen (BUN), creatinine, and other components. These tests, combined with information gained from urinalysis, can significantly aid in renal assessment.

Electrolytes

Electrolytes are ions (chemicals that carry a charge) found in blood and body fluids. They may be positively charged (cations) or negatively charged (anions). Electrolytes conduct electric impulses across cell membranes to maintain fluid and acid–base balance and aid in the functioning of nervous and muscle tissue.

Major body electrolytes include sodium, potassium, chloride, calcium, magnesium, phosphorus, and **bicarbonate** (dissolved form of carbon dioxide). The renal system helps regulate electrolytes and fluid and acid–base balance. In the presence of an electrolyte imbalance, electric impulses are not transmitted properly, resulting in fluid and acid–base imbalances and impaired functioning of nervous and muscle tissue. Table 48-1 summarizes common electrolyte imbalances, which are described below.

Sodium

Sodium (chemical symbol Na) is the major cation of the **extracellular** fluid (the fluid outside the cell). Normal serum levels range from 135 to 145 mEq/L. *Hyponatremia* (sodium level below 135 mEq/L) is one of

the most common electrolyte imbalances and can result from many factors, including gastrointestinal losses (vomiting, diarrhea), burns, cardiac or renal failure, and hypothyroidism. Symptoms of hyponatremia range in severity, depending on how low the value is. These may be manifested as subtle changes in energy levels and mental activity or, in severe forms, as neurologic malfunctions, including seizures.

Hypernatremia (sodium level above 145 mEq/L) can be caused by drug therapies, Cushing's syndrome, diabetes insipidus, and other pathologies. Typically, the kidneys help the body adjust to this more saline (salty) environment by not excreting as much water. In this way, sodium is diluted back to an acceptable level. Because water is retained in hypernatremia, the patient may present with signs of edema.

Potassium

Potassium (chemical symbol K) is the major cation of the **intracellular** fluid (fluid within the cell). Only 2% of potassium is extracellular; therefore, serum levels are much lower than sodium: 3.5 to 5.0 mEq/L. *Hypokalemia* (potassium level below 3.5 mEq/L) is seen with insulin therapy, gastrointestinal losses, and renal disease. *Hyperkalemia* (potassium level above 5.0 mEq/L) can occur with cell injuries and renal failure. **Artifactual** (caused by outside interference) hyperkalemia can result from red blood cell lysis, as in a traumatic venipuncture, or if the tourniquet is left on the arm too long or is applied too tightly. Abnormal blood levels of potassium can have profound effects on the neuromuscular system, resulting in muscle weakness, paralysis, and cardiac arrhythmias.

Chloride

Chloride (chemical symbol Cl) is the major anion of the extracellular fluid. The normal range for chloride is 96 to 110 mEq/L. *Hypochloremia* is a condition is which the serum chloride level is below 96 mEq/L. In *hyperchloremia* the serum chloride level is above 110 mEq/L. Chloride is closely associated with acid–base balance and is adversely affected in such conditions as diabetic ketoacidosis and **metabolic acidosis** (a condition of increased metabolic acids). Renal disease can alter chloride levels in either direction.

Calcium

Calcium (chemical symbol Ca) is a cation, with normal serum levels ranging from 8.5 to 10.5 mg/dL. *Hypocalcemia* (calcium level below 8.5 mg/dL) is associated with acute or chronic renal failure or electrolyte imbalances due to hypoparathyroidism. *Hypercalcemia* (cal-

---

Table 48-1

Terms Describing Electrolyte Imbalances

Imbalance	Definition
Hypernatremia	An excess of sodium in the blood
Hyponatremia	A deficit of sodium in the blood
Hyperkalemia	An excess of potassium in the blood
Hypokalemia	A deficit of potassium in the blood
Hyperchloremia	An excess of chloride in the blood
Hypochloremia	A deficit of chloride in the blood
Hyperphosphatemia	An excess of phosphate in the blood
Hypophosphatemia	A deficit of phosphate in the blood
Hypercalcemia	An excess of calcium in the blood
Hypocalcemia	A deficit of calcium in the blood
Hypermagnesemia	An excess of magnesium in the blood
Hypomagnesemia	A deficit of magnesium in the blood

(From Timby, B. K., Lewis, L. W., [1992]. Fundamental Skills and Concepts in Patient Care, 5th ed., p. 678. Philadelphia: J. B. Lippincott.)

cium level above 10.5 mg/dL) is associated with metabolic conditions such as hyperparathyroidism or excessive calcium intake or absorption due to medications or alterations in gastrointestinal metabolism.

Magnesium

Magnesium (chemical symbol Mg) is a cation found in intracellular fluid. Normal magnesium levels range from 1.3 to 2.1 mEq/L. *Hypomagnesemia* (magnesium level below 1.3 mEq/L) may result from shifts in body fluids and other electrolytes. *Hypermagnesemia* (magnesium level above 2.1 mEq/L) may also result from fluid and electrolyte shifts as well as from impaired excretion caused by kidney failure. Symptoms of hypermagnesemia are similar to those for hyperkalemia (see above).

Phosphorus

Phosphorus (chemical symbol P) is the major anion in the intracellular fluid. Normal phosphorus levels range from 2.5 to 4.5 mg/dL. *Hypophosphatemia* (phosphorus level below 2.5 mg/dL) can result from a number of factors, including inadequate absorption, gastrointestinal losses, electrolyte shifts, and endocrine disorders. *Hyperphosphatemia* (phosphorus level above 4.5 mg/dL) is associated with hypocalcemia, hypoparathyroidism, and renal impairment or failure. In patients with renal failure, soft-tissue calcification is seen as a long-term effect of hyperphosphatemia.

Bicarbonate

Bicarbonate (chemical symbol HCO_3) is formed when carbon dioxide (CO_2) dissolves in the bloodstream, providing another negatively charged ion to the extracellular fluid. Bicarbonate is the major factor in acid–base balance; increased levels result in *alkalosis* (the body pH is too basic) and decreased levels cause *acidosis* (the body pH is too acidic).

The acid–base system is extremely sensitive and cannot tolerate large pH fluctuations. The body's normal pH range is 7.35 to 7.45, very slightly basic from the neutral 7.0. The renal and respiratory systems work to regulate acid–base balance. Bicarbonate is breathed out in the form of CO_2 and is also excreted through the kidneys. Measurement of CO_2 is considered more useful for pH balance assessment than for measuring renal functioning, but it also aids in the overall assessment of renal function.

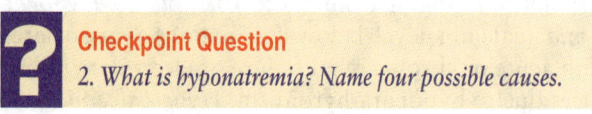

? Checkpoint Question
2. What is hyponatremia? Name four possible causes.

Nonprotein Nitrogenous Compounds

More than 15 different nonprotein **nitrogenous** (nitrogen-containing) compounds are recognized. Three that can be increased as a consequence of impaired renal function are urea, creatinine, and uric acid. However, other diseases can also affect the concentrations of these substances, making this a relatively nonspecific indicator.

Urea

Urea is the major end-product of protein and amino acid metabolism. Because urea is formed in the liver and excreted mainly by the kidneys, it can be an indicator for both liver and renal function. Typically, urea is measured as blood urea nitrogen (BUN) and ranges from 10 to 20 mg/dL. Various other factors affect BUN levels besides renal and liver functions, such as dietary intake of protein and state of hydration.

Creatinine

Creatinine is a breakdown product of **creatine**, which aids in delivering energy to cells. Creatine is a chemical compound that adds phosphorus to adenosine diphosphate (ADP) to make **adenosine triphosphate (ATP)**, the energy currency of the body. Normal range for creatinine is 0.8 to 1.7 mg/dL for men and 0.6 to 1.0 mg/dL for women depending on the muscle mass of the patient. Creatinine is more effective is assessing renal function than BUN. This is because only trace amounts of creatinine are reabsorbed in the renal tubules. Urinary excretion of this compound equals the amount produced in the body, whereas urea is reabsorbed to a certain extent. This is useful in determining the filtering ability of the kidneys.

A test called creatinine clearance is used for this purpose. A 24-hour urine sample is collected for a creatinine clearance because excretion of creatinine varies throughout the day. (See the procedure for 24-hour urine collection in Chap. 44, Urinalysis.)

The term used to describe elevated levels of urea and creatinine is **azotemia** (azo- means compounds containing nitrogen). A large increase in urea alone is called uremia. Liver and renal dysfunction can cause azotemia. Other conditions include dehydration, shock, trauma, congestive heart failure, skeletal muscle necrosis, starvation, and **muscular dystrophies** (diseases characterized by progressive atrophy of skeletal muscles). As levels of these toxins rise, systemic affects may include neurologic alterations (eg, memory loss, hallucinations, seizures, coma), cardiovascular alterations (eg, hypertension, congestive heart failure), and respiratory distress.

Uric Acid

Uric acid is a metabolic end-product of proteins containing purine. For men, the normal range is 4.0 to 8.5 mg/dL and for women it is 2.7 to 7.3 mg/dL. Like other nitrogen-containing compounds, uric acid is formed in the liver and excreted mostly by the kidneys; therefore, it can be an indicator of organ dysfunction. Clinically, increased amounts of uric acid are more significant than decreased amounts. *Hyperuricemia* is seen with renal failure, use of **diuretics** (substances that promote urine formation and excretion), obesity, and atherosclerosis. Diets high in proteins (meat, legumes, and yeast) can cause a mild case of hyperuricemia. The disease gout is characterized by a high uric acid accumulation in the joints; the joints become inflamed, producing significant discomfort. Typically, gout is due to an inborn error of metabolism (an inherited trait wherein an enzyme is missing or decreased so that a normal metabolic process is not fully functional). Gout can be treated with various drugs.

What If?

What if a patient is diagnosed with gout and asks you about dietary restrictions?

First and foremost, speak to the physician to determine if there are any other medical conditions that warrant a special diet. Patients with gout are usually placed on a low purine diet initially. Foods that are high in purine are liver, kidneys, sweetbreads, sardines, anchovies, and meat extracts. Diet and medications can often keep gout under control. Dietary retraining is usually done by the physician or a registered dietitian.

Checkpoint Question

3. What are the nonprotein nitrogenous compounds important for assessing renal function?

➤ LIVER FUNCTION

The liver is the largest gland of the body and one of the most complex. More than 500 of its functions have been identified. Among the major functions are the production of **bile** (bitter yellow-green secretion of the liver), metabolism of many compounds used by the body (glucose, fats, proteins, and vitamins), processing of bilirubin, and detoxifying substances found in the blood that could prove dangerous to the body.

Liver malfunction is an extremely serious condition. It can be brought on by disease, acute or chronic toxicities, cancer, or inherited abnormalities. Discussed below are some of the commonly tested chemistries that help determine liver function. Many laboratories offer a panel of tests often called liver function tests (LFTs). Typically included in this panel would be bilirubin, alkaline phosphatase, alanine aminotransferase, aspartate aminotransferase, total protein, and albumin. Table 48-2 shows how these tests are affected by abnormal liver conditions.

Bilirubin

When red blood cells break down, hemoglobin is released into the plasma. Hemoglobin, through a series of steps, is then converted into bilirubin. At this stage it is unconjugated (not attached to another compound) and is insoluble in water. It travels through the bloodstream until it enters the liver. Here it is converted into conjugated bilirubin, which is water soluble and excreted into the bile. Testing for serum bilirubin provides valuable information for diagnosis and evaluation of liver disease, biliary obstructions (blockage of bile ducts), and hemolytic anemias. Bilirubin has a yellow-orange color; if excess amounts settle into the skin and sclera, its presence will make the patient appear yellow (jaundiced).

Note: Bilirubin is extremely sensitive to light and will break down readily when exposed to ultraviolet rays. Testing should be performed within 1 hour of collection or the specimen should be placed in an area where it will be protected from light.

Enzymes

An enzyme is a protein produced by living cells and **catalyzes** (speeds up) chemical reactions. The liver has many enzymes to speed up its various processes. Some of these can be found in the serum and in quantities sufficient for analysis.

Alkaline Phosphatase

Alkaline phosphatase (ALP or AP) is present in the bones, liver, intestines, kidneys, and placenta. Circulating ALP is primarily from the liver and bone. Levels of ALP will rise in disorders such as Paget's disease (bone) or hepatitis (liver).

Normal values vary with age. Increased levels of ALP are considered normal during periods of bone growth activity, such as childhood growth spurts and third trimester pregnancy. These elevated levels are not indicators of a disease process.

Table 48-2
Chemistry Tests Affected By Abnormal Liver Conditions

Chemistry Test	Normal Values	Acute Hepatitis	Cirrhosis	Obstructive Jaundice	Liver Cancer
Albumin	3.5–5.0 g/dL	NL/↓	↑	NL/↓	↓
Bilirubin	Direct: 0.4 mg/dL Total: 1.0 mg/dL	↑↑	↑	↑	NL/↓
Alkaline phosphatase	30–115 IU/L	↑	NL/↑	↑	NL/↓
Aspartate aminotransferase	0–41 IU/L	NL/↑	NL/↑	NL/↑	NL/↑
Alanine aminotransferase	0–45 IU/L	↑↑	NL/↑	↑	NL/↑

NL, normal; ↑, increased; ↑↑, marked increase; ↓, decreased

Alanine Aminotransferase (ALT) and Aspartate Aminotransferase (AST)

These enzymes are present in the liver. AST, however, is present in many other organs as well. Increased levels of ALT and AST are seen with liver damage; AST also rises in myocardial infarctions.

Albumin

Albumin is the major protein in the blood. The liver is responsible for its manufacture. Albumin serves as a transport protein linking up with other chemical compounds that otherwise could not be processed. When liver function is impaired, albumin values decrease. The normal range for albumin is 3.6 to 5.2 g/dL.

Other Tests

Other laboratory tests used to evaluate liver function are total protein (normal range, 6–8 g/dL), cholesterol (discussed in the section "Lipids and Lipoproteins," below), and the prothrombin time (see Chap. 46, Hematology, for a discussion of prothrombin time). Techniques such as imaging (eg, ultrasound) and biopsies also help in diagnosis.

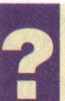

Checkpoint Question

4. What are three diseases that can be diagnosed by testing bilirubin levels?

➤ THYROID FUNCTION

The thyroid gland regulates metabolism by secreting the hormones triiodothyronine (T_3) and thyroxine (T_4). Its primary function is to establish the **basal metabolic rate**, which is the amount of energy used in a unit of time to maintain vital functions. The thyroid gland is controlled by another hormone, thyroid-stimulating hormone (TSH), which is produced in the anterior pituitary gland.

Thyroid-Stimulating Hormone

In the absence of a disease process, when additional thyroid hormones are needed, more TSH is secreted to stimulate the thyroid gland. In the same manner, when lesser amounts of the hormones are required, less TSH is secreted so the thyroid gland will reduce its production. However, many situations can cause an imbalance in this delicate endocrine system. There may be a malfunction in the anterior pituitary gland so that it over- or undersecretes TSH. If the thyroid gland is malfunctioning, it cannot be stimulated, regardless of the amount of TSH secreted. TSH levels may be quite high in cases such as this.

Triiodothyronine and Thyroxine

The thyroid hormones, T_3 and T_4, target many organs to control various processes (see above). For T_3 and T_4 to be present in sufficient quantities, a functional thyroid gland and adequate amounts of **iodine** (an essential micronutrient) are required. Elevations of one or both hormones along with TSH levels aid in the diagnosis of various conditions.

➤ CARDIAC FUNCTION

Several enzymes can be analyzed for the diagnosis of a myocardial infarction (MI). When an MI occurs, these enzymes are released in large quantities by the damaged heart muscle into the bloodstream.

Lactate Dehydrogenase

Lactate dehydrogenase (LDH or LD) is widely distributed in body tissues but concentrated in the myocardium, liver, kidney, and muscle. LDH is markedly increased within 24 hours of an MI; elevations usually return to normal in 8 to 14 days. Elevations are also seen with certain leukemias, pulmonary infarctions, hemolytic anemias, and progressive muscular dystrophy. LDH has five isoenzymes, LDH-1 to LDH-5. Isoenzymes are similar but not identical structures that have the same function but originate in different organs. In a normal profile, LDH-2 is in greater quantity than LDH-1, but an MI causes LDH-1 to be much higher.

Creatine Kinase

Creatine Kinase (CK) is found almost exclusively in skeletal muscle and myocardium. Within 2 to 8 hours of an MI, CK levels will increase. CK will also be increased in crushing injuries to muscles, such as those sustained in car accidents. CK has three isoenzymes, designated MM (muscle), MB (hybrid), and BB (brain). Most of the normal levels of CK consist of the MM fraction. The MB fraction rises with an MI.

Note: The aspartate aminotransferase level (see section on "Liver Function") will also rise after an MI but takes longer to detect (2–3 days). Other techniques, such as electrocardiograms, are also used for assessing cardiac function (Table 48-3).

> **Checkpoint Question**
> 5. Which enzyme will assist the physician in the diagnosis of a myocardial infarction (MI) within 3 hours of onset? Why?

➤ LUNG FUNCTION

The lungs are the organs that bring oxygen into contact with the circulatory system and aid in the removal of the waste product carbon dioxide. The lungs, along with the kidneys, help regulate acid–base balance. There are many methods of assessing lung function using respiratory therapy; in the laboratory, assessment is accomplished with blood gases.

Blood Gases

Specimens for blood gases are usually drawn from an artery; therefore, they are typically termed arterial blood gases (ABGs). However, venous or capillary spec-

Table 48-3

Enzymes Elevated After a Myocardial Infarction

Enzyme	Timing of Release	Special Notation
Lactate dehydrogenase	• Begins rise at 24 h. • Peaks at 3–6 days. • Reaches baseline at approximately 2 weeks.	Isoenzyme LDH-1 is greater in relation to LDH-2.
Creatine kinase	• Begins rise at 2–8 h. • Peak is variable. • Reaches baseline at 4 days.	Isoenzyme CK-MB is the increased fraction.
Aspartate amino transferase	• Begins rise at 8 h. • Peaks at 18–36 h. • Reaches baseline at 4 days.	

Table 48-4

Blood Gases in Relation to Acid–Base Balance in the Body

Condition in the Body	pH	Oxygen Tension	Oxygen Saturation	Carbon Dioxide Tension	Bicarbonate
Normal	7.35–7.45	75–100 mm Hg	96–100%	35–45 mm Hg	22–26 mEq/L
Respiratory acidosis	<7.35			>45 mm Hg	
Metabolic acidosis	<7.35				<22 mEq/L
Respiratory alkalosis	>7.45			<35 mm Hg	
Metabolic alkalosis	>7.45				>26 mEq/L

imens are used on occasion. Blood gases consist of oxygen, carbon dioxide, and nitrogen. These gases are given as percentages and partial pressures. By comparing blood gas values to the normal ranges, the physician can assess a patient's ventilatory status (how well the patient is oxygenated). Also included in the determination is the patient's acid–base balance or pH (Tables 48-4 and 48-5). The blood gas determination is often used to aid in the evaluation of cardiac failure, hemorrhage, kidney failure, diabetes, shock, and drug overdose.

➤ PANCREATIC FUNCTION

The pancreas functions in both the endocrine and exocrine systems and produces many secretions. Amylase and **lipase**, two of its exocrine system products, are released as excretory enzymes into the intestines to aid in digestion. Insulin and glucagon are hormonal products of its endocrine function and are released into the bloodstream to regulate carbohydrate metabolism.

Pancreatic Enzymes

Amylase

Amylase is markedly increased with **pancreatitis** (inflammation of the pancreas). The salivary glands also produce amylase, which accounts for the elevated levels found with sialoadenitis and other inflammatory diseases of the salivary glands such as mumps.

Lipase

Lipase levels also rise with pancreatitis. For a differential diagnosis of pancreatitis, it is recommended that both of the enzymes be quantitated.

Table 48-5

Causes of Acid-Base Imbalance

Condition	Possible Causes
Respiratory acidosis	Obstructive lung disease, respiratory depression due to drug toxicity or disease, other causes of hypoventilation
Metabolic acidosis	Diarrhea (bicarbonate loss), diabetic acidosis, renal failure, aspirin toxicity, ammonium chloride therapy, starvation, diabetes, heart failure, shock
Respiratory alkalosis	Hypoxia, anxiety, pulmonary embolus, pregnancy, other causes of hypoventilation
Metabolic alkalosis	Diuretic therapy, severe gastrointestinal losses, Cushing's syndrome, excessive ingestion of antacids

Pancreatic Hormones

Glucose is one of the main energy sources for the body. When foods are broken down by the metabolic processes, many nutrients are released. Sugars, mainly glucose, provide energy by entering a complex biochemical pathway called the **Krebs's cycle**, also known as the citric acid cycle. As glucose works through this metabolic chain of events, one of the co-events in the breakdown of glucose into carbon dioxide (CO_2) and water is the generation of adenosine triphosphate (ATP).

For glucose to be used for stored energy in the form of glycogen, it must be brought into the cells where the Krebs's cycle occurs. Two hormones regulate this process: insulin and glucagon. Blood glucose levels need to be maintained within narrow limits so that there are no adverse physical effects. By their actions, insulin and glucagon keep these levels within the approximate range.

Glucose-Regulating Hormones

Insulin brings the glucose used for energy into cells for immediate use or for storage. If there is sufficient energy available for cell use, the glucose is stored as either glycogen (long chains of glucose) in the liver and muscles or as fat. Insulin is an important hormone; cells would starve if insulin were not available or were not able to bring glucose in for energy. By arranging for glucose storage, insulin keeps glucose levels down, thereby stabilizing it within a normal range.

Glucagon is a hormone that causes glucose stored in the form of glycogen to be released into the bloodstream, thereby raising glucose levels. Whenever blood glucose levels drop, glucagon acts on glycogen to break it apart so molecules of glucose are available for cellular use.

Common Glucose Tests

The time during which a blood sample is taken for glucose testing can assist in the diagnostic or monitoring process. The tests described below are the most frequently ordered.

The glucose reflectance photometer (glucose meter) is often used as a quick, accurate, easy-to-perform in-office procedure to measure a patient's blood glucose level. Glucose meters are commercially available under different names: the Glucometer made by Ames, the Accu-Chek by Boeringer Mannheim, and the Glucosan by Lifescan. The basic testing principle involves the application of whole blood to a reagent strip, which is read optically by the instrument after a designated time period. The amount of color change (to

Charting Example

| 03/05/99 | 1500 | Lancet skin puncture right index finger. Glucose tested with Gluco-meter — results: 60 mg/dL. Dr. Peters was notified. Pt. was given a glass of orange juice. —————— Sue Rogers, CMA |

blue) correlates with glucose concentration and a value is reported.

FASTING BLOOD GLUCOSE (SUGAR)

A fasting blood sugar (FBS) can be obtained from the patient after a 12- to 14-hour fast (nothing but water is taken in during the fast). Procedure 48-1 describes the process for obtaining a FBS using a Glucometer. The normal range for an FBS is typically 50 to 110 mg/dL, but there may be a slight interlaboratory variation depending on the population used to establish the normal range.

The main purpose of an FBS is to detect either diabetes mellitus or hypoglycemia. Fasting glucose levels of 140 mg/dL or greater are considered indicative of diabetes. Further testing by either another FBS, a 2-hour postprandial glucose test, or a glucose tolerance test is used to corroborate the initial high result. Hypoglycemia is a syndrome characterized by FBS levels below 45 mg/dL and a variety of symptoms: sweating, weakness, dizziness, headache, trembling, lethargy, and other nervous manifestations.

RANDOM BLOOD GLUCOSE

Although a random glucose is not as diagnostically useful as a fasting test, it is a good **screening** tool (preliminary test) on otherwise healthy patients. A random glucose can be drawn anytime during the day and has a slightly broader range: 45 to 130 mg/dL.

2-HOUR POSTPRANDIAL GLUCOSE

A 2-hour postprandial (designated 2 hr pp) is usually used for individuals already diagnosed with diabetes. The patient must eat a high carbohydrate meal after a 12-hour fast. Patients who may not be compliant are given a glucose solution to drink as a substitute for the meal for better control of the testing results. Two hours after the meal, a blood sample is drawn and

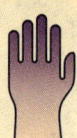

Procedure 48-1   Determining Blood Glucose Using the Glucometer

Equipment/Supplies

- Glucometer (or glucose meter of the physician's choice)
- glucose reagent strips
- lancet
- alcohol pad
- sterile gauze
- paper towel
- appropriate biohazard barrier devices (eg, gloves, impervious gown, face shield)

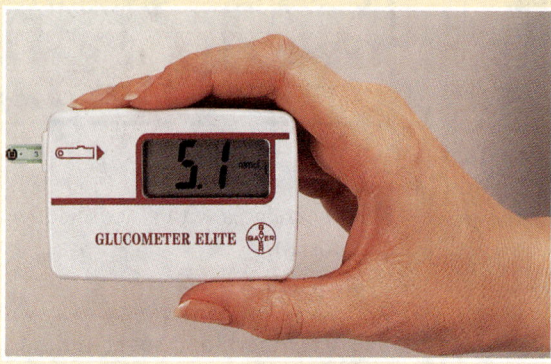

Glucometer Elite blood glucose monitoring device. (Courtesy of Bayer Corporation, Ekhart, Indiana)

Steps	Purpose
1. Wash your hands.	1. Handwashing aids infection control.
2. Assemble the equipment and supplies.	2. This ensures that everything you need is available.
3. Put on gloves before removing reagent strip.	3. Standard Precautions must be observed when handling blood or body fluids. Sugar residues on hands can falsely elevate glucose results if the strip is contaminated by touching.
4. Turn the Glucometer on and ensure that it is calibrated. The digits 888 appear on the display screen followed by the code of the strips being used.	4. Calibration of the glucose meter is essential for accurate test results.
5. Remove one reagent strip, lay it on the paper towel, and recap the container.	5. The strip is ready for testing. The paper towel will serve as a disposable work surface and will absorb excess blood added to the strip. The strips are sensitive to humidity and will deteriorate if allowed to absorb moisture.
6. Greet and identify the patient. Explain the procedure. Ask for and answer any questions.	6. Identifying the patient prevents errors. Explaining the procedure helps ease anxiety and ensure compliance.

(continued)

glucose is measured. Timing of the specimen collection is extremely important in this test result. "Good control" of diabetes has been defined as a 2 hr pp of less than 130 mg/dL.

GLUCOSE TOLERANCE TEST

The glucose tolerance test (GTT) is used for diagnosing diabetes and hypoglycemia. The patient is challenged (tested) with a large dose of glucose, then blood glucose levels are checked at intervals to see how the body is metabolizing the glucose. Many conditions can affect a GTT. Strict control should be maintained where possible to minimize extraneous factors. A diet of 150 g of carbohydrate per day is usually ordered for 3 days before the test. Other carbohydrate levels will be calibrated by body weight if the weight is not what is expected for a

Procedure 48-1 Determining Blood Glucose Using the Glucometer *(continued)*

Steps	Purpose
7. Have the patient wash hands.	7. Washing removes sugar residues from the skin and the warm water stimulates blood flow.
8. Cleanse the selected site (finger) with alcohol and puncture with a lancet, following the steps described in Chapter 45, Phlebotomy. Wipe away the first drop of blood. Turn the patient's hand palm down and gently squeeze the finger to form a large drop of blood.	8. Alcohol removes bacteria from the site. Gentle squeezing obtains a blood specimen without diluting the sample with tissue fluid.
9. Bring the reagent strip up to the finger and touch the pad to the blood. Do not touch the finger. Completely cover the pad with blood.	9. The entire pad must be covered for accurate reading. There is no chance of contamination by oils or other residue remaining on the finger if this surface is not touched.
10. Immediately press the TIME button. The Glucometer counts up to 60 seconds. (Meanwhile, apply pressure to the puncture wound with gauze.) At the end of 60 seconds, firmly wipe the blood off with a clean gauze. The Glucometer continues to count for another 60 seconds. During this time, the reagent strip is inserted into the chamber with the pad side down.	10. This time frame allows the reaction changes to occur.
11. At 120 seconds, the Glucometer reads the reaction strip and displays the result on the screen in mg/dL. If the glucose level is higher or lower than expected, refer to the troubleshooting guide provided by the manufacturer.	11. The reaction is now complete. The color change is photo-optically measured and reported in mg/dL.
12. Thank the patient and give appropriate instructions.	12. Courtesy encourages the patient to have a positive attitude about the laboratory or physician's office.
13. Properly care for or dispose of equipment and supplies. Clean the work area. Remove gloves and wash your hands.	13. Standard Precautions must be followed throughout the procedure.
14. Record the results.	14. Procedures are considered not to have been done if they are not recorded.

Quality assurance measure: *Controls are available in the low, normal, and high range to ensure that the glucose meter is functioning properly. These controls should be run daily or every time a patient glucose test is performed if the meter is not used daily.*

normal adult. The day of the test, the patient should fast for 12 hours and should not smoke or exercise before the test. Also, the patient should have been free of illnesses during the previous 2 weeks. These precautions are taken because glucose utilization is affected by many factors and can interfere with an accurate picture of how the body would normally metabolize glucose.

Briefly, the GTT is performed by administering an amount of glucose calculated by the patient's weight. Blood is obtained ½, 1, 2, and 3 hours after the glucose has been administered. Blood sampling *must* occur at the precise times indicated for valid diagnosis. Urine specimens may also be collected during the timed intervals.

Procedure 48-2 — Glucose Tolerance Testing (GTT)

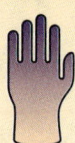

Equipment/Supplies

- calibrated amount of glucose per the physician's order
- urine specimen cups
- urine dipsticks for glucose determination
- glucose meter equipment
- alcohol wipes
- stopwatch
- appropriate biohazard barrier devices (eg, gloves, impervious gown, face shield)

Steps	Purpose
1. Wash your hands.	1. Handwashing aids infection control.
2. Assemble the equipment and supplies.	2. To ensure that everything you need is available. A stopwatch is necessary because the timing of the collections is important to the test results.
3. Greet and identify the patient. Explain the procedure. Ask for and answer any questions.	3. Identifying the patient prevents errors. Explaining the procedure helps ease anxiety and ensure compliance.
4. Put on gloves, gown, and face shield.	4. Standard Precautions must be observed when handling blood and body fluids.
5. Obtain a fasting glucose (FBS) specimen and urine from the patient. (See Procedure 48-1 and Chap. 44, Urinalysis, for the steps for performing these procedures.) It is recommended that laboratories test the blood sample before you administer the glucose drink; if the FBS exceeds a certain reading (eg, greater than 140 mg/dL), do not perform the GTT. Notify the physician.	5. Fasting glucose gives a baseline for further interpretation. Giving more glucose to a patient whose blood glucose level is already too high could cause serious harm.
6. Give the glucose drink to the patient ideally to consume within a 5-minute period. Note the time the patient finishes the drink; this is the "START" of the test.	6. The body begins to metabolize the glucose immediately, so rapid ingestion of the drink is necessary.
7. Exactly 30 minutes after the patient has finished the glucose drink, obtain blood sugar and urine specimens. (See Procedure 48-1 and Chap. 44, Urinalysis, for the steps for performing these procedures.) LABEL THE SPECIMENS WITH THE PATIENT'S NAME AND TIME OF COLLECTION.	7. Precise timing of specimen collection is vital for accurate interpretation of results. Many specimens will be received from this patient, making proper notation of the sequence extremely important.

(continued)

Blood may be drawn by venipuncture (see Chap. 45, Phlebotomy). If the blood is to be stored for processing, it should be centrifuged as soon as possible and the testing should be performed on either serum or plasma. This procedure stabilizes the glucose, which might otherwise be destroyed by the red blood cells in whole blood. Sodium fluoride may be added to the tube if it is not to be centrifuged to prevent glucose destruction.

Blood also may be drawn using capillary puncture (see Chap. 45, Phlebotomy). The number of samples required make capillary collection more acceptable to the patient and the accuracy of the glucose meter makes this method a viable option. Procedure 48-2 describes the steps to follow when performing a GTT.

Interpretation of GTT Results. The medical assistant does not interpret the results of the GTT. However, knowledge of how patients with various conditions (diabetes, hypoglycemia) will respond to this testing can be useful.

Numerous methods can be used to interpret the values obtained from a GTT. The criteria proposed by the National Diabetes Data Group and the World Health

Procedure 48-2   Glucose Tolerance Testing (GTT) (continued)

Steps	Purpose
8. Exactly 1 hour after the glucose drink, repeat step 7.	
9. Exactly 2 hours after the glucose drink, repeat step 7.	
10. Exactly 3 hours after the glucose drink, repeat step 7. Unless a GTT of longer than 3 hours has been requested, the testing is complete at this time. (For a longer GTT, continue specimen collection in the same manner for as many additional hours as required.)	
11. Thank the patient and give appropriate instructions.	11. Courtesy encourages the patient to have a positive attitude about the laboratory or the physician's office.
12. If the specimens are to be tested by an outside laboratory, package as required and arrange for transportation.	12. Careful handling and transport helps ensure accurate testing.
13. Properly care for or dispose of equipment and supplies. Clean the work area. Remove gloves, gown, and face shield and wash your hands.	13. Standard Precautions must be followed throughout the procedure.
14. Record the data.	14. Procedures are considered not to have been done if they are not recorded.

Note: *Ensure that the patient remains fairly sedentary throughout this procedure (eg, no long walks between blood draws); exercising will alter the glucose level by burning it for more energy. The patient also should avoid smoking because it may artificially increase the glucose level. Only water should be ingested. Encourage the patient to drink water to increase the blood volume and make it easier to draw blood from venipuncture and to collect urine specimens. If the patient experiences any severe symptoms (eg, headache, dizziness, vomiting), end the test and notify the physician. These symptoms could be the result of glucose levels that are too high or too low for the patient to tolerate.*

Organization, and endorsed by the American Diabetes Association, recommend that a diagnosis of diabetes be established if the fasting glucose level is greater than 140 mg/dL and the 2-hour measurement is equal to or above 200 mg/dL. Some sources recommend as well that another value between fasting and the 2-hour (ie, either the ½ or 1 hour) be above 200 mg/dL.

Hypoglycemia can also be diagnosed by the GTT, but it is often not as useful. Symptoms of hypoglycemia include headaches, weakness, shakiness, fatigue, sweating, and light-headedness. Whenever any of these occur during a GTT, it is important to obtain a blood specimen from the patient even if it is not at an appointed time. Unfortunately, many times a lower-than-normal range glucose level does not correspond to the symptoms presented. Different authors noting this theorize that emotional states and anxieties may be causing the symptoms, not lowered glucose levels. Frequently, these same patients will improve when their food intake is divided so that they eat many small meals (thereby introducing smaller glucose loads) rather than several large ones. This leads to the consideration that an imbalance of glucose levels has some merit in explaining why these symptoms appear.

Charting Example

09/15/99	0800 *GTT test:*
	0800 *FBS — 100 mg/dL. Urine specimen sent to the laboratory.*
	0810 *glucose drink given to patient.* 0815 *glucose drink finished.*
	0845 *glucose — 125 mg/dL, urine sent to lab.* 0915 *glucose — 132*
	mg/dL, urine sent to lab. 1015 *glucose — 120 mg/dL, urine sent to lab.*
	1115 *glucose — 110 mg/dL, urine sent to lab. Pt. tolerated procedure*
	well, d/c by Dr. Lynch. ———————————— Sue Collins, RMA

Checkpoint Question

6. What is hypoglycemia? List the symptoms associated with this disorder.

DIABETIC GLUCOSE TESTING

Although blood glucose levels are used to detect and monitor the diabetic patient, the test of choice is hemoglobin A_{1C}. This allows the physician to get a more accurate picture of the diabetic's physiologic state over long periods of time (weeks to several months).

Glucose converts the A portion of hemoglobin into A_{1C}, which is simply the glucose attached to a portion of hemoglobin A. As glucose levels increase over long periods of time, increasing amounts of hemoglobin A are converted to A_{1C}. A certain amount of conversion is considered to be in the "good control" range. Above a certain level of hemoglobin A_{1C} indicates to the physician that the patient has "poor control" of the condition even if the fasting blood sugar at the time is acceptable.

Patient Education: Using a Glucometer

Many diabetic patients are discharged with instructions for using a Glucometer. As a medical assistant, you can help the patient learn to perform this procedure. Here are points to stress:

- Teach patients about the need to regularly test and document glucose levels.
- Offer instructions in the proper technique for obtaining a blood sample (eg, do not "milk" the finger, cleanse the area well before beginning).
- Caution patients against "self-regulating" insulin. Have patients call the physician for abnormal glucose levels.
- Alert patients to the signs and symptoms of high and low glucose levels and the treatments for each.

Most pharmacies and surgical supply stores that sell Glucometers will be able to educate patients in their use. The strips for Glucometers are expensive and may be covered by certain insurance companies if the physician clearly documents the need.

OBSTETRIC GLUCOSE TESTING

An increase of glucose intolerance has been noted among pregnant patients in the second and third trimesters. Because **gestational diabetes** can endanger the fetus, the pregnant patient's glucose level needs to be monitored. The widely accepted screening method used for this purpose is to administer a 100-g glucose load in drink form and draw blood samples 1 hour later. If the value exceeds 155 mg/dL, a glucose tolerance test is indicated for a diagnosis of gestational diabetes. This screening method is usually done during the second trimester.

➤ LIPIDS AND LIPOPROTEINS

Cholesterol and associated **lipids** (free fatty acids) and **lipoproteins** (substances composed of lipids and proteins) have long been implicated as the culprits in heart disease. It is important to remember, however, that these compounds are part of the important building blocks of our bodies and in proper quantities are vital to health maintenance. They are a component of every cell membrane and of the myelin sheath around the nerves. They also cushion and support organs. Testing for these quantities aids the physician in assessing the risk of heart disease and assesses liver function because many of these compounds are formed and stored in the liver.

Cholesterol

Bile acids, formed partially by cholesterol, are produced in the liver and stored in the gallbladder, and are then released into the intestine as needed for the digestion of fats. Vitamin D is formed from cholesterol at the skin's surface when exposed to sunlight. Various hormones such as **cortisol**, testosterone, and estrogen are synthesized from cholesterol as well. Only in proportions not necessary for cell maintenance and other body functions should cholesterol be considered a health hazard.

Measurement of cholesterol is done on a 12- to 14-hour fasting specimen. The ideal range for cholesterol is 140 to 200 mg/dL (as recommended by the American Heart Association). Anyone with a cholesterol level greater than 200 mg/dL is considered to be at increased risk of developing atherosclerosis.

Low-Density Lipoprotein

Low-density lipoprotein (LDL) is a plasma protein that transports cholesterol, carrying it from the liver and depositing it on the walls of large and medium-sized arteries. Atherosclerotic plaques form causing the vessel to thicken and become more rigid. Circulation is then reduced to the organs and other areas normally supplied by this artery. Atherosclerosis is the major cause of coronary heart disease, angina pectoris, myocardial infarctions, and other cardiac disorders. When LDL values are above normal range, the risk of heart disease is greater.

High-Density Lipoprotein

High-density lipoprotein (HDL) is the protein molecule that carries cholesterol that has been deposited on arterial walls back to the liver. HDL typically exists in lesser quantities than LDL does. Much research has

---

Table 48-6
Risk Factors for Premature Atherosclerosis and Coronary Heart Disease

Chemistry Test	Low Risk	Moderate Risk	High Risk
Cholesterol	Levels at or below 200 mg/dL	Levels above 200 mg/dL	Levels above 200 mg/dL
HDL	Levels within or above normal range	Levels within or above normal range	Levels below normal range
LDL	Levels within or below normal range	Levels within or below normal range	Levels above normal range
Triglycerides	Levels within or below normal range	Levels within or below normal range	Levels above normal range

Note: *Frequently, a patient's chemistry tests will fall into two of the categories, so that the patient's risk group is not clearly defined. The physician decides the degree of risk for the patient based on these tests and other risk factors, such as life-style and family history. Normal range will vary by age and sex.*
HDL, high-density lipoprotein; LDL, low-density lipoprotein

Table 48-7

Common Chemistry Panel Tests

Test	Function in the Body	Normal Values	Increases Seen With	Decreases Seen With
Blood urea nitrogen (BUN)	Metabolic by-product	10–20 mg/dL	Kidney disease, kidney obstructions, dehydration	Liver failure, malnutrition
Calcium	Structural element for bones, teeth, and muscles	8.5–10.5 mg/dL	Hyperparathyroidism, hyperthyroidism, Addison's disease, bone cancer, multiple myeloma, other malignancies	Hypoparathyroidism, renal failure
Chloride	Acid–base balance, component of stomach acid	96–110 mEq/L	Dehydration, Cushing's syndrome, hyperventilation	Severe vomiting, severe diarrhea, severe burns, pyloric obstruction, heat exhaustion
Cholesterol	Building block for cell membranes, steroid hormones, and bile acids	120–200 mg/dL	Atherosclerosis, heart disease, certain liver diseases with obstruction, hypothyroidism	Liver disease, hyperthyroidism, malabsorption syndromes
Creatinine	Metabolic by-product	0.6–1.7 mg/dL	Kidney disease, muscle disease	Muscular dystrophy
Glucose	Energy source for body	70–110 mg/dL	Diabetes mellitus, Cushing's syndrome, liver disease	Excess insulin, Addison's disease, bacterial sepsis, hypothyroidism
Phosphorus	Used in bone and endocrine processes	2.5–4.5 mg/dL	Renal disease, hypoparathyroidism, hypocalcemia, Addison's disease	Hyperparathyroidism, bone disease
Potassium	Acid–base balance	3.5–5.0 mEq/L	Kidney disease, cell damage, Addison's disease	Diarrhea, starvation, severe vomiting, severe burns, some forms of liver disease
Sodium	Fluid balance	135–145 mEq/L	Dehydration, Cushing's syndrome, diabetes insipidus	Severe burns, diarrhea, vomiting, Addison's disease
Triglycerides	Energy source, lipid deposits for stored energy and organ support	40–170 mg/dL	Atherosclerosis, liver disease, poorly controlled diabetes, pancreatitis	Malnutrition
Uric acid	Metabolic by-product	Men: 4.0–8.5 mg/dL Women: 2.7–7.3 mg/dL	Renal failure, gout, leukemia, eclampsia	Drug therapy to lower uric acid levels

been directed along the lines of increasing HDL because higher levels of this correlate with decreased risk of heart disease. In contrast, decreased HDL levels correlate with increased risk of heart disease.

Triglycerides

Triglycerides are the principal lipids in blood. They also are the lipids in all vegetable and animal fats. Adipose (fatty) tissue is composed almost entirely of triglycerides. The normal range for men is 40 to 160 mg/dL and for women, 35 to 135 mg/dL. Research is implicating triglycerides as a risk factor in heart disease (Table 48-6).

A summary of the common chemistry tests is presented in Table 48-7.

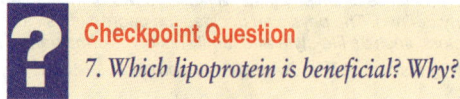

Checkpoint Question
7. Which lipoprotein is beneficial? Why?

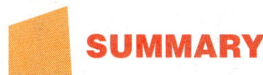

SUMMARY

Testing for the many chemical substances found in the blood is an important diagnostic and monitoring tool. Such tests help the physician to determine the functioning of various organs, including the kidneys, liver, thyroid, heart, pancreas, and lungs. Certain tests, such as glucose tests and tests of lipids and lipoproteins, also assist the physician in assessing a patient's general health status.

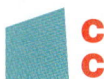

CRITICAL THINKING CHALLENGES

1. A patient with edema is told by her physician to restrict her salt intake. Why may this help improve her condition?
2. A diabetic patient gave herself too much insulin by mistake. Would you expect her glucose to be very high or very low? Why?
3. A patient's amylase level is very high but her lipase level is in the normal range. What might she have?
4. A medical assistant draws a red top tube for a number of chemistry tests. Unfortunately, the tube is left on the counter for several hours before being centrifuged and refrigerated. Which chemistries may be affected by this? Why?

ANSWERS TO CHECKPOINT QUESTIONS

1. Chemical components tested include ions (K^+, Na^+, C^-), metabolic by-products (urea, creatinine), proteins (albumin, globulin), or hormones (testosterone, thyroid-stimulating hormone).
2. Hyponatremia is a sodium deficiency that can be caused by gastrointestinal losses (vomiting, diarrhea), burns, cardiac or renal failure, and hypothyroidism.

3. Urea, creatinine, and uric acid are important for assessing renal function.
4. Testing of bilirubin levels aids in the diagnosis of liver disease, biliary obstructions, and hemolytic anemias.
5. Creatine Kinase (CK) can help diagnose myocardial infarction within 3 hours of onset because CK levels increase within 2 to 8 hours of an infarction.
6. Hypoglycemia is a syndrome characterized by fasting blood sugar levels below 45 mg/dL. Symptoms include sweating, weakness, dizziness, headache, trembling, lethargy, and other nervous manifestations.
7. High density lipoprotein is beneficial because higher levels of this correlate with a lower risk of heart disease.

SUGGESTIONS FOR FURTHER READING

Bauer, J., & Ackerman, G. (1982). *Clinical Laboratory Methods,* 9th ed. St. Louis: C. V. Mosby.

Bishop, M. L. (Ed.). (1996). *Clinical Chemistry: Principles, Procedures, Correlations,* 3rd ed. Philadelphia: Lippincott-Raven Publishers.

Bullock, B. (1996). *Pathophysiology Adaptations and Alterations in Function,* 3rd ed. Glenview IL: Scott Foresman.

Fishbach, F. (1996). *A Manual of Laboratory and Diagnostic Tests,* 5th ed. Philadelphia: Lippincott-Raven Publishers.

Henry, J. (1991). *Todd-Sanford-Davisohn Clinical Diagnosis and Management by Laboratory Methods,* 18th ed. Philadelphia: W. B. Saunders.

Memmler, R. L., Cohen, B. J., & Wood, D. L. (1996). *The Human Body in Health and Disease,* 8th ed. Philadelphia: Lippincott-Raven Publishers.

Porth, C. M. (1994) *Pathophysiology: Concepts of Altered Health States,* 4th ed. Philadelphia: J. B. Lippincott.

Rubin, E., Farber, J. L. (1994). *Pathology,* 2nd ed. Philadelphia: J. B. Lippincott.

Tietz, N. (1990). *Clinical Guide to Laboratory Tests,* 2nd ed. Philadelphia: W. B. Saunders.

Unit

8

Working With Special Patient Populations

Pediatric Patients

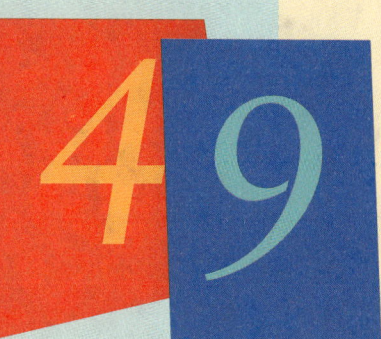

Chapter Outline

The Pediatric Practice
The Office Environment
   Safety
   Types of Office Visits
Psychological Aspects of Care
   Psychosocial Development
   Role of the Parents
Physiologic Aspects of Care
   Growth and Development
   Well-Child Visits
   Immunizations
   Sick-Child Visits
The Physical Examination
   Pediatric Histories
   Preparing for the Physical Examination
   Using Restraints
Procedure: Restraining a Child
   Obtaining Measurements
Procedure: Measuring Height
Procedure: Measuring Length

Procedure: Measuring Head Circumference
Procedure: Measuring Chest Circumference
Procedure: Weighing an Infant
   Graphic Charts
   Pediatric Vital Signs
Procedure: Measuring Pediatric Blood Pressure
Administering Medications
   Oral Medications
   Injections
Collecting a Urine Specimen
Procedure: Applying a Pediatric Urine Collection Device
Understanding Child Abuse
Summary
Critical Thinking Challenges
Answers to Checkpoint Questions
Suggestions for Further Reading

DACUM Components

1.3 Practice within the scope of education, training, and personal capabilities
1.6 Conduct oneself in a courteous and diplomatic manner
2.2 Treat all patients with empathy and impartiality
4.1 Apply principles of aseptic technique and infection control
4.2 Take vital signs
4.5 Prepare and maintain examination and treatment area
4.10 Collect and process specimens
4.13 Prepare and administer medications as directed by physician
5.0 Document accurately
7.3 Teach patients methods of health promotion and disease prevention

Learning Objectives

Upon successfully completing this chapter, you will be able to:

1. Spell and define the Key Terms.
2. List safety precautions to use in the pediatrician's office.
3. Explain the differences between a well-child and a sick-child office visit.
4. List types and schedule of immunizations.
5. Describe the role of the parent during the office visit.
6. Describe the kinds of feelings a child might experience during an office visit.
7. List the anthropometric measurements obtained in preparation for a pediatric physical examination.
8. Explain how to record anthropometric measurements on a graphic chart.
9. Identify two sites for intramuscular injections in an infant.
10. Identify two sites for intramuscular injections in a child.

Performance Objectives

Upon successfully completing this chapter, you will be able to:

1. Restrain a pediatric patient (Procedure 49-1).
2. Obtain measurements on an infant or child, including height (Procedure 49-2), length (Procedure 49-3), head circumference (Procedure 49-4), chest circumference (Procedure 49-5), and weight (Procedure 49-6).
3. Measure pediatric blood pressure (Procedure 49-7).
4. Apply a pediatric urine collection device (Procedure 49-8).

Key Terms

(See Glossary for definitions.)

aspiration	pediatrician
autonomous	pediatrics
congenital anomalies	psychosocial
humidifier	restrain
immunization	sick-child visit
malaise	varicella zoster
neonatologist	well-child visit

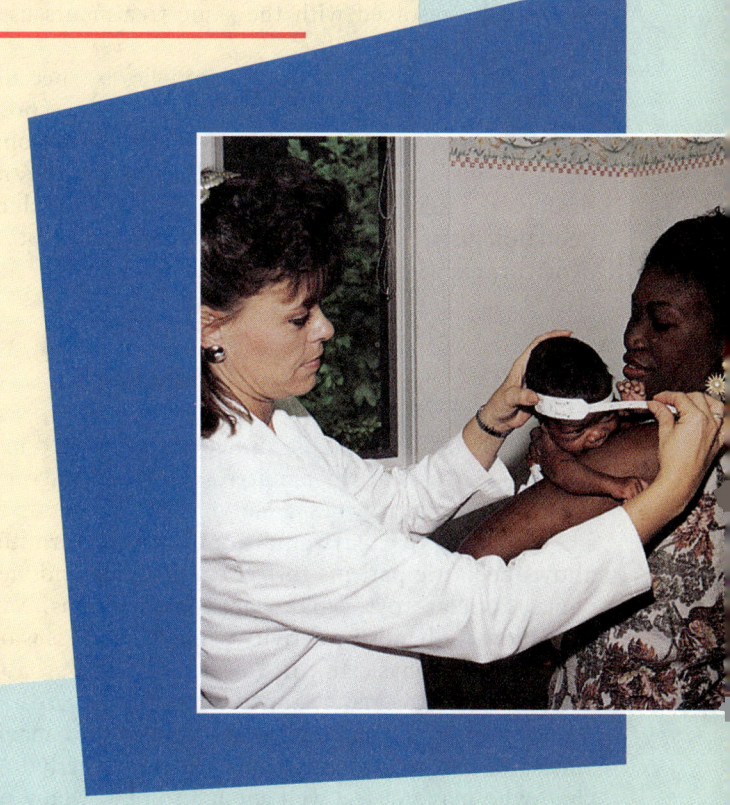

Medical assistants who work in a pediatric practice must understand that the needs of children and adolescents are typically different from those of adult patients. This chapter discusses special considerations in caring for pediatric patients. It also addresses the particular skills needed by medical assistants working with this distinct patient population.

➤ THE PEDIATRIC PRACTICE

Pediatrics is the medical specialty devoted to the care of infants, children, and adolescents. This care involves the diagnosis and treatment of childhood diseases as well as monitoring the physical and **psychosocial** (mental and emotional) development of the child.

Pediatric patients are not simply small adults; they are susceptible to a unique array of illnesses and problems not present in adults. The acute illnesses suffered by children are typically not encountered in adulthood. Some young patients will present with **congenital anomalies** (abnormalities present from birth) that are life-threatening or debilitating. Because of their increased metabolism, immature nervous systems, and accelerated growth patterns, pediatric patients often experience complications that may not occur in adult patients. There are few routine medical concerns related to infants and children that can be resolved with the same treatments used for adult patients.

A **pediatrician** is a physician who is specially trained to care for the well child and the diseases present in infants, children, and adolescents. Traditional pediatricians treat children of all ages, up to and through the teen years. Pediatric subspecialists include **neonatologists**, who treat only newborns, and other pediatricians who treat only adolescents.

➤ THE OFFICE ENVIRONMENT

A pediatric office that is decorated and furnished in a manner appropriate to children's physical and psychosocial needs provides a nonthreatening and possibly even inviting environment. Child-size furniture allows pediatric patients to feel comfortable and welcome. Popular toys evoke happy associations. Safe toys allow for hands-on activity while the child is waiting to see the physician. All toys should be washable and should be cleaned frequently to reduce the risk of disease transmission. Popular storybooks and magazines give parents an opportunity to read quietly to a child who may not feel well enough to play. Many offices are designed with separate waiting areas for sick children and well children.

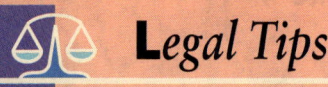

Legal Tips

Before treating a minor (persons under age 18), parental permission must be obtained. The **exceptions** to this rule include treatment for:

- pregnancy (testing or prenatal care)
- sexually transmitted diseases
- rape
- life- or limb-threatening injuries.

Emancipated minors (persons under 18 who support themselves financially), minors enlisted in the armed services, or minors who are married may obtain treatment without parental consent. You are responsible for knowing your state's laws regarding treatment of minors.

Safety

Medical assistants who care for children must always protect them from injury and accidents. Providing a "safe world" demands an awareness of children's insatiable curiosity and need to explore their surroundings. Never leave children unattended in the reception area.

Safety is a prime concern when considering toys and equipment in a pediatric office. Toys should be examined frequently and replaced when damaged or soiled. Try to see the office from a child's viewpoint. If necessary, get down to a child's level to discover potential danger areas—sharp table corners or uncovered, exposed electrical outlets—that an adult might overlook.

The examination room presents special concerns for children's safety. Keep all medical equipment out of a child's reach, and never leave a child alone in the examining room. Follow these tips to ensure your pediatric patient's safety:

- Place infant scales on a sturdy table, and never leave a child alone on a scale.
- Store any disinfection solutions away from patient care areas.
- Dispose of all sharps in proper containers.
- Practice stringent handwashing and standard precautions with every patient. Many childhood illnesses are highly contagious and can be transmitted by poor medical asepsis. These practices protect both the patient and the medical assistant from the spread of infection (see Chap. 19, Asepsis and Infection Control, for more information).

Types of Office Visits

The two types of pediatric patient office visits are the well-child visit and the sick-child visit. Well-child visits are regularly scheduled checkups designed to maintain the child's optimum health. **Sick-child visits** occur whenever the child requires medical treatment for symptoms or signs of illness or injury. (See Physiologic Aspects of Care, below, for more specific information about these types of visits.)

Checkpoint Question

1. What are three safety precautions that should be used in a pediatric practice?

➤ PSYCHOLOGICAL ASPECTS OF CARE

Psychosocial Development

Understanding a child's psychological needs and development will enable you to provide safe and effective care. During an office visit, the pediatric patient may experience many of the same feelings that adults do, depending on the child's age and ability to understand. These feelings might include:

- Fear that something painful and frightening might be done
- Anxiety that a previous bad experience may be repeated at the current visit
- Guilt and feelings of being punished for "being bad" or "misbehaving"
- Powerlessness and loss of physical autonomy
- Curiosity about new surroundings and experiences

Some children may be able to verbalize these feelings. Others may only be able to express them physically by crying and resisting the approach of the medical staff. As a medical assistant, you can reassure the pediatric patient and family by demonstrating your understanding of the child's feelings and displaying a kind and gentle manner. Include the child in the explanation of procedures on an age-appropriate level. Children who are helped to feel part of the examination will frequently be more cooperative.

Role of the Parents

Parents are a source of support and comfort to a child. Their presence minimizes stress in unfamiliar surroundings. Encourage parents to remain with the child and to assist in care when appropriate. For instance,

Focus on the Patient: Communicating With Children

Pediatric patients require special communication techniques. Here are a few tips to help you speak to children:

- Ask the child how he or she feels, then speak to the parent. Make the child feel part of the communication.
- Use simple and concrete terms.
- Explain all procedures to both the parent and child, using age-appropriate explanations.
- Avoid using confusing medical terms.
- Avoid condescending language.
- Be honest. If a procedure is going to hurt, say so. Do not lie. Keep in mind that children may view pain as punishment. If a procedure is painful, explain that the procedure is necessary to promote the child's health.
- If you need to communicate with an adolescent about sexual history or other intimate circumstances, ask the parents if they feel comfortable leaving the room.

ask the parent to stand beside the child during the weight measurement as you adjust the scales. Many children are more compliant if much of the preliminary workup is performed while the parent holds the child.

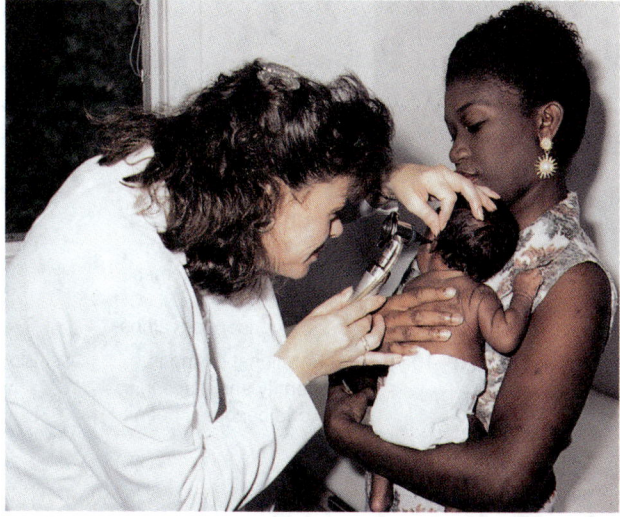

FIGURE 49-1
Much of the examination can be performed while the mother holds the baby.

The child may be less anxious if the parent **restrains**, or holds, the head for ear examinations and is within the child's sight, rather than having the medical assistant in this position (Fig. 49-1).

As a child develops and becomes more **autonomous (independent)**, a parent's immediate presence may be less meaningful as long as the child knows that the parent is close by. Many adolescent patients prefer to be alone with the physician to demonstrate their independence and to discuss matters that they may not be comfortable talking about with the parent present. Depending on the maturity of the adolescent, ask the patient, not the parent, if the parent is needed during the examination.

> **? Checkpoint Question**
> 2. *What kinds of feelings might a pediatric patient experience during an office visit?*

PHYSIOLOGIC ASPECTS OF CARE

Growth and Development

To anticipate age-appropriate behavior and to provide proper psychological support and physical care, the medical assistant must have a broad knowledge of child growth and development patterns. Never expect a child to react or respond beyond his or her developmental age. For example, a 2-year-old is naturally reluctant to be examined and may resist your advances. Many 4- or 5-year-olds are curious and willing to cooperate if you turn the examination into a game. Children older than 4 or 5 should have the reasoning capacity to understand the need to comply.

A normal child's growth and development follows an orderly progression involving mind, body, and personality. Table 49-1 describes the stages of growth and development and lists special considerations for the medical assistant.

Table 49-1
Pediatric Growth and Developmental Stages, With Considerations for the Medical Assistant

Age	Growth	Development	Considerations for the Medical Assistant
Infancy (0–1 y)	• Triples birth weight • Increases physical control of body • Sits and stands • May walk by 1st birthday	Trust versus mistrust	• Involve the parent. • Keep the parent in the child's view. • Approach the child slowly. • Use a soft, soothing voice. • Verbalize reassurance.
Toddler (1–3 y)	• Growth rate slows • Body proportions change • Language skills begin	Autonomy	• Use all of the skills listed above. • Explain procedures in terms the child can understand. • Expect resistance. • Use a firm, direct approach. • Ignore negative behavior. • Restrain to maintain the child's safety. • Allow the child to hold a "security object."
Preschool (3–6 y)	• Language and self-control develop • Motor skills increase	Initiative	• Use all of the skills listed above. • Encourage the child to verbalize feelings • Explain why the procedure is being done. • Have the child help as much as possible (eg, hold equipment.)
School-age (6–12 y)	• Social skills develop • Peer group becomes important • Self-concept develops	Industry	• Involve the child in decision making. • Involve the child in care, such as collecting specimens or choosing which procedure to do first. • Encourage and support questions.
Adolescent (12–18 y)	• Emotional changes • Identity and place in the world becomes defined.	Biologic and identity	• Discuss procedures in terms an adolescent can understand. • Be aware that adolescents may resist authority figures. • Be sure patient education includes information regarding smoking, alcohol, and, in some cases, birth control and sexually transmitted diseases. At the physician's discretion, this information may be discussed without the parent present.

One of the most popular tools for evaluating early childhood development is the Denver Development Screening Test (DDST) II. This tool is designed to assess fine motor, gross motor, language, and social development. The DDST II evaluates from the most basic reflexes to complex interpersonal reactions. The medical assistant who will perform the assessment should be educated in proper testing to evoke the most diagnostic response.

The indicators are registered in a vertical line drawn at the child's current age. Children should register within the normal range for age (Fig. 49-2).

Well-Child Visits

Well-child visits are scheduled at regular intervals, depending on the child's age. The goal of these visits is to maintain the child's optimum health, which is accomplished by a complete physical examination and an evaluation of the child's neurologic and psychosocial development. During an infant's first few well-child visits, for example, the pediatrician will check reflexes. Responses are predictors of neurologic health and development (Table 49-2).

The physician discusses the examination results with the child's parents and prescribes treatment for any problems found. Guidance and answers are offered for any questions parents may have about their child's health and development. Parents also are counseled about what to expect as part of the child's upcoming stages of growth and maturation. A child who is old enough to understand should also be included in the discussion. As the child matures, these visits become less frequent (Table 49-3).

Immunizations

Immunizations are a scheduled, routine part of the well-child visit and have dramatically improved children's health over the past 50 years. Immunizations

Stage	Caution
The newborn can see, hear, smell, feel pain, and communicate. Protective mechanisms are in place, such as a blink reflex, pulling in for warmth, or pulling away from pain or restraint. Development is from cephalic to caudal. Head control comes first, then gradually evolves into full body control (eg, rolling over, crawling, walking) and, finally, fine motor development (eg, picking up small objects). The most phenomenal growth and development occurs during this time, from total dependence to walking and talking.	Advise the parents to call the physician if the child has a temperature over 100.5°F rectally; has breathing difficulties, diarrhea, or jaundice; is crying inconsolably or vomiting; or is failing to nurse.
Growth levels off but exploration and social development continue. Negativism precedes autonomy. The child will begin to seek relationships and is acutely aware of strangers.	Advise parents to report any of the appropriate signs of illness as before, but also instruct them to be aware of the increased incidence of accidents with the need to explore. Children at this stage may indicate what hurts and how they feel, so you should not only talk with the parents, but also include the child when asking questions.
Socialization continues with fairly clearly marked stages of social development through the next 10 y. Many of the early-stage problems have resolved and, with the exception of the usual communicable diseases, this is generally a time of good health. Diseases such as leukemia, Hodgkin's, and various sarcomata may present in these next stages, but these years are usually spent establishing relationships with peers, exercising autonomy, and completing the growth process.	

protect children from diseases that in the past caused early death or long-term health problems. Immunizations produce immunity by slowly introducing into the body an altered form of the disease-causing bacteria or virus, which in turn stimulates the body to produce an-tibodies to protect against the specific disease. Currently, immunizations are available for:

- Hepatitis B (HBV)
- Diphtheria, tetanus, and pertussis (DTP)

text continues on page 996

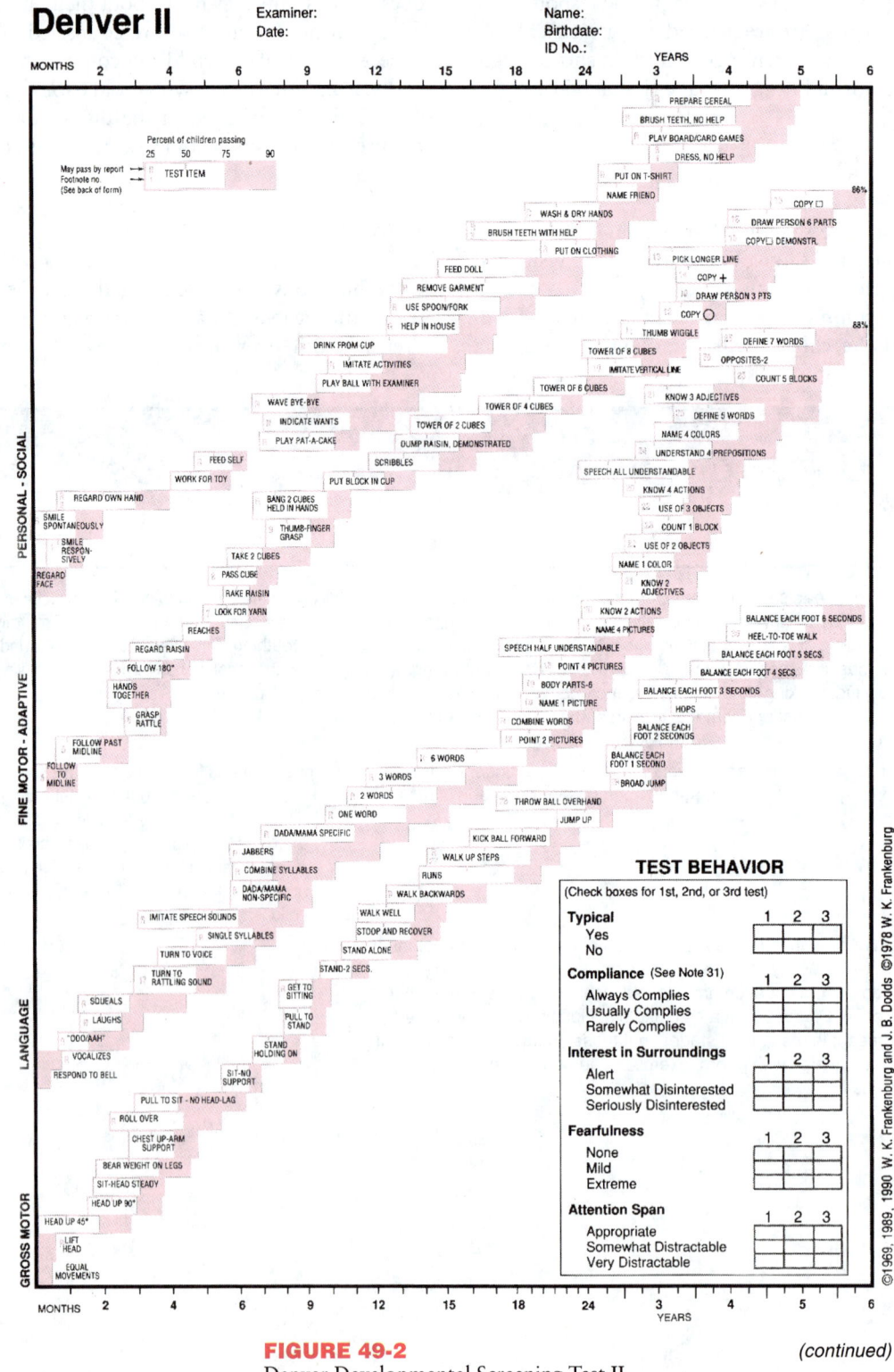

FIGURE 49-2 *(continued)*
Denver Developmental Screening Test II.

DIRECTIONS FOR ADMINISTRATION

1. Try to get child to smile by smiling, talking or waving. Do not touch him/her.
2. Child must stare at hand several seconds.
3. Parent may help guide toothbrush and put toothpaste on brush.
4. Child does not have to be able to tie shoes or button/zip in the back.
5. Move yarn slowly in an arc from one side to the other, about 8" above child's face.
6. Pass if child grasps rattle when it is touched to the backs or tips of fingers.
7. Pass if child tries to see where yarn went. Yarn should be dropped quickly from sight from tester's hand without arm movement.
8. Child must transfer cube from hand to hand without help of body, mouth, or table.
9. Pass if child picks up raisin with any part of thumb and finger.
10. Line can vary only 30 degrees or less from tester's line.
11. Make a fist with thumb pointing upward and wiggle only the thumb. Pass if child imitates and does not move any fingers other than the thumb.

 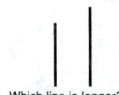 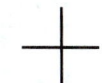 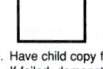

12. Pass any enclosed form. Fail continuous round motions.
13. Which line is longer? (Not bigger.) Turn paper upside down and repeat. (pass 3 of 3 or 5 of 6)
14. Pass any lines crossing near midpoint.
15. Have child copy first. If failed, demonstrate.

When giving items 12, 14, and 15, do not name the forms. Do not demonstrate 12 and 14.

16. When scoring, each pair (2 arms, 2 legs, etc.) counts as one part.
17. Place one cube in cup and shake gently near child's ear, but out of sight. Repeat for other ear.
18. Point to picture and have child name it. (No credit is given for sounds only.) If less than 4 pictures are named correctly, have child point to picture as each is named by tester.

 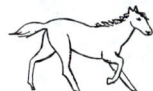 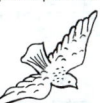 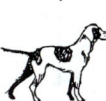 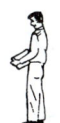

19. Using doll, tell child: Show me the nose, eyes, ears, mouth, hands, feet, tummy, hair. Pass 6 of 8.
20. Using pictures, ask child: Which one flies?... says meow?... talks?... barks?... gallops? Pass 2 of 5, 4 of 5.
21. Ask child: What do you do when you are cold?... tired?... hungry? Pass 2 of 3, 3 of 3.
22. Ask child: What do you do with a cup? What is a chair used for? What is a pencil used for? Action words must be included in answers.
23. Pass if child correctly places and says how many blocks are on paper. (1, 5).
24. Tell child: Put block **on** table; **under** table; **in front of** me, **behind** me. Pass 4 of 4. (Do not help child by pointing, moving head or eyes.)
25. Ask child: What is a ball?... lake?... desk?... house?... banana?... curtain?... fence?... ceiling? Pass if defined in terms of use, shape, what it is made of, or general category (such as banana is fruit, not just yellow). Pass 5 of 8, 7 of 8.
26. Ask child: If a horse is big, a mouse is __? If fire is hot, ice is __? If the sun shines during the day, the moon shines during the __? Pass 2 of 3.
27. Child may use wall or rail only, not person. May not crawl.
28. Child must throw ball overhand 3 feet to within arm's reach of tester.
29. Child must perform standing broad jump over width of test sheet (8 1/2 inches).
30. Tell child to walk forward, ⊂●⊃●⊃●⊃➜ heel within 1 inch of toe. Tester may demonstrate. Child must walk 4 consecutive steps.
31. In the second year, half of normal children are non-compliant.

OBSERVATIONS:

FIGURE 49-2 *(continued)*

Table 49-2
Infant Reflexes and Responses

Reflex	Response
Sucking or rooting	Stroking the cheek causes the infant to turn toward the stroke with its mouth open to suck. This reflex subsides by 3–6 months.
Moro or startle	A loud noise or sudden change in position causes the infant to look startled; the back arches, the arms and legs fly out and then are quickly brought back close to the body, and the infant cries. The Moro reflex results in the thumbs and forefingers forming a "C" while the other fingers spread open. (In the startle reflex, the fingers remain clenched.) Both reflexes disappear by 6 months.
Grasp	Stroking the infant's palm causes the fingers to grasp; stroking the plantar surface causes the toes to flex to grasp. The palmar grasp disappears by 3 months. The plantar grasp disappears by 9–12 months.
Tonic neck or fencing	With the infant in a supine position, the physician turns the head to either side. The arm and leg on the side the infant is facing will flex and the limbs on the opposite side will extend. This reflex disappears by 3–4 months.
Placing or stepping	The physician holds the infant at the edge of the examining table with the feet just below the edge. When the tops of the feet touch the table edge, the infant will place each foot up on the table and make walking movements. This reflex disappears by 6 weeks.
Babinski	When the plantar surface is stroked, the toes flare outward. This reflex disappears by 12 months.

Note: The absence of a response or a hyperresponse may indicate a neurologic deficit.

Table 49-3
Recommendations for Preventive Pediatric Health Care

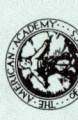

American Academy of Pediatrics

RECOMMENDATIONS FOR PREVENTIVE PEDIATRIC HEALTH CARE

Committee on Practice and Ambulatory Medicine (RE 9535)

Each child and family is unique; therefore, these **Recommendations for Preventive Pediatric Health Care** are designed for the care of children who are receiving competent parenting, have no manifestations of any important health problems, and are growing and developing in satisfactory fashion. **Additional visits may become necessary if circumstances suggest variations from normal.**

These guidelines represent a consensus by the Committee on Practice and Ambulatory Medicine in consultation with national committees and sections of the American Academy of Pediatrics. The Committee emphasizes the great importance of **continuity of care** in comprehensive health supervision and the need to avoid **fragmentation of care.**

A **prenatal visit** is recommended for parents who are at high risk, for first-time parents, and for those who request a conference. The prenatal visit should include anticipatory guidance and pertinent medical history. Every infant should have a newborn evaluation after birth.

	INFANCY							EARLY CHILDHOOD						MIDDLE CHILDHOOD				ADOLESCENCE											
AGE[4]	NEWBORN[1]	2–4d[2]	By 1mo	2mo	4mo	6mo	9mo	12mo	15mo	18mo	24mo	3y	4y	5y	6y	8y	10y	11y	12y	13y	14y	15y	16y	17y	18y	19y	20y	21y
HISTORY Initial/Interval	•	•	•	•	•	•	•	•	•	•	•	•	•	•	•	•	•	•	•	•	•	•	•	•	•	•	•	•
MEASUREMENTS Height and Weight	•	•	•	•	•	•	•	•	•	•	•	•	•	•	•	•	•	•	•	•	•	•	•	•	•	•	•	•
Head Circumference	•	•	•	•	•	•	•	•	•	•	•																	
Blood Pressure												•	•	•	•	•	•	•	•	•	•	•	•	•	•	•	•	•
SENSORY SCREENING Vision	S	S	S	S	S	S	S	S	S	S	S	•	•	•	•	•	•	S	•	S	•	S	•	S	•	S	•	S
Hearing[6]	S/O	S	S	S	S	S	S	S	S	S	S	•	•	•	•	•	•	S	•	S	•	S	•	S	•	S	•	S
DEVELOPMENTAL/ BEHAVIORAL ASSESSMENT[7]	•	•	•	•	•	•	•	•	•	•	•	O[5]	O	O	O	O	O	•	O	•	•	•	•	•	O	O	•	•
PHYSICAL EXAMINATION[8]	•	•	•	•	•	•	•	•	•	•	•	•	•	•	•	•	•	•	•	•	•	•	•	•	•	•	•	•
PROCEDURES – GENERAL[9] Hereditary/Metabolic Screening[10]	• ←→																											
Immunization[11]	•		•	•	•	•		•	•	•			•					←	•	→								
Hematocrit or Hemoglobin[12]				←	•			→											←		•			→				
Urinalysis														•														
PROCEDURES – PATIENTS AT RISK Lead Screening[12]							*	*																				
Tuberculin Test[15]	*	*	*	*	*	*	*	*	*	*	*	*	*	*	*	*	*	*	*	*	*	*	*	*	*	*	*	*
Cholesterol Screening[16]														*	*	*	*	*	*	*	*	*[13]	*	*	*	*	*	*
STD Screening[17]																		*	*	*	*	*[14]	*	*	*	*	*	*
Pelvic Exam[18]																		*	*	*	*	*	*	*	* ←→ [18]			→
ANTICIPATORY GUIDANCE[19] Injury Prevention[20]	•	•	•	•	•	•	•	•	•	•	•	•	•	•	•	•	•	•	•	•	•	•	•	•	•	•	•	•
INITIAL DENTAL REFERRAL[21]												•																

1. Breastfeeding encouraged and instruction and support offered.
2. For newborns discharged in less than 48 hours after delivery.
3. Developmental, psychosocial, and chronic disease issues for children and adolescents may require frequent counseling and treatment visits separate from preventive care visits.
4. If a child comes under care for the first time at any point on the schedule, or if any items are not accomplished at the suggested age, the schedule should be brought up to date at the earliest possible time.
5. If the patient is uncooperative, rescreen within six months.
6. Some experts recommend objective appraisal of hearing in the newborn period. The Joint Committee on Infant Hearing has identified patients at significant risk for hearing loss. All children meeting these criteria should be objectively screened. See the Joint Committee on Infant Hearing 1994 Position Statement.
7. By history and appropriate physical examination; if suspicious, by specific objective developmental testing.
8. At each visit, a complete physical examination is essential, with infant totally unclothed, older child undressed and suitably draped.
9. These may be modified, depending upon entry point into schedule and individual need.
10. Metabolic screening (eg, thyroid, hemoglobinopathies, PKU, galactosemia) should be done according to state law.
11. Schedule(s) per the Committee on Infectious Diseases, published periodically in *Pediatrics*. Every visit should be an opportunity to update and complete a child's immunizations.
12. Blood lead screen per AAP statement "Lead Poisoning: From Screening to Primary Prevention" (1993).
13. All menstruating adolescents should be screened.
14. Conduct dipstick urinalysis for leukocytes for male and female adolescents.
15. TB testing per AAP statement "Screening for Tuberculosis in Infants and Children" (1994). Testing should be done upon recognition of high risk factors. If results are negative but high risk situation continues, testing should be repeated on an annual basis.
16. Cholesterol screening for high risk patients per AAP "Statement on Cholesterol" (1992). If family history cannot be ascertained and other risk factors are present, screening should be at the discretion of the physician.
17. All sexually active patients should be screened for sexually transmitted diseases (STDs).
18. All sexually active females should have a pelvic examination. A pelvic examination and routine pap smear should be offered as part of preventive health maintenance between the ages of 18 and 21 years.
19. Appropriate discussion and counseling should be an integral part of each visit for care.
20. From birth to age 12, refer to AAP's injury prevention program (TIPP®) as described in "A Guide to Safety Counseling in Office Practice" (1994).
21. Earlier initial dental evaluations may be appropriate for some children. Subsequent examinations as prescribed by dentist.

Key: • = to be performed   * = to be performed for patients at risk   S = subjective, by history   O = objective, by a standard testing method   ←→ = the range during which a service may be provided, with the dot indicating the preferred age.
NB: Special chemical, immunologic, and endocrine testing is usually carried out upon specific indications. Testing other than newborn (eg, inborn errors of metabolism, sickle disease, etc.) is discretionary with the physician.
The recommendations in this publication do not indicate an exclusive course of treatment or serve as a standard of medical care. Variations, taking into account individual circumstances, may be appropriate.

Pediatrics Vol. 96 No. 2 August 1995
Pediatrics (ISSN 0031 4005). Copyright 1995 by the American Academy of Pediatrics.

Educating Parents About Possible Side Effects of Childhood Immunizations

- **Diphtheria-pertussis-tetanus (DPT)** may produce discomfort, swelling and redness at the site of injection, slight fever, and **malaise** (a feeling of generalized weakness and discomfort) within 24–48 h. Parents can administer acetaminophen for discomfort and fever. The pertussis component may cause loss of consciousness, seizures, inconsolable crying, hyperpyrexia, and systemic allergic reactions. If these symptoms occur, parents should notify the physician immediately.
- **Trivalent oral polio vaccine (TOPV)** usually causes no side effects, although vaccine-associated paralysis has been documented within 2 months of immunization. Be sure to question parents about the immune status of the family members and caregivers; immune suppression may lead to vaccine-induced polio.
- **Measles-mumps-rubella (MMR)** may cause fever, rash, malaise, lymphadenopathy, and arthralgia. A delay in symptom onset may occur in some children. Antipyretics for discomfort may be ordered.
- **Hemophilus B vaccine (HiB)** causes a low-grade fever with only a mild local reaction. Parents may give acetaminophen for discomfort.

Patient's Name _____ Sex _____ D.O.B. _____

VACCINE	DATE GIVEN			Name of Physician and/or Local H.D. Stamp	DATE NEXT DOSE DUE
	Mo.	Day	Yr.		
DTP DT					
DTP DT¹ (Diphtheria, Tetanus, Pertussis) 1 2 3 4 5²					
HEMOPHILUS INFLUENZA b (Hib) 1 2 3 4					
OPV IPV					
Polio, Oral Trivalent Polio,¹ Inactivated 1 2 3 4² 5					
Hepatitis B 1 2 3					
MMR #1					
MMR #2					
MEASLES					
RUBELLA					
MUMPS					
Td					
Tetanus, Diphtheria					
BOOSTER EVERY 10 YEARS					

¹Check the appropriate box for the specific vaccine administered.

²Administered on or after the fourth birthday and before enrolling in school (K-1).

VACCINE	Date Given	Administered By	Date Given	Administered By	Date Given	Administered By
INFLUENZA						

VACCINE	DATE GIVEN	ADMINISTERED BY	DATE NEXT DOSE DUE
PNEUMOCOCCAL (one dose only)			
HEPATITIS B: Recommended for persons at risk 1			
2			
3			

Medical Notes:

NORTH CAROLINA
DEPARTMENT OF ENVIRONMENT, HEALTH, AND NATURAL RESOURCES

LIFETIME IMMUNIZATION RECORD

Patient's Full Name _____
First   Middle   Last

Birthdate _____
Month/Day/Year   Sex ___   SS# ___

Name of Parent/Guardian _____

Address _____

If properly completed this record can be used to comply with Immunization Laws for day care, primary school entry, and entry into N.C. colleges and universities. This card can also be used to comply with immunization requirements of various employers.

Present this record at each visit to your doctor or clinic. The date each dose was given and the name of the physician and/or local health department stamp are required as proof of immunization.

DEHNR 1065 (Revised 6/93)
Immunization (Review 6/95)

FIGURE 49-3
A standard form for recording immunizations.

Table 49-4
Recommended Childhood Immunization Schedule

Recommended Childhood Immunization Schedule
United States, January - June 1996

Vaccines are listed under the routinely recommended ages. Bars indicate range of acceptable ages for vaccination. Shaded bars indicate catch-up vaccination: at 11-12 years of age, hepatitis B vaccine should be administered to children not previously vaccinated, and Varicella Zoster Virus vaccine should be administered to children not previously vaccinated who lack a reliable history of chickenpox.

Age ▶ Vaccine ▼	Birth	1 mo	2 mos	4 mos	6 mos	12 mos	15 mos	18 mos	4-6 yrs	11-12 yrs	14-16 yrs
Hepatitis B[1,2]	Hep B-1									Hep B[2]	
			Hep B-2		Hep B-3						
Diphtheria, Tetanus, Pertussis[3]			DTP	DTP	DTP	DTP[3] (DTaP at 15+ m)			DTP or DTaP	Td	
***H. influenzae* type b**[4]			Hib	Hib	Hib[4]	Hib[4]					
Polio[5]			OPV[5]	OPV	OPV				OPV		
Measles, Mumps, Rubella[6]						MMR				MMR[6] or MMR[6]	
Varicella Zoster Virus Vaccine[7]						Var				Var[7]	

Approved by the Advisory Committee on Immunization Practices (ACIP), the American Academy of Pediatrics (AAP), and the American Academy of Family Physicians (AAFP).

- Poliomyelitis (polio, both oral vaccine [OPV or TOPV] and injectable forms)
- Measles, mumps, and rubella (MMR)
- *Haemophilus influenzae* type B (Hib)
- **Varicella zoster** (VZV)—also known as chickenpox

Vaccine manufacturers have trade names for each product and have established protocols that must be followed to ensure full immunity to the specific diseases. As a medical assistant, you are responsible for reading all package inserts to become familiar with the adverse effects and cautions for each vaccine and to alert parents to potential problems they might observe after routine immunizations. Manufacturers of vaccines require that parents read and sign a consent form regarding the possible side effects of routine immunizations (Box 49-1).

Immunization schedules, which are developed by the American Academy of Pediatrics (AAP), change periodically as new vaccines become available for current diseases or as information regarding vaccines requires an altered pattern. Immunization schedules should be posted prominently in the office and replaced as suggested by the AAP (Table 49-4).

For various reasons, some children may not be kept on the suggested immunization schedule. However, all children must be current with their immunizations before they are allowed to attend public school (Fig. 49-3).

Sick-Child Visits

Sick-child visits are made on an as-needed basis. The goal of these visits is the diagnosis and treatment of the child's immediate illness or injury. The pediatrician examines the child and prescribes treatment that may include x-rays, laboratory tests, medication, or simply the reassurance that the illness will run a predictable and manageable course. Table 49-5 lists three common childhood illnesses and their causes, symptoms, and treatments. (No immunizations for these illnesses are available at this time.)

¹ **Infants born to HBsAg-negative mothers** should receive 2.5 µg of Merck vaccine (Recombivax HB) or 10 µg of SmithKline Beecham (SB) vaccine (Engerix-B). The 2nd dose should be administered ≥1 mo after the 1st dose.
Infants born to HBsAg-positive mothers should receive 0.5 mL Hepatitis B Immune Globulin (HBIG) within 12 hr of birth, and either 5 µg of Merck vaccine (Recombivax HB) or 10 µg of SB vaccine (Engerix-B) at a separate site. The 2nd dose is recommended at 1-2 mos of age and the 3rd dose at 6 mos of age.
Infants born to mothers whose HBsAg status is unknown should receive either 5 µg of Merck vaccine (Recombivax HB) or 10 µg of SB vaccine (Engerix-B) within 12 hr of birth. The 2nd dose of vaccine is recommended at 1 mo of age and the 3rd dose at 6 mos of age.

² Adolescents who have not previously received 3 doses of hepatitis B vaccine should initiate or complete the series at the 11-12 year-old visit. The 2nd dose should be administered at least 1 mo after the 1st dose, and the 3rd dose should be administered at least 4 mos after the 1st dose and at least 2 mos after the 2nd dose.

³ DTP4 may be administered at 12 mos of age, if at least 6 mos have elapsed since DTP3. DTaP (diphtheria and tetanus toxoids and acellular pertussis vaccine) is licensed for the 4th and/or 5th vaccine dose(s) for children aged ≥15 mos and may be preferred for these doses in this age group. Td (tetanus and diphtheria toxoids, adsorbed, for adult use) is recommended at 11-12 years of age if at least 5 years have elapsed since the last dose of DTP, DTaP, or DT.

⁴ Three *H. influenzae* type b (Hib) conjugate vaccines are licensed for infant use. If PRP-OMP (PedvaxHIB [Merck]) is administered at 2 and 4 mos of age, a dose at 6 mos is not required. After completing the primary series, any Hib conjugate vaccine may be used as a booster.

⁵ Oral poliovirus vaccine (OPV) is recommended for routine infant vaccination. Inactivated poliovirus vaccine (IPV) is recommended for persons with a congenital or acquired immune deficiency disease or an altered immune status as a result of disease or immunosuppressive therapy, as well as their household contacts, and is an acceptable alternative for other persons. The primary 3-dose series for IPV should be given with a minimum interval of 4 wks between the 1st and 2nd doses and 6 mos between the 2nd and 3rd doses.

⁶ The 2nd dose of MMR is routinely recommended at 4-6 yrs of age or at 11-12 yrs of age, but may be administered at any visit, provided at least 1 mo has elapsed since receipt of the 1st dose.

⁷ Varicella zoster virus vaccine (Var) can be administered to susceptible children any time after 12 months of age. Unvaccinated children who lack a reliable history of chickenpox should be vaccinated at the 11-12 year-old visit.

Immunization Protects Children

Regular checkups at your pediatrician's office or local health clinic are an important way to keep children healthy.

By making sure that your child gets immunized on time, you can provide the best available defense against many dangerous childhood diseases. Immunizations protect children against: hepatitis B, polio, measles, mumps, rubella (German measles), pertussis (whooping cough), diphtheria, tetanus (lockjaw), *Haemophilus influenzae* type b, and chickenpox. All of these immunizations need to be given before children are 2 years old in order for them to be protected during their most vulnerable period. Are your child's immunizations up-to-date?

The chart on the other side of this fact sheet includes immunization recommendations from the American Academy of Pediatrics. Remember to keep track of your child's immunizations—it's the only way you can be sure your child is up-to-date. Also, check with your pediatrician or health clinic at each visit to find out if your child needs any booster shots or if any new vaccines have been recommended since this schedule was prepared.

If you don't have a pediatrician, call your local health department. Public health clinics usually have supplies of vaccine and may give shots free.

The information contained in this publication should not be used as a substitute for the medical care and advice of your pediatrician. There may be variations in treatment that your pediatrician may recommend based on individual facts and circumstances.

Table 49-5
Common Childhood Illnesses

Illness	Symptoms	Cause	Treatment
Common cold	• Congestion • Cough • Malaise • Sore throat • Fever	Virus	• Increased fluids • Rest • Cold steam **humidifier** • Antihistamines • Decongestants
Gastroenteritis	• Vomiting or diarrhea • Fever	Virus or bacteria	• Increased fluids (especially electrolyte-replacement fluids) • Medication may be ordered to relieve symptoms
Otitis media (middle ear infection)	• Earache (may accompany or follow a cold) • Reduced hearing in affected ear • Fever	Virus or bacteria	• Increased fluids • Antihistamines • Decongestants • Antibiotics

Sick-child visits occur frequently during early childhood. Because children do not have well developed immune systems, they are more susceptible to viruses and bacterial infections. High fevers in young children may trigger seizures because of the child's immature nervous system. This does not mean that the child will be prone to seizures as he or she matures because the tendency to have seizures is usually outgrown fairly early. The physician will determine the course to follow in the event of childhood febrile seizures.

Never give aspirin to young children with viral fevers. Aspirin has been associated with Reye's syndrome after cases of varicella zoster (chickenpox) and viral illnesses. Reye's syndrome, a condition of acute encephalopathy and fatty infiltration of the internal organs, may be fatal.

As children grow older and receive the full schedule of immunizations, and as parents become more knowledgeable about certain disorders, communicable diseases as well as common childhood illnesses occur less often.

Children are inquisitive, adventurous, and unaware of dangers that can lead to many of the accidents and injuries that account for a large percentage of visits to the pediatrician's office. As a child's reasoning abilities mature, accidents diminish as well. Closely supervising a child's diet, rest, and exercise as well as teaching stress reduction techniques will help to promote good health habits for a lifetime.

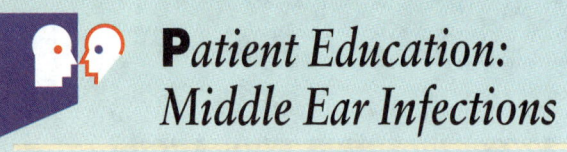

*P*atient Education: *Middle Ear Infections*

Explain to your pediatric patient's parents that children have short, straight eustachian tubes. Upper respiratory infections, particularly with coughing, may force microorganisms into the middle ear spaces. As the infection grows, the child's eustachian tubes swell and eventually close. Exudate from the mucous membrane continues to be produced, causing fluid to build with resulting pressure and pain.

Bacterial otitis media (middle ear infection) has been associated with, and may be caused by, putting the child to bed with a milk bottle. The milk and bacteria set up a medium for growth within the eustachian tube.

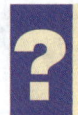

Checkpoint Question
3. What is the difference between well-child and sick-child visits?

➤ THE PHYSICAL EXAMINATION

Typically, the medical assistant prepares the pediatric patient for examination by the pediatrician and may also assist with the examination by restraining the child. The medical assistant usually is responsible for documenting much of the history and chief complaint information and for collecting appropriate specimens for diagnostic testing.

Pediatric Histories

A pediatric patient's medical history differs greatly from an adult patient's history. During the early years of a patient's life, it is important to know the history of the pregnancy, labor, and delivery. The length of the pregnancy, maternal illnesses or complications, neonatal complications, or risk factors must be recorded as predictors of infant health and development. Most newborn charts will contain a copy of the delivery record or birth summary outlining the delivery with the Apgar score and progress notes from the newborn nursery (Box 49-2).

As the child grows, the information needed will expand to include childhood illnesses, developmental milestones, immunizations, and nutritional status.

Figure 49-4 displays the kinds of forms used for documenting pediatric histories at various ages.

Preparing for the Physical Examination

You should approach the pediatric patient in a calm and cheerful manner and use a firm but gentle touch to increase the patient's feeling of security. Involve the parents as much as possible and keep them in the patient's view to reduce anxiety for both the child and parents.

Prepare the pediatric patient for physical examination by obtaining some or all of the following measurements: height or length, head and chest circumference, weight, temperature, pulse and respiratory rate, and blood pressure. Many of the measurements needed will depend on the child's age. The schedule preferred by the physician should be listed in the procedures manual.

BOX 49-2   The Apgar Score

Named for pediatrician Dr. Virginia Apgar, the Apgar score is a method for describing the general health of the newborn at 1 minute and 5 minutes after delivery. Signs assessed include:

- Heart rate
- Respiratory effort
- Muscle tone
- Response to a suction catheter in the nostril
- Color

A perfect score for each sign is 2; a total absence of any sign is 0. A perfect score of 10 indicates:

- Heart rate is greater than 100 beats per minute.
- Respirations are eupneic or the baby is crying.
- Muscle tone is good and the baby is active.
- Cough or sneeze occurs in response to suction catheter.
- Skin is completely pink with no acrocyanosis.

Most babies have 1-minute scores of 7 to 9 because many have a bit of acrocyanosis until respirations are established. Babies with 1-minute scores below 4 usually require assistance, particularly respiratory interventions such as oxygen.

The Apgar score is not considered an indicator of future intelligence or health problems. Rather, it is used by the obstetrician, pediatrician, and delivery room personnel to assess newborns who may require closer observation.

Using Restraints

During the examination, the physician may need the medical assistant to help restrain the child. Restraining is sometimes necessary to protect the child from injury and to help the physician complete the examination in a timely manner. Children understandably resist the physician because they are frightened and do not want to be touched. Calm and gentle restraint is in the best interest of everyone involved.

In hospitals, many forms of restraints are used including elbow, clove hitch, or abdominal. In the pediatrician's office, the medical assistant will most likely assist by using the papoose or mummy wrap (Fig. 49-5), or simply by holding the child in a position that the physician directs (Procedure 49-1).

Obtaining Measurements

During a well-child visit, **anthropometric** measurements commonly obtained include height or length, head and chest circumference, and weight. These mea-surements show the child's growth and development patterns and are good indicators of the child's health status and of the parent–child bonding. For example, parents who are not bonding well may either over- or underfeed a child, resulting in either significantly above- or below-average measurements. Head versus chest measurements may alert the pediatrician to intracranial abnormalities.

Height is measured when the child is standing; length, when the child is lying down. Weight is the most frequently obtained measurement in pediatric practices. The way in which weight is measured depends on the child's ability to remain still. For instance, a young child can either sit or recline on an infant scale while an older child can stand on a larger scale (Procedures 49-2 through 49-6).

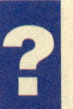

Checkpoint Question

4. Why is it important to track a child's anthropometric measurements?

text continues on page 1007

P.E. CODE:
Abnormalities described
✓ Normal
⊃ Not done
Att: attempted

REVIEW OF SYSTEMS:	DEVELOPMENT:	PERCENTILES:
Recent illness: _____	☐ Sits well	Ht. _____
	☐ Crawls/creeps	
☐ Crosses eyes	☐ Pulls to stand	Wt. _____
☐ Head tilt / Squints	☐ Cruises	H.C. _____
☐ Problems with hearing	☐ Pincer grasp	
☐ Problems with vision	☐ Finger feeds self	Daycare Y / N
☐ Perceived developmental delay	☐ 1-2 meaningful vocalization	Where? _____
☐ Problems with siblings	☐ Peek-a-boo	
☐ Fails to have strong voiding stream	☐ Pat-a-cake	Pleased? _____
Favorite toy _____	☐ Reacts to stranger with anxiety	Babysitters _____
Ipecac at home? _____	☐ Imitates gestures	
		Problems or changes at home? _____
	✓ - pass / circle if failed	

3. PHYSICAL EXAMINATION/ASSESSMENT	Normal for Age	Abnormal	Not Eval.	Concerns _____ Problems
a. General Appearance				
b. Posture, Gait				Assessment/Plan:
c. Speech				
d. Head				
e. Skin				
f. Eyes: (1) External Aspects ____				
(2) Optic Fundiscopic____				
(3) Cover Test				
g. Ears: (1) External & Canals ____				
(2) Tympanic Membranes				
h. Nose, Mouth, Pharynx				
i. Teeth				
j. Heart				
k. Femoral Pulses				
l. Lungs				
m. Abdomen (include hernia)				
n. Genitalia				
o. Bones, Joints, Muscles				
p. Neurological/Social				☐ ViDaylin/F 0.25
(1) Gross Motor _____				☐ Hgb
(2) Fine Motor _____				☐ Hgb electrophoresis
(3) Communication Skills ____				☐ Nutrition/diet counseling
(4) Cognitive				☐ Start using cup
q. Glands (Lymphatic/Thyroid)				☐ Change car seat at 20 pounds
r. Hips - R.O.M. / Click				☐ Accidents/safety discussed
s. Other Clavicles/Hernia				☐ Teething
				☐ Discipline/autonomy
				☐ Sleep: anticipate night awakening
Vision Screening				DATE:
Hearing Screening				
Other: Bonding:				**9 Months**

A

FIGURE 49-4

(**A**) Pediatric history form, age 9 months. (**B**) Pediatric history form, age preschool/5 years.

P. E. CODE:
Abnormalities described
⌐ Normal
ↄ Not done
Att: attempted

REVIEW OF SYSTEMS:
☐ Developmental concerns
☐ Behavioral problems
☐ Need for dental referral
☐ Vision/Hearing concerns

☐ Discuss parental activities/expectations.
☐ Promote interaction with other children.
☐ Encourage help with chores and tidy up of child's room.

DEVELOPMENT:
☐ Dresses without supervision
☐ Separates from mom easily
☐ Opposite analogies
☐ Defines 6-9 words
☐ Balances on one foot-10 seconds
☐ Catches bounced ball
☐ Interactive play
☐ Identify coins
☐ States age
☐ Tells simple story
☐ Right/wrong   Fair/unfair
☐ Copies "☐"
☐ Imitates a demonstration of ☐
☐ Draws man - 3 parts
☐ Draws man - 6 parts
☐ Hops on one foot

☐ Backward heel/toe
☐ Cut/paste
☐ Reading
☐ Crossing of eyes?
☐ Voids w/good stream
☐ Daycare
☐ School
☐ TV
⌐ - pass/circle if failed

PERCENTILES:

Ht. _____

Wt. _____

---

3. PHYSICAL EXAMINATION/ASSESSMENT

	Normal for Age	Abnormal	Not Eval.
BP /			
a. General Appearance			
b. Posture, Gait			
c. Speech			
d. Head			
e. Skin			
f. Eyes: (1) External Aspects _____			
(2) Optic Fundiscopic_____			
(3) Cover Test			
g. Ears: (1) External & Canals _____			
(2) Tympanic Membranes			
h. Nose, Mouth, Pharynx			
i. Teeth			
j. Heart			
k. Femorol Pulses			
l. Lungs			
m. Abdomen (include hemia)			
n. Genitalia			
o. Bones, Joints, Muscles			
p. Neurological/Social			
(1) Gross Motor _____			
(2) Fine Motor _____			
(3) Communication Skills _____			
(4) Cognitive			
q. Glands (Lymphatic/Thyroid)			
r. Spine			
s. Other Clavicles/Hernia			

Vision   (R)   (L)   ☐ Snellen
Hearing Screening Audiometry   ☐ Passed   ☐ Failed
Color Vision   ☐ Passed   ☐ Failed

Concerns _____
Problems

Assessment/Plan:

☐ Vi Daylin/F 1.0 Chewable
☐ Hgb
☐ U/A _____
☐ Urine culture - females
☐ Monovac
☐ DPT: Here   /   PHD
☐ OPV: Here   /   PHD
☐ Dental referral
☐ Safety-bicycle/water/fire
☐ Home telephone no. memorization
☐ T.V.
☐ Other

DATE:

Preschool/5 yr.

B

FIGURE 49-4 (continued)

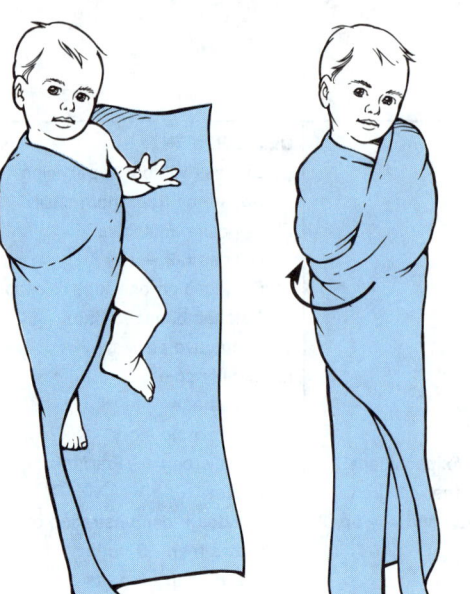
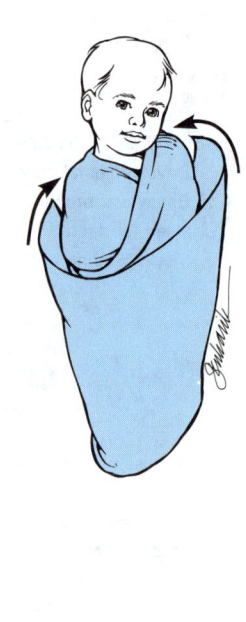

FIGURE 49-5
Mummy restraint. (A) Place the child diagonally on a small receiving blanket. (B) Wrap the right corner across the torso, covering the right arm and shoulder. Pull it snugly under the child's left arm and tuck it under the child's body. (C) Pull the left corner across the child's left arm and shoulder and tuck it snugly under the torso at the back so that the child's weight secures the end.

A   B   C

Procedure 49-1	Restraining a Child

Steps	Purpose
1. Wash your hands.	1. Handwashing aids infection control.
2. Identify the patient.	2. Identifying the patient prevents errors in treatment.
3. Explain the purpose of the restraints to the child's parents.	3. Parents may become concerned that their child may be injured by the restraint. Explaining the need for the restraint and how it increases treatment safety will ease parents' fears.
4. Approach the child in a calm and purposeful manner. Speak softly close to the child's ear.	4. This will reassure the child and decrease anxiety.
5. Stabilize the child's joints.	5. This will eliminate leverage that might allow the child to break from the proper restraint position. For instance, to keep the thigh still for an injection, hold the child's knee rather than the lower leg.
6. Guard against excessive pressure on the area of the child's body that is being restrained.	6. This will avoid injury. In many instances, the restraint may be more frustrating for the child than the actual procedure.
7. Observe the child for any signs of respiratory distress or pain.	7. Adjust the restraint or the holding position to provide for the child's physical comfort.
8. Wash your hands.	

Procedure 49-2 Measuring Height

Equipment/Supplies

- wall-mounted measuring unit
- growth chart

Steps	Purpose
1. Wash your hands.	1. Handwashing aids infection control.
2. Greet and identify the child.	2. Identifying the patient prevents errors in treatment.
3. Explain the procedure to the parent or to the child in an age-appropriate manner.	3. This will help ensure cooperation.
4. Have the child stand as tall as possible against a wall-mounted measuring unit. Make sure the child's heels are together and that the heels, buttocks, and shoulders are against the wall unit. Have the child look straight ahead. Place a horizontal bar against the crown of the child's head to determine the measurement.	4. Full extension to the child's tallest stature ensures a correct measurement.
5. Record the child's height on the growth chart and in the patient chart.	5. Procedures are considered not to have been done if they are not recorded.
6. Wash your hands.	

Procedure 49-3 Measuring Length

Equipment/Supplies

- examining table with clean paper
- tape measure
- growth chart

Steps	Purpose
1. Wash your hands.	1. Handwashing aids infection control.
2. Identify the patient.	2. Identifying the patient prevents errors in treatment.
3. Place the child on a firm examining table covered with clean paper. If using a measuring board, cover with a clean paper.	3. Measurements may not be correct if the surface is not firm. Clean paper prevents cross-infection.
4. Fully extend the child's body by holding the head in the midline. Grasp the knees and press flat onto the table. Mark the top of the head and the heel of the feet. Measure between the marks in either inches or centimeters.	4. Full extension is necessary because infants and some small children may assume a flexed position. If you need assistance, ask the parent or a coworker to hold the child in position. A foot board against the soles will give the most accurate measurement.
5. Record the child's length on the growth chart and in the patient chart.	5. Procedures are considered not to have been done if they are not recorded.
6. Wash your hands.	

Procedure 49-4

Measuring Head Circumference

Equipment/Supplies

- paper or cloth measuring tape
- growth chart

Steps	Purpose
1. Wash your hands.	1. Handwashing aids infection control.
2. Identify the patient.	2. Identifying the patient prevents errors in treatment.
3. Place the child supine on the examining table, or ask the parent to hold the child. Measure around the head above the eyebrow and posteriorly at the largest part of the occiput.	3. For an accurate reading, measure the largest circumference.

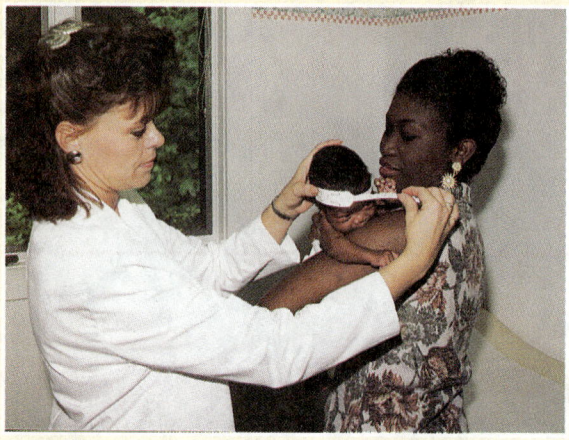 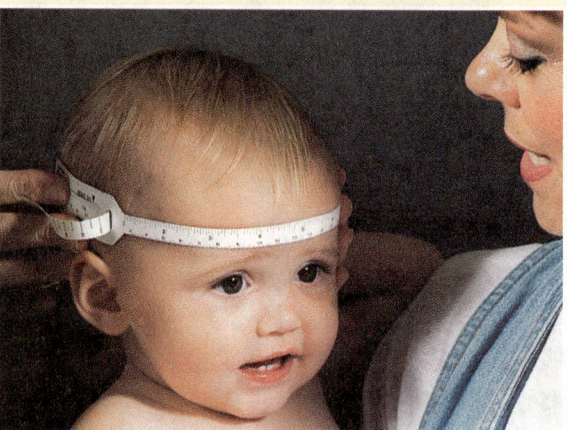

Step 3: Ask the parent to hold the child. Measure around the head above the eyebrow and posteriorly at the largest part of the occiput.

4. Record the child's head circumference on the growth chart and in the patient chart.	4. Procedures are considered not to have been done if they are not recorded.
5. Wash your hands.	

Note: If head and chest growth are within normal limits, this measurement is not usually required after 12 months.

Procedure 49-5   Measuring Chest Circumference

Equipment/Supplies

- paper or cloth measuring tape
- growth chart

Steps	Purpose
1. Wash your hands.	1. Handwashing aids infection control.
2. Identify the patient.	2. Identifying the patient prevents errors in treatment.
3. Place the child supine on the examining table, or ask the parent to hold the child. Measure around the chest at the nipple line, keeping the measuring tape at the same level anteriorly and posteriorly.	3. The tape should be at the same level to ensure the most accurate reading.

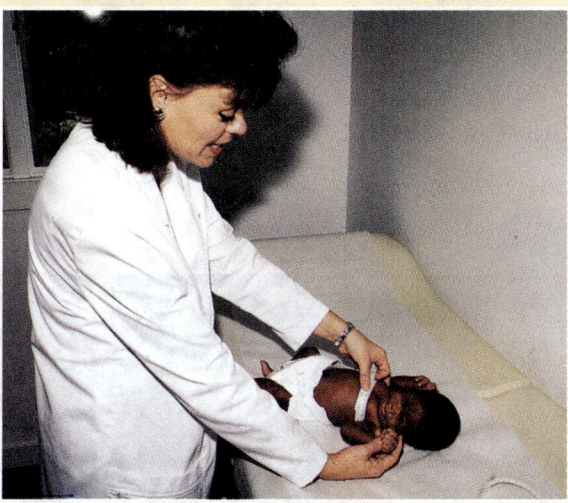

Step 3: Measure around the chest at the nipple line, keeping the measuring tape at the same level anteriorly and posteriorly.

4. Record the child's chest circumference on the growth chart and in the patient chart.	4. Procedures are considered not to have been done if they are not recorded.
5. Wash your hands.	

Note: If head and chest growth are within normal limits, this measurement is not usually required after 12 months.

<table>
<tr><td>Procedure
49-6</td><td>Weighing an Infant</td></tr>
</table>

Procedure 49-6 — Weighing an Infant

Equipment/Supplies

- infant scale
- protective paper for the scale
- growth chart

Steps	**Purpose**
1. Wash hands.	1. Handwashing aids infection control.
2. Identify the child.	2. Identifying the patient prevents errors in treatment.
3. Explain the procedure to the parent or to the child in an age-appropriate manner.	3. This will help gain cooperation.
4. Place a protective paper on the scale.	4. Protective paper prevents transmission of micro-organisms.
5. Balance the scale.	5. The balance beam must be centered before each use.
6. Place the child gently on the scale or have the parent place the child. Infants are weighed lying down. Children who can sit may be weighed in a sitting position if this is less frightening for them. Have the parent stand in the child's view. Keep one of your hands near the child at all times.	6. The child may feel insecure on the scale and seeing a parent is reassuring. Having a hand near the child reduces the risk of falling.

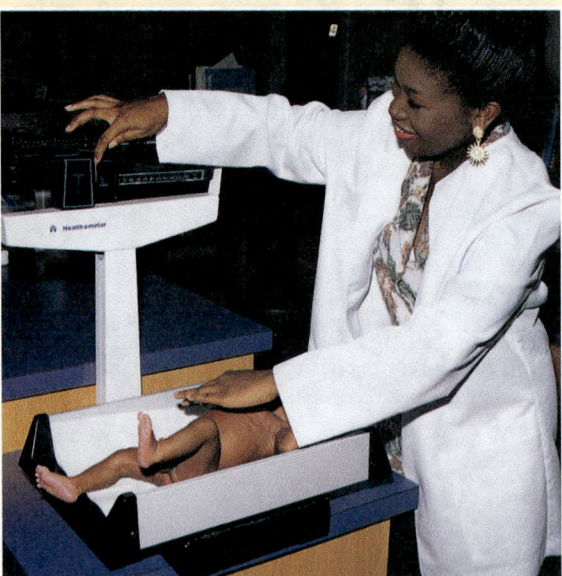

Step 6A.: Infants are weighed lying down.

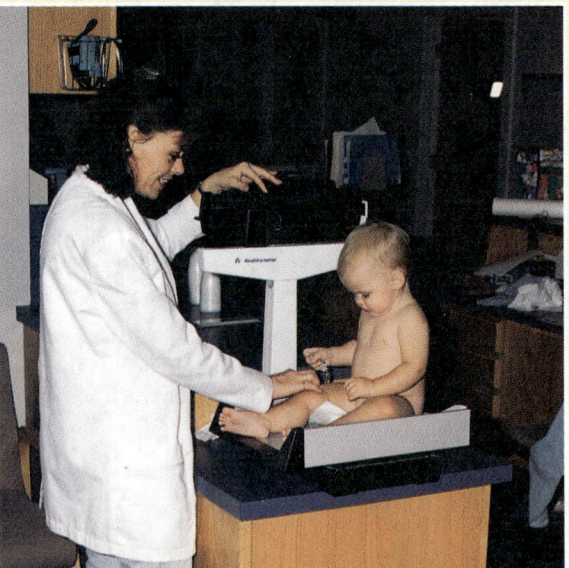

Step 6B.: Children who can sit may be weighed in a sitting position if this is less frightening for them.

7. Remove the infant's diaper just before balancing the scale. *Note:* Gloves should be worn to handle diapers. Feces have been implicated in the transmission of disease. (Children may be weighed while wearing undergarments.)	7. For the most accurate measurement, infants should be weighed without any clothing. Note that cool air against the infant's skin often causes voiding.

(continued)

Procedure 49-6 · Weighing an Infant *(continued)*

Steps	Purpose
8. Balance the scale quickly but carefully, moving the counterbalances to the proper places on the weight bar to exactly balance the apparatus. Have the parent pick up and soothe the child.	8. This will ensure accurate measurement.
9. Record the child's weight on the growth chart and in the patient chart.	9. Procedures are considered not to have been done if they are not recorded.
10. Wash your hands.	

Graphic Charts

Graphic charts are designed to show the child's growth patterns at a glance. The child's measurements commonly are plotted on percentile charts, then compared with those of children of the same age (Fig. 49-6).

Growth charts typically include the child's age, length or height, and weight. Notice that head circumference is not included on growth charts for children older than 36 months. Chest circumference usually is not graphed.

To use a growth chart, find the child's measurement (for length or height, in either inches or centimeters; for weight, in either pounds or kilograms), then move in that line across to the age column. Find the month or year opposite the measurement and make a mark at the point where the two values intersect. Moving a straight edge across the page helps keep within the proper lines. If you make an error, mark through it with an **X** and initial it. Then make the correction in the proper lines.

Checkpoint Question

5. Using the chart in Figure 49-6B, find the mark for a 4-month-old girl whose head circumference is 43 cm. What is this child's percentile?

Checkpoint Question

6. Using the chart in Figure 49-6A, find the mark for a 3-year-old girl who is 91 cm tall. What is this child's percentile?

Checkpoint Question

7. Using the chart in Figure 49-6B, find the weight/length percentile for a 7-month-old baby girl who weighs 16½ lb. What is this baby's percentile?

Pediatric Vital Signs

Temperature

Infants and children have immature heat-regulating mechanisms, resulting in more temperature fluctuations than in adults. Factors that can influence a child's temperature include:

- Illness
- Infection
- Activity
- Dehydration
- Environmental temperature
- State of dress

Temperatures may be measured by the axillary, oral, rectal, or tympanic methods. If the child is compliant, the axillary route is a viable choice and is more acceptable to most children than rectal (Fig. 49-7). The oral route may be used for a child over 5 to 6 years of age if the child is not seriously ill or septic and is cooperative. Oral measurement should not be used if the child is congested, coughing, vomiting, or uncooperative. The rectal route should not be used if the child has diarrhea or objects strenuously to the procedure. The tympanic method is gaining popularity because it is rapid, reliable, and most readily accepted by all ages. (See Chap. 21, Vital Signs and Anthropometric Measurements, for more information about temperature.)

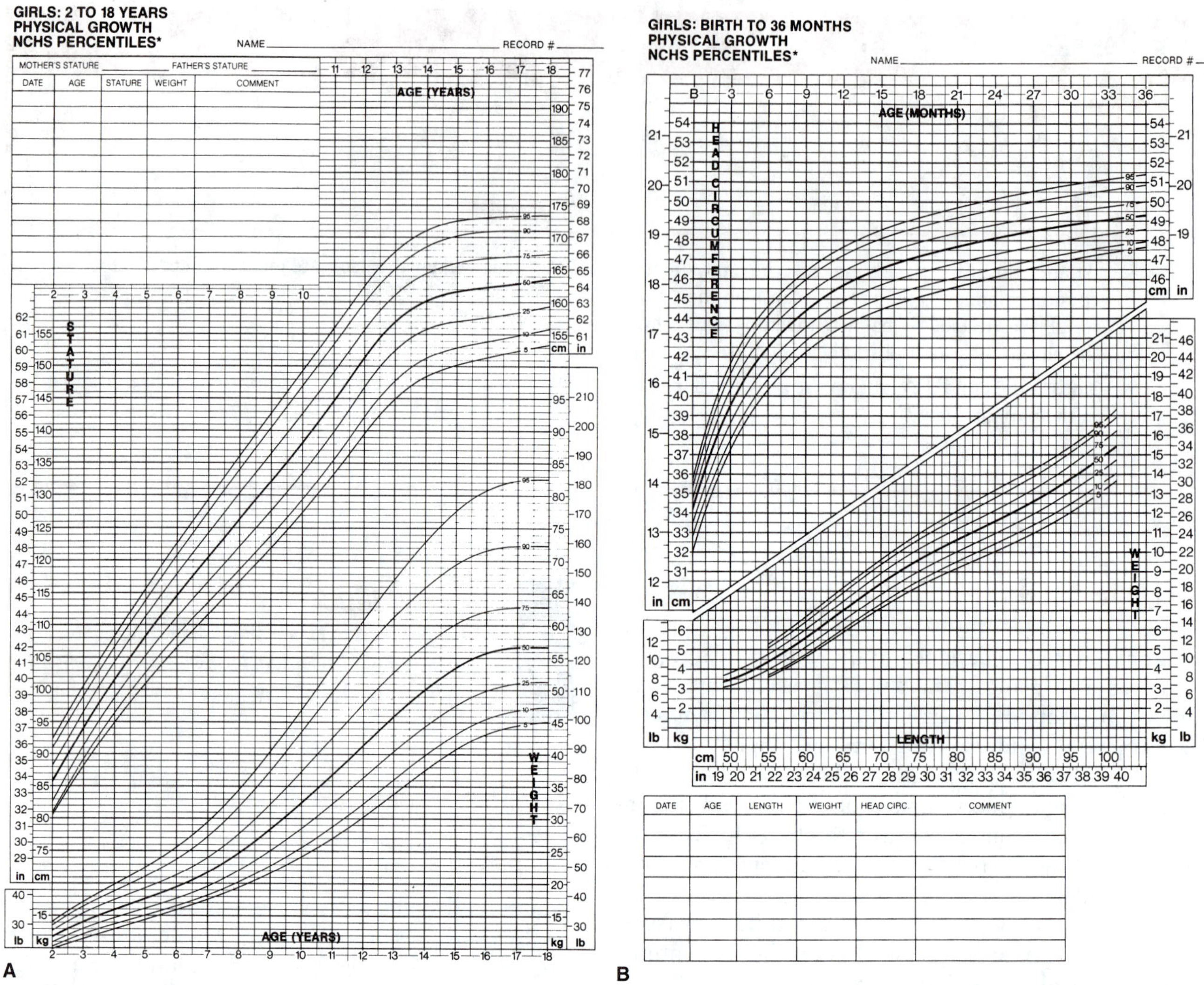

GIRLS: 2 TO 18 YEARS
PHYSICAL GROWTH
NCHS PERCENTILES*

GIRLS: BIRTH TO 36 MONTHS
PHYSICAL GROWTH
NCHS PERCENTILES*

FIGURE 49-6

Pediatric growth charts (**A**) for girls 2–18 years—height and weight and (**B**) for girls birth to 36 months—length, weight, and head circumference. Adapted from: Hamill PVV, Drizd TA, Johnson CL, Reed RB, Roche AF, Moore WM: Physical growth: National Center for Health Statistics percentiles. AM J CLIN NUTR 32:607-629, 1979. Data from the National Center for Health Statistics (NCHS), Hyattsville, Maryland (Part A). Data from the Fels Longitudinal Study, Wright State University School of Medicine, Yellow Springs, Ohio (Part B). © 1982 Ross Laboratories

Checkpoint Question

8. Besides illness and infection, what other factors can affect a child's temperature?

Pulse

The pulse rate reflects the heart rate and is usually easily measured. Pulse rate can be affected by activity, temperature, emotions, and illness. For children under 2 years of age, measure the pulse apically. To do this, place the stethoscope on the chest between the sternum and left nipple. Count the heart rate for 1 full minute. For children older than 2, obtain the heart rate using the radial pulse site (see Chap. 21, Vital Signs and Anthropometric Measurement).

Expect a child's pulse to be considerably higher than an adult's. A newborn may have a pulse rate of 100 to 180 beats/min; with fever, a rate of 200 beats/min or more is not unusual. As the child matures, the rate will slow. By age 2, a child's rate may range from 70 to 110 beats/min; with fever or exercise, it may possibly reach 200 beats/min. By puberty, the rate is comparable to an adult's rate (Table 49-6).

Respiration

Measure respiratory rate by observing the rise and fall of the child's chest. It is not necessary to disguise the fact that you are counting respirations, as you would with an adult patient. Because infants breathe by using the abdominal muscles more than the chest, observe abdomi-

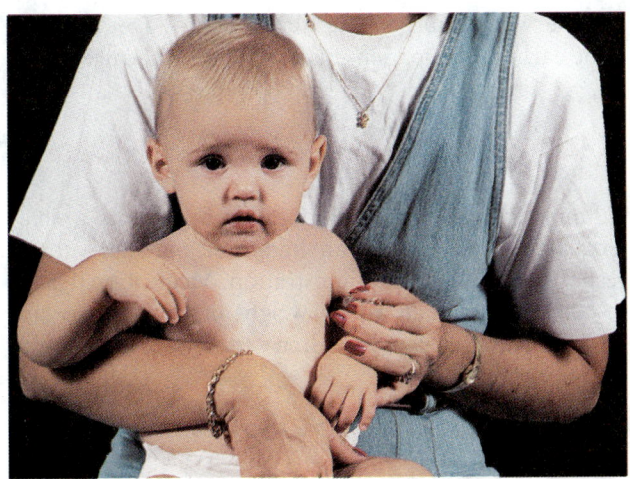

FIGURE 49-7
The axillary temperature is readily acceptable to most children and is considered accurate if the child is compliant.

nal movements and count 1 full minute. For children over age 2, use the same method as for adults. Count the respiration rate for 30 seconds and multiply by two.

Expect a newborn's respiratory rate to be as high as 35/min (Table 49-7). As with the pulse, the respiratory

---

Table 49-6	
Normal Pulse Rates for Children	
Age	**Rate/Minute**
Newborn	100–180 (may be over 200 with illness or crying)
3 months–2 y	80–150 (may be up to 200 with illness or crying)
2–10 y	65–130
10 y and older	60–100

rate will slow as the child matures. At age 2, it will be about 25; by puberty, it will be comparable to an adult's.

Checkpoint Question
9. *How does a child's pulse and respiratory rate differ from an adult's?*

Blood Pressure

Blood pressure measurements are not required for most pediatric examinations but may be appropriate at times (Procedure 49-7). Blood pressure is the most difficult measurement to obtain in an infant or child because it is so difficult to prevent movement. Infants and children have smaller extremities than adults and require a smaller cuff. Select a cuff by the same method recommended in Chapter 21, Vital Signs and Anthropometric Measurements.

Because of their soft, nonresistant vessels and smaller bodies, children have lower blood pressures than adults. You may have problems determining a diastolic pressure in some children using standard sphygmomanometers. In children less than 1 year of age, expect a blood pressure of about 90/50. The blood pressure will gradually rise as the child matures. By age 10, a child's blood pressure will be in the low normal range of 110/60 (Table 49-8). Blood pressure checks become

---

Charting Example

04/12/99	11:30 AM
	S: "My baby is doing great. He is now 10 months old."
	O: 10-month-old infant. Ht-79.5 cm Wt-26 lb HC-46 cm T-98.4F P-100 R-22 Child very alert, babbling various sounds, able to crawl and is able to pull self up. Child appears well nourished.
	A: Healthy 10-month-old. 95 percentile on growth chart.
	P: Educate parent on preventing ear infections and household safety tips. Physician in to see patient.
	————— Marie Gonzalez, MA

Table 49-7	
Normal Respiratory Rates for Children	
Age	**Rate/Minute**
Newborn	30–35
1–2 y	25–30
4–6 y	23–25
8 y and older	16–20

Table 49-8

Normal Blood Pressure for Children

Age	Systolic (mm Hg)	Diastolic (mm Hg)
Newborn	<90	<70
1–5 y	<110	<70
10 y and older	<120	<84

routine when children are about school age; they are done earlier if the patient history suggests the need.

➤ ADMINISTERING MEDICATIONS

Administering medication to children presents a challenge to the medical assistant and to the parents, who are responsible for home administration. Medication dosage in children is calculated by weight or by body surface area. However, because children vary in weight, age, and

---

Procedure 49-7

Measuring Pediatric Blood Pressure

Equipment/Supplies
- stethoscope
- sphygmomanometer

Steps	**Purpose**
1. Wash your hands.	1. Handwashing aids infection control.
2. Select the appropriate size cuff.	2. Infants and children require a smaller cuff than adults. Choose the proper size cuff to accurately assess the child's blood pressure. (See Chap. 21, Anthropometric Measurements and Vital Signs, for an explanation of choosing cuff size.)
3. Identify the patient.	3. Identifying the patient prevents errors in treatment.
4. Explain the procedure to the child's parent or to the child in an age-appropriate manner. For instance, you might say, "This may squeeze your arm a little bit."	4. This will help gain cooperation.
5. Expose the child's arm and determine the systolic pulse as described for adults (see Chap. 21, Vital Signs and Anthropometric Measurements).	5. Doing this helps identify the proper site. Determining the systolic pulse will avoid pumping the cuff too high and causing discomfort, or not pumping it high enough and missing the first systolic sounds.
6. Wrap the cuff around the arm ½ to 1 inch above the antecubitus.	6. To avoid environmental noises, the cuff must not be against the area covered by the stethoscope.
7. Palpate the brachial pulse. Pump the cuff about 30 mm Hg above the last pulse felt.	7. Pumping higher than necessary will cause discomfort; not pumping high enough may cause the systolic to be missed.
8. Release the pressure 2–4 mm Hg per second and note the first return of the pulse. This will be the systolic measurement. The diastolic will not be assessed by palpation.	8. Releasing more slowly will interfere with circulation; releasing more quickly may cause the systolic to be measured too low.
9. Thank the child for cooperating.	9. By providing praise and reassurance, you will help the child to develop a positive attitude about the pediatrician's office.
10. Record the blood pressure measurement.	10. Procedures are considered not to have been done if they are not recorded.
11. Care for the equipment as appropriate.	11. To maintain a clean work environment.
12. Wash your hands.	

fat/muscle ratio, they metabolize and absorb medication at varying rates. TO AVOID ERRORS, ALWAYS CHECK DRUG DOSAGE CALCULATIONS FOR A CHILD WITH ANOTHER STAFF MEMBER. Formulas for calculating pediatric dosages are discussed in Chapter 26, Preparing and Administering Medications.

You should be knowledgeable about the safe dosage amount, action, side effects, and signs of toxicity of any medications you administer. In most pediatric practices, the physician limits the choices to 50 or so medications that are suitable for children, making it relatively easy for you to learn all that is necessary about each medication. As for any medication, the seven "rights" of drug administration remain the same. These are: *right patient, right drug, right dose, right route, right time, right method, and right documentation.*

Oral Medications

Use caution when administering oral medications to a child to prevent aspiration (inhaling the medication). Hold infants in a semi-reclining position, not lying. Place the medication in the mouth on either side of the tongue. Depending on the child's age, use a medication spoon, syringe, dropper, or medicine cup. Many children will suck medication from a syringe easily and safely. Administer small amounts of medication, allowing the child time to swallow. Older children who resist may need to be strongly encouraged to take medications. Always explain to children who are old enough to understand why medications are important, then proceed in a swift and safe manner to give the medication.

Injections

Medications are given to infants and children via the injection route when there is no other choice. Children commonly fear injections more than any other medical procedure. You should approach the child in a calm and firm manner. Never lie to the child or say that it will not hurt. For example, you might say, "You'll feel a prick, but it will hurt for only a few seconds. You can say 'ouch' but don't move."

Although it is important for the child to know that an injection is about to be given, some anxiety may be alleviated if the child does not see the syringe. Offer the child an age-appropriate explanation, then quickly give the medication. After administering any medication, praise and comfort the child. Childhood injections are more commonly given in the vastus lateralis, at least until age 2 (Fig. 49-8). The ventrogluteal site may be used if you are familiar with the landmarks. The dorsogluteal site is not used for children under age 2 because the muscles have not developed well.

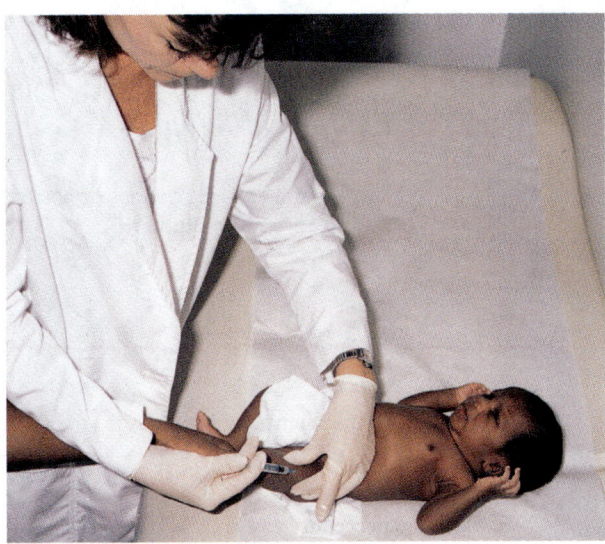

FIGURE 49-8
The vastus lateralis is the site of choice for infant injections.

The specific steps for administering an intramuscular injection are discussed in Chapter 26, Preparing and Administering Medications.

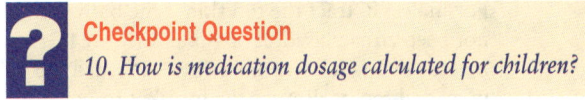

Checkpoint Question
10. How is medication dosage calculated for children?

➤ COLLECTING A URINE SPECIMEN

You may need to obtain a urine specimen from an infant or young child for urinalysis. Because infants and young children cannot void on command into a specimen container, you will need to apply a pediatric urine collection device (Procedure 49-8). Ask parents to entertain or distract the child while waiting for the child to void.

➤ UNDERSTANDING CHILD ABUSE

A child's social and physical well-being may be compromised by physical or emotional abuse or neglect or by sexual abuse. Abuse is thought to be the second most common cause of death in children under the age of 5. More die by the hands of their parents than by accidents, fires, falls, or drowning. Many are permanently disabled or seriously injured; many more carry emotional scars that will never heal.

According to the National Center on Child Abuse and Neglect (NCCAAN), the following 1993 statistics

Procedure 49-8   Applying a Pediatric Urine Collection Device

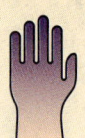

Equipment/Supplies

- gloves
- personal antiseptic wipes or cotton balls and antiseptic solution
- pediatric urine collection bag
- completed laboratory request slip
- transport container

Steps	Purpose
1. Wash your hands.	1. Handwashing aids infection control.
2. Assemble the equipment and supplies.	2. Doing this ensures that all of the materials are available.
3. Identify the patient.	3. Identifying the patient prevents errors in treatment.
4. Explain the procedure to the child's parents..	4. This will help gain cooperation.
5. Place the child in a supine position and ask for help from the parent, as needed.	5. The urine collection bag must be properly attached to obtain the specimen. The child may be more cooperative if a parent is available to help.
6. Put on gloves.	6. Standard Precautions must be followed when handling body fluids.
7. Clean the genitalia with the wipes or solution.	
a. For females: Cleanse front to back with separate wipes for each downward stroke on the outer labia. The last clean wipe should be between the inner labia (or labia minora).	a. Cleansing front to back will remove debris from the area and avoid introducing bacteria into the urethra.
b. For males: Retract the foreskin if the baby has not been circumcised, if possible. Cleanse the meatus in an ever-widening circle. Discard the wipe and repeat. Return the foreskin to position.	b. Cleansing outward will avoid introducing bacteria into the urethra. Returning the foreskin to position will prevent constriction of the penis.
8. Holding the collection device, remove the upper portion of the paper backing and press it around the mons pubis. Remove the second section and press it against the perineum. Loosely attach the diaper.	8. The collection device must be securely attached to ensure collection of the next voiding. Reattaching the diaper will avoid soiling if the child has a stool.
9. Give the baby fluids unless contraindicated and check the diaper frequently for the specimen.	
10. When the child has voided, remove the device, clean the skin of residual adhesive, and rediaper.	10. Adhesive may be irritating to the skin.
11. Perform a routine urinalysis (see Chap. 44, Urinalysis) or route the specimen as required.	
12. Remove gloves and wash your hands.	
13. Record the procedure.	13. Procedures are considered not to have been done if they are not recorded.

represent the incidence of child abuse in the United States:

Emotional neglect	3.2/1000
Emotional abuse	3.0/1000
Physical neglect	8.1/1000
Physical abuse	4.9/1000
Sexual abuse	2.1/1000

The best available statistics only partially reflect the true incidence of child abuse and neglect.

The Federal Child Abuse Prevention and Treatment Act mandates that threats to a child's physical and mental welfare must be reported. Some states require that all professionals report suspected child abuse or neglect to the proper authorities. Health care workers, teachers, and social workers who report in good faith will not be identified to the parents and will be protected against liability.

Medical assistants should be aware of the signs of abuse—either obvious indications or subtle warnings—that must be pursued for the child's safety.

Obvious Indications

- Reports of physical or sexual abuse by the child
- Previous reports of abuse in the family with current indicators
- Conflicting stories about the "accident" or injury from the parents and the child
- Injuries inconsistent with the history
- Injury blamed on siblings or someone other than the parent
- Repeated emergency room visits for injuries
- Fractures, burns, or skeletal injuries of a suspicious nature

Hidden Indicators

- Dislocations
- Nervous system trauma, particularly "shaken baby syndrome"
- Internal injuries, particularly to the abdominal area

Behavioral Indicators

- Overly compliant, too eager to please
- Passive avoidance, such as refusing to make eye contact, shrinking from contact
- Extremely aggressive, demanding, rage-filled behavior
- Role reversal, "parenting" the parent
- Developmental delays (the child may be using energy needed for maturation to protect himself from abuse)

Warning Signs

- Malnutrition
- Poor growth pattern
- Poor hygiene
- Gross dental disorders
- Unattended medical needs

What If?

What if you notice bruises and burn marks on the chest and back of the 3-year-old girl you are assessing?

If you suspect a child is being abused, approach the child and the parent in a calm and supportive manner. Any suspicions about the cause of a child's injuries should be discussed privately with

the pediatrician right away. State laws vary regarding the procedure for reporting abuse; local regulations should be outlined in the policies and procedures manual. As a medical assistant, you have an ethical and moral responsibility to report suspected cases of abuse or neglect.

SUMMARY

Pediatrics reflects the special needs and unique physiology of children. Participating in their care offers many rewards and challenges. This chapter has focused on the skills necessary to assist the pediatrician. Knowing childhood psychosocial and physiologic growth and development helps you meet the needs of the child and family during the office visit.

The principles and structure of the well-child and sick-child visits provide guidelines for obtaining the necessary information about the child in preparation for the physical examination.

CRITICAL THINKING CHALLENGES

During years of practice, Dr. Hernandez has found that many new parents are unfamiliar with basic child care needs. He decides to publish a short booklet for his new patients describing various aspects of child care. The booklet should be informative, professional, and show genuine concern for children. Topics to be covered include:

- General safety tips
- Types of office visits
- Immunizations (what they are, why they are important, at what ages they are given)
- What a parent can expect during an office visit
- Brief explanation of child development
- Tips for administering oral medications

Using your creativity and your knowledge of child care, write a sample booklet for Dr. Hernandez's patients.

ANSWERS TO CHECKPOINT QUESTIONS

1. Safety precautions that should be used in a pediatric practice include:
   Keeping all medical equipment out of a child's reach
   Never leaving a child alone in the examining room
   Placing infant scales on a sturdy table and never leaving a child alone on a scale

Storing disinfection solutions away from patient care areas

Disposing of all sharps in proper containers

Practicing stringent handwashing and standard precautions with every patient

2. A pediatric patient might experience fear, anxiety, guilt, powerlessness, or curiosity during an office visit.

3. Well-child visits are scheduled at regular intervals, depending on the child's age, and are designed to maintain the child's optimum health. During a well-child visit, the pediatrician conducts a physical examination of the child and evaluates neurologic and psychosocial development. Sick-child visits are scheduled as needed. The goal of these visits is diagnosis and treatment of the child's immediate illness or injury.

4. A child's anthropometric measurements show growth and development and are good indicators of the child's health status and parent–child bonding.

5. 75%

6. 25%

7. 10%

8. A child's temperature can be affected by activity, dehydration, environmental temperature, and state of dress.

9. In a child, both the pulse and respiratory rate are higher than in an adult.

10. Medication dosage in children is calculated by weight or by body surface area.

SUGGESTIONS FOR FURTHER READING

Brown, J. L. (1994). *Pediatric Telephone Medicine: Principles, Triage, and Advice,* 2nd ed. Philadelphia: J. B. Lippincott.

Castiglia, P. T. & Harbin, R. E. (1992). *Child Health Care: Process and Practice.* Philadelphia: J. B. Lippincott.

Kozier, B., & Erb, G. (1993). *Techniques in Clinical Nursing,* 4th ed. California: Addison Wesley.

Marks, M. G. (1994). *Broadribb's Introductory Pediatric Nursing,* 4th ed. Philadelphia: J. B. Lippincott.

Pilliteri, A. (1995). *Maternal and Child Health Nursing: Care of the Childbearing and Childraising Family,* 4th ed. Philadelphia: J. B. Lippincott.

Schuster, C. S., & Ashburn, S. S. (1992). *The Process of Human Development. A Holistic Life-span Approach,* 3rd ed. Philadelphia: J. B. Lippincott.

Whaley, L. F., & Wong, D. L. (1991). *Nursing Care of Infants and Children,* 4th ed. St. Louis: C. V. Mosby.

Geriatric Patients

Chapter Outline

Concepts of Aging
Memory Enhancement to Reinforce
  Medical Compliance
Reinforcing Mental Health
Coping With Aging
  Alcoholism
  Suicide
Long-Term Care
Elder Abuse
  Risk Factors for Abuse
  Signs of Elder Abuse
Medications and the Elderly

Systemic Changes in the Elderly
Diseases of the Elderly
  Parkinson's Disease
  Alzheimer's Disease
Maintaining Optimum Health
  Exercise
  Diet
  Safety
Summary
Critical Thinking Challenges
Answers to Checkpoint Questions
Suggestions for Further Reading

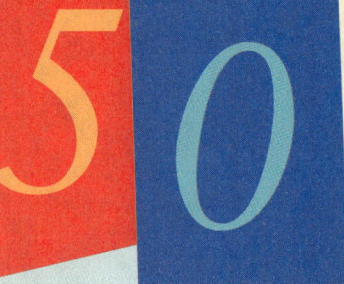

DACUM Components

1.3 Practice within the scope of education, training, and personal capabilities
1.6 Conduct oneself in a courteous and diplomatic manner
2.2 Treat all patients with empathy and impartiality
2.3 Adapt communication to individuals' abilities to understand
2.6 Evaluate understanding of communication
7.2 Instruct patients with special needs

Chapter Competencies

Learning Objectives

Upon successfully completing this chapter, you will be able to:

1. Spell and define the Key Terms.
2. Describe the changing concepts of the aging process.
3. Describe how aging affects the ability to remember and reason and how these changes affect thought processes.
4. List ways to ensure compliance with health maintenance programs among the elderly and give reasons for noncompliance.
5. Outline steps to maintain open communication with the elderly patient.
6. Describe the coping mechanisms used by the elderly to deal with multiple losses and ways to recognize and alleviate the stressors.
7. List risk factors and signs of elder abuse and give the responsibility of the medical office in suspected abuse.
8. Define the types of long-term care facilities available and the responses expected of the elderly at confinement.
9. Describe the affects aging will have on medication as it is processed in the body and the medical assistant's responsibility in patient education.
10. List and describe physical changes and diseases common to the aging process and how the medical assistant may alleviate the symptoms.

Key Terms

(See Glossary for definitions.)

activities of daily living (ADL)
biotransforming
bradykinesia
cataracts
cerebrovascular accident (CVA)
degenerative joint disease (DJD)
dementia
dowager's hump (kyphosis)
dysphagia
glaucoma
keratoses (senile)

lentigines
osteoporosis
positron emission tomography (PET)
potentiation
presbycusis
presbyopia
syncope
transient ischemic attack (TIA)
vertigo

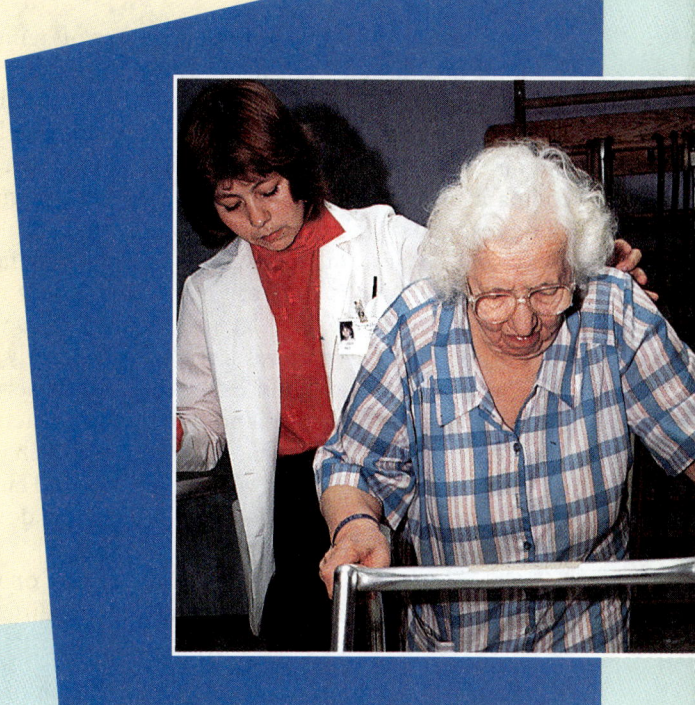

The elderly are the fastest growing segment of our population. They bring to the medical profession needs and concerns not generally faced by younger patients. Caring for these patients will test your skills in communication and will require the greatest degree of caring, compassion, and patience. The challenge of caring for the elderly may be one of the most rewarding aspects of the profession.

➤ CONCEPTS OF AGING

As the elderly population has increased, established concepts of the aging process have changed. It is no longer expected that older relatives will be dependent on family members or that they will become incompetent by a specific age. Many are healthy enough to maintain homes well into their eighties and nineties. With many years spent in retirement, some are starting second careers at an age that their parents were either no longer alive or were incapacitated by ill health. College degrees are sought and earned, volunteering becomes a way of life, and hobbies become businesses. The greeting card image of the cozy, gray-haired grandmother in her rocking chair is more likely in reality to be a trim, active woman rushing out the door with a briefcase or tennis racket under her arm.

Compare these myths and stereotypes to the reality of the aging population (Box 50-1). How many of these are true? How many are far from typical of this age group?

Stereotyping the elderly, based on fear of aging, is a subtle and usually unconscious way to dissociate ourselves from the prospect of growing old. If these people are seen as somehow different, we may feel we can never be as they are now. This is striking when we compare the way children without preconceptions of aging respond to the elderly as opposed to the pulling away and separation adults may adopt when faced with someone who is not very many years older than they are themselves.

Although other cultures revere their elderly for their wealth of wisdom and experience, the American media perpetuate the myths and stereotypical reactions to the elderly by implying that graying hair and character lines are repulsive and should be avoided at all costs. Those "costs" range in the billions of dollars spent on delaying the physical signs of aging.

Consider how the following situations take on new meaning when applied through prejudice to different age groups.

- You are running late again. Dashing out of the door, locking it behind you, you remember that you left the keys to the house and car on the kitchen table . . . again.

BOX 50-1 **Myths and Stereotypes About the Elderly**

Myths

Old people are weak and sick.
Old people can no longer learn.
Old people have no more contributions to make.
Old people are boring.
Old people are a drag on the economy.
Old people are always lonely.
Old people cannot live alone.
Old people cannot be trusted to make rational decisions.
Old people have lost all interest in life.

Stereotypes

Old people have sensory losses.
Old people have erratic sleep patterns and nap a lot.
Old people do everything slower.
Old people have lost stature and slump a lot.
Old people cannot remember what happened this morning but can recall everything that happened 40 years ago.

- You stride purposefully from the bedroom into the kitchen with a specific goal in mind, only to reach the kitchen without any idea why you were in such a hurry to get there.

We have all done these things and will no doubt do them again. However, if these thing are done by an elderly person, they are considered to be a sign of approaching senility simply because the elderly are perceived as more forgetful than younger adults.

➤ MEMORY ENHANCEMENT TO REINFORCE MEDICAL COMPLIANCE

Considering the differing functions of the aging mind and the interference that disease processes and medications can work with thought processes, it will be a challenge to help the patient work through methods of memory reinforcement. You might try these approaches:

1. Write out instructions in easy-to-understand terms. Use large print if the patient is vision impaired.
2. Have the patient repeat instructions to you for reinforcement.

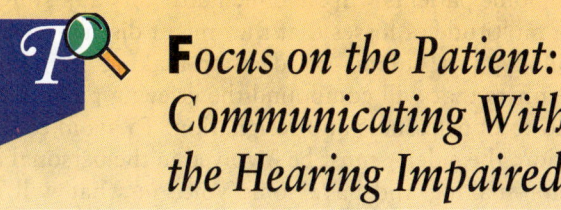

Focus on the Patient: Communicating With the Hearing Impaired

When giving instructions to an elderly patient who is hearing impaired, do not shout. Instead, decrease the distance between you and the patient, face the patient directly, and speak slowly and distinctly. Consider calling the patient the day after the office visit to assess compliance with and understanding of the instructions and to provide additional information if needed.

3. Have the patient show you how he or she will perform a procedure before leaving the office.
4. Give the patient a large calendar or photocopy pages of a large appointment calendar and list times and days for treatments and medications to be crossed off as completed.

If a good rapport exists between the patient and the office staff, the patient is more likely to be truthful regarding the need for memory aids. If the importance of prescribed treatments and medications is explained in terms the patient can understand, compliance is more likely.

Many of the illnesses presented will be long-term chronic situations that will require medication for the remainder of the patient's life. In these situations, little improvement, if any, will be noticed by the patient, making compliance over a long period of time less probable. It may be explained in some circumstances that there is little chance for a return to former health, but that the prescribed treatment will maintain health at a manageable level. This is especially important for patients with disorders such as diabetes or chronic heart disease. These patients will never be free of these diseases, but treatment will maintain a reasonable standard of health and independence. The patient may be helped to understand this with assistance from counselors and support groups.

Ask each time the patient visits the office for a complete account of all medications, prescribed and over-the-counter, and all current treatments. Ask the patient to list them. If you ask, "Mrs. Jones, are you still taking your heart medicine?", she may answer "Yes" whether or not she is actually taking this medication. Many patients pick and choose what adjustments they make in their lives to comply with health restrictions, some grow tired of the constraints that ill-

ness and medications impose on their lives, some must choose between medication and food on the table, some forget, and some simply rebel. A stronger effort at remembering and adhering to treatment plans may depend on reinforcement of the patient's self-esteem and the will to be in control of one's own health status.

Assisting the patient to find ways to fit health requirements into a fairly normal life-style will help to ensure that treatment plans are followed and that the best level of health possible is achieved.

Checkpoint Question
1. *What memory enhancement techniques could you use to reinforce compliance?*

► REINFORCING MENTAL HEALTH

With the recognized correlation between physical and mental health, we must be acutely aware of the patient's mental status. Elderly patients are adapting to new roles of dependency after a lifetime of social interaction, career objectives, and family development. Some have been relieved of social responsibility whether this is welcomed or not, and if they are ill, they must take on a dependent role. The presenting disease may be socially isolating, as in oxygen-assisted chronic obstructive pulmonary disease, a laryngostomy, or **dysphagia** (difficulty swallowing) requiring tube feedings.

Adjusting to pain or disability is often easier than adjusting to loss of social interaction. As we are better able to assist patients back to a semblance of health with advanced technology, more patients will have to make the adjustment to diseases that are not conducive to socialization. These patient will experience all of the stages of grief as they lose their previous identities and will lash out at the very people who are trying to help them. Their family members will be dealing with stress, anger, frustration, and fear at the same time the patient will be testing the patience of all caregivers.

Paradoxically, if you open yourself to the patient and are accessible and caring, you are more likely to be the object of anger and abuse simply because you will be seen as safe. A suffering patient is less likely to release pent up rage at someone who may respond with hostility or corresponding anger; consequently, the rage is held in and the problem is compounded. Making yourself available to field these emotions can be as therapeutic as any treatment that might be administered to this patient. To do this effectively:

1. Maintain open communication, freely discussing hopes and fears realistically with the patient.

2. Help the patient to cope with and express feelings of guilt for being ill, anger at self and all nearby, and the loss of health and independence.
3. Work toward maintaining the patient's positive self-image.
4. Assist family members to maintain positive support.
5. Prepare the patient for the possibility that a return to the previous state of health may not be feasible.
6. Direct the patient and family to specific support groups, such as the American Heart Association, the American Cancer Society, or other groups specific to the patient's problem.

Checkpoint Question
2. How can you help promote good mental health in your elderly patients?

➤ COPING WITH AGING

Although the majority of the elderly are generally healthy and satisfied with their lives, those who are consigned to long-term care facilities or whose health and economic situations are precarious have every right to feel overwhelming stress and grief. Stress will compromise the immune system, raise the blood pressure and blood sugar level, and strain the heart and lungs—all at a time when the patient needs all available resources to fight debilitating disease processes. Help patients to cope with stress by listening to their fears and concerns, respecting their right to have these feelings, and by helping them to reduce the stressors in their lives.

The coping mechanisms used to protect ourselves from stress become more pronounced with age. Young adults who handle stress by retreating into themselves will become withdrawn and stoical as older adults; young adults who handle stress by aggressive release will continue to be outspoken and vocal as older adults. The ability of patients to cope with the losses that confront them will be in direct relation to the importance of the losses. For instance, an artist with severe arthritis will mourn the loss of artistic ability and may scarcely notice sags and wrinkles. Conversely, an actor who loses physical beauty will mind that loss and may not notice fingers stiff with arthritis.

Be aware of the loss of specifics such as sight, hearing, movement, perception, health, employment, home, and spouse. Also be alert to the loss of non-specifics—life purpose, goals, a sense of achievement, self-worth, recognition, security.

Some patients will have such difficulty adjusting to the multitude of losses that they might disengage emotionally and submit to decision-making by family members that will compound the grieving process and lead to hopelessness and resignation. To avoid this reaction, the elderly must be involved in the personal decision-making and have some voice in what will become of them. The elderly who are encouraged to make decisions and take responsibility for themselves are happier, more sociable, and live longer.

Alcoholism

If coping fails, some elderly will turn to alcohol as an escape. Alcohol slows brain activity and impairs mental processes, coordination, and judgment at a time that every available resource is needed. Alcohol may mask pain until the source of the pain becomes a danger. Alcohol abuse may be mistaken for **dementia** (mental deterioration), **transient ischemic attacks (TIAs)** (acute episodes of cerebrovascular insufficiency), or central nervous system impairment, and so may either be left untreated or be treated incorrectly. Many of the medications used to treat the central nervous system will react badly with alcohol and compound the problem. Alcohol will increase the effect of narcotics, barbiturates, and depressants of all types and the reason for the **potentiation** may go unrecognized.

The alcoholic patient will be manipulative and convincing. The presenting symptoms may be explained away with no indication that alcohol is the problem. It will require the perception of the entire office working as a team with the patient's family or caregiver to search for the cause of the symptoms and will demand that the patient and all who are involved in the case work toward a solution to the addiction.

Suicide

When ill health, multiple losses, and deep depression become too much for the patient to bear, suicide may seem preferable to life. Unlike suicide among younger people, suicide among the elderly is more likely to be well planned and successful. Approximately one-fifth of all suicides are persons over the age of 60. Most of those suicides are white men over the age of 65 who have recently lost a spouse. These suicides are not usually a cry for help, but a genuine effort to end life. Watch for these signs of intent:

- Deepening confusion and scattered attention span
- Increasing anger, hostility, or isolation
- Increase in alcoholism or requests for narcotics or sedatives
- Marked loss of interest in matters of health
- Secretive behavior
- Sharp mood swings from deep depression to euphoria
- Giving away favored objects

Checkpoint Question

3. What are seven signs of suicidal intent?

Believe the patient who expresses an intent to commit suicide and communicate this to the physician. Work with the health care team to restore mental health as aggressively as to restore physical health.

➤ LONG-TERM CARE

More than 90% of the elderly live within the community, as many as 75% in their own homes. A small minority find that long-term care is the only option available if a return to health and independence is not possible.

Long-term care is divided into three main categories:

- *Group homes* for the elderly who are able to tend to their own **activities of daily living (ADL)** (eg, bathing, dressing, self-feeding), but who need companionship and mild supervision for safety purposes. Bed and board is usually provided along with a variety of other options.
- *Long-term care facilities* for those who need help with most areas of personal care as well as moderate medical supervision. Many are ambulatory and suffer from chronic diseases that make living at home alone impossible.
- *Skilled nursing facilities* are for those who are gravely or terminally ill and need constant supervision. If the illness is acute and short term, the patient may return to an intermediate stage of care after recovery.

Expect the elderly patient's move to long-term care to be met with sorrow and a deep sense of loss. The patient will probably show symptoms of bereavement: poor appetite, headaches, insomnia, deep depression, and vague aches and pains. All of these must be referred to the physician.

Many physicians will continue to care for long-time patients who may be residing in long-term care facilities. As the medical assistant, you may be responsible to block time in the daily schedule for visits to patients in such facilities. You must direct calls from the facility to the physician regarding the patient's status and offer assistance to the family as they call with concerns about the care and physical condition of the patient.

Checkpoint Question

4. What is the difference between long-term care facilities and skilled nursing facilities?

What If?

What if a patient's relative asks you about options for home care for an elderly parent?

You can explain that many options are available that allow patients to remain in the home. One option is the use of home health aides. Some insurance plans will pay for this service. The home health aides do light housecleaning, cooking, and will promote patient safety. A second option is community resource centers. Some communities have senior citizen programs that provide transportation for shopping, doctor appointments, or entertainment. These programs get the older patient out of the house, preventing boredom and enhancing self-esteem. A third option is placing the patient in a day-care program for the elderly. These programs keep the patient safe, entertained, and cared for during daytime hours. The advantage of day care is that it relieves the caregiver of the need to place a parent in a long-term care facility, yet provides for patient safety during the day and allows the relative the freedom to continue employment or attend to personal needs. Community programs for senior citizens are good sources of information for caregivers or for relatives searching for respite or permanent care.

➤ ELDER ABUSE

Although elder abuse is not as well researched or as widely publicized as child abuse, it is thought to be almost as prevalent.

Risk Factors for Abuse

The following are common risk factors for elder abuse:

- Multiple chronic illnesses that stress the family's physical, emotional, and financial resources
- Senile dementia that precludes reasoning or interaction
- Bladder or bowel incontinence
- Age-related sleep disturbances that interfere with the caretaker's rest patterns
- Dependence on the caretaker for activities of daily living

Elder abuse may take several different forms depending on the caretaker's need to exact punishment on the victim and the victim's access to resources.

Passive neglect may simply be ignorance on the part of the caretaker regarding the physiologic and psychological needs of the patient. The caretaker may be ill or elderly also and unable to supply the needs to the patient.

Active neglect may take many forms, including overmedicating (to render the patient passive and easier to care for) or purposely depriving the victim of adequate nutrition (to decrease physical resources).

Psychological abuse may include threatening imprisonment or physical abuse, withholding food or medication, or physical isolation.

Financial abuse may involve only small amounts of money or entire substantial estates. Financial resources may be embezzled, squandered, or frankly stolen, leaving the victim destitute.

Physical abuse may be as simple as pinches and slaps or may be life-threatening, may be sexual in nature, and may be so well concealed as to be missed even by perceptive health care providers.

Checkpoint Question

5. What are the different types of elder abuse? Describe each one.

Signs of Elder Abuse

Be aware of these signs of elder abuse:

- Wounds of suspicious origins in various stages of healing
- Signs of restraint (wrist or ankle abrasions or bruising)
- Large, deep, neglected decubital ulcers
- Large amounts of physical debris and poor hygiene
- Poor nutrition with no efforts at correction
- Dehydration without related disease process
- Untreated injuries or medical conditions
- Excessive and unwarranted agitation or apathetic resignation

If you suspect abuse, you are responsible for bringing it to the attention of the physician, who should then assess the situation. If abuse is confirmed, referral should be made to the proper authorities. The majority of the states now require that all suspected cases be reported to the Department of Social Services just as required for child abuse. Regulations for elder abuse are contained in statutes that address the concerns of the disabled adult. The entire medical staff may be held responsible if the abuse is not reported immediately.

The elderly fear reprisal or abandonment by their caregivers just as children do and are reluctant to complain of any improprieties. Separate the caregiver from the patient for the examination, if possible, and treat the patient with the utmost care and compassion. Document all findings with full descriptions. It may be necessary to photograph the suspected injuries to present with the documentation.

► MEDICATIONS AND THE ELDERLY

Educating the elderly in self-medication is a challenge that will become increasingly common as the population ages. At the time that more medications are needed, the body is coping with the stress of illness or injury and a slowing down of all functions. The gastrointestinal system is no longer moving medications along as efficiently now that peristalsis has slowed. The circulatory system is not absorbing the dissolved medication from the intestines or the injection site and delivering it to the target tissue as quickly. The liver is not **biotransforming** (converting) the medication, causing it to remain in effect longer than might be desirable and possibly adding to a cumulative effect. And, lastly, the kidneys are receiving less blood, thus less medication is being filtered, making the kidneys less effective at removing the medications from the system, with possible toxic effects.

The fact that the patient is ill adds to the problems of providing an education that will contribute to a return to an acceptable health status. Patients will frequently have trouble understanding what is being explained to them because of their age-related barriers to understanding (poor hearing, slow response); these barriers are compounded by illness.

Your responsibility as a medical assistant is to elicit information regarding any and all of the prescribed and over-the-counter substances the patient is taking. Emphasize that the physician must be made aware of any change, addition, or deletion to the current list of substances. If the concept of interaction is understood, most patients will choose to adhere to suggestions made for their benefit.

Follow these guidelines to help ensure that your elderly patient adheres to the prescribed medication regimen:

1. Explain all side effects, precautions, interactions, and expected action in a manner that is appropriate for the patient's level of understanding.
2. Explain the proper dosage and how to measure. Mark plastic measuring cups with indelible ink at the appropriate level to be more easily read by patients with failing eyesight.
3. Write out a schedule and suggest methods for adherence. Suggestions may include daily dose packs available at pharmacies, egg cartons with hours of medication marked on the cups and filled with the proper medications each morning or evening, or calendars marked with the medications and hours to be checked off when the medication is taken.
4. Tell the patient to take the most important medication first. If it is not possible to take the other medications at this time, it may be acceptable to skip a dose of the less vital medications.
5. Help the patient understand not to rush taking the medication. The patient should be sitting or standing, not reclining. One pill should be taken at the time with lots of water. If the medication is difficult to swallow, have the patient try putting the pill on the back of the tongue and drinking with a straw.
6. Have the patient ask the pharmacist for large print on the label so that medication errors are less likely. Child-proof containers may not be necessary if there are no children in the home and the patient finds these hard to open.
7. Explain that the medication must be taken until it is gone (if this is the case) and must not be passed through the family or saved for another illness just like this one.
8. Encourage patients to take an active role in their therapy. Teach them to apply ointments or transdermal patches, even to give injections. A patient who feels in charge will more likely make the decision to complete a course of medication or to remain on the medication if its use is to be long term.

As a medical assistant, you will be in control of the medication administration that occurs in the office, but responsibility to patients does not end there. To ensure that medications are used to their best benefit, emphasize to patients the importance of proper medication administration in their return to health.

Checkpoint Questions

6. What are eight things you can do to make sure your elderly patient follows the prescribed medication regimen?

➤ SYSTEMIC CHANGES IN THE ELDERLY

Although longevity is considered largely hereditary, environmental factors play a considerable part in how long and how well we will live. The obese, physically inactive smoker is less likely to maintain a state of optimum health than the nonsmoker whose diet is well balanced and who is actively involved in an exercise program. In addition, certain occupational hazards, such as black lung disease or radiation exposure, may shorten a life that should have lasted for decades longer.

The aging changes are thought to be programmed into our cells along with our DNA. Theories now suggest that when cells have reached their allotted reproduction level, they either will not replace themselves or will replicate more slowly or ineffectively. These changes will manifest themselves at varying rates for all persons, but will follow a recognized order as outlined in Table 50-1.

➤ DISEASES OF THE ELDERLY

The degenerative conditions noted in Table 50-1 are part of the aging process. Many of the changes present problems that must be managed by the health care team; others are only inconveniences for the patient. Diseases specific for aging are covered in the chapters presenting each system. Below are two others commonly associated with aging, but they may present in the middle years as well.

Parkinson's Disease

Parkinson's disease is a slow, progressive neurologic disorder. It may take 10 years or more for complete debilitation or death. The initial presenting symptoms will frequently be muscle rigidity, involuntary tremors, and difficulty walking. It affects men more than women and is estimated to be present in some form in approximately 1 in 100 persons over the age of 60.

The cause is unknown but is thought to be a loss of dopamine in the brain cells. Normally dopamine and acetylcholine are in balance to inhibit involuntary movements of muscles. With the loss of normal levels of

text continues on page 1027

Table 50-1
Effects of Aging on Body Systems

	Systemic Changes	*Manifestations*	*How the Medical Assistant Can Help*
Integumentary System	Loss of subcutaneous fat	Wrinkling, sagging, decreased ability to maintain hydration, less protection against temperature changes	Encourage the patient to drink plenty of fluids and dress appropriately for climate changes.
	Loss of pigment	Less protection against sun damage, paler skin, graying hair	Encourage the use of sunscreens with appropriate UV protection.
	Loss of elasticity	Increased incidence of trauma	Suggest using good lubricating lotions and bathing less often. Caution the patient to guard against injuries.
	Receding capillaries	Sallow skin, thicker nails	
	Slower reproduction of hair and skin cells	Balding; thin, fine hair; slower healing	Suggest ways to guard against injuries.
	Diminished oil and sweat production	Dry, fragile skin; intolerance to heat	Encourage the patient to use good lubricating lotions and bathe less often. Suggest ways to avoid becoming overheated.
	Erratic pigment and cell production	Senile **lentigines** (liver spots) and **keratoses** (skin thickening)	Show the patient how to conduct skin checks and consult a dermatologist with any concerns.
Musculoskeletal System	Loss of muscle strength and size	Loss of strength, flexibility, and endurance	Suggest frequent exercise appropriate to the patient's age and ability.
	Loss of bone density	Vertebral compression with diminished height and a **dowager's hump** (abnormal spinal curvature); **osteoporosis** (abnormal bone porosity) with frequent fractures	Educate the patient regarding weight bearing exercises. Encourage the patient to conduct a home safety check to avoid falls. The physician may recommend calcium supplements, dietary consultations, or estrogen replacement.

continued

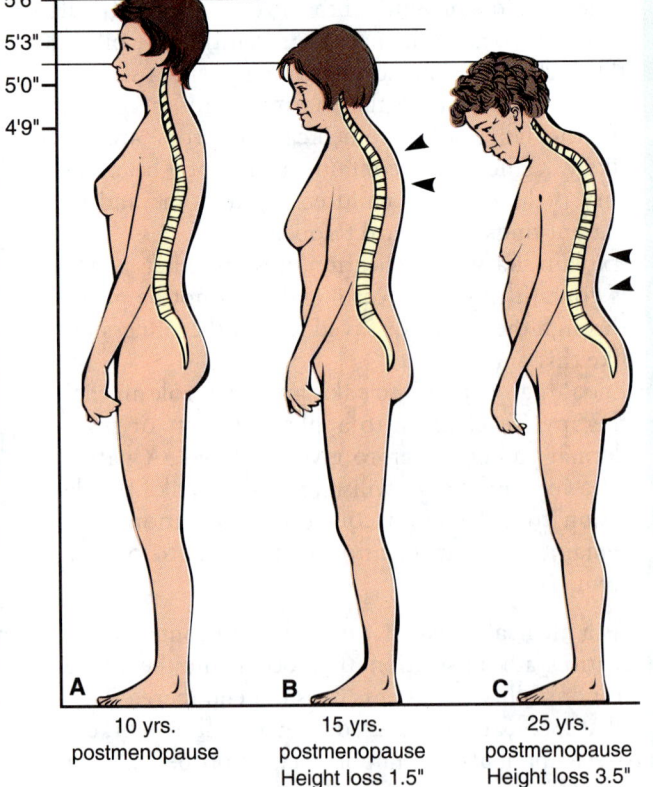

Typical loss of height associated with osteoporosis and aging. (Courtesy of Wilson Research Foundation.)

A 10 yrs. postmenopause

B 15 yrs. postmenopause Height loss 1.5"

C 25 yrs. postmenopause Height loss 3.5"

Table 50-1

Effects of Aging on Body Systems (Continued)

	Systemic Changes	*Manifestations*	*How the Medical Assistant Can Help*
	Degenerative joint cartilage	Less clear margins with spurs of bone that restrict movement, **degenerative joint disease (DJD)**, arthritis	The physician may limit phosphorus intake.
Nervous System	Slower nerve conduction	Slower reaction time, slower learning, slower perception of pain with resulting increase in injuries	Allow extra time as needed and educate the patient about possible hazards of delayed reaction times. Aim teaching at comprehension level. Encourage the patient to conduct home safety checks.
	Reduced cerebral circulation	Loss of balance and **vertigo** (whirling sensation), frequent falls	Have the patient install bath rails, remove throw rugs, conduct a home safety check. Encourage the patient to use ambulatory aids.
	Referred circulatory problems	Increase in cardiovascular diseases (atherosclerosis, arteriosclerosis) reflected as **cerebrovascular accidents (CVA)** (brain ischemia due to vessel occlusion), cerebral hypoxia, and transient ischemia attacks	Educate the patient and family about the danger signs for cerebrovascular accidents and transient ischemic attacks.
Eyes	Less time spent in deep sleep	Less restful sleep, more frequent naps	Allow the patient rest periods as needed.
	Diminished adjustment of lens to accommodation	**Presbyopia** (farsightedness)	Obtain a referral to an ophthalmologist. Provide adequate lighting and use large print books.
	Lens cloud	**Cataracts** (lens opacity) that dim vision as less light reaches the retina	Obtain a referral to an ophthalmologist. Provide adequate lighting.
	Loss of ciliary function	**Glaucoma** (increased intraocular pressure as the pupils press on the canal of Schlemm), intolerance to light or glare, poor night vision	Obtain a referral to an ophthalmologist. Provide adequate lighting and have the patient avoid night driving.
Ears	Loss of auditory hair cells (organ of Corti)	Hearing loss in upper frequencies, problems distinguishing Ch, S, Sh, and Z	Obtain a referral to an otologist. Speak clearly, facing the patient, in an area with few distractions.
	Ossicle becomes fixed	**Presbycusis** (hearing loss), strains to hear, misses cues, inappropriate responses	Obtain a referral to an otologist. Speak clearly, facing the patient, in an area with few distractions.
Other Senses	Diminished sense of smell	Loss of appetite, poor nutrition	Suggest dietary consultation.
	Diminished sense of taste	Loss of appetite, poor nutrition, may increase use of salt or spices	Suggest dietary consultation. Encourage use of spices rather than salt.
Cardiovascular System	Atherosclerosis and arteriosclerosis, narrowing of vessels	Loss of peripheral circulation, fatty plaques with resulting myocardial infarctions and CVAs, cold extremities, slower healing time, hypertension	Encourage the patient to exercise and to eat a balanced, low-fat, low-salt diet. Have the patient dress appropriately for temperature changes and conduct a home safety check.
	Slower response time to demands for increased output	Complaints of fatigue on exertion	Help the patient pace exercise and exertion.
	Diminished function	Pulmonary involvement with edema, dyspnea	Educate the patient regarding low-salt diets and orthopneic position.

continued

Table 50-1

Effects of Aging on Body Systems (Continued)

	Systemic Changes	Manifestations	How the Medical Assistant Can Help
Respiratory System	Stiffening costal cartilage	Decreased expansion and contraction, barrel chest, decreased lung capacity	Educate the patient about smoking hazards and emphysema. Encourage moderate exercise.
	Decreased gas exchange	Fatigue and breathlessness on exertion, impaired healing due to insufficient oxygen, **syncope** (sudden drop in blood pressure)	Encourage the patient to exercise, as appropriate, and to use ambulatory aids. Caution the patient to guard against upper respiratory infections and to conduct a home safety check.
	General loss of muscle mass	Difficulty coughing deeply (may lead to pneumonia)	Encourage the patient to drink adequate fluids to liquefy respiratory secretions.
Gastrointestinal System	Drying of secretions, including saliva	Dry mouth, dysphagia (difficulty swallowing)	Educate the patient regarding oral hygiene and adequate fluid intake.
	Decreased enzyme activity	Incomplete digestion, poor conversion of nutrients with malnourishment	Encourage the patient to eat small, frequent, well balanced meals.
	Slower peristalsis	Constipation, flatulence, indigestion	Suggest the patient increase fluid and fiber intake. Have the patient avoid laxative dependency.
	Loss of teeth	Poor chewing function, choking on large pieces, loss of appetite, poor nutrition	Refer the patient to dentist and provide instruction regarding good oral hygiene. Suggest dietary counseling.
Urinary System	Decreased bladder capacity	Urinary frequency	Encourage the patient to respond to the initial urge to void.
	Decreased bladder muscle tone	Urinary retention with resulting urinary tract infections or incontinence	Suggest exercises for strengthening the pelvic floor. Urge the patient to completely empty the bladder with each voiding.
	Fewer functioning nephrons	Less blood flowing through the kidneys to be cleaned of wastes, creating possible lethal levels of medications or normal body wastes	Have the patient increase fluid intake to maintain hydration.
Endocrine System	Decreased enzyme activity	Menopause, glucose intolerance with non–insulin-dependent diabetes mellitus, slower metabolism	The physician will supplement as needed.
Immune System	Diminished production and function of T cells and B cells	Less resistance to illness	Encourage the patient to obtain immunizations as age appropriate.
	Diminished ability to distinguish self from other	Increase in autoimmune diseases	Educate the patient regarding symptoms of autoimmunity.
	Diminished defenses elsewhere (eg, gastrointestinal enzymes)	Overload on compromised immune system and more frequent serious illnesses	Encourage the patient to obtain immunizations as age appropriate and to guard against communicable diseases.
Female Reproductive System	Decreased egg production	Menopause or climacteric	The physician may prescribe supplemental estrogen.
	Decreased estrogen production	"Hot flashes"; thinner, drier vaginal walls with vaginal itching and painful intercourse; osteoporosis	The physician may prescribe supplemental estrogen.
	Poor perineal muscle tone	Rectocele, cystocele, stress incontinence	Suggest exercises for strengthening the pelvic floor.
Male Reproductive System	Decreased penile and testicle size	Loss of libido	The physician may refer the patient for counseling.
	Atherosclerosis and arteriosclerosis	Impotence	The physician may refer the patient for counseling. Educate the patient regarding good nutrition to avoid atherosclerosis.
	Benign prostatic hypertrophy (BPH)	Urgency, frequency, nocturia, retention	Encourage the patient to have yearly checks for BPH and provide instruction regarding testicular self-examination.

dopamine, acetylcholine has no counterbalance. This imbalance can be precipitated by cerebral injury or by cerebrotoxic medications in addition to idiopathic disease.

Signs and symptoms of Parkinson's disease include:

- Muscle rigidity
- **Bradykinesia** (abnormally slow voluntary movements)
- Difficulty walking with a shuffling, mincing gait
- Forward-bending posture with no normal arm swing
- Laryngeal rigidity with a resulting monotone voice
- Pharyngeal rigidity with resulting dysphagia and drooling
- Facial muscle rigidity with resulting mask-like, expressionless face and infrequent blinking reflex, causing eye infections
- Small tremors in the fingers in a characteristic "pill-rolling" action. These start unilaterally and stop with purposeful action in the affected hand. Tremors are greater during times of stress and anxiety and are diminished at sleep or at rest. Muscles will resist passive stretching and will become rigid with passive manipulation (Fig. 50-1).

Diagnosis is usually made by excluding other possible causes. Testing may show decreased levels of dopamine in the urine. Symptomatic history remains the primary method of diagnosis after all other possibilities have been ruled out.

Parkinson's disease has no cure. Treatment is symptomatic, supportive, and palliative. Medications include:

- Levodopa (L-dopa). Dopamine replacement crosses the blood–brain barrier to restore the balance with acetylcholine. Individualized doses are gradually increased as the disease symptoms progress. Levodopa is fairly effective for a period of time but will gradually lose its effectiveness. Unfortunately, levodopa has serious side effects that include nausea and vomiting, tachycardia, and arrhythmias. It has severe adverse reactions with alcohol.
- Anticholinergics. By decreasing the levels of acetylcholine, depleted levels of dopamine are not so out of balance. This method works best in mild, early stages.
- Antihistamines with anticholinergic actions. In the early, mild stages, this method of lowering acetylcholine to balance with low levels of dopamine will alleviate symptoms.

Neurosurgery exactly pinpointing the appropriate area of the thalamus involved will help to prevent involuntary movement. This method of treatment is rarely

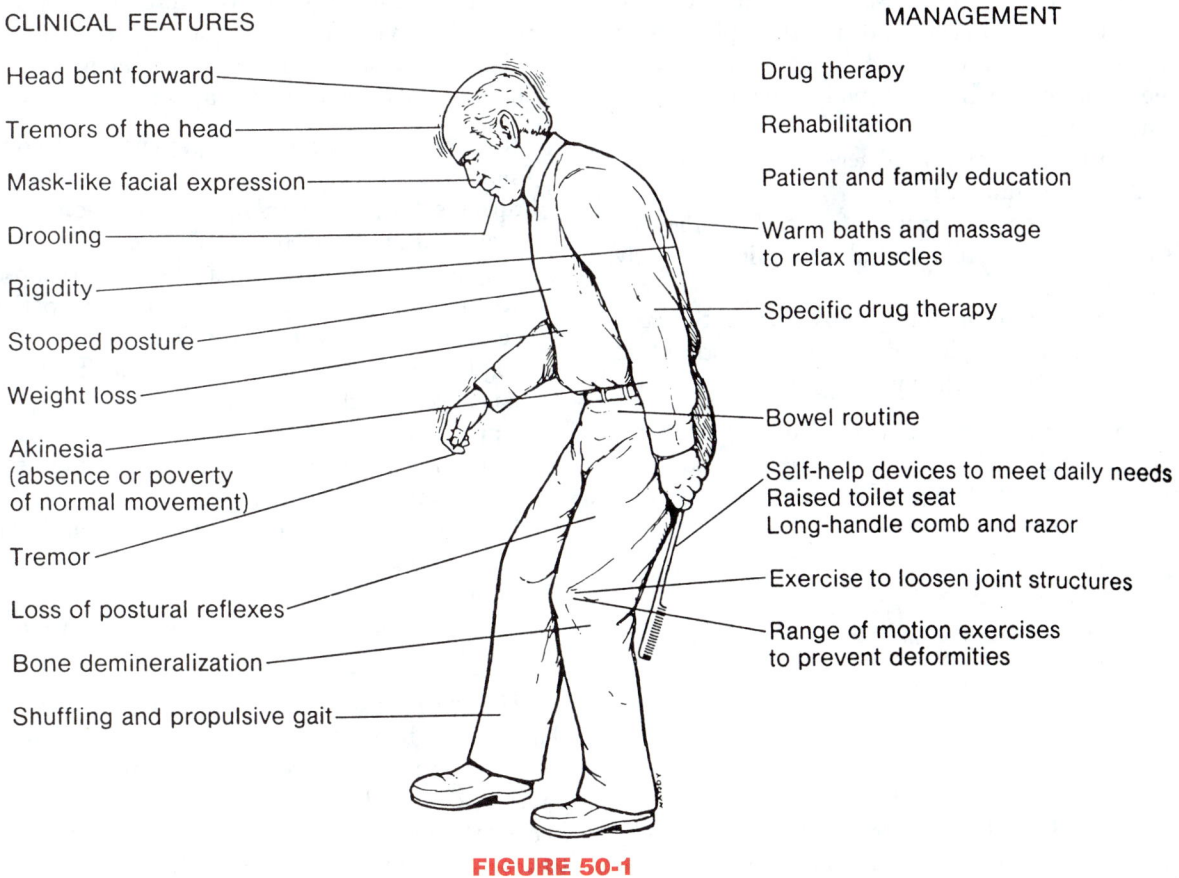

CLINICAL FEATURES

Head bent forward
Tremors of the head
Mask-like facial expression
Drooling
Rigidity
Stooped posture
Weight loss
Akinesia (absence or poverty of normal movement)
Tremor
Loss of postural reflexes
Bone demineralization
Shuffling and propulsive gait

MANAGEMENT

Drug therapy
Rehabilitation
Patient and family education
Warm baths and massage to relax muscles
Specific drug therapy
Bowel routine
Self-help devices to meet daily needs
Raised toilet seat
Long-handle comb and razor
Exercise to loosen joint structures
Range of motion exercises to prevent deformities

FIGURE 50-1
The Parkinson's patient.

used except in young, otherwise healthy patients. As with all other methods, this is palliative and not curative.

Passive range-of-motion and active range-of-motion exercises will help to maintain a level of muscle tone and flexibility. Regular walking schedules, heat, and massage will help to keep muscle tissue supple. Parkinson's patients tire easily and must rest often but will ultimately benefit from regular schedules of moderately challenging exercise.

Parkinson's patients will retain their former level of intelligence unless an organic brain disturbance is also present. They are aware of the outward signs of the disease and are embarrassed and depressed. They will require great psychological support from the medical staff, family, and support groups. As a medical assistant, you can:

1. Encourage the patient to participate in all activities of daily living (ADL).
2. Encourage independence; do not infantilize the patients.
3. Be aware that rigidity extends to the gastrointestinal tract, so expect dysphagia and constipation. Suggest that the patient increase fluids, watch nutrition, and increase fiber intake.
4. Tell the patient that a decreased cough reflex can lead to choking.
5. Encourage the patient to use aids for safety and assistance in eating, such as no-spill cups, plates with high sides, and special utensils. Raised toilet seats and handrails in the bath will increase independence and safety.
6. Listen to the patient. Intelligence is still intact and needs to be stimulated.
7. Educate the patient about safety factors; the forward-bending posture and altered gait frequently lead to falls.
8. Enlist the help of support groups. Include the caregiver and urge respite care when exhaustion and stress become overwhelming.

Death is usually the result of aspiration pneumonia, falls, accidents, or opportunistic diseases secondary to the effects of long-term stress.

Checkpoint Question

7. How can you assist a patient with Parkinson's disease?

Alzheimer's Disease

Roughly half of the dementia seen in the elderly can be traced to Alzheimer's disease. Alzheimer's may masquerade as transient ischemic attacks, cerebral tumors, and dementias other than Alzheimer's. There is no clearly defined cause for this disease at this time.

Symptoms may begin as early as age 40 with gradual loss of memory function and slight personality changes. The changes may cover a period as long as 15 years and are frequently so gradual that diagnosis is difficult and may only be made on the basis of symptoms. If swift and early diagnosis is necessary, **positron emission tomography (PET)** has been used with varied success. (PET is computerized radiography using radioactive substances to assess metabolic or physiologic functions within the body.)

Later diagnosis may sometimes be made by electroencephalography or computed tomography. However, diagnosis is generally made by excluding or ruling out all other possibilities. No reliable treatment is available at this time. On autopsy, organic brain changes are seen with loss of neurons and neurotransmitters. Plaques or deposits may be present as a residue of the neural cell deterioration.

Alzheimer's disease has seven recognized stages. The progression from one stage to the next may be gradual. Some stages may last for years, and some stages may be passed through so quickly that the progression may go unnoticed. Expect varying levels of response from patients as they present at each of these levels (Table 50-2).

As a medical assistant, your responsibility will be to remember that anger and hostility are symptoms of this disease and should not be taken personally. When caring for patients with Alzheimer's disease, be sure to:

- Respond with the utmost patience and compassion.
- Speak calmly and without condescension.
- Never argue with the patient, even if you are blamed unfairly for the patient's memory lapses.
- Reintroduce yourself. Do not expect the patient to remember the staff from previous visits.
- Explain even common procedures as if the patient has never had them explained.
- Approach quietly and professionally in a nonthreatening manner and remind the patient of who you are and what you must do.
- Use short, simple, direct statements, and explain only one action at the time rather than a sequence of directions.
- Keep a list of support contacts for family members to call.

Home care agencies usually offer the respite care that is vital to the caregiver if mental and physical health are to be maintained. Remember that an exhausted, distraught family member may not be thinking clearly. The most therapeutic action may be for you to assist the family with the proper contacts to make the diagnosis of this devastating disease less traumatic.

Table 50-2
Levels of Alzheimer's Disease

Level	Description
I and II	Presenile dementia may end here with no further progression. Brain changes are not significant and the only remarkable symptom may be forgetfulness. Patients at this level still perform all activities of daily living (ADL) with reasonable ease.
III	At this level, there will be an increased inability to remember facts, faces, and names. The patient will still have enough awareness to recognize the problem and will become increasingly frustrated and angry. Most ADL are still performed reasonably well.
IV	Late confusional or mild Alzheimer's. The patient at this level will begin to misplace things, has increasing difficulty remembering, and will neglect ADL. Most patients will be aware that a problem exists but will deny that it is a concern.
V	Early dementia or moderate Alzheimer's. By this level, the patient must have custodial care. There will be severe lapses in memory, disorientation, anger, and great frustration.
VI	Middle dementia or moderately severe Alzheimer's. The patient now has severe memory loss, is incapable of self-care at any level, and is disoriented most of the time. There is immense anger, hostility and combativeness. At this level, a fear of water is present.
VII	Late dementia. The patient requires full-time care and will rarely be seen in the office setting. Unless home care is an option, the physician will probably make calls to the long-term care facility. The patient at this stage rarely speaks and almost never speaks intelligibly. There will be incontinence and the patient may require tube feedings.

➤ MAINTAINING OPTIMUM HEALTH

No one realistically expects to maintain at age 70 the same strength and agility that is taken for granted at age 20. It is possible, however, to achieve a level of fitness that adds a dimension to life not possible if proper nutrition and exercise are neglected.

Exercise

Exercise plays a vital role in maintaining over-all physical and mental health (Table 50-3). Patients beginning an exercise program should only do so after a thorough physical examination and should proceed at the physician's recommendation.

Provide the following guidelines for elderly patients who are starting an exercise program:

1. Always warm up cold muscles for at least 10 minutes. Slow and rhythmic movements, such as walking, raise the heart rate and increase metabolism before beginning slow, easy stretching to lengthen sluggish muscles.
2. Begin by exercising for brief time periods. Expect to exercise 5 to 10 minutes a day the first week, then progress to 10 or 15 minutes a day the next week, and gradually work up to about 30 to 45 minutes of pleasantly challenging strength and cardiovascular/endurance activity after about a month. This routine will reduce the chance of injury and is more likely to be an attainable goal.

Table 50-3
Benefits of Exercise

System Targeted	Benefits
Cardiovascular	Increases endurance
	Lowers cholesterol to avoid atherosclerosis
	Maintains vascular elasticity to delay arteriosclerosis
Musculoskeletal	Increases bone mass to reduce osteoporosis
	Decreases fat/muscle ratio to maintain metabolism
	Retains strength and flexibility to ensure mobility and improve posture
Nervous	Improves mental health by reducing stress, fatigue, tension, and boredom
	Maintains or restores balance to reduce falls

3. Stop if you feel pain, shortness of breath, or dizziness. Never try to work through pain.

4. Breathe deeply and evenly. If you cannot carry on a conversation, slow down. Never hold your breath while you exercise.

5. Rest when you get tired. Do not try to work to the point of exhaustion.

6. Keep a record of your progress. It helps to see how much your performance has improved.

7. Exercise with a friend, with a group, or to music that you enjoy.

8. Make exercise a part of your daily routine, do not make it a chore. Do something vigorous every day and take pride in it.

Diet

The elderly have several factors that interfere with good nutrition. A decrease in activity will mean a corresponding decrease in hunger. Decaying teeth or poorly fitting dentures cause pain, making it hard to chew. Saliva production decreases, making it harder to swallow. The sense of smell diminishes, interfering with the cephalic phase of digestion. Taste buds do not work well, so nothing tastes good. Many eat alone or cannot enjoy the socialization that adds immeasurably to the joy of eating.

A balanced diet is vital to good health at any age. Although activity levels are lower among the elderly, decreasing the need for a certain amount of calories, vitamin and mineral requirements are not lowered with age. Efforts must be made to increase the nutritional level of the elderly. The food should be easy to chew but offer texture and variety. There should be a decrease in sugar, salt, and fat intake and an increase in vitamins, protein, and fiber consumption. Smaller, more frequent meals may be easier to digest than infrequent large meals. Water should be offered frequently to maintain hydration and to aid digestion and elimination.

Talk to patients or their families about valuable services such as Meals On Wheels. Nutritious meals are delivered to the home either daily or 5 days a week (some do not operate on weekends). This ensures that at least one well balanced meal a day is available. Most will prepare meals to meet special dietary needs such as low sodium, low fat, and so on. In addition to the meals, contact with a caring volunteer is a daily occurrence. The volunteer will be alert to the needs of the patient and will report to a coordinator if the patient does not answer the door or seems ill or confused. This resource is reassuring to the patient and the family that nutritional and socialization needs are being met.

Safety

Alert the patient and caregivers to areas of concern for safety and offer the following suggestions:

- Avoid scatter rugs, especially on highly polished floors.
- Never allow electrical cords across passageways.
- Remove or reduce clutter as much as possible.
- Strengthen handrails on stairs and install them in tubs and near the commode.
- Install a telephone by the bedside and near a favorite chair. Consider having a telephone in the bathroom also.
- Install and frequently maintain smoke alarms and carbon monoxide detectors throughout the house.
- Establish a system for calling and checking every day. Many communities have available systems in which volunteers call the sick or elderly daily to check on needs and to offer a few minutes of conversation. If the patient fails to answer, someone is sent to the home to check on the patient. This service ensures that the patient will never be without contact for long periods of time. Lifeline, an emergency service contact worn by the patient, is also an option that increases the feeling of safety for patients who live alone.

SUMMARY

In the early 1900s, the leading causes of death were infant mortality and infectious diseases. Currently, the major causes of death are cardiovascular disease, trauma, and homicide. The median age of the population has steadily increased, with the average life span growing by about 25 years since the turn of the last century. The generation that matured in this country during World War II is the healthiest, longest lived in its history. With the advances being made in all areas of health care, each succeeding generation will likely exceed the life span of the preceding generations. This will be a major force in shaping the health care in this country for many years to come and will significantly change many medical specialties to accommodate a large population of adults who present with diseases not common to younger adults. Medical assistants who are actively involved in the care of the elderly will find this a challenging, rewarding, ever-changing career direction.

CRITICAL THINKING CHALLENGES

1. Mrs. Moss, age 78, lives with her son and daughter-in-law and their two school-age children. She has dysphagia and requires tube feedings, so she misses family

mealtimes. Identify ways in which Mrs. Moss could participate in a family meal.
2. Mr. Brown is 90 and his wife is 86. They live alone and Mrs. Brown is the primary caregiver. During the physical examination, Mr. Brown is found to have several large, deep decubital ulcers. Summarize the various types of elder abuse or neglect. What is likely the problem in this case?

ANSWERS TO CHECKPOINT QUESTIONS

1. To reinforce compliance, you could write out instructions in easy-to-understand terms (using large print if the patient is vision impaired); have the patient verbalize instructions and demonstrate a procedure; or list times and days for treatments on a large calendar.
2. You can help your elderly patients maintain good mental health by encouraging open communication, helping them deal with their feelings, promoting a positive self-image, helping family members to be supportive, preparing the patient for the future, and suggesting support groups as needed.
3. The seven signs of suicidal intent are deepening confusion, increasing anger, increased alcohol or narcotic use, lack of interest in health, secretive behavior, sharp mood swings, and giving away personal possessions.
4. Long-term care facilities are for individuals who need help with personal care and some medical supervision. Skilled nursing facilities are for gravely or terminally ill individuals who need constant supervision.
5. Elder abuse can take the form of passive or active neglect or it can be psychological, financial, or physical in nature. Passive neglect refers to the caregiver's inability to identify the patient's needs; active neglect involves the caregiver's refusal to supply the patient's needs. Psychological abuse includes threats, withholding food or medication, or forced isolation. Financial abuse involves de-

priving the patient of material resources. Physical abuse includes varying degrees of physical injury.
6. To help your elderly patient follow the prescribed medication regimen: provide a full explanation of the medication in a way that the patient understands; explain the proper dosage and techniques for measuring; develop a written schedule for taking the medication; instruct the patient to take the most important medication first; tell the patient not to rush when taking the medication; have the patient ask the pharmacist for large print on the label; explain the appropriate use of the medication (eg, do not give it to others or save it); encourage patients to take an active role in their therapy.
7. To assist a patient with Parkinson's disease, encourage activity and independence, promote good nutrition and hydration, caution the patient about the potential for choking, educate the patient about safety, use therapeutic communication skills, and enlist the help of support groups.

SUGGESTIONS FOR FURTHER READING

Birchenall, J. M. & Streight, M. E. (1992). *Care of the Older Adult*, 3rd ed. Philadelphia: J. B. Lippincott.

Craven, R. F., & Hirnle, C. J. (1996). *Fundamentals of Nursing: Human Health and Function*, 2nd ed. Philadelphia: Lippincott-Raven.

Memmler, R. L, Cohen, B. J., & Wood, D. L. (1996). *The Human Body in Health and Disease*, 8th ed. Philadelphia: Lippincott-Raven.

Miller, C. A. (1995). *Nursing Care of Older Adults*, 2nd ed. Philadelphia: J. B. Lippincott.

(1992). *Professional Guide to Diseases*, 4th ed. Springhouse, PA: Springhouse.

Staab, A. S. & Hodges, L. C. (1995). *Essentials of Geriatric Nursing*. Philadelphia: J. B. Lippincott.

Career Strategies

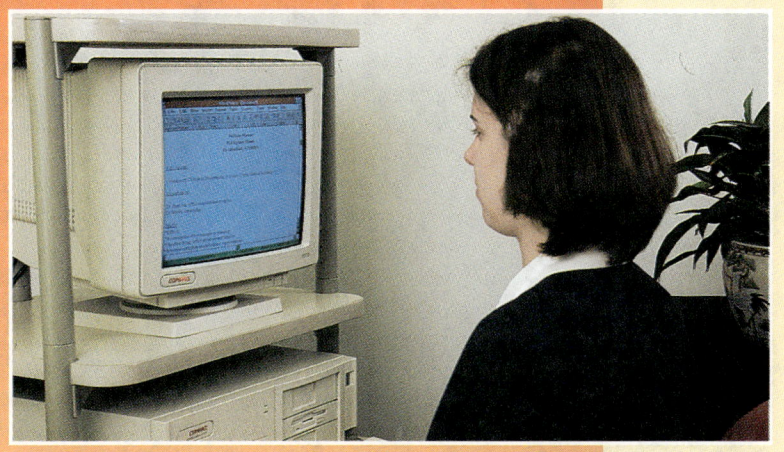

Unit 9

Competing in the Job Market

Medical assisting is a fascinating and exciting career that requires constant adjustment and upgrading of skills. This section will help ease your transition from student to professional, and prepare you for a lifetime of growth, challenges, and rewards.

Externship

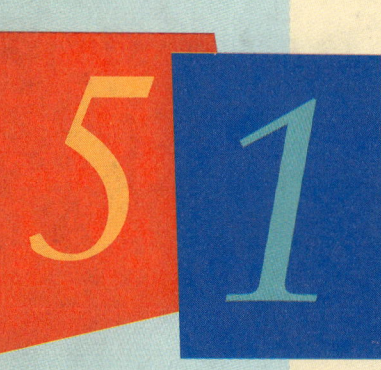

Chapter Outline

Externship Scheduling
Types of Facilities
Site Selection
Benefits of Externship
    Benefits to the Student
    Benefits to the Medical Assisting
      Program
    Benefits to the Externship
      Site
Responsibilities of Externship
    Responsibilities of the Student
    Responsibilities of the Medical
      Assisting Program
    Responsibilities of the Externship
      Site

Student Evaluation Criteria for the
    Preceptor
Guidelines for a Successful Externship
    Preparedness
    Attendance
    Appearance
    Attitude
Time Records and Site Evaluations for
    the Student
    Time Records
    Site Evaluation
    Self-evaluation
Summary
Critical Thinking Challenges
Answers to Checkpoint Questions

DACUM Components

1.1   Project a positive attitude
1.2   Perform within ethical boundaries
1.3   Practice within the scope of education, training, and personal capabilities
1.4   Maintain confidentiality
1.5   Work as a team member
1.6   Conduct oneself in a courteous and diplomatic manner
1.7   Adapt to change
1.8   Show initiative and responsibility
1.9   Promote the profession

Learning Objectives

Upon successfully completing this chapter, you will be able to:

1. Spell and define the Key Terms.
2. Explain the purpose of the externship experience.
3. Understand the benefits of externship to the school, facility, and to the medical assistant student.
4. List the professional responsibilities of a medical assistant student during externship.
5. Understand the evaluation process for the extern student.
6. List attributes necessary to ensure a successful externship.

Key Terms

(See Glossary for definitions.)

affiliation
attribute
criteria
evaluation
externship
preceptor
transition

Students of a formal training program for medical assistants probably have heard their instructors say: "In the real world, it will be done like this...." In this chapter, you will discover that the introduction to the real medical world is through the **externship** component of the curriculum.

Most medical assistant programs provide an externship as part of the course requirement. An externship is a training program that gives students the experience of a professional medical office under the supervision of a **preceptor**, or supervisor, who will help them apply the theories and procedures learned during classroom training. This is the opportunity for you to perform the skills perfected during the many weeks and months of study in the academic portions of the program.

Externship will help ease the **transition**, or change, from the classroom into the first graduate medical assisting position. You will use this time to discover areas of interest in certain types of practices or health care specialties. Rotating through clinical sites will expose you to specific offices that can be pursued as possible opportunities for future employment.

EXTERNSHIP SCHEDULING

The externship period may be as short as 3 to 4 weeks or may extend to one or more full quarters or semesters. The time required to complete the externship may be based around the regular 40-hour work week. Externing students may be scheduled for 8 hours a day for 5 days a week or any variation that meets the requirements of the curriculum.

Most medical offices do not provide evening and weekend hours for students; those that have evening or weekend hours may not have staff to spare to precept students. These hours also do not provide the normal heavy flow of patients that will allow the student the optimum office experience.

TYPES OF FACILITIES

In recent years, the health care industry has developed into a diversified profession with a wide variety of specialty offices and clinics. As a medical assisting student, you will experience an extensive scope of procedures when assigned to a general or family practice clinic or office. These facilities have physicians who are more frequently called the primary care provider. Patients will range in age from newborns to the elderly. These patients will also have a broad range of complaints and illnesses. General practice facilities will provide the best exposure to all types of the procedures performed by a medical assistant (Fig. 51-1).

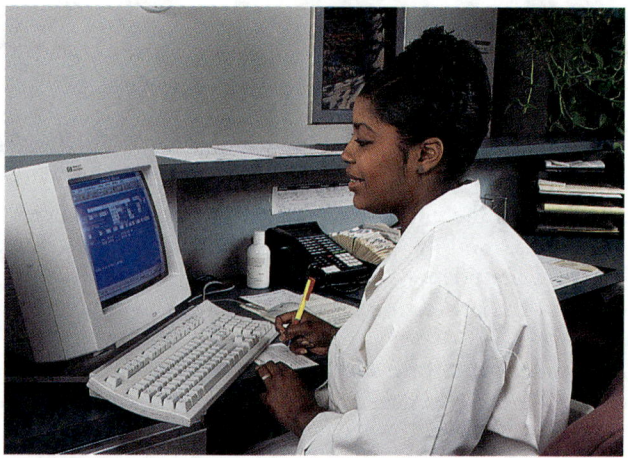

FIGURE 51-1
The general practice office will provide the best exposure to all types of procedures performed by a medical assistant.

The responsibilities for the medical assistant are sometimes limited in specialty practices. For example, staff members in obstetric offices usually do not perform electrocardiograms, nor do staff members in orthopedic offices perform gynecologic examinations. However, working in these types of practices will provide experience in the special examinations and procedures specific to those areas that might not be observed in the general practice setting. Each specialty has advantages and disadvantages as a site, but all will offer invaluable experience that cannot be adequately simulated in the classroom.

 Checkpoint Question
1. What is an externship and why is it beneficial to have an externship at a general practice office?

SITE SELECTION

Most schools have extern sites available that have had students assigned before and that understand what the student must do to complete the clinical experience. These sites have been chosen and continue to be used based on the experience of former students. An ideal site should provide a variety of experiences, both in administrative (front office) and clinical (back office) procedures.

A preceptor will be assigned to work with students as the instructor did in the classroom. Although students will be expected to perform procedures with at least entry-level proficiency, a preceptor must be present to supervise. Preceptors typically are graduate medical assistants who have been through the same type of externship program and understand how eager to learn and how ready students are to begin the medical assisting experience.

The school is careful to choose externship sites with preceptors who are willing to work with students and help them feel comfortable in the medical setting and who understand that all experiences up to this point have been with fellow students in the protected arena of the classroom. They will understand how nervous students may be and will ease the transition from classroom to medical office.

Clinical sites are usually within easy travel distance to avoid unreasonable expense to the students.

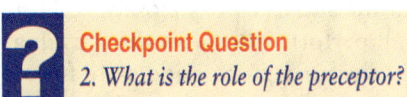

Checkpoint Question
2. What is the role of the preceptor?

➤ BENEFITS OF EXTERNSHIP

Benefits to the Student

Externship serves as a vital part of medical assisting training. You will develop self-confidence and professionalism during the externship portion of your training. No amount of classroom training can compare to the experience of applying skills and knowledge in a medical facility.

Benefits to the Medical Assisting Program

As you gain experience from the externship, the school also benefits from the **affiliation**, or connection, with the medical community. Many sites have a long history of training students. Schools rely on good training sites for the students to enhance the medical assisting curriculum. Medical assisting programs rely on the medical profession to aid in updating and revising the curriculum and course content to ensure that the methods and procedures presented to the students from year to year are current.

The school, the program director, and externship preceptors will review the extern experiences to plan for changes in the program to reflect the needs of the community and the profession as health care constantly changes its technologic needs. If students are routinely required to perform a procedure or examination that is not currently a part of the curriculum, it will usually be considered as an addition to future lectures and laboratory experience in the classroom. If the accepted practice of a procedure has changed from the method taught within the curriculum, changes will need to be made in the way it is taught to

ensure that students are kept abreast of health care advances.

Benefits to the Externship Site

The student and the school are not the only ones to benefit from the externship period. The site also gains information about how well different areas of the facility are functioning. It may be discovered through the presence and questions of students that there should be a review of certain policies or the addition of others that could help the office to run more smoothly. Medical facilities must be updated on a continuing basis. The policy and procedures manual may need items deleted or added, or parts may need to be revised to provide clearer instructions.

As a student, you will be looking at the office as a newcomer, with a fresh perspective, and you may have many questions for the staff. As you become more familiar with the office routine, you will be more comfortable asking questions without the fear of appearing as inexperienced as you feel. These questions may help point out things to the office personnel that need to be changed or clarified.

The externship benefits everyone involved and is a vital, irreplaceable part of the total educational experience.

➤ RESPONSIBILITIES OF EXTERNSHIP

Responsibilities of the Student

You will develop many **attributes**, or characteristics, of a professional health care worker during the externship program. These characteristics must be fostered during this time to ensure that you will continue to grow professionally and will be an asset to the profession.

You must be dependable. Dependability is a good sign of maturity in the development of a professional health care provider. Students who are not at the site on time, who take excessive numbers of breaks, or who do not follow through on assignments cannot properly provide for the needs of the patients who rely on the medical staff of the facility.

You must act professionally. There are many interpretations of professionalism, but all include a positive, pleasant, confident attitude, with a sincere desire to help the physician, the patient, and the staff.

You must be well groomed and dressed in compliance with the program's dress code. If the medical facility requires clothing that differs from the requirements of the school, you will usually have permission to comply with the site.

These desirable attributes of a health care worker are discussed further in "Guidelines for a Successful Externship," below.

Checkpoint Question

3. What are three important attributes of a health care worker?

Responsibilities of the Medical Assisting Program

The primary responsibility of the program is to arrange for the best possible clinical experience for students. The program will usually have a coordinator who matches students to appropriate sites. Once a site has been chosen for a student, the student will meet with the clinical coordinator to discuss the particulars of the medical facility. An interview is sometimes required to acquaint the student and preceptor before the externship begins.

After the site rotation has begun, the program's clinical coordinator will visit or call frequently to follow the student's progress. If there are any concerns from either the student or the site, the coordinator will mediate to eliminate problems or concerns as they arise.

The clinical coordinator will maintain an **evaluation,** or appraisal, of the student from the site. Sites evaluations are usually completed on a form that contains detailed areas to be graded and are equivalent to a grade that might be received in class on a test or examination. These evaluations will be used to determine if the student is prepared for the profession or if skills are deficient and need to be reinforced. The clinical coordinator is responsible for compiling evaluations and keeping the student abreast of progress. This is usually accomplished by frequent student–coordinator conferences.

The school also is responsible for maintaining liability insurance for the student during clinical hours. Students are required in most instances to provide proof of general immunizations and vaccination for hepatitis B. Some schools may provide the vaccine for students. Most programs require a current physical examination, a serology profile, and a tuberculin skin test before students are admitted to the program or before they make patient contact.

Responsibilities of the Externship Site

The medical facility is, of course, responsible for providing opportunities for training. The staff will need to orient students to the office and the procedures. In some sites, students are only allowed to observe certain procedures but are given permission for performing some of the more basic or routine procedures. Even if the student is not allowed to perform specific procedures, every opportunity to observe and ask questions will be a learning, growing experience. In this way, the student will become as familiar as possible with all areas and functions of the clinical sites.

Students are ultimately working under the physician's supervision and direction even though the physician has delegated the role of supervisor to the preceptor. Errors or lack of professionalism on the part of the student during externship will reflect directly on the physician.

The preceptor at the site will work closely with the student, observing all performances. A written evaluation is completed by the preceptor periodically for review by the clinical coordinator and student. Most programs request at least a midpoint and a final evaluation; some require more frequent reports. The preceptor will keep in mind the entry-level status of the student and will not require proficiency expected of an experienced graduate. Even with that in mind, there is no room for hesitancy in performing procedures and certainly no room for error. The preceptor must see satisfactory improvement as the rotation progresses. As competency improves, the preceptor will allow the student to become independent during procedures, but at no time should the student be considered able to perform procedures independent of the preceptor's knowledge and approval.

What If?

What if you have a personality conflict with the preceptor assigned to you at your externship site?

First, discuss the issue with your preceptor. Determine if the problem is due to miscommunication or if it is truly a personality clash. If you are unable to come to a mutual understanding with your preceptor, speak to your externship coordinator at the school for guidance. The externship coordinator can help mediate the situation and visit the site if necessary.

➤ STUDENT EVALUATION CRITERIA FOR THE PRECEPTOR

Criteria are standards, rules, or tests by which something can be judged. The persons evaluating students while on externship are professional medical personnel who know the standards for the health care field as they relates to medical assisting.

You will be judged on your ability to measure up to the standard of care for an entry-level medical assistant. This means you will be expected to perform at the level of a new employee in the field. Of course, you will not know immediately all the things that an experienced medical assistant knows. It may be some time, even years, before you are highly confident and competent in some areas. You will be gathering experiences each day that will help you to grow in the profession.

The major areas of evaluation are:

- Procedural performance
- Professionalism
- Personal attributes

The procedures performed may vary from one facility to another; therefore, evaluations will concentrate on comments regarding how you perform any procedures assigned. This can be referred to as work habits. Students are expected to accept responsibility for their performance and to demonstrate initiative when asked to perform various tasks. The tasks should be performed in an efficient, timely fashion, and of course, above all, must be performed accurately.

A professional must be well groomed at all times and will look as fresh for the last patient of the evening as for the first patient in the morning. Appearance is noticed immediately and many judgments are made on first impressions.

Dependability is a major point in evaluating professionalism. If the office opens at 8:00 AM, the office staff is depended on to be ready to greet patients and answer the phone by 8:00 AM, not 8:05 or 8:10. You will be expected to arrive at the time scheduled, not when it is convenient for you. Dependable persons can be trusted to follow through on assignments, to perform well, and to be reliable from day to day.

A medical assistant should also display enthusiasm while performing daily office tasks, no matter how routine the task may be. Medical assisting students are frequently assigned to perform repetitive tasks, such as filing (see Chap. 10, Medical Records and Records Management). For some facilities, this could be an all day task. Even a chore such as filing can be a learning experience if approached as a challenge. To approach a task such as filing as an extension of the classroom experience, use this time to become familiar with the format of the medical records used in the clinic. For example, note how they are arranged, what type of filing system is used, how the filing system is set up, and what safeguards are in place to ensure quick retrieval of information.

Each job in the medical office has its importance. Most students would prefer to perform more exciting tasks than filing, but much of the work in an office involves procedures that are vitally important for the support of the practice, however routine and mundane they may seem to be. If the patient's medical record is improperly filed and is unavailable for the physician, time will be lost, resulting in delayed care for the patient and frustration for the physician and staff.

Integrity is a vital component of professionalism. The dictionary defines integrity as a quality of honesty and sincerity. In the medical profession, this also includes patient confidentiality. Everything concerning the patient and the functions of the office should be held in strictest confidence and not shared with others from outside the facility unless you are told to divulge the information by legal directive or by the physician. Students will be entrusted to hold in confidence the matters pertaining to each patient. Students will be regarded as a member of the facility staff while assigned to the site and are held to the same degree of confidentiality as any other employee of the facility.

Good working relations are a sign of a mature professional (Fig. 51-2). The office staff must be treated with respect and an effort must be made to develop a good rapport with each level and position within the facility. Interaction with staff and patients will be judged for appropriateness. For example:

- Do you treat the patient with respect and warmth, with too much familiarity, or with an uncaring attitude?
- Do you volunteer for tasks that might be seen as unpleasant?
- Are you team player or are you more likely to resist attempts at inclusion by the staff?

Clinical preceptors and office employees may provide references for you as you seek your first position

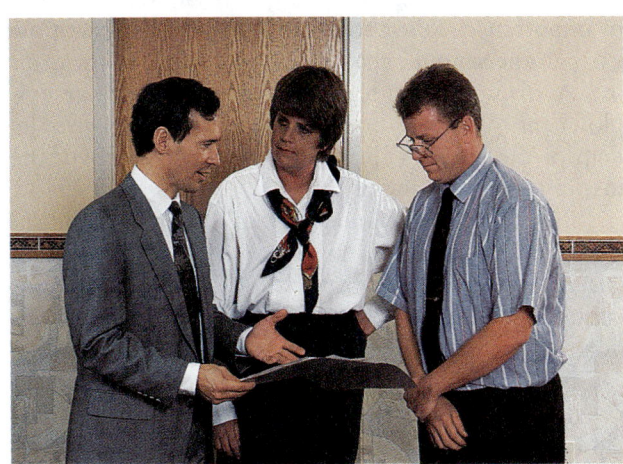

FIGURE 51-2
Good working relationships are a sign of a mature professional.

in medical assisting. If the association was pleasant and positive, the references will be pleasant and positive as well. It is in the best interest of all concerned— you, staff members, patients—for you to make every effort to become a part of the functioning unit of the office during the rotation. Evaluations are designed to reflect the rapport established by you with both the physician and staff. Cooperation is the key to building this relationship.

Checkpoint Question

4. Why is it important to maintain good working relations with the staff at the externship site?

➤ GUIDELINES FOR A SUCCESSFUL EXTERNSHIP

Preparedness

Preparation is the best insurance for success, no matter the goal. Personal preparation during this part of the curriculum will help to avoid time lost to extracurricular obligations.

Many medical assistant externs have to manage a full home life in addition to handling school responsibilities. Some are parents of small children and will need to arrange day care for the extra hours spent in externship. This may mean enlisting family members and relatives to help during hours that day care may not be available. It will be impossible to anticipate all of the problems that an active family life can cause for the student, but careful planning and alternatives can keep to a minimum the distractions caused by unforeseen difficulties.

Finances during externship may be another issue of importance. Many students work at least part time early in the school experience. The longer hours spent in externship may interfere with extracurricular employment. A budget should be set up, possibly with the help of the school's financial aid officer, to cover the loss in wages during this time.

Reliable transportation may fall under the financial aspect of externship. Arrangements must be made to ensure a backup if transportation is unreliable. Students must arrive daily and on time at scheduled sites; no one is impressed by students who have failed to plan for this possibility. It may help to network through classmates and offer to trade driving days with others who are scheduled in sites nearby.

After the family, financial, and transportation situations have been arranged, the personal attributes necessary for success must be considered. These are the three As of professional success: attendance, appearance, and attitude.

Attendance

If transportation, family considerations, and finances are in line, students are more likely to be in attendance as scheduled at the clinical sites. Students must be healthy enough to attend. A good diet, regular exercise, and proper rest will help maintain good health. Careful attention to hygiene and medical asepsis will help ensure that illnesses are not brought home from the clinical sites.

If at any time you will be late or will not be able to attend the site for whatever reason, you must notify both the clinical coordinator and the site preceptor. At no time should you be considered a "no call, no show." Almost all sites have an answering service for leaving messages as do most schools. There is no excuse for not notifying all parties involved when you will be unavoidably late or will not be able to attend the scheduled site.

Office hours will vary from site to site; however, it is a good practice to arrive a few minutes before the scheduled opening. This allows time to check for telephone messages, arrange the day's appointments, turn on office equipment, and generally get oneself into the routine of the office. Plan to leave home in plenty of time to allow for all manner of problems. Arriving in a flurry, frustrated by traffic and home problems, with no time to ease into the morning, will begin the day with a high level of tension and anxiety. It will be harder to show the caring and compassion necessary to deal with the complex problems in the medical office if the day gets off to a bad, late start.

Appearance

There is only one opportunity to make a first impression, and first impressions are usually based on appearance. Appearance is much more than "looks." A beautiful face with a poorly groomed appearance will not be seen as professional and will not inspire trust and confidence in patients or coworkers. The key to a professional appearance is careful preparation and planning.

If uniforms are worn for externship, they must be freshly laundered and pressed before wearing; clean but wrinkled is not acceptable. Wardrobes should be planned for ease of care and a professional appearance. Fad or trendy clothing, suggestive clothing, or flashy clothing will not be appropriate for the clinical sites. All clothing should be in good repair, with no missing buttons, hanging hems, tears, rips, or stains. Duty shoes should be clean and polished frequently and kept in good condition. Laced shoes will look better with fresh, clean shoe laces. Nylon hose should be checked for runs and snags and should be replaced if not serviceable. Lab coats may be worn in some programs; uniforms may be worn in others. The clinical preceptor or the clinical coordinator will clarify the dress code before the rotation begins.

Professional appearance includes hair and makeup. Hair should be conservatively styled, and if long, must be kept away from the face. It should be washed frequently so that it is fresh and clean. Makeup should be kept at a minimum and should be tastefully applied. Perfume and cologne are never worn as part of the uniform; it may be irritating to coworkers and patients. Nails should be kept short to avoid the transfer of pathogens or ripping gloves if procedures are performed.

Jewelry must be tasteful and should be kept at a minimum. Rings and bracelets should never be worn for examining room procedures; therefore, it is a good idea to avoid wearing them in the clinical site.

Attitude

Attitude is also part of appearance. Most patients and coworkers will easily see emotions in facial expressions and body language. Anyone who looks eager is usually perceived as a good worker and will be diligent in completing assigned tasks. Much of attitude is determined by how well a person handles change and direction and how adaptable and flexible he or she is during difficult assignments.

The medical profession is constantly changing, making it imperative that all professionals allow for flexibility. Students will be taught in the classroom the generic methods for treatments and procedures. With the constantly changing technology, they will have to adjust to other methods in the field. If the student has learned a procedure one way in the classroom training and finds in the clinical site that it is performed differently, the new method must be accepted and performed as well as possible. Frequently there will be more than one right way to do any procedure and the classroom method may have been just one of the accepted or generic methods. The next physician or clinical site may have another preferred, and equally correct, procedural method.

"*Your attitude determines your altitude.*" This means that students who work with a positive attitude during externship are more likely to reach higher levels of the profession than those who see the externship as an imposition or a burden.

Box 51-1 offers some additional suggestions to follow during the externship.

➤ TIME RECORDS AND SITE EVALUATIONS FOR THE STUDENT

Time Records

Most programs require a time sheet or record of some sort to document the hours spent in externship (Fig. 51-3). There will be a form to record the beginning and ending hours of each day. Breaks will be handled individually by the clinical coordinator or program requirements and the specific sites. Some sites allow only one-half hour for lunch and others allow an hour; some close for an hour or more midday, others are open and staffed from morning until evening. Some programs require the student to be responsible for time sheet signatures; others delegate the responsibility to

BOX 51-1 Tips for a Successful Externship

You will be more likely to have a successful externship if you follow these tips:

- Be a team player. Workers in any office have been together for a while, so they know how to function as a unit. Learning to work with a well adjusted team is a valuable experience in office relationships.
- Offer to assist in as many tasks as possible because each one will be a learning experience. It is easier to learn by doing than by watching.
- Never hesitate to ask for help from coworkers. Trying to perform procedures for the first time in the clinical setting is a challenge. Asking for assistance will help avoid potentially dangerous errors.
- Always admit errors when they occur. It is easier to correct a problem when it happens rather than try to cover it up and have it discovered later when it may not be reversed or changed.
- Be willing to accept correction and suggestions from the office staff. Many will have invaluable experience and are delighted to share years of hard-earned wisdom.
- Remember that if you are uncertain about a procedure, the preceptor is always available for clarification and to guide and assist with the difficult transition from class to clinic.

CLINICAL EXPERIENCE
STUDENT'S TIME REPORT

To obtain proper credit, an account of time and days in attendance must be recorded by each intern student. This report must be verified by the job supervisor and attached to the final 55-day roster. This information is kept strictly confidential.

Student's Name: _____   Course No.: _____

Program: _____   Course Title: _____

Minimum Contact Hrs. Required: _____   Quarter/Year: _____

WEEK OF (DATES)	M	T	TIME OF DAY W	TH	F	S	TOTAL HOURS	SITE SUPERVISOR

TOTAL HOURS FOR QUARTER: _____

I certify that the above time report is a true statement of the hours worked

I approve this statement of hours in attendance for the quarter covered.

_____   _____
Student's Signature   Date

_____   _____
Curriculum Coordinator's Signature   Date

FIGURE 51-3
Sample student time report used to document attendance and hours worked.

the site preceptor. However the form is handled, it is used to validate the time spent in externship and is a requirement for completion from most programs.

Site Evaluation

The site evaluation form is used by most schools to gather the impressions of the sites and externship experiences for future consideration (Fig. 51-4). It is used to determine the effectiveness of the site for training and if any issues need to be addressed before assigning other students. Students should be objective and honest about the site. When completing a site evaluation, consider these questions:

- Was the overall experience positive or negative?
- Were opportunities for learning abundant and freely offered or hard to obtain?

- Was the staff open and caring or unwelcoming?
- Was the preceptor available and easily approachable or preoccupied and distant?

If the site is not providing a positive learning experience, it should be eliminated.

Checkpoint Question
5. What is the purpose of the site evaluation?

Self-evaluation

The self-evaluation form helps the student identify personal and professional skills that need to be developed or enhanced. These forms encourage introspection and personal honesty for you to begin a lifelong program

CLINICAL SITE EVALUATION
STUDENT QUESTIONNAIRE

Name of Clinical Site: _____

Department/Unit Worked: _____

Dates Worked: From _____   To _____

Name of Preceptor _____

SCALE CODES: 1 = Disagree; 2 = Agree; 3 = No opinion

1. The clinical experience was worthwhile.

   1   2   3

   Comments: _____

2. The objectives of the clinical experience seemed adequately understood and followed by the clinical site.

   1   2   3

   Comments: _____

3. Would you recommend this clinical site for future externs?

   1   2   3

   Comments: _____

4. Was the preceptor helpful?

   1   2   3

   Comments: _____

5. The routines of the department/unit were clearly explained throughout the clinical experience.

   1   2   3

   Comments: _____

6. The clinical site provided sufficient educational experiences.

   1   2   3

   Comments: _____

7. Did you receive constructive feedback, both verbal and written, on your clinical performance?

   1   2   3

   Comments: _____

8. What part of the clinical experience did you like the best?

   Comments: _____

9. What part of the clinical experience did you like the least?

   Comments: _____

10. What changes would you recommend for future clinical experiences at this clinical site?

    Comments: _____

11. Upon completion of your clinical experience, did you feel like a part of the team?

    Comments: _____

12. Were you offered a position at this site?

    Yes _____   No _____

    If yes, fill in the blank spaces.

    FT _____   PT _____   Starting salary _____

Date Completed: _____   Signature: _____

FIGURE 51-4
Sample site evaluation form.

of self-improvement. There should be components that encourage you to outline those things that were done well and that were sources of pride, as well as areas that need improvement.

The self-evaluation and the site evaluation may be included on one form or may be two separate forms.

SUMMARY

Externship is an extension of the classroom learning experience. You will learn from the experience in direct ratio to the effort you put into it. If you feel comfortable with yourself and the skills you bring to the sites, if you are confident in *your professional appearance and have a good attitude, externship will be a fitting conclusion to a program of study that will lead to a career to last a lifetime.*

CRITICAL THINKING CHALLENGES

1. The method used to complete a procedure in your site differs significantly from what your classroom instructor has taught you. How would you handle this?
2. Your preceptor does not follow Standard Precautions on several occasions in your presence. Discuss why this is dangerous, then explain what you would do.

ANSWERS TO CHECKPOINT QUESTIONS

1. An externship is the part of the medical assisting course requirement that allows the student to perform the skills learned in the classroom in a clinical site. A general practice facility will provide you with the best exposure to a wide range of medical assisting procedures.

2. The preceptor acts as the instructor in the clinical site, providing supervision and technical direction to the medical assisting student.

3. Among the attributes required for success, a health care worker should be dependable, professional, and well groomed.

4. The ability to interact positively and pleasantly with coworkers is a sign of professionalism. Also, coworkers may provide you with job references.

5. The medical assisting program uses information obtained in the site evaluation to determine how well a particular site provided training and if it should be used again for future students.

Employment

Chapter Outline

Establish the Job for You
  Setting Goals
  Self-Analysis
Finding the Right Job
Applying for the Job
  Answering Newspaper
    Advertisements
  Preparing Your Resumé
  Preparing Your Cover Letter
  Completing an Employment
    Application

Interviewing
  Preparing for the Interview
  Crucial Questions
Follow-up
  Why Some Applicants Fail to Get
    the Job
Keep the Job or Move on?
Summary
Critical Thinking Challenges
Answers to Checkpoint Questions
Suggestions for Further Reading

DACUM Components

1.1 Project a positive attitude
1.2 Perform within ethical boundaries
1.3 Practice within the scope of education, training, and personal capabilities
1.4 Maintain confidentiality
1.5 Work as a team member
1.6 Conduct oneself in a courteous and diplomatic manner
1.7 Adapt to change
1.8 Show initiative and responsibility
1.9 Promote the profession
2.11 Compose written communication using correct grammar, spelling, and format

Chapter Competencies

Learning Objectives

Upon successfully completing this chapter, you will be able to:

1. Spell and define the Key Terms.
2. Define personal strengths and weaknesses.
3. Determine the best career direction to reflect skills and strengths.
4. Know the steps necessary to apply for the right position and be able to accomplish those steps.
5. Draft an appropriate cover letter.
6. List guidelines for an effective interview resulting in employment in the desired position.
7. Understand the steps to take to ensure proper career advancement.
8. List steps to exit a previous position with a positive reference.

Performance Objectives

Upon successfully completing this chapter, you will be able to:

1. Write a resumé to properly communicate skills and strengths.
2. Complete an employment application.

Key Terms

(See Glossary for definitions.)
flextime
networking
portfolio
resumé

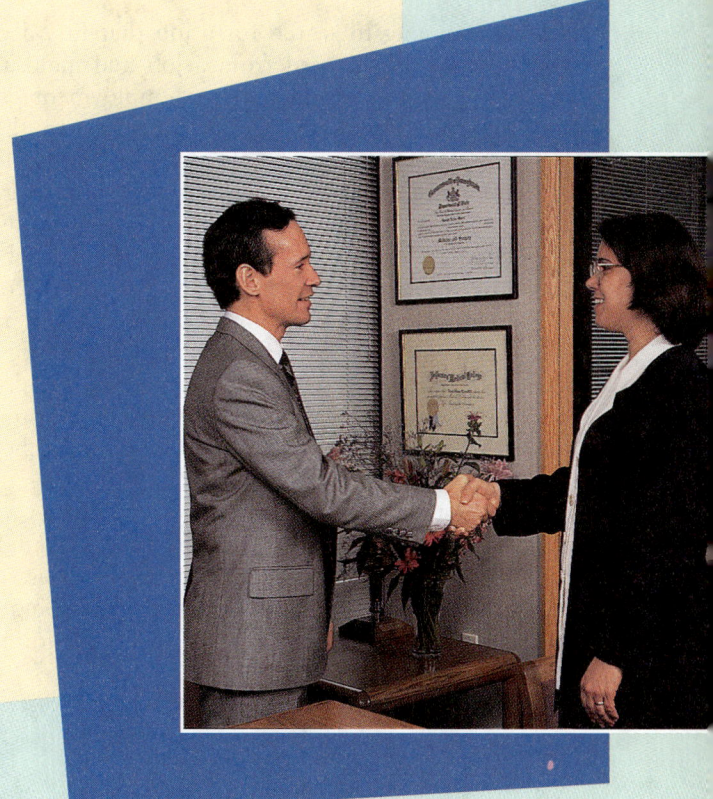

As the medical profession continues to expand, so obviously will the job opportunities available within it. Forecasts predict that the allied health professions will continue the present growth well into the next century. Some experts estimate that the demand for medical assistants will grow by 70% by the year 2010.

Classified advertising in newspapers has reflected the growing need for medical personnel, and in some areas a separate section is set aside for the needs of the medical field. Personnel search agencies have expanded into the area of health care and are trying now to staff medical facilities with trained medical assistants rather than filling positions with business-trained secretaries. Well prepared graduates will know how to take advantage of this trend to acquire the best position possible for their interests and skills.

This chapter will help you discover how to determine the right position, how to apply for that position, how to prepare for the interview, how to interview successfully, and how to secure the position.

➤ ESTABLISH THE JOB FOR YOU

Setting Goals

Before beginning to search for a job that fits, decide what you want and need from a job and make that your goal. People who do not set employment goals must eventually accept what is presented to them. They are often unhappy in their work because they have not chosen their job in the first place. The average person approaches the job search with the attitude, "I wonder what is available," rather than, "Here is what I would like to do, and here is the facility where I would like to work." THAT is setting a goal. It is also a positive, proactive approach to the job market, rather than a reactive position to what is available. In general, the medical field is looking for proactive people. You will work harder and more enthusiastically if you choose your workplace.

The best way to set a goal and eventually get what you want is to study your strengths and weaknesses and from these strengths and weaknesses design the best job for you. Goal setting means describing the ideal job for you and deciding that this is the job that you will someday have.

On a sheet of paper, describe the best job for you if you had your choice. For example, you might describe such elements as:

- Specialty area (eg, obstetrics, pediatrics, surgery)
- Duties (clinical or administrative)
- Type of employer and supervisor
- Other employees and coworkers
- Type of facility
- Desired atmosphere (casual or regimented)
- Ideal hours
- Availability of **flextime** (a system of scheduling that allows for a personal choice in hours or days worked)

Next, write down where you expect to be in 2 years and in 5 years, both by position and income. Now you can decide with more focus where you want to work, what you want to do, and the direction you want to be going. The next question is how to get there.

To win the position you want, you have to learn to sell yourself. Generally speaking, employers will not come looking for you—you will have to go to them. You will be compared with all the other equally qualified candidates who are interested in the same position. If 25 people interview for a job and you are second best, you still lose. The one who is chosen is the one who interviews best. It is not necessarily the one who is best suited for a job who gets the job; it is frequently the one who performs best in the interview. To market yourself takes real effort.

Self-Analysis

A good presentation of your qualifications begins with "self-analysis." You must know what strengths you have to offer a potential employer as well as your weaknesses. Make an honest list of all of your strengths and weaknesses. (If you skipped this exercise, please note that one of your weaknesses is failure to follow through, looking for a short cut, and perhaps procrastination.)

Keep in mind that every strength you have presents an opportunity, a chance to sell yourself and your value as an employee. When you are interviewing for a position, concentrate on projecting your strengths to the interviewer.

Just as your strengths give you a special advantage, each weakness represents a reason someone may not want to offer you the position. Weaknesses must be recognized and resolved. Recognizing your weaknesses as a threat to securing the position you want will help you develop strategies to eliminate these problems or turn them into strengths. As long as you are aware of your weaknesses, you will be prepared to handle them.

Now that you know the type of job you want and have identified your positive and negative qualities, it is time to begin to look for the right job.

➤ FINDING THE RIGHT JOB

Everybody begins with the newspaper, and you should too. But there are other opportunities that might work for you. Keep in mind that many of the most desirable job openings are never advertised—they are posted internally and filled from within.

From a random survey recently conducted at Commonwealth College in Richmond, Virginia, it was discovered that fully 60% of all available positions are never advertised in mass media. They are filled by referral, by word of mouth, or by **networking**. Networking is a way to build personal contacts and share information.

Open positions that are posted internally are often filled with current employees or referrals from current employees. Any organization that looks within itself and is able to obtain a recommendation from a current employee to fill an available position accomplishes two things: the cost of advertising is saved, and the recommendation itself is usually a good one because it comes from someone who presumably knows the demands and special needs of that particular organization.

Questions can be asked at the time of a personal recommendation that might be difficult during an interview. It is important for someone seeking employment in the medical field to build as many contacts within the field as possible. It is impossible to have too many contacts. Everyone with whom you associate should know that you are looking for employment. Friends and acquaintances cannot tell you about a job or recommend you for a job if they do not know that you are searching.

Traditional sources of information for job openings include:

- *Local, state, or federal government employment offices.* These agencies are designed to find work for the unemployed. They frequently have listings of positions that will not be found anywhere else. Rather than calling the office with inquiries, make an appointment to visit. Register with the service. Get to know a contact person whom you will feel comfortable contacting frequently.
- *School placement office.* If your school has a placement office, contact the coordinator or personnel officer and outline what you are looking for and where you want to work. Their job is to assist you in securing the position you want. If you establish a working relationship with a contact person, you will probably have better results.
- *Medical facilities.* Do not wait for an advertisement. Go to the office or facility where you would like to work and leave a **resumé**—a document summarizing your professional qualifications—and a cover letter explaining how much you want

to work there. It helps to know the name of the office manager or personnel officer and to call first for an appointment. This shows better planning and foresight and is more professional than dropping by unannounced.

- *Private agencies.* Many medical facilities solicit privately to avoid being swamped by unqualified applicants. A fee is charged for the service but is usually paid by the employer. Call to make an appointment with a representative who will interview you and tell you what steps to follow for the agency.
- *Temporary services.* These agencies work well to scout for sites with no pressure. If you are new to an area, this is a good way to learn which facilities would be good choices for you. You may be assigned for several days or several weeks. If you work well as a temporary replacement and like the site, leave your resumé and let the proper individuals know that you would like to work in this place if an opening develops. Check with the temporary agency regarding fees attached if you are hired as a result of a placement through the agency.

Checkpoint Question

1. Besides the newspaper and networking, where else can you find information about job openings?

➤ APPLYING FOR THE JOB

Answering Newspaper Advertisements

When responding to a newspaper advertisement, be sure that you do exactly what the advertisement asks you to do; one of the qualities that many interviewers look for is the ability to follow directions. At the same time, try to make your response more distinctive (yet still professional) than the others. The medical profession rarely responds well to those who do not fit its image and almost never accepts someone who will not conform at the entry level. A well prepared resumé and cover letter are essential to the job-hunting process.

Preparing Your Resumé

Many good books on preparing resumés are available. Find one in your school library and style your resumé directly after one that appeals to you. Resumé texts include many examples and hints for making yours outstanding. Put your resumé on a computer disk and be sure to personalize it for the position you are seeking (Fig. 52-1). For example, if you use a "career objec-

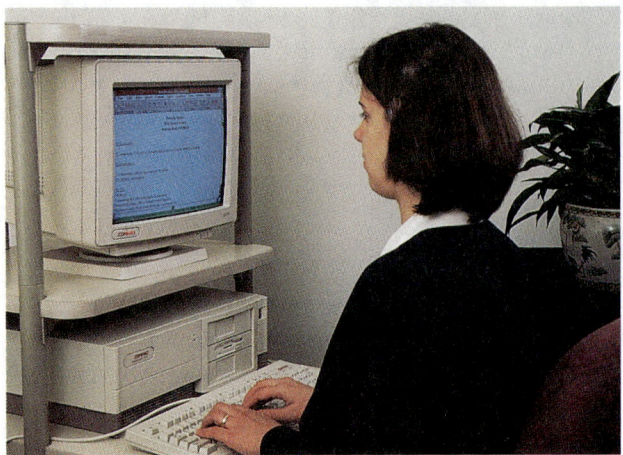

FIGURE 52-1
Have your resume on a computer disk so you can personalize it for the position you are seeking.

tive," try putting in the title or description of the particular job you are seeking. Keep changing this for every different position so that your resumé is personalized for each interview.

The resumé is a flash picture of yourself; if it is neat and professional, the reviewer will presume that it is a reflection of you. Remember these guidelines as you prepare to capture the reviewer's interest:

1. Evaluate your list of your skills, goals, and what you have to offer. With this list in hand, you can better concentrate on highlighting your strengths.

2. Confine your resumé to one page, selecting carefully what you want to include. The resumé must state just what the reviewer needs to know and no more.

3. Do include the following key pieces of information:

   - *Name, address, and telephone number.* Include these at the top of your resumé (usually centered). (Because you are including your telephone number, you should expect calls from prospective employers. Box 52-1 offers some tips for handling such calls.)
   - *Education.* Start with the most recent and work back in reverse order. List only relevant courses.
   - *Affiliations or volunteer work (if appropriate).* If this information will show that you have good organizational skills or have held an office for the group, it should be included.
   - *Experience.* This may be listed in either of two standard resumé forms: functional or chronological. A functional resumé focuses on skills and qualifications rather than employment and works well for those who recently gradu-

ated or who are re-entering the job market after a period of years (Fig. 52-2). A chronological resumé is useful for those who have an employment history, particularly if the history is relevant to the position being sought. Start with the most recent employment and work backward. Include your title, position, and a few of your responsibilities (see Figure 52-3). Explain any gaps such as pregnancy, schooling, relocations, and so on.

   - *References.* You may or may not include your references on a separate sheet. When you have chosen your references, be sure to ask permission to use their names. Prospective employers are not interested in your neighbors or pastor and are certainly not interested in your relatives as references. They are more impressed by good recommendations from previous employers.

4. Do not include hobbies and personal interests unrelated to work. It is not relevant that you play the guitar, but it would be impressive to know that you volunteer at a free clinic.

5. Use action words (Box 52-2).

6. Center the resumé on white or off-white heavy bond or high rag content paper, 8½ by 11 inches. (Colors are not acceptable and cheap paper will not convey the professional impression you hope to make.) Keep a 1-inch margin around the text. Single space within the sections of information but double space between the sections.

7. Use regular type. Do not use italics, script, or other unusual type fonts. A right unjustified margin is easier to read through quickly than a right justified one.

8. Have someone proofread your work. It is difficult to find your own errors or see areas that are not clearly worded.

9. If you are using a computer or word processor, print your resumé on a letter-quality printer. A dot matrix printer is not acceptable.

Jane Q. Smith, C.M.A.
123 Main Street
Mountain Laurel, CE 00000
111-222-3333

Organization/Coordination:
- Organized yearly fund raising event for civic group
- Maintained lists of volunteers and sponsors
- Coordinated advertising and solicited contributions
- Supervised and scheduled volunteers during festival

Teaching:
- Taught Sunday school for preteens for three years
- Assisted in selecting curriculum for Sunday school class

Professional Externships:
- American Association of Medical Assistants
  Professional Experience Externship (160 hours),
  Dr. Walter Scott, Mountain Laurel, CE

Education:
- Diploma, Medical Assisting
  Mountain Laurel College, Mountain Laurel, CE
- Mountain Laurel High School
- Mountain Laurel, CE

Certifications:
- Certified Medical Assistant, American Association of Medical Assistants
- Cardiopulmonary Resuscitation Certificate, American Heart Association

Skills:
- Clinical and Laboratory Skills
- Administrative Skills
- Office Equipment

FIGURE 52-2
Sample functional resumé.

10. Mail the resumé in an 8½ by 11 inch manila envelope. This will present the interviewer with a resumé and cover letter that are smooth, with no fold lines. Many prefer to work with resumés that have not been folded to an envelope.

Checkpoint Question
2. How does a functional resumé differ from a chronological one?

BOX 52-2 Action Words for Your Resume

achieved	organized
attained	operated
assisted	performed
conducted	planned
completed	prepared
developed	processed
directed	scheduled
ensured	selected
filed	systemized
handled	screened
generated	solved
maintained	

Preparing Your Cover Letter

When contacting a prospective employer about a job, you not only need to send a resumé, you must also include a cover letter. Keep your cover letter brief and meaningful. You want it to be read, and you want the reader to be impressed by what it says. Be sure that you mention the job itself in your letter. You may even consider a statement such as, "This is the type of position I would prefer." If you know something favorable about the facility, include that in your letter. If you know anyone who works for the company, mention it. DO NOT mention the person by name unless you have secured his or her permission.

Make sure you address your letter to the right person. Call the personnel department or office manager and ask the name of the person handling the applica-

Jane Q. Smith, C.M.A.
123 Main Street
Mountain Laurel, CE 00000
111-222-3333

Employment Objective:
To apply medical assisting skills to a challenging position in the medical profession.

Education:
199_ –199_ Mountain Laurel College
Certificate in Medical Assisting

199_ –199_ Mountain Laurel High School
Tech Prep Program

Work Experience:
199_ –199_ Country General Hospital, Mountain Laurel, CE
Volunteer in Patient Reception
Assisted patients to destinations within the hospital, assisted
receptionists with duties, completed errands required by admission procedures.

199_ –199_ Cashier/Clerk, FoodStuff Groceries
567 Maple Lane, Mountain Laurel, CE
Worked at check-out counter, handled cash flow, helped maintain
inventory, trained new employees

Skills:
Clinical and Laboratory Procedures
Administrative Procedures
Computer and Office Equipment Skills
Cardiopulmonary Resuscitation Certificate

Activities and Honors:
Student Government Representative
Who's Who in American Colleges
Honors Recipient

References:
Available upon request

FIGURE 52-3
Sample chronological resumé.

tions. Determine the correct spelling of the name and the preferred address, such as Mr., Ms., or Mrs.

The standard form for a cover letter recommends three brief paragraphs:

- First paragraph: State the position you are applying for.
- Second paragraph: Stress your skills. Do not be redundant because you will also send a resume but mention or highlight specifically those skills needed for this job.
- Third paragraph: Request an interview. Offer to call in a week to set up an interview (then do so). Keep a copy of your letter to refer to when calling.

Use the same good quality paper for the cover letter that you used for your resume. Include your name, address, and telephone number at the top of the page, centered or in block form. Single space the letter and double space between paragraphs. Block form or modified block form are both acceptable (Fig. 52-4).

Checkpoint Question
3. What should you include in a cover letter?

Completing an Employment Application

Some sites will have you prepare an employment application while you wait; others may have mailed one to you earlier. **Although resumés have their place and are indispensable, many facilities rely more on an application form to clearly pinpoint their needs.** Practice filling out several types, following these guidelines:

1. Read through completely before beginning.
2. Follow instructions exactly. Prospective employers notice neatness, erasures, evasions, and indecision.
3. Answer thoroughly. If the question does not apply to you, draw a line or write N/A so that the interviewer will know that the question was not overlooked.

Jane Q. Smith, C.M.A.
123 Main Street
Mountain Laurel, CE 00000
111-222-3333

June 1, 199_

Ms. Joan Z. Brown, Office Manager
Medical Park Practice
987 Hospital Road
Mountain Laurel, CE 00000

Dear Ms. Brown:

I understand from my Medical Assisting instructor, Ms. Ann P. Tidy, that an opening is anticipated in your office in the very near future.

I am a recent graduate of the Medical Assisting Program at Mountain Laurel College and am interested in working in the area of orthopedics, the medical specialty served by your physicians. My educational experience exposed me to many areas of medicine and allowed me to develop skills that will be required to carry out both the clinical and administrative responsibilities encountered in your practice. In addition, I completed an externship in an orthopedic practice, where I gained experience assisting with examinations and procedures specific to this area of practice.

My resume is enclosed for your review. May I speak with you about this opening? I will call in a week to schedule an interview.

Sincerely,

Jane Q. Smith, C.M.A.
Enclosure

FIGURE 52-4
Sample cover letter.

4. In the line for wage or salary desired, write "negotiable" or find out before the interview what is usual for the area for this type of position.
5. In spaces requiring the reason for leaving a previous position, try to sound positive. Answers such as "To explore a new career direction" are ambiguous enough to fill many needs. If the reason for leaving was due to relocation, schooling, or pregnancy, say so.
6. Write your very best, being as neat as possible.

You may attach your résumé to the application if one has not been mailed before this time.

➤ INTERVIEWING

Interviewing well is a skill and it takes effort to develop it. Like any skill, if you want to stay proficient and keep your skills in good working order, you have to practice. Ask friends or family members to work with you to develop a relaxed approach to answering the questions most often asked during an interview. Have them try to trip you up or confuse you by throwing in questions that are tricky to answer. Although the effect will not be the same with a friend or family member as it will be with an interviewer, the practice can mean the difference between getting this job or losing the chance. You can also rehearse your answers to questions in front of a mirror.

It is usually the person who interviews best who is hired for the position. **An excellent interview is absolutely crucial for obtaining any job.** It is highly unlikely that you will get the job you want without being skilled in the interviewing process.

Preparing for the Interview

Before the day of the interview, find out all that you can about the facility. What is its local reputation? Does it have a big turnover of employees? Review your textbooks that cover the specialty so that you can ask informed questions about procedures performed on site. Think of questions to ask and write them down. Anticipate questions that might be asked of you. Find out the name of the interviewer; if it is a difficult name, practice saying it. Drive to the site to time the distance and to be sure of its location so that you will not be late for the appointment. This should ideally be done about the same time of day as the appointment to judge traffic delays, parking problems, and so on.

Dress well for the interview. The general rule is to dress one step above that which is required for the job. Do not overdress, as if for a party; make sure your outfit is professional. Your personal hygiene must be above reproach. If you normally smoke, try to avoid smoking before the interview. Those who do not smoke are acutely aware of the odor of smoke on clothes and breath. Avoid overlarge jewelry and apply makeup carefully. Avoid perfumes because some people are very sensitive to scents.

Arrive on time or a few minutes early. Go alone; do not take a friend or family member for moral support. When you are introduced to the interviewer, offer your hand for a handshake and sit only when and where you are directed. Do not fidget, swing your foot, play with your hair, or tap your fingers on the chair arm. Make eye contact when the interviewer speaks

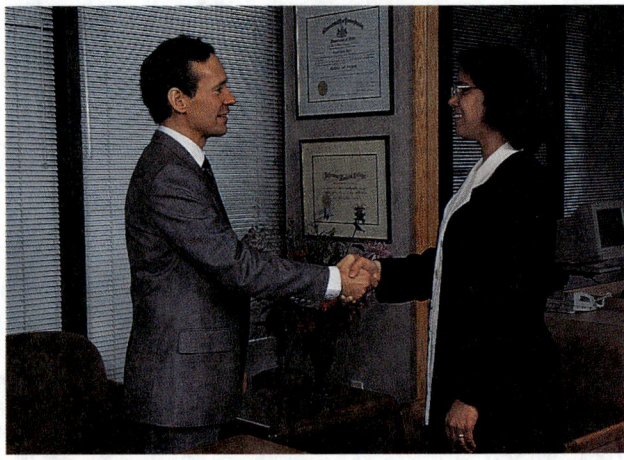

FIGURE 52-5
During an interview, be sure to use correct posture and to make eye contact with the interviewer.

with you and when you respond to the comments (Fig. 52-5). Sit up straight but relaxed, with your **portfolio** on your lap. A portfolio is a folder containing all of the information you will need to impress the interviewer. If you do not have a special folder or brief case, a neat, new manila folder will be adequate. This folder or portfolio will contain items crucial to your interviewing process (Box 52-3).

BOX 52-3 The Interview: Come Prepared

At the interview, be sure to have with you:

- At least one good pen that writes well (preferably black ink) and a backup (borrowing the interviewer's pen is unprofessional)
- A #2 pencil with a good eraser
- A note pad with a list of questions about the job
- Your Social Security card and any certification that you hold
- Your portfolio containing:
    at least two copies of your resumé
    letters of reference
    typed list of references (if not included with the resumé previously mailed)
    copies of awards received
    honors/certificates from schools and colleges
    special projects you have completed in your field
    list of any special credits or continuing education
    club/organization membership information
    list of graduation dates and credits earned
    list of previous employment dates and work experience not reflected on
        the resumé
    any other information that demonstrates your abilities and successes

Crucial Questions

There are three basic questions every interviewer must have answered. When you respond to the interviewer's questions, you need to keep these in mind:

1. Do you have the necessary skills to do the job?
2. Do you have the necessary drive, energy, and commitment to get the job done?
3. Will you work well with the rest of the team?

A positive answer to all of these questions is not a guarantee that you will be offered the job, but a negative answer to any one of these will most assuredly mean that you will NOT get the job. Make sure that your comments will ensure a positive impression regarding these three questions.

In the medical field, the interviewer will need to establish your level of confidentiality and professionalism. The interviewer will also want to know how interested you are in increasing and continuing your education and skills. Be sure that your answers will satisfy the interviewer.

Many interviewers will have a standard, prepared list of questions to direct the flow of the interview. Box 52-4 contains some commonly asked interview questions and guidance for responses. Be prepared with answers that will reflect well on your professionalism and qualifications.

What If?

What if you become "tongue-tied" while being interviewed?

It's not unusual to feel nervous during the interview. To stay calm, take a deep breath and count to three before answering a question. Doing this also gives you time to think before you begin speaking. Remember: Believe in yourself and your skills. Say to yourself, "I am going to get this job."

When the interviewer finishes asking questions, he or she will usually ask if you have any questions. Refer to the note pad on which you have listed questions, such as:

*   What are the responsibilities of the position offered?
*   If it is not personal, why is the current employee leaving?
*   What are the opportunities for advancement?

BOX 52-4 Commonly Asked Interview Questions

1. **Tell me something about yourself.** Here you might stress how much you enjoy taking care of others and why you are interested in allied health. Talk about having the characteristics that the interviewer is looking for. Emphasize the good points that you wrote down in your self-analysis.
2. **What do you like most about yourself?** Again, stress the items listed in your self-analysis.
3. **What is there about yourself that you do not like or would like to change?** Answer this one carefully. You must be honest but certainly do not want to mention anything that might jeopardize your chance for this position.
4. **I see that you went to ABC high school. What was your favorite subject?** Your answer here should mention a subject that can be directly related to doing your job well. Math, English, and health sciences are good responses, while subjects such as art or history are not relevant.
5. **I see that you worked for the ABC Hospital. What was that like? Why did you leave? What were your responsibilities? What did you like or dislike about**

it? Any good interviewer will check with your previous employer before asking you to come in for an interview and will know as much about you as possible from previous employers even if they are not listed as references. You must answer honestly, as always, but answer with positive comments about any previous positions. This is one of the questions that will tell the interviewer if you are likely to work well with the rest of the team. Never criticize any previous employer or coworker, even if there were aspects of the job that you disliked. Rather than reflecting badly on the former work situation, you will make yourself look bad.

6. **Describe the perfect position. Which interests you most, the administrative or clinical area?** Answer this one in a way that reflects your ability to adapt to many working conditions, with varying personality types and with a wide range of duties. Stress that your training was in both areas of assisting and that you enjoyed many aspects of each and would like the opportunity to try all facets of the profession.

- How long is the training or probation period?
- How does the facility feel about continuing education? Is time offered to upgrade skills? Does the facility subsidize the expense?
- Is there a job performance or evaluation process?
- What is the benefit package? Is there access to a 401(k) plan or other retirement plan? Health insurance? Life insurance?

Make notes on your pad about the answers for future reference. Avoid asking about time off or vacations during the interview. These questions imply that you are more interested in being paid to avoid work than you are in contributing to the work at hand.

Make sure the interviewer knows how important continuing education is to you. Talk about the types of continuing education courses you would like to attend and the subjects you would like to study. Let the interviewer know that you are aware that the only constant in medicine is "change" and that you expect to keep abreast of your area.

Thank the interviewer for the opportunity to apply for the position and ask the time frame for a decision. As you leave, offer your hand for a handshake and ask if you might call again before the decision date to clear up any questions that might occur to the interviewer during the decision-making process.

Checkpoint Question

4. What are the three basic questions an interviewer needs to have answered?

➤ FOLLOW-UP

The day of the interview or no later than the day after, write a short thank you note for the opportunity to apply and restate how interested you are in the job (Fig. 52-6). Remind the interviewer that you are available for additional questions.

Jane Q. Smith, C.M.A.
123 Main Street
Mountain Laurel, CE 00000
111-222-3333
June 21, 199_

Ms. Joan Z. Brown, Office Manager
Medical Park Practice
987 Hospital Road
Mountain Laurel, CE 00000

Dear Ms. Brown:

Thank you for giving me the opportunity to interview for the position with your agency. I enjoyed meeting you and touring the facility.

The information regarding the operation of your physician s' practice confirmed my opinion that I have been trained in all of the skills required to fill the position being offered. My background in anatomy, physiology, medical terminology, and administrative and clinical procedures would address your needs. I believe this position would offer me an opportunity to use the education and training I received in my Medical Assisting courses and to grow in my professional career.

I am very interested in the position. This is the type of career opportunity that I have hoped to find. If you have any questions, please feel free to call me at 000-000-0000.

Sincerely,

Jane Q. Smith, C.M.A.

FIGURE 52-6
Sample thank you letter.

Call several days after the interview. Re-introduce yourself politely and add any new information or ask any questions that might have occurred to you after the interview. Thank the interviewer again for this opportunity.

Why Some Applicants Fail to Get the Job

The first reason is simple: They do not have the abilities needed (Box 52-5). Every employer is looking for something special from each employee. The field of medicine has special needs. The employer must believe that you possess a number of skills necessary to do the job:

- Technical skills—You must have the necessary proficiency to get the job done.
- Confidentiality—The field of medicine exposes you to sensitive information about patients. Is the interviewer convinced that you are someone who can be relied on to keep those confidences?
- Human relations skills—Are you someone who will get along with the others in the workplace?
- Communication skills—Do you have the necessary level of verbal and writing skills that the job demands? Remember the importance of correct English skills. You will not be hired if your English and grammar are not exemplary.

If you fail to impress the interviewer with your grasp of these skills, you will never be considered for the position.

Another major reason an applicant is not hired is lack of professionalism. Watch the way you are dressed and the manner in which you speak. The interviewer knows that whatever is displayed in the interview will also be displayed to the patients.

➤ KEEP THE JOB OR MOVE ON?

Almost everyone comes to this question at some point in his or her career. Should I look for a new place to work and leave this place where I am safe and comfortable? Would another job be better or more satisfying? Would benefits be better?

An important factor in many relocations is salary. But beyond the financial aspects, employees today are looking for other elements that will result in job satisfaction. These include:

- A sense of achievement
- Recognition
- Opportunity for growth and advancement
- Harmonious peer group relationships
- A good working relationship with supervisors
- Status
- Job security
- Comfortable working conditions
- Fair company policies

BOX 52-5 Sure Fire, No Hire

Here are several reasons why an applicant may not get the job:

- Poor personal appearance or personal hygiene
- Inarticulate or rambling responses
- Inappropriate demeanor (eg, unenthusiastic or overly aggressive)
- Lack of purpose or direction
- Lack of poise and self-confidence
- Lack of tact, diplomacy, maturity, or humor
- Failure to research the position
- Failure to make eye contact
- Poorly prepared application form
- Poorly prepared questions about the facility (or no questions at all)
- Overemphasis on time off or wages

BOX 52-6 When You Leave Your Job

- *Always give adequate notice.* Facilities have no surplus staff and your position will need to be filled. One month is traditional. This gives the office time to find your replacement and finalize the hiring process. Offer to stay long enough to train your replacement.
- *Write a letter of resignation.* The letter will be placed in your personnel file. State a positive reason for leaving—this is no time to air grievances in a letter that will be part of your permanent record. State the date you need to leave. Express your appreciation for the experience and skills you gained while working in this position.
- *Be positive during an exit interview.* Some agencies have an exit conference for employees. Do not use this interview as an opportunity to criticize former coworkers. Instead, end on a positive note and ask for a letter of reference.

If you are no longer happy in your job, the answer lies in one of these elements. At least one of the items listed above must be missing for you. Before you make the decision to change jobs, make sure you are not ending one problem just to start another. Make a checklist of the above items, then score your current position. If it makes sense to move on, then begin the process that gained this position for you.

If you make the decision for whatever reason that this job is not the one you want, then you must also make the decision that the one you have chosen to pursue is better or more satisfying. If you decide to leave, you must leave with positive feelings all around. Box 52-6 offers some guidelines to follow when leaving your job.

SUMMARY

A job should be fulfilling and rewarding, and the rewards are not always monetary. To secure the right job will take careful planning. Set a goal. Decide the position you want and what you must do to secure it. Learn all you can about your own strengths and weaknesses. Learn how to promote yourself and earn the position you want. If this is the right job for you, and if you truly enjoy what you are doing, you will arrive early and work late. You will work hard and with great pleasure. Your enjoyment will be your reward, but so also will be the benefits that come to valued and irreplaceable employees.

CRITICAL THINKING CHALLENGES

1. Read the classified section of the Sunday newspaper and select a job advertisement that interests you. Write a cover letter and resumé tailored to this position. Assume that you have been called for an interview. What questions would you ask the prospective employer? What questions would you expect to be asked? Explain your responses.

2. Obtain two employee application forms from the human resources department of your local hospital. Complete one application form yourself and invite a fellow student to complete the other form. Swap applications and evaluate one another's work. Determine which areas are appropriately addressed and which need further attention.

ANSWERS TO CHECKPOINT QUESTIONS

1. Other sources of job information include government employment offices, your school placement office, medical facilities, private agencies, and temporary services.

2. A functional resumé stresses skills and qualifications rather than employment history. A chronological resumé lists positions held, starting with the most recent and working backward.

3. In a cover letter, you should state the position you are applying for, highlight pertinent skills, and ask for an interview.

4. The interviewer needs to know: Do you have the required skills for the job? Can you get the job done? Will you work well with the people currently employed at the facility?

SUGGESTIONS FOR FURTHER READING

Becklin, K. J., & Sunnarborg, E. M. (1992). *Medical Office Procedures*, 3rd ed. Lake Forest IL: Glencoe Publishers.

What You Should Know About Getting a Job. (1990). Channing L. Bete Co., Inc., South Deerfield, MA.

Zedlitz, R. (1987). *Getting a Job in Health Care*. Cincinnati, OH: South-Western Publishing Co.

Appendices

Appendix

I

1990 DACUM Analysis of the Medical Assisting Profession†

1.0 Display Professionalism	2.0 Communicate	3.0 Perform Administrative Duties	4.0 Perform Clinical Duties
1.1 Project a positive attitude	2.1 Listen and observe	3.1 Perform basic secretarial skills	4.1 Apply principles of aseptic technique and infection control
1.2 Perform within ethical boundaries	2.2 Treat all patients with empathy and impartiality	3.2 Schedule and monitor appointments	4.2 Take vital signs
1.3 Practice within the scope of education, training, and personal capabilities	2.3 Adapt communication to individuals' abilities to understand	3.3 Prepare and maintain medical records	4.3 Recognize emergencies
1.4 Maintain confidentiality	2.4 Recognize and respond to verbal and nonverbal communication	3.4 Apply computer concepts for office procedures	4.4 Perform first aid and CPR
1.5 Work as a team member	2.5 Serve as liaison between physician and others	3.5 Perform medical transcription	4.5 Prepare and maintain examination and treatment area
1.6 Conduct oneself in a courteous and diplomatic manner	2.6 Evaluate understanding of communication	3.6 Locate resources and information for patients and employers	4.6 Interview and take patient history
1.7 Adapt to change	2.7 Receive, organize, prioritize, and transmit information	3.7 Manage physician's professional schedule and travel	4.7 Prepare patients for procedures
1.8 Show initiative and responsibility	2.8 Use proper telephone technique		4.8 Assist physician with examinations and treatments
1.9 Promote the profession Enhance* skills through continuing education	2.9 Interview effectively		4.9 Use quality control
	2.10 Use medical terminology appropriately		4.10 Collect and process specimens
	2.11 Compose written communication using correct grammar, spelling, and format Develop* and conduct public relations activities to market professional services		4.11 Perform selected tests that assist with diagnosis and treatment
			4.12 Screen and follow-up patient test results
			4.13 Prepare and administer medications as directed by physician
			4.14 Maintain medication records Respond* to medical emergencies

5.0 Apply Legal Concepts to Practice	*6.0 Manage the Office*	*7.0 Provide Instruction*	*8.0 Manage Practice Finances*
5.1 Document accurately 5.2 Determine needs for documentation and reporting 5.3 Use appropriate guidelines when releasing records or information 5.4 Follow established policy in initiating or terminating medical treatment 5.5 Dispose of controlled substances in compliance with government regulations 5.6 Maintain licenses and accreditation 5.7 Monitor legislation related to current health care issues and practice Develop* and maintain policy and procedure manuals Establish* risk management protocol for the practice	6.1 Maintain the physical plant 6.2 Operate and maintain facilities and equipment safely 6.3 Inventory equipment and supplies 6.4 Evaluate and recommend equipment and supplies for a practice 6.5 Maintain liability coverage 6.6 Exercise efficient time management Supervise* personnel Develop* job descriptions Interview* and recommend new personnel Negotiate* leases and prices for equipment and supply contracts	7.1 Orient patients to office policies and procedures 7.2 Instruct patients with special needs 7.3 Teach patients methods of health promotion and disease prevention 7.4 Orient and train personnel Provide* health information for public use Supervise* student practicums Conduct* continuing education activities Develop* educational materials	

Appendix

II *Key English-to-Spanish Healthcare Phrases*

Although English is the major language spoken in North America, a variety of languages are used in certain areas. Prominent among them is Spanish, representing Spain, the Caribbean Islands, Central and South America, and the Philippines. Rapport can be more easily established, and the patient and family will be at ease and feel more relaxed, if someone on the staff speaks their language. Some health care facilities, especially in areas with a large population of Spanish-speaking people, provide interpreters. In smaller hospitals or smaller communities this may not be possible.

It is to your advantage to learn the second most prominent language in your community. For this reason, the following table of English-to-Spanish has been prepared. Instructions for using it are simple. Look for the phrase in English in the first column of the table. The second column gives the phrase in Spanish. You can write this or point to it. The third column gives a phonetic pronunciation. The syllable in each word to be accented is printed in italic type. Even if you are not proficient in English-to-Spanish, your Spanish-speaking patients will appreciate your trying to converse in their language. Begin with "Buenos dias. ¿Como se siente?" And remember "por favor."*

Introductory Phrases

Please*	Por favór	Por fah-*vor*
Thank you	Grácias	*Grah*-see-ahs
Good morning	Buénos días	*Bway*-nos *dee*-ahs
Good afternoon	Buénas tárdes	*Bway*-nas *tar*-days
Good evening	Buénas nóches	*Bway*-nas *Noh*-chays
My name is	Mi nómbre es	Me *nohm*-bray ays
Yes/No	Si/No	See/No
What is your name?	¿Cómo se llama?	¿koh-moh say *jah*-mah?
How old are you?	¿Cuántos años tienes?	¿*kwan*-tohs ahn-yos tee-*ayn*jays?
Do you understand me?	¿Me entiende?	¿Me ayn-tee-*ayn*-day?
Speak slower	Habla más despacio	*Ah*-blah mahs days-*pah*-see-oh
Say it once again	Repítalo, por favor	Ray-*pee*-tah-loh, por fah-*vor*
How do you feel?	¿Cómo se siente?	¿*Koh*-moh say see-*ayn*-tay?
Good	Bien	bee-ayn
Bad	Mal	*mah*l
Physician	Medico	*May*-dee-koh
Hospital	Hospital	*Ooh*-spee-tall
Midwife	Comadre	Koh-*mah*-dray
Native healer	Curandero	Ku-ren-*day*-roh

You should begin or end any request with the word PLEASE (POR FAVOR).

General

English	Spanish	Pronunciation
Zero	Cero	*Se*-roh
One	uno	*oo*-noh
Two	dos	dohs
Three	tres	trays
Four	cuatro	*kwah*-troh
Five	cinco	*sin*-koh
Six	seis	says
Seven	siete	see-*ay*-tay
Eight	ocho	oh-choh
Nine	nueve	new-*ay*-vay
Ten	diez	*dee*-ays
Hundred	ciento, cien	see-*en*-toh, see-*en*
Hundred and one	ciento uno	see-*en*-toh oo-noh
Sunday	domingo	doh-*ming*-goh
Monday	lunes	*loo*-nays
Tuesday	martes	*mar*-tays
Wednesday	miercoles	mee-*er*-cohl-ays
Thursday	jueves	*hway*-vays
Friday	viernes	vee-*ayr*-nays
Saturday	sabado	*sah*-bah-doh
Right	derecha	day-*ray*-chah
Left	izqierda	ees-kee-*ayr*-dah
Early in the morning	temprano por la mañana	tehm-*prah*-noh por lah mah-*nyah*-na
In the daytime	en el dia	ayn el *dee*-ah
At noon	a mediodía	ah meh-dee-oh-*dee*-ah
At bedtime	al acostarse	al ah-kos-*tar*-say
At night	por la noche	por la *noh*-chay
Today	Hoy	oy
Tomorrow	Mañana	mah-*nyah*-nah
Yesterday	Ayer	ai-*yer*
Week	Semana	say-*may*-nah
Month	mes	mace

Parts of the body

The head	la cabeza	lah kah-*bay*-sah
The eye	el ojo	el *o*-hoh
The ears	los oídos	lohs o-*ee*-dohs
The nose	la nariz	lah nah-*reez*
The mouth	la boca	lah *boh*-kah
The tongue	la lengua	la *len*-gwah
The neck	el cuello	el koo-*eh*-joh
The throat	la garganta	lah gar-*gan*-tah
The skin	la piel	lah pee-el
The bones	los huesos	lohs hoo-*ay*-sos
The muscles	los músculos	lohs *moos*-koo-lohs

The nerves	los nervios	lohs *nayhr*-vee-ohs
The shoulder blades	las paletillas	lahs pah-lay-*tee*-jahs
The arm	el brazo	el *brah*-soh
The elbow	el codo	el *koh*-doh
The wrist	la muñeca	lah moon-*yeh*-kah
The hand	la mano	lah *mah*-noh
The chest	el pecho	el *pay*-choh
The lungs	los pulmones	lohs *puhl*-moh-nays
The heart	el corazón	el koh-rah-*son*
The ribs	las costillas	lahs kohs-*tee*-jahs
The side	el flanco	el *flahn*-koh
The back	la espalda	lay ays-*pahl*-dah
The abdomen	el abdomen	el *ahb*-doh-men
The stomach	el estómago	el ays-*toh*-mah-goh
The leg	la pierna	lah pee-ehr-nah
The thigh	el muslo	el *moos*-loh
The ankle	el tobillo	el toh-bee-joh
The foot	el pie	el *pee*-ay
Urine	urino	u-*re*-noh

Diseases

Allergy	Alergia	Ah-*layr*-hee-ah
Anemia	Anemia	ah-*nay*-mee-ah
Cancer	Cancer	Kahn-sayr
Chicken pox	Varicela	Vah-ree-*say*-lah
Diabetes	Diabetes	Dee-ah-bay-tees
Diphtheria	Difteria	Deef-*tay*-ree-ah
German measles	Rubéola	Roo-*bay*-oh-lah
Gonorrhea	Gonorrea	Gun-noh-*ree*-ah
Heart disease	Enfermedad del corazón	Ayn-*fayr*-may-*dahd* dayl koh-rah-*sohn*
High blood pressure	Presión alta	Pray-see-*ohn al*-ta
Influenza	Gripe	*Gree*-pay
Lead poisoning	Envenenamiento con plomo	Ayn-vay-nay-nah-mee-*ayn*-toh kohn *ploh*-moh
Liver disease	Enfermedad del hígado	Ayn-*fayr* may-dahd del ee-*gah*-doh
Measles	Sarampion	Sah-rahm-pee-*ohn*
German measles	Rubeola	roo-be-*oh*-lah
Mumps	Paperas	Pah-*pay*-rahs
Nervous disease	Enfermedades nerviosa	Ayn-fayr-may-*dahd*-days nayr-vee-*oh*-sah
Pleurisy	Pleuresía	Play-oo-ray-*see*-ah
Pneumonia	Pulmonia	Pool-*moh*-nee-ah
Rheumatic fever	Reumatismo (fiebre reumatica)	Ray-oo-mah-*tees*-moh (fee-*ay*-bray ray-oo-*mah*-tee-kah)
Scarlet fever	Escarlatina	Ays-kahr-lah-*tee*-nah
Syphilis	Sifilis	See-fee-lees
Tuberculosis	Tuberculosis	Too-*bayr*-koo-lohs-sees

Signs and Symptoms

Do you have stomach cramps?	¿Tiene calambres en el estómago?	¿Tee-*ay*-nay kah-*lahm*-brays ayn el ays-*toh*-mah-goh?
Chills?	Escalofrios	Ays-kah-loh-*free*-ohs
An attack of fever?	Un ataque de fiebre	Oon ah-*tah*-kay day fee-*ay*-bray
Hemorrhage?	Hemoragia	Ay-moh-*rah*-hee-ah
Nosebleeds?	Hemoragia por la nariz	Ay-moh-*rah*-hee-ah por-lah nah-*rees*
Unusual vaginal bleeding?	Hemoragia vaginal fuera de los periodos	Ay-moh-*rah*-hee-ah *vah*-hee-nahl foo-*ay*-rah day lohs pay-ree-*oh*-dohs
Hoarseness?	Ronquera	Rohn-*kay*-rah
A sore throat?	¿Le duele la garganta?	¿Lay doo-*ay*-lay lah gahr-gahn-tah?
Does it hurt to swallow?	¿Le duele al tragar?	¿Lay doo-ay-lay ahl trah-gar?
Have you any difficulty in breathing?	¿Tiene difficultad al respirar?	¿Tee-*ay*-nay dee-fee-kool-*tahd* ahl rays-*pee*-rahr?
Does it pain you to breathe?	¿Le duele al respirar?	¿Lay doo-*ay*-lay ahl rays-*pee*-rahr?
How does your head feel?	¿Cómo siente la cabeza?	¿*Koh*-moh see-*ayn*-tay lah Kah-*bay*-sah?
Is your memory good?	¿Es buena su memoria?	¿Ays *bway*-nah soo may-moh-*ree*-ah?
Have you any pain in the head?	¿Le duele la cabeza?	¿Lay doo-*ay*-lay lah Kah-*bay*-sah?
Do you feel dizzy?	¿Tiene udsted vértigo?	¿Tee-*ay*-nay ood-*stayd* vehr-tee-goh?
Are you tired?	¿Está udsted cansado?	¿Ay-*stah* ood-*stayd* kahn-*sah*-doh?
Can you eat?	¿Puede comer?	¿*pway*-day koh-*mer*?
Have you a good appetite?	¿Tiene udsted buen apetito?	¿Tee-*ay*-nay ood-*stayd* bwayn ah-pay-*tee*-toh?
How are your stools?	¿Cómo son sus heces fecales?	¿*Koh*-moh sohn soos *bay*-says fay-*kal*-ays?
Are they regular?	¿Son regulares?	¿Sohn ray-goo-*lah*-rays?
Are you constipated?	¿Está estreñido?	¿Ay-*stah* ays-trayn-*yee*-do?
Do you have diarrhea?	¿Tiene diarrea?	¿Tee-*ay*-nay dee-ah-*ray*-ah?
Have you any difficulty passing water?	¿Tiene dificultad en orinar?	¿Tee-*ay*-nay dee-fee-kool-*tahd* ayn oh-ree-*nahr*?
Do you pass water involuntarily?	¿Orina sin querer?	¿Oh-*ree*-nah seen kay-rayr?
How long have you felt this way?	¿Desde cuándo se siente asi?	¿*Days*-day *Kwan*-doh say see-*ayn*-tay ah-see?
What diseases have you had?	¿Qué enfermedades ha tenido?	¿Kay ayn-fer-may-*dah*-days hah tay-*nee*-doh?
Do you hear voices?	¿Tiene los voces?	¿Tee-*ay*-nay los *vo*-ses?

Examination

Remove your clothing	Quítese su ropa	*Key*-tay-say soo *roh*-pah
Put on this gown	Pongáse la bata	Pohn-*gah*-say lah *bah*-tah
Need a urine specimen	Es necesário una muéstra de su orina	Ays nay-say-*sar*-ee-oh oo-nah moo-*ay*-strah day oh-*ree*-nah
Be seated	Siéntese	See-*ayn*-tay-say
Recline	Acuestése	Ah-cways-*tay*-say
Sit up	Siéntese	See-*ayn*-tay-say
Stand	Parése	Pah-*ray*-say

Bend your knees	Dóble las rodíllas	*Doh*-blay lahs roh-*dee*-yahs
Relax your muscles	Reláje los músculos	Ray-*lah*-hay lohs *moos*-koo-lohs
Try to	Aténte	Ah-*tayn*-tay
Try again	Aténte ótra vez	Ah-*tayn*-tay *oh*-tra vays
Do not move	No se muéva	Noh say moo-*ay*-vah
Turn on (or to) your left side	Voltése a su ládo izquiérdo	Vohl-*tay*-say ah soo *lah*-doh is-key-*ayr*-doh
Turn on (or to) your right side	Voltése a su ládo derécho	Vohl-*tay*-say ah soo *lah*-doh day-*ray*-choh
Take a deep breath	Respíra profúndo	Ray-*speer*-rah pro-*foon*-doh
Hold your breath	Deténga su respiración	Day-*tayn*-gah soo ray-speer-ah-see-*ohn*
Don't hold your breath	No deténga su respiración	Noh day-*tayn*-gah soo ray-speer-ah-see-*ohn*
Cough	Tosa	*toh*-sah
Open your mouth	Abra la boca	*ah*-brah lah *boh*-kah
Show me . . .	Enséñeme . . .	ayn-*sayn*-yay-may
Here There	Aquí Allí	Ah-kee ah-jee
Which side?	¿En qué lado?	Ayn kay *lah*-doh?
Let me see your hand	Enséñeme la mano	Ayn-*sehn*-yay-may lah *mah*-noh
Grasp my hand	Apriete mi mano	Ah-*pree*-it-tay mee *mah*-noh
Raise your arm	Levante el brazo	Lay-*vahn*-tay el *brah*-soh
Raise it more	Más alto	Mahs *ahl*-toh
Now the other	Ahora el otro	Ah-*oh*-rah el *oh*-troh

Treatment

It is necessary	Es necesario	ays neh-say-*sah*-ree-oh
An operation is necessary	Una operación es necesaria	oo-nah oh-peh-rah-see-*ohn* ays neh-say-*sah*-ree-ah
A prescription	una receta	oo-na ray-*say*-tah
Use it regularly	tómelo con regularidad	*toh*-may-loh kohn ray-goo-*lah*-ree-dad
Take one teaspoonful three times daily (in water)	Toma una cucharadita tres veces al dia, con agua	*Toh*-may oo-na koo-chah-rah-*dee*-tah trays *vay*-says ahl *dee*-ah, kohn ah-gwah
Gargle	Haga gargaras	*Ah*-gah gar-*gah*-rahs
Use injection	use una inyección	oo-say oo-nah in-*yek*-see-ohn
Oral contraceptives	una pildora	oo-nah peel-*doh*-rah
A pill	una pastilla	oo-nah pahs-*tee*-yah
A powder	un polvo	oon *pohl*-voh
Before meals	antes de las comidas	*ahn*-tays day lahs koh-*mee*-dahs
After meals	despues de las comidas	*days*-poo-ehs day lahs koh-mee-dahs
Every day	todos los dia	*toh*-dohs lohs *dee*-ah
Every hour	cada hora	*kah*-dah *oh*-rah
Breathe slowly—like this (in this manner)	respire despacio—asi	rays-*pee*-ray days-*pah*-see-oh—ah-*see*
Remain on a diet	estar a dieta	ays-*tar* a dee-*ay*-tah

General

How do you feel?	¿Como se siénte?	¿*Koh*-moh say see-*ayn*-tay?
Do you have pain?	¿Tiéne dolór?	¿Tee-*ay*-nay doh-*lorh*?
Where is the pain?	¿Adónde es el dolór?	¿Ah-*dohn*-day ays ayl doh-*lorh*?
Do you want medication for your pain?	¿Quiére medicación para su dolór?	¿Kay-*ay*-ray may-dee-kah see-*ohn pak*-rah soo doh-*lorh*?
Are you comfortable?	¿Está comfortáble?	¿Ay-*stah* kohn-for-*tah*-blay?
Are you thirsty?	¿Tiéne sed?	¿Tee-*ay*-nay sayd?
You may not eat/drink	No cóma/béba	Noh *koh*-mah/bay-*bah*
You can only drink water	Solo puéde tomár água	Soh-loh *pway*-day toh-mar *ah*-gwah
Apply bandage to . . .	Ponga una vendaje a . . .	*pohn*-gah *oo*-nah vehn-*dah*-hay ah . . .
Apply ointment	Aplíquese unguento	ah-*plee*-kay-say oon-goo-*ayn*-toh
Keep very quiet	Estése muy quieto	ays-*tay*-say moo-ay key-*ay*-toh
You must not speak	No debe hablar	noh *day*-bay ha-*blahr*
It will be uncomfortable	Séra incomódo	*Say*-rah een-koh-*moh*-doh
It will sting	Va ardér	Vah ahr-*dayr*
You will feel pressure	Vá a sentír presión	Vah ah sayn-*teer* pray-see-*ohn*
I am going to . . .	Voy a:	Voy ah:
Count (take) your pulse	Tomár su púlso	Toh-*marh* soo *pool*-soh
Take your temperature	Tomár su temperatúra	Toh-*marh* soo taym-pay-rah-*too*-rah
Take your blood pressure	Tomar su presión	Toh-*mahr* soo pray-see-*ohn*
Give you pain medicine	Dárle medicación para dolór	*Dahr*-lay may-dee-kah-see-*ohn* pah-rah doh-*lohr*
You should (try to) . . .	Tráte de:	*Trah*-tay day:
Call for help/assistance	Llamár para asisténcia	Yah-*marh* pah-rah ah-sees-*tayn*-see-ah
Empty your bladder	Orínar	Oh-*ree*-narh
Do you still feel very weak?	¿Se siente muy débil todavía?	Say see-*ayn*-tay moo-ee *day*-beel toh-dah-*vee*-ah
It is important to . . .	Es importánte de:	Ays eem-por-*tahn*-tay day
Walk (ambulate)	Caminár	Kah-mee-*narh*
Drink fluids	Bebér líquidos	Bay-*bayr* lee-kay-dohs

(From Rosdahl, C.B. [1995]. Textbook of Basic Nursing, 6th ed. Philadelphia: J.B. Lippincott.)

Appendix

III

Two-Letter State and Possession Abbreviations

Alabama	AL	Nebraska	NE
Alaska	AK	Nevada	NV
Arizona	AZ	New Hampshire	NH
Arkansas	AR	New Jersey	NJ
American Samoa	AS	New Mexico	NM
California	CA	New York	NY
Colorado	CO	North Carolina	NC
Connecticut	CT	North Dakota	ND
Delaware	DE	Northern Mariana Islands	MP
District of Columbia	DC	Ohio	OH
Federated States of Micronesia	FM	Oklahoma	OK
Florida	FL	Oregon	OR
Georgia	GA	Palau	PW
Guam	GU	Pennsylvania	PA
Hawaii	HI	Puerto Rico	PR
Idaho	ID	Rhode Island	RI
Illinois	IL	South Carolina	SC
Indiana	IN	South Dakota	SD
Iowa	IA	Tennessee	TN
Kansas	KS	Texas	TX
Kentucky	KY	Utah	UT
Louisiana	LA	Vermont	VT
Maine	ME	Virginia	VA
Marshall Islands	MH	Virgin Islands	VI
Maryland	MD	Washington	WA
Massachusetts	MA	West Virginia	WV
Michigan	MI	Wisconsin	WI
Minnesota	MN	Wyoming	WY
Mississippi	MS	Armed Forces of the Americas	AA
Missouri	MO	Armed Forces Europe	AE
Montana	MT	Armed Forces Pacific	AP

Appendix

IV Abbreviations Commonly Used in Documentation

Abbreviation	Meaning	Abbreviation	Meaning
ā	before	NG	nasogastric
abd	abdomen	NKA	no known allergies
ac	before meals	noc	night
ADL	activities of daily living	NPO	nothing by mouth
ad lib	as needed	os	mouth
adm.	admitted, admission	OOB	out of bed
amp.	ampule	oz	ounce
ant.	anterior	p̄	after
AP	anterior–posterior	p.c.	after meals
ax.	axillary	post	posterior
b.i.d.	twice a day	prep	preparation
BP	blood pressure	prn	when necessary
BR	bed rest	q̄, q	every
BRP	bathroom privileges	q̄ 2 (3, 4, etc.) hours	every 2 (3, 4, etc.) hours
C	Centigrade	qd	every day
c̄	with	qh	every hour
caps	capsule	q.i.d.	four times a day
C.C.	chief complaint	q.o.d.	every other day
cc	cubic centimeter (1 cc = 1 mL)	q.s.	quantity sufficient
		R/O	rule out
CVP	central venous pressure		
c/o	complains of	ROM	range of motion
D/C	discontinue	s̄	without
disch; DC	discharge	SBA	stand by assistance
drsg	dressing	SC	subcutaneous
dr	dram	SL	sublingual
elix	elixir	SOB	shortness of breath
ext	extract or external	sol, soln	solution
F	Fahrenheit	spec	specimen
fx.	fracture, fractional	S/P	status post
gm	gram	sp. gr.	specific gravity
gr	grain	S.S.E.	soapsuds edema
gt/gtt	drop/drops	ss	one-half
"H," SC, or sub q	hypodermic or subcutaneous	stat	immediately
		tab	tablet
h	hour		
HOB	head of bed	t.i.d.	three times a day
h.s.	bedtime (hour of sleep)		
hx	history	tinct or tr.	tincture
I & O	intake & output	TKO	to keep open
		TPN	total parenteral nutrition hyperalimentation
IM	intramuscular		
		TPR	temperature, pulse, respiration
IV	intravenous		
kg	kilogram	tsp	teaspoon
KVO	keep vein open	TO	telephone order

(continued)

Abbreviation	Meaning	Abbreviation	Meaning
L	left; liter	TWE	tap water enema
lat	lateral	VO	verbal order
MAE	moves all extremities	VS	vital signs
mg	milligram	VSS	vital signs stable
ml, mL	milliliter (1 mL = 1 cc)	W/C	wheelchair
NAD	no apparent distress	WNL	within normal limits

Selected Abbreviations Used for Specific Descriptions

Abbreviation	Meaning	Abbreviation	Meaning
AKA	above-knee amputation	O.D.	right eye
ASCVD	arteriosclerotic cardio-vascular disease	O.S.	left eye
ASHD	arteriosclerotic heart disease	O.U.	each eye
BKA	below-knee amputation	OPD	outpatient department
ca	cancer	ORIF	open reduction internal fixation
chest clear to A & P	chest clear to auscultation &* percussion	Ortho	orthopedics
CMS	circulation movement sensation	OT	occupational therapy
		PE	physical examination
CNS	central nervous system	PERRLA	pupils equal, round, & react to light and accommodation
DJD	degenerative joint disease		
DOE	dyspnea on exertion	PID	pelvic inflammatory disease
DTs	delirium tremens	PI	present illness
D_5W	5% dextrose in water	PM & R	physical medicine & rehabilitation
FUO	fever of unknown origin		
GB	gall bladder	Psych	psychology; psychiatric
GI	gastrointestinal	PT	physical therapy
GYN	gynecology	RL (or LR)	Ringer's lactate; lactated Ringer's
H_2O_2	hydrogen peroxide		
HA	hyperalimentation headache	RLE	right lower extremity
		RLQ	right lower quadrant
HCVD	hypertensive cardiovas-cular disease	RR, PAR, PACU	recovery room, post-anesthesia room, post-anesthesia care unit
HEENT	head, ear, eye, nose, throat		
HVD	hypertensive vascular disease	RUE	right upper extremity
		RUQ	right upper quadrant
ICU	intensive care unit	Rx	prescription
I & D	incision and drainage	SOB	short of breath
		STD	sexually transmitted disease
LLE	left lower extremity	STSG	split-thickness skin graft
LLQ	left lower quadrant		
LOC	level of consciousness; laxatives of choice	Surg	surgery, surgical
		T & A	tonsillectomy & adenoid-ectomy
LMP	last menstrual period		
LUE	left upper extremity	THR, TJR	total hip replacement; total joint replacement
LUQ	left upper quadrant	URI	upper respiratory infection
MI	myocaridal infarction		
Neuro	neurology; neurosurgery	UTI	urinary tract infection
NS	normal saline	vag	vaginal
Nys.	nursery	WNWD	well-nourished, well-developed
NWB	non–weight-bearing		

(continued)

Abbreviation	Meaning	Abbreviation	Meaning

Selected Abbreviations Related to Common Diagnostic Tests

Abbreviation	Meaning	Abbreviation	Meaning
BE	barium enema	hct	hematocrit
B.M.R.	basal metabolism rate	Hgb	hemoglobin
Ca^{++}	calcium	IVP	intravenous pyelogram
CAT	computed axial tomography	K^+	potassium
		LP	lumbar puncture
CBC	complete blood count	MRI	magnetic resonance imaging
Cl^-	chloride		
C & S	culture & sensitivity	Na^+	sodium
Dx	diagnosis	RBC	red blood cell
ECG, EKG	electrocardiogram	UGI	upper gastrointestinal x-ray
EEG	electroencephalogram		
FBS	fasting blood sugar	UA	urinalysis
		WBC	white blood cell

Commonly Used Symbols

Symbol	Meaning	Symbol	Meaning
>	greater than	@	at
<	less then	+	positive
=	equal to	−	negative
≈	approximately equal to	±	positive or negative
≤	equal to or less than	F_1	first filial generation
≥	equal to or greater than	F_2	second filial generation
↑	increased	PO_2	partial pressure of oxygen
↓	decreased	PCO_2	partial pressure of carbon dioxide
♀	female		
♂	male	:	ratio
°	degree	∴	therefore
#	number or pound	%	percent
×	times	2°	secondary to
		Δ	change

(From Craven, R.F. & Hirnle, C.J. (1996). Human Health and Function, 2nd ed. Philadelphia: Lippincott-Raven.)

Appendix
V

Metric Measurements

Unit	Abbreviation	Metric Equivalent	U.S. Equivalent
Units of weight			
Kilogram	kg	1000 g	2.2 lb
Gram*	g	1000 mg	0.035 oz.; 28.5 g/oz
Milligram	mg	1/1000 g; 0.001 g	
Microgram	µg	1/1000 mg; 0.001 mg	
Units of length			
Kilometer	km	1000 meters	0.62 miles; 1.6 km/mile
Meter*	m	100 cm; 1000 mm	39.4 inches; 1.1 yards
Centimeter	cm	1/100 m; 0.01 m	0.39 inches; 2.5 cm/inch
Millimeter	mm	1/1000 m; 0.001 m	0.039 inches; 25 mm/inch
Micrometer	µm	1/1000 mm; 0.001 mm	
Units of volume			
Liter*	L	1000 mL	1.06 qt
Deciliter	dL	1/10 L; 0.1 L	
Milliliter	mL	1/1000 L; 0.001 L	0.034 oz., 29.4 mL/oz
Microliter	µL	1/1000 mL; 0.001 mL	

*Basic unit

(From Memmler, R.L., Cohen, B.J., and Wood, D.L. (1996). *The Human Body in Health and Disease, 8th ed.* Philadelphia: Lippincott-Raven.)

Appendix

VI *Celsius–Fahrenheit Temperature Conversion Scale*

Celsius to Fahrenheit

Use the following formula to convert Celsius readings to Fahrenheit readings:

$$°F = 9/5°C + 32$$

For example, if the Celsius reading is 37°:

$$°F = (9/5 × 37) + 32$$
$$= 66.6 + 32$$
$$= 98.6°F \text{ (normal body temperature)}$$

Fahrenheit to Celsius

Use the following formula to convert Fahrenheit readings to Celsius readings:

$$°C = 5/9 (°F − 32)$$

For example, if the Fahrenheit reading is 68°:

$$°C = 5/9 (68 − 32)$$
$$= 5/9 × 36$$
$$= 20°C \text{ (a nice spring day)}$$

(From Memmler, R.L., Cohen, B.J., and Wood, D.L. (1996). The Human Body in Health and Disease, 8th ed. Philadelphia: Lippincott-Raven.)

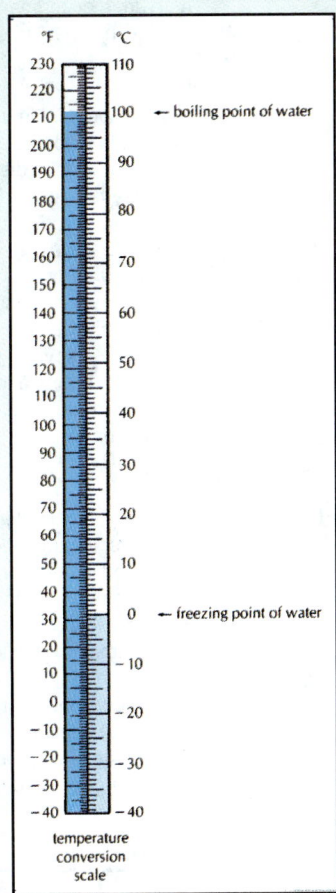

temperature conversion scale

Table 1
Routine Urinalysis

Test	Normal Value	Clinical Significance
General characteristics and measurements		
Color	Pale yellow to amber	Color change can be due to concentration or dilution, drugs, metabolic or inflammatory disorders
Odor	Slightly aromatic	Foul odor typical of urinary tract infection, fruity odor in uncontrolled diabetes mellitus
Appearance (clarity)	Clear to slightly hazy	Cloudy urine occurs with infection or after refrigeration; may indicate presence of bacteria, cells, mucus, or crystals
Specific gravity	1.003–1.030 (first morning catch; routine is random)	Decreased in diabetes insipidus, acute renal faiure, water intoxication; increased in liver disorders, heart failure, dehydration
pH	4.5–8.0	Acid urine accompanies acidosis, fever, high protein diet; alkaline urine in urinary tract infection, metabolic alkalosis, vegetarian diet
Chemical determinations		
Glucose	Negative	Glucose present in uncontrolled diabetes mellitus, steroid excess
Ketones	Negative	Present in diabetes mellitus and in starvation
Protein	Negative	Present in kidney disorders, such as glomerulonephritis, acute kidney failure
Bilirubin	Negative	Breakdown product of hemoglobin; present in liver disease or in bile blockage
Urobilinogen	0.2–1.0 Ehrlich units/dL	Breakdown product of bilirubin; increased in hemolytic anemias and in liver disease; remains negative in bile obstruction
Blood (occult)	Negative	Detects small amounts of blood cells, hemoglobin, or myoglobin; present in severe trauma, metabolic disorders, bladder infections
Nitrite	Negative	Product of bacterial breakdown of urine; positive result suggests urinary tract infection and needs to be followed up with a culture of the urine
Microscopic		
Red blood cells	0–3 per high-power field	Increased due to bleeding within the urinary tract from trauma, tumors, inflammation, or damage within the kidney
White blood cells	0–4 per high-power field	Increased in infection of the kidney or bladder
Renal epithelial cells	Occasional	Increased number indicates damage to kidney tubules
Casts	None	Hyaline casts normal; large number of abnormal casts indicates inflammation or a systemic disorder
Crystals	Present	Most are normal; may be acid or alkaline
Bacteria	Few	Increased in infection of urinary tract or contamination from infected genitalia
Others		Any yeasts, parasites, mucus, spermatozoa, or other microscopic findings would be reported here

(continued)

Table 2
Complete Blood Cound (CBC)

Test	Normal Value*	Clinical Significance
Red blood cell count (RBC)	Men: 4.2–5.4 million/µL Women: 3.6–5.0 million /µL	Decreased in anemia; increased in dehydration, polycythemia
Hemoglobin (HGB)	Men: 13.5–17.5 g/dL Women: 12–16 g/dL	Decreased in anemia, hemorrhage and hemolytic reactions; increased in dehydration, heart and lung disease
Hematocrit (HCT) or packed cell volume (PCV)	Men: 40%–50% Women: 37%–47%	Decreased in anemia; increased in polycythemia, dehydration
Red blood cell indices (examples)		These values, calculated from the RBC, HGB, and HCT, give information valuable in the diagnosis and classification of anemia
Mean corpuscular volume (MVC)	87–103 µL/red cell	Measures the average size or volume of each red blood cell: Small size (microcytic) in iron-deficiency anemia; large size (macrocytic) typical of pernicious anemia
Mean corpuscular hemoglobin (MCH)	26–34 pg/red cell	Measures the weight of hemoglobin per red blood cell; useful in differentiating types of anemia in a severely anemic patient
Mean corpuscular hemoglobin concentration (MCHC)	31–37 g/dL	Defines the volume of hemoglobin per red blood cell; used to determine the color or concentration of hemoglobin per red cell
White blood count (WBC)	5,000–10,000/µL	Increased in leukemia and in response to infection, inflammation, and dehydration; decreased in bone marrow suppression
Platelets	150,000–350,000/µL	Increased in many malignant disorders; decreased in disseminated intravascular coagulation (DIC) or toxic drug effects; spontaneous bleeding may occur at platelet counts below 20,000
Differential (Peripheral blood smear)		A stained slide of the blood is needed to perform the differential. The percentages of the different white cells are estimated, and the slide in microscopically checked for abnormal characteristics in WBCs, RBCs, and platelets.
White cells		
Segments neutrophils (SEGs, POLYs)	40%–74%	Increased in bacterial infections; low numbers leave person very susceptible to infection
Immature neutrophils (BANDs)	0%–3%	Increase when neutrophil count increases
Lymphocytes (LYMPHs)	20%–40%	Increased in viral infections; low numbers leave a person dangerously susceptible to infection
Monocytes (MONOs)	2%–6%	Increased in specific infections
Eosinophils (EOs)	1%–4%	Increased in allergic disorders
Basophils (BASOs)	0.5%–1%	Increased in allergic disorders

*Values vary depending on instrumentation and type of test.

Table 3
Blood Chemistry Tests

Test	*Normal Value*	*Clinical Significance*
Basic panel: An overview of electrolytes, waste product management, and metabolism		
Blood urea nitrogen (BUN)	7–18 mg/dL	Increased in renal disease and dehydration; decreased in liver damage and malnutrition
Carbon dioxide (CO_2) (includes bicarbonate)	23–30 mmol/L	Useful to evaluate acid–base balance by measuring total carbon dioxide in the blood: Elevated in vomiting and pulmonary disease; decreased in diabetic acidosis, acute renal failure, and hyperventilation
Chloride (Cl)	98–106 mEq/L	Increased in dehydration, hyperventilation, and congestive heart failure; decreased in vomiting, diarrhea, and fever
Creatinine	0.6–1.2 mg/dL	Produced at a constant rate and excreted by the kidney; increased in kidney disease
Glucose	Fasting: 70–110 mg/dL Random: 85–125 mg/dL	Increased in diabetes and severe illness; decreased in insulin overdose or hypoglycemia
Potassium (K)	3.5–5 mEq/L	Increased in renal failure, extensive cell damage and acidosis; decreased in vomiting, diarrhea, and excess administration of diuretics or IV fluids
Sodium (Na)	101–111 mEq/L or 135–148 mEq/L (depending on test)	Increased in dehydration and diabetes insipidus; decreased in overload of IV fluids, burns, diarrhea, or vomiting
Additional blood chemistry tests		
Alanine aminotransferase (ALT)	Men: 7–24 U/L Women: 7–17 U/L	Used to diagnose and monitor treatment of liver disease and to monitor the effects of drugs on the liver, increased in myocardial infarction
Albumin	3.8–5.0 g/dL	Albumin holds water in blood; decreased in liver disease and kidney disease
Albumin–globulin ratio (A/G ratio)	Greater than 1	Low A/G ratio signifies a tendency for edema because globulin is less effective than albumin at holding water in the blood.
Alkaline phosphatase (ALP)	20–70 U/L (varies by method)	Enzyme of bone metabolism; increased in liver disease and metastatic bone disease
Amylase	21–160 U/L	Used to diagnose and monitor treatment of acute pancreatitis and to detect inflammation of the salivary glands
Aspartate aminotransferase (AST)	0–41 U/L (varies)	Enzyme present in tissues with high metabolic activity; increased in myocardial infarction and liver disease
Bilirubin, total	0.2–1.0 mg/dL	Breakdown product of hemoglobin from red blood cells; increased when excessive RBCs are being destroyed or in liver disease
Calcium (Ca)	8.8–10.0 mg/dL	Increased in excess parathyroid hormone production and in cancer; decreased in alkalosis, elevated phosphate in renal failure, and excess IV fluids
Cholesterol	120–220 mg/dL desirable range	Screening test used to evaluate risk of heart disease; levels of 200 or above indicate increased risk of heart disease and warrant further investigation
Creatinine phosphokinase (CPK or CK)	Men: 38–174 U/L Women: 96–140 U/L	Elevated enzyme level indicates myocardial infarction or damage to skeletal muscle. When elevated, specific fractions (isoenzymes) should be tested
Gamma glutamyl transferase (GGT)	Men: 6–26 U/L Women: 4–18 U/L	Used to diagnose liver disease and test for chronic alcoholism
Globulins	2.3–3.5 g/dL	Proteins active in immunity; help albumin keep water in blood
Iron, serum (Fe)	Men: 75–175 µg/dL Women: 65–165 µg/dL	Decreased in iron deficiency and anemia; increased in hemolytic conditions
High-density lipoproteins (HDLs)	Men: 30–70 mg/dL Women: 30–85 mg/dL	Used to evaluate the risk of heart disease

(continued)

Table 3

Blood Chemistry Tests (Continued)

Test	*Normal Value*	*Clinical Significance*
Lactic dehydrogenase (LDH or LD)	95–200 U/L (normal ranges vary greatly)	Enzyme released in many kinds of tissue damage; including myocardial infarction, pulmonary infarction, and liver disease
Lipase	4–24 U/L (varies with test)	Enzyme used to diagnose pancreatitis
Low-density lipoproteins (LDLs)	80–140 mg/dL	Used to evaluate the risk of heart disease
Magnesium (Mg)	1.3–2.1 mEq/L	Vital in neuromuscular function; decreased levels may occur in malnutrition, alcoholism, pancreatitis, diarrhea
Phosphorus (P) (inorganic)	2.7–4.5 mg/dL	Evaluated in response to calcium; main store is in bone: elevated in kidney disease; decreased in excess parathyroid hormone
Protein, total	6–8 g/dL	Increased in dehydration, multiple myeloma; decreased in kidney disease, liver disease, poor nutrition, severe burns, excessive bleeding
Serum glutamic oxalacetic transaminase (SGOT)		See Aspartate aminotransferase (AST)
Serum glutamic pyruvic transaminase (SGPT)		See alanine aminotransferase (ALT)
Thyroxin (T_4)	5–12.5 µg/dL (varies)	Screening test of thyroid function; increased in hyperthyroidism; decreased in myxedema and hypothyroidism
Thyroid stimulating hormone (TSH)	0.5–6 mIU/L	Produced by pituitary to cause thyroid gland to function; elevated when thyroid gland is not functioning
Triiodothyronine (T_3)	120–195 mg/dL	Elevated in specific types of hyperthyroidism
Triglycerides	Men: 40–160 mg/dL Women: 35–135 mg/dL	An indication of ability to metabolize fats; increased triglycerides and cholesterol indicate high risk of atherosclerosis
Uric acid	Men: 3.5–7.2 mg/dL Women: 2.6–6.0 mg/dL	Produced by breakdown of ingested purines in food and nucleic acids; elevated in kidney disease, gout, and leukemia

(From Memmler, R.L., Cohen, B.J., and Wood, D.L. (1996) *The Human Body in Health and Disease*, 8th ed. Philadelphia: Lippincott-Raven.)

Glossary

abdominal regions   divisions of the abdomen into nine regions by two horizontal and two vertical lines; used to identify specific locations

ablation   removal or excision of a part; laser ablation is destruction/removal of tissue by use of laser

abortion   termination of pregnancy or products of conception prior to fetal viability and/or 20 weeks gestation

abscess   an inflamed cavity filled with pus as a result of infection

accounts payable   a record of all monies owed

accounts receivable   a record of all monies due

acquired immunodeficiency syndrome (AIDS)   a cluster of disorders caused by the Human Immunodeficiency Virus (HIV) that specifically destroys cell-mediated immunity

acrosome   the superior surface of the head of the spermatozoon

activities of daily living (ADL)   activities usually performed in the course of the day, ie, bathing, dressing, feeding oneself

Addison's Disease   partial or complete failure of the adrenal cortex functions, causing general physical deterioration

adenosine triphosphate (ATP)   the energy currency used by the body; breaking down the phosphate bond of the compound releases high energy potential

adipose   of or pertaining to fat

adjustments   changes in a posted account

adnexa   any part added to a main structure; an accessory part

administrative   pertaining to administration (eg, office procedures and nonclinical tasks that a medical assistant will perform)

advance directive   a statement of a patient's wishes regarding health care prior to a critical medical event

aerobe   microorganism that requires oxygen to live

aerosol   suspended particles in gas or air

afferent   carrying impulses towards the center

affiliation   to connect or associate with, as a medical site would associate with a school to assist in completion of student training

agar   a type of seaweed or algae that helps solidify culture media; the media may be referred to as agar

age of majority   age at which an individual is considered to be an adult (usually 18–21 years of age)

agglutination   clumping of cells due to the presence of antibodies called agglutinins

aging schedule   a form used to track outstanding balances

agranulocytes   white blood cells that do not contain visible granules when stained

allergen   any substance that causes manifestations of an allergy, usually a protein to which the body has built antibodies

allergy   an acquired, abnormal response to a substance (allergen) that does not ordinarily cause a reaction

alphabetic filing   arranging of names or titles according to the sequence of letters in the alphabet

alphafetoprotein   substance produced by the embryonic yolk sac

alveolar-capillary membrane   the structure in the lung fields through which oxygen and carbon dioxide diffuse during the respiratory process

amenorrhea   condition of not menstruating, without menses

American Medical Technologist Institute for Education (AMTIE)   professional organization for medical assistants, medical laboratory technicians, and dental technicians

American Association of Medical Assistants (AAMA)   professional organization for medical assistants

Americans with Disabilities Act (ADA)   a law designed to meet the needs of people with physical and mental challenges

ammonia   a substance produced by decomposition of organic matter containing nitrogen

amniocentesis   puncture of the amniotic sac in order to remove fluid for testing

amphiarthroses   slightly movable joints

ampule   a small glass container that can be sealed and its contents sterilized

anaerobe   microorganism that lives without oxygen

anaphylaxis   a severe systemic reaction resulting from an allergic reaction

anatomical position   a position used for reference in which the subject is standing erect, facing forward, feet are slightly apart and pointing forward, the hands are down at the sides with palms forward and thumbs outward

anatomy   the study of the structure of the body

aneurysm   a localized dilatation on a vessel wall

angina pectoris   paroxysmal chest pain usually caused by myocardial anoxia due to coronary artery occlusion

angiotensin   a substance occurring in the blood that works with renin to affect the blood pressure, usually increasing the pressure by vasoconstriction

anisocytosis   blood abnormality in which red blood cells are not equal in size (aniso = unequal)

ankylosing spondylitis   stiffening of the spine with inflammation

annotation   the process of reading, highlighting and summarizing a document for another person

anovulation   condition of not ovulating

antagonism   mutual opposition or contrary action with something else; opposite of synergism

antagonist   any muscle that opposes the action of the prime mover to balance movement. (Example: When the biceps contact and pull the forearm upward, the triceps oppose the motion and relax.)

antecubital space   inner surface of the bend of the elbow where the major veins for venipuncture are located

antepartum   period of time prior to labor

anthropometric   pertaining to measurements of the human body

antibiotic   a drug that inhibits or destroys pathogenic microorganisms

antibodies   complex glycoproteins produced by B-lymphocytes in response to the presence of an antigen

anticoagulant   anything that prevents or delays the clotting of blood

antigens   protein markers on cells that cause the formation of antibodies and react specifically with those antibodies

antihistamine   medication that opposes the action of a histamine

antiseptic   any substance that inhibits the growth of bacteria; used on skin before any procedure that breaks the integumentary barrier

anuria   failure of the kidneys to produce urine

appeal   process by which a higher court reviews the decision of a lower court

appendicular skeleton   the parts of the skeleton added to the axial skeleton, including the shoulder and pelvic girdles and all of the bones of the upper and lower extremities

applicator   a device used for making local applications

approximate   to bring tissue surfaces together as closely as possible to their original positions

arachnoid   web-like membrane covering the brain and spinal cord

arrector pili   involuntary muscle attached to the hair follicle that when contracted causes "goose bumps"

arteriole   a small arterial branch that joins a capillary to an artery

arthrogram   X-ray of a joint

arthroplasty   repair of a joint

artifact   activity recorded on an electrocardiogram caused by patient movement, loose leads or electrical interference

artifactual   something added to a substance or structure, not belonging to it; in medicine, generally implies a negative connotation

artificial insemination   the insertion of sperm into a woman's vagina by artificial means

ascites   the accumulation of serous fluid in the peritoneal cavity

asepsis   a state of being sterile; a condition free from germs, infection, and any form of life, including spore forms

aspiration   drawing in or out by suction; as in breathing objects into the respiratory tract or suctioning substances from a site

assault   an attempt or threat to touch another person without his or her consent

assessment   the process of gathering information about the patient and the presenting condition

astigmatism   unfocused refraction of light rays on the retina

asymmetry   lack or absence of symmetry; inequality in size or shape on opposite sides of the body

asymptomatic   without any symptoms

atelectasis   collapsed lung fields; incomplete expansion of the lungs, either partial or complete

atraumatic   without injury; may pertain to treatments or instruments that are not likely to cause further damage

atria (plural)   the upper chamber of each half of the heart; the atria receive blood from the great vessels (singular: atrium)

atrioventricular (AV) node   located on the floor of the right atrium on or close to the septum; receives the electrical impulse from the SA node after it is transmitted through the upper half of the heart; transmits the impulse to the bundle of His

attenuated   diluted or weakened; pertaining to reduced virulence of a pathogenic organism

attribute   a characteristic or quality of a person; usually considered a positive feature

audit   a review of an account

auscultation   the act of listening for sounds within the body, usually with a stethoscope, to evaluate the heart, lungs, pleura, intestines, or fetal heart sounds

autoclave   an appliance used to sterilize medical instruments or other objects by steam under pressure

autolet   small, sharp, spring-loaded instrument for quick capillary puncture

autonomic   self controlling, spontaneous

autonomous   existing or functioning independently

axial skeleton   the bones forming the main skeleton around which the appendicular skeleton moves, including bones of the head, thorax, and trunk

axon   part of the neuron that transmits impulses away from the cell body

Azidothymidine (AZT)   a drug used to treat AIDS by blocking the growth of the virus after it enters the T-cell lymphocyte

azotemia   from the Latin azote meaning nitrogen plus -emia, meaning blood; the condition of having excessive amounts of nitrogen in the blood

B-cells   lymphoid stem cells from the bone marrow that migrate to and become mature antigen-specific cells in the spleen and lymph nodes

bacilli   rod-shaped or cylindrical organisms

back-up   (noun) a duplicate file made to a separate disk to protect information; (verb) to make a duplicate file

bacteriology   the science and study of bacteria

balance   remainder; amount due

bandage   (noun) soft material applied to a body part for treatment purposes; usually a soft, absorbent gauze to hold a dressing, immobilize or support a part, aid in controlling bleeding. (verb) to apply a wrapping material for treatment purposes

Bartholin's glands   small mucous glands bilaterally in the vaginal vestibule

basal ganglia   pertaining to the gray matter in the cerebral hemispheres

basal metabolic rate   the amount of energy used in a unit of time to maintain vital functions by a fasting, resting subject

baseline   the original or initial measure by which other judgments will be made

battery   actual touching of a person without his or her consent

beliefs   ideas that are held to be true

bench trial   trial in which the judge hears the case and renders a verdict; no jury is present

benign   not cancerous or malignant

bias   formation of an opinion without foundation or reason; prejudice

bibulous   very absorbent

bicarbonate   the dissolved form of carbon dioxide; it combines with water to make carbonic acid, $H2CO_3$. Carbonic acid loses one of its hydrogen (H) ions to then form bicarbonate, HCO_3-.

bile   a bitter, yellow-green secretion of the liver stored by the gallbladder; derived from bilirubin, cholesterol, and other substances. Emulsifies fats in the small intestine so they can be further digested and absorbed.

biliary obstruction   blockage of one of the bile ducts (the tubes leading from liver and gallbladder into duodenum); common causes included cysts, tumors, and stones

bilirubinuria   bilirubin in the urine

bimanual   pertaining to the use of both hands; performed by both hands

bioethics   moral issues and concerns that affect a person's life

biotransforming   conversion of the molecules of a substance from one form to another, as in medications within the body

blister   a collection of fluid in or beneath the epidermis; a vesicle

block   a type of letter format in which the date, subject line, closing and signatures are to the right margin; all other lines are justified left

body fluids   any of the fluids that accumulate in the compartments of the body, such as the blood plasma, and the intracellular and extracellular spaces

boil   an abscess of the subcutaneous tissues of the skin; a furuncle

bolus   a mobile mass, for instance, a mass of food that passes into the upper gastrointestinal tract in one swallow, or a dose of medication injected intravenously

boot   to start up the computer

bradykinesia   abnormally slow voluntary movements

Braxton Hicks   uterine contractions that occur during pregnancy

bruit   an abnormal sound or murmur heard in the blood vessels while auscultating an organ, gland, or blood vessel

budget   financial planning tool that helps an organization estimate its anticipated expenditures and revenues

bulla   a large blister or vesicle

BUN   abbreviation for Blood Urea Nitrogen

bundle of His   A band of specialized cardiac muscle fibers that receive the electrical impulse from the AV node and transmit it through right and left branches to the Purkinje fibers

bursae   small, pad-like sacs filled with clear synovial fluid that surround some joints

byte   a unit of symbolic transfer; each character equals one byte

caduceus   a symbol using a wand or staff with two serpents coiled around it; sometimes used as the sign of the medical profession (the more appropriate symbol has only one snake)

calibrated   measured against a standard

calibrations   measurements for size or volume, as in calibrations on a syringe or pipette

callus   in the musculoskeletal system, a deposit of new bone tissue that forms between the healing ends of broken bones; in the integumentary system, a thickened area of the epidermis caused by pressure or friction

calyx (pl. calyces)   a cup-like collecting structure of the kidney

cancellous   porous, spongy bone inside the medulla of the bone, usually filled with marrow

capillary action   the raising or lowering of a liquid at the point of contact with a solid; used to pull blood into a capillary tube or small pipette

cardiac cycle   the period from the beginning of one heart beat to the beginning of the next; includes the systole and the diastole

cardiac output   the amount of blood ejected from either ventricle per minute, either to the pulmonary or to the systemic circulation

cardinal signs   usually refers to the vital signs and signifies their importance in the assessment process

cardiogenic shock   a type of shock in which the left ventricle fails to adequately pump enough blood for the body to function

carina   a ridge-like structure; that part of the trachea that projects from the lower end of the trachea

carrier   asymptomatic or unaffected person who can transmit infection to another person

cassette   the lightproof holder in which film is exposed

catalyzes   increases the rate at which a chemical reaction takes place. Example: Amylase found in saliva catalyzes (speeds up) the rate at which starches are broken down.

cataracts   progressive loss of transparency of the lens resulting in opacity and loss of sight

catheterization   introducing a tube into the body; urinary catheterization involves the removal of urine from the bladder

cautery   a means, device or agent that destroys or coagulates tissue; may be electrical current, freezing or burning agents, or chemical solutions (caustics)

cell   the most basic unit of all living organisms

cellular telephone   a telephone that works by electronic signals and does not require attachment to a telephone plug

Celsius, centigrade (C)   a temperature scale on which 0 degrees is the freezing point of water and 100 degrees is the boiling point of water at sea level

censure   a verbal or written reprimand from a professional organization regarding a specific incident

centesis   surgical puncture made into a cavity

central processing unit (CPU)   circuitry imprinted on a silicon chip that processes information; the "brain" of the computer

centrifugal force   a spinning motion to exert force outward, heavier components of a solution are spun downward

cerebellum   located in the posterior part of the brain, responsible for balance and muscle coordination

cerebrovascular accident (CVA)   ischemia of the brain due to an occlusion of the vessels supplying the brain, resulting in varying degrees of debilitation

cerebrum   largest part of the brain, divided into two hemispheres, responsible for thought processes, sensory and motor functions, speech, writing, memory, and emotions

certification   voluntary process that involves a testing procedure to prove an individual's baseline competency in a particular area

cerumen   the yellowish or brownish waxlike secretion found in the external ear canal; earwax

Chadwick's sign   sign of early pregnancy in which the vaginal, cervical, and vulvular tissues develop a bluish-violet color

challenge   a method of testing a patient's sensitivity or response to a substance by introducing it into the body and watching its effects

chancre   a hard ulcer that appears two to three weeks after exposure to syphilis, near the site of infection

check register   place to record checks that have been written

check stub   indicates to whom a check was issued, in what amount, and on what date

chemical name   the exact chemical structure of a drug

chlamydia   a parasitic microorganism with properties common to bacteria but unable to sustain life without a host, in the manner of a virus

chronic obstructive pulmonary disease (COPD)   a progressive, irreversible condition with diminished respiratory capacity

chronological order   placing in the order of time; usually the most recent is placed foremost

chyle   milky, fatty product of digestion absorbed through the small intestines and returned to circulation by the lymphatics

chyme   the thick, semi-liquid mass of ingested food mixed with gastric juices as it passes from the stomach

cilia   hair-like projections on cells that either propel the cell or objects that come in contact with the cell

circumcision   surgical removal of the prepuce

civil law   a branch of law that focuses on issues between private citizens

clarification   explanation

climacteric period   menopause; developmental phase in which a woman's reproductive ability ceases

Clinical Laboratory Improvement Amendments (CLIA)   guidelines established by Congress in 1988 to standardize and improve laboratory testing

clinical   pertaining to direct patient care (eg, nonadministrative tasks that a medical assistant will perform)

closing   a one to two word phrase that precedes the sender's signature and indicates the end of the letter

coagulate   to change from a liquid form to a solid or semi-solid mass

coerce   to force or compel a person to do something against his or her wishes

collagen   protein substance that gives structure to the connective tissue

collection   a process of acquiring funds that are due

colpocleisis   surgery to occlude the vagina

colporrhaphy   suture of the vagina

colposcopy   visual examination of the vagina and cervix under magnification

comedo   a blackhead

common law   traditional laws that were established by the English legal system

comparative negligence   a percentage of damage awards based on the contribution of negligence between two parties

complement   a group of proteins in the blood that influence the inflammatory process and serve as the primary mediator in the antigen-antibody reactions of the B-cell-mediated response

concussion   injury to the brain due to trauma

conference call   a telephone call between two or more people that occurs at a designated time and is used for discussing a topic of mutual concern

confidentiality   protection of patient data from unauthorized personnel

congenital anomalies   abnormalities, either structural or functional, that are present from birth

conjugate   joined or paired

consent   an agreement between a patient and physician to do a given medical procedure

consideration   the exchange of fees for a service

contract   an agreement between two or more parties for a given act

contracture   abnormal shortening of muscles around a joint caused by atrophy of the muscles and resulting in flexion and fixation

contributory negligence   a defense strategy in which the defendant admits to negligence but claims that the plaintiff assisted in promoting the damages

contusion   collection of blood in tissues after an injury; also known as a bruise

convoluted tubules   the twisted portion of the nephron that connects the glomerulus to the collecting tubules; consists of a proximal and a distal portion connected by the Loop of Henle

convulsion   sudden, involuntary muscle contractions of voluntary muscle groups

coping mechanisms   unconscious methods of alleviating intense stressors

corpora cavernosa   the erectile bodies of the penis or clitoris

corpus spongiosum   erectile tissue around the male urethra

corticoid   any of the hormonal steroid substances obtained from the adrenal cortex

cortisol   a naturally occurring steroidal hormone that regulates metabolism and acts as an anti-inflammatory agent

coumarin   an anticoagulant prescribed for persons likely to form blood clots, such as valve replacement recipients; also called Coumadin (trade name) or warfarin

cranium   the portion of the skull that encloses the brain

crash   "lock up" of the computer central processing unit as a result of a system breakdown

creatine   a chemical compound in the body that adds phosphorus to ADP (adenosine diphosphate) to make ATP (adenosine triphosphate) that is the energy currency of the body

creatinine   the substance formed when creatine (an important compound in metabolic processes) is used

credit   balance in one's favor on an account; promise to pay a bill at a later date

cretinism   severe congenital hypothyroidism; signs include dwarfism, low intelligence, puffy features, dry skin, macroglossia, and poor muscle tone

criteria   the standard, rule, or test by which something or someone can be judged

cross examination   questioning of a witness by the opposing attorney

cross-reference   notation in a file telling that a record is stored elsewhere and giving the reference

cul-de-sac   blind pouch or cavity, as in the cul-de-sac that lies between the rectum and the posterior uterus

culdocentesis   surgical puncture of and aspiration of fluid from the vaginal cul-de-sac for diagnostic/therapeutic purpose

culture   a laboratory process whereby microorganisms are grown in a special medium often for the purpose of identifying a causative agent in an infectious disease; also means the way of life, including commonly held beliefs, of a group of people

curettage   scraping of a cavity

Current Procedural Terminology (CPT)   a comprehensive list of codes used by physicians to bill for procedures and services

cursor   flashing line on the monitor indicating where data input will occur

cyanotic   a bluish discoloration of the skin due to the lack of oxygen

cyst   a sac of fluid or semisolid material under the skin

cystocele   herniation of the urinary bladder into the vagina

cystoscopy   direct visualization of the bladder for diagnostic purposes

cytology   study of cells

DACUM   a code of educational standards for medical assisting students developed by the American Association of Medical Assistants

damages   the resulting injury or suffering that resulted from negligence

data   information that is stored and processed by the computer

database   accumulation of files on the computer

day sheet/daily journal   a daily business record of charges and payments

debit   a charge or money owed on an account

decibel (db)   a unit for measuring the intensity of sound

deciduous   to fall or shed; deciduous teeth: the set of 20 teeth appearing during infancy and shedding during childhood

decongestant   substance that reduces congestion or swelling

defamation of character   making false or malicious statements about a person's character or reputation

defendant   the party that is accused

degenerative joint disease (DJD)   also known as osteoarthritis; arthritis characterized by degeneration of the bony structure of the joints, usually noninflammatory

deglutition   the act of swallowing

demeanor   the way a person looks, behaves and conducts himself or herself

dementia   progressive organic mental deterioration with loss of intellectual function

demographic   relating to the statistical characteristics of populations

dendrite   part of the neuron that transmits impulses toward the cell body

denial   saying that something is not true; refusing to acknowledge

dentin   the main component of the tooth structure, surrounds the inner pulp and lies just below the enamel

depolarization   progressive wave of stimulation causing contraction of the myocardium

deposition   a process in which one party questions another party under oath

dermatitis inflammation of the skin

dermatophytosis a fungus infection of the skin

dermis layer of skin under the epidermis

dextrocardia the condition of having the heart in the right side of the thoracic cavity

diabetes insipidus a disorder of metabolism characterized by polyuria and polydipsia; caused by a deficiency in ADH or an inability of the kidneys to respond to ADH

diagnosis the art of identifying a disease or condition by evaluating physical signs and symptoms, health history, and laboratory tests; the term denoting the name of a disease or condition

Diagnostic Related Groups (DRG) categories used to determine hospital and physician reimbursement for Medicare patients' inpatient services

dialysis removal of urine wastes by passing fluid through a semipermeable barrier that allows normal electrolytes to remain in the general circulation; may be performed either using a machine with circulatory access or by passing a balanced fluid through the peritoneal cavity

diaphragmatic excursion the movement of the diaphragm during respiration

diarthroses freely-movable joints; also called synovial joints

diastole the relaxation phase of the cardiac cycle

diazo a double nitrogen compound that reacts with bilirubin

diction the style of speaking and enunciating words

dideoxycytidine (DDC) a drug used to treat AIDS by blocking the growth of the virus after it enters the T-cell lymphocytes

dideoxyinosine (ddI) a drug used to treat AIDS by blocking the growth of the virus after it enters the T-cell lymphocytes

diencephalon part of the brain lying beneath the hemispheres, containing the thalamus and hypothalamus

digital pertaining to, resembling, or performed with a finger; expressed in digits (0–9)

diluent an agent that dilutes the substance or solution to which it is added

diplococci spherical microorganisms in pairs

diplomacy the art of handling people with tact and genuine concern

direct examination questioning of a witness by the attorney for the individual the witness is representing

directory a "table of contents" of a file system

discrimination making a difference in favor of or against someone

disease a definite pathological process having a descriptive set of symptoms and a general course of progression

disinfectant a chemical that can be applied to objects to destroy microorganisms; will not destroy bacterial spores

disinfection the process of killing or rendering inert most, but not all, pathogenic organisms

disk drive a device that gets information on and off a floppy disk

diuretics substances that promote the formation and excretion of urine

documentation the process of recording patient information

donor one who contributes something to another

dowager's hump exaggerated cervical curve with prominence of the top thoracic vertebrae found in some osteoporotic elderly women; a type of kyphosis

downtime computer malfunction or any time when the machine is not operational

dress to apply a covering to a wound

dressing a covering applied directly to a wound to apply pressure or support, to absorb secretions, to protect from trauma or microorganisms, to stop or slow bleeding, or to hide disfigurement

drug any substance that when taken into the living organism may modify one or more of its functions

due process a formal proceeding in which the accused is considered not guilty until a verdict is reached

dura mater the outer covering of the brain

durable power of attorney a legal document giving another person the authority to act in one's behalf

duress the act of compelling or forcing someone to do something that they do not want to do

dwarfism (endocrine or pituitary) abnormal underdevelopment of the body with extreme shortness but normal proportions; achondroplastic dwarfism is an inherited growth disorder characterized by shortened limbs and a large head but almost normal trunk proportions

dysmenorrhea painful menstruation

dyspareunia painful coitus or sexual intercourse

dysphagia inability or difficulty in swallowing

dysphasia impairment of speech

dyspnea difficulty breathing

ecchymosis an accumulation of blood at a bruise site that causes the skin to become black and blue

edema an accumulation of fluid within the tissues

efferent carrying impulses away from the center

elastin protein substance that gives elasticity and flexibility to the connective tissues

electrode a medium for conducting or detecting electrical current

electroencephalogram tracing of the electrical activity in the brain

electrolytes certain chemical substances dissolved in the blood and having numerous basic functions such as conducting electrical currents; the principal electrolytes are sodium, potassium, chloride, and bicarbonate

electromyography the process of recording electrical nerve transmission in skeletal muscles

element a substance that cannot be separated or broken down into substances with properties other than its own; a primary substance

ELISA enzyme-linked immunosorbent assay. A test used to screen blood for the antibody to the AIDS virus

elliptocytosis a condition in which all or almost all of the red blood cells are elliptical or oval in shape; typically asymptomatic

emancipated minor a patient under the age of majority but who is legally considered to be an adult

embolus a mass of matter free-floating in the circulatory system, such as a thrombus that has broken free, an air mass, or a fat globule

empathy the ability to understand or to some extent share what someone else is feeling

emulsify to disperse a liquid into another, usually incompatible, liquid

enclosure indication for the reader that an item is accompanying the letter

endemic a disease that occurs continuously in a particular population but has a low mortality; used in contrast to epidemic

endocardium the innermost part of the heart wall; it lines the heart chamber and covers the connective tissue skeleton of the heart valves

endogenous having its origin within an organism

endotracheal tube a large instrument usually inserted through the mouth (may use the nose) and into the trachea to the point of the tracheal division to deliver oxygen under pressure

enumerated counted

enuresis bed wetting

enzyme a protein that begins (catalyzes) a chemical reaction

epicardium the inner or visceral layer of the pericardium that forms the outermost layer of the heart wall

epidermis outer layer of the skin

epiglottis   the leaf-like flap that closes down over the glottis during swallowing

epiphyseal end plate   a thin layer of cartilage at the end of long bones where new growth takes place

episiotomy   incision of the perineum to accommodate vaginal delivery of fetus

Erlich units   a unit of measurement for urobilinogen

erythema   redness of the skin

erythematous   characterized by redness (erythema)

erythropoietin   a hormone produced mainly by the kidney in response to lowered oxygen levels; stimulates the production of red blood cells to increase blood oxygen levels

ester   compound formed by combining alcohol and acid; fats are esters

esterase   an enzyme that splits esters

ethics   guidelines for moral behavior that are enforced by peer groups

ethylene oxide   a gas used to sterilize surgical instruments and other supplies

etiology   cause of disease

eunuchoidism   deficient production of male hormone by the testes, resulting in loss of the secondary male characteristics

eustachian tubes   a mucous membrane-lined tube between the nasopharynx and the middle ear bilaterally that equalizes the internal and external otic air pressure

euthanasia   allowing a patient to die with minimal medical interventions

evaluation   the process of indicating how well the patient or person is progressing toward a particular goal; to appraise; to determine the worth or quality of something or someone

exercise   performed activity of the muscles, voluntary or otherwise, to maintain fitness

exogenous   having its origin outside of the organism; its opposite is endogenous

exophthalmic goiter   abnormal protrusion of the eyeballs accompanied by goiter

expected threshold   a numerical goal

expert witness   a professional who testifies on the standard of care in a trial

expressed consent   a statement of approval from the patient for the physician to perform a given procedure after the patient has been educated about the risks and benefits of the particular procedure; also referred to as informed consent

expulsion   formal discharge from a professional organization

externship   an educational course that allows the student to obtain hands-on experience

extracellular   outside of the cell

extraocular   pertaining to outside the eye, as in extraocular eye movement

exudate   drainage from an inflammatory lesion, such as pus or serum

familial   a disorder that tends to occur more often in a family than would be anticipated solely by chance

Family and Medical Leave Act   a law designed to allow an employee up to 12 weeks of unpaid leave from his or her job to meet family needs

fascia   fibrous membrane tissue that covers and supports the muscles and joins the skin with underlying tissue

febrile   exhibiting an elevated temperature

fee-splitting   sharing of fees between physicians for patient referrals

feedback   in communication, the response to input from another

femtoliter   one quadrillionth of a liter

file   grouping of data that is given a name for easy access

filing system   a method for organizing records so that they can be found when needed

film   the raw material prior to processing; does not contain a visible image (similar to photographic film)

filtration   removal of particles from a solution by passing the solution through a membrane

fissure   a groove, cleft, slit or crack-like lesion

fixative   a chemical substance used to bind, fix or stabilize specimens of tissue to slides for later examination

flagella   hair-like extremity of a bacterium or protozoan; used to facilitate movement

flextime   a system of scheduling that allows for a personal choice in hours or days worked

flocculation   condition of having a consistency of loose woolly masses

floppy disk   thin magnetic film on which to store data

folate   a salt of folic acid; it acts to help enzymes that build structures such as blood cells

forceps   a surgical instrument used to grasp, handle, compress, pull or join tissues, equipment or supplies

fraud   a deceitful act with the intention to conceal the truth

fructose   a simple sugar; a monosaccharide

full block   a type of letter format in which all letter components are justified left

full-thickness burn   a burn that has destroyed all skin layers

gait (gat)   the manner or style of walking

galactosuria   condition in newborns lacking an enzyme that metabolizes galactose; increased levels of galactose appear in the blood and urine (If proper therapy is not initiated, mental retardation and other difficulties will occur).

gastroenteritis   inflammation of the gastrointestinal tract caused by bacteria or viruses

gauge   a standard of measurement; a device for measuring size, capacity, amount, or power of an object or substance

gel separator   a non-reacting substance located in an evacuated tube that forms a physical barrier between the cells and serum or plasma after the specimen has been centrifuged

generic   the official name given to a drug that is no longer owned by the company that developed it

germicide   a chemical or drug that kills most pathogenic microorganisms

gestation   period of time from conception to birth; usually 37–41 weeks

gestational diabetes   a disorder characterized by an impaired ability to metabolize carbohydrates, usually due to insulin deficiency occurring in pregnancy and usually disappearing after delivery

gigantism   excessive size and stature caused most frequently by hypersecretion of the Human Growth Hormone (HGH)

gingiva   the gums; the mucous membrane covered tissues that support the teeth

glaucoma   abnormal increase in the fluid within the eye usually as a result of obstructed outflow of aqueous humor resulting in degeneration of the intraocular components

glomerulus   a small cluster of blood vessels within the Bowman's Capsule

glucocorticoid   an adrenal cortex hormone that increases the conversion of fatty acids and proteins to glucose for energy

glycosuria   the presence of glucose in the urine

goiter   an enlargement of the thyroid gland

gonads   a generic term referring to the sex glands of both sexes, either ovaries or testes

goniometer   an instrument used to measure the angle of joints for range of motion. Goniometry is the act of measuring the angle of range of motion

Goodell's sign   softening of cervix that occurs in early pregnancy

granulocytes white blood cells that have visible granules when stained

Graves' disease pronounced hyperthyroidism with signs of enlarged thyroid and exophthalmos

gravid pregnant

gravida a pregnant woman

gravidity pregnancy

grief great sadness caused by loss

gross income the amount of money earned by an employee before taxes are withheld

guaiac substance used in laboratory tests for occult blood in the stool

gyri the convolutions of the brain tissue

hard copy printed copy on paper

hard drive a place where the computer stores programs and data files

hardware equipment on the computer system, e.g., keyboard, disk drive, monitor, printer

HCFA see Health Care Financing Administration

HCPCS see Health Care Financing Administration Common Procedures Coding System

Health Care Financing Administration Common Procedures Coding System (HCPCS) a numerical system used by HCFA for services not covered by the CPT coding system

Health Care Financing Administration (HCFA) a federal agency that regulates health care financing and the procedural classification (Volume 3 of the ICD-9-CM coding book)

healthcare surrogate a patient's representative who makes health care decisions for the patient

heat exhaustion a type of hyperthermia that causes an altered mental status due to inadequate fluid replacement

heat cramps a type of hyperthermia that causes muscle cramping due to high sodium losses

heat stroke the most serious type of hyperthermia in which the body is no longer able to compensate for the elevated temperatures

hematemesis vomiting blood or bloody vomitus

hematocytometer (hemocytometer) device for counting blood cells

hematoma a blood clot at an injury site

hematuria bloody urine

hemoglobin C disease a genetic blood disorder in which the red blood cells contain an abnormal hemoglobin C, which reduces the elasticity of the red cells causing them to hemolyze easily

hemoglobinuria presence of free hemoglobin in urine

hemolysis rupture of erythrocytes with the release of hemoglobin into the plasma or serum causing the specimen to appear pink or red in color

hemolytic anemia a disorder characterized by premature destruction of the red cells; this may be brought on by an infectious process, inherited red cell disorder, or as a response to certain drugs or toxins

hemoptysis coughing up blood from the respiratory tract

hemostat a surgical instrument with slender jaws used for grasping blood vessels

heparin a naturally occurring anticoagulant given to prevent clot formation

hepatomegaly liver enlargement

hepatotoxin a substance that can be damaging to the liver

hereditary traits or disorders that are transmitted from parent to offspring

hernia the protrusion of an organ through the muscle wall of the cavity that normally surrounds it

hiatus an opening or gap; hiatal hernia: a protrusion of part of the stomach upward through the diaphragm

Hippocratic Oath a code of ethics written by Hippocrates

hirsutism abnormal or excessive growth of hair in women

histamine a substance found normally in the body in response to injured cells, resulting in the inflammatory process with dilation of capillaries, increased gastric secretions and contraction of smooth muscles

homeostasis maintaining a constant internal environment by balancing positive and negative feedback

hormone a substance that is produced by an endocrine gland and travels through the blood to a distant organ or gland where it acts to modify the structure of function of that gland or organ

human chorionic gonadotropin (HCG) hormone secreted by the placenta

humidifier appliance that increases the moisture content in the air

hydrogen ion hydrogen that is missing an electron and therefore readily binds with substances having extra electrons; it is an important constituent of acids

hypercalcemia an excessive amount of calcium in the blood

hyperglycemia an increase in blood sugar, as in diabetes mellitus

hyperopia farsightedness

hyperosmolarity a condition of having increased numbers of dissolved substances in the plasma

hyperplasia excessive proliferation of normal cells in the normal tissue arrangement of an organism

hypertension abnormally elevated blood pressure

hyperthermia an elevated body temperature

hypoglycemia deficiency of sugar in the blood

hypothalamus part of the diencephalon; activates and controls the peripheral nervous system, endocrine system, and certain involuntary functions

hypothermia a below-normal body temperature

hypovolemic shock a type of shock caused by fluid loss

hysterosalpingogram radiograph of the uterus and fallopian tubes after injection of contrast media

hysteroscopy visual examination with magnification of the uterus

iatrogenic a condition caused by treatment or medical procedures

identification line a series of initials indicating who dictated the letter and who composed it

idiopathic unknown etiology

immune globulins proteins produced by plasma cells in response to foreign antigens; they provide immediate antibody protection, which lasts for a few weeks to a few months

immunization act or process of rendering an individual immune to specific diseases

immunohematology the study of the antigen-antibody reaction including the study of autoimmunity

implementation the process of initiating and carrying out an action such as a teaching plan or patient treatment

implied consent an informal agreement of approval from the patient to perform a given task

impotence inability to achieve or retain an erection

incident report a form used by an organization to document an unusual occurrence to a patient, visitor or employee

incontinence inability to control elimination, either urine or feces or both

indices (sing. index) numbers expressing a property or ratio

informed consent a statement of approval from the patient for the physician to perform a given procedure after the patient has been educated about the risks and benefits of the procedure; also referred to as expressed consent

inguinal pertaining to the regions of the groin

inpatient a medical setting in which patients are admitted for diagnostic, radiographic, or treatment purposes

insertion a place of attachment, usually the freely movable portion of a muscle

inspection   the act or process of inspecting; visual examination

institutional review board   internal committee that reviews ethical issues

instrument   a surgical tool or device designed to perform a specific function, such as cutting, dissecting, grasping, holding, retracting, or suturing

insufflator   a device for blowing air, gases or powders into a cavity

insula   fifth lobe of the cerebrum

insulin dependent diabetes mellitus (IDDM)   a deficiency in insulin production that leads to an inability to metabolize carbohydrates

interferon   a group of proteins released by white blood cells and fibroblasts when the invading organism is a virus

intermittent   occurring at intervals

Internal Revenue Service (IRS)   a federal agency that regulates and enforces various taxes

International Classification of Diseases (ICD)   a classification system used to assign a numerical code to a disease

interosseous   between bones

interstitial   the spaces between the cells

intracellular   inside of the cell

intraocular pressure   pressure within the eyeball

intrauterine pregnancy (IUP)   pregnancy located in the uterus

intravascular coagulation   clot formation within the vessels; strands of fibrin may form from one wall of the vessel to the other and shear red cells as they pass by

intravenous pyelogram (IVP)   An x-ray using contrast medium to evaluate kidney function

intrinsic   found within a structure

introitus   vaginal orifice

iodine   an element that is an essential micronutrient used in the thyroid gland to manufacture its hormones; present in seafood, foods grown in iodized soil, iodized salt and some dairy products

ion   an atom or group of atoms that has become electrically charged by the loss or gain of one or more electrons

iontophoresis   introducing various chemical ions into the skin by means of electrical current

job description   a statement that informs an employee about the duties and expectations for a given job

Joint Commission on Accreditation of Health Care Organizations (JCAHO)   a voluntary organization that sets and evaluates the standards of care for health care institutions; based on the JCAHO evaluation, an accreditation title will be given to the organization.

Kaposi's sarcoma   multiple areas of cell proliferation initially in the skin and eventually in other body sites; this condition is frequently related to the immunocompromised state that accompanies AIDS

keratin   a tough, insoluble protein substance of the stratum corneum, hair and nails

keratoses (senile)   premalignant overgrowth or thickening of the upper layer of epithelium or horny layer of the skin

ketoacidosis   acidosis accompanied by an accumulation of ketones in the body

ketones   the end products of fat metabolism

kinesics   a form of non-verbal communication including gestures, body movements, facial expressions

Krebs cycle   a sequence of reactions within cells that metabolizes sugars and other energy sources, such as carbohydrates, proteins and fats, into carbon dioxide, water and ATP

kyphosis   abnormally deep dorsal curvature of the thoracic spine; also known as humpback or hunchback

labor   normal physiological process involving involuntary contractions of the uterine muscle resulting in cervical dilation and effacement (thinning)

laparoscopy   process of viewing the internal abdominal cavity and its contents

laparotomy   incision of the abdominal cavity

laryngectomy   removal of the larynx, either partial or total

laser ablation   destruction or removal of tissue by use of laser

lead   an electrode or electrical connection attached to the body to record electrical impulses in the body, especially the heart or brain

learning objectives   steps that needed to be achieved to accomplish the learning goal

learning goal   an agreed upon outcome of the teaching process

ledger card   a record of the patient's financial activities

ledger   a continuous record of business transactions with debits and credits

lentigines   tan or brown macule found on elderly skin after prolonged sun exposure; also known as liver spots

leukocytosis   abnormal increase of leukocytes (white blood cells)

libel   written statements that defame a person's reputation or character

licensure   the strictest form of professional accreditation

ligament   a flexible band of tissue that holds joints together

lightening   the descent of the fetus further into the pelvis

lipase   any of several enzymes that begin the breakdown of fats in the digestive tract

lipids   any of the free fatty acids (fats) in the body

lipoproteins   a substance made up of a lipid and a protein

lithotripsy   crushing a stone

litigation   process of filing or contesting a lawsuit

lochia   uterine discharge following childbirth, composed of some blood, mucus and tissue

login   use of a password to gain access to the computer

loop of henle   a portion of the renal tubule, shaped like a U and consisting of a thick ascending and thin descending vessels

lordosis   an abnormally deep ventral curve at the lumbar flexure of the spine; also known as swayback

lubricant   an agent that reduces friction between parts

Luer adapter   a device for connecting a syringe or evacuated holder to the needle to promote a secure fit

lyse   to cause disintegration; ie, destruction of adhesions, or the breakdown of red blood cells

macrophage   a monocyte that has left the circulation and settled and matured in tissue; macrophages process antigens and present them to T-cells, activating the immune specific response

macule   small, flat discoloration of the skin

mainframe   central computer to which individual computers are connected; used in large institutions

malaise   general feeling of illness without specific signs or symptoms

malignant   cancerous

malocclusion   abnormal contact between the teeth in the upper and lower jaw

malpractice   a tort in which the patient is harmed by the actions of a health care worker

manipulation   the skillful use of the hands in diagnostic procedures

Mantoux   tuberculin skin test using a purified protein derivative (PPD) of tuberculin bacillus given intradermally to establish exposure to tuberculosis

masticate   the act of chewing or grinding, as in chewing food

Material Safety Data Sheet (MSDS)   a detailed record of all hazardous substances kept within a site

matrix   a system for blocking off unavailable patient appointment times

mediastinum   the mid-portion of the thoracic cavity containing the heart, the great vessels, the upper esophagus and the trachea

medical history   record containing information about a patient's complete past and present health status

medical assistant   a multiskilled health professional who performs a variety of clinical and administrative tasks in a medical setting

medical asepsis   destruction of organisms after they leave the body

medical setting   a place that is designed to meet the health care needs of patients; may be inpatient or outpatient.

medulla oblongata   part of the brain that controls breathing, heart rate, and blood pressure

megabyte   one million bytes; a way to measure the quantity of computer information that a particular device can hold

megaloblastic anemia   a disorder characterized by production of large, dysfunctional erythrocytes; folate deficiency is considered a cause

meiosis   the cell division specific to sperm and ova that results in 23 chromosomes rather than 46 (23 pairs)

melanin   dark pigment that gives color to the skin, hair and eyes

melanocyte   cell that produces melanin

melena   black, tarry stools caused by digested blood from the GI tract

memorandum   a type of written documentation used for interoffice communication

menarche   age at which the first menstruation occurred

meninges   membranes of the spinal cord and brain

meningocele   meninges protruding through the spinal column

meniscus   the curved upper surface of a liquid in a container

menorrhagia   excessive or heavy menstruation

menses   menstruation; bloody discharge that occurs monthly or cyclically

mensuration   the act or process of measuring

message   words sent from one person to another; information sent through spoken, written, or body language

metabolic acidosis   an acidic condition of the body caused when excess acids are produced in the body's fluids (as in the metabolism of fats instead of glucose) or when the body's natural bicarbonates are lost or diminished

metabolism   the total of all chemical processes that result in growth, energy production, elimination of waste and all body functions as digested nutrients are distributed

metrorrhagia   irregular uterine bleeding

microbiology   the study of microscopic organisms

microfiche   sheets of microfilm

microfilm   photographs of records in a reduced size

microorganisms   microscopic living organisms

microprocessor   a chip that allows the computer to function

micturition   also known as voiding or urination

midbrain   part of the brain stem, responsible for relaying messages

migraine   a type of severe headache, usually unilateral, may appear in clusters

mission statement   a statement describing the goals of the medical office and those it serves

modem (modulator/demodulator)   a communication device that connects a computer to the standard telephone system, allowing information exchange with other computers off site

monitor   visual display terminal (VDT) that shows information being input via the keyboard

monosaccharide   a simple sugar that cannot be broken down further

mordant   a substance used to fix, or bind, dyes or stains

morphology   the science and study of structure and form

motherboard   fiberglass board that contains the central processing unit (CPU), memory, and other pieces of circuitry

mourning   to demonstrate signs of grief; grieving

mouse   a device that allows the user to control cursor movement on the monitor

multidisciplinary   involving many disciplines; a group of healthcare professionals from various specialties brought together to meet the patient's needs

multimedia   various forms of communication available on the computer, eg, stereophonic sound, animation, full-motion video, photographs

multipara   woman who has given birth to more than one viable fetus

multiskilled health professional   an individual with versatile training in the healthcare field

muscular dystrophies   a group of genetically transmitted diseases characterized by progressive atrophy of skeletal muscles

mycology   the science and study of fungi

myelofibrosis   a disorder in which bone marrow tissue develops in abnormal sites such as the liver and spleen; signs include immature cells in the circulation, anemia, and splenomegaly

myelogram   invasive radiologic test in which dye is injected into the spinal fluid

myelomeningocele   protrusion of the spinal cord through the spinal defect called a spina bifida

myocardium   the middle layer of the walls of the heart, composed of cardiac muscle

myofibrils   a slender light/dark strand of muscle tissue in striated muscle

myopia   nearsightedness

myxedema   the most severe form of hypothyroidism; signs include edema of the extremities and the face

nasal septum   the wall or partition dividing the nostrils

National Committee for Clinical Laboratory Standards (NCCLS)   a committee appointed to establish rules to ensure the safety, standards and integrity of all testing performed on human specimens

nebulizer   an instrument for administering a fine spray of medication, usually used in the respiratory tract

needle holder   a surgical forceps used to hold and pass a suture through tissue

negative feedback   a decrease in function in response to a stimulus

negative stress   stress that does not allow for relaxation periods

negligence   performance of an act that a reasonable health care worker would not have done or the omission of an act that a reasonable person would have done

neoplasm   an abnormal growth of new tissue; a tumor

nephron   the portion of the kidney responsible for the production of urine

nephrostomy   an opening into the kidney

net pay   the amount of money an employee is paid after all taxes are withheld

networking   a system of personal and professional relationships through which to share information

neurogenic shock   a type of shock caused by a dysfunction of the nervous system

neuron   a nerve cell

neurotransmitter   chemical needed to transmit an message between synapses

nitrogenous   pertaining to or containing nitrogen, usually the end-product of protein metabolism

nitroprusside   a nitrogen cyanic compound that reacts with ketones

nocturia   excessive urination at night

nodule   a small node, mass or swelling

non compos mentis   mental incompetence

non-insulin dependent diabetes mellitus (NIDDM)   a type of diabetes in which patients do not require insulin to control the blood sugar

noncompliance   the patient's inability or refusal to follow prescribed orders

nonlanguage   not expressed in spoken language, eg, laughing, sobbing, grunting, sighing.

normal value   acceptable range as established for an age, a population, or a sex; variations usually indicate a disorder

normal flora   organisms normally found in an area; also known as resident or indigenous flora

nosocomial infection   infection acquired in a medical setting, generally presumed to be in a hospital setting but may also refer to the medical office

nulligravida   woman who has never been pregnant

nullipara   woman who has never given birth to a viable fetus

numeric filing   arranging files by a numbered order

nutrition   the study of food and how it is used for growth, nourishment, and repair

obligate   to require; a parasite that has no choice but to attach to a living organism

obstipation   extreme constipation

obturator   a smooth, rounded, removable inner portion of a hollow tube, such as an anoscope, that allows for easier insertion

occult   hidden or concealed from observation

olecranon fossa   the depression in the posterior surface of the humerus that allows the arm to extend by receiving the olecranon process

olecranon process   the proximal end of the ulna that becomes the point of the elbow that fits into the olecranon fossa

oliguria   scanty urine formation

on-line   direct link to off-site computers

oophorectomy   excision of an ovary

operating system   the program that tells the computer how to interface with hardware and software

ophthalmoscope   lighted instrument to visually examine the inner surfaces of the eye

opportunistic infection   infections that result from a defective immune system that cannot defend against pathogens normally found in the environment

optician   a trained specialist who grinds lens to fit refraction corrective lens prescriptions written by ophthalmologists and optometrists

optometrist   a trained specialist who can measure for errors of refraction and prescribe lens for refraction errors but who cannot treat eye disorders

organ   the source or starting point; (muscle) any part that is made up of cells and tissues that cause it to perform its specified function in conjunction with a body system

organizational chart   a flow sheet depicting the members of a team in a structured or hierarchical manner

origin   the source or starting point; (muscle) the more fixed end of a muscle, usually the proximal end

OSHA   Occupational Safety and Health Administration

osteoporosis   abnormal porosity of the bone found in the elderly and predisposing the affected bony tissue to fracture

otoscope   instrument used to visually examine the ear canal and tympanic membrane

outlier   a patient whose hospital stay is longer than allowed by the DRG

outpatient   a medical setting in which patients receive care but are not admitted

over-the-counter   medications that are available without prescriptions

overdraft protection   protection against having insufficient funds to cover checks

ovulation   the periodic rupture of the mature ovum from the ovary

ovum (pl. ova)   the female reproductive cell; sex cell or egg

packing slip   a document that accompanies a supply order and lists the enclosed items

Paget's disease   degenerative bone disease usually in older persons with bone destruction and poor repair

palliative   to relieve or reduce but not to cure

palmar   the palm surface of the hand

palpation   a technique used in physical examination in which the examiner feels the texture, size, consistency, and location of parts of the body with the hands

pancreatitis   an inflammation of the pancreas that may be brought on by alcohol, trauma, infection, or certain drugs

Papanicolaou test or smear (Pap test)   a simple smear method of examining tissue cells for cancer, especially of the cervix; named for George N. Papanicolaou, a Greek physician, anatomist, and cytologist in the United States, 1883–1962

papilla (pl. papillae)   a small nipple shaped projection

papillae lingua   the taste buds

papilloma virus   virus that causes papillomas or warts

papilloma   a benign form of skin tumor

papule   small, red, solid elevation of the skin

paralanguage   factors connected with, but not essentially part of language, e.g., tone of voice, volume, pitch.

parameters   values used to describe or measure a set of data representing a physiologic function or system

parasitology   the science and study of parasites

parasympathetic   the part of the autonomic nervous system involved in periods free from stress

parity   pregnancies that resulted in a viable birth

partial thickness burn   a burn that involves the epidermis and varying levels of the dermis

particulate matter   a material composed of particles

passive range of motion   assisted range-of-motion movements

pathogens   disease-causing microorganisms

patient education   active participation of the patient in a process that will yield a change in behavior

payroll journal   a method for keeping track of payroll data using the pegboard system

payroll   the process of calculating employee salary

pediatrician   medical doctor who specializes in the care of infants, children, and adolescents

pediatrics   specialty of medicine that deals with the care of infants, children and adolescents

pediculosis   infestation with lice

percussion   the act of striking parts of the body with the hands to evaluate the size, borders, consistency, and presence of fluid in some of the internal organs

pericardium   the double-layered serous, membranous sac that encloses the heart and the origins of the great vessels

peripheral   pertaining to or situated away from the center

peristalsis   rhythmic waves of smooth muscle contractions that force substances to points of elimination

PERRLA   abbreviation used in documentation to denote pupils equal, round, reactive to light and accommodation if all findings are normal; refers to the size and shape of the pupils, their reaction to light, and their ability to adjust to distance

pessary   device that supports the uterus when inserted into the vagina

petri plate   a shallow glass or plastic dish with a lid to hold solid media for cultures

pH   abbreviation for potential hydrogen, pH is a scale representing the relative acidity or alkalinity or a substance in which 7.0 is neutral; numbers lower than 7.0 are acid and numbers above 7.0 are basic

phagocyte   a cell that has the ability to ingest and destroy particular substances such as bacteria, protozoa, cells and cell debris by ingesting them

phagocytosis   the process by which certain cells engulf and dispose of microorganisms; to eat or ingest

pharmacodynamics   the study of how drugs act within the body

pharmacokinesis   the study of the action of drugs within the body from administration to excretion

pharmacology the study of drugs and their origin, nature, properties, and effects upon living organisms

phimosis narrowing or tightening of the prepuce that prevents retraction over the glans penis

phonophoresis an ultrasound treatment used to force medications into tissues

phosphates a compound containing phosphorus and oxygen; they are very important in living organisms, especially for the transfer of genetic information

physiology the study of the function of the body

pia mater thin vascular covering that adheres to the surface of the brain

plaintiff the party who initiates a lawsuit

planes a point of reference made by a straight cut through the body at any given angle

planning the process of using information gathered during the assessment phase to organize learning or patient care objectives in order to accomplish the specific learning or treatment goal

pleura the serous membrane enclosing the lungs; (visceral pleura: the layer that covers the lungs most closely; parietal pleura: the layer that follows the contours and lines the chest wall, the diaphragm, and the mediastinum)

poikilocytosis abnormal variations in the shapes of red blood cells (poikilo = variation)

policy a statement that reflects the organization's rules on a given topic

polydipsia excessive thirst

polymenorrhea abnormally frequent menstrual periods

polyphagia abnormal hunger

polyuria excessive excretion and elimination of urine

pons part of the brain stem, responsible for communication within the central nervous system

portfolio a portable case containing documents

positive stress stress that allows a person to perform at peak levels and then relax afterward

positive feedback an increase in function in response to a stimulus

positron emission tomography (PET) computerized radiography using radioactive substances to assess metabolic or physiological functions within the body rather than anatomical structures

posting listing financial transactions in a ledger

postural hypotension sudden drop in blood pressure upon standing

potentiation the synergistic action of two substances, such as hormones or drugs, in which the total effects are greater than the sum of the independent effects of the two substances

precedent the use of previous court decisions as a legal foundation

preceptor a teacher; one who gives direction, as in a technical matter

precipitation the settling out of a substance in a solution

quantitative the measuring of an amount

prepuce a fold of skin that forms a cover

presbycusis loss of hearing associated with aging

presbyopia vision changes associated with age

preservative a substance that delays decomposition

primary survey an initial assessment of an emergency patient for life-threatening problems

prime mover the muscle most responsible for the desired muscle action or movement

primigravida woman who is pregnant for the first time

printer a device that transfers information on the computer into hard copy

procedure a series of steps required to perform a given task

professional courtesy a discount fee given to healthcare professionals

proofreading a part of editing a document in which the writer reads the draft for accuracy and clarity and corrects errors

proprietary private school with preset curricula

prostate-specific antigen a normal protein produced by the prostate that usually elevates in the presence of cancer

prosthesis any artificial replacement for a missing body part, such as false teeth or an artificial limb

proteinuria the presence of large quantities of protein in the urine; usually a sign of renal dysfunction

proxemic having to do with the degree of physical closeness tolerated by humans

pruritus itching

psychogenic of psychological origin

psychosocial relating to mental and emotional aspects of social encounters

puerperium period of time (about 6 weeks) from childbirth until reproductive structures return to normal

purchase order a document that lists the required items to be purchased

Purkinje fibers extensions of the Bundle of His that branch through the myocardium to end the transmission of the electrical impulse and cause the ventricles to contract

pustules vesicle filled with pus

pyosalpinx pus in the fallopian tube(s)

pyuria pus in the urine

quadrants a division of the abdomen into four equal parts by one horizontal and one vertical line dissecting at the umbilicus

quality control method to evaluate the proper performance of testing procedures, supplies or equipment in a laboratory

quality improvement a plan that allows an organization to scientifically measure the quality of its product and service

quantification the process of ascertaining the amount of something

Queckenstedt test test to determine the presence of an obstruction in the CSF flow

radiograph processed film that contains a visible image

radiographer technical specialist who works to assist the radiologist in the performance of procedures and who is responsible for producing routine examination images for the radiologist to interpret

radiography the art and science of producing diagnostic images to be used in the care of patients

radioimmunoassay (RIA) the introduction of radioactive substances into the body to determine the concentration of a substance in the serum, usually the concentration of antigens, antibodies, or proteins

radiologist a medical doctor who specializes in radiology; performs some procedures and interprets images to provide diagnostic information to physicians

radiology the branch of medicine including diagnostic and therapeutic applications of x-rays and other techniques

radiolucent permitting the passage of x-rays

radionuclide a radioactive material used in small amounts in nuclear medicine studies; has a short life

radiopaque not permeable to the passage of x-rays

random access memory (RAM) temporary memory; data is lost when the computer is turned off if it is not backed up on disk

range of motion (ROM) the range, measured in degrees, through which a joint can be extended and flexed

ratchets notched mechanisms, usually at the handle end of an instrument, that click into position to maintain tension on the opposing blades or tips of the instrument

read only memory (ROM) permanent memory inside the computer

reagent a substance used to react in a certain manner in the presence of specific chemicals to obtain a diagnosis

rectocele herniation of the rectum into the vaginal area

rectovaginal pertaining to the rectum and vagina

reduction   correcting a fracture by realigning the bone; may be closed (corrected by manipulation) or open (requires surgery)

reflux   a return or backward flow of fluid

refract, refraction   bending the light rays that enter the pupil to reflect exactly on the fovea centralis, the area of greatest visual acuity

remittent   fluctuating

renal pelvis   the funnel-shaped upper portion of the ureters that collects urine from the kidneys

renal medulla   the inner portion of the kidney that contains the collecting structures

renal cortex   the portion of the kidney that contains the structures that form urine

renal pyramids   situated in the renal medulla, part of the collecting structures

renin   enzyme formed in the kidney that works with angiotensin to affect the blood pressure

repolarization   the active process of restoring the cardiac fibers to the resting (polarized) state. Re-establishment of the electrical polarized state in a muscle or nerve fiber following contraction or conduction of a nerve impulse

res ipsa loquitur   "the thing speaks for itself"

res judicata   "the thing has been decided"

Resource-Based Relative Value Scale (RBRVS)   a value scale designed to decrease Medicare Part B costs and establish national standards for coding and payment

respiration   the exchange of oxygen and carbon dioxide (external respiration: the exchange between the alveoli and the bloodstream; internal respiration: the exchange between the cells and the bloodstream)

respondeat superior   "let the master answer"

restrain   control or confine movement

resume   document summarizing an individual's work experience or professional qualifications

retinal degeneration   pathological changes in the cell structure of the retina that impairs or destroys its function (blindness may result)

retrograde pyelogram   an x-ray of the urinary tract using contrast medium injected through the bladder and ureters; useful in diagnosing obstructions

retroperitoneal   the space behind the peritoneal cavity that contains the kidneys

retrovirus   viruses containing reverse transcriptase, which allows the viral cell to replicate its DNA into the DNA of the host cell, thereby taking over the substance of the cell

rickettsia   organism that is smaller than bacteria, larger than viruses

ringworm   lay term for tinea, a group of fungal diseases

risk factors   any issue that possesses a safety or liability concern for an organization

Romberg test   inability to maintain body balance when eyes are closed and feet are together, an indication of spinal cord disease

rugae   ridges or folds in the skin or mucous membranes that allow for expansion of a part

salpingectomy   excision of the fallopian tube

salpingo-oophorectomy   excision of both an ovary and fallopian tube

salutation   a introductory phrase that greets the reader of a letter

sanitation   the science of maintaining a healthful, disease-free environment

sanitizing   the practice of lowering the number of microorganisms on a surface by use of low-level disinfectant practices

scale   a thin, dried flake of skin

scalpel   a small, pointed knife with a convex blade edge for surgical procedures

scanner   a piece of office equipment that transfers a written document into a computer

scissors   a sharp instrument composed of two opposing cutting blades, held together by a central pin on which the blades pivot

sclera   the white fibrous tissue that covers the eye

scoliosis   a lateral curve of the spine, usually in the thoracic area with a corresponding curve in the lumbar region, causing uneven shoulders and hips

screening   a preliminary procedure, such as a test or exam, to detect the more characteristic signs of a disorder

sebaceous gland   oil gland

seborrhea   over-production of sebum with excessive oiliness or dry scales

sebum   fatty secretion of the sebaceous gland

secondary survey   an assessment of an emergency victim for head to toe injuries

seizure   involuntary contractions of voluntary muscles; an abnormal discharge of electrical activity in the brain

semi-block   a type of letter format that is styled the same as block, except the first sentence of each paragraph is indented five spaces

sensitivity   susceptibility to a certain substance

septic shock   a type of shock that is caused by a generalized infection in the body

septicemia   presence of pathogenic bacteria in the blood

serology   the study of the nature and properties of serum

serrations   grooves, either straight or criss-cross, etched or cut into the blades or tips of an instrument to more firmly hold the tissue in its grasp

service charge   a charge by a bank for various services

sesamoid   resembling the shape of a sesame seed

shock   a lack of oxygen to individual cells of the body

sick child visit   a pediatric visit for the treatment of illness or injury

sickle cell anemia   a condition in which the patient has both copies of the gene for hemoglobin S; the red cells become sickle shaped and non-flexible causing obstruction of small vessels and capillaries. Necrosis due to tissue hypoxia occurs beyond the obstruction. Most commonly seen in African-Americans.

signs   objective indications of disease or bodily dysfunction

sinoatrial (SA) node   considered the pacemaker of the heart, located in the upper portion of the right atrium; a specialized group of cells that initiate the electrical impulse of the heart

slander   oral statements that defame a person's reputation or character

smegma   a cheesy secretion of the sebaceous glands either in the labia or prepuce

software   application programs that direct the hardware to perform given tasks

specific gravity   the relative density of a substance (eg, urine)

specificity   relating to a definite result

specimen   a small portion of anything used to evaluate the nature of the whole

speculum   an instrument that enlarges and separates the opening of a cavity to expose its interior for examination

spherocytosis   a condition where all or almost all of the red cells are spherocytes; typically asymptomatic

spicules   sharp points

spina bifida occulta   a congenital defect in the spinal column caused by lack of union of the vertebrae

spinal   pertaining to the spine

spirochete   long, flexible, motile microorganisms

staff privileges   hospital approval for a physician to admit patients for treatment

staghorn   stone formation in the renal pelvis that fills the chamber and assumes the shape of the calyces

staphylococci   spherical microorganism found in grapelike clusters

Staphylococcus a genus of bacteria, some of which are causative agents for skin infections

stare decisis "the previous decision stands"

status asthmaticus an asthma attack that is not responsive to treatment

statute of limitations a legal time limit; eg, the length of time in which a patient may file a lawsuit

statutes laws that are written by federal, state or local legislators

stereotyping to place in a fixed mold, without consideration of differences

sterile field a specific area, such as within a tray or on a sterile towel, that is considered free of microorganisms

sterilization a process, act or technique for destroying microorganisms using heat, water, chemicals or gases

stoma an opening to the surface; suggests that it is surgically created

stratum corneum outer layer of the epidermis

stratum germinativum innermost layer of the epidermis

streptococci spherical microorganism clustered in chains

Streptococcus a genus of bacteria that are commonly implicated in diseases of the skin

striated having a striped appearance with alternating light and dark bands

subcutaneous beneath the skin

subject filing arranging files according to their title, grouping similar subjects together

subpoena duces tecum a court order requiring medical records to be submitted to the court at a given date and time

subpoena a court order requiring an individual to appear at court at a given date and time

substrate an underlying layer; a substance acted upon, as by an enzyme or reagent

sudoriferous gland sweat gland

sulci a groove in the brain tissue

sulfosalicylic acid an acid used to test for protein

superbill preprinted patient bill that lists a variety of procedures

superficial burn a burn that is limited to the epidermal layers

surgical asepsis destruction of organisms before they enter the body

surrogate mother a women who carries a baby to term for another female who is unable to carry a pregnancy to term

suspension temporary removal of privileges

swab (noun) stick topped with cotton or other absorbent man-made fiber for cleaning areas, applying treatments or for obtaining specimens

swab (verb) to wipe with a swab

swaged needle a metal needle fused to a suture material

symmetry equality in size or shape or position of parts on opposite sides of the body

sympathetic the part of the autonomic nervous system involved in stress reaction

sympathy feeling sorry for or pitying someone

symptoms subjective indications of disease or bodily changes as sensed by the patient

synapse the junction of two neurons

synarthroses immovable joints

syncope a sudden fall in blood pressure or cerebral hypoxia resulting in loss of consciousness

synergism the harmonious action of two agents, such as drugs or organs, producing an effect that neither could produce alone or an effect that is greater than the total effects of each agent operating by itself

synergist muscles that work together for more efficient movement

system a collection of organs that perform a certain function

systole the contraction phase of the cardiac cycle

T cells lymphoid cells from bone marrow that migrate to the thymus gland where they mature into differentiated lymphocytes that circulate between blood and lymph

tab the projection on a file folder on which the patient name or title is written

tactile pertaining to the sense of touch

task force a group of employees that works together to solve a given problem

tax withholding the amount of tax that is withheld from a paycheck

tendons tough, flexible fibers that bind muscle to bone

tetany severe cramping, convulsions or muscle spasms due to an abnormality of calcium metabolism

thalamus part of the diencephalon, responsible for sorting messages

thalassemia a hemolytic anemia caused by deficient hemoglobin synthesis; more commonly found in those of Mediterranean heritage

therapeutic having to do with treating or curing disease; curative

thoracentesis a surgical puncture into the pleural cavity for aspiration of serous fluid or for the injection of therapeutic medications

thromboplastin a complex substance found in blood and tissues that aids the clotting process

thyrotoxicosis excess quantities of thyroid hormone in the tissues

tickler file a file that provides a reminder to do a given task at a particular date and time

tine test skin test for exposure to tuberculosis, involves pricking the skin with sharp tines coated with the tuberculin bacillus

tinnitus an extraneous noise heard in one or both ears, described as whirring, ringing, whistling, roaring, etc.; may be continuous or intermittent

tissues a group of cells that function together for a specific purpose

titer a measure of the amount of an antibody in serum

tomography procedure in which the x-ray tube and film move in relation to each other during the exposure, blurring out all structures except those in the focal plane; used frequently in excretory urography

tonsils a small mass of lymphoid tissue; includes the palatine, nasopharyngeal and lingual tonsils

tonus the steady, partial contraction of skeletal muscles that allows the body to remain upright

tort the righting of wrongs or injuries suffered by someone because of another person's wrongdoing

toxoid a toxin that has been treated to destroy its toxicity, but is still capable of inducing formation of antibodies on injection

tracheostomy a permanent surgical stoma in the neck with an indwelling tube

tracheotomy incision into the trachea below the larynx to circumvent a blockage superior to this point; suggests an emergency situation and a reversible procedure

trade name the name given to a medication by the company that owns the patent

transient flora organisms that do not normally reside in an area; the presence of transient flora in an area may or may not produce disease

transient ischemic attack (TIA) acute episode of cerebrovascular insufficiency usually as a result of narrowing of an artery by artherosclerotic plaques, emboli, or vasospasm; usually passes quickly but should be considered a warning for predisposition to cerebrovascular accidents

transillumination the passage of light through body tissues for the purpose of examination

transition passing from one place or activity to another

traumatic causing or relating to tissue damage

trigone the triangle formed in the base of the bladder by the entrance of the two ureters and the exit of the urethra

truss   a device of pressing against a hernia to keep it in place

turbid   cloudy

turbinates   mucous membrane-covered conchae, the three scroll-shaped bones that project into the nasal cavity bilaterally from the lateral walls, each covers a sinus meatus

turgor   normal tension in a cell or the skin; normal skin turgor resists deformation and will resume its former position after being grasped or pulled

tympanic membrane   thin, semitransparent membrane in the middle ear that transmits sound vibrations; also called the eardrum

unemployment tax   federal tax paid by the employer based on each employee's gross income

unit   each part of a name or title that is used in indexing; a quantity of a standard measurement

upcoding   billing more for a patient care service than it is worth by selecting a code that is higher on the coding scale; this is an illegal practice

urates   a nitrogenous compound derived from protein use and is excreted in the urine

urea   the final product of protein metabolism in the body and the main nitrogenous component in the urine

uremic frost   a frost-like deposit of uremic compounds on the skin of patients whose kidneys are no longer functional

ureterostomy   an opening in a ureter

ureters   the pair of tubes designed to carry urine from the kidneys to the bladder

urethra   the short tube that carries urine from the bladder to the outside of the body

URI   Upper Respiratory Infection

uric acid   a by-product of protein metabolism present in the blood and excreted by the kidneys

urinalysis   chemical analysis of urine for diagnostic purposes

urinary frequency   the urge to urinate occurring more often than is required for normal bladder elimination

urticaria   hives

vaccine   a suspension of infectious agents, or some part of them, given for the purpose of establishing resistance to an infectious disease

values   established ideals of life, conduct, customs, etc., of an individual person or members of a society

varicella zoster   viral infection manifested by characteristic rash of successive crops of vesicles that scab before resolution; also called chicken pox

vasopressin   a hormone formed in the hypothalamus and transported to the posterior lobe of the pituitary through the hypothalamo-hypophyseal tract. It has an antidiuretic and a pressor effect that elevates the blood pressure.

vector   (biological) a living, nonhuman carrier of disease, usually an arthropod; (mechanical) a carrier of disease that does not support growth but will transmit disease; examples include inanimate objects or asymptomatic carriers

ventricle   either of the two lower chambers of the heart that when filled with blood contract to propel it into the arteries

venule   the small vessel that joins a capillary to a vein

verdict   a decision of guilty or not guilty based on evidence presented in a trial

verruca   wart

vertigo   sensation of whirling of oneself or the environment

vesicle   a small sac containing fluid; blister

vial   a small bottle for medicines or chemicals

villus (pl. villi)   tiny, almost microscopic projections in the mucous membrane of the small intestines

virology   the science and study of viruses

virulent   highly pathogenic

visualization   a relaxation technique that allows the mind to wander and the imagination to run free and focus on positive and relaxing situations

wave scheduling   a flexible scheduling method that allows time for procedures of varying lengths and the addition of unscheduled patients, as needed

well child (or baby) visit   visit for evaluation of growth and development

Western Blot   A specific, confirmatory antibody test for the presence of HIV in the blood

wheal   small round itchy elevation of the skin with a white center and red border; a hive

whorls   a spiral arrangement, as in the ridges on the finger that make up a fingerprint

withdrawing   the act of terminating a medical treatment that has already been initiated

withholding   not initiating certain medical treatments

Wood's light   ultraviolet light used to detect fungal diseases

write off   cancellation of an unpaid debt

yolk sac   a structure that develops in the inner zygotic cell mass and supplies nourishment for the embryo until the 7th week when the placenta takes over the function

INDEX

Note: Page numbers in *italics* indicate figure; those followed by *t* indicate tables; those followed by *b* indicate boxed material; and those followed by *p* indicate procedures

A

AAMA (American Association of Medical Assistants), 9, *9*, 10, 11
Abbreviations, 133b
  drug, 428t
  in electrocardiography, 677b
  obstetric, 806
Abdominal aortic aneurysm, 672
Abdominal cavity, 513, *513*
Abdominal examination, 349
  emergency, 492–493
Abdominal muscles, 555, *556*, 557t
Abdominal quadrants, 514
Abdominal regions, 513, *514*
Abdominal thrusts, *487*, 487–488, 489p
Abducens nerve, 587, *588*, 588t
Abduction, 547, *548*
ABO group, 961
  testing for, 962, *962*, 963t
Abortion, 804, 805t
  bioethical issues in, 25
Abrasions, 494b
Abruptio placentae, 805–806
Abscess, 520
  incision and drainage of, 391, 412p
Abuse
  child, 1011–1013
  elder, 526, 1021–1022
  reporting of, 42
Accessioner, 825b
Accessory nerve, 587, *588*, 588t
Accounting, 216–227. *See also* Bookkeeping
  cash-basis, 206
Accounting cycle, 218
Accounts payable, 206, 219–221
Accounts receivable, 206
  collection of, 199–202
    bookkeeping and, 210–211
Accreditation, Joint Commission on Accreditation of Health Care Organizations (JCAHO), 170–171, 171b, 172t
Acetabulum, 553
Acetest, for urinary ketones, 872, 887p
Achilles reflex, assessment of, 599, 599t, *600*
Acid-base balance, 970
  blood gases and, 974, 974t
  disturbances in, causes of, 974t
Acidosis, 970
  causes of, 974t
  metabolic, 969
    causes of, 969, 974t
  respiratory, causes of, 974t
Acid precipitation test, for proteinuria, 872–873, 888p
Acne vulgaris, 524
Acoustic nerve, 587, *588*, 588t
  tumors of, 617
Acquired immunodeficiency syndrome (AIDS), 701–703
  history of, 700b
  history taking in, 704t
  opportunistic infections in, 701, 701t
  prevention of, 703
  signs and symptoms of, 702, 702b
  stages of, 702
  testing for
    ELISA in, 704–705
    legal aspects of, 704
    Western blot in, 705
  transmission of, 702
  treatment of, 702–703
Acromegaly, 649, *649*
Acrosome, 768, 768–769
ACTH (adrenocorticotropic hormone), 643t, 644
  deficiency of, 651
  excess of, 652
Acute renal failure, 756
Acute rhinitis, 715
Adam's apple, 710

Addison's disease, 652
Addressing envelopes, 136, *136*, 137b
Adduction, 547, *548*
Adenoids, 694
Adipose tissue, 520
Adjustments, fee, 198
  bookkeeping and, 207, 210–211
Administrative law, 34
Adnexa, 609, *609*
Adolescents, dealing with, 520
Adrenals, 643t, 646
Adrenergic blocking agents, 417t
Adrenergics, 417t
Adrenocorticotropic hormone (ACTH), 643t, 644
  deficiency of, 651
  excess of, 652
Adson forceps, *355*, *356*
Advance directives, 28, *45*, 45–46, 593b
Adverse reactions, to drugs, 423t
Advertisements, employment, 1051
Advocacy, 21
Aesculapius, 6, *6*
Afferent nerves, 582
African Americans
  beliefs and practices of, 62t
  dietary preferences of, 88t
Agar, 846
Agendas, composition of, 139, *140*
Age of majority, 40
Agglutination test, 952–953, 953b
  for blood typing, 962–963
  for C-reactive protein, 958
  for infectious mononucleosis, 957–958
  for rheumatoid factor, 957
  for rubella, 958
  for syphilis, 958–959
Aging. *See also* Elderly
  concepts of, 1018
  systemic changes in, 1023, 1024t–1206t
Aging accounts, 200–201
Agranulocytes, 661, 662t, 926
AIDS. *See* Acquired immunodeficiency syndrome (AIDS)
Airborne precautions, 273–274, 274t
Airway management
  in anaphylaxis, 498
  in emergencies, *487*, 487–488, 489p–491p
  in seizures, 497
Airways, structure and function of, *708*, *709*, 709–711
Alanine aminotransferase (ALT), 972, 972t
ALARA concept, 474
Albinism, 526
Albumin, 972, 972t
Alcohol, as disinfectant, 365t
Alcohol abuse, 92, 93t
  in elderly, 1020
  patient teaching for, 92–94, 93t
Aldosterone, 643t, 646
Alkaline phosphatase, 971–972, 972t
Alkalosis, 970
  causes of, 974t
Allergens, 497–498
  skin tests for, 530–531
Allergic rhinitis, 623
Allergies, 497–498, 700
  acute rhinitis and, 715
  anaphylaxis and, 493, 497, 498
  drug, 423t, 424
  latex, 897
  nasal polyps and, 624
  skin testing for, 530b, 530–531, 704
Allied health professionals, 14, 15t
Allis hemostatic forceps, 355
Allis tissue forceps, *356*
Alopecia, tinea capitis and, 522, 526
Alphabetic filing, 151, 151b, 152b
Alpha cells, 647

Alpha-fetoprotein, prenatal measurement of, 600, 808
Alveolar-capillary membrane, 713, *714*
Alveoli, 711, 713
Alzheimer's disease, 1028, 1029t
Ambulance transport, 486
Ambulatory aids, 570–578
  cane, 577
  crutches, 571–577
  safety tips for, 570b
  walker, 577–578
Ambulatory surgery, HCPCS codes for, 238
American Association of Medical Assistants (AAMA), 9, *9*, 10, 11
  Code of Ethics, 21
  Medical Assistant's Creed, 21
American Hospital Association's Patient Bill of Rights, 36, 37–38
American Hospital Formulary Service, 424
American Medical Association (AMA)
  Code of Ethics, 20
  Council on Ethical and Judicial Affairs, 23–29
American Medical Technologists, 10, *10*, 11
American Medical Technologists Institute for Education (AMTIE), 10
Americans with Disabilities Act (ADA), 192
Ammonia, urinary, 871
Amniocentesis, 600, 808
Amobarbital, abuse of, 93t, 94
Amphetamines, abuse of, 93t, 94
Amphiarthroses, 546
Ampules, 439, *439*
  syringe filling from, 452p–454p
Amputation, 564
  traumatic, 494b, 495
Amylase, 974
Amyotrophic lateral sclerosis (ALS), 594
Anabolism, 729
Anaerobic bacteria, culture media for, 846, *847*
Analgesics, 417t
Anal specula, 361t
Anaphylaxis, 493, 497, 498
Anatomic position, 511
Anemia, 672–673
  diagnosis of, 928
  iron deficiency, patient education for, 928
    diagnosis of, 928, 929
  sickle cell, 672, 672–673
Aneroid sphygmomanometer, 312, *312*
Anesthesia codes (CPT), 233
Anesthetics, 417t
  local, 381
Aneurysm, 672
Angel dust, 93t, 94
Angina, Vincent's, 734
Angina pectoris, 665
  vs. myocardial infarction, 667b
  nitroglycerin for, 666
Angiogram, 476t
Angioplasty
  balloon, 478
  laser, 478
Angiotensin, 753
Animal bites
  rabies and, 592
  reporting of, 592
Anisocytosis, 928
Ankle, structure and function of, 554
Ankle reflex, assessment of, 599, 599t, *600*
Ankylosing spondylitis, 569
Annotation, of letters, 139
Anoscope, 340
  Hirschman, *361*
Anoscopy, 743, 744p–745p
Answering services, 109
Antacids, 417t
Antagonism, drug, 424
Antagonist muscle, 554

Anterior pituitary
  disorders of, 647–648
  structure and function of, 643t, 643–644
Anthropometric measurements, 302
  in children, 999, 1003p–1007p
Antiadrenergics, 417t
Antianginal agents, 417t
Antianxiety agents, 417t
Antiarrhythmics, 417t
Antibiotics, 417t
  sensitivity testing for, 851
Antibodies, 695, 696–697, 697, 697t, 698t
  in acquired immunity, 699, 699t
  function of, 952
Antibody titer, 697t
Anticholinergics, 418t
  for Parkinson's disease, 1027
Anticoagulants, 417t
  coagulation tests and, 931
  prothrombin time for, 931
Anticonvulsants, 417t
Antidepressants, 417t
Antidiarrheals, 417t
Antidiuretic hormone, 643t, 644
  in diabetes insipidus, 649
Antiemetics, 417t
Antifungals, 417t
Antigens, 696–697
  blood group, 961–962
    testing for, 962, 962–963, 963t
  function of, 952
Antihelminthics, 417t
Antihistamines, 417t, 700
  for Parkinson's disease, 1027
Antihypertensives, 417t
Antiinflammatory agents, 417t
Antimicrobials, sensitivity testing for, 851
Antineoplastic agents, 417t
Antinuclear antibody (ANA), 960
Antiparkinsonian agents, 417t
Antipsychotics, 418t
Antipyretics, 418t
Antisepsis. See Asepsis
Antistreptolysin-O test (ASOT), 960
Antithyroid agents, 418t
Antitussives, 418t
Antivirals, 418t
  for AIDS, 703
Anxiolytics, 417t
Aortic aneurysm, 672
Aortic semilunar valve, 663, 663
Aortic stenosis, 669
Apgar score, 999b
Apical pulse, 308–310, 327p–328p. See also Pulse
  in children, 1008, 1009t
  pulse deficit and, 328p
Apical/radial pulse, 328p
Aplastic anemia, 672, 672–673
Aponeurosis, 555
Apothecary measurements, 430, 430, 431t
  conversion of, 431t, 431–432, 432t
Apparel
  for medical assistant, 102, 1041, 1042–1043
  protective, 274, 275, 832
    decontamination and laundering of, 285
Appeal, legal, 49
Appearance and dress, 102–104, 1041, 1042–1043
Appendicular skeleton, 544, 544
Application, employment, 1054–1055
Applicators, cotton-tipped, 339, 340, 842
  for serology specimens, 955
Appointment(s), 112–124
  cancelling of, 123
  flexible hours for, 114
  missed, 122–123
  open hours for, 114
  patient reminders for, 120–121, 121
  return, scheduling of, 119–120
  scheduled, 114
  scheduling of, 114–123
    in acute illness, 121
    appointment book for, 114–116, 115–116, 117
    computerized, 117
    on daily/weekly basis, 120–121

double booking in, 119
in emergencies, 108, 121
facilities and, 118
factors affecting, 117–118
guidelines for, 118–120
for new patients, 118–119, 119b
open time slots for, 118
patient needs and, 117
physician delays and, 122
physician's preferences and needs and, 117–118
problem solving for, 124
for return appointments, 119–120
for tardy patients, 122
for walk-in patients, 121–122
wave, 119
Appointment book, 114–116, 115–116
  as legal documents, 117
Appointment cards, 120, 120
Aquathermia (Aqua-K) pad, 531
Aqueous humor, 608, 609
Arachnoid, 584
Areas, body, 513b, 513–514
Arm
  assessment of, in emergencies, 493
  muscles of, 557t
Arm sling, 562, 563b
Arrector pili, 519
Arrhythmias, 670
  electrocardiogram for, 675–683, 679p–683p
Arterial blood gases, 724–725, 973–974, 974t
Arterial blood sample, 724, 897
Arterial occlusive disease, 666. See also Atherosclerosis
Arteries, 658–660, 659
  aneurysms of, 672
  coronary, 663, 663
  laceration of, 494b
Arteriography, coronary, 674t, 689
Arterioles, renal, 754
Arteriosclerosis. See Atherosclerosis
Arthritis
  degenerative, 569
  rheumatoid, 569
    test for, 957
Arthrography, 476t, 570
Arthropods, 845
Artificial insemination, bioethical issues in, 25
Artificial pacemaker, 665b
Ascites, 739
Asepsis, 266–286. See also Infection control
  definition of, 268
  medical, 270–271, 271b, 276t, 363
    handwashing for, 271, 272–273
    patient education for, 274
  for phlebotomy, 897–898
  principles of, 363
  surgical, 276, 276t, 363
Asians
  beliefs and practices of, 62t
  dietary preferences of, 88t
ASOT (antistreptolysin-O test), 960
Asparatate aminotransferase (AST)
  after myocardial infarction, 973, 973t
  liver function and, 972, 972t
Aspergillus, 844
Aspiration
  foreign body, 487, 487–488, 489p
  suprapubic, for urine collection, 869
Aspirin, Reye's syndrome and, 998
Assault, 48
Assessment. See Patient assessment
Assets, 206
Assignment of benefits, 244, 244b, 250, 261
Assisted suicide, 27, 27b
Assumption of risk, 50
Asthma, 717
Astigmatism, 612
Atherosclerosis
  arterial occlusion and, 666
  heart disease and, 665, 665–666
    myocardial infarction in, 666–667, 667b
    surgery for, 668b
  hypertension and, 667
  premature, risk factors for, 981t
  stroke and, 671

Athlete's foot, 523, 844
Atlas, 552, 552
Atoms, 506, 507, 507
Atraumatic needles, 383
Atria, 658, 659
Atrioventricular node, 664, 664
Atrioventricular valves, 662, 662–663, 663
Attitude transmission, 102
Audiometry, 619–620, 620
Audioscope, 337, 362t
Audit, 227
  Medicare, 239–240
  tax, 218
Auditory tube, 616, 619
Auricle, 615, 619
Auscultation, 341
  in blood pressure measurement, 312, 313, 326p–328p
  of breath sounds, 720, 721t
  of heart sounds, 674, 675b
  of respirations, 311, 329p
Auscultatory gap, 313
Autoclave, 365–370, 367
  loading of, 367–368, 370, 371p
  operation of, 369–370, 371p
  records for, 372
  wrapping equipment for, 368b–369b
Autoclave tape, 367, 370, 380b
Autoimmunity, 700–701
Automated blood cell counter, 925, 925b
Automated files, 153
Automated front desk, 165
Autonomic nervous system, 582, 587–590, 590, 591t
AVPU system, 490–491
Avulsion, 494b
Avulsion fracture, 560t, 561
Axial skeleton, 544, 544
Axillary crutches, 571, 571–577. See also Crutches
  fitting of, 572p–573p
Axillary temperature, 303, 304b, 307, 323p, 1007, 1009. See also Temperature
Axis, 552, 552
Axon, 582, 583
Ayre spatula, 339, 340
Azotemia, 970

B
Babcock forceps, 355
Babinski reflex, 993t
Baby. See Children; Infant
Baby blues, 807–808
Bacilli, 842, 843
Back, assessment of, in emergencies, 492
Backhaus towel clamp, 358
Back pain, posture and, 566b
Back strain, prevention of, 552, 553p
Bacteria, 842t, 842–843, 843. See also Microorganisms
  aerobic, 842
  anaerobic, culture media for, 846, 847
  classification of, 842, 842t
  morphology of, 842, 842t
  non-spore-forming, 365
  spore-forming, 365, 842–843, 843
Bacterial meningitis, 590–591
Bacterial pneumonia, 717
Bacterial skin infections, 520–522
Bacteriology, 842
Bacteriuria, nitrite test for, 873, 874
Bailey foreign body remover, 362
Balance, 206
  assessment of, 349–350
Balance billing, 244, 247, 261
Baldness, tinea capitis and, 522
Ballenger sponge forceps, 356
Balloon angioplasty, 478
Band, 924, 927
Bandages, 386–389
  application of, 389, 390, 407p–410p
  roller, 388, 390
  sterile dressings with, 386, 403p–407p
  tubular gauze, 388–389, 407p–410p
  types of, 388–389
Bandage scissors, 354, 357
Banking, 212–214

Bank statement, *213*, 214
Barbiturates, abuse of, 93t, 94
Barium studies, 471–472, *475*, 475–476, 476t
Barrett's esophagus, 734, 735b
Bartholin glands, 768, 781
Barton, Clara, 8
Basal cell carcinoma, *528*, 528–529
Basal ganglia, 585
Basal metabolic rate, 972
Base. *See* Acid-base balance
Baseline data, 302, 336
Basilic vein, blood collection from, *896*, 896. *See also* Blood sample, collection of
Basophils, *924*, 927
Battery, 48
Battery back-up units, 161
B cells, 697–698, *924*, 927
Beakers, 828, *829*
Bedsores, *525*, 525–526
Behavioral emergencies, 500–501
Belching, 739
Bench trial, 49
Benign prostatic hypertrophy, 769–770, 770b, 1026t
Bereavement, 67–68, 68b
Berry aneurysm, 672
Beta cells, 647
Bias, 66
Bicarbonate, 970. *See also* Acid-base balance
Biceps reflex, assessment of, 599, 599t, *600*
Bile, 733, 971
Bilirubin, 971, 972t
Bilirubinuria, 873, 889p
Bill collection, 199–202
    bookkeeping and, 210–211
Billing
    balance, 244, 247
    monthly, 200
Billing inquiries, 106–107
Bill paying, 220–221
Bimanual pelvic examination, 793p
Bioethics, 23–29. *See also* Ethics
    abortion and, 25
    allocation of resources and, 23–24, 28b
    AMA Council on Ethical and Judicial Affairs and, 23–29
    artificial insemination and, 25
    assisted suicide/euthanasia and, 27b
    genetic testing and, 25
    office management issues and, 28–29
    professional conduct and behavior and, 27–28
    social policy issues and, 23–27
    surrogate mothers and, 25–26
    treatment withdrawal/witholding and, 27
Biohazard waste disposal, 394b
Biologic spills, handling and prevention of, *833*, 833–834
Biopsy
    cervical, 795, 796p–797p
    of female reproductive tract, instruments for, *360*
    punch, instruments for, *362*, 362t
    skin, 529
    specimen handling for, *393*, 393
Birth certificates, 42
Birth control implants, 809t, 810–811
Birth control pills, 809t
Birthday rule, 244b, 250
Birth defects. *See* Congenital anomalies
Birthmarks, 526
Bites, animal
    rabies and, 592
    reporting of, 592
Blackheads, 524
Blacks
    beliefs and practices of, 62t
    dietary preferences of, 88t
Blackwell, Elizabeth, 8
Bladder, 752, *752*
    catheterization of, 760, 760b–761b
        for urine specimen, 869
    examination of, in males, 776
    structure and function of, 756
    tumors of, 760
Bladder stones, 875, 876p
Blades, scalpel, 357, *358*, 381–382, *382*
    handling and disposal of, 285–286, *286*, 359–363, 382, *382*, 898

Blastomycosis, 844
Bleach, as disinfectant, 285, 365t, 897–898
Bleeding
    coagulation tests for, 930–932, 947p–948p
    dysfunctional uterine, 784
    gastrointestinal, occult blood test for, 349, 746–749, 7438p
    nasal, 624
    occult, 349, 738, 746–749, 748p
    from soft tissue injuries, 494–495
    thrombocytopenia and, 930
Bleeding time, 931–932, 947p–948p
Blisters, 522
Block letter format, 130, *130*
Blood
    cleaning and decontamination procedures for, 285
    constituents of, 659–660, 924–925
    occult, tests for, 349, 738, 746–749, 748p
    in urine, 873, 874
Blood agar, 846
Blood bank, 823–824
Blood cells. *See also* Platelets; Red blood cells; White blood cells
    formation of, 924–925
    types of, 924–925
Blood clot. *See also* Coagulation
    formation of, 930–931
Blood donation, 963–964
Blood drawing station, 897, *897*
Blood gases, 973–974, 974t
    arterial, 724–725, 973–974, 974t
Blood group antigens, 961–962
    testing for, 962–963
Blood pressure, 312–314
    diastolic, 313
    elevated. *See* Hypertension
    factors influencing, 314
    measurement of, 313–314
        auscultatory gap in, 313
        in children, 1009–1010, 1010p, 1010t
        cuffs for, 314, *314*
        in dialysis patient, 314
        errors in, 314, 315b
        Korotkoff sounds in, 312–313
        palpatory method of, 332p
        procedure for, 329p–332p
    phases of, 313t
    systolic, 313
Blood pressure cuff, 314, *314*
Blood sample
    arterial, 724, 897
    capillary, 896
    collection of, 724
        butterfly system for, 901, *901*, 902
        complications of, 905–913
        disinfection and asepsis for, 897–898
        equipment for, 897, 897–899, 898
        evacuated tube system for, 899, 899–900, 900t, 901
        fainting during, 905
        labeling of, 905
        needle position for, 905, *905*
        order of draw in, 901
        patient identification for, 905
        patient preparation for, 903–905
        sites for, 896–897
        by skin puncture, 901–903, 913–919, 914p–918p
        syringe system for, 899, 900, 901
        by venipuncture, 898–899, 905–913, 906p–912p, 913t
        winged infusion set for, 901, *901*, 902
    slides for, 898
    storage and handling of, 724, 849t
    venous, 896–897, 897
Blood smear, 924
Blood spills, handling and prevention of, *833*, 833–834
Blood transfusion
    blood typing for, 961–963, *962*, 963t
    donation for, 963–964
Blood typing, 961–963, *962*, 963t
Blood urea nitrogen (BUN), 760, 970, 982t
Blood vessels, *658*, 659, *659*
Blood work, for male reproductive disorders, 776
Bloody show, 798, 806
Blue Cross and Blue Shield, 244
Blues, postpartum, 807–808

Body
    locations and positions on, 512
    organization of, 506–511
Body areas, 513b, 513–514
Body cavities, 513, *513*
Body fluids, cleaning and decontamination procedures for, 285
Body language, 57, 58t, *59*
Body planes, 511–512, *512*
Body regions, 513b, 513–514
Body substance isolation, 273
Body surface area
    in children, 433, *433*, 496, *496*
    rule of nines for, 496, *496*
Body systems, 511, 511t
Body temperature. *See* Temperature
Body weight. *See* Weight
Boiling, of equipment, 370–372
Boils, incision and drainage of, 391
Bone. *See also* Musculoskeletal system
    age-related changes in, *1024*, 1024t
    cancellous, 545
    compact, 545, *545*
    function of, 545–546
    landmarks of, 546t
    structure of, 544–545, *545*, 546t
    tumors of, 570
    types of, 544
Bookkeeping, 206–212
    accounting cycle and, 218
    accounts payable, 219–221
    audits and, 227
    banking and, 212–214
    computerized
        for accounts payable, 220–221, *221*
        for accounts receivable, 212
    double-entry, 206
    payroll, 221–227
    pegboard system for
        for accounts payable, 220, *220*
        for accounts receivable, *206*, 206–208
    petty cash, 190, 214
    posting in
        to cash paid out section of day sheet, 211–212
        of charge, 208
        of credit, 210
        of credit adjustment, 210–211
        of debit adjustment, 211
        of payment, 208–210
    record-keeping components in, 218–219
    report preparation in, 227, 229
    single-entry, 206
    taxes, 224–227
    tips for, 207b
Booster shots, 700
Booting, 162
Bounced checks, 212
Bowel. *See also* Intestinal
Bowel studies, patient preparation for, 743b, 744p–745p
Bowman's capsule, 754, 755
Boyle's law, 712
Bozeman forceps, 355
Brachial pulse, *310*. *See also* Pulse
    in blood pressure measurement, 330p–331p
Brachioradialis reflex, 599t
Bradycardia, 670
Bradypnea, 311
Brain
    divisions of, 584–587, *585*, *586*
    injury of, 596–597, 597t, *598*
    structure and function of, 583–587, *585*, *586*
    tumors of, 597–598
Brain stem, 586–587
Braxton-Hicks contractions, 798
Breast
    examination of, 349
        by patient, 788, *790*
        by physician, 790
        schedule for, 350
    structure and function of, 781, *782*
Breast cancer, 788, 789t, *790*
    mammography for, 478, 478b
Breast feeding, 807b
Breast self-examination, 788, *790*

Breathing, 713. *See also* Respiration(s)
  Cheyne-Stokes, 311–312
  stertorous, 721t
Breathing patterns, abnormal, 720t
Breathing techniques, for stress management, 92
Breath sounds, abnormal, 720, 721t
Bronchi, 711
Bronchioles, 711
Bronchiolitis, 716t
Bronchitis, 717
  chronic, 718–719
Bronchodilators, 418t
Bronchogram, 476t
Bronchopulmonary dysplasia, 716t
Bronchoscopy, 724
Bruise, 494
Bubbling, 721t
Buck ear curet, *362*
Buck neurologic hammer, 336, *336*, 599
Budget, 190
Buffy coat, 827, *828*
Bullae, 520, *521*
Bulletin boards, staff, 183
Bundle branches, 664, *664*
Bundle of His, 664, *664*
Bunions, 568
Burns, 495–496
  body surface area calculation for, 496, *496*
  classification of, 495, 495t
  depth of, 495, 495t
  extent of, assessment of, 496, *496*
  management of, 496
  types of, 495
Burping, 739
Bursae, 547
Bursitis, 567
Business checking account, 212–214
Business letters. *See* Letters
Business manager. *See* Office manager
Butterfly collection system, 901, *901*, *902*
Bypass graft, coronary artery, 668b
Byte, 158

C
Caduceus, 6, *6*
Calcitonin, 643t, 644
Calcium balance, 969–970, 982t
  renal regulation of, 753
Callus
  bone, 564
  skin, 525, 568
Calories, expended in exercise, 90t
Calyces, renal, 754, *754*
Canadian crutches, *571*, 571–577. *See also* Crutches
Cancellous bone, 545
Cancer
  bone, 570
  breast, 788, 789t, *790*
    mammography for, 478, 478b
  cervical, 788, 789t
    Pap smear for, *339*, 339–340, 350, 788, 790–791, 791t, 792p–795p
  colorectal, 738, *738*
  early warning signs of, 342
  endometrial, 788, 789t
  esophageal, 735
  gallbladder, 741
  gastric, 736
  gynecologic, 788, 789t
  laryngeal, 719
  liver, 741
  lung, 719
  lymphatic, 696
  oral, 734
  ovarian, 788, 789t
  pancreatic, 742
  prostate, 769, 770b
  radiation therapy for, 479
  reporting of, 42
  skin, 527–629
    basal cell, 527–528, *528*
    malignant melanoma, *526*, 527b, *528*, 528–529
    squamous cell, 528, *528*

testicular, 775
urinary tract, 760
Candida albicans, 844, *844*
Candidiasis, 733–734, 844
  vaginal, 784, 784b
Canes, *577*, *577*
Capillaries
  blood, 659, *659*, *660*
  lymphatic, 692, *693*
Capillary blood sample, 896
Capital budget, 190
Capitalization rules, 133b
Capitation, 244b, 258
Carbuncle, 520, *520*
  incision and drainage of, 391
Cardiac. *See also* Heart
Cardiac arrhythmias, 670
  electrocardiogram for, 675–683, 679p–683p
  Holter monitor for, 683, 685b, 686p–688p
Cardiac catheterization, 674t, 688–689
Cardiac conduction system, 663–664, *664*
Cardiac cycle, 313, 675
Cardiac disease
  atherosclerotic, *665*, 665–666
    myocardial infarction in, 666–667, 667b
  diagnosis of, 673–689, 674t. *See also* Cardiovascular examination
  risk factors for, 981t
  valvular, 669
Cardiac enzymes, 973, 973t
Cardiac function, assessment of, 973, 973t
Cardiac muscle, 554–555, *555*
Cardiac radiography, 476t
Cardiac stress test, 674t, 685, *688*
Cardiac surgery, 668b
Cardiac valves, 662, 662–663, *663*
  disorders of, 669
Cardiac veins, 663, *663*
Cardinal signs, 302–333
Cardiogenic shock, 493
Cardiopulmonary resuscitation (CPR), 488, 490p–491p
  advance directives for, 28, 44–45, *45*
  termination/witholding of, 27, 44–45
Cardiotonics, 418t
Cardiovascular disorders, 664–673
  diagnosis of. *See* Cardiovascular examination
  emergency care in, 497
  history in, 673b
  physical examination in, 673–674
  symptoms of, 664–665
Cardiovascular examination
  cardiac catheterization in, 674t, 688–689
  chest x-ray in, 674t, 683–684
  coronary arteriography in, 674t, 689
  electrocardiogram in, 674t, 675–683, 679p–683p
  history in, 673, 673b
  Holter monitor in, 674t, 683, 685b, 686p–688p, 688–689
  physical examination in, 673–675
Cardiovascular system
  age-related changes in, 1025t
  structure and function of, 658–664
Carditis, 671–672
Cards
  appointment, 120, *120*
  reminder, 120–121, *121*
Career opportunities, 1048–1060. *See also* Employment
Carotid pulse, *310*. *See also* Pulse
Carpal tunnel syndrome, 568
Carrier, insurance, 244b
Carriers, disease, 268
Cartilage, types of, 547b
Cartilaginous joints, 548t
Cartridges, *439*, 439–440
  data, 161
Case review, 178–179
Cash, petty, 190, 214
Cash-basis accounting, 206
Cash deposits, 213–214
Cast knife, 562, *562*
Casts, 559–562
  application of, 559–562
  injury from, 562
  removal of, 562
  types of, 561b

urinary, 875
Catabolism, 729
Cataracts, 610, *610*, 1025t
Catheterization
  cardiac, 674t, 688–689
  urinary, 760, 760b–761b
    for specimen collection, 869
CD4 count, in HIV infection, 703
Cecum, 732
Celiac sprue, 736–737
Cell, structure and function of, 507–508, *508*, 509t
Cell counter, 825
Cell-mediated immunity, 698
Cell membrane, 508, *508*, 509t
Cellular phones, 109
Cellulitis, 520–521
Celsius scale, 269, 303, *303*
Censure, 20
Centesis, 842
Centigrade scale, 269, 303, *303*
Centimeters-inches conversion, 318p
Central nervous system. *See also* Brain; Spinal cord
  structure and function of, 583–587
Central processing unit (CPU), 158
Centrifuge, 827, *828*
Cephalic vein, blood collection from, 896, *896*. *See also* Blood sample, collection of
Cerebellum, 587
Cerebral cortex, *585*, 585–586, *586*
Cerebral palsy, 596
Cerebrospinal fluid, 584, *585*
  hydrocephalus and, 596
  lumbar puncture for, 599–600, *601*, 602p–603p
Cerebrovascular accident, 671, 1025t
Cerebrum, 584–585, *585*
Certification, 10–11, 43–44
Certified mail, *137*, 138, *138*
Certified Medical Assistant (CMA), 9–10
Cerumen, 348, 615
  impacted, 617
  removal of, 617, *619*, 634p–635p
Ceruminosis, 617
Cervical cancer, 788, 789t
  Pap smear for, 788, 790–791, 791t, 792p–795p
    equipment for, *339*, 339–340
    schedule for, 350
Cervical intraepithelial neoplasia, 788
Cervical spine, fractures of, 564
  spinal cord injury and, 564, 597, 597t, 598
Cervix, *780*, 781
  biopsy of, 795, 796p–797p
  in pregnancy, 798
Cervix scraper, 339, *340*
Cesarean section, 806b
Chadwick's sign, 798
CHAMPUS, 249
CHAMPVA, 249
Chancre, syphilitc, 773
Charges. *See* Fees
Charting. *See also* Documentation; Medical records
  focus, 146, *146*
  for missed appointments, 122
  of vital signs, 314–315, *316*
Charts
  growth, 1007, *1008*
  preparation of, 103
  for vital signs, 314–315, *316*
Check, endorsement of, 212–213, *213*
Checking account, 212–214
Check payments, for accounts receivable, 212–213, *213*, 220
Check register, 219
Checkups. *See also* Physical examination
  pediatric, 989, 991
  schedule for, 350
Cheekbones, 551, *551*
Chemical burns, 495–496
Chemical names, drug, 416, 416b
Chemical reagent strip analysis, 871, 883p–884p
Chemicals, 506–507, 507t
Chemical spills, handling and prevention of, *833*, 833–834
Chemistry. *See* Clinical chemistry
Chemistry analyzer, 827
Chest
  auscultation of, 720, 721t

examination of, 348, 720
    in emergencies, 492
    inspection of, 720
    palpation of, 720
    percussion of, 720
Chest circumference, measurement of, 1005p
Chest pain
    in heart disease, 665, 667b
        nitroglycerin for, 666
    in pericarditis, 671
    telephone reports of, 108, 121
Chest x-ray
    in cardiovascular disease, 674t, 683
    in respiratory disease, 721
Cheyne-Stokes breathing, 311–312
Chickenpox
    herpes zoster and, 522
    Reye's syndrome and, 592–593
Chief complaint, 294, 296–297
Chief technologist, 825b
Child abuse and neglect, 1011–1013
    reporting of, 42
Children, 986–1013. See also Pediatric practice
    anthropometric measurements for, 999, 1003p–1007p
    blood pressure in, 1009–1010, 1010p, 1010t
    body surface area in
        nomogram for, 433, 433
        rule of nines for, 496, 496
    cancer in, early warning signs of, 342
    common illnesses in, 997t
    communication with, 66, 989
    congenital anomalies in. See Congenital anomalies
    developmental delay in, diagnosis of, 601–604, 991,
        992–993
    drug actions in, 422b
    drug dosages for, calculation of, 433, 433–434
    febrile seizures in, 594–595
    growth and development of, 990t–991t, 990–991, 992–993
    growth charts for, 1007, 1008
    hypothyroidism in, 649–650, 650
    medications for, administration of, 1010–1011
    neurologic assessment in, 601–604
    physical examination in, 998–1010
    psychosocial development of, 989
    pulse in, 1008, 1009t
    in reception area, 105
    respiratory disorders in, 716t
    respiratory rate in, 1008–1009, 1009t
    restraints for, 999, 1002, 1002p
    temperature taking in, 1007, 1009
Chlamydia
    in females, 786, 843–844
    in males, 772
Chloral hydrate, 93t
Chlordiazepoxide, abuse of, 93t, 94
Chloride balance, 969, 982t
Chlorine bleach, as disinfectant, 285, 365t, 897–898
Choking, 487, 487–488, 489p
Cholangiogram, 476t
Cholangitis, 741
Cholecystitis, 741
Cholecystogram, 476t
Choledocholithiasis, 741
Cholelithiasis, 741, 741
Cholesterol, 981, 981t
Cholinergic blocking agents, 418t
Cholinergics, 418t
Chondromalacia patella, 568
Choroid, 608, 608
Chromatographic assay, 954
Chronic bronchitis, 718–719
Chronic obstructive pulmonary disease (COPD), 711, 718–719
Chronic renal failure, 756
Chyle, 733
Chyme, 729, 731, 733
Cicatrix, 524–525
Cigarette smoking
    chronic obstructive pulmonary disease and, 718
    lung cancer and, 719
    respiratory effects of, 715b
Cilia, tracheal, 710
Ciliary body, 608, 608
Circular files, 153
Circulation, 662–663

age-related changes in, 1025t
assessment of, in emergencies, 488
Circumcision, 768
Circumduction, 547, 549
Cirrhosis, 740
Civilian Health and Medical Program of the Uniformed
    Services (CHAMPUS), 249
Civilian Health and Medical Program of the Veterans
    Administration (CHAMPVA), 249
Civil law, 34
Claims. See Health insurance claims
Claims administrator, 244b, 246
Clamp
    Kelly, 354, 355
    towel, 357, 358
Clark's rule, for pediatric drug dosage, 434
Classified ads, 1051
Clean-catch urine specimen, 868–869, 877p–878p
Clean technique, 270–271, 271b, 276t, 363
Cleft lip, 624
Cleft palate, 623–624
Climacteric, 812–815
Clinical chemistry, 966–983. See also Laboratory tests
    for cardiac function, 973, 973t
    definition of, 968
    glucose tests in, 975–981
    instruments and methods in, 968
    for lipids and lipoproteins, 981–982
    for liver function, 971–972
    for pancreatic function, 974–981
    for pulmonary function, 973–974, 974t
    for renal function, 968–971
    for thyroid function, 654, 654t, 972–973
Clinical chemistry department, 823
Clinical Laboratory Improvement Amendments, 192, 824,
    834–839
Clinical procedures, written guidelines for, 188–189
Clinical trials, bioethical issues in, 24
Clinitest, 871–872, 885p–886p
Clips, skin, 383–384
    removal of, 385–386, 402p–403p
Clitoris, 781
Closed fracture, 560t
Clot, formation of, 930–931
Clothing
    for medical assistant, 102, 1042–1043
    protective, 274, 275
        decontamination and laundering of, 285
Clotting tests, 930–932, 947p–948p
Cluster headaches, 598
Coagulation, 930–931
Coagulation department, 823
Coagulation tests, 930–932, 947p–948p
Cocaine, 93t, 94
Coccidiomycosis, 844
Cochlea, 616, 619
Cochlear implants, 617
Codeine, 93t, 94
Code of Ethics
    of American Association of Medical Assistants, 20
    of American Medical Association, 20
Coding
    diagnostic, 228–232
        diagnostic related groups and, 239
    fraudulent, 239–240
    procedural, 232–238
COD mail, 138
Coinsurance, 244b, 255
Cold agglutinins, 960–961
Cold applications, 531–540, 532t, 533t, 534p–536p
Cold-related emergencies, 499
Colds, 715
    in children, 997t
    otitis media and, 618
Cold sores, 522, 733–734
Colitis, ulcerative, 737
Collagen, 519
Collateral ligaments, 554
    injuries of, 558
Collection agencies, 202, 210
Collections, 198, 199–202
    bookkeeping and, 198, 210–211
Colon. See also under Intestinal; Rectal
    cancer of, 738, 738

disorders of, 737–739
    lazy, 739
    spastic, 737–738
    structure and function of, 732
Colonic polyps, 738
Colonoscopy, 743, 743, 744p–745p
Colorectal cancer, 738, 738
Color vision, 609
    assessment of, 614, 614, 629p
    deficits in, 612
Colposcopy, 788, 795, 796p–797p
Coma, diabetic, 653, 653t
Comedos, 524
Comminuted fracture, 560t
Common cold, 715
    in children, 997t
    otitis media and, 618
Common law, 34
Communicable diseases, reporting of, 42
Communication, 54–68
    active listening and, 59
    with children, 66, 989
    clarification in, 60, 61t
    confidentiality and, 68b
    cultural differences in, 57–59, 61–64, 62t–64t
    definition of, 56
    with elderly, 1019–1020
    elements of, 56
    factors affecting, 61–66
    feedback in, 56
    flow of, 56, 56
    with foreign language speakers, 64–65
    forms of, 56–59, 58t
    in grief support, 67–68, 68b
    with hearing impaired, 65–66, 1019
    nonverbal, 57–59, 58t, 59
    open-ended questions in, 60, 61t
    oral, 56–57
    paralanguage and, 57, 57b
    paraphrasing in, 60, 61t
    in patient teaching, 68
    reflecting in, 60, 61t
    with sight impaired, 66
    silence in, 61
    summarizing in, 60–61, 61t
    verbal, 56–57, 58t
    via telephone, 105–109
    written, 57, 127–141. See also Letters; Memorandum
Communication notebook, 183
Compact bone, 545, 545
Comparative negligence, 50
Compendium of Drug Therapy, 425
Complement, 698
Complement fixation test, 697t
Complete blood count (CBC), 925–930
    parameters of, 925
Compound fracture, 560t
Compound microscope, 825–827, 826
Compresses
    hot/cold, 531–540, 532t, 533t, 535p–536p
Compression fracture, 560t
Computed tomography (CT), 477, 477
Computer(s), 156–166
    accessories for, 161
    administrative applications of, 161, 163–164
    care and maintenance of, 161–162, 162b
    clinical applications of, 161, 164–165
    hardware, 158–159
    literature searches on, 165
    mainframe, 161
    operation of, 162–163
    privacy safeguards for, 144
    secondary storage systems for, 159–160
    selection of, 165–166
    software for, 161
    training for, 163
Computer graphics, 164
Computerized bill paying, 220–221, 221
Computerized bookkeeping
    for accounts payable, 220–221, 221
    for accounts receivable, 212
Computerized charting, 146–147
Computerized scheduling, 117
Computer viruses, 163

Computer word processing, 164
Conchae, 551, *551*
Concussion, 596
Condom, 809t
Conductive hearing loss, 617
Condylomata acuminata, 786–787
Cones, retinal, 609
Conference calls, 109
Confidentiality, 21, 48, 68b
  of computerized information, 144b, 165
Congenital anomalies
  causes of, 799–800, 800b, 801b
  neural tube defects, 595–596, *596*
  prenatal diagnosis of, 600, 808
  prenatal screening for, 600–601
Congenital heart disease, 669
Congestive heart failure, 669–670
Conjunctivitis, 610
Connective tissue, 509, 509t, *510*
Consent, 36
  age of majority for, 40
  of emancipated minor, 40
  expressed, 40
  form for, 40, *41*
  implied, 40
  informed, 36, 40
  for minor office surgery, 379, *380*
  refusal of, 40–42
  requirements for, 40
Consolidated Omnibus Budget Reconciliation Act (COBRA),
    46
Constipation, 739
Contact precautions, 273–274, 274t
Contamination, management of, 285, 833–834
Continuing education units (CEUs), 10, *11*
Contraception, 809t, 809–812, 811p–812p
Contract, physician-patient
  express, 35
  implied, 35
  rights and responsibilities under, 35–36
  termination/withdrawal of, 36–39, *39*
Contractions
  Braxton-Hicks, 798
  uterine, 806
Contraction stress test, 808
Contracture
  Dupuytren's, 568
  joint, 567
Contraindications, drug, 423t
Contrast media examinations, 475–476, 476t
  barium studies, 471–472, *475*, 475–476, 476t
Contributory negligence, 50
Controlled substances, 416–420, 419t
Controlled Substances Act, 44
Control sample, 835–837
Contusion, 494
  brain, 596
Convulsions. *See* Seizures
Coordination, assessment of, 349–350
Coordination of benefits, 244b
Co-payment, 245b
Copper reduction test, 871–872, 885p–886p
Cornea, 608, *608*
Corneal reflex, 599t
Corneal ulcer, 610–611
Corns, 525, 568
Coronary angioplasty, percutaneous transluminal, 668b
Coronary arteries, 663, *663*
Coronary arteriography, 674t, 689
Coronary artery bypass graft, 668b
Coronary artery disease, *665*, 665–666. *See also* Athero-
    sclerosis
  myocardial infarction in, 666–667, 667b
  risk factors for, 981t
Corpora cavernosa, 768
Corpus spongiosum, 768
Correspondence. *See* Letters; Mail
Corticoids, 643t, 646
Cortisol
  deficiency of, 651
  excess of, 652
Cortisone, for Addison's disease, 652
Cotton-tipped applicators, 339, *340*, 842
  in serology specimen collection, 955

Coudé catheter, *760*, 761b
Cough, in bronchitis, 717
Coumadin
  coagulation tests and, 931
  prothrombin time for, 931
Courtesy
  telephone, 106
  toward patients, 102
Cover letter, 1053–1054, *1055*
Cowper's glands, 767, 768
CPT-4 codes, 232–238
  fraud and, 239–240
  modifiers for, 236b, 236–238
Crack cocaine, 93t, 94
Crackles, 721t
Cramps, heat, 499
Cranial nerves, 587, *588*, 588t
Crash diets, 89
C-reactive protein (CRP), 958
Creatine clearance, 970
Creatine kinase, after myocardial infarction, 973, 973t
Creatinine, 970, 982t
Credit, 199, 206
  posting of, 210
Credit adjustment, posting of, 210–211
Credit bureaus, 202
Credit card payments, 198
Cretinism, 649–650, *650*
Crile hemostatic forceps, *355*
Crile-Wood needle holder, *356*
Crohn's disease, 737
Cross examination, 49
Crossover claim, 245b, 248
Croup, 716t
Cruciate ligaments, 554
  injuries of, 558
Crush injuries, 494
Crutches, 571–577
  fitting of, 572p–573p
  gaits for, 574p–576p
  patient education for, 572
  safety tips for, 570b, 571b
  types of, *571*
Cryptorchidism, 771, *771*
Crystals, urine, 875, 879p
Culdocentesis, 787, 795
Cultural issues
  in communication, 57–59, 61–64, 62t–64t
  language and, 64–65
  in nutrition, 88t
  stereotyping and bias and, 66
  values and, 61
Culture
  blood, specimen collection for, 845
  microbiologic inoculation for, 850–851, *851*
  mixed, 845
  pure, 845
  secondary, 845
  specimen collection for. *See also* Specimen(s)
  sputum, 720–721, 723p
    specimen collection for, 845–846
  stool, 745, 746b, 747p
  throat, 720, 722p
  urethral, 776
  urine. *See also* Urinalysis
    specimen collection for, 760, 868–869
    specimen storage and handling for, 849t
  wound, 529, *529*, *530*
    specimen collection for, 846
Culture inoculation, 850–851, *851*, 861p–864p
Culture media
  care of, 847
  transport, 847–848, *848*, 853p
  types of, 846, *847*
Culture test, for sterilization, 367
Cumulative problem list, 296–297
Curet(s), 362, 362t
  ear, 362, 362t
  nasal, 362t
  uterine, *360*
Curie, Marie, 8
Current Procedural Terminology (CPT) codes, 232–238
  fraud and, 239–240
  modifiers for, 236b, 236–238

Cursor, 159
Curved scissors, 354, *357*
Cushing's syndrome, 652
Cystic fibrosis, 716t
Cystitis, 758
Cystocele, uterine prolapse and, 785
Cystoscopy, 761
  in males, 776
Cystourethrogram, voiding, 476t
Cystourethroscopy, 761
Cysts
  acne, *521*, 524
  ovarian, 788
Cytogram, 476t
Cytologist, 825b
Cytology department, 824
Cytoplasm, 508, *508*, 509t
Cytotoxic T cells, 698

D

Dacryocystitis, 612
DACUM, 9, 10
Daily journal, 206–207
Data base, for medical history, 290
Day sheet, 206–207
D & C (dilatation and curettage), 797
Deafness. *See* Hearing loss
Death and dying
  advance directives for, 28, *45*, 45–46
  assisted suicide/euthanasia in, 27b
  debt collection from estate and, 199b
  ethical issues in, 27, 27b
  grief and, 67–68, 68b
  treatment withdrawal/witholding in, 27, 27b
Death certificates, 42
Debakey forceps, *356*
Debit, 206
Debit adjustment, posting of, 211
Debt collection, 198, 199–202
  bookkeeping and, 198, 210–211
Debt collection agencies, 202, 210
Deciduous teeth, 730
Decongestants, 418t
Decubitus ulcers, *525*, 525–526
Deductible, 245b, 247
Deep, 512
Deep-vein thrombosis, 670–671
Defamation of character, 48
Defecation, 732
Defendant, 47
Defibrillation, 497
Defibrillator, 670
Degenerative joint disease, 569
Deglutition, 730
Delivery, obstetric, 806
  abbreviations used in, 807b
  cesarean, 806b
Delivery services, 138
Deltoid muscle, injection in, *442*, 443
Demeanor, 59
Dementia, Alzheimer's, 1028–1029, 1029t
Demographic problems, 145
Dendrite, 582, *583*
Denial, in grief, 67
Dental caries, 733
Denver Developmental Screening Test, 604, 991, *992–993*
Deoxyribonucleic acid (DNA), 508
Dependents, insurance for, 245b
Depolarization, in cardiac cycle, 664, *675*
Deposit, bank, 213–214
Deposition, 49b
Deposit slip, 206, 213
Depressants, abuse of, 93t, 94
Depressed fracture, 560t, *561*
Depression, postpartum, 807–808
Dermal drug administration, 437–438, 450p, 451p
Dermatitis. *See also* Skin disorders
  seborrheic, 524
Dermatology. *See* Skin
Dermatomes, spinal, 589
Dermatophytosis, 522–523
Dermis, *518*, 518–519
Desktop publishing, 164

Desmarres lid retractor, 362
Development
  assessment of, 604, 991, 992–993
  charting of, 1007, 1008
  prenatal, 802, 804
Developmental delay, diagnosis of, 601–604, 991, 992–993
Developmental disorders, neurologic, 595–596
Dextrocardia, 683
Diabetes insipidus, 649
Diabetes mellitus, 652–653
  diet in, 85
  in elderly, 653
  gestational, 981
  glucose monitoring in, 980
  glucose tests in, 975–980, 980. See also Glucose tests
  glucose tolerance test in, 654, 976–979, 978p–979p
  insulin-dependent, 652–653
  insulin for, syringe for, 441, 441
  non–insulin-dependent, 652–653
Diabetic coma, 653, 653t
Diabetic ketoacidosis, 652, 653
Diagnostic coding, 228–240, 230–232
  diagnostic related groups and, 239
  fraud and, 239–240
Diagnostic imaging, 468–481
  computed tomography, 477, 477
  fluoroscopy, 477
  interventional, 478
  magnetic resonance imaging, 477
  mammography, 478
  medical assistant's role in, 479–480
  nuclear medicine, 477–478
  outpatient, 470–471
  patient education in, 479
  radiography, 470–478. See also Radiography
  sonography, 477, 477
  teleradiology, 478
Diagnostic related groups (DRGs), 238–239
Diagnostic set, 613, 613
Diagnostic tests. See Clinical chemistry; Laboratory tests
Dialysis, 756, 757b
  blood pressure measurement in, 314
Diaphragm, 712–713
  contraceptive, 809t
Diaphragmatic excursion, 720
Diaphysis, 545, 545
Diarrhea, 739
  in irritable bowel syndrome, 737–738
  malabsorption and, 736–737
Diarthroses, 546
Diazepam, abuse of, 93t, 94
Diazo tablet method, 873, 889p
Dictation, 140–141
Diction, 106
Didanosine, for AIDS, 703
Dideoxycytidine, for AIDS, 703
Diencephalon, 584
Diet. See also Nutrition
  constipation and, 739
  cultural factors in, 88t
  diabetic, 85
  in elderly, 1030
  fad, 89
  gas and, 739
  gout and, 971
  in iron deficiency anemia, 928
  physician-ordered, 86, 87t
  weight loss, 89
Dietary guidelines, 82, 83, 84, 85t–87t
  Food Guide Pyramid and, 82, 83
  Guide to Good Eating, 82, 84
Digestion, 729, 730t
Digital palpation, 341
Digital rectal examination (DRE), 769, 776
Digoxin
  excretion of, 423
  toxicity of, 423
Dilatation and curettage (D & C), 797
Dilators, uterine, 360
Diluents, for powdered drugs, 439
Diphtheria, Shick test for, 531
Diphtheria-pertussis-tetanus immunization, 592, 699t
  schedule for, 994, 996
  side effects of, 995b

Diplococci, 842, 843
Diplomacy, 103
Dipstick, urine, 871, 883p–886p
Direct examination, 49
Directors, 357, 358
Directory, computer, 160
Disciplinary action, staff, 186, 186–187
Disclosures. See Reporting
Discovery, 49, 49b
Discrimination, 66
Disease(s)
  carriers of, 268
  familial, 290
  hereditary, 290
Disease transmission
  direct, 270
  hosts for, 270, 270b
  indirect, 270
  infection cycle and, 269, 269–270
  methods of, 271b
  vector in, 270
  vehicle of, 269–270
Disease updates, computerized, 165
Disinfection, 284–285, 363–364, 365t, 897–898
  environmental, 393
  for phlebotomy, 897–898
  of thermometer, 307–308, 325p–326p
Disk, herniated, 564–567
Disk drive, 159
Dislocations, 559
  emergency management of, 496–497
Disposable thermometer, 306, 307
Dissecting aneurysm, 672
Distal, 512
Dittel urethral sound, 361
Diuretics, 418t
Diverticulitis, 738
Diverticulosis, 738
DNA, 508
Documentation. See also Legal documents; Medical records;
        Written communication
  in emergencies, 485–486
  of equipment maintenance, 836, 837, 837–838
  guidelines for, 147–148
  incident reports and, 174–178
  of medication errors, 429b
  of patient teaching, 74–75
  of prescriptions, 420
  of telephone messages, 108
Documents
  legal. See Legal documents
  storage of, 154
Domestic needles, 383
Doppler ultrasonography
  in pregnancy, 808
  in pulse measurement, 310, 310
Dorsal cavity, 513, 513
Dorsalis pedis pulse, 310
Dorsal position, 343, 344t
Dorsiflexion, 547, 550
Dorsogluteal injection, 442, 443
Dosimeter, 474, 474
Double booking, 119
Dowager's hump, 1024
Drainage
  abscess, 391, 412p
  wound, 386b
Draping, 379–381
Drawer files, 153, 153
Dress, for medical assistant, 102, 1041, 1042–1043
Dressing, sterile, 386, 403p–405p
Dressing forceps, 356
DRGs (diagnostic related groups), 238–239
Droplet precautions, 273–274, 274t
Drug abuse
  controlled substances and, 416–420, 419t
  patient teaching for, 92–94, 93t
Drug Enforcement Agency (DEA), 416–420, 419t
Drug names, 416, 416b
Drugs. See Medications
Dry smear, 848, 854p–856p
Duchenne's muscular dystrophy, 569
Ductus deferens, 767, 767
Due process, 23

Duodenal ulcers, 736
Duodenum, 731, 731
Duplay tenaculum forceps, 356, 360
Dupuytren's contracture, 568
Durable power of attorney for health care, 45–46, 46
Dura mater, 584
Duress, 48
Dwarfism, 648
Dysfunctional uterine bleeding, 784
Dysmenorrhea, 785
Dyspareunia, 785
Dysphagia
  in rabies, 592
  in tetanus, 592
Dysphasia, in multiple sclerosis, 593
Dyspnea, in pneumonia, 717
Dysrhythmias, 670
  electrocardiogram for, 675–683, 679p–683p

E
Ear
  age-related changes in, 1025t
  disorders of, 617–621. See also Hearing loss
    diagnosis of, 619–621
    patient education for, 621
  examination of, 348, 619, 719–720
    instruments for, 336–337, 337
  external, 615
    infection of, 618
  foreign objects in, 621, 634p–635p
  inner, 616
  instruments for, 362, 362t
  irrigation of, 619, 621, 634p–635p
  middle, 615–616
    infection of, 618, 997t, 998
  structure and function of, 615–617, 619
  swimmer's, 618
Eardrum. See Tympanic membrane
Ear forceps, 362, 362t
Ear medications, instillation of, 621, 635p–637p
Ear syringe, 619
Earwax, 348, 615
  impacted, 617
  removal of, 617, 619, 634p–635p
Ecchymosis, 494
Echocardiography, 674t, 685–688
Eclampsia, 804
Ectopic pregnancy, 803
Eczema, 523–524
Editing, of letters, 132–135, 133b, 134t
Education
  for laboratory personnel, 838–839
  manager, 191–192
  for medical assistants, 10
  patient. See Patient education
  staff, 191
Educational videos, 105
Efferent nerves, 582
Elastic bandages, 388, 390
Elastic cartilage, 547b
Elastin, 519
Elbow
  nursemaid's, 559
  structure and function of, 552
  subluxation of, 559
  tennis, 567–568
Elderly
  abuse of, 526, 1021–1022
  alcoholism in, 1020
  Alzheimer's disease in, 1028, 1029t
  communication with, 1019–1020
  coping with loss by, 1020–1021
  diabetes in, 653
  diet in, 1030
  diseases of, 1023–1028
  drug therapy in, 422b, 1022–1023
  exercise for, 1029t, 1029–1030
  fracture healing in, 564, 565b
  health maintenance in, 1029–1030
  home care for, 1021
  long-term care for, 1021
  Medicaid for, 249
  Medicare for, 247–249. See also Medicare

Elderly, (*continued*)
  memory aids for, 1018–1019
  mental health of, 1019–1020
  myths and stereotypes about, 1018, 1018b
  osteoporosis in, 569–570
  Parkinson's disease in, 1023–1028, *1027*
  presbyopia in, 612
  psychosocial needs of, 1019–1020
  safety for, 1030
  suicide in, 1020–1021
  systemic changes in, 1023, 1024t–1026t
Electrical burns, 495–496
Electrocardiogram, 674t, 675–683
  abbreviations for, 677b
  artifacts on, 682, 684t
  baseline, 350
  cardiac cycle and, 675
  in cardiac stress test, 685
  equipment for, 678
  interpretation of, 678–683
  intervals and segments on, 675, 677
  leads for, 675, 676–678, 677, 678b, 678t
    placement of, 680p–681p
  paper for, 675, 676
  preparation for, 678
  procedure for, 679p–683p
  rhythm strip and, 683
  strip mounting for, 683p
Electrocautery, 391–392
Electrodesiccation, 391
Electroencephalography, 599
Electrolytes, 969t, 969–970
Electromyography, 570
Electronic mail, 136
Electronic thermometer, 305, *306*, 324p
Electrons, 506, 507, *507*
Electrosection, 392
Electrosurgery, *391*, 391–392
  assisting with, 411p
Elements, 506–507, 507t
Elephantiasis, 695
Eligibility, insurance, 245b
ELISA, 953–954, 954b
  for HIV, 704–705
E-mail, 136
Emancipated minor, 40
Embolism, pulmonary, 670–671
Embolization, therapeutic, 478
Embryo, 783b
E/M codes, 232–233
Emergency care, 482–501, 484, 494–501
  action plan for, 484
  airway management in, 487–488
  for allergic reactions, 497–498
  for allergies, 497
  ambulance transport in, 486
  assessment in, 486–493
    of airway, 487–488
    of breathing, 488
    of circulation, 488
    personal protective equipment in, 486
    physical examination in, 492–493
    primary survey in, 486–488
    of responsiveness, 487
    scene survey in, 486
    secondary survey for, 488–493
  for behavioral and psychiatric emergencies, 500–501
  for bleeding, 494b, 494–495
  for burns, 495t, 495–496, *496*
  cardiopulmonary resuscitation in, 488, 490p–491p
  for cardiovascular disorders, 497
  for cold-related disorders, 499–500
  computerized information for, 165
  documentation in, 485–486
  first aid kit for, 484, 485b
  Good Samaritan Act and, 44
  for heart disease, 497
  for heat-related disorders, 499
  for musculoskeletal injuries, 496–497
  for myocardial infarction, 497
  for neurologic disorders, 497
  office procedures for, 484–486
  for poisoning, 498
  for seizures, 497, 595t
    for shock, 493b, 493–494, 497, 498
    for soft tissue injuries, 494b, 494–495
    for stroke, 497
    supplies for, 484, 485b
    telephone communication in, 108, 121, 484, 715
Emergency medical services (EMS), 484
  telephoning of, 108, 121, 484
Emetics, 418t
Emotional crisis, 500–501
Emotional distress, intentional infliction of, 48
Empathy, 13, 67
Emphysema, 718–719
Employee Retirement Security Act (ERISA), 247
Employees. *See* Staff
Employment, 1048–1060
  application for, 1051–1055, *1054–1055*
  goals for, 1050
  interview for, 1055–1059, 1056b, 1057b
  networking and, 1051
  resignation from, 1059b, 1059–1060
  resumé for, *105*, 1051–1054, *1054*
  self-analysis for, 1050–1051
  sources of information for, 1051
  temporary, 1051
Employment agencies, 1051
EMS. *See* Emergency medical services (EMS)
Encephalitis, 591
Encounter form, 208, *209*
Endemic goiter, 649
Endocarditis, 672
Endocardium, 659
Endocrine system
  age-related changes in, 1026t
  disorders of, 647–654
    diagnosis of, 654, 654t
  structure and function of, *642*, 642–647, 643t
End-of-life issues
  advance directives, 28, *45*, 45–46
  treatment refusal, 48
  treatment withdrawal/witholding, 27
Endometrial cancer, 788, 789t
Endometriosis, 784–785
Endometritis, postpartum, 807
Endometrium, 781
Endorsement, check, 212–213, *213*
Endoscopic retrograde cholangiopancreatogram, 476t
Endoscopy, 742–743, *743*
Enema
  barium, 471–472, *475*, 475–476, 476t
  drug administration via, 436–437, *437*
Envelopes
  addressing of, 136, *136*, 137b
  postage for, 136–137, *137*, 137b
Environmental contamination, management of, 285
Enzyme(s)
  cardiac, 973, 973t
  definition of, 971
  digestive, 729, 730t
  hepatic, 971–972, 972t
  pancreatic, 974
Enzyme immunoassays (EIAs), 704–705, 953–954, 954b
  for pregnancy, 959
Enzyme-linked immunosorbent assay (ELISA), for HIV, 704–705
Eosinophils, *924*, 927
Epidermis, *518*, 518–519
Epididymis, *767*, 767
Epididymitis, 771–772
Epigastric region, 513, *514*
Epiglottis, 710
Epiglottitis, 716t
Epilepsy, 594–595, 595t
  reporting of, 42
Epinephrine, 643t, 646
  for allergic reactions, 498
Epiphyseal end plate, *545*, 545
Epiphysis, 545, *545*
Episiotomy, 781
Epistaxis, 624
Epithelial cells, in urine, 874–875
Epithelial tissue, 509, 509t, *510*
Equipment. *See also* Instruments
  boiling of, 370–372
  disinfection of, 284–285, 363–364, 365t, 897–898
    emergency, 484, 485b
    laboratory, 824–828
    maintenance of, 191, 372, *836*, 837–838
    personal protective, 274, *275*, 832
      decontamination and laundering of, 285
      in emergency care, 486
    for physical examination, 336–341, 345p
    purchasing of, 219–221
    recordkeeping for, 372
    service contracts for, 191
    specialist, 359, 360t–362t
    sterilization of, 284, 365–372, *367*, 368b–370b, 371p
    storage of, 372
    wrapping of, for sterilization, 368b–369b
Equity, 206
Erection, 768
Erect position, *343*, 344t
ERISA (Employee Retirement Security Act), 247
Eructation, 739
Erythema, 524
Erythrocte (RBC) count, 928, 941p–942p
Erythrocytes, 659, *660*, 661, *924*
  abnormalities of, 929t
  formation of, 924–925, 928
  function of, 928
  mean cell volume for, 929
  in urine, 873, 874
Erythrocyte sedimentation rate (ESR), 930, *931*, 946p–947p
Erythropoiesis, 928
Erythropoietin, 928
Esophageal cancer, 735
Esophageal varices, 735
Esophagitis, 734, 735b
Esophagus
  Barrett's, 734, 735b
  disorders of, 734–735
  structure and function of, 730–731
ESR (erythrocyte sedimentation rate), 930, *931*, 946p–947p
Estate, patient's, collection from, 199b
Estimated date of delivery (EDD), 798–799, 800b
Estrogen, 643t, 647
Estrogen replacement therapy, 813–815
Ethical decision making, 22, 28b
Ethics, 20–30
  bioethics and, 23–29. *See also* Bioethics
  controlled substances, 420
  honesty and, 22
  insurance fraud, 250
  laws and, 22
  patient advocacy and, 21
  patient confidentiality and, 21
  patients' views on, 21b
  problem solving in, 22, 28b
  unprofessional conduct and, 22–23
Ethmoidal sinuses, 551, 622, 709, *709*
Ethmoid bone, 551, *551*
Ethnic groups. *See also under* Cultural
  beliefs and practices of, 62t–64t
Ethylene oxide, as sterilant, 365, 366
Eunuchoidism, 648
Eustachian tube, 616, *619*, 709
Euthanasia, 27, 27b
Evacuated tube system, for blood collection, *899*, 899–900, 900t, 901
Evaluation, employee, *185*, 186
Evaluation and management (E/M) codes (CPT), 232–233, 234t
Eversion, 547, *550*
Ewing's sarcoma, 570
Examination light, 337
Examination table, cleaning of, 393
Excisional surgery, 390–393
  assisting with, 411p
  electrosurgery, 391–392
  laser, 392–393
Excision biopsy, of skin, 529
Excretory urogram, 476t
Exercise
  benefits of, 89b
  calorie use in, 90t
  for elderly, 1029t, 1029–1030
  patient teaching for, 89b, 89–90
  for stress management, 92
  types of, 89b

Exercises
  Kegel, 786
  range-of-motion, 90
  stretching, 92
Exit interview, 1059b
Exophthalmic goiter, 650, 651
Expectorants, 418t
Expert witness, 47
Expiration, 713
Explanation of benefits, 245b, 255, 256
Expressed contract, 35
Express mail, 137
Expulsion, 20
Extension, 547
External ear, 615
  infection of, 618
Externship, 10, 1036–1045
  attendance and, 1042
  benefits of, 1039
  definition of, 1038
  evaluation in, 1040
    criteria for, 1040–1042
  in general practice, 1038
  length of, 1038
  preceptors for, 1038–1039
    evaluations by, 1040–1042
    problems with, 1040
  preparedness and, 1042
  responsibilities of, 1039–1040
  scheduling of, 1038
  self-evaluation in, 1044–1045
  site evaluation in, 1044, 1045
  site selection for, 1038–1039
  in specialty practice, 1038
  successful, guidelines for, 1042–1043
  time records for, 1043–1044, 1044
  types of, 1038
Extraocular movements, assessment of, 348
Extremities. See Arm; Leg
Eye
  adnexa of, 609, 609
  age-related changes in, 1025t
  disorders of, 610–615
    diagnosis of, 612–6152
  examination of, 348
    instruments for, 337, 337, 362, 362t
  irrigation of, 615, 631p–632p
    eye wash basin for, 833
  medication administration for, 614–615, 630p–631p
  movements of, assessment of, 348
  muscles of, 609
    strabismus and, 612
  pink, 610
  preventive care for, 616
  structure and function of, 608, 608–610, 609
Eye chart, 613, 628p
Eye contact, cultural aspects of, 64
Eye drops, administration of, 614–615, 630p–631p
Eyelid, 609, 609
  sty of, 610
Eyelid retractor, 362, 362t
Eye wash basin, 833

F
Face shield, 274, 275
Facet joint, 552
Facial bones, 549–551, 551
Facial expressions, 57, 58t, 59
Facial nerve, 587, 588, 588t
Facioscapulohumeral dystrophy, 569
Facsimile machines, 136
Fad diets, 89
Fahrenheit scale, 303, 303
Fainting, during venipuncture, 905
Fair Debt Collection Act, 202
Fallopian tube
  in ectopic pregnancy, 803
  infection of, 787
  structure and function of, 780, 780–781
False imprisonment, 48
False labor, 806
False-negative results, 957
False-positive results, 957

Familial diseases, 290
Family and Medical Leave Act, 192
Family history, 290
Farsightedness, 611
Far vision, testing of, 613, 614
Fascia, superficial, 520
Fasciitis, plantar, 568
Fasting blood glucose, 975
Fat, malabsorption of, 736–737
Fax machines, 136
Fax modem, 161
FDA (Food and Drug Administration), 416
Febrile seizures, 594–595, 998
Feces. See Stool
Federal unemployment tax (FUTA), 224
Feedback
  in communication, 56
  in homeostasis, 514
Fee-for-service, 245b, 258
Fees, 198
  adjustment of, bookkeeping and, 207, 210–211
  collection of, 198
  Medicare reimbursement for, 247–249
  posting of, 208
  professional courtesy, 198
  setting of, 198
  write off for, 198
Fee schedule, 245b, 258
Fee-splitting, 43
Feet. See Foot
Female condom, 809t
Femoral pulse, 310. See also Pulse
Fencing reflex, 993t
Fertility awareness, 809t
Fertilization, 782, 783b
Fetal heart rate, measurement of, 808
Fetal ultrasonography, 601, 808
  α-Fetoprotein, prenatal measurement of, 600, 808
Fetotoxins, 799–800, 800b, 801b
Fetus, 783b
  development of, 802, 804
Fever, 304. See also Temperature
  causes of, 304
  as defense mechanism, 696
  intermittent, 304, 305t
  patient education for, 304
  patterns of, 305t
  relapsing, 304, 305t
  remittent, 304, 305t
  seizures and, 594–595, 998
  stages of, 304
  sustained, 304, 305t
  temperature measurement in, 303, 305–308
Fever blisters, 522, 733–734
Fiberglass casts, 559. See also Casts
Fibrocartilage, 547b
Fibrous joints, 548t
Filariasis, 695
File, tickler, 121, 121b
Files
  computer, 160
  types of, 153
Filing
  alphabetic, 151, 151b, 152b
  numeric, 151–152, 152b
  procedures for, 150–151
  subject, 153
  systems for, 151b, 151–153, 152b
Film, x-ray, handling and storage of, 480
Filter paper devices, for microcollection, 903
Financial records, 218–219
Fine-point splinter forceps, 356
Finger puncture. See Skin puncture
Firing, of employees, 187
First aid. See also Emergency care
First aid kit, 484, 485b
First-class mail, 137
Fissures, 521, 523
Fixative, 339
Fixator muscle, 554
Flagellum, 768, 768–769
Flashlight, 338
Flasks, 828, 829
Flatulence, 739

Fleming, Alexander, 8
Flexion, 547, 549
Floppy disks, 160, 162b
Flora
  normal, 268
  transient, 268
Flow sheets, 146, 147
Fluid balance, 753
Fluorescent antibody test, 697t
Fluoroscopy, 477
Focal seizures, 595
Focus charting, 146, 146
Folate deficiency, neutrophils in, 927
Foley catheter, 760, 761b
Follicles
  hair, 519
  nail, 519
Follicle-stimulating hormone, 643t, 644, 781–782
Folliculitis, 520, 520
Food
  digestion of, 729
  transport of, 728–729
Food and Drug Administration (FDA), 416
Food Guide Pyramid, 82, 83
Foot
  athlete's, 523, 844
  deformities of, 568–569
  muscles of, 557t
  structure and function of, 554
Foot drop, 554
Forceps, 354, 355, 356
  ear, 362, 362t
  nasal, 362, 362t
  sterile transfer, 297p, 377, 377, 378, 378
  wide ear, 362
Forearm crutches, 571, 571–577. See also Crutches
Foreign body
  in ear, 621, 634p–635p
  in eye, 615, 631p–632p
  in upper airway, 487, 487–488, 489p
Foreign language speakers, 64–65
Formaldehyde
  as disinfectant, 365t
  as sterilant, 366
Formula method, for dosage calculation, 433
Four-point gait, 574p–576p
Fourth-class mail, 138
Fovea centralis, 608, 609
Fractures, 559–564
  ambulatory aids for, 570–578
  casts for, 559–562
  of cervical spine, 564
    spinal cord injury and, 564, 597, 597t, 598
  emergency management of, 496–497
  healing of, 564
    in elderly, 564, 565b
  reduction of, 559
  types of, 560t, 561
Fraud, insurance, 34, 43, 48, 239–240, 250, 255
  coding and, 239–240
Freezer, laboratory, 827–828
Fresh frozen plasma, 963
Friction rub, 721t
Fried's rule, for pediatric drug dosage, 434
Frontal lobe, 585, 585–586, 586
Frontal plane, 512, 512
Frontal sinuses, 551, 551, 622, 709, 709
Frostbite, 500
Frozen shoulder, 567
Full block letter format, 129, 130
Functional ovarian cysts, 788
Functional position, for instruments, 384, 384
Fungal infections, of skin, 522–523
Fungi, 844, 844
Furuncle, 520, 520
  incision and drainage of, 391

G
Gait
  assessment of, 349–350, 599
  crutch, 574p–576p
Galactosuria, 871–872
Galen, 7

Gallbladder, 733, *733*
    disorders of, 741
Gallstones, 741
Gamma globulins, 699, 699t
Gardnerella vaginitis, 784, 784b
Gas, 739
Gas exchange, pulmonary, 713–714, *714. See also* Arterial
        blood gases
Gastric cancer, 736
Gastric disorders, 735–736
Gastric function, 731, *731*
Gastric ulcers, 735–736
Gastritis, 735
Gastroenteritis, 736
    in children, 997t
Gastroesophageal reflux, 734, 735b
Gastrointestinal bleeding, occult blood test for, 349, 738,
        746–749, 748p
Gastrointestinal disorders
    assessment in, 742
    blood tests in, 742
    diagnosis of, 742–749
    endoscopy in, 742–743, *743*
    history in, 742
    radiologic studies in, 742
Gastrointestinal system
    accessory organs of, 732–733, *733*
    age-related changes in, 1026t
    food transport in, 728–729
    layers of, 728–729
    structure and function of, 728–733, *729*
Gauze bandages
    roller, 388, *390*
    tubular, 388–389, 407p–410p
Gel separator, 900
Generic names, drug, 416, 416b
Genetic immunity, 698
Genetic testing, bioethical issues in, 25
Genital herpes
    in females, 787
    in males, 773
Genitals. *See also* Reproductive system
    examination of, 349
Genital warts, 786–787
Geographical practice cost index (GPCI), 239
Geriatrics. *See* Elderly
German measles, tests for, 958
Gestation, 783b. *See also* Pregnancy
Gestational diabetes, 981
Gestational wheel, 800b
Gestures, 57, 58t, *59*
Gingiva, 730
Gingivitis, 734
Glassware, laboratory, 828, *829,* 830p
Glaucoma, 611, 1025t
    tonometry for, 614, *615*
Glomerulonephritis, 756–757
Glomerulus, 754, *755*
Glossopharyngeal nerve, 587, *588,* 588t
Gloves, 274, 274t, *275, 275,* 275b, 338, 897
    donning of, 280p–282p
    latex allergy and, 897
    removal of, 283p–284p
Glucagon, 647, 975
Glucocorticoids, 643t, 646
Glucometer, 975, 976p–977p, 980
Glucose. *See also* Hyperglycemia; Hypoglycemia
    function of, 982t
    normal values for, 982t
    production and metabolism of, 647
    urinary, 871–872, 885p–886p
Glucose meter, 975, 976p–977p, 980
Glucose reflectance photometer, 975, 976p–977p, 980
Glucose-regulating hormones, 975
Glucose regulation, insulin in, 975
Glucose tests, 975–981
    in diabetes, 980
    fasting blood glucose, 975
    glucose tolerance test, 654, 976–979, 978p–979p
    in pregnancy, 981
    random blood glucose, 975
    2-hour postprandial glucose, 975–976
Glucose tolerance test, 654, 976–979, 978p–979p

Glutaraldehyde, as disinfectant, 365t
Glutaraldehyde, as sterilant, 366
Gluteus maximus, injection in, *442,* 443–444
Glycosuria, 871–872, 872b
    in diabetes, 652
Goiter, 649
    exophthalmic, 650, *651*
Gonadotropic hormone, 643t, 644
Gonads, 643t, 647
Goniometer, 570
Gonioscopy, 614
Gonococcal urethritis, 772–773
Gonorrhea
    in females, 787
    in males, 772–773
Goodell's sign, 798
Good Samaritan Act, 240
Gooseneck lamp, 338
Gout, 569, 971
Gowns, 274, 274t, *275*
Graafian follicle, 782
Graduated cylinder, 828, *829*
Grammar tips, 133b
Gram stain, 849–850, 850b, 856p–860p
Grand mal seizures, 594, 595t. *See also* Seizures
Granulocytes, 661, 662t, 926
Graph, for vital signs, 314–315, *316*
Graphic charts, 1007, *1008*
Grasp reflex, 993t
Graves disease, 650–651, *651*
Graves vaginal speculum, *360*
Gravidity, 799b
Gray cells, neural, 582
Gray matter
    cerebral, 584
    spinal cord, 587
Great vessels, 658
Greenstick fracture, 560t
Greeting, of patients and visitors, 103
Grief, 67–68, 68b
    in elderly, 1020
Gross income, 222
Group A streptococcus, tests for, 851–852, 960
Group health insurance, 246–247. *See also*
        Health insurance
Group homes, for elderly, 1021
Growth and development
    assessment of, 604, 991, 992–993
    charting of, 1007, *1008*
    prenatal, *802, 804*
Growth charts, 1007, *1008*
Growth hormone, 643t, 643–644
    deficiency of, 647–648
    excess of, 648–649
Guaiac, stool, 349, 738, 746–749, 748p
Guide to Good Eating, 82, *84*
Gynecologic cancer, 788, 789t
Gynecologic disorders, 784–797
Gynecologic examination
    instruments for, *360,* 360t
    routine, 349, 350, 788, 789–795, 792p–795p
Gyri, 584, *585*

H

Haemophilus influenzae, immunization for, 699t, 996,
        996–997
Hair, structure and function of, 519
Hair follicles, 519
Hair loss, 526
    tinea capitis and, 522
Hair removal, preoperative, 381, 399p–400p
Hallucinogens, 93t, 94
Hallux valgus, 568–569
Halsted hemostatic forceps, *355*
Hammer, percussion, 336, *336*
Hand
    muscles of, 557t
    structure and function of, 553
Handwashing, 271, 272p–273p
    by patient, 274
    in surgical scrub, 277p–279p
Hanging drop method, 848, *850*

Hank uterine dilator, *360*
Hard drive, 159
Hard palate, 549–551, *551,* 730
Hare lip, 624
Harvey, William, 7
Hashish, 93t, 94
Hay fever, 715
Hazardous materials, Material Safety Data Sheets for, 366
HCFA (Health Care Financing Administration), Common
        Procedure Coding System of, 238
HCPCS codes, 238
Head
    examination of, 344
        in emergencies, 492
    muscles of, 557t
Headaches, 598
Head circumference, measurement of, 1004p
Headlight, 338, *338*
Head mirror, 338, *338*
Head tilt/chin thrust, 487, *487*
Head trauma, 596–597, 597t, 598
Healing, wound, 387b–388b
Health care
    allocation of resources in, 23–24, 28b
    costs of, 255
Health Care Financing Administration (HCFA), 230
    Common Procedure Coding System of, 238
Health care surrogate, 40, 593b
Health care system, patient education about, 12b
Health care team, 13–14, 14t, 15t
Health insurance
    assignment of benefits and, 244, 244b, 250, 261
    birthday rule and, 244, 250
    CHAMPUS, 249
    claims administrator for, 244, 246
    coinsurance and, 244b, 255
    coordination of benefits and, 244, 250
    deductible in, 245, 247
    denial of claims and, 250–251
    dependent benefits and, 244, 247, 250
    eligibility for, 247
    fee adjustments and, 198
    filing claims for, 250–255
    fraud and, 34, 43, 239–240, 250, 255
    government-sponsored, 247–248
    group, 246–247
    individual, 247
    malpractice, 51
    managed care and, 255–261
    Medicaid, 249
    Medicare, 247–249. *See also* Medicare
    payments from, 198
    pre-existing conditions and, 244, 250
    self-funded, 246, 247
    terms and concepts for, 244b–246b
    third-party administrator for, 244, 246
    worker's compensation, 149, 249
Health insurance carrier, 244b
Health insurance claims, 244b
    confidentiality of, 255
    denial of, 250–251
    explanation of benefits for, 245b, 255, *256*
    filing of, 250–255
        electronic, 251–254
    processing of
        diagnostic coding for, 230–232
        procedural coding for, 232–238
    required information for, 252b–254b
    usual, customary and reasonable (UCR) tables for, 261
Health insurance companies, 244b
    overpayment by, 211
    refunds to, 211
Health maintenance, teaching for, 80–96
Health maintenance organizations (HMOs), 245b, 257–258
    payments from, 198
Hearing, process of, 616–617
Hearing aids, 617–618
Hearing assessment
    audioscope for, 337
    tuning fork for, 336, *337*
Hearing loss, 617
    age-related, 1025t
    ceruminosis and, 617

communication in, 65–66, 1019
conductive, 617
otosclerosis and, 618–619
perceptual, 617
tests for, 619–621
Heart. See also under Cardiac
structure and function of, 658, 658–659, 663, 664
Heart disease
atherosclerotic, 665, 665–666
myocardial infarction in, 666–667, 667b
surgery for, 668b
chest pain in, 665, 666–667, 667b
diagnosis of, 673–689, 674t. See also Cardiovascular examination
risk factors for, 981t
valvular, 669
Heart murmurs, 675b
Heart rate, fetal, measurement of, 808
Heart sounds, 674, 675b
Heat applications, 531–540, 532t, 533t, 535p–538p
Heat cramps, 499
Heat exhaustion, 499
Heat-related emergencies, 499
Heat stroke, 499
Heat transfer, mechanisms of, 303t
Heel puncture, 915p. See also Skin puncture
Hegar uterine dilator, 360
Height
age-related loss of, 1024t
charting of, 1007, 1008
measurement of, 302, 318p
in children, 999, 1003p
Heimlich maneuver, 487, 487–488, 489p
Helicobacter pylori
gastritis and, 735
peptic ulcers and, 735–736
Helminths, 844–845
Hematemesis, 735
Hematocele, 770
Hematocrit, 928, 944p–945p
Hematocytometer, 925, 926
Hematologic testing, 925–949
Hematology, 922–949
Hematology department, 823
Hematoma, 494
Hematopoiesis, 925
Hematuria, 873, 874
Hemiplegia, 597t
Hemoccult test, 349, 738, 746–749, 748p
Hemocytoblasts, 659
Hemocytometer, 925, 926, 933, 935
Hemodialysis, 756, 757b
blood pressure measurement in, 314
Hemoglobin
mean corpuscular, 929–930
measurement of, 928, 942p–943p
types of, 928
Hemoglobin A, in diabetes, 980
Hemoglobinuria, 873, 874
Hemogram, 925
Hemolytic anemia, 672, 672–673
Hemophilus B vaccine, 994, 995b, 996, 996–997
Hemorrhage, intracranial, 596
Hemorrhagic shock, 493
Hemorrhoidal ligator, 361t
Hemorrhoids, 738
Hemostasis, process of, 930–931
Hemostat, 354
Heparin, coagulation tests and, 931
Hepatic. See also Liver
Hepatic cancer, 741
Hepatic cirrhosis, 740
Hepatic disorders, 739–741
Hepatic enzymes, 971–972
Hepatic fibrosis, 740
Hepatitis, 740, 740t
Hepatitis B, immunization for, 699t, 996, 996–997
Hepatomegaly, 739
Hepatotoxic drugs, 739–740
Hereditary diseases, 290
Hernia, 349
hiatal, 734
inguinal, 771

Herniated disk, 564–567
Heroin, 93t, 94
Herpes genitalis
in females, 787
in males, 773
Herpes labialis, 522, 733–734
Herpes simplex infections, of skin, 522
Herpes stomatitis, 522, 733–734
Herpes zoster, 522
Hiatal hernia, 734
Hierarchy of needs, 75, 75
High blood pressure. See Hypertension
High-density lipoproteins, 981, 981t
Hip
prosthetic, 565b
structure and function of, 553
Hippocrates, 6, 20
Hippocratic Oath, 20
Hiring. See also Employment
staff, 186
Hirschman anoscope, 361
Hispanics
beliefs and practices of, 63t–64t
dietary preferences of, 88t
Histamine, 700
Histamine H₂ antagonists, 418t
Histobrush, 339, 340
Histologist, 825b
Histology department, 824
Histoplasmosis, 844
History, 147, 148b, 290. See also Interviewing
elements of, 290
family, 290
form for, 292–293
interviewing for, 59–61, 60b, 61t, 290, 291–294, 295p. See also Interview
legal aspects of, 290
past, 290
pediatric, 998, 1000–1001
social, 290
techniques for, 59–61, 60b, 61t
HIV. See Human immunodeficiency virus (HIV)
Hives, 524
HMOs, 257–258
payments from, 198
Hodgkin's disease, 696
Holter monitor, 674t, 683, 685b, 686p–688p
Home care, for elderly, 1021
Homeostasis, 514
Home oxygen therapy, in chronic obstructive pulmonary disease, 719
Honesty, 22
Hordeolum, 610
Hormone implants, contraceptive, 809t, 810–811, 814p
Hormone replacement therapy, 813–815
Hormones, 642, 643t
classification of, 648t
functions of, 643t, 648t
organs secreting, 643t
pancreatic, 975–981
pharmacologic, 418t
tests for, 654, 654t
Hospital laboratory, 821
Hospitals, staff privileges at, 28
Host
reservoir, 269
susceptible, 270, 270b
Hot water bottle, 531–540, 532t, 533t, 536p–538p
Household measurements, for medications, 430, 430t, 431t
Human chorionic gonadotropin (HCG), 782
in pregnancy testing, 877, 959, 960
Human growth hormone, 643t, 643–644
deficiency of, 647–648
excess of, 648–649
Human immunodeficiency virus (HIV), 701. See also Acquired immunodeficiency syndrome (AIDS)
testing for
ELISA in, 704–705
Western blot in, 705
Human immunodeficiency virus (HIV) infection
history taking in, 704t
testing for, legal aspects of, 704
Human papillomavirus, condylomata and, 787

Human resources policy, 188, 190b
statement of, 188, 190b
Humoral immunity, 698
Hunter, John, 7
Hyaline cartilage, 547b
Hydrocele, 770, 770
Hydrocephalus, 596
Hydrochloric acid, in digestion, 731
Hydrocortisone, for Addison's disease, 652
Hydrogen ions, in urine, 871
Hydrogen peroxide, as disinfectant, 365t
Hydronephrosis, 758
Hyoglycemia, glucose tolerance test for, 979
Hyoid bone, 551, 551
Hyperadrenocorticalism, 652
Hyperbilirubinemia, 971
Hypercalcemia, 651, 969–970, 982t
Hyperchloremia, 969, 982t
Hyperemesis gravidarum, 803–804
Hyperextension, 547
Hyperglycemia, 647
diabetic, 652
diagnosis of. See Glucose tests
Hyperkalemia, 969, 982t
Hypermagnesemia, 970
Hypernatremia, 969, 982t
Hyperopia, 611
Hyperparathyroidism, 651
Hyperphosphatemia, 970, 982t
Hyperpituitarism, 648–649
Hyperpyrexia, 303
Hypersegs, 927
Hypersensitivity. See Allergies
Hypertension, 667–669
auscultatory gap in, 313
blood pressure measurement in, 313, 314
pregnancy-induced, 804
Hyperthermia, 499
Hyperthyroidism, 650, 651
Hyperuricemia, 971, 982t
Hypnotics, 418t
Hypoadrenocorticalism, 651
Hypocalcemia, 969, 982t
Hypochloremia, 969, 982t
Hypogastric region, 513, 514
Hypoglossal nerve, 587, 588, 588t
Hypoglycemia, 647
diagnosis of. See Glucose tests
Hypokalemia, 969, 982t
Hypomagnesemia, 970
Hyponatremia, 969, 982t
Hypoparathyroidism, 650–651
Hypophosphatemia, 970, 982t
Hypophysis. See Pituitary
Hypopituitarism, 647–648
Hypotension
postural, 312
supine, 801–802
Hypothalamus, 586
Hypothermia, 499–500
Hypothyroidism, 649–650, 650
Hypovolemic shock, 493
Hysterectomy, for endometriosis, 785
Hysterosalpingogram, 476t, 795–796
Hysteroscopy, 788

I

ICD-9-CM coding, 230–232
diagnostic related groups and, 239
fraud and, 239–240
resource-based relative value scale and, 239
Ice packs, 531–540, 532t, 533t, 534p
Icotest, 873, 889p
Identification card, insurance, 247, 248, 250
Idiosyncratic reaction, to drugs, 423t, 424
IgA, 698t
IgD, 698t
IgE, 698t
IgG, 698t
IgM, 698t
Ileostomy, 737, 737
Ileum, 731

Ilium, 553
Imaging, 468–481. *See also* Diagnostic imaging
Immobilization, in emergency care, 496–497
Immune globulin Rh₀, 699t
Immune response, allergic reactions and, 497
Immune serum globulin, 699t
Immune system. *See also* Lymphatic system
  age-related changes in, 1026t
  antibodies in, 696–697
  antigens in, 696–697
  assessment of, serology in, 952–961
  defenses in
    nonspecific, 696
    specific, 697–698, 698t
  disorders of, 700–703
    diagnosis of, 704–705
  functions of, 696–700
Immunity
  acquired, 699t, 699–700
  cell-mediated, 698
  genetic, 698
  humoral, 698
  legal, 50
Immunization(s), 600, 699, 699t, 699–700, 991–996, 994–996
  adult, 350
  booster shots in, 700
  CPT-4 codes for, 235–236
  Haemophilus, 699t, 996, 996–997
  hepatitis B, 699t, 740
  influenza, 699t
  measles, mumps, rubella, 699t
  poliomyelitis, 592, 699t
  rabies, 592
  record of, 995
  schedule for, 350, 994, 996
  side effects of, 995b
  tetanus, 592, 699t, 994, 995b, 996
  vaccines for, 418t, 699, 699t, 700
Immunodeficiency diseases, 700b, 701–704. *See also* Acquired
    immunodeficiency syndrome (AIDS)
Immunoglobulins, 695, 696–697, 697, 697t, 698t
Immunohematology, 961–963
  definition of, 952
Immunohematology department, 823–824
Impacted fracture, 560t, 561
Impaled object, 495
Impedance audiometry, 620
Implantation, 783b
Implied contract, 35
Impotence, 772
Impress account, 214
Inches-centimeters conversion, 318p
Incident reports, 174–178, 175b, 176–177
Incision and drainage, 391, 412p
Incus, 615, 619
Independent practice association, 245b, 258
Indications, drug, 423t
Indicator tapes/strips, sterilization, 367, 370, 370b, 377
Induced abortion, 804, 805t
Infant. *See also* Children
  Apgar score for, 999b
  breast feeding of, 807b
  chest circumference in, 1005p
  congenital anomalies in. *See* Congenital anomalies
  head circumference in, 1004p
  heel puncture for, 915p. *See also* Skin puncture
  length measurement for, 999, 1003p
  pyloric stenosis in, 736
  reflexes in, 993t
  weight measurement for, 999, 1006p–1007p
Infantile hypogammaglobulinemia, 701
Infant respiratory distress syndrome, 716t
Infection. *See also* specific sites and types
  opportunistic, in AIDS, 701, 701t
Infection control, 266–286, 276–287. *See also* Asepsis
  contamination management in, 285, 833–834
  disinfection in, 284–285, 363–364, 365t, 897–898
  handwashing in, 271, 272–273
  isolation precautions for, 271–274
  levels of, 284–285
  medical asepsis for, 270–271, 271b
  sterilization in, 284, 363, 365–372, 368b–369b
Infection control policies, statement of, 189
Infection cycle, 269, 269–270

Infectious diseases, reporting of, 42
Infectious hepatitis, 740, 740t
Infectious mononucleosis, 957
  test for, 957–958
Infectious waste, disposal of, 285–286
Infertility
  bioethical issues in, 25–26
  female, 788–789
    endometriosis and, 785
  male, 773–774, 774b
Inflammation, as defense mechanism, 696
Influenza, immunization for, 699t
Informed consent, 36, 40. *See also* Consent
Infundibulum, 643
Inguinal hernia, 771
Inguinal lymph nodes, 349
Inhalant drugs, 445, 445
Injections, 438–444, 452p–466p
  in children, 1011
  equipment for, 438b, 438–441, 439–441
    sterility of, 438b. *See also* Sterilization
  filling syringe for, 452p–457p
  intradermal, 441, 441–442, 458p–459p
  intramuscular, 438, 443–444, 443–444, 464p–466p
    Z-track, 444, 444, 466p
  subcutaneous, 441, 442–443, 462p–463p
  types of, 441–444
Inoculation, culture, 850–851, 851, 861p–864p
Inpatient settings, 14–15
Inspection, 341
Inspiration, 712–713
Institutional review board, 23, 23
Instrument pouches, 368b
Instruments, 354–363. *See also* Equipment
  boiling of, 370–372
  calibration of, 837, 837–838
  care and handling of, 359–363
  dermatology, 362, 362t
  disinfection of, 284–285, 363–364, 363–365, 364p, 365t
  functional position for, 384, 384
  maintaining supplies of, 372
  obstetric/gynecologic, 360, 360t
  ophthalmology, 362, 362t
  orthopedic, 361, 361t
  otology, 362, 362t
  for physical examination, 336–341, 345p
  proctology, 361, 361t
  recordkeeping for, 372
  rhinology, 362, 362t
  sanitation of, 363, 364p, 365–370
  specialist, 359, 360t–362t
  sterilization of, 284, 363, 365–372, 367, 368b–370b, 371p
  storage of, 372
  urology, 361, 361t
  wrapping of, for sterilization, 368b–369b
Insula, 586
Insulin, 418t, 643t, 647
  in glucose regulation, 975
Insulin-dependent diabetes mellitus. *See also* Diabetes mellitus
Insulin shock, 653, 653t
Insulin syringe, 441, 441
Insurance. *See* Health insurance
Integumentary system. *See also* Skin
  age-related changes in, 1024t
  disorders of, 520–540
  function of, 518
  structure of, 518, 518–520
Interferon, 696, 697b
Interleukin, 698
Intermittent fever, 304, 305t
Internal Revenue Service (IRS), 218
  audits by, 227
  tax returns for, 218, 224–227, 225–226
  tax witholding for, 222, 224
International Classification of Diseases, 9th Revision, Clinical
    Modification (ICF-9-CM) coding, 230–232
  diagnostic related groups and, 230
  fraud and, 239–240
  resource-based relative value scale and, 239
International mail, 138
Interpreters, 66
Interrogatory, 49b
Interstital cells, 766
Interstitial cell-stimulating hormone, 643t, 644

Intertrigo, 526
Interventional radiographic techniques, 478
Intervertebral disk, herniated, 564–567
Interview, 291–294. *See also* Communication; Medical history
  of children, 66
  employment, 186, 1055–1059, 1056b, 1057b
  exit, 1059b
  of hearing impaired, 65–66
  procedure for, 295p
  of sight impaired, 66
  techniques for, 59–61, 60b, 61t, 291–294
Intestinal disorders, 736–739
Intestinal gas, 739
Intestinal studies, patient preparation for, 743b, 744p–745p
Intestines. *See also* Colon; Small intestine
  structure and function of, 731–732, 732
Intra-arterial drug administration, 445
Intra-articular drug administration, 445
Intracranial hemorrhage, 596
Intradermal injections, 441, 441–442, 458p–459p
Intradermal tests, 530, 704
Intramuscular injections, 442–444, 443–444, 464p–466p
  Z-track, 444, 444, 466p
Intraocular pressure, 609
  elevated, in glaucoma, 611
  measurement of, 614, 615
Intrathecal drug administration, 445
Intrauterine device (IUD), 810, 811p–812p, 813p
Intravenous drug administration, 445
Intravenous pyelogram (IVP), 762
Intrinsic muscles, 553
Introitus, 781
Invasion of privacy, 48
Inventory
  of controlled substances, 419–420
  maintenance of, 191, 372, 836, 837–838
Inversion, 547, 550
Invoices, payment of, 220–221
Iodinated contrast media, 475
Iodine
  deficiency of, goiter and, 649
  as disinfectant, 365t
  thyroid hormones and, 643t, 644
Iontophoresis, 567
Iris, 608, 608–609
Iron deficiency anemia
  diagnosis of, 928, 929
  patient education in, 928
Irrigation
  of ear, 619, 621, 634p–635p
  of eye, 615, 631p–632p
    eye wash basin for, 833
Irritable bowel syndrome, 737–738
Ischium, 553
Ishihara color plate, 614, 614, 629p
Islets of Langerhans, 643t, 647
Isolation precautions, 271–274, 274t, 275b
  standard, 273, 274, 275b
  transmission-based, 273–274, 274t
Itching
  in diabetes, 652
  in eczema, 524
  in urticaria, 524
IUD (intrauterine device), 810, 811p–812p, 813p
Ives rectal speculum, 361

J

Jacksonian seizures, 595
Jaeger tests, 613–614
Jaundice, 971
Jaw, 549–551, 551
Jaw thrust, 487, 487
Jejunum, 731
Jenner, Edward, 7
Job description, 183, 184, 185
Job opportunities, 1048–1060. *See also* Employment
Jock itch, 522
Joint(s), 546–549
  age-related changes in, 1025t
  cartilaginous, 548t
  contractures of, 567
  dislocations of, 559
  fibrous, 548t

injuries of, emergency management of, 496–497
movement of, 547
prosthetic, 564, 565b
range of motion of, 547–549, 549–550
sprains of, 558
synovial, 547, 548t
types of, 546–547, 548t
Joint Commission on Accreditation of Health Care Organizations (JCAHO), 170–171m171b, 172t, 192
Jones cross-action towel clamp, 358
Juvenile myxedema, 650

K

Kegel exercises, 786
Keith needles, 383
Kelly clamp, 354, 355
Kelly hemostatic forceps, 355
Keloids, 525
Keratin, 519
Ketoacidosis, diabetic, 652, 653
Ketones, 652
   urinary, 872, 887p
Keyes cutaneous punch, 362, 362t
Kidney. See also under Renal
   age-related changes in, 1026t
   in blood pressure maintenance, 753
   in calcium and vitamin D metabolism, 753
   in erythropoietin production, 753
   filtration in, 753
   in fluid balance, 753
   functions of, 753, 754–755, 968–969
   in pH regulation, 753
   structure of, 754, 754–755, 755
   tumors of, 760
Kidney stones, 757, 758b, 875, 876p
Killer T cells, 698
Kilograms-pounds conversion, 317p
Kinesics, 57, 58t, 59
Kits, reagent, 955–956
Knee
   ligaments of, 554
      injuries of, 558
   structure and function of, 554
Knee-chest position, 343, 344t
Knee replacement, 565b
Korotkoff sounds, 312–313, 313t
Krause's end bulbs, 627t
Krebs's cycle, 975
Kyphosis, 564, 566b

L

Labor and delivery, 806
   abbreviations used in, 807b
Laboratory, 818–839
   hospital, 821
   physician's office, 821–823
      testing in, guidelines for, 824, 825b
   reference, 820–821
   safety in, 828–834
   types of, 820–823
Laboratory codes, 235
Laboratory data sheet, 822
Laboratory departments, 823–824
   blood bank, 823–824
   clinical chemistry, 823
   coagulation, 823
   hematology, 823
   immunohematology, 823–824
   microbiology, 824
   pathology, 824
   serology, 824
   toxicology, 823
   urinalysis, 823
Laboratory equipment, 824–828. See also Equipment
Laboratory manager, 825b
Laboratory personnel, 824, 825b
   education and training standards for, 838–839
   proficiency testing for, 838–839
Laboratory request forms, 340, 821, 821, 822b
Laboratory safety, government standards for, 192
Laboratory technician, 825b
Laboratory tests. See also Clinical chemistry; Microbiology

complexity of, 834–835
errors in, detection of, 838, 838
government standards for, 192, 824, 834–839
medical assistant's role in, 845
package insert instructions for, 824, 825b
quality assurance for, 838
quality control for, 835–838
requests for, 107
results of, reporting of, via telephone, 107
scheduling of, 123
specimens for. See under Specimen(s)
Lacerations, 494b
Lacrimal apparatus, 609, 609
   infection of, 612
Lacrimal bone, 551, 551
Lactate dehydrogenase, after myocardial infarction, 973, 973t
Lahey retractor, 359
Lamp, gooseneck, 338
Lancets, 902–903, 903
Laparoscopy, 785, 797, 798
Large intestine. See Colon; Rectum
Laryngeal mirror, 338, 339
Laryngectomy, 710
Laryngitis, 715–716
Laryngoscope, 339
Laryngotracheobronchitis, 716t
Larynx
   cancer of, 719
   structure and function of, 710
Laser angioplasty, 478
Laser surgery, 392–393
   assisting with, 411p
Late patients, scheduling of, 122
Lateral, 512
Lateral epicondylitis, 567–568
Lateral files, 153
Latex agglutination test, 952–953
   for infectious mononucleosis, 957–958
   for rheumatoid factor, 957
   for rubella, 958
Latex allergy, 897
Law. See also under Legal
   administrative, 34
   branches of, 34
   common, 34
   ethics and, 22
   private (civil), 34
   public, 34
   sources of, 34
   statutory, 34
   tort, 47–49
Law of agency, 50–51
Lawsuits, 34, 48–51, 49, 49b. See also Malpractice; Negligence; Tort(s)
   prevention of, 51b
   rise in, 35
Lazy colon, 739
Leads, electrocardiogram, 675, 676–678, 677, 678b, 678t
Learning goals and objectives, 73
Ledger, 207
Ledger card, 206, 207–208, 208
Leeuwenhoek, Anton von, 7
Left bundle branch, 664, 664
Leg
   assessment of, in emergencies, 493
   examination of, 349
   muscles of, 557t
Legal documents
   appointment book as, 117
   day sheets as, 207
   ledger cards as, 207–208
   medical records as, 117, 290
Legal issues, 34–51. See also Law
   abandonment, 39
   Americans with Disabilities Act, 192
   child abuse, 1012–1013
   coding, 239–240
   consent, 39–42
   contracts, 35–39
   controlled substances, 44, 44b, 416–420
   credit, 199
   debt collection, 199–200, 202
   disclosures, 42–43
   elder abuse, 1022

emergency care
   duty to provide, 46–47
      liability for, 44
employee firing, 187
employee hiring, 186
employee references, 187
Family and Medical Leave Act, 192
health insurance claims, 255
HIV testing, 704
laboratory safety, 192
litigation process, 49, 49b
medical practice acts, 43–44
medical records, 147–148, 149
Medicare fraud, 239–240
negligence and malpractice, 47–48
   defenses to, 49–51
in office management, 192
physician-patient relationship, 35–39
radiography, 480
sexual harassment, 192
telephone consultation, 715
torts, 47–49
Leiomyomas, 787–788
Length
   charting of, 1007, 1008
   measurement of, 999, 1003p
Lens, 608, 608
   Morgan, 632
   opacities of, 610, 610
Letters
   addressing of, 136, 136, 137b
   annotation of, 139
   components of, 128–130, 129
   cover, for resumé, 1053–1054, 1055
   dictation and transcription of, 140–141, 141b
   editing of, 132–135, 133b, 134t
   formats for, 130, 130, 131, 132b
   grammar tips for, 133b
   postage for, 136–137, 137
   post-interview, 1058, 1058–1059
   proofreading of, 132–134, 134t
   receiving and handling of, 138–139, 139b
   of resignation, 1059b, 1059–1060
   sending of, 135–138, 136–138, 137b
   spelling tips for, 133b
   writing of, 57, 131–135, 132b, 134b
Leukocyte esterase reaction, 873
Leukocytes, 659, 660, 661, 662t
   formation of, 924–925
   measurement of, 925–927, 932p–936p
   types of, 924, 927
Leukocytosis, causes of, 925–926
Leukoderma, 526
Leukopenia, causes of, 925
Levodopa, for Parkinson's disease, 1027
Liabilities, financial, 206
Liability, 47–48
   defenses to, 49–50
   Good Samaritan Acts and, 44
   incident reports and, 175b
Libel, 48
Lice, 523
Licensed practical nurse (LPN), 13
Licensure, 43
Ligaments, 547
   injuries of, 558
   of knee, 554
      injuries of, 558
Light, examination, 337
Lightening, 806
Limb-girdle dystrophy, 569
Limbs. See Arm; Leg
Linens, soiled, handling of, 285
Lingual tonsils, 694, 710
Lip, cleft, 624
Lipase, 974–975
Lipids, 981t, 981–982
Lipoprotein
   high-density, 981, 981t
   low-density, 981, 981t
Listening, active, 59
Lister, Joseph, 8
Lister bandage scissors, 354, 357
Literature searches, computerized, 165

Lithotomy position, *343, 344t*
Lithotripsy, 757, *758b*
Litigation, 34
Liver, 732–733, *733. See also under* Hepatic
  cancer of, 741
  disorders of, 739–741
  drug metabolism in, 421–423
  enlargement of, 739
  functions of, 971
Liver function tests, 740, 971–972, 972t
Living will, *593b*
Load records, 372
Local anesthesia, 381
Lochia, 807
Lockjaw, 592
Lofstrand crutches, *571, 571–577. See also* Crutches
Log, quality control, *835, 839*
Log-in screen, *162, 162*
Long, Crawford Williamson, 8
Long-term care, for elderly, 1021
Loop of Henle, *755, 755*
Lordosis, 564, *566b*
Lou Gehrig's disease, 594
Low-density lipoproteins, 981, 981t
Lower respiratory disorders, 716–719
LSD, 93t, 94
Lubb, dubb, in blood pressure measurement, 312–313, *328p*
Lubricant, 340
Lucae bayonet forceps, *362*
Lumbar puncture, 599–600, *601, 602p–603p*
Lung. *See also under* Pulmonary
  alveoli of, 711
  cancer of, 719
  structure and function of, 711–712, *712*
Luteinizing hormone, 643t, 644, 782
Luxation, 559
Lymph, 692
Lymphadenitis, 695
Lymphangitis, 695
Lymphatic system
  disorders of, 695–696
  spleen in, 694
  structure and function of, 692–695, *693*
  thymus in, 694–695
  tonsils in, 694
Lymph nodes, 692, *693*, 694t
  inguinal, 349
Lymphocytes, *924*
  assessment of, 927
  B, 697–698
  function of, 927
  T, 698
Lymphogram, 476t
Lymphogranuloma venereum, 772–773
Lymphoma, 696
Lymphosarcoma, 696
Lymph vessels, 692
Lysergic acid diethylamide (LSD), 93t, 94

M
Macrophages, 692, 696
Macules, 520, *521*
Magnesium balance, 970
Magnetic resonance imaging (MRI), 477
Mail, 136–138. *See also* Letters
  certified, *137, 138, 138*
  COD, 138
  express, 137
  first–fourth class, 137–138
  international, 138
  postage for, 136–137, *137, 137b*
  priority, 137
  receiving and handling of, 138–139, *139b*
  registered, 138
Mailed reminders, 120–121, *121*
Malabsorption syndromes, 736–737
Malignant melanoma, 526, *527b, 528, 528–529*
  urine melanin test for, 530
Malleus, 615, *619*
Malocclusion, 733
Malpractice, 47–48
  defenses to, 49–50
  Good Samaritan Acts and, 44

incident reports and, *175b*
  rise in claims for, 35
Malpractice insurance, 51
Mammogram, 478, *478b*
  schedule for, 350
Managed care, 245b–246b, 255–261
  future of, 260b–261b
  health maintenance organizations and, 257–258
  peer review organizations and, 257
  physician hospital organizations and, 259
  preferred provider organizations and, 258–259
  ultilization review in, 255–257
Mandible, 549, *551*
Mandl, D.M., 9
Manipulation, 341
Mantoux test, 441–442, *460p–461p*, 531
Manuals, policies and procedures, 187–189
Marie-Strumpell disease, 569
Marijuana, 93t, 94
Mask, 274, 274t, *275*
Maslow's hierarchy of needs, *75, 75*
Mastication, 730
Material Safety Data Sheets, 366, 828, *832b*
Matrix, appointment book, 115, *116*
Maxilla, 549, *551*
Maxillary sinuses, 622, 709, *709*
Meals on Wheels, 1030
Mean cell volume, 929
Mean corpuscular hemoglobin, 929–930
Mean corpuscular hemoglobin concentration, 929–930
Measles-mumps-rubella immunization, 699t, *994, 995b, 996,*
  996–997
Measurements
  anthropometric, 302
    in children, 999, *1003p–1007p*
  apothecary, 430, *430, 431t*
  conversion methods for, 431t, 431–432, 432t
  for medications, 429–432, 430t, 431t
  metric, 431t, 431–432, 432t
    for drug dosages, 430, 431t
Media. *See* Culture media
Medial, 512
Median cubital vein, blood collection from, *896, 896. See also*
  Blood sample, collection of
Mediastinum, 658
Medicaid, 249
Medical asepsis, 270–271, 271b, 276t, 363. *See also* Asepsis;
  Infection control
  handwashing for, 271, 272–273
  patient education for, 274
Medical assistant
  appearance of, 12, *12*, 1042–1043
  as attitude transmitter, 102, 1043
  certification of, 10–11, 43–44
  characteristics of, 12–13, 1041–1043
  definition of, 9
  duties of
    administrative, 11
    clinical, 11–12
  education of, 10
  employment opportunities for, 14–15, 1048–1060
  externships for, 10, 1036–1045
  first impression of, 103
  professional image of, 102–103, 1041, 1042–1043
  professional organizations for, 9, 9–10, 11
  as role model, 102
Medical assistant's creed, 21
Medical assisting
  history of, 9
  inpatient settings for, 14–15
  outpatient settings for, 14–15
Medical ethics, 20–30. *See also* Bioethics; Ethics
Medical examiner reports, 42
Medical history. *See* History
Medical laboratory. *See* Laboratory
Medical office. *See* Office
Medical Office Management Association, 191
Medical practice acts, 43–44
Medical records, 142–155. *See also* Documentation
  active, 153
  additions to, 149
  charting by exception in, 146
  classification of, 153
  closed, 153

computerized, 146–147
  confidentiality of, 21
  contents of, 144
  copying of, 154
  correction of, 149
  documentation forms for, 145–147
  filing of, 150–153
  flow sheets for, 146, *147*
  history in, 147
  immunization, 995
  inactive, 153
  as legal documents, 147–148, 149
  making entries in, 147–149
  as negligence defense, 49–50
  organization of, 144–145
  problem-oriented, 144–145
  progress notes for, *145,* 145–146, *146,* 148b
  radiography in, 480
  release of, *154,* 154–155
  reporting requirements for, 42–43, 43b, 155
  source-oriented, 144
  standard, 144
  storage of, 144, 144b, 153–154
  subpoena for, 49b, 154
  tampering with, 149
  transcription of, 140–141, *141b*
  for worker's compensation, 149
Medical research, bioethical issues in, 24
Medical technologist, *825b*
Medicare, 247–249
  diagnostic related groups (DRGs) for, 238–239
  fraud in, coding and, 239–240
  Medigap coverage for, 248–249
  resource-based relative value scale (RBRVS) for, 239
Medicare fraud, 34, 43, 250
Medicare taxes, 224
Medication(s), 414–425
  absorption of, 421
  administration of
    buccal, 435, *449p*
    in children, 1010–1011
    in ear, 621, *635p–637p, 636p–638p*
    in eye, 614–615, *630p–631p, 630p–632p*
    by inhalation, 445, *445*
    intra-arterial, 445
    intra-articular, 445
    intrathecal, 445
    intravenous, 445
    mucosal, 435–436
    nasal, *639p–640p*
    oral, 435, 436t, *446p–449p*
    parenteral, 438–444, *452p–466p. See also* Injections
    rectal, 436–437, *437, 438*
    routes of, 434–445, *446p–466p*
    safety guidelines for, 428–429
    seven rights for, 429
    topical, 437–438, *451p*
    transdermal, 438, *450p*
    vaginal, 437, *437*
  allergy to, 423t, 424
  in ampules, 439, *439*
  in cartridges, *439,* 439–440
  classification of, 416, 417t–418t
  common abbreviations for, 428, 428t
  distribution of, 421
  dosage of
    calculation of, 432–433
      for children, *433,* 433–434
    measurement systems for, 429–432, *430,* 431b, 431t
  drug interactions with, computerized information on, 164
  for elderly, 1022–1023
    compliance with, 1018–1019
  excretion of, 423
  hepatotoxic, 739–740
  information sources for, 424–425
  interactions of, 423–424
  legal aspects of, 416–420
  local effects of, 421
  metabolism of, 421–423
  names of, 416, *416b*
  patient teaching for, 94–96, *95*
  pharmacodynamics of, 420–421, *422b*
  pharmacokinetics of, 421–423
  in pregnancy, 800, *800b*

prescriptions for, 420, *421*
  telephone refills for, 107
scheduling tool for, 94, *95*
sensitivity testing for, 851
sources of, 420, 422t
systemic effects of, 421
terminology for, 423t
in vials, 439, *439*
Medication errors
  documentation of, 429b
  incident reports for, 174–178
  prevention of, 428–429
Medicine, history of, 6–9
Medicine codes, 235–236
Medigap coverage, 248–249
Meditation, 92
Medulla oblongata, 586–587
Meetings
  agenda for, 139, *140*
  minutes of, 139
Megabytes, 158
Melanin, 519
  urine, 530
Melanocytes, 519
Melanocyte-stimulating hormone, 643t, 644
Melanoma, 526, 527b, *528*, 528–529
  urine melanin test for, 530
Melatonin, 647
Melena, 735
Membrane, cell, 508, *508*, 509t
Memorandums, 135, *135. See also* Written communication
Memory aids, for elderly, 1018–1019
Memory cells, 698, 700
Meniere's disease, 618
Meninges, 583–584
Meningitis, 590–591
Meningocele, 595–596, *596*
  prenatal screening for, 600, 808
Meniscus, tears of, 558
Menopause, 812–815, 1026t
Menorrhagia, 784
Menstrual cycle, 781–783, *783*
  proliferative (follicular) phase of, 781–783
  secretory (luteal) phase of, 782
Menstruation, 782–783
Mensuration, 341
Mental health, in elderly, 1019–1020
Meperidine, 93t, 94
Mercury sphygmomanometer, 312, *312*
Mercy killing, 27b
Mescaline, 93t, 94
Messages
  checking for, 104
  recording of, 108
Metabolic acidosis, 969, 970
  causes of, 974t
Metabolic alkalosis, 970
  causes of, 974t
Metabolism, 729
  drug, 421–423
Metaphysis, 545, *545*
Metazoa, 844–845
Metered mail, 136–137, *137*
Methadone, 93t, 94
Methamphetamine, 93t, 94
Methaqualone, 93t
Metric measurements
  conversion methods for, 431t, 431–432, 432t
  for drug dosages, 430, 431t
Metrorrhagia, 784
Mexican Americans
  beliefs and practices of, 63t
  dietary preferences of, 88t
Microbiologic inoculation, 850–851, *851*, 861p–864p
Microbiologic testing
  culture inoculation in, 850–851, *851*, 861p–864p
  culture media for, 846–847
  medical assistant's role in, 845
  microscopy in, 848–851, 854p–860p
  sensitivity testing in, 851
  smears for
    preparation of, 848, *850*, 854p–856p
    staining of, 849, 850b, 856p–860p
  specimens for. *See also* Specimen(s)

collection and handling of, 845–848, 849t
  transport of, 847–848, 853p
  staining in, 849–850, 856p–860p
  streptococcal testing in, 851–852
Microbiology, 840–864. *See also under* Laboratory; Specimen(s)
Microbiology department, 824
Microcollection, blood, 901–903, 913–919, 914p–918p
Microcytosis, 929
Microfiche, 144
Microfilm, 144
Microhematocrit, 928, 944p–945p
Microorganisms
  bacteria, 842t, 842–843, *843. See also* Bacteria
  beneficial, 268
  defenses against, 268
  exogenous, 268
  fungi, 844, *844*
  growth of, requirements for, 269
  in infection cycle, *269*, 269–270
  pathogenic, 268
  specimens of. *See* Specimen(s)
  staining of, 849–850
  virulent, 268
  viruses, 844
Micropipet dilution systems, 903, *904*
Microprocessor, 158
Microscope, 825–827, *826*, 827b
Microscopy
  slide preparation for, 848, *850*
  urine examination on, 874–875, 890p–891p
Micturition, 752
Midbrain, 586
Middle ear, 615–616
  infection of, 618, 997t, 998
Miessner's corpuscles, 627t
Migraine headaches, 598
Military time, 148, *148*
Mineralocorticoids, 643t, 646
Minerals, sources and functions of, 85t
Ministroke, 671
Minor
  consent of, 40, 42
  emancipated, 40
  release of medical records to, 155
Minor office surgery
  assisting with, 374–412, 411p–412p
  clean-up after, 393, 394b
  consent for, 379, *380*
  draping for, 379–381
  electrosurgery in, *391*, 391–392
  equipment setup for, 376–379
  for incision and drainage, 390
  instruments for, 381–382
  laser surgery in, 392–393
  local anesthesia for, 381
  patient instructions for, 379, 392
  patient positioning for, 379–380
  patient preparation for, 379–381
  postsurgical procedures in, 393
  for skin lesions, 389–390, 411p–412p
  skin preparation for, 381, 399p–400p
  specimen collection in, 393
  sterile field for, 376–379
Minutes, of meetings, 139
Mirror
  head, 338, *338*
  laryngeal, 338, *339*
Miscarriage, 804, 805t
Missed appointments, 122–123
Mission statement, 188, *188*
Mitosis, 508
Mitral stenosis, 669
Mitral valve, 662, *663*
Mixed culture, 845
Mixed deafness, 617
Mobile radiographic units, 470, *471*
Modem, 161
Molds, 844
Molecules, 507
Moles, 526
Monitor, computer, 159
Monocytes, *924*, 927
Mononucleosis, 695

Montgomery straps, 389, *391*
Morgan lens, 632
Morning sickness, 803–804
Moro reflex, 993t
Morphine, 93t, 94
Motherboard, 158
Motor function, assessment of, 599
  in children, 604
Mourning, 67–68, 68b
Mouse, 161
Mouth
  disorders of, 733–734
  examination of, 348
  structure and function of, 730
MRI (magnetic resonance imaging), 477
Mucolytics, 418t
Mucosal drug administration, 435–436, 449p
Mucous membranes, gastrointestinal, 728, *728*
Mucous plug, 798, 806
Mucus, urinary, 875
Multidisciplinary health care team, 13–14, 14t, 15t
Multimedia upgrades, 161
Multiple sclerosis, 593b, 593–594
Mummy wrap, 999, *1002*, 1002p
Mumps, immunization for, 699t, *994*, 995b, 996, 996–997
Mumps orchitis, 772
Murmurs, 675b
Muscle(s)
  abdominal, 557t
  antagonist, 554
  cardiac, 554–555, *555*
  fixator, 554
  function of, 555–556, 557t
  of head and neck, 557t
  insertion of, 556
  intrinsic, 553
  of lower extremities, 557t
  ocular, 609
    strabismus and, 612
  origin of, 556
  prime mover, 554
  smooth, 554, *555*
  striated (skeletal), 554, *555*
  structure of, 554–555, *555*, *556*
  of trunk, 557t
  of upper extremities, 557t
Muscle tonus, 556
Muscular atrophy, postpoliomyelitis, 592
Muscular dystrophy, 569
Muscular tissue, 509, 509t, *510*
Musculoskeletal disorders, 556–570
  ambulatory aids in, 570–578
  diagnostic studies in, 570
  pain in, 558b
  physical examination in, 570
Musculoskeletal pain, 558b
Musculoskeletal system
  age-related changes in, 1024t
  structure and function of, 544–556
Mycology, 844
Mycoses, 844
Myelin sheath, 582, *583*
Myelography, 476t, 599
Myelomeningocele, 595–596, *596*
  prenatal screening for, 600, 808
Myocardial infarction, 666–667, 667b
  cardiac enzymes after, 973t, 973t
  emergency care in, 497
Myocarditis, 671–672
Myocardium, 659
Myoglobin, in urine, 873, 874
Myometrium, 781
Myopia, 611–612, *612*
Myxedema, 650

N

Nail follicles, 519
Nails, fungal infection of, 523
Narcotics, 93t, 94
  as controlled substances, 44, 416–420, 419t
  dispensing of, 44
Narrative documentation, 145, *145*
Nasal bones, 551, *551*

Nasal disorders, 623–625
    diagnosis and treatment of, 624–625
Nasal forceps, 362, 362t
Nasal medications, administration of, 639p–640p
Nasal polyps, 624
Nasal septum, 348
Nasal speculum, 336, 337, 362, 362t
Nasal turbinates, 551, 551, 622, 709
National Center for Health Statistics, 230
National Committee for Clinical Laboratory Standards, 837
National Council on Patient Information and Education
    (NCPIE), 95–96
Native Americans, beliefs and practices of, 64t
Natural immunity, 698
Nausea and vomiting, in pregnancy, 803–804
Nearsightedness, 611–612, 612
Near vision, testing of, 613–614
Nebulizers, 445, 445
Neck. See also under Spinal
    assessment of, in emergencies, 492
    examination of, 344–348
    fractures of, 564
    muscles of, 557t
Needle holder, 354, 356
Needles, 440, 440. See also Sharps
    disposal of, 285–286, 286, 359–363, 898
    gauge of, 899
    phlebotomy, 898–899
    recapping of, 898
    suture, 382–383
    venipuncture, 898–899
Needle sticks, prevention of, 275b, 285–286, 286
Negative feedback, 514
Neglect
    child, 1011–1013
    of elderly, 526, 1021–1022
    reporting of, 42
Negligence, 47–48
    comparative, 50
    contributory, 50
    defenses to, 49–50
    Good Samaritan Acts and, 44
    incident reports and, 175b
Nematodes, 845
Neonate. See Infant
Nephron, 754, 754, 755
Nephrostomy, 758
Nerves
    afferent, 582
    cranial, 587, 588, 588t
    disorders of, 580–604. See also Neurologic disorders
    efferent, 582
    spinal, 587, 589
Nervous system
    age-related changes in, 1025t
    autonomic, 582, 587–590, 590, 591t
    central. See also Brain; Spinal cord
        structure and function of, 583–587
    communication in, 582–583
    parasympathetic, 589, 591t
    peripheral, 587, 588, 588t, 589
    structure and function of, 582–590
    sympathetic, 587–589, 591t
Nervous tissue, 509, 509t, 510
Net pay, 222
Networking, 1051
Neubauer hemocytometer, 925, 933, 935
Neural tube defects, 595–596, 596
    prenatal screening for, 600, 808
Neurogenic shock, 493
Neuroleptics, 418t
Neurologic assessment, in infant, 993t
Neurologic disorders, 580–604, 590–604
    degenerative, 593–594
    developmental, 595–596
    diagnosis of
        in children, 601–604, 993t
        prenatal, 600–601
    infectious, 590–593
    physical examination in, 598–599
    traumatic, 596–597, 597t, 598
Neurologic emergencies, 497
Neurologic hammer, 336, 336

Neuron, structure of, 582, 583
Neurotransmitters, 582–583
Neutron, 506, 507
Neutrophil band, 924, 927
Neutrophils, 927
    function of, 927
Nevus, 526
    melanoma and, 526, 527b
Newspaper advertisements, employment, 1051
Nicotine, 92–94, 93t
Nightingale, Florence, 8, 8
911 system, 108, 121, 484
Nitrite test, for bacteriuria, 873
Nitroglycerin, patient education for, 666
Nitroprusside reaction, for urinary ketones, 872, 887p
Nodule, 520, 520
Nomogram, body surface area, for children, 433, 433
Non-A, non-B hepatitis, 740
Noncompliance, 74
Non compos mentis, 40
Non-English speakers, 65–66
Non–insulin-dependent diabetes mellitus, 652–653. See also
    Diabetes mellitus
Nonlanguage sounds, 57
Nonprotein nitrogenous compounds, renal function and,
    970–971
Nonstress test, 808
Nonverbal communication, 57–59, 58t, 59. See also Commu-
    nication
Norepinephrine, 643t, 646
Norplant, 809t, 810–811, 814p
Nose. See also under Nasal
    disorders of, 623–625
    examination of, 348, 719–720
    instruments for, 362, 362t
    structure and function of, 622–623, 623, 709
Nosebleed, 624
No shows, 122–123
Nostrils, examination of, 348
Notebook, communication, 183
Notice, of resignation, 1059b
Nuclear medicine, 477–478
Nucleus, atomic, 506, 507
Numbers, in written communication, 133b
Numeric filing, 151–152, 152b
Nurse
    licensed practical, 13
    registered, 13
Nursemaid's elbow, 559
Nurse practitioner (NP), 13–14
Nursing homes, 1021
Nutrition, 82–89. See also Diet
    cultural factors in, 88t
    in diabetes, 85
    dietary guildelines for, 82, 83, 84, 85t–87t
    in elderly, 1030
    Food Guide Pyramid for, 82, 83
    patient teaching for, 82–89
Nutritional anemia, 672, 672–673

O
Obesity
    diabetes and, 652–653
    intertrigo and, 526
Obligate intracellular parasites, 843–844
Oblique fracture, 560t, 561
Obstetric care, 797–808. See also Pregnancy
    abbreviations used in, 807b
    bioethical issues in, 24–26
    instruments for, 360t
    postpartum, 806–808
    prenatal, 798–806
Obstipation, 738
Occipital bone, 551, 551
Occipital lobe, 585, 586, 586
Occlusive arterial disease, 666. See also Atherosclerosis
Occult blood test, 349, 738, 746–749, 748p
Occupational Safety and Health Administration (OSHA), 172,
    192
    laboratory safety and, 832, 834
Occurrence reports, 174–178, 175b, 176–177
Oculomotor nerve, 587, 588, 588t

Office
    automated front desk in, 165
    organizational structure of, 182, 182
    in pediatric practice, 988–989
    policy and procedure manuals for, 187–189
    preparation of, 103
    reception area in, 104–105
Office emergencies, 482–501. See also Emergencies
Office hours, 114
Office management, 180–192
    banking in, 212–214
    bioethical issues in, 28–29
    bookkeeping in, 206–212
    legal issues in, 192, 202
Office management software, 164
Office manager, 182–183
    professional organizations for, 191
    qualities of, 182
    responsibilities of, 182–191
        communication, 183
        discipline, 186, 186–187
        educational, 191
        employee evaluations, 185, 186
        financial, 190–191
        firing, 187
        policy and procedure manuals, 187–189
        promotional materials, 189–190
        staff-related, 184–187
        staff scheduling, 187
Office manuals, 187–189
Office supplies
    maintenance and inventory of, 191
    purchasing of, 219–221
Office visits
    appointments for, 114–123. See also Appointments
    fees for, 198
    greeting patients in, 103
    hours for, 114
    pediatric, 989
    sign-in sheets for, 114
    termination of, 105
Ointment, eye, administration of, 614–615, 630p–631p
Olecranon, 552
Olfactory nerve, 587, 588, 588t, 622–623
Oligospermia, 773, 774b
Oliguria, 756
Onychomycosis, 523
Open fracture, 560t
Operating budget, 190
Operating system, 159
Ophthalmology, instruments for, 362, 362t
Ophthalmoscope, 337, 337, 612–613, 613
Opportunistic infections, in AIDS, 701, 701t
Optic disk, 608, 609
Optician, 612
Optic nerve, 587, 588, 588t, 608, 609
Optometrist, 612
Oral cavity
    disorders of, 733–734
    examination of, 348
    structure and function of, 730
Oral contraceptives, 809t
Oral drug administration, 435, 436t, 446p–449p
Oral hypoglycemics, 418t
Oral temperature, 303, 303, 304b. See also Temperature
Orchitis, 772
Organ donor card, 26, 26
Organic impotence, 772
Organizational chart, 182, 182
Organ of Corti, 616, 619
Organs, 509–511, 511t
Organ transplantation. See Transplantation
Oropharynx. See also Oral cavity; Pharynx
    structure and function of, 730
Orthopedics, instruments for, 361, 361t
Oscillating plaster saw, 361
Ossicles, 615, 619
Osteoarthritis, 569
Osteoporosis, 569–570, 1024, 1024t
Osteosarcoma, 570
Otis/Dittel urethral sound, 361
Otitis externa, 618
Otitis media, 618, 997t, 998

Otology, instruments for, 362, 362t
Otosclerosis, 618–619
Otoscope, 336–337, 337, 613, 613
Outlier, 239
Outpatient settings, 14–15
Outpatient surgery, HCPCS codes for, 238
Oval window, 616, 619
Ovary, 643t, 647
    cancer of, 788, 789t
    cysts of, 788
    disorders of, 653
    polycystic, 788
    structure and function of, 780, 780
Overdraft protection, 212
Overdue accounts
    bookkeeping and, 210–211
    collection of, 201–202
Overdue notices, 201, 201
Oviducts, 780, 780–781
Ovulation, 780, 782
Ovum, 780
    fertilization of, 782, 783b
    release and transport of, 782
Oxygen therapy, in chronic obstructive pulmonary disease, 719
Oxytocin, 643t, 644

P
Pacemaker
    artificial, 665b
    sinoatrial node as, 664, 670
Pacinian corpuscles, 627t
Package insert instructions, for laboratory tests, 824, 825b
Packed red cells, 863
Packing slip, 219
Paget's disease, 560t
Pain
    back, posture and, 566b
    chest
        in heart disease, 665, 667b
            nitroglycerin for, 666
        in pericarditis, 671
        telephone reports of, 108, 121
    musculoskeletal, 558b
    perception of, 626
    referred, 626–627
    treatment of, 627
Palate, 549–551, 551, 730
    cleft, 623–624
Palatine bones, 549–551, 551
Palatine tonsils, 694, 710
Palpation, 341
    of chest, 720
    of pulse, 308, 310
    of uterus, 792p–795p
Pancreas, 643t, 647, 733, 733
    disorders of, 742. See also Diabetes mellitus
Pancreatic cancer, 742
Pancreatic enzymes, 974
Pancreatic function, assessment of, 974–981
Pancreatic hormones, 975–981
Pancreatitis, 742
Panhypopituitarism, 648
Paper drapes, 380–381
Papillae lingua, 730
Papillary layer, dermal, 519
Papillomas, 522
Papoose wrap, 999, 1002, 1002p
Pap smear, 788, 790–791, 791t, 792p–795p
    equipment for, 339, 339–340
    schedule for, 350
Papules, 521, 522
Paralanguage, 57, 57b
Paralysis
    in poliomyelitis, 591–592
    in spinal cord injury, 596, 596t, 597
    types of, 596t
Paraplegia, 597t
Parasites

metazoal, 844–845
obligate intracellular, 843–844
protozoal, 844
of skin, 522–523
stool examination for, 745, 746b, 747p
Parasitology, 844
Parasympathetic nervous system, 589, 591t
Parathormone, 645
Parathyroid hormone, 645
Parathyroids, 643t, 644–645
    disorders of, 650–651
Parenteral drug administration, 438–444, 452p–466p. See also Injections
Parietal bones, 551, 551
Parietal lobe, 585, 586, 586
Parity, 799b
Parkinson's disease, 1023–1028, 1026
Parotid glands, 730
Partial thromboplastin time (PTT), 931
Pasteur, Louis, 7–8
Patch, drug, 438, 450p
Patch tests, 530–531, 704
Patellar reflex, assessment of, 599, 599t, 600
Pathogens, 268. See also Microorganisms
Pathologic fracture, 560t
Pathologist, 825b
Pathology and laboratory codes, 235
Pathology department, 824
Pathology specimens. See Specimen(s)
Patient(s)
    abandonment of, 40
    proper form of address for, 67
    reception of, 103–105
    registration and orientation of, 103–104
    rights and responsibilities of, 35–39, 37–38
Patient advocacy, 21
Patient appointments. See Appointments
Patient assessment, 294–298
    anthropometric measurements in, 302
    baseline data for, 302
    chief complaint in, 294, 296–297, 297
    in emergencies, 486–493
    present illness in, 294–298
    reference points for, 302
    signs and symptoms in, 294
    vital signs in, 302–333
Patient Bill of Rights, 36, 37–38
Patient care notes, 145, 145–146, 146
Patient confidentiality, 21, 48, 68b
    of computerized information, 144b, 165
Patient education, 70–78
    about health care system, 12b
    assessment in, 72–73
    communication in, 68
    demonstrations in, 74
    for diagnostic imaging, 479
    documentation in, 74–75
    evaluation in, 74
    general topics for, 294
    for health maintenance, 80–96. See also Health maintenance
    implementation in, 73b, 73–74
    learning ability and, 75–76
    for legally required disclosures, 43b
    Maslow's hierarchy of needs and, 75, 75
    materials for, in reception area, 104
    for medical asepsis, 274
    for medication therapy, 94–96, 95
    nutritional, 82–89
    planning in, 73
    for stress management, 90–92
    for substance abuse, 92–94, 93t
    teaching materials for, 76–78, 78
    teaching plans in, 76–78, 77
    topics for, 72b
    videos for, 105
Patient history. See History
Patient information sheet, 103
Patient-physician relationship
    contractual aspects of, 35–39
    ethical aspects of. See Bioethics; Ethics
    legal aspects of, 35–43. See also under Law; Legal
    rights and responsibilities in, 35–36
    termination of, 36–39, 39

Patient positioning, 342, 343, 344t, 349
    for minor office surgery, 379–380
    for pelvic examination, 791–795, 792p
    for prenatal examination, 801–803
    for radiography, 471, 472, 473b
Patient relationships, 66–68
    professional distance in, 67
Patient reminders, 120–121, 121
Patient transport, for emergency care, 486
Patient visits. See Appointments; Office visits
Payments
    fees and, 198
    forms of, 198
    by insurance companies, 198
    posting of, 208–210
Payroll, 190, 218–219, 221–227
    computerized, 223
    earnings calculations for, 223b
    manual systems for, 222
    outside services for, 221–222, 222b
    pegboard systems for, 222, 222–223
Payroll journal, 222, 222
Payroll taxes, 224–227, 225–226
PCP, 93t, 94
Peak flowmeter, 717, 717
Pederson vaginal speculum, 360
Pediatric practice, 986–1013. See also Children
    child abuse and, 1011–1013
    growth charts in, 1007, 1008
    history taking in, 998, 1000–1001
    immunizations in, 991–996, 994–996. See also immunization(s)
    injections in, 1011, 1011
    medication administration in, 1010–1011
    office environment in, 988–989
    parents' role in, 989–990
    physical examination in, 998–1010
    preventive care in, 991–996, 994–996
    psychological aspects of, 989–990
    sick-child visits in, 989, 996–998, 997t
    urine specimen collection in, 1011
    well-child visits in, 989, 991
Pediculosis, 523
Peel-back packages, sterile, 378, 378–379, 379
Peer review organization, 246b, 257
Pegboard system. See also Bookkeeping
    for accounts payable, 220, 220
    for accounts receivable, 206–212
    day sheet in, 206–207
    ledger card in, 206, 207–208, 208
    superbill in, 206, 208
Pelvic cavity, 513, 513
Pelvic examination, 349
    routine, 788, 789–795, 792p–795p
Pelvic inflammatory disease (PID), 787
Pelvic muscle exercises, 786
Penis
    cleansing of, 773
    structure and function of, 767, 768
Penlight, 338
Pentobarbital, abuse of, 93t, 94
Peptic ulcers, 735–736
Perceptual hearing loss, 617
Percival, Thomas, 20
Percussion, 341
    of chest, 720
Percussion hammer, 336, 336
Percutaneous transluminal coronary angioplasty (PTCA), 478, 668b
Performance appraisals, 186
Pericarditis, 671–672
Pericardium, 658–659
Perimenopause, 813
Perimetrium, 781
Perineal resection, for prostatic hypertrophy, 770b
Perineum, 781
Periosteum, 545, 545
Peripheral blood smear
    preparation of, 926, 936p–938p
    staining of, 926, 938p
Peripheral nervous system, 587, 588, 588t, 589
Peripheral vision, assessment of, 348
Peristalsis, 729

Peritoneal dialysis, 756, 757b
  blood pressure measurement in, 314
Peritoneum, 729, 729
Pernicious anemia, 672, 672–673
PERRLA, 348
Personal protective equipment, 274, 275, 832
  decontamination and laundering of, 285
  in emergency care, 486
Personnel. See also Staff
Personnel file, 223–224
Pertussis immunization, 699t
  schedule for, 994, 996
  side effects of, 995b
Pessary, 785–786
Petit mal seizures, 594. See also Seizures
Petri plate, 828, 829, 846, 847, 847
Petty cash, 190, 214
pH
  regulation of, 753
  urine, 871
Phagocytosis, 268, 692, 696, 927
Pharmaceutical representatives, 118
Pharmacodynamics, 420–421, 422b
Pharmacokinetics, 421–423
Pharmacology. See also Medication(s)
  definition of, 416
Pharyngeal tonsils, 694, 710
Pharyngitis, 715
  streptococcal, rapid test for, 851–852
Pharynx, 730
  examination of, 719–720
  specimen collection from, 720, 722p
  structure and function of, 709–710
Phencyclidine (PCP), 93t, 94
Phenols, as disinfectant, 365t
Phenylketonuria test, 42–43
Phimosis, 773
Phlebotomist, 825b
Phlebotomy, 894–919. See also Blood sample
Phone. See Telephone
Phonophoresis, 568
Phosphorus balance, 970, 982t
Physical examination, 336–350
  abdomen in, 349
  assisting physician with, 342, 345p–347p
  auscultation in, 341
  balance in, 349–350
  baseline information in, 336
  breasts in, 349
  chest in, 348
  components of, 336
  coordination in, 349–350
  format for, 342–350
  gait in, 349–350
  genitalia in, 349
  head in, 344
  inspection in, 341
  instruments and supplies for, 336–341, 345p
  legs in, 349
  manipulation in, 341
  medical assistant's responsibilities in, 341–342
  mensuration in, 341
  neck in, 344–348
  palpation in, 341
  patient positioning in, 342, 343, 344t, 349
  patient preparation for, 341–342
  pediatric, 998–1010
    blood pressure in, 1009–1010, 1010p, 1010t
    growth charts in, 1007, 1008
    history in, 998, 1000–1001
    patient preparation for, 998
    pulse in, 1008, 1009t
    respiratory rate in, 1008–1009, 1009t
    restraints in, 999, 1002, 1002p
    temperature in, 1007, 1009
    vital signs in, 1007–1010
  percussion in, 341
  postexamination duties in, 342
  posture in, 349–350
  purpose of, 336
  rectum in, 349
  reflexes in, 348–349
  room preparation for, 341
  routine, schedule for, 350

  strength in, 349–350
  techniques of, 341
Physician(s)
  abandonment by, 40
  AMA Code of Ethics for, 20
  dispensing of controlled substances by, 44
  education and training of, 13
  insurance fraud and, 34, 43, 48, 239–240, 250, 255
  medical practice acts for, 43
  professional ethics for, 27–29. See also Bioethics
  specialties of, 14t
  staff privileges of, 28
  unprofessional conduct by, 43
Physician-assisted suicide, 27, 27b
Physician hospital organizations, 246b, 259
Physician-patient relationship
  contractual aspects of, 35–39
  ethical aspects of. See Bioethics; Ethics
  legal aspects of, 35–43. See also under Law; Legal
  rights and responsibilities in, 35–36
  termination of, 36–39, 39
Physician referrals, 123
Physician's assistant (PA), 13
Physician's Current Procedural Terminology (CPT) codes, 232–238
  fraud and, 239–240
Physician's Desk Reference (PDR), 424
Physician's office laboratory (POL), 821–823
  testing in, guidelines for, 824, 825b
Pia mater, 584
Picture chart, 613, 614
PIE format, 146, 146
Pigmentation disorders, 526
Pigmented nevus, 526
Pimples, 524
Pineal body, 647
Pink eye, 610
Pinna, 615, 619
Pinworms, stool examination for, 746b
Pipette
  RBC, 941
  Thoma, 933
Pituitary
  disorders of, 647–649
  structure and function of, 642–644, 643t, 644, 645
Pityriasis versicolor, 523
PKU test, 42–43
Placental abruption, 805–806
Placenta previa, 804–805
Placing reflex, 993t
Plaintiff, 47
Planes, body, 511–512, 512
Plan maximum, 246b
Plantar fasciitis, 568
Plantar flexion, 547, 550
Plaques, 521, 524
Plasma, 661
  fresh frozen, 963
Plasma cell, 698
Plaster casts, 559. See also Casts
Plaster knife, 562, 562
Plaster saw, 361
Plaster shears, 361
Plaster spreader, 361
Platelet concentrates, 863
Platelet count, 930
Platelets, 662, 924
  formation of, 924–925
  function of, 930
Pleura, 711–712
PMNs, 927
Pneumonia, 717
Poikilocytosis, 928
Poison control center, 498
Poisoning, 498
  computerized information on, 165
Policy and procedure manuals, 187–189
Poliomyelitis, 591–592
  immunization for, 699t, 994, 995b, 996, 996
Polycystic ovary syndrome, 788
Polydipsia, in diabetes insipidus, 649
Polymenorrhea, 784
Polymorphonuclear neutrophils, 927
Polyphagia, in diabetes, 652

Polyps
  colonic, 738
  nasal, 624
Polys, 927
Polyuria, in diabetes insipidus, 649
Pons, 586
Popliteal pulse, 310. See also Pulse
Portfolio, 1056
Position(s)
  anatomic, 511
  body, 512
Positioning. See Patient positioning
Position of function, for instruments, 384, 384
Positive feedback, 514
Positive reinforcement, 74
Positron emission tomography (PET), 478
Posnatal care, 806–808
Postage, 136–137, 137, 137b
Postage meters, 136–137, 137
Postal Service, 136–138
Postcards, reminder, 120–121, 121
Posterior pituitary
  disorders of, 648
  structure and function of, 643t, 644
Posterior tibial pulse, 310. See also Pulse
Posting, 208–212
  to cash paid out section of day sheet, 211–212
  of credit adjustment, 210–211
  of debit adjustment, 211
Postpartum care, 806–808
  abbreviations used in, 807b
Postpartum depression, 807–808
Postpoliomyelitis muscular atrophy, 592
Postural hypotension, 312
Posture
  assessment of, 349–350
  back pain and, 566b
Potassium balance, 969, 982t
Potentiation, drug, 424
Potts-Smith dressing forceps, 356
Pouches, instrument, 368b
Pounds-kilograms conversion, 317p
Power of attorney, 45–46, 46
Pratt rectal speculum, 361
Precautions, isolation, 271–274, 274t, 275b
  standard, 273, 274, 275b
  transmission-based, 273–274, 274t
Precedent, 34
Precipitation tests, for proteinuria, 872–873, 888p
Preeclampsia, 804
Pre-existing condition, 246b
Preferred provider organizations, 246b, 258–259
Pregnancy, 783b, 797–808, 797–815. See also under Obstetric
  abbreviations used in, 807b
  abortion in, 25, 804, 805t
  abruptio placentae in, 805–806
  artificial insemination for, 25
  cesarean section in, 806b
  complications in, 803–806
  diagnosis of, 798, 799t
    tests for, 808
  due date in, 798–799, 800b
  eclampsia in, 804
  ectopic, 803
  ethical issues in, 24–26
  fetal development in, 802, 804
  fetotoxins in, 799–800
  fundal height in, 804
  genetic testing in, bioethical issues in, 25
  gestational diabetes in, 981
  glucose testing in, 981
  gravidity and, 799b
  hyperemesis gravidarum in, 803–804
  hypertension in, 804
  intrapartum care in, 806
  labor and delivery in, 806
  parity and, 799b
  placenta previa in, 804–805
  postpartum care and, 806–808
  preeclampsia in, 804
  prenatal visits in
    first, 798–801
    subsequent, 801–803, 803t

radiography in, 473, 474
Rh status and, 963
signs and symptoms of, 798, 799t
supine hypotension in, 801–802
surrogate, 25–26
teratogens in, 799–800
tests for, 808, 959
urine test for, 877
Pregnancy-induced hypertension, 804
Prejudice, 66
Premenstrual syndrome (PMS), 784, 785b
Prenatal care, 798–806. See also Pregnancy
    bioethical issues in, 24–26
Prenatal screening, 600–601
    bioethical issues in, 25
Prepuce, 768
    tightening of, 773
Presbycusis, 617, 1025t
Presbyopia, 612, 1025t
Prescription pad, safety tips for, 44b
Prescription refills, telephone requests for, 107
Prescriptions, 420, 421
Preservative, specimen, 393, 393
Pressure sores, 525, 525–526
Preventive maintenance record form, 836
Prime mover, 554
Printers, 159, 160
PR interval, 675, 677
Priority mail, 137
Privacy, computerized information and, 144b, 165
Privacy rights, 48
Private law, 34
Probes, 357, 358
Problem-oriented medical records, 144–145
Procedural coding, 232–238
    fraud and, 239–240
Proctology, instruments for, 361, 361t
Proctoscope, 340, 361t
Proctoscopic examination, routine, 349, 350
Professional Association of Health Care Office Managers,
    191
Professional conduct and behavior
    ethical issues in, 27–28
    in externship, 1041–1043
Professional courtesy, 198
Professional distance, 67
Professional image, 102–103, 1041, 1042–1043
Professional liability, 47–48
    defenses to, 49–50
Professional organizations, 9, 9–10, 11
    censure by, 20
    expulsion by, 20
    suspension by, 20
Proficiency testing, for laboratory personnel, 838–839
Progress notes, 145, 145–146, 146, 148b
Progress reports, requests for, 107
Prolactin, 643t, 644
Promotional materials, development of, 189–190
Pronation, 547, 550
Prone position, 343, 344t
Proofreading, of letters, 132–134, 134t
Propoxyphene, 93t, 94
Proprietary schools, 10
Prostate
    cancer of, 769, 770b
    examination of, 769, 776
    structure and function of, 767, 767–768
Prostatectomy
    retropubic, 770b
    suprapubic, 770b
Prostate-specific antigen (PSA), 770
Prostatic fluid, 768
Prostatic hypertrophy, benign, 769–770, 770b, 1026t
Prostatitis, 772
Protective equipment, 274, 275, 832
    decontamination and laundering of, 285
    in emergency care, 486
Protective equipment and clothing, 274, 275
    decontamination and laundering of, 285
Proteinuria, tests for, 872–873, 888p
Prothrombin time (PT), 931
Proton, 506, 507
Protozoa, 844
Proxemics, 57–59, 58t

Proximal, 512
PR segment, 675, 677
Pruritus
    in diabetes, 652
    in eczema, 524
    in urticaria, 524
Psoriasis, 524
Psychiatric emergencies, 500–501
Psychogenic impotence, 772
Psychosocial needs, of elderly, 1019–1020
Pubic lice, 523
Public law, 34
Puerperium, 806
Puerto Ricans
    beliefs and practices of, 63t–64t
    dietary preferences of, 88t
Pulmonary. See also Lung
Pulmonary circulation, 662, 662–663
Pulmonary embolism, 670–671
Pulmonary function
    age-related changes in, 1025t–1026t
    assessment of, 724, 973–974, 974t
Pulmonary semilunar valve, 663
Pulse, 308–310
    apical, 308–310, 327p–328p
    averages and ranges for, 308, 308t
    brachial, in blood pressure measurement, 330p–331p
    characteristics of, 308
    in children, 1008, 1009t
    factors affecting, 308–310, 310t
    palpation of, 308, 310
    radial, 308, 309, 310, 326p
Pulse deficit, 328
Punch biopsy
    instruments for, 362, 362t
    of skin, 529
Punctuation, 133b
Puncture tests, for allergens, 530
Puncture wound, 494b
Pupil, 608, 608–609
    assessment of, 348
    in emergencies, 492
Purchase order, 219
Purchasing, 219–221
Pure culture, 845
Purkinje fibers, 664, 664
Pustules, 520, 521
Pyelography
    intravenous, 762
    retrograde, 476t, 762
Pyelonephritis, 758
Pyloric stenosis, 736
Pyrexia, 303. See also Temperature
Pyuria, 758

Q
QT interval, 675, 677
Quad cane, 577, 577
Quadrants, abdominal, 514
Quadriplegia, 597t
Quality assurance, 838
    serology, 956–957
Quality control
    for laboratories, 835, 835–839
    log book for, 835, 839
    serology, 956–957
Quality improvement, 168–179
    benefits of, 170
    case review for, 178–179
    definition of, 170
    Occupational Safety and Health Administration (OSHA)
        and, 172
    policy statement for, 188
    problems requiring, 173t
    program development for, 172–174
    regulatory agencies and, 170–171
Queckenstedt test, 600
Questions, open-ended, 60, 61t

R
Rabies, 592
Rabies antiserum, 699t

Radial pulse, 308, 309, 310, 326p. See also Pulse
    pulse deficit and, 328p
Radiation burns, 495–496
Radiation safety guidelines, 472–474
Radiation therapy, 479
Radioallergosorbent test (RAST), 961
Radiograph, 470, 470
Radiographic units, 470, 470, 471
Radiography
    ALARA concept in, 474
    barium studies in, 471–472, 475, 475–476, 476t
    in cardiovascular disease, 674t, 683
    chest, in respiratory disease, 721
    common procedures in, 476t
    contrast media examinations in, 475–476, 476t
    film storage and handling in, 480
    fluoroscopy, 477
    interventional, 478
    legal issues in, 480
    mammography, 478
    medical assistant's role in, 479–480
    in neurologic assessment, 599
    outpatient, 470–471
    patient positioning for, 471, 472, 473b
    in pregnancy, 473, 474
    principles of, 471
    routine, 474–475, 475t
    safety guidelines, 472–474
    scheduling of, 123
    sequence of procedures in, 471–472
    teleradiology, 478
    terminology for, 473b
    transfer of information for, 480
    upper GI studies in, 472
    x-ray machines and, 470, 470
    x-rays and, 470–471
Radioimmunoassay, in endocrine disorders, 654
Radiology codes, 235
Radionuclide scanning, 477–478
Rales, 721t
Random access memory (RAM), 158
Random blood glucose, 975
Range of motion, 547–549, 549–550
Range-of-motion exercises, 90
Rapid plasma reagin test, for syphilis, 958–959
RAST, 961
Ratio method, for dosage calculation, 432–433
RBC pipette, 941
RBCs. See Red blood cell(s)
Read only memory (ROM), 158
Reagents
    quality contol for, 837
    serology, storage and handling of, 955–956
Rebound phenomenon, 531
Receipts, 219
Receiving, of supplies, 219
Receptionist, duties of, 103–104
Records. See also Documentation
    financial, 218–219
    medical. See Medical records
    sterilization, 372
    time, for externship, 1043–1044, 1044
Rectal cancer, 738, 738
Rectal examination, 349
    in males, 769, 776
    routine, 350
Rectal specula, 361, 361t
Rectal suppositories, 436–437, 437, 438
Rectal temperature, 303, 304b, 307, 321p–322p. See also Tem-
    perature
Rectal thermometer, 303, 305, 306, 306, 307
Rectocele, uterine prolapse and, 785
Rectovaginal examination, 349
Rectum, 732. See also under Colon; Intestinal
Rectus femoris, injection in, 443, 443
Recumbent position, 343, 344t
Red blood cell(s), 659, 660, 661, 924
    abnormalities of, 929t
    formation of, 924–925, 928
    function of, 928
    mean cell volume for, 929
    in urine, 873, 874
Red blood cell agglutination test, 952–953
    for blood typing, 962–963

Red blood cell agglutination test, (continued)
  for infectious mononucleosis, 957–958
  for rubella, 958
Red blood cell (RBC) count, 928, 941p–942p
Reference laboratory, 820–821
Reference points, 302
References, employee, 186
Referrals, 123
Referred pain, 626–627
Reflecting, 60, 61t
Reflex arc, 583, 584
Reflexes
  assessment of, 348–349, 599, 599t, 600
  in infants, 993t
  testing of, 583
Reflex hammer, 336, 336
Reflux, gastroesophageal, 734, 735b
Refractive errors, 611–612
Refractometer, 870, 882p
Refrigerator, laboratory, 827–828
Refunds, 210
Regions, body, 513b, 513–514, 514
Registered mail, 138
Registered Medical Assistant (RMA), 10–11, 11
Registered nurse (RN), 13
Registration, patient, 103–104
Reimbursement, diganostic related groups (DRGs) for,
      238–239
Relapsing fever, 304, 305t
Relaxation techniques, 92
Release form, for medical records, 154, 154–155
Reminders
  mailed, 120–121, 121
  of overdue accounts, 201, 201
  telephone, 120
Remittent fever, 304, 305t
Renal. See also Kidney
Renal arteriolese, 754
Renal calculi, 757, 758b, 875, 876p
Renal cortex, 754, 754
Renal dialysis, 756, 757b
Renal failure, 756
Renal function
  age-related changes in, 1026t
  assessment of, 968–971
  electrolyte balance and, 969–970
  nonprotein nitrogenous compounds and, 970–971
Renal medulla, 754, 754
Renal pelvis, 754, 754
Renal pyramids, 754, 754
Renal tubules, 754, 755
Renin, 753
Repolarization, in cardiac cycle, 675
Reporting
  of child abuse, 1012–1013
  of elder abuse, 526, 1022
  requirements for, 42–43, 43b, 155
Reproductive system
  female
    age-related changes in, 1026t
    disorders of, 784–797
    structure and function of, 780, 780–781
  genital examination and, 349
  male, 764–777
    age-related changes in, 1026t
    disorders of, 769–777
      diagnosis of, 769, 776–777
    evolution and differentiation of, 766
    organs of, 766–769, 767
Rescue breathing, 490p
Research, bioethical issues in, 24
Reservoirs, of infection, 268
Resignation, 1059b, 1059–1060
Res ipsa loquitur, 47
Res judicata, 50
Resource-Based Relative Value Scale (RBRVS), 198, 239
Respiration(s)
  abnormal, 311–312, 720t
  assessment of, 310–312, 329p
    in emergencies, 488
  averages and ranges for, 311t, 311–312
  characteristics of, 311
  Cheyne-Stokes, 311–312
  counting of, 311, 329p

  definition of, 310
  external, 713
  internal, 713–714
  regulation of, 310–311
Respiratory acidosis, causes of, 974t
Respiratory alkalosis, causes of, 974t
Respiratory distress syndrome, infant, 716t
Respiratory rate, in children, 1008–1009, 1009t
Respiratory system
  age-related changes in, 1026t
  defense mechanisms of, 714, 714t
  disorders of, 715–719
    in children, 716t
    diagnosis of, 719–725
  respiration and, 712, 713–714
  smoking and, 715b
  structure and function of, 708, 708–712
  ventilation and, 712, 712–713
Respondeat superior, 50–51
Restraints, 48
  for children, 999, 1002, 1002p
Resumé
  chronological, 1052, 1054
  cover letter for, 1053–1054, 1055
  distribution of, 1051
  functional, 1052, 1053
  preparation of, 1051–1053, 1053
Resuscitation
  advance directives for, 28, 44–45, 45
  termination/witholding of, 27, 44–45
Retina, 608, 609
Retinal degeneration, 611
Retinopathy, 611
Retractors, 357–359, 359
  Desmarres lid, 362
  eyelid, 362, 362t
Retrograde pyelography, 476t, 762
Retropubic prostatectomy, 770b
Retrovirus, 701
Return appointments, scheduling of, 119–120
Returned check fee, 212
Review of systems, 290
Reye's syndrome, 592–593, 998
Rh blood group, 961–962
  testing for, 963
Rheumatic fever, heart disease and, 669
Rheumatoid arthritis, 569
  test for, 957
Rheumatoid factor, test for, 957
Rhinitis
  acute, 715
  allergic, 623
Rhinology, instruments for, 362, 362t
RhoGAM, 961
Rhonchi, 721t
Rhythm method, 809t
Rhythm strip, 683
Ribonucleic acid (RNA), 508
Rickettsias, 843–844
Right bundle branch, 664, 664
Ringworm, 522–523
Rinne test, 621
Risk management, 174–178
  case review for, 178–179
  incident reports in, 174–178, 175b, 176–177
  policy statement for, 188
RNA, 508
Rochester-Ochsner forceps, 355
Rochester-Pean forceps, 355
Rods, retinal, 609
Roentgen, Wilhelm Konrad, 8
Role model, medical assistant as, 102
Roller bandages, 388, 390
Romberg test, 599
Rooting reflex, 993t
Rotary files, 153
Rotation, 547, 549
Rotator cuff, 552
  injury of, 567
Rubella
  immunization for, 699t, 994, 995b, 996,
      996–997
  tests for, 958
Ruffini's corpuscles, 627t

Rule of nines, 496, 496
Rush, Benjamin, 7

S
Sabin, Albert, 8
Sacculated aneurysm, 672
Sacrum, 553
Safety
  for ambulatory aids, 570b
  for elderly, 1030
  laboratory, 828–834
  in pediatric practice, 988–989
  radiation, 472–474
Sagittal plane, 512, 512
Sales calls, 118
  telephone, 107
Saliva, 730
Salivary glands, 730
Salk, Jonas, 8
Salpingitis, 787
Salpingo-oophorectomy, for endometriosis, 785
Same-day surgery, HCPCS codes for, 238
Sandwich method, 953–954, 954b
Sanitation, 363, 364p
Scabies, 523
Scale, 302, 302, 317p, 521, 523
Scalp, lice infestation of, 523
Scalpel, 357, 358
Scalpel blades, 357, 358, 381–382, 382
  handling and disposal of, 285–286, 286, 359–363, 382,
      382, 898
Scars, 524–525
Schamberg comedone extractor, 362, 362t
Scheduling, 114–123
  in acute illness, 121
  appointment book for, 114–116, 115–116, 117
  of appointments, 114–123. See also Appointments
  for cancelled appointments, 123
  computerized, 117
  on daily/weekly basis, 120–121
  double booking in, 119
  in emergencies, 108, 121
  facilities and, 118
  factors affecting, 117–118
  guidelines for, 118–120
  for laboratory tests and x-rays, 123–124
  for new patients, 118–119, 119b
  of nonpatient visitors, 117–118
  open time slots for, 118
  at other facilities, 123
  patient needs and, 117
  of patients with unpaid accounts, 202
  physician delays and, 122
  physician's preferences and needs and, 117–118
  problem solving for, 124
  for referrals, 123
  for return appointments, 119–120
  staff, 187
  for surgery, 124
  for tardy patients, 122
  for walk-in patients, 121–122
  wave, 119
Schick test, 531
School placement office, 1051
Schroeder tenaculum forceps, 360
Scissors, 354, 357
Sclera, 348, 608, 608
Scoliosis, 564, 566b
Scratch test, 530, 704
Scrotum, 766
  assessment of, 349
  examination of, 776
Sebaceous glands, 519–520
Seborrheic dermatitis, 524
Sebum, 519
Secobarbital, abuse of, 93t, 94
Secondary culture, 845
Secondary sexual characteristics, female, 780
Second-class mail, 138
Sedatives, 418t
Sed rate, 930, 931, 946p–947p
Segmented neutrophils (segs), 924, 927
Seizures, 594–595, 595t

emergency care for, 497
febrile, 594–595, 998
focal (Jacksonian), 595
grand mal, 594, 595t
petit mal, 594
Self-analysis, for career choices, 1050–1051
Self-Determination Act, 45
Semen, 769
specimen of, 774b
Semiblock letter format, 130, *131*
Semicircular canals, 616, *619*
Semi-Fowler's position, *343*, 344t
Semilunar valves, *662, 662, 663, 663*
Seminal fluid, *767, 767*
Seminal vesicles, *767, 767*
Semmelweiss, Ignaz, 8
Senn retractor, *359*
Sensitivity testing, 851, *851, 852*
Sensorineural hearing loss, 617
Sensory disorders, 606–638
Sensory examination, 599
Sensory receptors, 625, *625–627*, 626t
dermal, 519
Sensory system, age-related changes in, 1025t
Septicemia, 695
Septic shock, 493
Serology, definition of, 952
Serology department, 824
Serology tests, 952–961
agglutination test, 952–953, 953b
for antinuclear antibodies, 960
antistreptolysin-O, 960
chromatographic assay, 954
cold agglutinins, 960–961
for C-reactive protein, 958
enzyme immunoassays, 953–954, 954b
external controls for, 956–957
false-negative results for, 957
false-positive results for, 957
for group A streptococcus, 960
for infectious mononucleosis, 957–958
internal controls for, 956–957
methods and principles of, 952–954
for pregnancy, 959
procedures for, 956
quality assurance and control for, 956–957
radioallergosorbent test, 961
reagent and kit storage and handling for, 955–956
for rheumatoid factor/rheumatoid arthritis, 957
for rubella, 958
specimen collection and handling for, 954–955
for syphilis, 958–959
troubleshooting for, 956b
Serum hepatitis, 740, 740t
Service charges, bank, 212
Service contracts, 191
Sesamoid bones, 544
Setups, surgical, 376–377
Sexual harassment, 192
Sexual history, in AIDS diagnosis, 704t
Sexually transmitted diseases
in females, 786–787
in males, 772–773
Sharps, handling and disposal of, 285–286, 286, 359–363,
382, *382*, 898
Shave biopsy, of skin, 529
Shaving, preoperative, 381, 399p–400p
Shelf files, 153
Shingles, 522
Shock, 493b, 493–494
anaphylactic, 493, 497, 498
cardiogenic, 493
hypovolemic, 493
insulin, 653, 653t
management of, 493–494
neurogenic, 493
septic, 493
signs and symptoms of, 493b
types of, 493
Shoulder
frozen, 567
muscles of, 557t
rotator cuff injury of, 567
structure and function of, 552

Sialogram, 476t
Sick-child visits, 996–998, 997t
Sickle cell disease, *672,* 672–673
Sight. *See* Vision
Sigmoidoscopy, 340, 361t, 743, *743,* 744p–745p
Sign-in sheets, 114
Signs and symptoms, assessment of, 294
Simple fracture, 560t
Simpson uterine sound, *360*
Sims position, *343,* 344t
Sims uterine curet, *360*
Sims uterine sound, *360*
Single photon emission spectroscopy (SPECT), 478
Sinoatrial node, *664, 664,* 670
Sinuses, 551, *551,* 622, 709, *709,* 710t
examination of, 348
infection of, 624, 715
Sinusitis, 624, 715
Sitting position, *343,* 344t
Sitz bath, 538p–540p, 540
Skeletal system, *544,* 544–546, *545*546t. *See also under* Bone;
Musculoskeletal
Skene's glands, 781
Skilled nursing facilities, for elderly, 1021
Skin
abnormal color of, 492t
age-related changes in, 1024t
biopsy of, 529
in emergency assessment, 492, 492t
examination of, 529–531
function of, 518
inflammations of, 523–524
structure of, *518,* 518–520
sun damage to, 528b
Skin cancer, 527–629
basal cell, 527–528, *528*
malignant melanoma, 526, 527b, *528,* 528–529
prevention of, 528b
squamous cell, 528, *528*
Skin clips, 383–384
removal of, 385–386, 402p–403p
Skin closure
with staples, 383–384, 385–386, 402p–403p
with Steri-strips, 384, *385*
with sutures, 382–384, *383, 384*
Skin disorders, 520–540
diagnostic procedures for, 529–531
infectious, 520–523
inflammatory, 523–524
instruments for, *362,* 362t
of pigmentation, 526
Skin infections
bacterial, 520–522
fungal, 521–522
parasitic, 522
viral, 521
Wood's light for, 523, 530
Skin lesions, 520, *521*
diagnosis of, 529–531
excision of, 389–390
assisting with, 411p
electrosurgery for, *391,* 391–392
laser surgery for, 392–393
pressure-induced, 525–526
types of, *521*
Skin preparation, for minor surgery, 381, 399p–400p
Skin puncture, for blood collection, 901–903, 913–919,
914p–918p
complications of, 913–919
procedure for, 914p–919p
sources of error in, 919t
Skin tests
for allergens, 441–442, 460p–461p, 530b, 530–531, 704
intradermal injection for, *441,* 441–442, 458p–461p
for tuberculosis, 441–442, 460p–461p, 531
Skull, 549–551, *551*
Slander, 48
Slide covers, 340
Slides, 340, 828, *829*
for blood smear, 898
fixative for, 339
preparation of, 848, *850*
Sling, 562, 563b
Small bowel series, 476t

Small claims court, 202
Small intestine, structure and function of, 731, *732*
Smallpox, 7
Smears, 848, *850,* 854p–856p
blood, slides for, 898
peripheral blood
preparation of, 926, 936p–938p
staining of, 926, 938p
staining of, 849–850, *850b,* 856p–860p
Smegma, 773
Smell
process of, 622–623, 625
taste and, 625
Smoking
chronic obstructive pulmonary disease and, 718
lung cancer and, 719
respiratory effects of, 715b
Snellen chart, 613, *614,* 628p
Soaks, 538p–540p, 540
SOAP format, 145, 146, *146,* 148b
Social history, 290
Social Security taxes, 224
Sodium balance, 969, 982t
Soft tissue injuries, 494b, 494–495
Software, 161
desktop publishing, 164
graphics, 164
office management, 164
selection of, 165–166
word processing, 164
Soiled linens, handling of, 285
Solution, sterile, pouring of, 378, 397p–398p
Somatotropin hormone, 643t, 643–644
Sonography, 477, *477*
fetal, 601
Sore throat, 715
tests for, 851–852, 960
Sound, transmission of, 617
Sounds, urethral, 361
Source-oriented medical records, 144
Spastic colon, 737–738
Spatula, Ayre, 339, *340*
Specific gravity, urine, 870, 881p, 882p
Specimen(s). *See also* Clinical chemistry; Laboratory tests
blood. *See* Blood sample
collection of, 393, *393. See also* Biopsy
guidelines for, 846b, 849t
for Pap smear, 792p–795p
patient education for, 820
for serology tests, 954–955
control sample for, 835–837
culture of. *See* Culture
microbiologic, storage and handling of, 845–848, 849t
mounting of, 848, *850*
quality control for, 835–838
semen, 774b
serum, for serology tests, 954–955
smears of, 848, *850,* 854p–856p
sputum, 720, 723p, 845–846
staining of, 849–850, *850b,* 856p–860p
stool, 745, 746b, 748p
storage and handling of, 849t
storage and handling of, for serology tests, 954–955
swab, for serology tests, 955
for throat culture, 720, 722p
transport of, *820,* 847–848, 853p
types of, 845–846
urine, 760, 849t, 868–869. *See also* Urine specimen
wound, 529, *529, 530,* 846
Specimen processor, 825b
SPECT (single photon emission spectroscopy), 478
Spectrophotometer, 968, *968*
Speculum
nasal, 336, *337, 362,* 362t
rectal, *361*
vaginal, 339, *339, 360,* 791
Speech, production of, 710
Speech audiometry, 620
Spelling tips, 133b
Spencer stitch scissors, *357*
Sperm, abnormalities of, infertility and, 773, 774b
Spermatogenesis, 766–767
Spermatozoa, *768,* 768–769
Spermicides, 809t

Sphenoidal sinuses, 622, 709, *709*
Sphenoid bone, 551, *551*
Sphygmomanometer, 312, *312*
Spills, handling and prevention of, *833*, 833–834
Spina bifida, 595–596, *596*
    prenatal screening for, 600, 808
Spinal cord, structure and function of, 587
Spinal cord injury, 564, 597, 597t, 598
Spinal dermatomes, *589*
Spinal nerves, 587, *589*
Spinal tap, 599–600, *601*, 602p–603p
Spine
    cervical, fractures of, 564
    curvature of, abnormal, 564, 566b
    rheumatoid arthritis of, 569
    structure and function of, 551–552, *552*
Spiral fracture, 560t, *561*
Spirochetes, 842, *843*
Spleen, structure and function of, 694
Splenomegaly, 695–696
Splinter forceps, *356*
Splints, 496, *497*
Spontaneous abortion, 804, 805t
Spores, bacterial, 842–843, *843*
Sprains, 558
    emergency management of, 496–497
Spreadsheets, 163–164
Spring forceps, 354
Sputum culture, specimen collection for, 845–846
Squamous cell carcinoma, 528, *528*
Stab, 927
Staff
    communication with, by office manager, 183
    hiring and interviewing of, 186
    infection control procedures for, 270–271
    job descriptions for, 183, *184*, 185
    laboratory, 824, 825b
        education and training standards for, 838–839
        proficiency testing for, 838–839
    payroll for, 190, 221–227. *See also* Payroll
    personnel file for, 223–224
    policies for, 188, 190b
    policy and procedure manuals for, 187–189
    references for, 186
    scheduling of, 187
    termination of, 187
Staff meetings, 183
    agenda for, 139, *140*
    minutes of, 139
Staff privileges, 28
Staghorn calculi, 757
Stains, 849–850, 850b, 856p–860p
    for peripheral blood smear, 926, 938p
Standard precautions, 273, 275b
Stapes, 615, *619*
Staphylococcal skin infections, 520–521
Staphylococci, 842, *843*
Staples, skin, 383–384
    removal of, 385–386, 402p–403p
Stare decisis, 34
Startle reflex, 993t
Stasis ulcers, 670
Status asthmaticus, 717
Statute of limitations, 50, 154
Statutes, 34. *See also under* Law; Legal
Stein-Leventhal syndrome, 788
Stent, vascular, 478
Stepping reflex, 993t
Stereotyping, 66
Sterile drapes, 379–381
Sterile dressings, 386, 403p–407p
Sterile field, 357
    preparation and maintenance of, 376–379
Sterile gloving, 280–282
Sterile items, handling of, 376, 377–379
Sterile peel-back packages, *378*, 378–379, *379*
Sterile solution, pouring of, 378, 397p–398p
Sterile surgical packs, 376–377
    opening of, 376–377, 395p–396p
Sterile technique, 276, 276t
Sterile transfer forceps, 377, *377*, 378, *378*, 397p
Sterilization
    autoclave for, 365–370, *367*
    by boiling, 370–372

culture test for, 367
    in infection control, 284, 363, 365–370
    wrapping equipment for, 368b–369b
Sterilization indicators, 367, *370*, 370b, 377
Sterilization records, 372
Sterilizer forceps, 354
Steri-strips, 384, *385*
Steroids, for Addison's disease, 652
Stertorous breathing, 721t
Stethoscope, *313*, 338. *See also* Auscultation
Stillbirths, reporting of, 42
Stimulants, 418t
    abuse of, 93t, 94
Stitches. *See* Sutures
Stoma, tracheal, 711
Stomach. *See also under* Gastric
    cancer of, 736
    disorders of, 735–736
    structure and function of, 731, *731*
Stomatitis, 733–734
Stones
    gallbladder, 741, *741*
    urinary tract, 875, 876p
Stool, occult blood in, 349, 738, 746–749, 748p
Stool culture, 745, 746b, 747p
Stool guaiac, 349, 738, 746–749, 748p
Stool sample, 745, 746b, 748p
    storage and handling of, 849t
Strabismus, 612
Straight digit filing, 152
Straight scissors, 354, *357*
Strain
    back, prevention of, 552, 553p
    emergency management of, 496–497
Stratum corneum, *518*, 519
Stratum germinativum, *518*, 519
Strength, assessment of, 349–350
Strep throat, tests for, 851–852, 960
Streptococcal skin infections, 520–521
Streptococci, 842, *843*
    tests for, 851–852, 960
Stress, 90–92
    coping mechanisms for, 91, 91t
    definition of, 90
    in elderly, 1020
    negative, 91
    positive, 90–91
    relaxation techniques for, 92
Stress test, 674t, 685, 688
Stretching exercises, 92
Stridor, 721t
Strips, sterilization indicator, 367, *370*, 370b, 377
Stroke, 671, 1025t
ST segment, 675, *677*
Sty, 610
Subcutaneous injections, *441*, 442–443, 462p–463p
Subcutaneous tissue, *518*, 520
Subdermal hormone implants, 809t, 810–811, 814p
Subject filing, 153
Sublingual drug administration, 435, 449p
Sublingual glands, 730
Subluxation, 559
Submandibular glands, 730
Subpoena, 49b
Subpoena *duces tecum,* 49b
Substance abuse
    controlled substances regulations and, 44
    in elderly, 1020
    patient teaching for, 92–94, 93t
Sucking reflex, 993t
Sudoriferous glands, 520
Suicide
    assisted, 27, 27b
    in elderly, 1020–1021
Sulci, cerebral, 584, *585*
Sulfosalicylic acid, for proteinuria, 872–873, 888p
Sunlight, skin cancer and, 528b
Sunscreens, 528b
Superbill, 206, 208
Superficial, 512
Supination, 547, *550*
Supine hypotension, 801–802
Supine position, *343*, 344t
Supplies. *See also* Equipment; Instruments

first aid, 484, 485b
    maintenance and inventory of, 191, 372, *836*, 837–838
    office
        maintenance and inventory of, 191
        purchasing of, 219–221
Suppositories, rectal, 436–437, *437*, 438
Suppressor T cells, 698
Suprapubic aspiration, for urine specimen, 869
Suprapubic prostatectomy, 770b
Surgery
    ambulatory, HCPCS codes for, 238
    electrosurgery, *391*, 391–392
    excisional, 390–393
        assisting with, 411p
    laser, 392–393
    minor office, 374–412. *See also* Minor office surgery
    for prostatic hypertrophy, 770b
    scheduling of, 124
Surgery codes (CPT), 233–234
Surgical asepsis, 276, 276t, 363
Surgical packs, sterile, 376–377
    opening of, 376–377, 395p–396p
Surgical scrub, 276, 277p–279p
Surgical specialties, 14t
Surrogate, health care, 40
Surrogate mothers, bioethical issues in, 25–26
Suspension, 20
Sustained fever, 304, 305t
Sutures, 382–384, *383*, *384*
    removal of, 384–385, *385*, 400p–401p
Suture scissors, 354, *357*
Swab, 339, *340*, 842
Swab specimens, for serology tests, 955
Swaged needles, 383
Swimmer's ear, 618
Swing-through gait, 576p
Swing-to gait, 576p
Sympathetic nervous system, 587–589, 591t
Sympathy, 67
Synapse, 582–583
Synarthroses, 546
Syncope, during venipuncture, 905
Synergism, drug, 423
Synovial fluid, 547
Synovial joints, 547, 548t
Syphilis, 958
    in females, 787
    in males, 773
    rapid plasma reagin test for, 958–959
Syringe(s), 440, *440*, *441*
    ear, 619
    filling of, 452p–457p
    hypodermic, 440, *440*
    insulin, 441, *441*
    prefilled, *439*, 439–440
    tuberculin, 440–441, *441*
Syringe system, for blood collection, *899*, 900, 901

T

Tachypnea, 311
Tactile organs, 625, 625–627, 626t
Tape, sterilization indicator, 367, *370*, 370b, 377
Tape measure, 338
Tardiness, scheduling and, 122
Taste, 625
Taste buds, 730
Tax audits, 227
Tax returns, 218, 224–227, *225–226*
Tax witholding, 222, 224
T cells, 698, *924*, 927
TDD telephone, 66
Teaching. *See* Education
Teaching plans, 76–78, *77*
Tears, 609, *609*
Tear sac, 609, *609*
    infection of, 612
Teeth, 730
    caries of, 733
Telephone, 105–109
    answering services, 109
    cellular, 109
    conference calls, 109
    in debt collection, 201

guidelines for, 106
    in emergencies, 108, 121, 484, 715
    for obstetric patients, 797
incoming calls, 106–108
modem for, 161
outgoing calls, 108–109
poison control center, 498
services, 109
TDD, for hearing impaired, 65
Telephone reminders, 120
Teleradiology, 478
Television, educational videos for, 105
Temperature, 302–308.
    axillary, 303, 304b, 307, 323p–324p, 1007, 1009
    centrigrade (Celsius), 269, 303, 303, 304b
    elevated, 304, 305t. See also Fever
    in emergency assessment, 491–492
    factors affecting, 302, 302, 304
    Fahrenheit, 303, 303, 304b
    measurement of, 302–308. See also Thermometer
        in children, 1007, 1009
        oral, 303, 303, 304b, 319p–320p, 1007
        rectal, 303, 303, 304b, 307, 321p–322p, 1007
    regulation of, 304
    tympanic, 306, 306, 307, 325p, 1007
Temporal bone, 551, 551
Temporal lobe, 585, 586, 586
Temporary services, 1051
Tendinitis, 567
Tendons, 544, 555
Tennis elbow, 567–568
Tension headaches, 598
Teratogenic category, 423t
Teratogens, 799–800, 800b, 801b
Terminal digit filing, 152
Terminal illness
    advance directives for, 28, 45, 45–46
    assisted suicide/euthanasia in, 27b
    ethical issues in, 27, 27b
    treatment withdrawal/witholding in, 27
Testicular cancer, 775
Testicular self-examination, 775
Testis
    assessment of, 349
    development of, 766
    infection of, 772
    structure and function of, 766–767, 767
    undescended, 771, 771
Testosterone, 643t, 647, 766
Tests. See Laboratory tests
Test tubes, 828, 829
Tetanus, 592
Tetanus immune globulin, 699t
Tetany, 650–651
Thalamus, 586
Thallium scan, in cardiac stress test, 685
Thank you letter, for interview, 1058, 1058–1059
T-helper cells, 698
Therapeutic classification, 423t
Therapeutic soaks, 538p–540p, 540
Therapeutic touch, 59, 59
Thermal burns, 495–496
Thermometer
    cleaning of, 307–308, 325p–326p
    disposable, 306, 307
    electronic, 305, 306, 324p
    glass, 305, 306
    oral, 303, 303, 305–306, 306, 319p–320p
    rectal, 303, 303, 305, 306, 306, 307, 321p–322p
    sheath for, 306, 307
    tympanic, 306, 306, 307, 325p
Third-class mail, 138
Third-party administrator, 244, 246b
Thixotropic gel separator, 900
Thoma pipette, 933
Thomas uterine curet, 360
Thoracic cavity, 513, 513
Three-point gait, 574p–576p
Throat, 730
    examination of, 348, 719–720
    structure and function of, 709–710
Throat culture, 720, 722p
Thrombocyte count, 930
Thrombocytes, 662, 924

formation of, 924–925
function of, 930
Thrombocytopenia, 930
Thrombolytics, 417t
Thrombosis, venous, 670–671
Thrombus, atherosclerotic, 665, 665
Thumb, structure and function of, 553
Thumb forceps, 354
Thymosin, 646
Thymus, 646
    disorders of, 651
    structure and function of, 694–695
Thyroid, 643t, 644
    assessment of, 972–973
    disorders of, 649–650
    examination of, 344
    goiter and, 649
    hyperplasia of, 649
Thyroid agents, 418t
Thyroid cartilage, 710
Thyroid function tests, 654, 654t, 972–973
Thyroid hormones, 972–973
    deficiency of, 649–650, 650
    excess of, 650
Thyroid-stimulating hormone, 643t, 644, 972
    measurement of, 654, 654t
Thyrotoxicosis, 650
Thyrotropin. See also Thyroid hormones
Thyroxine, 643t, 644, 972–973
    measurement of, 654, 654t
Tickler file, 121, 121b
Time, military, 148, 148
Time records, externship, 1043–1044, 1044
Tinea, 844
Tinea capitas, 522
Tinea circinata, 522
Tinea corporis, 522
Tinea cruris, 522
Tinea pedis, 523, 844
Tinea unguium, 523
Tinea versicolor, 523
Tine test, 441–442, 460p–461p, 531
Tinnitus, 617
Tissues, 509, 509t, 510
Tomography, 477
Tongue
    airway obstruction by, 488
    structure and function of, 730
Tongue depressor, 338
Tonic-clonic seizures, 594, 595t
Tonic neck reflex, 993t
Tonometer, Schiotz, 362
Tonometry, 614, 615
Tonsillitis, 715
Tonsils, 694, 710
Tooth decay, 733
Topical medications, 437–438, 451p
Tort(s), 34. See also Malpractice; Negligence
    definition of, 47
    intentional, 48–49
    unintentional, 47–48
Tort law, 47–49
Tort of outrage, 48
Total hip replacement, 565b
Total knee replacement, 565b
Touch, 625–626
    therapeutic, 59, 59
Tourniquet, venipuncture, 898, 907p–908p
Towel clamps, 357, 358
Toxic exposures, 498
    computerized information on, 165
    poison control center for, 498
Toxic hepatitis, 740
Toxicology, computerized information on, 165
Toxicology department, 823
Toxoid, 700
Trachea, structure and function of, 710–711
Tracheostomy, 710–711, 711
Tracheotomy, 710
Trade names, drug, 416, 416b
Transcription, 140–141, 141b
Transcutaneous electrical nerve stimulation (TENS), 627
Transdermal drug administration, 438, 450p
Transfer forceps, sterile, 377, 377, 378, 378, 397p

Transfusions
    blood donation for, 963–964
    blood typing for, 961–963, 962, 963t
Transient flora, 268
Transient ischemic attack, 671
Transillumination, 338
    of sinuses, 348
    of testis, 770
Transmission-based precautions, 273–274, 274t
Transplantation
    ethical issues in, 26
    organ donor card for, 26, 26
    Uniform Anatomical Gift Act for, 44–45
Transport
    ambulance, 486
    of specimens, 847–848, 848, 853p
Transport containers, 820
Transport media, 847–848, 848, 853p
Transurethral resection, of prostate, 770b
Transverse fracture, 560t, 561
Transverse plane, 512, 512
Trauma. See also Emergency care
    assessment in, 486–493
    bleeding in, 494–495
    head, brain injury in, 596–597, 597t, 598
    physical examination in, 492–493
    shock in, 493–494
    soft tissue injuries in, 494b, 494–495
    violent, reporting of, 42
Traumatic needles, 383
Treadmill test, 674, 685, 688
Treatment
    emergency. See Emergency care
    refusal of, 48
        advance directives and, 28, 45, 45–46
    withdrawal/witholding of, 27
        advance directives for, 28, 45, 45–46
Trend reports, 42
Treponema pallidum, 773, 843
    rapid plasma reagin test for, 958–959
Trial, 49
Triangular sling, 562, 563b
Triceps reflex, assessment of, 599, 599t, 600
Trichomonas vaginalis, in urine, 875
Tricuspid valve, 662, 663
Trigeminal nerve, 587, 588, 588t
Triglycerides, 981t, 982
Trigone, 756
Triiodothyronine, 643t, 644, 972–973. See also Thyroid hormones
    measurement of, 654, 654t
Tripod crane, 577, 577
Trochlear nerve, 587, 588, 588t
Tubal ligation, 809t
Tuberculin syringe, 440–441, 441
Tuberculosis
    Mantoux test for, 441–442, 460p–461p, 531
    tine test for, 441–442, 460p–461p, 531
Tubular gauze bandages, 388–389, 407p–410p
Tumors. See also Cancer
    acoustic nerve, 617
    bone, 570
    brain, 597–598
    urinary tract, 760
    uterine, 787–788
Tuning fork test, 336, 337, 621
Turbidity tests, for proteinuria, 872–873, 888p
Turbinates, 551, 551, 622, 709
24-hour urine collection, 868, 869, 879p
2-hour postprandial glucose, 975–976
Two-point gait, 574p–576p
Tympanic membrane, 336–337, 348, 615, 619
Tympanic temperature, 306, 306, 307, 325p, 1007
Tympanic thermometer, 306, 306, 307
Tympanometry, 362t, 621, 621

U
UCR concept, for fees, 198
Ulcerative colitis, 737
Ulcers
    corneal, 610–611
    decubitus, 525, 525–526
    duodenal, 736

Ulcers, (continued)
  gastric, 735–736
  stasis, 670
Ultilization review, 255–257
Ultrasonography, 477, 477
  with cortisone, 568
  Doppler, in pulse measurement, 310, 310
  fetal, 601, 808
  urinary tract, 762
Umbilical region, 513, 514
Unbundling, 255
Undescended testis, 771, 771
Undue influence, 49
Uniform Anatomical Gift Act, 44–45
United States Pharmacopeia Dispensing Information, 424
United States Postal Service, 136–138
Universal precautions, 273
Unopette system, 830p, 903, 904
Unprofessional conduct, 22–23
Upper airway obstruction, 487, 487–488, 489p
Upper GI series, 471–472, 476t
Upper respiratory disorders, 715–716
Upper respiratory infections, otitis media and, 618
Urea, 752, 970
Uremia, 970
Uremic frost, 756
Ureter, 752, 752
  structure and function of, 755–756
Ureterostomy, 758
Urethra, 752, 752
  structure and function of, 756
Urethral culture, 776
Urethral sounds, 361
Urethritis, 758
  gonococcal, 772–773
Uric acid, 752, 971, 982t
Urinalysis, 760, 866–892
  in children, 1011
  for drug abuse, 877
  in endocrine disorders, 654
  in males, 776
  in pregnancy, 877
  specimen collection for, 760, 868–869
  specimen storage and handling for, 849t
Urinalysis department, 823
Urinary catheterization, 760, 760b–761b
  for specimen collection, 869
Urinary system
  age-related changes in, 1026t
  disorders of, 756–762
    diagnosis of, 760–762
    prevention of, 759
    symptoms of, 759t
  structure and function of, 752–756
  tumors of, 760
Urinary tract infections, 758
  bacteriuria in, 873, 874
  leukocyte esterase reaction in, 873–874
  in males, 771–772
Urinary tract stone formation, 875, 876p
Urination, voiding reflex and, 756
Urine
  ammonia in, 871
  bacteria in, nitrite test for, 873, 874
  bilirubin in, 873, 879p
  blood in, 873
  casts in, 875
  chemical properties of, 870–874
  clarity of, 869–870, 870t, 880p
  cloudy, 870, 870t, 880p
  color of, 869, 870t, 880p
  crystals in, 875, 879p
  dipsticks for, 871, 883p–886p
  epithelial cells in, 874–875
  formation and transport of, 752–755
  glucose in, 871–872, 885p–886p
  hazy, 870, 870t
  ketones in, 872, 887p
  leukocytes in, 873–874
  microscopic examination of, 874–875, 890p–891p
  mucus in, 875
  nitrites in, 873
  pH of, 871

  physical properties of, 869–870, 870t
  protein in, tests for, 872–873, 888p
  specific gravity of, 870, 881p, 882p
  Trichomonas vaginalis in, 875
  turbidity of, 869–870, 870t, 880p
  yeast in, 875
Urine melanin, 530
Urine sediment
  preparation of, 874, 890p–891p
  structures in, 874–875, 875
Urine specimen
  catheter, 869
  from children, 1011
  clean-catch, 868–869, 877p–878p
  collection of, 760, 868–869
  for drug testing, 877
  for serology tests, 955
  storage and handling of, 849t
  suprapubic, 869
  24-hour, 868, 869, 879p
Urine tests, 760. See also Urinalysis
  for drug abuse, 877
  for pregnancy, 877, 959
Urinometer, 870, 881p
Urobilinogen, 873
Urogram, excretory, 476t
Urolithiasis, 875, 876p
Urology, instruments for, 361, 361t
Urticaria, 524
Usual, customary and reasonable (UCR) tables, 246b, 261
Uterine bleeding, dysfunctional, 784
Uterine contractions, 806
  Braxton-Hicks, 798
Uterine curets, 360
Uterine dilators, 360
Uterine displacement, 786, 786
Uterine fibroids, 787–788
Uterine prolapse, 785, 785–786
Uterus, structure and function of, 780, 781
Utilization review, 246b, 255–257

V
Vaccines, 418t, 699, 699t, 700. See also Immunization
Vagina
  examination of, 349
  structure and function of, 780, 781
Vaginal drug administration, 437, 437
Vaginal speculum, 339, 339, 791
Vaginitis, 784, 784b
Vagus nerve, 587, 588, 588t
Values, cultural differences in, 61
Valves, cardiac, 662, 662–663, 663
  disorders of, 669
Valvular heart disease, 669
Varicella
  immunization for, 996, 996–997
  Reye's syndrome and, 592–593
Varicella zoster, 522
Varices, esophageal, 735
Varicose veins, 670
Vascular stent, 478
Vas deferens, 767, 767
Vasectomy, 777, 809t
Vasopressin, 643t, 644
  in diabetes insipidus, 649
Vastus lateralis, injection in, 443, 443
  in children, 1011, 1011
Vector, 270
Veins, 659, 659, 661
  cardiac, 663, 663
  varicose, 670
Vena cava, 658, 659
Venipuncture, 896, 896–897. See also Blood sample
  complications of, 905–913
  equipment for, 898, 898–899
  needle positioning for, 905
  patient preparation for, 903–905
  procedure for, 905, 906p–912p
  sources of error in, 913t
Venous blood sample, 896, 896–897
Venous thrombosis, 670–671
Ventilation, 712, 712–713. See also Respiration(s)

Ventilatory status, 974
Ventral cavity, 513, 513
Ventricles, 658, 659, 662, 662–663, 663
Ventricular activation time, 677
Ventricular fibrillation, 670
Ventricular tachycardia, 670
Ventrogluteal injection, 442, 443
Venules, 659, 659
Verbal communication, 56–57, 58t. See also Communication
Verdict, 49
Verruca, 522
Vertebrae. See also Spine
  cervical, fractures of, 564
    spinal cord injury and, 564, 597, 597t, 598
  structure and function of, 551–552, 552
Vesalius, 7
Vesicles, 520, 521
Vessels
  blood, 658, 659, 659
  lymph, 692, 693
Vestibular apparatus, 616, 619
Vials, 439, 439
  syringe filling from, 454p–457p
Videos, educational, 105
Vienna nasal speculum, 362
Villi, intestinal, 731, 732
Vincent's anginga, 734
Violent injuries, reporting of, 42
Viral hepatitis, 740, 740t
Viral infections, of skin, 522
Viral meningitis, 590–591
Viral pneumonia, 717
Virology, 844
Virulent microorganisms, 268
Viruses, 844
Vision
  age-related changes in, 1025t
  assessment of, 348, 613–614, 628p
  color, 609
    assessment of, 614, 614, 629p
    deficits in, 612
  process of, 610
  refractive errors and, 611–612, 612, 628p
Vision-impaired patient
  assistance for, 611
  communication with, 66
Visitors, nonpatient, scheduling of, 117–118
Visual acuity testing, 613–614, 628p
  assessment of, 348, 628p
Visualization, 92
Vital signs, 302–333
  blood pressure, 312–314
  charting of, 314–315, 316
  in emergency assessment, 491
  pulse, 308–310
  respiration, 310–312
  temperature, 302–308
Vital statistics, reporting of, 42
Vitamin D, renal regulation of, 753
Vitamins, functions and sources of, 86t–87t
Vitiligo, 526
Vitreous humor, 608, 609
Vocal cords, 710
Voice box. See Larynx
Voiding cystourethrogram, 476t
Voiding reflex, 756
Volkman retractor, 359
Vomer, 551, 551
Vomiting
  in pregnancy, 803–804
  in pyloric stenosis, 736
Von Leeuwenhoek, Anton, 7
Voucher, petty cash, 214, 214
Vulva, structure and function of, 780, 781
Vulvovaginitis, 784, 784b

W
W-2 forms, 224–227
W-4 form, 224, 225–226
Waiting room, 104–105
Waiting time, management of, 104
Wald, Lillian, 9

Walkers, *577*, 577–578
Walking
  with cane, 577
  with crutches, 571–577
  with walker, 577
Warfarin, coagulation tests and, 931
Warm applications, 531–540, 532t, 533t,
    535p–538p
Warming devices, for microcollection, 903
Warts, 522
  genital, 786–787
Waste disposal, 285–286, 394b
Water bath, 538p–540p, 540
Wave scheduling, 119
WBCs. *See* White blood cell(s)
Weber test, 621
Weight
  charting of, 1007, *1008*
  measurement of, 302, *302*, 317p
    in children, 999, 1006p–1007p
Weight loss
  diets for, 89
  exercise for, 90t
Welcoming, of patients and visitors, 103
Well-child visits, 989, 991
Westergren erythrocyte sedimentation rate, 930, *931*
Western blot, 705
Wet mount, 848, *850*
Wheals, *521*, 524
Wheezing, 721t
White blood cell (WBC) count and differential, 925–927,
    932p–940p

White blood cells, 659, *660, 661–662*, 662t
  formation of, 924–925
  types of, 924, 927
  in urine, 873–874
White cells, neural, 582
White matter
  cerebral, 585
  spinal cord, 587
Windpipe. *See* Trachea
Winged infusion set, 901, *901, 902*
Wintrobe erythrocyte sedimentation rate, 930, 946p–947p
Wood's light, 523, 530
Word processing, 164
Worker's compensation, 249
  records for, 149
Wound(s)
  banaging of, 386–389
  closure of
    assisting with, 384
    with staples, 383–384, 385–386, 402p–403p
    with Steri-strips, 384, *385*
    with sutures, 382–385, *383–385,* 400p–401p
  drainage from, 386b
  healing of, 387b–388b
  soft tissue, 494, 494b
  sterile dressings for, 386, 403p–407p
Wound cultures, 529, *529, 530*
  specimen collection for, 846
Wound healing, disorders of, 524–525
Wrist
  carpal tunnel syndrome of, 568
  structure and function of, 552–553

Write offs, 198
Written communications, 57, *58*, 127–141
  delivery services for, 138
  dictation and transcription of, 140–141, 141b
  grammar tips for, 133b
  letters, 128–134. *See also* Letters; Mail
  memorandums, 134
  sending of, 135–138, *136–138,* 137b
  spelling tips for, 133b

X
X-ray film, handling and storage of, 480
X-ray machines, 470, *470*
X-rays, 470. *See also* Radiography
  safety of, 472–474

Y
Yeast, 844
  in urine, 875
Yeast infection, 784, 784b
Young's rule, for pediatric drug dosage, 434

Z
Zalcitadine, for AIDS, 703
Zidovudine, for AIDS, 703
Z-track injection, 444, *444,* 466p
Zygomatic bones, 551, *551*

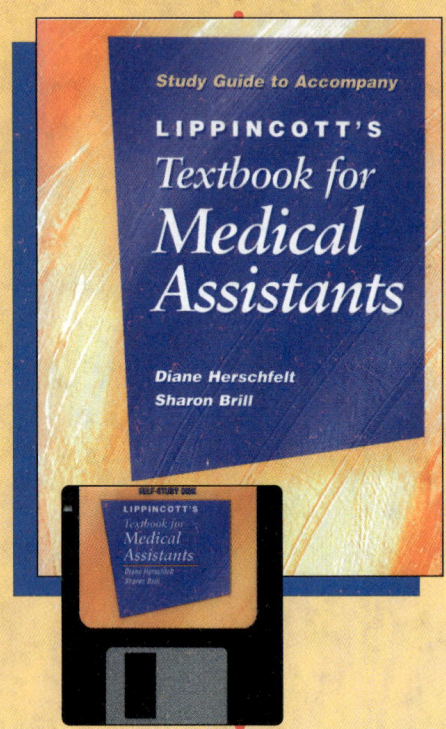
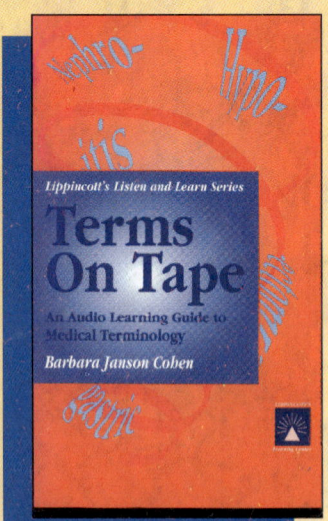
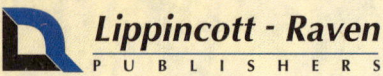

Performance Objectives

Chapter 8
Appointments 112
1. Schedule an appointment for a new patient. 118
2. Schedule an appointment for a patient's return visit. 119

Chapter 9
Written Communications 126
1. Create a business letter. 134
2. Create a memorandum. 135
3. Address and send written communication. 137
3. Open and sort mail. 139
4. Annotate a document. 139
5. Transcribe a document. 141

Chapter 10
Medical Records and Records Management 142
1. Prepare a medical record file folder (Procedure 10-1). 150

Chapter 11
Computers in the Medical Office 156
1. Turn on a computer. 162
2. Shut off a computer. 162

Chapter 12
Quality Improvement and Risk Management 168
1. Complete an incident report. 175

Chapter 13
Management of the Medical Office Team 180
1. Write a job description. 185
2. Create policy and procedure manuals. 187

Chapter 14
Credit and Collections 196
1. Use an aging schedule. 200
2. Write a collection letter. 201

Chapter 15
Bookkeeping and Banking 204
1. Record financial transactions, such as charges, payments, credits, and adjustments to patient ledger cards. 208
2. Complete a bank deposit slip and make a deposit. 212
3. Maintain a petty cash account. 214

Chapter 16
Accounts Payable and Payroll 216
1. Issue a payroll check using the pegboard system. 222
2. Calculate the amount of an employee's payroll check for a given pay period. 223

Chapter 18
Health Insurance 242
1. Fill out a HCFA 1500 claim form. 250

Chapter 19
Asepsis and Infection Control 266
1. Perform a medical aseptic handwashing (Procedure 19-1). 272
2. Perform a surgical scrub (Procedure 19-2). 277
3. Put on sterile gloves (Procedure 19-3). 280
4. Remove gloves after a procedure (Procedure 19-4). 283
5. Clean and decontaminate spills of blood or body fluids. 285

Chapter 20
Medical History and Patient Assessment 288
1. Interview a patient and correctly complete appropriate sections of the medical history form (Procedure 20-1). 294

Chapter 21
Anthropometric Measurements and Vital Signs 300
1. Auscultate a patient's pedal pulse using a Doppler. 310
2. Measure and record a patient's weight (Procedure 21-1). 317
3. Measure and record a patient's height (Procedure 21-2). 318
4. Measure and record a patient's oral temperature using a glass mercury thermometer (Procedure 21-3). 319

5. Measure and record a patient's rectal temperature using a glass mercury thermometer (Procedure 21-4). 321
6. Measure and record a patient's axillary temperature using a glass mercury thermometer (Procedure 21-5). 323
7. Measure and record a patient's temperature using an electronic thermometer (Procedure 21-6). 324
8.7. Measure and record a patient's temperature using a tympanic thermometer (Procedure 21-7). 325
9. Disinfect a glass thermometer (Procedure 21-8). 325
10. Measure and record a patient's radial pulse (Procedure 21-9). 326
11. Measure and record a patient's apical pulse (Procedure 21-10). 327
12. Count a patient's respirations (Procedure 21-11). 329
13. Measure a patient's blood pressure (Procedure 21-12). 329

Chapter 22
Physical Examination 334
1. Assist the physician in all aspects of the physical examination (Procedure 22-1). 345

Chapter 23
Instruments and Equipment 352
1. Sanitize equipment for disinfection or sterilization (Procedure 23-1). 364
2. Properly wrap equipment in preparation for sterilization in an autoclave. 368
3. Operate an autoclave observing protocol for pressure, time, and temperature appropriate for the material to be sterilized (Procedure 23-2). 371

Chapter 24
Assisting with Minor Office Surgery 374
1. Add the contents of peel-back packets to the sterile field. 378
2. Open sterile surgical packs (Procedure 24-1). 395
3. Use sterile transfer forceps (Procedure 24-2). 397
4. Add sterile solution to a sterile field (Procedure 24-3). 397
5. Perform skin preparation and hair removal (Procedure 24-4). 399
6. Attach a surgical blade to a scalpel handle. 381
7. Remove sutures (Procedure 24-5). 400
8. Remove staples (Procedure 24-6). 402
9. Apply a sterile dressing (Procedure 24-7). 403
10. Change an existing sterile dressing (Procedure 24-8). 405
11. Wrap roller bandages using various techniques. 390
12. Apply tubular gauze bandage (Procedure 24-9). 407
13. Assist with excisional surgery (Procedure 24-10). 411
14. Assist with incision and drainage (Procedure 24-11). 412

Chapter 26
Preparing and Administering Medications 426
1. Administer oral medications (Procedure 26-1). 446
2. Administer sublingual or buccal medications (Procedure 26-2). 449
3. Apply transdermal medications (Procedure 26-3). 450
4. Apply topical medications (Procedure 26-4). 451
5. Prepare an injection (Procedure 26-5). 452
6. Administer an intradermal injection (Procedure 26-6). 458
7. Administer and read a tine or Mantoux Test (Procedure 26-7). 460
8. Administer a subcutaneous injection (Procedure 26-8). 462
9. Administer an intramuscular injection (Procedure 26-9). 464
10. Administer an intramuscular injection using the Z-track method (Procedure 26-10). 466
11. Administer rectal medications. 437
12. Administer vaginal medications. 438

Chapter 28
Medical Office Emergencies 482
1. Manage an adult with a foreign body airway obstruction (Procedure 28-1). 489
2. Perform one-rescuer adult cardiopulmonary resuscitation (Procedure 28-2). 490

Chapter 30
Caring for Patients With Integumentary Disorders 516
1. Obtain a wound culture. 529
2. Apply cold packs (Procedure 30-1). 534
3. Apply warm or cold compresses (Procedure 30-2). 536
4. Use a hot water bottle or commercial hot pack (Procedure 30-3). 536
5. Assist with therapeutic soaks (Procedure 30-4). 538